Essentials of Paramedic Care

VOLUME 2

Care

Canadian Edition

BRYAN E. BLEDSOE

D.O., F.A.C.E.P., EMT-P

Emergency Department Staff Physician
Baylor Medical Center—Ellis County
Waxahachie, Texas
and
Clinical Associate Professor of Emergency Medicine
University of North Texas Health Sciences Center
Fort Worth, Texas

ROBERT S. PORTER

M.A., NREMT-P

Senior Advanced Life Support Educator
Madison County Emergency Medical Services
Canastota, New York
and
Flight Paramedic
AirOne, Onondaga County Sheriff's Department
Syracuse, New York

RICHARD A. CHERRY

M.S., NREMT-P

Clinical Assistant Professor of Emergency Medicine
Assistant Residency Director
SUNY Upstate Medical University
Syracuse, New York

DWAYNE E. CLAYDEN

M.E.M., Paramedic

Assistant to the Medical Director
The City of Calgary Emergency Medical Services
Calgary, Alberta

PEARSON

Prentice
Hall

Toronto

Library and Archives Canada Cataloguing in Publication

Essentials of paramedic care/Bryan E. Bledsoe ... [et al.]. — Canadian ed.

Includes index.
ISBN 0-13-120305-3 (vol. 1)
ISBN 0-13-120306-1 (vol. 2)

1. Emergency medicine—textbooks. 2. Emergency medical technicians—handbooks, manuals, etc.
I. Bledsoe, Bryan E., 1955–

RC86.7.E88 2006   616.02'5   C2004-906406-1

0-13-120306-1

Vice President, Editorial Director: Michael J. Young
Executive Editor: Samantha Scully
Executive Marketing Manager: Cas Shields
Developmental Editor: Pamela Voves
Production Editor: Marisa D'Andrea
Copy Editor: Rohini Herbert
Proofreader: Dawn Hunter
Production Coordinator: Patricia Ciardullo
Manufacturing Coordinator: Susan Johnson
Literary Permissions and Photo Researcher: Amanda McCormick
Indexer: Belle Wong
Page Layout: Jansom
Art Director: Julia Hall
Interior and Cover Design: Anthony Leung
Cover Image: Mike Powell, Getty Images

9 10 11   14 13 12

Printed and bound in the United States.

Notices

It is the intent of the authors and publisher that this textbook be used as part of a formal paramedic education program taught by a qualified instructor. The care procedures presented here represent accepted competencies and practices in Canada. They are not offered as a standard of care.

Paramedic-level prehospital care in Canada is to be performed under the specific paramedic competencies available in each province and territory. These competencies are specific for Primary Care Paramedics (PCP), Advanced Care Paramedics (ACP), and Critical Care Paramedics (CCP). Medically delegated acts can only be performed by a paramedic certified by a licensed medical physician or base hospital physician. It is the reader's responsibility to know and follow local protocols and follow their scope of practice associated to the system to which they belong. Also, it is the reader's responsibility to remain current of emergency care procedures and changes to their scope of practice.

NOTICE ON DRUGS AND DRUG DOSAGES

Every effort has been made to ensure that the drug dosages presented in this textbook are in accordance with nationally accepted standards. When applicable, the dosages and routes have been taken from the American Heart Association's Advanced Cardiac Life Support Guidelines. It is the responsibility of the reader to be familiar with the drugs used in his or her system, as well as the dosages specified by medical direction. The drugs presented in this book should only be administered by direct order of a licensed physician, whether verbally or through accepted orders.

NOTICE ON GENDER USE

The authors have made a great effort to treat the use of the two genders equally. The chapters alternate in their use of gender by applying male pronouns in one chapter and female pronouns in the next. (Exceptions exist in situations that are specifically related to only one gender.)

NOTICE ON PHOTOGRAPHS

Please note that many of the photographs contained in this book are of actual emergency situations. As such, it is possible that they may not accurately depict current, appropriate, or advisable practices of emergency medical care. They have been included for the sole purpose of giving general insight into real-life emergency settings.

DEDICATION

This book is respectfully dedicated to the paramedics who toil each day in an environment that is unpredictable, often dangerous, and constantly changing. They risk their lives to aid the sick and the injured, driven only by their love of humanity and their devotion to this profession we call emergency medical services.

We remember the EMS, fire, and law enforcement personnel who have made the ultimate sacrifice for their communities and our nation. May they never be forgotten.

Brief Contents

DIVISION 3   Trauma Emergencies   1

CHAPTER 16   Trauma and Trauma Systems   2
CHAPTER 17   Blunt Trauma   12
CHAPTER 18   Penetrating Trauma   44
CHAPTER 19   Hemorrhage and Shock   64
CHAPTER 20   Soft-Tissue Trauma   93
CHAPTER 21   Burns   134
CHAPTER 22   Musculoskeletal Trauma   167
CHAPTER 23   Head, Facial, and Neck Trauma   204
CHAPTER 24   Spinal Trauma   247
CHAPTER 25   Thoracic Trauma   275
CHAPTER 26   Abdominal Trauma   308

DIVISION 4   Medical Emergencies   327

CHAPTER 27   Pulmonology   328
CHAPTER 28   Cardiology   442
CHAPTER 29   Neurology   568
CHAPTER 30   Endocrinology   606
CHAPTER 31   Allergies and Anaphylaxis   622
CHAPTER 32   Gastroenterology   633
CHAPTER 33   Urology and Nephrology   657
CHAPTER 34   Toxicology and Substance Abuse   680
CHAPTER 35   Hematology   723
CHAPTER 36   Environmental Emergencies   741
CHAPTER 37   Infectious Disease   780
CHAPTER 38   Psychiatric and Behavioural Disorders   833
CHAPTER 39   Gynecology   857
CHAPTER 40   Obstetrics   867

DIVISION 5   Special Considerations   905

CHAPTER 41   Neonatology   906
CHAPTER 42   Pediatrics   937
CHAPTER 43   Geriatric Emergencies   1021
CHAPTER 44   Abuse and Assault   1074
CHAPTER 45   The Challenged Patient   1088
CHAPTER 46   Acute Interventions for the Chronic-Care Patient   1106

Appendix A   PCP and ACP Competencies   1141

Glossary   1148

Index   1168

Detailed Contents

DIVISION 3   TRAUMA EMERGENCIES   1

CHAPTER 16   TRAUMA AND TRAUMA SYSTEMS   2

✳Introduction to Trauma and Trauma Care 3   ✳Trauma 3
✳The Trauma Care System 4   ✳Trauma Centre Designation 5
✳Your Role as a Paramedic 6

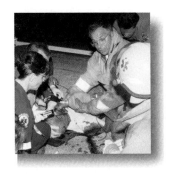

CHAPTER 17   BLUNT TRAUMA   12

✳Introduction to Blunt Trauma 13   ✳Kinetics of Blunt Trauma 13
✳Types of Trauma 15   ✳Blunt Trauma 16

CHAPTER 18   PENETRATING TRAUMA   44

✳Introduction to Penetrating Trauma 45   ✳Physics of Penetrating Trauma
45   ✳Specific Tissue/Organ Injuries 55   ✳Special Concerns with
Penetrating Trauma 59

CHAPTER 19   HEMORRHAGE AND SHOCK   64

✳Introduction to Hemorrhage and Shock 65   ✳Hemorrhage 66
✳Shock 82

CHAPTER 20   SOFT-TISSUE TRAUMA   93

✳Introduction to Soft-Tissue Injuries 95   ✳Pathophysiology of Soft-Tissue
Injury 95   ✳Dressing and Bandage Materials 111   ✳Assessment of
Soft-Tissue Injuries 113   ✳Management of Soft-Tissue Injury 118

CHAPTER 21   BURNS   134

✳Introduction to Burn Injuries 136   ✳Pathophysiology of Burns 136
✳Assessment of Thermal Burns 151   ✳Management of Thermal
Burns 156   ✳Assessment and Management of Electrical, Chemical,
and Radiation Burns 160

CHAPTER 22   MUSCULOSKELETAL TRAUMA   167

✳Introduction to Musculoskeletal Trauma 168   ✳Prevention Strategies 169
✳Pathophysiology of the Musculoskeletal System 169   ✳Musculoskeletal
Injury Assessment 177   ✳Musculoskeletal Injury Management 183

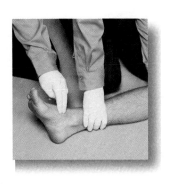

CHAPTER 23   HEAD, FACIAL, AND NECK TRAUMA   204

✳Introduction to Head, Facial, and Neck Injuries 206   ✳Pathophysiology
of Head, Facial, and Neck Injury 206   ✳Assessment of Head, Facial, and
Neck Injuries 225   ✳Head, Facial, and Neck Injury Management 232

CHAPTER 24 SPINAL TRAUMA 247

*Introduction to Spinal Injuries 248 *Pathophysiology of Spinal Injury 249 *Assessment of the Spinal Injury Patient 256 *Management of the Spinal Injury Patient 261

CHAPTER 25 THORACIC TRAUMA 275

*Introduction to Thoracic Injury 277 *Pathophysiology of Thoracic Trauma 278 *Assessment of the Thoracic Trauma Patient 296 *Management of the Chest Injury Patient 302

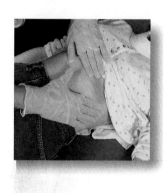

CHAPTER 26 ABDOMINAL TRAUMA 308

*Introduction to Abdominal Trauma 310 *Pathophysiology of Abdominal Injury 310 *Assessment of the Abdominal Injury Patient 318 *Management of the Abdominal Injury Patient 324

DIVISION 4 MEDICAL EMERGENCIES 327

CHAPTER 27 PULMONOLOGY 328

Part 1 Pathophysiology and Respiratory Disorders 331
*Introduction 331 *Pathophysiology 334 *Assessment of the Respiratory System 338 *Management of Respiratory Disorders 347 *Specific Respiratory Diseases 348

Part 2 Airway Management and Ventilation 370
*Respiratory Problems 370 *Respiratory System Assessment 372 *Basic Airway Management 380 *Advanced Airway Management 387 *Managing Patients with Stoma Sites 431 *Suctioning 432 *Gastric Decompression 434 *Oxygenation 435 *Ventilation 437

CHAPTER 28 CARDIOLOGY 442

Part 1 Cardiovascular Anatomy and Physiology, ECG Monitoring, and Dysrhythmia Analysis 448
*Introduction 447 *Review of Cardiovascular Anatomy and Physiology 448 *Electrocardiographic Monitoring 452 *Dysrhythmias 465

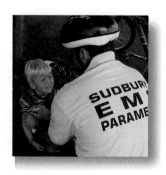

Part 2 Assessment and Management of the Cardiovascular Patient 511
*Assessment of the Cardiovascular Patient 511 *Management of Cardiovascular Emergencies 521 *Managing Specific Cardiovascular Emergencies 536 *Prehospital ECG Monitoring 564

CHAPTER 29 NEUROLOGY 568

*Introduction 569 *Pathophysiology 570 *General Assessment Findings 572 *Management of Specific Nervous System Emergencies 581

CHAPTER 30   ENDOCRINOLOGY   606

*Introduction 607   *Endocrine Disorders and Emergencies 608

CHAPTER 31   ALLERGIES AND ANAPHYLAXIS   622

*Introduction 623   *Pathophysiology 624   *Assessment Findings in Anaphylaxis 628   *Management of Anaphylaxis 629 *Assessment Findings in Allergic Reaction 631   *Management of Allergic Reactions 631

CHAPTER 32   GASTROENTEROLOGY   633

*Introduction 634   *General Pathophysiology, Assessment, and Treatment 634   *Specific Illnesses 639

CHAPTER 33   UROLOGY AND NEPHROLOGY   657

*Introduction 659   *General Mechanisms of Nontraumatic Tissue Problems 660   *General Pathophysiology, Assessment, and Management 660   *Renal and Urological Emergencies 665

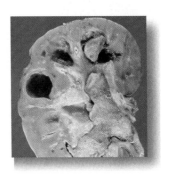

CHAPTER 34   TOXICOLOGY AND SUBSTANCE ABUSE   680

*Introduction 681   *Epidemiology 681   *Poison Control Centres 682 *Routes of Toxic Exposure 682   *General Principles of Toxicological Assessment and Management 685   *Ingested Toxins 688   *Inhaled Toxins 690   *Surface-Absorbed Toxins 691   *Specific Toxins 691   *Injected Toxins 707   *Substance Abuse and Overdose 715   *Alcohol Abuse 719

CHAPTER 35   HEMATOLOGY   723

*Introduction 724   *General Assessment and Management 727 *Managing Specific Patient Problems 732

CHAPTER 36   ENVIRONMENTAL EMERGENCIES   741

*Introduction 743   *Homeostasis 743   *Pathophysiology of Heat and Cold Disorders 744   *Heat Disorders 747   *Cold Disorders 753 *Near-Drowning and Drowning 761   *Diving Emergencies 764 *High-Altitude Illness 771   *Nuclear Radiation 775

CHAPTER 37   INFECTIOUS DISEASE   780

*Introduction 782   *Public Health Principles 782   *Public Health Agencies 783   *Microorganisms 783   *Contraction, Transmission, and Stages of Disease 787   *Infection Control 790   *Assessment of the Patient with Infectious Disease 795   *Selected Infectious Diseases 797 *Preventing Disease Transmission 831

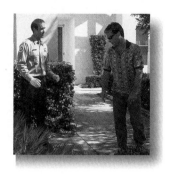

CHAPTER 38   PSYCHIATRIC AND BEHAVIOURAL
              DISORDERS   833

✳Introduction 834 ✳Behavioural Emergencies 834 ✳Pathophysiology
of Psychiatric Disorders 835 ✳Assessment of Behavioural Emergency
Patients 836 ✳Specific Psychiatric Disorders 840 ✳Management of
Behavioural Emergencies 851 ✳Violent Patients and Restraint 853

CHAPTER 39   GYNECOLOGY   857

✳Introduction 858 ✳Assessment of the Gynecological Patient 858
✳Management of Gynecological Emergencies 860 ✳Specific Gynecological
Emergencies 861

CHAPTER 40   OBSTETRICS   867

✳Introduction 868 ✳The Prenatal Period 868 ✳General Assessment
of the Obstetric Patient 875 ✳General Management of the Obstetric
Patient 878 ✳Complications of Pregnancy 878 ✳The Puerperium 889
✳Abnormal Delivery Situations 896 ✳Other Delivery Complications 899
✳Maternal Complications of Labour and Delivery 901

DIVISION 5   SPECIAL
              CONSIDERATIONS   905

CHAPTER 41   NEONATOLOGY   906

✳Introduction 907 ✳General Pathophysiology, Assessment, and
Management 908 ✳The Distressed Newborn 915 ✳Specific Neonatal
Situations 926

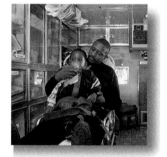

CHAPTER 42   PEDIATRICS   937

✳Introduction 939 ✳Role of Paramedics in Pediatric Care 939
✳General Approach to Pediatric Emergencies 940 ✳General Approach to
Pediatric Assessment 950 ✳General Management of Pediatric Patients 959
✳Specific Medical Emergencies 976 ✳Trauma Emergencies 1003 ✳Sudden
Infant Death Syndrome (SIDS) 1011 ✳Child Abuse and Neglect 1012
✳Infants and Children with Special Needs 1016

CHAPTER 43   GERIATRIC EMERGENCIES   1021

✳Introduction 1023 ✳Epidemiology and Demographics 1023 ✳General
Pathophysiology, Assessment, and Management 1025 ✳System
Pathophysiology in the Elderly 1035 ✳Common Medical Problems in the
Elderly 1041 ✳Trauma in the Elderly Patient 1068

CHAPTER 44   ABUSE AND ASSAULT   1074

✳Introduction 1075 ✳Partner Abuse 1075 ✳Elder Abuse 1078
✳Child Abuse 1079 ✳Sexual Assault 1084

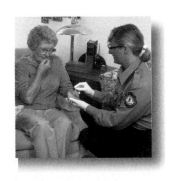

CHAPTER 45   THE CHALLENGED PATIENT   1088

*Introduction 1089   *Physical Disabilities 1089   *Mental Challenges and Emotional Impairments 1096   *Developmental Disabilities 1096 *Pathological Challenges 1098   *Other Challenges 1104

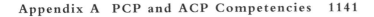

CHAPTER 46   ACUTE INTERVENTIONS FOR THE CHRONIC-CARE PATIENT   1106

*Introduction 1107   *Epidemiology of Home Care 1107   *General System Pathophysiology, Assessment, and Management 1113   *Specific Acute Home Health Situations 1118

Appendix A PCP and ACP Competencies 1141

Glossary 1148

Index 1168

Preface

Congratulations on your decision to further your EMS career by undertaking the course of education required for certification as a paramedic! The world of paramedic emergency care is one that you will find both challenging and rewarding. Whether you will be working as a volunteer or paid paramedic, you will find the field of advanced prehospital care very interesting.

This two-volume textbook program is derived from Brady's best-selling *Paramedic Care: Principles & Practice* (Volumes 1–5). Ideal for paramedic refresher and abbreviated paramedic programs, this book is based on the Canadian National Paramedic Competencies and is organized into five divisions.

The first division, entitled Introduction to Prehospital Care, addresses the medical-legal aspects of all levels of paramedic care in Canada as well as general ambulance operational systems. Included in this division are incident commands through mass casualty incidents, rescue awareness and operations, and hazardous material and crime scene incidents. The second division, Patient Assessment, builds on the patient assessment skills of a paramedic with special emphasis on advanced patient assessment at the scene. It also introduces the reader to basic anatomy and physiology, as well as pathophysiology, principles of pharamacology, and drug administration. Trauma Emergencies, the third division of the text, discusses advanced prehospital care from the mechanism of injury analysis to shock/trauma resuscitation. The fourth division of the text, Medical Emergencies, is the most extensive and addresses multiple levels of paramedic care involving medical emergencies. The last division addresses Special Considerations including neonatology, pediatrics, geriatric emergencies, chronic patients, the challenged patient, and assaulted or abused patients. An appendix that cross-references the text with the National Occupational Competency Profiles developed by the Paramedic Association of Canada concludes both volumes.

SKILLS

The psychomotor skills of fluid and medication administration, advanced airway care, electrocardiography (ECG) monitoring and defibrillation, and advanced medical and trauma patient care are best learned in the classroom, skills laboratory, and clinical and field settings. Common advanced prehospital skills are discussed in the text as well as outlined in the accompanying procedure sheets. Review these before and while practising the skill. It is important to point out that this or any other text cannot teach skills. Care skills are only learned under the watchful eye of a paramedic instructor and perfected during your clinical and field internship.

HOW TO USE THIS TEXTBOOK

Essentials of Paramedic Care, Canadian Edition, is designed to accompany a paramedic education program that includes ample classroom, practical laboratory, in-hospital clinical, and prehospital field experiences. These educational experiences must be guided by instructors and preceptors with special training and expertise in their areas of participation in your program.

It is intended that your program coordinator will assign reading from the text in preparation for each classroom lecture and discussion section. The knowledge gained from reading this text will form the foundation of the information you will need in order to function effectively as a paramedic in your EMS system. Your instructors will build on this information to strengthen your knowledge and understanding of advanced prehospital care so that you may apply it in your practice. The in-hospital clinical and prehospital field experiences will further refine your knowledge and skills under the watchful eyes of your preceptors.

The workbook that accompanies this text can also assist in improving classroom performance. It contains information, sample test questions, and exercises designed to assist learning, and can be very helpful in identifying the important elements of paramedic education, in exercising the knowledge of prehospital care, and in helping you self-test your knowledge.

Essentials of Paramedic Care presents the knowledge of emergency care in as accurate, standardized, and clear a manner as is possible. However, each EMS system is uniquely different, and it is beyond the scope of this text to address all differences. You must count heavily on your instructors, the program coordinator, and ultimately the program medical director to identify how specific emergency care procedures are applied in your system.

CHAPTER CONTRIBUTORS

We wish to acknowledge the remarkable talents and efforts of the following people who contributed to *Essentials of Paramedic Care*. Individually, they worked with extraordinary commitment on this new program. Together, they form a team of highly dedicated professionals who have upheld the highest standards of EMS instruction.

CANADIAN CONTRIBUTORS

Ronald Bowles, B.Ed., M.Ed. Technology, EMA II. Manager, Instructional Design, Paramedic Academy, Justice Institute of British Columbia, New Westminster, British Columbia. *All chapters, Volumes 1 and 2.*

Kevin Branch, BHSc., PHC, ACP Coordinator, Paramedic Programs, Cambrian College, Sudbury, Ontario. *All chapters, Volumes 1 and 2.*

Heather MacKenzie-Carey, B.Sc., EMT-P, M.Sc. (Disaster Management), Bridgewater, Nova Scotia. *Chapters 37 and 41*

U.S. CONTRIBUTORS

Beth Lothrop Adams, M.A., R.N., NREMT-P; ALS Coordinator, EHS Programs; Adjunct Assistant Professor, Emergency Medicine, The George Washington University. *Chapters 30, 39, 40*

J. Nile Barnes, B.S., NREMT-P; Associate Professor of EMS Professions, Austin Community College, Austin, Texas; Paramedic, Williamson County (Texas) EMS Department. *Chapter 1*

Brenda Beasley, R.N., B.S., EMT-P; EMS Program Director, Calhoun College, Decatur, Alabama. *Chapter 42*

Sandra Bradley, Pleasant Hill, California. *Chapter 45*

Lawrence C. Brilliant, M.D., F.A.C.E.P.; Clinical Assistant Professor, Department of Primary Care Education and Community Services, Hahnemann University; Emergency Physician, Doylestown Hospital, Doylestown, Pennsylvania. *Chapters 23, 28*

Eric C. Chaney, M.S. NREMT-P; Administrator, Office of the State EMS Medical Director, Maryland Institute for Emergency Medical Services Systems, Baltimore, Maryland. *Chapter 1*

Elizabeth Coolidge-Stolz, M.D., Medical Writer, Health Educator, North Reading, Massachusetts. *Chapters 30, 32, 33*

Robert A. De Lorenzo, M.D., F.A.C.E.P.; Lieut. Colonel, Medical Corps, US Army; Brooke Army Medical Center. *Chapters 20, 21*

Kate Dernocoeur, B.S. EMT-P, Lowell, Michigan. *Chapters 1, 5*

Clyde Deschamp, M.Ed., NREMT-P; Chairman and Assistant Professor, Department of Emergency Medical Technology; Director, Helicopter Transport, University of Mississippi Medical Center. *Chapter 37*

James W. Drake, B.S., NREMT-P; Instructor, Department of Emergency Medical Technology, School of Health Related Professions, University of Mississippi Medical Center, Jackson, Mississippi. *Chapter 15*

Robert Elling, M.P.A., NREMT-P; Professor, American College of Prehospital Medicine; Faculty Member, Institute of Prehospital Emergency Medicine, Hudson Valley Community College, Troy, New York. *Chapter 3*

Robert Feinberg, EMT-P, PA-C, Emergency Medicine, Wayne, Pennsylvania. *Chapter 24*

Joseph P. Funk, M.D., F.A.C.E.P.; Peachtree Emergency Associates, Piedmont Hospital, Atlanta, Georgia. *Chapter 28*

Kathleen G. Funk, M.D., F.A.C.E.P.; Emergency Medicine Physician, Atlanta, Georgia. *Chapter 28*

Eric W. Heckerson, R.N., M.A., NREMT-P; EMS Coordinator, Mesa Fire Department, Mesa, Arizona. *Chapters 1, 22, 29, 37, 38*

Chris Hendricks, NREMT-P, Field Instructor; Paramedic, Pridemark Paramedics, Boulder, Colorado. *Chapter 46*

Sandra Hultz, B.S., NREMT-P; EMS Instructor, University of Mississippi Medical Center, Jackson, Mississippi. *Chapter 1*

Jeffrey L. Jarvis, M.S., EMT-P; Medical Student, University of Texas Medical Branch, Galveston, Texas. *Chapter 14*

Deborah Kufs, R.N., B.S., C.C.R.N., C.E.N., NREMT-P; Clinical Instructor, Hudson Valley Community College, Institute for Prehospital Emergency Medicine, Troy, New York. *Chapters 35, 43*

Daniel Limmer, EMT-P, Frederick, Maryland. *Chapters 3, 38*

William Marx, D.O.; Associate Professor of Surgery and Critical Care; Director, Surgical Critical Care SUNY Upstate Medical University, Syracuse, New York. *Chapter 26*

Michael O'Keefe, NREMT-P; EMS Training Coordinator, Vermont Department of Health. *Chapter 1*

John M. Saad, M.D.; Medical Director of Emergency Services, Navarro Regional Hospital, Corsicana, Texas; Medical Director of Emergency Services, Medical Center at Terrell, Terrell, Texas. *Chapters 34, 36*

John S. Saito, M.P.H., EMT-P; Director, EMS/Paramedic Education; Assistant Professor, Oregon Health Sciences University, School of Medicine, Department of Emergency Medicine, Portland, Oregon. *Chapters 13, 37*

Jo Anne Schultz, B.A., NREMT-P; Paramedic, Lifestar Ambulance Inc., Salisbury, Maryland; Level II Emergency Medical Services Instructor, Maryland Fire and Rescue Institute, University of Maryland; Paramedic Instructor, Maryland Institute of Emergency Medical Services Systems, University of Maryland; ACLS, BTLS, and PALS instructor. *Chapters 11, 36, 41*

Craig A. Soltis, M.D., F.A.C.E.P.; Assistant Professor of Clinical Emergency Medicine, Northeastern Ohio Universities College of Medicine; Chairman, Department of Emergency Medicine, Forum Health, Youngstown, Ohio. *Chapters 25, 35*

Marian D. Streger, R.N., B.S.N., C.E.N., Cleveland, Ohio. *Chapters 11, 45*

Matthew R. Streger, M.P.A., NREMT-P; Deputy Commissioner, Cleveland Emergency Medical Services, Cleveland, Ohio. *Chapters 3, 44, 46*

Emily Vacher, Esq., M.P.A., EMT-CC; Associate Director of Judicial Affairs, Syracuse University, Syracuse, New York. *Chapter 2*

Kevin Waddington, EMT-P, MedStar, Fort Worth, Texas. *Chapter 28*

Gail Weinstein, M.A., EMT-P; Director of Paramedic Training, State University of New York Upstate Medical University, Syracuse, New York. *Chapter 43*

Howard A. Werman, M.D., F.A.C.E.P.; Associate Professor of Clinical Emergency Medicine, The Ohio State University College of Medicine and Public Health, Columbus, Ohio; Medical Director, Med-Flight of Ohio. *Chapter 27*

Matthew S. Zavarella, B.S.A.S., NREMT-P, CCTEMT-P; Director Prehospital Education, Medical College of Ohio, Toledo, Ohio. *Chapters 13, 32*

DEVELOPMENT AND PRODUCTION

The tasks of writing, editing, reviewing, and producing a textbook the size of *Essentials of Paramedic Care (Volumes 1 and 2)* are complex. Many talented people have been involved in developing and producing this new program.

First, the authors would like to acknowledge the support of Samantha Scully and Leslie Carson. We also thank Pamela Voves, Development Editor, for this project. Special thanks go to Patricia Ciardullo, Production Coordinator, and Marisa D'Andrea, Production Editor, who skillfully supervised all production stages to create the final product you now hold. We are grateful to Rohini Herbert and Dawn Hunter, Copyeditors, for their hard work on these volumes. In developing our art and photo program, we were fortunate to work with yet additional talent—leaders within their professions.

We also wish to thank John Fader, B.Sc., ACP (Professor and Coordinator, Fleming College Paramedic Program, Peterborough, Ontario) and Sean C. Fisher of the Manitoba Emergency Services College for their technical review of the volumes.

MEDICAL REVIEW BOARD

Our special thanks to the following physicians for their review of material in our paramedic program. Their reviews were carefully prepared, and we appreciate the thoughtful advice and keen insight each shared with us.

Dr. Robert De Lorenzo, Lieutenant Colonel, Medical Corps, U.S. Army; Associate Clinical Professor of Military and Emergency Medicine, Uniformed Services University of Health Sciences.

Dr. Edward T. Dickinson, Assistant Professor and Director of EMS Field Operations in the Department of Emergency Medicine, University of Pennsylvania School of Medicine in Philadephia.

Dr. Howard A. Werman, Associate Professor, Department of Emergency Medicine, The Ohio State University College of Medicine and Public Health, Columbus, Ohio.

INSTRUCTOR REVIEWERS

The reviewers of *Essentials of Paramedic Care* have provided many excellent suggestions and ideas for improving the text. The quality of the reviews has been outstanding, and the reviews have been a major aid in the preparation and revision of the manuscript. The assistance provided by these EMS experts is deeply appreciated.

Ron Bowles, Justice Institute of British Columbia
Kevin Branch, Cambrian College
Ian Dailly, Justice Institute of British Columbia
Carl Damour, The Michener Institute for Applied Health Sciences
John Fader, Fleming College
Sean C. Fisher, Manitoba Emergency Services College
Ralph Hofmann, Durham College of Applied Arts and Technology
Steve Pilkington, Southern Alberta Institute of Technology
Jim Whittle, Algonquin College

Prehospital emergency personnel, like all health-care workers, are at risk for exposure to bloodborne pathogens and infectious diseases. In emergency situations, it is often difficult to take or enforce proper infection control measures. However, as a paramedic, you must recognize your high-risk status.

Infection control is designed to protect emergency personnel, their families, and their patients from unnecessary exposure to communicable diseases.

Laws, regulations, and standards regarding infection control include:

* *Canadian Centre for Disease Guidelines.* The CCDC has published extensive guidelines regarding infection control. Proper equipment and techniques that should be used by emergency response personnel to prevent or minimize risk of exposure are defined.
* *The Canadian Occupational Safety and Health Administration Act.* This Act mandates that all employees within a workplace be protected from harm through lack of safety or lack of safety equipment. Each province and territory has variations to this Act and specifics associated with professions and trade occupations.
* *National Fire Protection Association Guidelines.* The NFPA is a national organization that has established specific guidelines and requirements regarding infection control for emergency response agencies, particularly fire departments in Canada.

BODY SUBSTANCE ISOLATION PRECAUTIONS AND PERSONAL PROTECTIVE EQUIPMENT

Emergency response personnel should practise body substance isolation (BSI), a strategy that considers all body substances potentially infectious. To achieve this, all emergency personnel should utilize personal protective equipment (PPE). Appropriate PPE should be available on every emergency vehicle. The minimum recommended PPE includes the following:

* *Gloves.* Disposable gloves should be donned by all emergency response personnel *before* initiating any emergency care. When an emergency incident involves more than one patient, you should change gloves between patients. When gloves have been contaminated, they should be removed as soon as possi-

ble. To remove gloves, first hook the gloved fingers of one hand under the cuff of the other glove. Then pull that glove off without letting your gloved fingers come in contact with bare skin. Then, slide the fingers of the ungloved hand under the remaining glove's cuff. Push that glove off, being careful not to touch the glove's exterior with your bare hand. Always wash your hands after gloves are removed, even when the gloves appear intact. Paramedics on the scene should utilize alcohol-based cleansers to wash their hands until a facility is readily available.

* *Masks and Protective Eyewear.* Masks and protective equipment should be present on all emergency vehicles and used in accordance with the level of exposure encountered. Proper eyewear and masks prevent a patient's blood and body fluids from spraying into your eyes, nose, and mouth. Masks and protective eyewear should be worn together whenever blood spatter is likely to occur, such as in arterial bleeding, childbirth, endotracheal intubation, invasive procedures, oral suctioning, and cleanup of equipment that requires heavy scrubbing or brushing. Both you and the patient should wear masks whenever the potential for airborne transmission of disease exists.
* *HEPA Respirators.* Due to the resurgence of tuberculosis (TB), prehospital personnel should protect themselves from TB infection through use of a high-efficiency particulate air (HEPA) respirator, a design approved by the National Institute of Occupational Safety and Health (NIOSH). It should fit snugly and be capable of filtering out the tuberculosis bacillus. The HEPA respirator should be worn when caring for patients with confirmed or suspected TB. This is especially important when performing "high-hazard" procedures, such as administration of nebulized medications, endotracheal intubation, or suctioning.
* *Gowns.* Gowns protect clothing from blood splashes. If large splashes of blood are expected, such as during childbirth, wear impervious gowns.
* *Resuscitation Equipment.* Disposable resuscitation equipment should be the primary means of artificial ventilation in emergency care. Such items should be used once and then disposed of.

Remember, the proper use of personal protective equipment ensures effective infection control and minimizes risk. Use *all* protective equipment recommended for any particular situation to ensure maximum protection.

Consider *all* body substances potentially infectious and *always* practise body substance isolation.

HANDLING CONTAMINATED MATERIAL

Many of the materials associated with emergency response become contaminated with possibly infectious body fluids and substances. These include soiled linen, patient clothing, dressings, and used care equipment, including intravenous needles. It is important that you collect these materials at the scene and dispose of them appropriately to ensure your safety as well as that of your patients, their family members, bystanders, and fellow caregivers. Properly dispose of any contaminated materials according to the recommendations outlined below.

* Handle contaminated materials only while wearing the appropriate personal protective equipment.
* Place all blood- or body-fluid-contaminated clothing, linen, dressings, patient-care equipment, and supplies in properly marked bio-hazard bags and ensure they are disposed of properly.
* Ensure that all used needles, scalpels, and other contaminated objects that have the potential to puncture the skin are properly secured in a puncture-resistant and clearly marked sharps container.
* Do not recap a needle after use, stick it into a seat cushion or other object, or leave it lying on the ground. This increases the risk of a needle-stick injury.
* Always scan the scene before leaving to ensure that all equipment has been retrieved and all potentially infectious material has been bagged and removed.
* Should you be exposed to an infectious disease, have contact with body substances with a route for system entry (such as an open wound on your hand when a glove tears while moving a soiled patient), or receive a needle-stick injury from a used needle, alert the receiving hospital and contact your service's infection control officer immediately.

Following these recommendations will help protect you and the people you care for from the dangers of disease transmission.

A Great Way to Learn and Instruct Online

The Pearson Education Canada Companion Website is easy to navigate and is organized to correspond to the chapters in this textbook. Whether you are a student in the classroom or a distance learner you will discover helpful resources for in-depth study and research that empower you in your quest for greater knowledge and maximize your potential for success in the course.

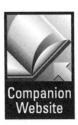

[www.pearsoned.ca/bledsoe]

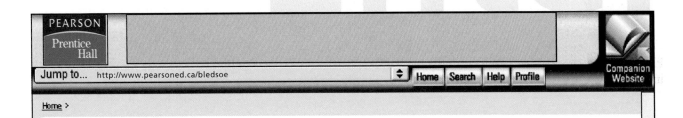

Jump to... http://www.pearsoned.ca/bledsoe   Home Search Help Profile

Home >

PH Companion Website

Essentials of Paramedic Care, Canadian Edition, Volumes 1 and 2, by Bledsoe/Porter/Cherry/Clayden

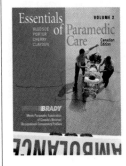

Student Resources

The modules in this section provide students with tools for learning course material. These modules include:

- Chapter Objectives
- Destinations
- Quizzes
- PowerPoint Presentations
- Glossary
- Flashcards

In the quiz modules, students can send answers to the grader and receive instant feedback on their progress through the Results Reporter. Coaching comments and references to the textbook may be available to ensure that students take advantage of all available resources to enhance their learning experience.

Instructor Resources

The modules in this section provide instructors with additional teaching tools. Downloadable PowerPoint Presentations and an Instructor's Manual are just some of the materials that may be available in this section. Where appropriate, this section will be password protected. To get a password, simply contact your Pearson Education Canada Representative or call Faculty Sales and Services at 1-800-850-5813.

EMPHASIZING PRINCIPLES

Chapter Objectives with Page References

Each chapter begins with clearly stated **Objectives** that follow the N.O.C.P. curriculum. Students can refer to these objectives while studying to make sure they fully understand the material. Page references after each objective indicate where relevant content is covered in the chapter.

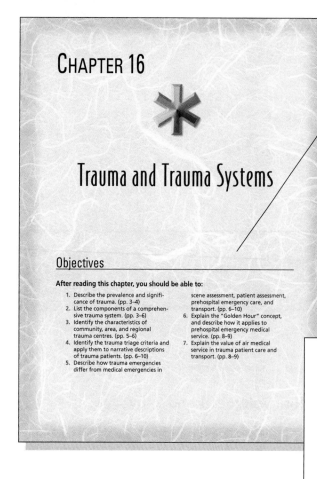

CHAPTER 16

Trauma and Trauma Systems

Objectives

After reading this chapter, you should be able to:

1. Describe the prevalence and significance of trauma. (pp. 3–4)
2. List the components of a comprehensive trauma system. (pp. 3–6)
3. Identify the characteristics of community, area, and regional trauma centres. (pp. 5–6)
4. Identify the trauma triage criteria and apply them to narrative descriptions of trauma patients. (pp. 6–10)
5. Describe how trauma emergencies differ from medical emergencies in scene assessment, patient assessment, prehospital emergency care, and transport. (pp. 6–10)
6. Explain the "Golden Hour" concept, and describe how it applies to prehospital emergency medical service. (pp. 8–9)
7. Explain the value of air medical service in trauma patient care and transport. (pp. 8–9)

Content Review

Content Review summarizes important content and gives students a format for quick review.

and the lumen does not constrict. The result is heavy and continued bleeding. Crush trauma often produces this type of damage. The vessels are not torn cleanly and do not withdraw. The actual hemorrhage site is lost in the disrupted tissue, resulting in severe, hard-to-control bleeding from a large wound area.

If a severe hemorrhage continues, frank hypotension reduces the blood pressure at the hemorrhage site. This limits the flow of blood and the dislodging of clots, thus improving the effectiveness of the clotting mechanism.

FACTORS AFFECTING THE CLOTTING PROCESS

The clotting process can be either helped or hindered by a variety of factors. For example, movement at or around the wound site, as in the manipulation of a fracture, may break the developing clot loose and disrupt the forming fibrin strands. For this reason, immediate wound immobilization (splinting) is beneficial.

Aggressive fluid therapy, which is often provided in cases of severe hemorrhage, may adversely change the effectiveness of clotting mechanisms. Aggressive fluid resuscitation may increase blood pressure, which, in turn, increases the pressure pushing against the developing clots. In addition, the water and salts used in fluid therapy dilute the clotting factors, platelets, and red blood cells, further inhibiting the clotting process.

The patient's body temperature also has an effect on the clotting process. As the body temperature begins to fall, as it may in shock states, clot formation is neither as rapid nor as effective as when the body temperature is 37°C (98.6°F). Thus, it is important to keep a patient with severe hemorrhage warm.

Medications may interfere with the body's ability to form a clot and halt both internal and external hemorrhage. Aspirin modifies the enzymes on the surface of platelets that cause them to aggregate after an injury. Ibuprofen and other NSAIDs (nonsteroidal anti-inflammatory drugs) may have a similar but temporary effect. Heparin and warfarin (Coumadin) interfere with the normal generation of protein fibres that produce a stable clot. While these drugs may prevent thrombosis and emboli in patients with heart disease, they may prolong or worsen hemorrhage when that patient is injured. Try to gather information on whether the patient uses such medications when taking the patient history.

HEMORRHAGE CONTROL

Hemorrhage is either internal or external. While there are a number of steps you can take to control external hemorrhage in the field, prehospital care of internal hemorrhage is more limited.

External Hemorrhage

External hemorrhage is easy to identify and care for. It presents with blood oozing, flowing, or spurting from the wound. Bleeding from capillary and venous wounds is easy to halt because the pressure driving it is limited (Figure 19-3). Usually, **direct pressure** on the wound or a combination of direct pressure and elevation work quite well in stopping the bleeding. Bleeding from an arterial wound, however, is powered by the arterial blood pressure, and the blood escapes from the blood vessel with significant force. The normal control and clotting mechanisms help reduce blood loss but do not stop it if the injured vessel is large. To stop bleeding from such a wound, pressure on the bleeding site must exceed the arterial pressure. Direct digital pressure on the site of blood loss, maintained by a dressing and pressure bandage, is most effective. Elevation of the wound area and use of pressure points may also be necessary if the bandage cannot bring about enough pressure directly to the hemorrhage site.

Content Review

FACTORS HINDERING THE CLOTTING PROCESS
Movement of the wound site
Aggressive fluid therapy
Low body temperature
Medications, such as aspirin, heparin, or warfarin

Immediate immobilization (splinting) of the wound site aids the clotting process.

✳ **direct pressure** method of hemorrhage control that relies on the application of pressure to the actual site of the bleeding.

Key Points

Key Points in the margins help students identify and learn the fundamental principles of paramedic practice.

Key Terms

Reinforcement of **Key Terms** helps students master new terminology.

Table 19-1	PATIENT SIGNS ASSOCIATED WITH STAGES OF HEMORRHAGE						
Stage	Blood Loss	Vasoconstriction	Pulse Rate	Pulse (Pressure) Strength	Blood Pressure	Respiratory Rate	Respiratory Volume
1	< 15%	↑	↑	→	→	→	→
2	15–25%	↑↑	↑↑	↓	→	↑	↑
3	25–35%	↑↑↑	↑↑↑	↓↓	↓	↑↑	↓
4	> 35%	↓↓	Variable	↓↓↓	↓↓↓	↓	↓↓

Tables and Illustrations

Tables and **illustrations** offer visual support to enhance students' understanding of paramedic principles and practice.

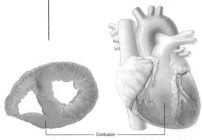

FIGURE 25-11 Myocardial contusion most frequently affects the right atrium and ventricle as they collide with the sternum.

The cardiac contusion is similar to a contusion in any other muscle tissue. The injury disrupts the muscle cells and microcirculation, resulting in muscle fibre tearing and damage, hemorrhage, and edema. The injury may reduce the strength of cardiac contraction and reduce cardiac output. Because of the automaticity and conductivity of the cardiac muscle, contusion may also disturb the cardiac electrical system. If the injury is serious, it may lead to hematoma, hemopericardium (blood in the pericardial sac), and necrosis and may result in cardiac irritability, ectopic (irregularly occurring) beats, and conduction system defects, such as bundle branch blocks and dysrhythmias. If the injury is extensive, it may lead to tissue necrosis (death), decreased ventricular compliance, congestive heart failure, cardiogenic shock, myocardial aneurysm, and acute or delayed myocardial rupture. In contrast to a myocardial infarction from coronary artery disease, the cellular damage from myocardial contusions heals with less scarring, and there is no progression of the injury in the absence of associated coronary artery disease.

The patient experiencing myocardial contusion will have a history of significant blunt chest trauma, most likely affecting the anterior chest. The patient will likely complain of chest or retrosternal pain, very much like that of myocardial infarction and may have associated chest injuries, such as anterior rib or sternal fractures. Cardiac monitoring most frequently reveals sinus tachycardia (though it may be caused by pain, hypovolemia, or hypoxia from associated chest injury). Other dysrhythmias associated with myocardial contusions are atrial flutter or fibrillation, premature atrial or ventricular contractions, tachydysrhythmias, bradydysrhythmias, bundle branch patterns, T-wave inversions, and ST-segment elevations. A pericardial friction rub and murmur may be auscultated over the **precordium** but is more likely to occur weeks after the injury and is associated with the development of an inflammatory pericardial effusion.

Pericardial Tamponade

Pericardial tamponade is a restriction to cardiac filling caused by blood (or other fluid) within the pericardial sac. It occurs in less than 2 percent of all serious chest

Content Review

SIGNS AND SYMPTOMS OF CARDIAC CONTUSION
Blunt injury to chest
Bruising of chest wall
Rapid heart rate—may be irregular
Severe nagging pain not relieved with rest but may be relieved with oxygen.

✴ **precordium** area of the chest wall overlying the heart.

✴ **pericardial tamponade** a restriction to cardiac filling caused by blood (or other fluid) within the pericardial sac.

Pathophysiology of Thoracic Trauma 291

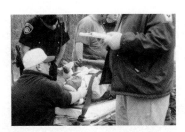

FIGURE 19-14 Emotional support for the seriously injured trauma patient is an important part of shock patient care.

associated with breathing and, in some cases, reducing chest excursion. Application of the garment also increases mortality when used in cases of penetrating chest trauma. In light of this information, it is imperative that you understand the limitations of the device and comply with your local protocols and medical direction when considering use of the PASG.

Pharmacological Intervention

In shock, pharmacological interventions are generally limited, especially in hypovolemic patients. The sympathetic nervous system efficiently compensates for low volume, and no agent, other than intravenous fluid and, in some cases, blood and blood products, has been shown to be effective in the prehospital setting. For cardiogenic shock, fluid challenge, vasopressors (e.g., dopamine), and the other cardiac drugs are indicated (see Chapter 28, "Cardiology"). For spinal and obstructive shock, consider intravenous fluids, such as normal saline and Ringer's Lactate solution. For distributive shock, consider IV fluids, dopamine, and use of the PASG.

The patient who has experienced trauma sufficient to induce hemorrhage and hypovolemia will be anxious and bewildered. As the care provider at the patient's side, it is your responsibility to be calm and reassuring, thus counteracting the natural "fight-or-flight" response (Figure 19-14). By acting in this manner, you not only help your patient deal with the event's emotional trauma but also combat some of the negative effects of sympathetic stimulation.

SUMMARY

Significant hemorrhage and its serious consequence, shock, are genuine threats to the trauma patient's life. The signs of these threats are often subtle or hidden, especially if bleeding is internal. Only through careful analysis of the mechanism of injury during the scene assessment and careful evaluation of the patient during the assessment process can you recognize and then treat these life-threatening problems. Treatment often involves rapidly bringing the patient to the services of a trauma centre and, while doing so, providing aggressive care—supplemental oxygen, positive pressure ventilations, and fluid resuscitation, aimed at maintaining vital signs, not necessarily improving them. With this approach, you afford your patient the best chance for survival.

End-of-Chapter Summary

Each end-of-chapter **Summary** reviews the main topics covered.

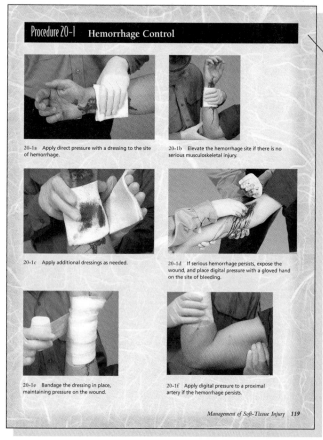

Procedure 20-1   Hemorrhage Control

20-1a   Apply direct pressure with a dressing to the site of hemorrhage.

20-1b   Elevate the hemorrhage site if there is no serious musculoskeletal injury.

20-1c   Apply additional dressings as needed.

20-1d   If serious hemorrhage persists, expose the wound, and place digital pressure with a gloved hand on the site of bleeding.

20-1e   Bandage the dressing in place, maintaining pressure on the wound.

20-1f   Apply digital pressure to a proximal artery if the hemorrhage persists.

Management of Soft-Tissue Injury   119

Procedure Scans

Newly photographed **Procedure Scans** provide step-by-step visual support on how to perform skills included in the DOT curriculum.

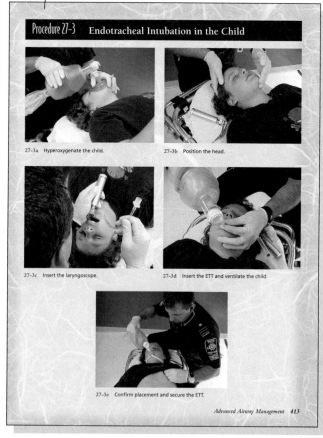

Procedure 27-3   Endotracheal Intubation in the Child

27-3a   Hyperoxygenate the child.

27-3b   Position the head.

27-3c   Insert the laryngoscope.

27-3d   Insert the ETT and ventilate the child.

27-3e   Confirm placement and secure the ETT.

Advanced Airway Management   413

Prehospital Care Report
FOR BLS FR USE ONLY

CHIEF COMPLAINT
SUBJECTIVE ASSESSMENT
PRESENTING PROBLEM
PAST MEDICAL HISTORY
VITAL SIGNS
OBJECTIVE PHYSICAL ASSESSMENT
COMMENTS
TREATMENT GIVEN
DISPOSITION
AGENCY COPY/WHITE

FIGURE 9-4 Complete both the narrative and check-box sections of every PCR.

Elements of Good Documentation 423

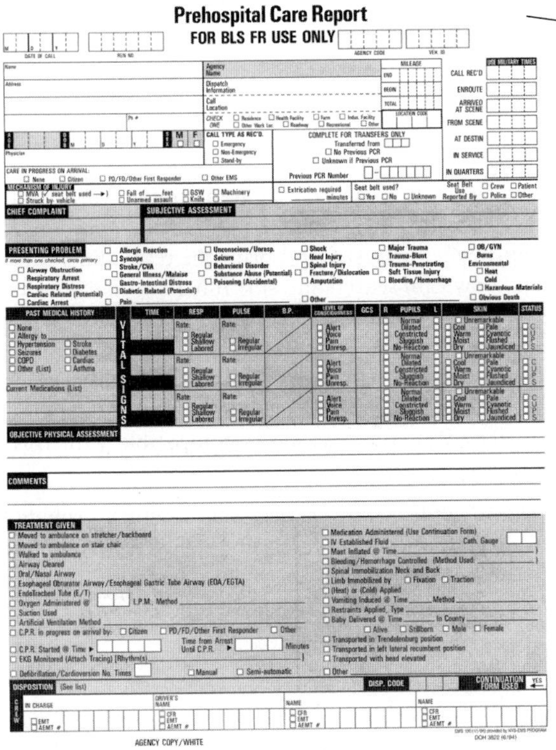

Documentation

Covered thoroughly throughout the text, **proper documentation techniques** are critical to ensuring provider protection on the job as well as patient safety during the transition of care.

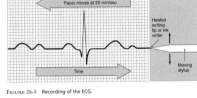

FIGURE 28-5 Recording of the ECG.

A single monitoring lead can provide considerable information:

- The rate of the heartbeat
- The regularity of the heartbeat
- The time it takes to conduct the impulse through the various parts of the heart

A single lead cannot provide the following information:

- The presence or location of an infarct
- Axis deviation or chamber enlargement
- Right-to-left differences in conduction or impulse formation
- The quality or presence of pumping action

ECG Graph Paper

ECG graph paper is standardized to allow comparative analysis of ECG patterns. The paper moves across the stylus at a standard speed of 25 mm/sec (Figure 28-5). The *amplitude* of the ECG *deflection* is also standardized. When properly calibrated, the ECG stylus should deflect two large boxes when one millivolt (mV) is present. Most machines have calibration buttons, and a calibration curve should be placed at the beginning of the first ECG strip. Many machines do this automatically when they are first turned on.

The ECG graph is divided into a grid of light and heavy lines. The light lines are 1 mm apart, and the heavy lines are 5 mm apart. The heavy lines thus enclose large squares, each containing 25 of the smaller squares formed by the lighter lines (Figure 28-6). The following relationships apply to the horizontal axis:

1 small box = 0.04 sec

1 large box = 0.20 sec (0.04 sec × 5 = 0.20 sec)

These increments measure the duration of the ECG complexes and time intervals. The vertical axis reflects the voltage amplitude in millivolts (mV). Two large boxes equal 1.0 mV.

Electrocardiographic Monitoring 455

Medical Calculations

Mathematical examples are provided to give students practice in medical calculations, a critical skill in prehospital care.

Teaching and Learning Package

For the Instructor

The following resources are available to aid instructors:

Instructor's Resource CD-ROM for Volume 1 and Volume 2 with Instructor's Resource Manual, TestGen, and PowerPoint Slides (ISBN 0-13-197285-5)

The Instructor's Resource CD-ROM contains all print and technology supplements on a single CD-ROM. Enjoy the freedom to transport the entire package to the office, home, or classroom. This enables you to customize any of the ancillaries, print only the chapters or materials that you wish to use, or access any item from the package within the classroom. This CD-ROM provides the following resources:

Instructor's Resource Manual The Instructor's Resource Manual contains everything needed to teach curriculum that is based on the Canadian National Paramedic Competencies. The manual provides a variety of teaching strategies for each chapter that are intended to help convey information to the broadest range of students. Included are:

- lecture outlines
- innovative teaching strategies
- suggestions for additional resources
- student activities handouts for reinforcement and evaluation

Pearson TestGen This special computerized test item file enables instructors to view and edit existing questions, add questions, generate tests, and print the tests in a variety of formats. Powerful search and sort functions make it easy to locate questions and arrange them in any order desired. TestGen also enables instructors to administer tests on a local area network, have the tests graded electronically, and have the results prepared in electronic or printed reports. The Pearson TestGen is compatible with IBM or Macintosh systems.

PowerPoint Slides PowerPoint Slides, which provide key points covered in each chapter, are included to aid instructors in the presentation of text material.

Downloadable Instructor Supplements The Instructor's Resource Manual and PowerPoint Slides are available for downloading at www.pearsoned.ca, Pearson's online catalogue. Search for this text within the catalogue and then click on "Instructor" to access the supplements in a protected area for instructors.

For the Student

Student Workbook (Volume 1: ISBN 0-13-120307-X; Volume 2: ISBN 0-13-120308-8)

A student workbook with review and practice activities accompanies *Essentials of Paramedic Care*. The workbook includes multiple-choice questions, fill-in-the-blank questions, labelling exercises, case studies, and special projects, along with an answer key with text page references.

Online Resources

Companion Website This free site, located at **www.pearsoned.ca/bledsoe**, is tied chapter by chapter to the text. It reinforces student learning through interactive online study guides, quizzes based on the new curriculum, and links to important EMS-related internet resources.

DIVISION 3
TRAUMA EMERGENCIES

Chapter 16   Trauma and Trauma Systems   2

Chapter 17   Blunt Trauma   12

Chapter 18   Penetrating Trauma   44

Chapter 19   Hemorrhage and Shock   64

Chapter 20   Soft-Tissue Trauma   93

Chapter 21   Burns   134

Chapter 22   Musculoskeletal Trauma   167

Chapter 23   Head, Face, and Neck Trauma   204

Chapter 24   Spinal Trauma   247

Chapter 25   Thoracic Trauma   275

Chapter 26   Abdominal Trauma   308

CHAPTER 16

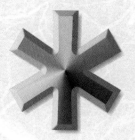

Trauma and Trauma Systems

Objectives

After reading this chapter, you should be able to:

1. Describe the prevalence and significance of trauma. (pp. 3–4)
2. List the components of a comprehensive trauma system. (pp. 3–6)
3. Identify the characteristics of community, area, and regional trauma centres. (pp. 5–6)
4. Identify the trauma triage criteria and apply them to narrative descriptions of trauma patients. (pp. 6–10)
5. Describe how trauma emergencies differ from medical emergencies in scene assessment, patient assessment, prehospital emergency care, and transport. (pp. 6–10)
6. Explain the "Golden Hour" concept, and describe how it applies to prehospital emergency medical service. (pp. 8–9)
7. Explain the value of air medical service in trauma patient care and transport. (pp. 8–9)

INTRODUCTION TO TRAUMA
AND TRAUMA CARE

Trauma is a physical injury or wound caused by external force or violence. It is the number-four killer in Canada today behind cardiovascular disease, stroke, and cancer. It is, however, the leading killer of persons under age 45. As such, trauma steals the greatest number of productive years from its victims. It also may be the most expensive medical problem because of the productivity losses it causes for its victims and the high cost of initial care, rehabilitation, and often lifelong maintenance of those victims.

Nearly all injuries are predictable and preventable. Drunk drivers kill well over twice as many Canadians as do murders. Firearms cause more than 1300 deaths in Canada each year. Other deaths are attributed to falls, blasts, stabbings, crush injuries, and sports injuries. In addition to the great death toll from trauma, many more of its victims are injured and carry lifelong physical reminders of their experiences with it.

Your role in trauma care, as a member of the Emergency Medical Services (EMS) team, is to understand the structure and objectives of the trauma care system, to promote injury prevention, and to provide the injured trauma patient with proper assessment, care, and rapid transport to the most appropriate facility. The remainder of this chapter will help you with these responsibilities as it further defines trauma, explains the components of trauma care systems, identifies the capabilities of different levels of trauma centres, and more fully defines your role as a care provider in the trauma system.

TRAUMA

The types of trauma can range from slight abrasions or scratches to the fatal, multiple-system injuries that might result from a collision between a high-speed automobile and a pedestrian. Trauma is broken down into two major categories; blunt and penetrating. **Penetrating trauma** occurs when an arrow, a bullet, a knife, or other object enters the body and exchanges energy with human tissue, thereby causing injury. **Blunt trauma** is injury that occurs as the energy and forces of collision with an object—not the object itself—enter the body and damage tissue. These two categories of trauma are discussed in greater detail in the next two chapters of this book.

Although trauma poses a serious threat to life, its presentation often masks the patient's true condition. Extremity injuries, for example, infrequently cause death. Yet they are often obvious and grotesque (Figure 16-1). On the other hand, life-threatening problems, such as internal bleeding and shock, may occur with only subtle signs and symptoms. When assessing a trauma patient, you must look beyond obvious injuries for evidence that suggests a life-threatening condition. When such a condition is found, you must ensure rapid access to the trauma system for your patient.

Serious and life-threatening injury occurs in fewer than 10 percent of trauma patients. In most patients with life-threatening injury, the injury is internal and is likely to involve the head or a body cavity hemorrhage. Prehospital care can neither properly nor definitively stabilize these patients and their injuries in the field. The best care you as a paramedic can offer is to secure the airway, ensure adequate respirations, control any significant external hemorrhage, and rapidly transport the patient to definitive trauma care. That care is only available at a specialized treatment facility with rapid access to surgery—a trauma centre.

Thus, 90 percent of trauma patients do not have serious, life-threatening injuries. Prehospital care for these patients includes providing thorough on-scene

* **trauma** a physical injury or wound caused by external force or violence.

Trauma is the leading killer of persons under age 45 in Canada.

* **penetrating trauma** injury caused by an object breaking the skin and entering the body.

* **blunt trauma** injury caused by the collision of an object with the body during which the object does not enter the body.

Life-threatening problems, such as internal bleeding and shock, may occur with only subtle signs and symptoms.

When assessing a trauma patient, look beyond obvious injuries for evidence that suggests a life-threatening condition.

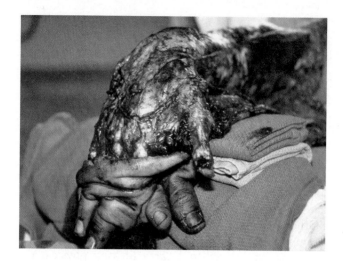

FIGURE 16-1 In prehospital care, it is essential that gruesome, non-life-threatening injuries do not distract you from more subtle, life-threatening problems.

assessment and stabilization, followed by conservative transport to the nearest general hospital or other appropriate health-care facility.

It is essential that you determine the difference between trauma patients with serious, life-threatening conditions and those less seriously injured patients during your assessment. You will be aided in making this determination by using guidelines known as trauma triage criteria. These criteria involve consideration of the mechanisms by which patients are injured and of the physical or clinical findings indicating internal injury. Using these criteria, which will be discussed in detail later in this chapter, will help you properly direct patients as they enter the trauma care system.

THE TRAUMA CARE SYSTEM

In the mid-to-late 1960s, several medically oriented groups investigated the death toll on American highways. (To date, similar studies have not been conducted in Canada at the national level.) Their studies revealed that victims of vehicle crashes suffered not only from the injuries received in the crashes but also from the lack of an organized approach to bringing these victims into the health-care system. The studies also demonstrated that most hospitals were inadequately equipped and staffed to care for the victims of these crashes.

More than two decades later, the American College of Surgeons, recognizing that the system of caring for severely injured trauma victims was still inadequate, successfully worked to achieve passage of the Trauma Care Systems Planning and Development Act of 1990. This act helped establish guidelines, funding, and state-level leadership and support for the development of trauma systems.

Serious trauma is a surgical disease; its proper care is immediate surgical intervention to repair internal hemorrhage sites.

The trauma system is predicated on the principle that serious trauma is a *surgical disease*. This means that the proper care for serious internal trauma is often immediate surgical intervention to repair internal hemorrhage sites. While patients with life-threatening injuries account for less than 10 percent of all trauma patients, immediate surgical care of these patients can drastically reduce trauma mortality and morbidity.

Care for seriously injured trauma patients is expensive and complicated. A well-designed EMS system will allocate limited resources in a way that provides the most efficient and effective care for these patients. Such a system utilizes hospitals with special resources and commitment to trauma patient care. These hospitals are designated as trauma centres.

TRAUMA CENTRE DESIGNATION

The current model for a trauma system includes three levels of **trauma centre**, with an increased ability and commitment to provide trauma care at each level (Table 16-1).

The tertiary trauma centre is a hospital, usually a university teaching centre, that is prepared and committed to handle all types of specialty trauma (Figure 16-2). These centres provide neurosurgery, microsurgery (limb reattachment), pediatric care, burn care, and care for multisystem trauma. They also provide leadership and resource support to other levels of the regional trauma system through system coordination and continuing medical and public education programs. When population density does not permit a commitment to the requirements of a tertiary trauma centre, a district trauma centre may act as the regional trauma centre.

The district trauma centre has an increased commitment to trauma care, but not as great as that of a tertiary trauma centre. It has surgical care capability available at all times for incoming trauma patients. District trauma centres can handle all but the most seriously injured specialty and multisystem trauma patients. Staff at these facilities can stabilize those patients in preparation for transport to a tertiary trauma centre.

The primary trauma centre is a general hospital with a commitment to special staff training and resource allocation for trauma patients. These centres are located in smaller cities situated in generally rural areas. They are well prepared to care for most trauma victims and to stabilize and triage more seriously injured ones for transport to higher level trauma centres.

The design of a trauma system should be flexible in order to meet the needs of the region it serves. In urban and suburban areas, there are just a few trauma centres to ensure that each receives adequate patient volume to maintain staff proficiency and to ensure that resources are being effectively used. In rural regions, a district trauma centre may act as the tertiary trauma centre because the incidence of serious trauma does not support any greater commitment. Consult your EMS system plan to determine the intended patient flow patterns in your region.

SPECIALTY CENTRES

Beyond classification as trauma centres, certain medical facilities may be designated as specialty centres. Such facilities may include neurocentres, burn centres,

The modern trauma system includes three levels of trauma centre, each with an increased ability and commitment to providing trauma care.

✳ trauma centre a hospital that has the capability to care for acutely injured patients; trauma centres must meet strict criteria to use this designation.

Table 16-1	CRITERIA FOR TRAUMA CENTRE DESIGNATION
Tertiary Trauma Centre (TTC)	
Commits resources to address all types of specialty trauma 24 hours a day, 7 days a week.	
District Trauma Centre (DTC)	
Commits the resources to address the most common trauma emergencies with surgical capability available 24 hours a day, 7 days a week; will stabilize and transport specialty cases to the tertiary trauma centre.	
Primary Trauma Centre (PTC)	
Commits to special emergency department training and has some surgical capability but will usually stabilize and transfer seriously injured trauma patients to a higher level trauma centre as needed.	

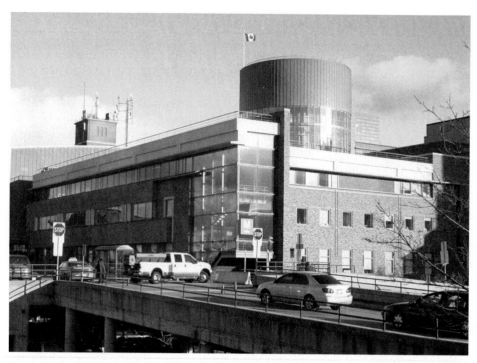

FIGURE 16-2   Toronto's Sunnybrook Hospital has a tertiary trauma facility.
Source: CP Photo/Boris Spremo

pediatric trauma centres, and centres specializing in hand and limb reattachment by microsurgery. One other specialty service is hyperbaric oxygenation, which is important in the treatment of carbon monoxide poisoning and problems related to SCUBA (self-contained underwater breathing apparatus) diving.

Specialty centres have made a commitment of trained personnel, equipment, and other resources to provide services not usually available at a general or trauma hospital. These centres are also more likely to provide a higher level of intensive care and state-of-the-art injury management than other facilities are able to. Be aware of the specialty services available in your system as well as the protocols defining when patients should be directed to them.

YOUR ROLE AS A PARAMEDIC

As a paramedic, your tasks in the trauma system are likely to include the triage of trauma patients against standards established by your medical direction authority (trauma triage criteria) and the rapid assessment, care, and transport of patients to the closest appropriate medical facility (Figure 16-3). For those patients who meet trauma triage criteria, the appropriate facility is the nearest trauma centre.

Trauma triage criteria are guidelines established to help you determine which patients require the services of a trauma centre and which do not. The presence of certain mechanisms of injury and clinical findings have been proven, by research, to accurately reflect the potential for serious injury and the need for the intensive services available only at a trauma centre. Compare your patient's mechanism of injury and any physical assessment findings with these pre-established criteria. These criteria are listed in detail later in this chapter. If your patient meets any of the criteria, rapid transport is required.

✳ **trauma triage criteria** guidelines to aid prehospital personnel in determining which trauma patients require urgent transportation to a trauma centre.

MECHANISM OF INJURY ANALYSIS

To help determine the **mechanism of injury,** mentally recreate the accident from evidence available at the scene. You should identify the forces involved in the incident, the direction from which they came, and the areas of the patient's body affected by these forces. In an automobile collision, for example, the mechanism of injury includes the energy exchange process between the auto and what it struck, between the patient and the auto's interior, and among the various tissues and organs as they collide one with another within the patient. Close inspection of the mangled auto reveals evidence about the collision and the forces at work in it. (See Chapter 17, "Blunt Trauma," and Chapter 18, "Penetrating Trauma.")

You will begin your consideration of the mechanism of injury during the scene assessment. Later, you should reconsider the mechanism of injury as the first step of the focused history and physical assessment of the trauma patient.

INDEX OF SUSPICION

The information you gather during your consideration and reconsideration of the mechanism of injury suggests an **index of suspicion** for possible injuries. This index is an anticipation of possible injuries based on analysis of the event. For example, a pedestrian struck by a car can be expected to have lower extremity fractures. Further, if the auto were moving at 30 km per hour, fracture severity would be less than if it were moving at 100 km per hour. Also, the probability of internal injury at lower speeds is less than it would be at higher speeds. By evaluating the force of the impact and its nature, you can anticipate the structures and organs damaged and the degree to which they have been damaged.

In addition to developing an index of suspicion for specific injuries, you will also examine the trauma patient for physical signs of injury, both during the initial assessment and during the rapid trauma assessment or the focused history and physical assessment. The physical signs suggesting serious trauma include the signs and symptoms of shock and those of internal head injury. Since shock and head injury are the principal killers in trauma, be alert for the earliest evi-

---

* **mechanism of injury** the processes and forces that cause trauma.

Consideration of the mechanism of injury begins during the scene assessment. The mechanism of injury should be reconsidered as the first step of the focused history and secondary assessment for trauma patients.

---

* **index of suspicion** the anticipation of injury to a body region, organ, or structure based on analysis of the mechanism of injury.

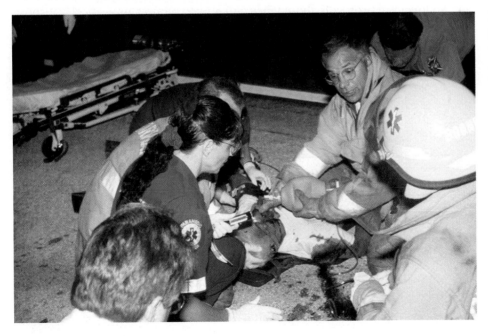

FIGURE 16-3 Your role as a paramedic attending a critical trauma patient is to ensure the ABCs and prepare the patient for rapid transport.

dence of their existence. Remember, the body compensates well for the internal loss of blood and hides serious signs of injury until late in the shock process. If you have any reason to suspect that a patient has sustained serious internal injury, move to enter that patient rapidly into the trauma system. Otherwise, provide frequent ongoing assessment to ensure that progressive signs of shock and internal head injury are discovered as early as possible.

THE GOLDEN HOUR

Time is a very important consideration in the survival of seriously injured trauma patients. Research has demonstrated that patient survival rates increase dramatically as time from the trauma incident to the beginning of surgery decreases. The current goal for incident-to-surgery time is one hour, often referred to as the **Golden Hour.**

 Golden Hour the 60-minute period after a severe injury; it is the maximum acceptable time between the injury and initiation of surgery for the seriously injured trauma patient.

Such factors as the location of the incident and the time needed to extricate a patient all consume a portion of the Golden Hour. Many of these factors will be beyond your control; for that reason, it is vital to keep to a minimum the time spent on factors over which you do have control. Ideally, you should provide the initial and rapid trauma assessments, emergency stabilization, patient packaging, and initiation of transport in under 10 minutes. When distances or traffic conditions present prolonged ground transport times, reduce transport times by using an air medical service if possible.

Air medical service, usually provided by helicopter, has added a weapon in the fight against time for the seriously injured trauma patient (Figure 16-4). The helicopter travels much faster than ground transport and in a straight line from the crash scene to the trauma centre.

Be aware, however, that air medical transport is not appropriate in all cases. Trauma patients must be in relatively stable condition for it to be utilized. Additionally, the limited space within the aircraft and its associated engine noise make in-flight care difficult. Further, combative patients may endanger the safety of the flight crew and the aircraft. Adverse weather conditions can also limit the use of air medical transport. Finally, air medical transport services are very expensive and can be used most effectively only as part of a comprehensive EMS trauma system. Follow local protocols about when and how to request air medical transport.

FIGURE 16-4 Air ambulance utilizes a helicopter to significantly reduce transport time from the accident scene to the nearest trauma centre.

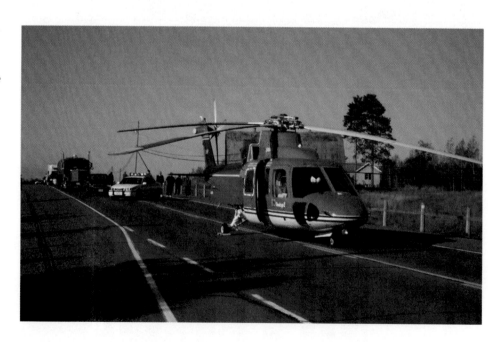

THE DECISION TO TRANSPORT

The decision either to transport a patient immediately or to attempt more extensive on-scene care is among the most difficult you must make. The trauma triage criteria are designed to help you with this decision. As a rule, quickly transport patients who experience certain mechanisms of injury or display key clinical findings, with intravenous access and other time-consuming procedures attempted en route. Indicators for immediate transport are given in Table 16-2.

Table 16-2	TRAUMA TRIAGE CRITERIA INDICATING NEED FOR IMMEDIATE TRANSPORT

Mechanism of Injury

- Falls greater than six metres (three times the victim's height)
- Pedestrian/bicyclist versus auto collisions
  - Struck by a vehicle travelling more than 10 km/h
  - Thrown or run over by vehicle
- Motorcycle impact at greater than 30 km/h
- Ejection from a vehicle
- Severe vehicle impact
  - Speed at impact greater than 60 km/h
  - Intrusion of more than 30 cm into occupant compartment
  - Vehicle deformity greater than 50 cm
- Rollover with signs of serious impact
- Death of another occupant in the vehicle
- Extrication time greater than 20 minutes

Significant mechanism of injury considerations with infants and children include the following:
- A fall of greater than three metres (three times the victim's height)
- A bicycle/vehicle collision
- A vehicle collision at medium speed
- Any vehicle collision in which the infant or child was unrestrained

Physical Findings

- Revised Trauma Score less than 11
- Glasgow Coma Scale less than 14
- Systolic blood pressure less than 90
- Respiratory rate less than 10 or greater than 29
- Pulse less than 50 or greater than 120
- Two or more proximal long-bone fractures
- Flail chest
- Pelvic fracture
- Limb paralysis
- Burns to more than 15 percent of body surface area
- Burns to airway or face
- Complete amputation of limb, thumb, or penis; eye avulsion; partial limb amputation (partial amputation of the thumb and penis, depending on severity of the injury)
- Tender, distended abdomen secondary to blunt/penetrating trauma
- Head injury with unilaterally dilated pupil, and/or patient unconscious or level of consciousness decreased or decreasing during assessment

In applying trauma triage criteria, it is best to err on the side of caution. If a patient does not fit the stated criteria, be suspicious. Remember, you often arrive at the patient's side only minutes after the accident. The patient may not yet have lost enough blood internally to exhibit signs of shock or progressive head injury. If in doubt, transport to a trauma centre without delay.

These criteria are designed for the "over-triage" of trauma patients. They ensure that patients with very subtle signs and symptoms, yet with significant and serious injuries, are not missed during assessment. Use of these criteria means that you will transport some patients to trauma centres unnecessarily. However, transporting a patient who may not need the resources of a trauma centre is far better than not transporting a patient who truly needs the care available only there.

INJURY PREVENTION

One of the best, most cost-effective ways of reducing mortality and morbidity is to prevent trauma in the first place. Programs promoting seat belt use and awareness of the dangers of drinking and driving have encouraged teenagers and adults to drive more safely and responsibly. Other programs increase society's awareness of trauma systems as well as appreciation for safety-oriented behaviours. Safety programs for users of boats and firearms also raise safety awareness and assist in injury prevention. The EMS system has a responsibility to support such programs and to promote their introduction and development where they do not exist. As an EMS provider, you should participate and encourage your peers to participate in these programs.

Technical developments, such as better highway design, airbag restraint systems, vehicles constructed to absorb the energy of crashes, and mandatory seat belt legislation have also played major parts in greatly reducing the yearly highway death toll. Paramedics have a responsibility to support the development and use of these new designs and technologies as a way of further reducing trauma deaths and injuries.

DATA AND THE TRAUMA REGISTRY

As with all emergency medical services, research is the only way to recognize those trauma care practices and procedures that benefit patients and those that do not. In the trauma system, the **trauma registry** is a uniform and standard set of data collected by regional trauma centres. These data are analyzed to determine how well the system is performing and to identify factors that may contribute to or lessen chances of patient survival.

It is important that you do all that you can to support this research effort by ensuring that your prehospital documentation accurately and completely describes the findings of your assessments, the care you provide to patients, the results of ongoing assessments, and the times associated with calls. You should also consider taking part in and supporting prehospital research projects if the opportunity presents itself.

QUALITY IMPROVEMENT

Trauma system quality improvement (QI) or quality management (QM) is another way of examining system performance with the aim of providing better patient care. In the QI process, committees look at selected care modalities (called indicators) to determine whether designated standards of care are being met. For trauma system QI, the committees study the application of trauma triage criteria, performance of field skills, and amounts of time spent in various aspects of response, care, and transport of patients. QI committees may also look at select calls to determine if their documentation accurately reflects the results of assessment and the care given. If the system standards are not being met, the committees may suggest such steps as continuing education programs or modification of protocols. As a member of the trauma system, you should become actively involved in such programs and encourage the participation of your peers.

SUMMARY

Trauma remains one of the greatest tragedies of our modern society. It accounts for large numbers of deaths and disabling injuries and often affects individuals who are in their most productive years of life. A well-designed and well-implemented trauma system offers a way of lessening the impact of these traumas.

As a paramedic, you are a part of the trauma system. You are charged with evaluating trauma patients by comparing their mechanisms of injury and the physical signs of their injuries with preestablished trauma triage criteria in order to determine which patients should enter the trauma system and which could be best cared for at a general hospital. In the presence of severe, life-threatening trauma, you must ensure rapid assessment, on-scene care, and appropriate transport to provide your patients with the best chances for survival.

CHAPTER 17

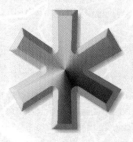

Blunt Trauma

Objectives

After reading this chapter, you should be able to:

1. Identify and explain by example the laws of inertia and conservation of energy. (pp. 13–14)
2. Define kinetic energy and force as they relate to trauma. (pp. 14–15)
3. Compare and contrast the types of vehicle impacts and their expected injuries. (pp. 16–19, 21–34)
4. Discuss the benefits of auto restraint and motorcycle helmet use. (pp. 19–21, 31–32)
5. Describe the mechanisms of injury associated with falls, crush injuries, and sports injuries. (pp. 40–43)
6. Identify the common blast injuries and any special considerations regarding their assessment and proper care. (pp. 34–40)
7. Identify and explain any special assessment and care considerations for patients suffering blunt trauma. (pp. 16–43)
8. Given several preprogrammed and moulaged blunt trauma patients, provide the appropriate scene assessment, initial assessment, rapid trauma or focused physical assessment and history, detailed assessment, and ongoing assessment, and provide appropriate patient care and transportation. (pp. 16–43)

INTRODUCTION TO BLUNT TRAUMA

Blunt trauma is the most common cause of trauma-related death and disability. It results from an energy exchange between an object and the human body, without intrusion of the object through the skin (Figure 17-1). The energy exchange causes a chain reaction among various body tissues that crushes and stretches their structures, resulting in injury beneath the surface. Blunt trauma is especially confounding because the true nature of the injury is often hidden, and evidence of the serious injury is very subtle or even absent.

To properly care for victims of blunt trauma, you should understand the injury process and its results. This study, called kinetics of trauma, gives insight into the events that produce injury, known as the mechanism of injury. This insight then helps you develop an index of suspicion, an anticipation of the nature and severity of likely injuries. Armed with an index of suspicion, you can then better focus your trauma patient assessment, triage, and care because you know what happened and the injuries the event is likely to have produced.

Let us look at the kinetics of blunt trauma, vehicular collisions, blast injuries, and other types of blunt trauma to better understand these prevalent mechanisms of injury and their physiologic results.

KINETICS OF BLUNT TRAUMA

Kinetics is a branch of physics dealing with forces affecting objects in motion and the energy exchanges that occur as objects collide. These collisions, or impacts, are the events that induce injury in patients. An understanding of kinetics helps you appreciate and anticipate the results of auto and other impacts. The two basic principles of kinetics are the law of inertia and the law of energy conservation. Further, the kinetic energy and force formulas quantify the energy exchange process between the moving object and the human body. These laws and formulas best describe what happens during impact and help in our understanding of blunt trauma.

INERTIA

The law of **inertia**, as described by Sir Isaac Newton and also known as Newton's first law, helps explain what happens during blunt trauma. The first part of his first law states: "A body in **motion** will remain in motion unless acted on by an outside force." As an example, think of identical autos moving at 100 km per hour. One car brakes for a red light; the other rams into a bridge abutment. An "outside force" stops the motion of both vehicles but with very different results. In the first case, the car's brakes absorb the energy of motion. In the second, the front bumper and grill, the frame, and eventually the occupants of the car absorb the energy as the car stops.

Blunt trauma is the most common cause of trauma-related death and disability.

Blunt trauma can be deceptive because the true nature of the injury is often hidden and evidence of the serious injury is very subtle or even absent.

Armed with an index of suspicion, you can then better focus your trauma patient assessment, triage, and care because you know what happened and the injuries the event is likely to have produced.

* **kinetics** the branch of physics that deals with motion, taking into consideration mass and force.

* **inertia** tendency of an object to remain at rest or remain in motion unless acted on by an external force.

* **motion** the process of changing place; movement.

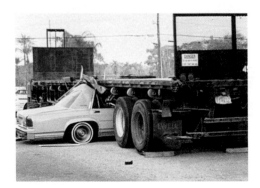

FIGURE 17-1 Blunt trauma is the most common cause of injury and trauma-related death. It is a physical exchange of energy from an object or surface transmitted through the skin into the body's interior.

The second part of the law states: "A body at rest will remain at rest unless acted on by an outside force." Examples of this include an auto accelerating from a stop sign or a stationary vehicle propelled forward by a rear-end collision. In the first case, the auto engine provides the force to initiate movement. In the second, the energy of the moving vehicle provides the force as the stationary car absorbs the energy and jolts ahead.

Conservation of Energy

✱ **energy** the capacity to do work in the strict physical sense.

The law of conservation of energy states: "**Energy** can neither be created nor destroyed. It only changes from one form to another." In an auto crash, as in other trauma, identifying probable energy changes helps you assess the impacts of various collisions. Kinetic energy, possessed by a moving car and its passengers, transforms into other energy forms whenever a car stops.

If an auto slows down gradually for a stop sign, the brakes develop friction against the turning wheels, producing heat. During an auto crash, however, the energy of motion is converted at a much faster rate into different forms. This conversion of energy is manifest in the sound of impact, the deformation of the auto's structural components, the heat in the twisted steel, and the injuries to passengers as they collide with the vehicle interior. When all the kinetic energy converts to other energy forms, the auto and its passengers come to a stop.

Kinetic Energy

✱ **kinetic energy** the energy an object has while it is in motion. It is related to the object's mass and velocity.

✱ **mass** a measure of the matter that an object contains; the property of a physical body that gives the body inertia.

✱ **velocity** the rate of motion in a particular direction in relation to time.

Kinetic energy is the energy of motion. It is a function of an object's **mass** and its **velocity** (Figure 17-2). (While mass or weight and velocity or speed are not identical, we will consider them as such for these discussions.) The kinetic energy of an object while in motion is measured by the following formula:

$$\text{Kinetic Energy} = \frac{\text{Mass} \times \text{Velocity (or speed)}^2}{2}$$

This formula illustrates that if you double an object's weight, you double its kinetic energy. It is twice as damaging to be hit by a two-kilogram baseball as to be hit by a one-kilogram ball. It is three times as damaging to be hit by a three-kilogram ball, and so on.

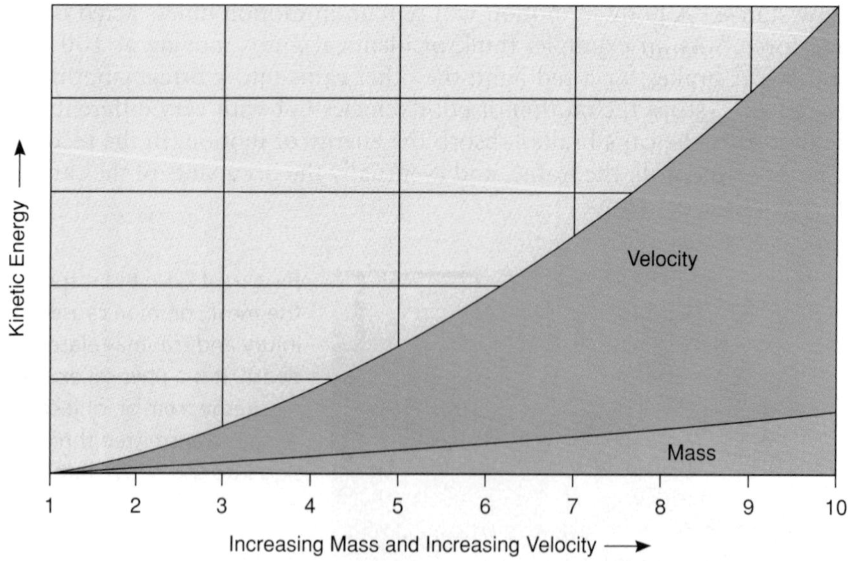

FIGURE 17-2 Increasing mass directly increases kinetic energy, while increasing velocity exponentially increases kinetic energy.

As speed (velocity) increases, there is a larger (squared) increase in kinetic energy. Being hit with a one-kilogram baseball travelling at 20 kmph is four times as injurious as being hit with the same ball moving at 10 kmph. If speed increases to 30 kmph, trauma is nine times worse. This concept plays a key role in understanding the devastating effects of a gunshot wound in which a small bullet can do great damage (as discussed in Chapter 18, "Penetrating Trauma").

Kinetic energy is the measure of how much energy an object in motion has, not necessarily how much injury occurs. Two autos travelling at 100 kmph have about the same kinetic energy. The same two autos would have the same kinetic energy once they have stopped, even if one came to rest by hitting a bridge. The difference between these two events is the rate of slowing. This rate is proportional to the crash force.

FORCE

Newton's second law of motion explains the forces at work during a collision. It is summarized by the formula below:

$$\text{Force} = \text{Mass (Weight)} \times \text{Acceleration (or Deceleration)}$$

The formula emphasizes the importance of the rate at which an object changes speed, either increasing (**acceleration**) or decreasing (**deceleration**). Slow changes in speed are usually uneventful.

✷ **acceleration** the rate at which speed or velocity increases.

Each year, approximately 3000 people die in motor vehicle crashes in Canada, while many more are seriously or permanently disabled. Of these deaths, 40 percent (1200) are attributed to drunk driving accidents. Canadians spend up to $25 billion annually in emergency care, rehabilitation, and other costs resulting from traffic accidents.

✷ **deceleration** the rate at which speed or velocity decreases.

TYPES OF TRAUMA

When significant kinetic energy is applied to human anatomy, we call it trauma. Trauma is defined as a wound or injury that is externally and violently produced by some outside force. The injury may be either blunt (closed) or penetrating (open) (Figure 17-3).

Trauma can be categorized as either blunt or penetrating.

Blunt trauma occurs when a body area is struck by, or strikes, an object. The transmission of energy, rather than the object, damages the tissues and organs beneath the skin as they collide with one another. An example of this is hitting your thumb with a hammer. The thumb is compressed between the hammer (which pushes the tissue) and the board (which resists the motion). Tissue injury results as flesh and bone are trapped between these two forces (acceleration and deceleration). Skin and muscle cells stretch and are crushed, blood vessels tear, and bone may fracture.

Blunt trauma can also induce injury deep within the body cavity. Forces of compression cause hollow organs, such as the bladder or bowel, to rupture, spilling their contents and hemorrhaging. In the thorax, alveoli or small airways may burst, permitting air to enter the pleural space. Solid organs, such as the spleen, liver, pancreas, and kidneys, may contuse or lacerate, leading to swelling, blood loss, or both.

Other blunt trauma may result from the effects of rapid speed change on organ attachment. An example is the liver, which is suspended in the abdomen by the ligamentum teres. During severe deceleration, the liver may be sliced by the ligament in a way similar to cheese being cut by a wire cheese cutter. Similarly, the aorta may be injured as the chest slows and the heart, which is suspended from the great vessels, twists upon impact. Layers of the vessel are torn apart, and blood enters the injury with the force of the systolic blood pressure. The aorta balloons like a defective tire, leading to a tearing chest pain, circulatory compromise, and immediate or delayed **exsanguination** (severe blood loss).

✷ **exsanguination** the draining of blood to the point at which life cannot be sustained.

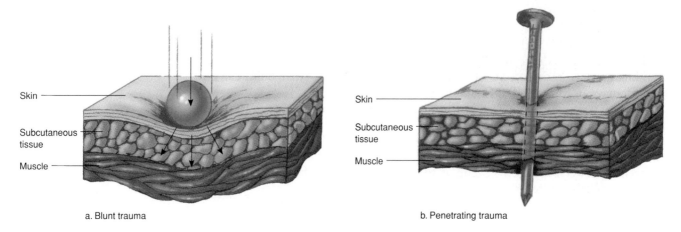

a. Blunt trauma

b. Penetrating trauma

FIGURE 17-3 Blunt trauma results when an object or force hits the body and kinetic energy is transferred to the involved body tissues. Penetrating injury is produced when an object enters the body resulting in direct injury.

Wounds that break the skin are classified as penetrating trauma. Penetrating trauma occurs when the energy source (such as a knife or bullet) progresses into the body. Energy may also be transmitted to surrounding body tissue, thus extending the trauma beyond the pathway of the object. This frequently happens with high-velocity gunshot wounds.

As a paramedic, you will encounter both blunt and penetrating trauma. The remainder of this chapter deals with examples of blunt trauma. Examples of penetrating trauma are discussed in Chapter 18.

BLUNT TRAUMA

Blunt trauma most commonly results from motor-vehicle collisions involving automobiles, motorcycles, pedestrians, or recreational vehicles (all-terrain vehicles, watercraft, snowmobiles). It can also result from explosions, falls, crush injuries, and sports injuries.

AUTOMOBILE COLLISIONS

Vehicular collisions (sometimes called motor-vehicle collisions, or MVCs) account for a large proportion of paramedic responses. Normal deceleration, such as slowing for a stop sign, covers about 5.76 m (from 90 kmph to 0 kmph at a breaking rate of 6.6 m to 16 m per hour). It therefore rarely results in injury. However, colliding with a bridge abutment and slowing from 90 kmph to 0 kmph in a matter of centimetres produces tremendous force and devastating injuries. As a paramedic, you must be prepared to offer rapid assessment and appropriate care to the victims of these crashes. To this end, you must recognize the various types of vehicular impacts, identify possible mechanisms of injury, and form a reasonable index of suspicion for specific injuries. Analysis of the types of impacts and the events associated with them help you form this index of suspicion.

Events of Impact

There are basically five types of vehicle impacts—frontal, lateral, rotational, rear-end, and rollover. Each type progresses through a series of five events (Figure 17-4). These events are:

Content Review

EVENTS OF VEHICLE COLLISION
Vehicle collision
Body collision
Organ collision
Secondary collisions
Additional impacts

1. *Vehicle Collision.* Vehicle collision begins when the auto strikes an object. Kinetic energy converts to vehicle damage or is transferred to the object hit by the auto. The force developed in the collision depends on the stopping distance. If the auto slides into a snow bank, damage is limited. If the auto strikes a concrete retaining wall, the damage is much greater. The degree of auto deformity is a good indicator of strength and direction of forces experienced by its occupants. The auto collision slows or stops the vehicle.

2. *Body Collision.* Body collision occurs when a vehicle occupant strikes the vehicle's interior. The vehicle and its interior have slowed dramatically during the crash, but an unrestrained occupant remains at or close to the initial speed. As the occupant contacts the interior, energy is transferred to the vehicle or is transformed into the initial tissue deformity, compression,

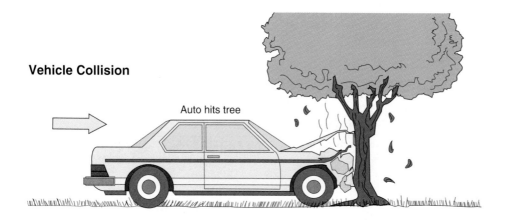

Vehicle Collision

Auto hits tree

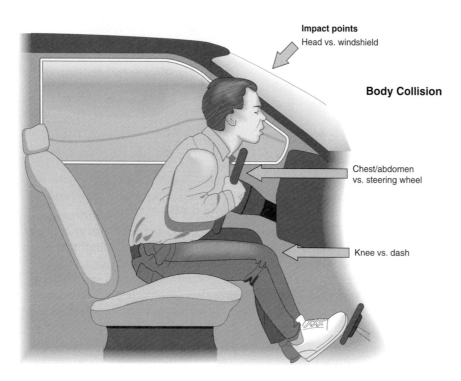

Impact points
Head vs. windshield

Body Collision

Chest/abdomen
vs. steering wheel

Knee vs. dash

FIGURE 17-4 An automobile crash generates four major collisions: the vehicle collision, the body collision, the organ collision, and secondary collisions.

Organ Collision

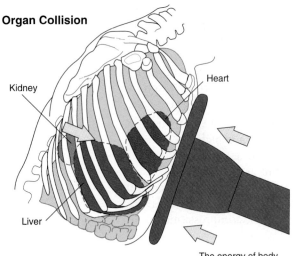

Kidney

Heart

Liver

The energy of body collision is transmitted to the interior.

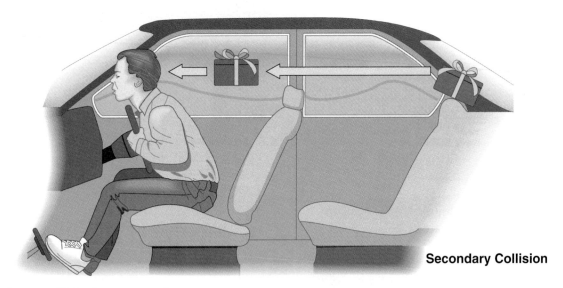

Secondary Collision

FIGURE 17-4 (CONTINUED)

stretching, and trauma. If the vehicle collision causes intrusion into the passenger compartment, this displacement may further injure occupants or otherwise worsen the injury process.

3. *Organ Collision*. Organ collision results as the occupant contacts the vehicle's interior and slows or stops. Tissues behind the contacting surface collide, one into another, as the occupant's body comes to a halt. This causes compression and stretching as tissues and organs violently press into each other. In the process, organs may also twist or decelerate and tear at their attachments or at blood vessels. The result is blunt trauma.

4. *Secondary Collisions*. Secondary collisions occur when a vehicle occupant is hit by objects travelling within the auto. During the crash, objects—such as those in the back seat, on the back window ledge, or in the back of a van—or other unrestrained passengers may continue to travel at the auto's initial speed. They

Secondary collisions may cause a patient's injuries or increase their severity.

then hit an occupant who has come to rest within the auto. It is important to consider the possibility of any secondary collisions and their effects on occupants when developing an index of suspicion for injuries.

5. *Additional Impacts.* Additional impacts occur when a vehicle receives a second impact—for example, when it hits a vehicle, is deflected, then hits a parked car. This second impact may induce additional patient injuries or increase the seriousness of those already received. Consider someone who sustains a femur fracture. It takes a great deal of energy to break the bone initially. Once the bone is broken, however, the energy now needed to move those bone ends around and cause further, possibly more severe, injury to nerves and blood vessels is small. It is important to consider what effect any additional impacts may have on the initial injuries and overall patient condition.

Restraints

Restraints, such as seat belts, shoulder straps, airbags, and child safety seats, have a profound effect on the injuries associated with auto collisions. Restraints have played a substantial role in reducing collision-related deaths. It is important that you determine whether restraints were used—and used properly—as you anticipate the possible results of an auto collision.

EMS workers should recognize the value of seat belts in reducing auto collision mortality and morbidity. Hence, all ambulance personnel must employ seat belts when in the patient care area of the vehicle and especially while driving. Securing the lap belt firmly provides positive positioning so that drivers and other crew-members are not as adversely affected by the gravitational forces (G forces) sometimes associated with emergency driving.

Seat Belts Use of seat belts and shoulder straps prevents the wearer's continuing and independent movement during a vehicle collision. The occupant slows with the auto, rather than moving rapidly forward and hitting the interior suddenly. The occupant's ultimate deceleration rate is thus reduced, lessening the likelihood of serious injury from collisions within the vehicle. Seat belts and shoulder straps also lessen the chances that the wearer will be ejected from the vehicle.

Although seat belts and shoulder straps significantly reduce injury severity, they may cause some, usually much less serious, injuries. A lap belt worn alone does not restrain the torso, neck, or head from continuing forward. These body regions may hit the dash or steering wheel, resulting in chest, neck, and head injuries. The sudden folding of the body at the waist during extreme impacts when only a lap belt is worn may result in intra-abdominal or lower spine injuries. If the lap belt is worn alone and too high, abdominal compression and spinal (T12 to L2) fractures may result. If worn too low, it may cause hip dislocations. If the shoulder strap is worn alone, it may cause severe neck contusions, lacerations, possible spinal injury, and even decapitation in more violent crashes. In very strong impacts, the shoulder strap may induce chest contusions and, in some cases, rib fractures. Further, the seat belt and/or shoulder strap do not protect against intrusions into the passenger compartment. In severe crashes, the dashboard may displace into the front seat, trapping or crushing the lower extremities of occupants.

Airbags Airbags, also called supplemental restraint systems (SRS), work much differently from seat belts and are extremely effective in frontal crashes. They inflate explosively on auto impact, producing a cushion to absorb the energy exchange. Their ignition is dependent on several detectors sensing a very strong frontal deceleration, as can only occur with serious vehicle impact. Only after

Restraints have had a profound effect in reducing collision-related deaths.

Seat belt use should be mandatory for all EMS personnel.

these detectors all agree does the explosive agent ignite. The ignition instantaneously fills the bag, slightly before or just as the occupant collides with it. The explosive gases escape quickly as the occupant compresses the bag, cushioning the impact much as the inflated bags used by pole-vaulters and movie stunt people do. Like seat belts, airbags are credited with dramatically reducing vehicular death and trauma (Figure 17-5).

Airbags are positioned in the steering wheel, and their presence is indicated by an "SRS" (supplemental restraint system) sticker on the windshield and/or on the steering wheel itself. They may also be located in the dash for the front seat passenger. Steering wheel and dash-mounted airbags offer significant protection only in frontal impact collisions. This protection is only for the first impact and not subsequent ones.

Airbags may induce injury during their ignition and rapid inflation. As the bag inflates, especially from the steering wheel, it may strike the driver's fingers, hands, and forearms, possibly causing dislocations and fractures. In persons of small stature seated very close to the steering wheel, airbag inflation may also cause nasal fractures, minor facial lacerations, and contusions. The residue from airbag inflation may cause some irritation of the eyes; this can be relieved with gentle irrigation. Whenever an airbag has deployed, check beneath it for steering wheel deformity, which is indicative of injury to the driver.

Passenger airbags have inflated in minor impacts and pushed infant and child safety seats into car seats with tremendous force. In some cases, infants and children have been severely injured or killed by inflation of the bags. For this reason, it is recommended that parents secure child carriers in the back seat when a passenger airbag system is in place.

Auto manufacturers are installing airbags in the seat sides, adjacent to the doors in some cars, for protection in lateral impact crashes. Some manufacturers also install airbags in the headliners above doors to provide protection for the head in such crashes. Since little experience has been gained with these types of restraints, their benefits and potential drawbacks are not well known. However, lateral impacts do account for a very high mortality rate that may be mediated with lateral-impact and head-protection airbags.

Like seat belts, airbags are credited with dramatically reducing vehicular death and trauma.

Although airbags can cause injury, they have, overall, greatly reduced injury and death in vehicular crashes.

FIGURE 17-5 Airbags cushion the driver from the forces of impact and significantly reduce mortality and morbidity in frontal impact crashes.

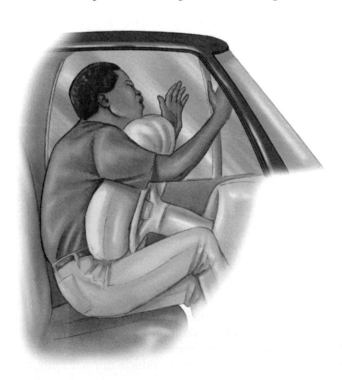

Child Safety Seats The child's anatomy makes protection in vehicle collisions difficult. Because a child's size changes so quickly with increasing age, normal restraint systems are designed for adults only. Small children should be placed in appropriate child safety seats to ensure their relative safety during an auto impact. With infants and very small children, the child safety seat is positioned facing the rear and held firmly to the seat with the seat belt. This positioning best distributes frontal impact forces and prevents unrestrained infant movement. As the child grows in size, the child carrier is turned facing forward and used as a small seat. The seat belt then crosses the child at the waistline.

Children held in an adult's lap or arms are not well protected during a crash. The holder may grasp them too tightly during impact or, more likely, will not (or cannot) hold on tightly enough. If the child is not held, she becomes an unrestrained moving object and will hit the vehicle interior suffering serious, possibly fatal, injury.

When evaluating the results of an auto impact, always be sure to examine for and ask questions about the use of restraints. Determine if seat belts and shoulder straps were used and used properly, if airbags deployed during the crash, and if child carriers were properly positioned and secured. If these restraints were properly employed, the severity of injuries to the vehicle occupants will very likely be reduced.

Properly used child safety seats provide the best protection for infants and small children riding in vehicles.

Types of Impact

As you have read, there are five general types of auto impacts:

- Frontal
- Lateral
- Rotational
- Rear-end
- Rollover

The following is a breakdown of the frequency of different types of motor-vehicle impacts (Figure 17-6). Figures reflect an urban setting. In a more rural area, anticipate a greater percentage of frontal impacts with corresponding reductions in other categories.

Frontal: 32 percent
Lateral: 15 percent
Rotational: 38 percent
Rear-end: 9 percent
Rollover: 6 percent

Note that rotational impact includes four subcategories: left front, right front, left rear, and right rear.

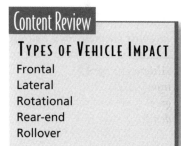

Content Review

TYPES OF VEHICLE IMPACT
Frontal
Lateral
Rotational
Rear-end
Rollover

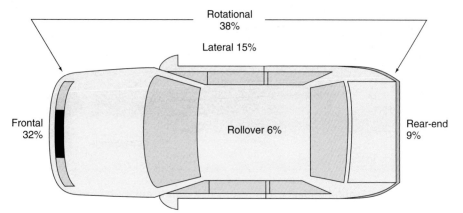

FIGURE 17-6 Incidence of motor vehicle impacts.

Frontal Impact Frontal impact is the most common type of impact (Figure 17-7) and produces three pathways of occupant travel:

1. *Down-and-under Pathway.* In the down-and-under pathway, the occupant slides downward as the vehicle comes to a stop. The knees contact the firewall, under the dash, and absorb the initial impact. Knee, femur, and hip dislocations or fractures are common. Once the lower body slows, the upper body rotates forward, pivoting at the hip, and crashing against the steering wheel or dash. Chest injuries like flail chest, myocardial contusion, and aortic tears result. If the neck contacts the steering wheel, tracheal and vascular injury may occur. An injury process frequently associated with steering wheel impact is "paper bag" syndrome (Figure 17-8). The driver takes a deep breath in anticipation of the collision. Lung tissue (alveoli, bronchioles, and larger airways) ruptures when the chest impacts the steering wheel, much like an inflated paper bag caught between clapping hands. Pneumothorax and pulmonary contusion may result.

2. *Up-and-over Pathway.* In the up-and-over pathway, the occupant tenses the legs in preparation for impact (Figure 17-9). With vehicle slowing, the unrestrained body's upper half pivots forward and upward. The steering wheel impinges the femurs, causing possible bilateral fractures. In addition, it compresses and decelerates the abdominal contents, causing hollow-organ rupture and liver laceration. Traumatic compression may also force abdominal contents against the diaphragm, causing it to rupture and allowing organs to enter the thoracic cavity. As the body continues forward, the lower chest strikes the steering wheel and may account for the same thoracic injuries seen with the down-and-under pathway.

The same forward motion propels the head into the windshield, leading to soft-tissue injury, skull or facial fractures, and internal head injury. Neck injury may result from hyperextension,

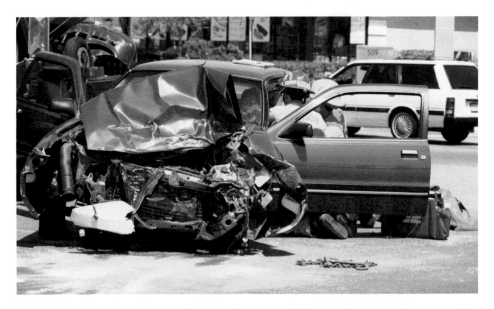

FIGURE 17-7   Frontal impact often results in a significant exchange of energy and serious injuries.

hyperflexion, or the compressional forces of windshield impact. As the body is thrown upward and forward, the head contacts the windshield. The rest of the body tries to push the head through the windshield. The result is a compressional force on

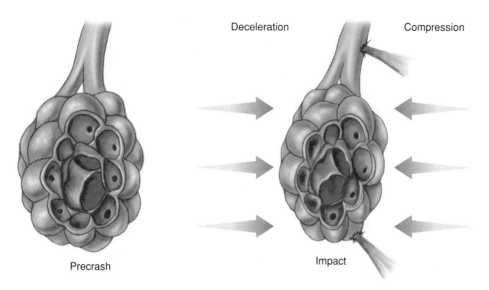

FIGURE 17-8   "Paper bag" syndrome results from compression of the chest against the steering column.

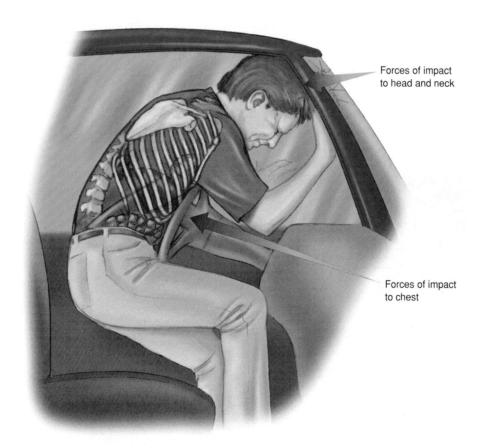

FIGURE 17-9   The up-and-over pathway is associated with frontal impact crashes.

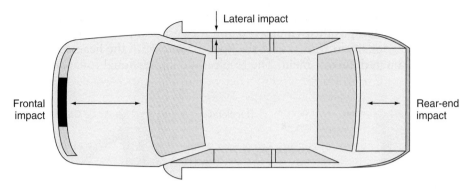

FIGURE 17-10   Crumple zones provide significant protection with both frontal and rear-end impacts but much less in cases of lateral impacts.

*✳ **axial loading** application of the forces of trauma along the axis of the spine; this often results in compression fractures of the spine.*

*✳ **crumple zone** the region of a vehicle designed to absorb the energy of impact.*

Occupants of a vehicle without a crumple zone may experience greater forces in a collision, even though damage to the vehicle itself may not appear as severe as damage to a vehicle with a crumple zone involved in a similar crash.

FIGURE 17-11   A lateral impact collision presents the least amount of crumple zone between the vehicle's exterior and its passenger compartment.

the cervical spine called **axial loading.** This loading may result in collapse of support elements of the vertebral column. More than half of vehicular deaths are attributed to the up-and-over pathway.

3. *Ejection.* The up-and-over pathway may lead to ejection of an unrestrained occupant. Such a victim experiences two impacts: (1) contact with the vehicle interior and windshield, and (2) impact with the ground, tree, or other object. This mechanism of injury is responsible for about 27 percent of vehicular fatalities. While ejection may occur with other types of impact, it is most commonly associated with frontal impact.

   Recognize that a frontal impact collision interposes more vehicle between the point of impact and the vehicle occupants. Modern vehicle design techniques use this area of the vehicle (called the **crumple zone**) to absorb the impact forces and limit occupant injury (Figure 17-10). Patients in such vehicle collisions as those involving vans and lateral impacts do not benefit from these energy-absorbing crumple zones. In these circumstances, the apparent vehicle damage may be less than in a frontal impact crash, even though the forces delivered to the occupants are greater.

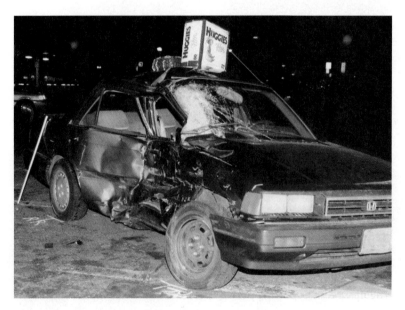

Lateral Impact The kinetics of lateral impact are the same as for frontal impact with two exceptions. First, occupants present a different profile (turned 90 degrees) to collision forces. Second, the amount of structural steel between the impact site and the vehicle interior is greatly reduced (Figure 17-11). Lateral impacts account for 15 percent of all auto accidents, and yet they are responsible for 22 percent of vehicular fatalities. When a lateral impact occurs, the index of suspicion for serious and life-threatening internal injuries must be higher than vehicle damage alone suggests.

With lateral impacts, there is an increase in upper extremity injuries (Figure 17-12). The ribs fracture laterally on the side of impact instead of anteriorly. The clavicle, humerus, pelvis, and femur may fracture on the impact side. Cervical spine injury occurs as the body moves laterally while the head remains stationary. Vertebrae may fracture with the rapid lateral motion as may the skull as it smashes into the window. Lateral compression, affecting the body cavity, may give rise to diaphragm rupture, pulmonary contusion, splenic injury (to the driver), and much more. Aortic aneurysm may occur with this injury mechanism. The heart, which is not firmly attached in the central thorax, moves violently toward the impact as the body accelerates. This twists the

Maintain a higher index of suspicion of serious injury when assessing lateral impact collisions because the degree of injury may be greater than the damage alone would indicate.

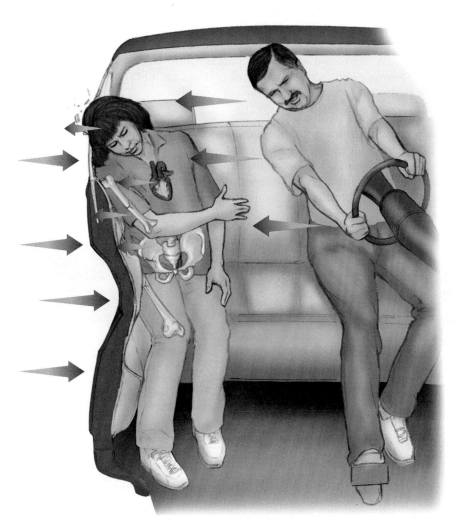

FIGURE 17-12 In a lateral impact collision, an occupant may experience lateral impact to the head, lateral bending of the neck, twisting of the heart and the aorta, and humeral, clavicular, pelvic, and femoral fractures.

aorta, tearing its inner layer, the intima. Blood seeps between the connective tissue layers, and the vessel begins to delaminate. The aorta may rupture immediately or in the next few hours.

Evaluation of lateral impact collisions should take into consideration any unrestrained passenger opposite the impact site. If the driver's side is struck and such a passenger is not belted, the passenger becomes an object that will strike and injure the driver shortly after initial impact.

* **oblique** having a slanted position or direction.

Rotational Impact In rotational impact, the auto is struck at an **oblique** angle and rotates as the collision forces are expended (Figure 17-13). The ensuing rotation causes injuries similar to those from frontal and lateral impacts. Acceleration (or deceleration) is greatest farther from the centre of the auto and closest to impact. Autos involved are deflected from their paths, rather than being stopped abruptly. While rotational impact injuries can be serious, they are often less than vehicle damage might suggest. With the deflection of the impact, the occupant's stopping distance is much greater, deceleration is more gradual, and injuries are generally less serious.

Rear-End Impact In rear-end impact, the collision force pushes the auto forward (Figure 17-14). Within the vehicle, the seat propels the occupant forward. If the headrest is not up, the head is unsupported and remains stationary. The neck extends severely, stretching the neck muscles and ligaments, while the head rotates backward. Once acceleration ceases, the head snaps forward, and the neck flexes. This rapid and extreme hyperextension followed by hyperflexion may result in severe connective tissue and cervical vertebra injuries (Figure 17-15). There is also risk of injury when the auto finally ends its acceleration and an unrestrained occupant is thrown forward.

Rollover Auto rollover is normally caused by a change in elevation and/or a vehicle with a high centre of gravity (Figure 17-16). As the vehicle rolls, it hits the ground at various points. The occupant experiences an impact with each impact of the vehicle. These impacts can be especially violent due to the absence of crumple zones and internal padding at the multiple points of impact (vehicle sides and

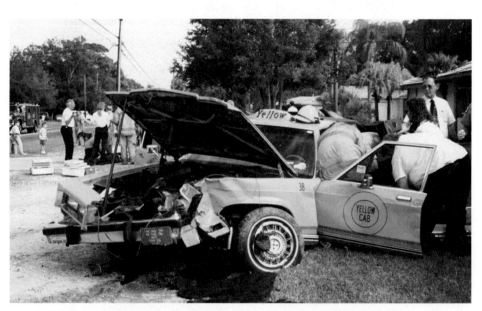

FIGURE 17-13 In rotational impacts, the energy exchange is more gradual, and there may be less injury than vehicle damage suggests. There may, however, be multiple impacts.

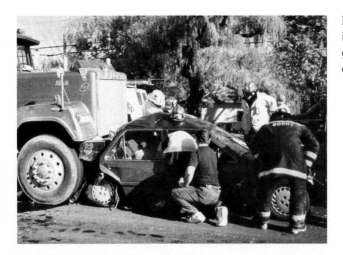

FIGURE 17-14 In rear-end impacts, there is generally good protection for the body, except for the head and neck.

roof). The type of injuries expected with a rollover relate to the specific vehicle impacts involved. Remember, any injury occurring with the first collision is likely to be compounded with subsequent impacts. A common result of rollover is ejection or partial ejection with a limb or head trapped between the rolling vehicle and the ground. Restraints are especially effective in reducing ejection and injury during rollover.

Vehicle Collision Analysis

Vehicle collisions often produce hazards not only to the vehicle occupants but also to bystanders and care providers. Be alert for these hazards during the scene assessment. Such hazards may include hot engine and transmission parts, hot fluids (such as radiator coolant or engine oil), caustic substances (such as battery acid and automatic transmission or steering fluids), and the sharp, jagged edges of torn metal or broken glass. Also remain aware of the potential danger from traffic moving near the collision site or from electrical power lines that may have been downed by the collision.

Be alert for these hazards during the scene assessment:
- *hot engine and transmission parts, hot fluids (such as radiator coolant or engine oil)*
- *caustic substances (such as battery acid and automatic transmission or steering fluids)*
- *sharp, jagged edges of torn metal or broken glass*

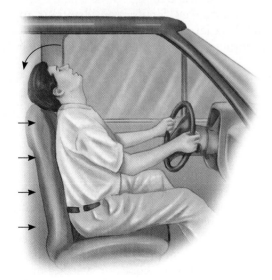

a. Victim moves ahead while head remains stationary. Head rotates backward. Neck extends.

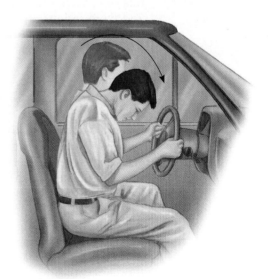

b. Head snaps forward. Head rotates forward. Neck flexes.

FIGURE 17-15 The effects of a rear-end collision on the occupant of a vehicle.

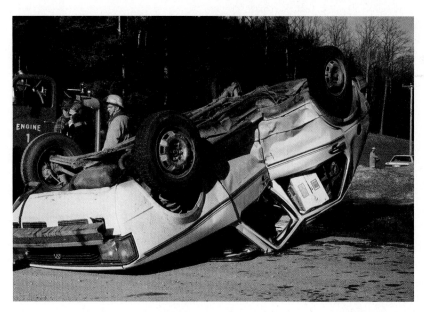

FIGURE 17-16 Rollover collisions result in multiple impacts and, possibly, multiple injury mechansims.

During the scene assessment, evaluate the vehicle to determine the direction of impact and the amount of vehicle damage. From the angle of impact, visualize the direction of forces expressed on the crash victims and the strength of those forces. Realize that the front and rear structures of the modern cars are designed to crumple during impact to absorb kinetic forces. While moderate-speed impacts may destroy the vehicle, the passengers may escape with minimal injury. Occupants in lateral and rollover impacts do not benefit from such crumple zones and frequently suffer injuries more directly related to the kinetic forces.

As you evaluate the collision, consider the relative sizes of the colliding vehicles or objects. A large, heavy vehicle colliding with a smaller, lighter one will experience lesser acceleration or deceleration forces than does the smaller vehicle. In this case, there is likely to be more severe vehicle damage to the smaller vehicle and more serious injuries to its occupants as well. Similar considerations apply with objects hit by vehicles. For example, a large, well-rooted tree that does not move will cause much more damage during an impact than will a telephone pole that shears off.

When evaluation of the outside of the vehicle is complete, look at the passenger compartment (Figure 17-17). Determine if there is any intrusion, which indicates the presence of forces greater than those that could be absorbed by the crumple zones. Quickly look for signs of occupant/interior impacts. A spider-webbed windshield suggests a severe impact between the occupant's head and the glass. A deformed steering wheel suggests injury to the driver's chest or upper abdomen. A dented dash suggests injury to the knees or injuries transmitted to the femur or hip. Deformities of the gas, brake, or clutch pedals suggest foot injury. Deployed and deflated airbags indicate possible chest, forearm, or hand injury.

In very severe impacts, collision forces may push the dashboard and firewall into the passenger compartment, entrapping and crushing the lower extremities of occupants against the seat. In such cases, parts of the vehicle, like the foot pedals, turn indicator arms, shift levers, and instrument panel knobs or switches may be imbedded in victims' bodies. This complicates extrication because the seat and the dash must be separated carefully to free the trapped victim. In these cases, the area should be carefully examined before and while any extrication equipment is used.

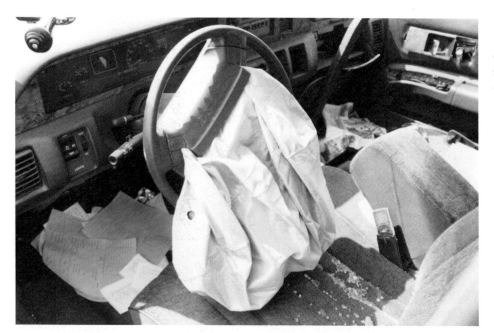

Ongoing examinations should be done frequently during extrication to ensure that the process does not result in further, unnecessary harm to the patient.

Assess whether restraints have been used or airbags deployed. Use of these devices may limit the severity of injuries in frontal impacts. Conversely, their nonuse may suggest more severe injuries. Check the positions of headrests in rear-impact collisions. Their proper positioning may limit neck hyperextension and injury.

Intoxication Whenever you evaluate motor-vehicle trauma, consider the possibility of alcohol intoxication. In 2001, there were 3021 deaths on Canadian highways, and 1103, or 36.5 percent, were alcohol related.[1] Alcohol also contributes to many recreational-vehicle accidents, boating accidents, and accidental drownings.

Alcohol intoxication is associated with most serious crashes.

Whenever you suspect alcohol intoxication, your assessment must be more diligent. Remember, alcohol interferes with the patient's level of consciousness and masks signs and symptoms of injury. Intoxication may be hard to differentiate from the signs of head injury. It also anesthetizes the patient somewhat to trauma pain. These factors make the mechanism of injury analysis and the resultant index of suspicion even more important. Otherwise, significant injuries may be overlooked or their effects brushed off as symptoms of alcohol intoxication.

Vehicular Trauma Examination of the effects of motor-vehicle trauma on the human anatomy reveals certain areas to be especially prone to life-threatening injury. A study of the incidence of associated trauma provides the findings in Table 17-1.

Head and body cavity injuries account for 67.2 percent of vehicular trauma. For this reason, the rapid trauma assessment should be directed at the head, neck, thorax, abdomen, and pelvis. Once you have assessed the airway, breathing, and circulation, proceed to rapid trauma assessment, looking at areas where your index of suspicion suggests injury. Examine the head, chest, and abdomen first to identify any evidence of life-threatening injuries.

Head and body cavity injuries account for 67.2 percent of all trauma due to vehicular trauma.

1. Canadian Council of Motor Transport Administrators. Available online at www.ccmta.ca. Downloaded July 16, 2004.

Table 17-1	MOTOR VEHICLE INJURIES	
(Incidence by Body Area)		
Head	4 067	26.2%
Orthopedic	3 944	25.4%
Superficial	3 847	24.8%
Internal	2 425	15.6%
Spinal Cord	337	2.2%
Blood Vessels	301	1.9%
Burns	223	1.4%
Nerves	194	1.3%
Other	158	1.0%

Source: NTR/CIHI, 2003. Percentages don't add to 100 due to rounding.

Collision Evaluation As a paramedic, you must be proficient in the assessment of trauma patients, especially because of the high incidence of serious injury associated with auto collisions. Whenever you respond to an accident, analyze the five types of collisions associated with vehicle impact. In each case, ask yourself these questions:

- How did the objects collide?
- From what direction did they come?
- At what speed were they travelling?
- Were the objects similarly sized or significantly different? (For example, did a car and a semi-truck collide?)
- Were any secondary collisions or additional transfers of energy involved?

In analyzing the mechanisms of injury, also consider the cause of the collision.

- Did wet roads or poor visibility contribute to the accident?
- Was alcohol involved?
- Is there an absence of skid marks? If so, what prevented the driver from braking?

Examine the auto interior for signs of areas struck by the moving occupant.

- Does the windshield show evidence of impact by the victim's head?
  - Is it bloody or broken in the characteristic spider-web or star shape?
  - Has it been penetrated by the patient's head or body?
- Is the steering wheel deformed or collapsed?
- Is the dash indented where the knees or head hit it?
- Has the impact damage extended into the passenger compartment (intrusion)?

Answers to such questions complement your mechanism of injury analysis and help you develop accurate indexes of suspicion.

MOTORCYCLE COLLISIONS

In addition to responding to auto collisions, as a paramedic you will respond to many motorcycle collisions. Because of the lack of protective vehicle structure, motorcycle collisions, even at low speeds, often result in serious trauma. The

Serious trauma is likely with even low-speed motorcycle crashes because of the lack of protective vehicle structure.

rider, rather than the structural steel, absorbs much of the collision energy (Figure 17-18). Injuries can be severe, with an especially high incidence of head trauma. The motorcycle collisions' impacts differ somewhat from those of an auto collision. The four types of motorcycle impacts are frontal, angular, sliding, and ejection.

In a frontal, or head-on impact, the bike dips downward, propelling the rider upward and forward. The handlebars catch the rider's lower abdomen or pelvis, causing abdominal and/or pelvic injury. Occasionally, the rider travels through a higher trajectory. In such cases, the handlebars can trap the femurs, often resulting in bilateral fractures.

An angular impact occurs when the bike strikes an object at an oblique angle. The rider's lower extremity is trapped between the object struck and the bike. This may fracture or crush the foot, ankle, knee, and femur. Open wounds often result.

Sliding impact occurs when an experienced rider, facing an imminent collision, "lays the bike down." The rider slides the bike sideways into the object, so that the bike hits the object first, absorbing much of the energy. Laying the bike down also reduces the chances of ejection. The result is an increase in lacerations, abrasions, and minor fractures, with a decrease in more serious injuries.

Ejection during a motorcycle collision is common and usually results in serious injury. It may occur with any of the mechanisms previously described and result in the following impacts:

- Initial bike/object collision
- Rider/object impact
- Rider/ground impact

Likely injuries include skull fracture and/or head injury, spinal fractures and paralysis, internal thoracic or abdominal injury, and extremity fractures.

In assessing a motorcycle collision, remember that protective equipment affects injury patterns. A helmet can reduce the incidence and severity of head

Ejection during a motorcycle collision is common and usually results in serious injury.

Helmets reduce the incidence and severity of head injuries in motorcycle collisions, but they have no effect on the incidence of spinal trauma.

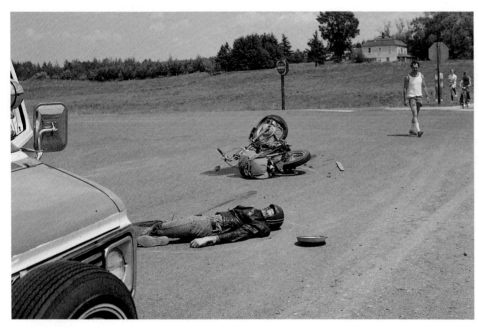

FIGURE 17-18 Motorcycle collisions result in serious trauma because the vehicle provides little protection for its rider.

injury by 50 to 66 percent. Use of a helmet, however, neither increases nor decreases the incidence of spinal trauma. Leather clothing and boots protect the rider against open soft-tissue injury, but they can also hide underlying contusions and fractures.

PEDESTRIAN ACCIDENTS

Some vehicular accidents involve pedestrians, who are often severely injured because of the mass and speed of the object hitting them and because of their lack of protection. Adults and children suffer different types of injuries because of differing anatomical sizes and differing responses to the impending accident. Recognition of these differences helps you assess injuries and provide the necessary treatment.

Adult pedestrians generally turn away from oncoming vehicles and present a lateral surface to impact. Anatomically, impact is low. The bumper strikes the lower leg first, fracturing the tibia and fibula. Energy transmitted to the opposing knee can lead to ligament injury. As the lower extremities are propelled forward with the car, the upper and lateral body crashes into the hood causing femur, lateral chest, or upper extremity fractures. The victim then slides into the windshield, leading to head, neck, and shoulder trauma. The adult may be further injured when thrown to the ground. This secondary collision may cause additional injury or compound those already received (Figure 17-19).

In contrast to adults, children usually turn toward an oncoming vehicle. Because of their smaller anatomy, injuries are located higher on children's bodies. The bumper strikes the femurs or pelvis, causing fracture. Children are frequently thrown in front of the vehicle because of their smaller size and lower centre of gravity. They may then be run over or pushed to the side by the vehicle. If a child is thrown upward, injuries are similar to those of an adult (Figure 17-20).

When evaluating the injuries associated with auto-versus-pedestrian accidents, look carefully at the scene. Try to determine the speed of the vehicle at time of impact and the distance the pedestrian was thrown. This information may be useful to the emergency department personnel in their determination of suspected injuries.

In pedestrian-versus-automobile collisions, adults tend to turn away from the oncoming vehicle before impact, while children turn toward it.

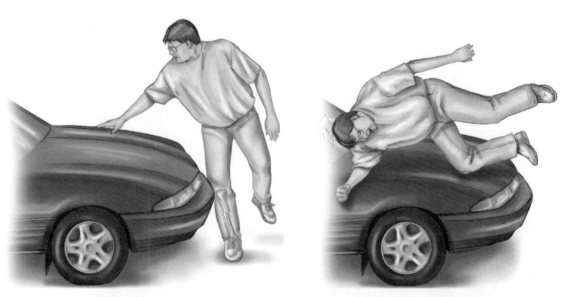

FIGURE 17-19 An adult frequently turns away from a collision with an automobile and thus hits the vehicle first with a leg. Because of a higher centre of gravity, adults are often thrown onto the hood and into the windshield.

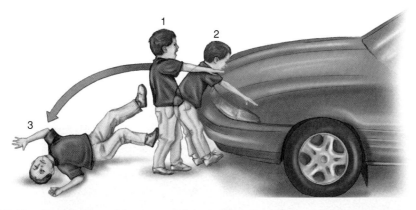

FIGURE 17-20 In collisions with autos, children often turn toward the impact and, because of their lower body heights, are frequently thrown in front of the vehicle.

RECREATIONAL VEHICLE ACCIDENTS

Over the past years, recreational-vehicle usage and, with it, the incidence of related trauma have increased. Recreational-vehicle collisions often cause injuries similar to those associated with auto collisions. Drivers and passengers of recreational vehicles, however, do not have the structural protections and restraint systems found in autos. Complicating injuries is the fact that recreational vehicles travel off-road, which means there is often difficulty in reaching and retrieving victims once collisions are reported. The major types of vehicles most often involved in recreational-vehicle collisions are snowmobiles, watercraft, and all-terrain vehicles (ATVs).

Snowmobile collisions can be extremely violent because the speeds at which snowmobiles travel can approach those of cars, but snowmobiles offer no crumple zones for impact absorption. These accidents commonly result in ejections, crush injuries secondary to rollover, and glancing blows against obstructions in the snow. Riders also experience severe head and neck injuries from collisions with other vehicles, including autos, other snowmobiles, or stationary objects, such as trees. Snowmobile trauma may include severe neck injury when the rider runs into an unseen wire fence. The anterior neck is deeply lacerated, causing airway compromise, severe bleeding, and, in some cases, complete decapitation. Injuries to snowmobilers may be compounded by the effects of cold exposure and hypothermia. When comparing winter sports activities, snowmobiling resulted in the most severe injuries, followed by downhill skiing and snowboarding. In fact, 16 percent of severe sports and recreational injuries in 2000–2001 were snowmobile related. The average age for those involved in snowmobile-related incidents in Canada is 33, and the majority (85 percent) of those injured were male. Of the 92 snowmobile-related severe injury admissions in 2000–2001 where the blood alcohol concentration was recorded, 26 percent involved prior consumption of alcohol.

Watercraft accidents commonly result from impact with other boats or obstructions, submerged or otherwise (Figure 17-21). These vehicles are not designed to absorb the energy of impacts, nor are the occupants provided with restraint systems. As a result, watercraft collisions can cause serious injuries, even though the speeds of typical watercraft are substantially lower than those of autos. Trauma in these collisions is further complicated by the potential for drowning if the occupants are thrown into the water or the boat sinks. In northern areas, water temperatures can also rapidly induce hypothermia. Alcohol is frequently associated with watercraft accidents.

The use of personal watercraft, commonly called jet skis, for water recreation has increased greatly in recent years, as has the incidence of watercraft

Recreational vehicles usually lack the structure and the restraint systems that offer significant protection to automobile drivers and passengers.

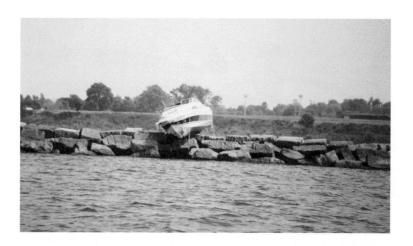

FIGURE 17-21 Watercraft accidents are common, may involve either objects on the surface or submerged, and present the risks of drowning or hypothermia.

accidents. Jet skis are especially dangerous in the hands of inexperienced riders. The high speeds attained by these watercraft contribute to the incidence and severity of injury associated with collisions. Although the craft's propulsion unit is protected and unlikely to cause trauma, collision with other watercraft, as well as objects and people in the water, lead to blunt trauma, again complicated by the potential for drowning.

There are two types of ATVs: the three- and four-wheeled versions (Figure 17-22). The three-wheeled ATV is notoriously unstable, especially when ridden by children, young adults, persons of lower body weight, or those with limited vehicle experience. The ATV's centre of gravity is relatively high, contributing to the likelihood of rollover during quick turns. As with snowmobiles, a significant incidence of frontal collision is common with both types of ATVs. The injuries expected might include upper and lower extremity fractures and head and spine injuries.

BLAST INJURIES

* **oxidizer** an agent that enhances combustion of a fuel.

Explosions can be caused by dust, as in a grain elevator, by fumes, such as gasoline or natural gas, or by explosive compounds (combustible and **oxidizer** mixes), such as dynamite, gun powder, and TNT. The explosion may be the result of an accident or intentional act of terrorism or warfare. The blast magnitude may range from that of a small firecracker in the hands of a teenager to a nuclear detonation.

FIGURE 17-22 All-terrain vehicles (ATVs) can cause a multitude of injuries due to their speed, instability, and lack of rider protection.

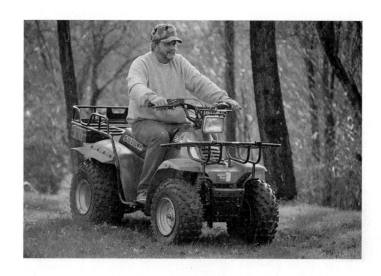

Explosion

An explosion occurs when an agent or environment combusts. During a conventional (nonnuclear) explosion, the fuel and oxidizing agent combine instantaneously. Chemical bonds are broken down and reestablished, releasing tremendous energy in the form of rapidly moving molecules, known to us as heat. This heat creates a great pressure differential between the exploding agent and the surrounding air. The heat and the pressure differential produce several mechanisms of injury including a pressure wave, blast wind, projectiles, displacement of persons near the blast, confined space explosions and structural collapse, and burns (Figure 17-23).

Pressure Wave

As the combustible agent ignites and burns explosively, it immediately heats the surrounding air. The molecules of heated air move very fast, increasing the pressure of the exploding cloud. The rapid increase in pressure compresses adjacent air. Adjacent air, in turn, pushes against air farther out from the point of ignition, and a **pressure wave** begins to move away from the blast epicentre. This is not a gross air movement but rather a narrow compression wave moving rapidly outward, similar to a wave through water (where the wave and not the water moves). This narrow wave, called **overpressure**, results in a drastic but brief increase and then decrease in air pressure as it passes. The blast overpressure wave moves outward slightly faster than the speed of sound through the air or water, and its strength decreases quickly.

When the explosion involves a dust, an aerosol, or a gas cloud, the result is an area, not a single point, of detonation. The exploding cloud's pressure is extremely lethal, and the area it involves can be extensive. A bomb's casing or confined spaces, such as a building interior, contain the pressure of an explosion until the structure ruptures. The ensuing rapid release of the pressure enhances the peak overpressure and the potential for injury and death.

Underwater detonation also greatly enhances the potential for injury and death associated with the pressure wave. Water is a noncompressible medium that transmits the overpressure efficiently. Any submerged portion of the victim is subject to the rapid compression and then decompression. The lethal range for an explosive charge increases threefold with an underwater detonation.

* **pressure wave** area of overpressure that radiates outward from an explosion.

Content Review

MECHANISMS ASSOCIATED WITH BLASTS
Pressure wave
Blast wind
Projectiles
Personnel displacement
Confined space explosions and structural collapses
Burns

* **overpressure** a rapid increase and then decrease in atmospheric pressure created by an explosion.

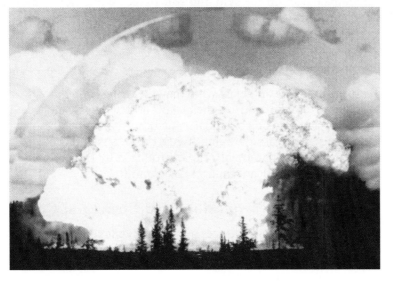

FIGURE 17-23 An explosion releases tremendous amounts of heat energy, generating a pressure wave, blast wind, and projection of debris.

On striking the body, the overpressure wave instantly compresses then decompresses the body's air-filled spaces, causing trauma. This rapid compression/decompression may produce injury to the middle ear, sinuses, bowel, or lungs. Because overpressure intensity diminishes rapidly as the wave travels outward, most life-threatening compression injuries are usually limited to people in close proximity to the detonation, with the exceptions of gas-cloud ignitions and underwater detonations.

A victim's orientation to the blast wave is also an important factor in the production of injuries. The greater the surface a victim presents to the blast wave, the greater are the impact and damage. People standing and facing directly toward or away from the blast experience the greatest pressure effect. People lying on the ground, with their heads away from or toward the blast, experience the least pressure effects. In water, the same is true, although the more deeply submerged a victim is, the greater the damaging effects of the overpressure.

Blast Wind

✱ blast wind the air movement caused as the heated and pressurized products of an explosion move outward.

Following the pressure wave and travelling just behind it is the **blast wind.** This is the actual outward movement of heated and expanding combustion gases from the explosion epicentre. The blast wind has less strength but greater duration than the pressure wave. It causes much less direct injury, although in powerful blasts, it may propel debris or displace victims, which will, in turn, produce injuries.

Projectiles

✱ ordnance military weapons and munitions.

If the exploding material is contained by a casing, as with military **ordnance** or a pipe bomb, or by a structure, as with a garage filled with gas fumes, the container holds the explosive force until the container breaks apart. The parts of the container then become high-speed projectiles, behaving much like bullets and bound by the same laws of physics. Although they are not as fast as bullets and lack good aerodynamic properties, they can cause serious injury beyond the injury zone of the blast's pressure wave itself. Some military ordnance contains special arrow-shaped missiles called **flechettes.** Their design gives the flechettes a greater following surface and aligns the missiles in flight, reducing their wind resistance and increasing their range and penetrating ability.

✱ flechettes arrow-shaped projectiles found in some military ordnance.

If the victim is in very close proximity to a strong blast, the casing and debris may move forcefully enough to tear off limbs or cause serious open wounds. The blast debris—glass fragments, building materials, or casing elements—may also impale itself in the skin and soft tissue. While the wounds caused by blast debris are normally small, large and heavy fragments may penetrate deeply into victims and cause serious tissue damage and hemorrhage.

Personnel Displacement

The pressure wave and blast wind may be strong enough to physically propel victims away from the centre of the blast. Those victims then become projectiles and strike the ground, objects, debris, or other personnel, resulting in blunt or, in some cases, penetrating trauma. While the effects of this mechanism of injury are limited when compared with those produced by the pressure wave, blast wind, or projectiles, significant injuries can occur.

Confined Space Explosions and Structural Collapses

The effects of explosive devices are usually limited in range because the pressure wave and debris radiate outward in all directions from a central point. This rapidly reduces the overpressure, the concentration, and, to a lesser degree, the velocity of projectiles. When an explosion occurs in a confined space, however, the pressure wave maintains its energy longer. There is also danger of structural collapse, and debris from the confining structure can increase the blast's projectile content. The blast overpressure also bounces off walls and, where pressure waves meet, the pressure greatly increases. The result can be extremely deadly overpressures. The most lethal blasts are those causing structural collapses, followed by those involving confined spaces.

Structural collapses may cause severe crush-type injuries. The collapses may also make victims difficult to locate and, once found, difficult to extricate because of the weight of the material entrapping them. Damage to structures may present further hazards to rescuers and victims, including the possibility of additional collapses, electrocution, fire, or secondary explosion due to gas or fuel leaks.

Burns

An explosion can create tremendous heat. This heat may cause flash burns to those very close to the detonation. These injuries are generally superficial or partial thickness burns and may occur in conjunction with other trauma. However, victims may also be burned as the heat of the blast ignites combustibles, such as clothing, debris, other munitions, or fuel. These secondary burns may be full thickness and extensive.

Some military and terrorist devices are designed to induce damage and injury through combustion. Napalm, for an example, is a highly **incendiary**, jelly-like substance that clings to people or structures when spread by a blast. It can produce severe or fatal full thickness burns. Other ordnance uses materials, such as phosphorus, that spontaneously combust when exposed to air.

✱ **incendiary** an agent that combusts easily or creates combustion.

Blast Injury Phases

The injuries produced by explosions are usually classified into three types, depending on the phase of the blast that caused them: primary, secondary, and tertiary (Figure 17-24).

Primary Blast Injuries Primary blast injuries are caused by the heat of the explosion and the overpressure wave. The pressure injuries are the most serious and life-threatening injuries associated with the explosion. Burn injuries are generally limited unless caused by secondary combustion.

Secondary Blast Injuries Secondary blast injuries include trauma caused by projectiles. These injuries may be as severe as or more severe than the primary blast injuries. Projectiles from an explosive blast do have the ability to extend the range of injury beyond those caused by the blast wave and wind. High concentrations of projectiles may also create multiple body penetrations and impalements over large areas of a victim's body. The resulting injuries may produce severe bleeding.

Tertiary Blast Injuries Tertiary blast injuries include those injuries resulting from personnel displacement and structural collapse. Blast victims may be thrown against walls, the ground, or other obstructions and suffer blunt and/or penetrating trauma. When the blast results in a structural collapse, crush injuries may also result. These injuries can be extensive and result in soft-skeletal, nervous, and vascular tissue and organ destruction.

Blast Injury Assessment

Blast injuries produce extreme trauma in those who are close to the blast epicentre. Blasts in densely populated areas may also involve large numbers of victims. Your role as a paramedic is to survey and assess the scene and do what you can to secure it for further EMS operations. This normally involves implementing the incident command system and ensuring overall scene management. Once command is established and operational, you will likely begin caring for patients by applying the normal assessment priorities (the ABCs of the initial assessment) and then focusing on the seriously injured but salvageable blast victims. If the number of victims exceeds the immediate capabilities of your EMS system, employ disaster triage.

Determine, if possible, whether the blast was the result of terrorist action. If you suspect that it was, be alert to the possibility that more explosive devices may be set or the area booby-trapped to endanger rescuers. Ensure that police and bomb squad personnel have swept the area before you and your team enter it.

Carefully evaluate the scene for secondary hazards. Look for such things as gas leaks, disrupted electrical wiring, sharp debris, and the possibility of further structural collapse. During the scene assessment, determine the location of the epicentre of the blast. Note the presence of greater destruction and injury as you progress toward the epicentre. As you get closer, your index of suspicion for serious injury increases.

The most common and serious trauma associated with explosions is lung injury. Pulmonary injury may not manifest itself immediately; anticipate it in anyone with any other significant signs or symptoms of blast trauma. Evaluate breathing and breath sounds frequently, carefully watching and listening for any dyspnea and crackles or other signs of respiratory congestion. At the first sign of breathing problems, arrange for high-flow oxygen and rapid transport.

Some blast victims may experience hearing loss caused by the pressure wave. After experiencing the emotional impact of the blast itself, this injury can produce extreme anxiety in victims. Do your best to calm and reassure these pa-

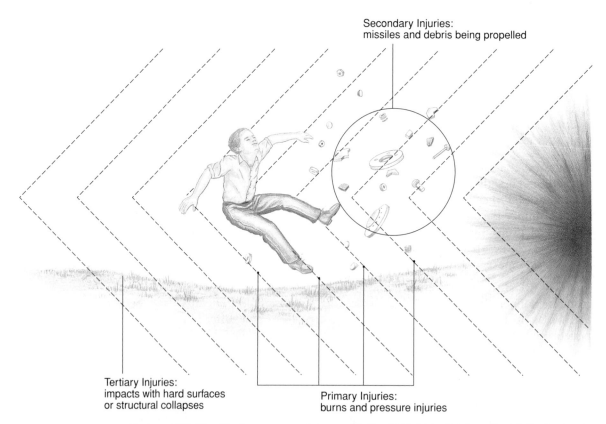

Secondary Injuries: missiles and debris being propelled

Tertiary Injuries: impacts with hard surfaces or structural collapses

Primary Injuries: burns and pressure injuries

FIGURE 17-24 Blasts can cause injury with the initial blast, when the victim is struck by debris, or when the victim is thrown by the blast or injured by structural collapse.

tients. Remember that they will find it difficult to understand what others are saying and will not be able to follow spoken instructions.

Blast Injury Care

The effects of a serious explosion can produce injuries to the lungs, abdomen, and ears that involve special care considerations. Otherwise, care for blunt trauma, punctures/penetrations, and burns as you would for these injuries if they were produced by other mechanisms.

Lungs Pulmonary blast trauma is the most frequent and life-threatening pressure injury associated with an explosion. The blast-induced pressure wave rapidly and forcefully compresses and distorts the chest cavity, individual air passages, and the alveoli. During compression/decompression, the air pressures in these areas do not have time to equalize, as they do with normal respiration. The extreme pressure damages or ruptures the thin and delicate alveolar walls, resulting in fluid accumulation, hemorrhage, and possibly even the entry of air directly into the bloodstream from the alveoli. Fluid accumulation (pulmonary edema) makes the lungs less elastic and air movement more difficult. The victim finds it more laborious and energy consuming to breathe. Alveolar wall rupture releases blood into the alveoli and may allow air to enter the capillaries. The victim may spit or cough up blood or a frothy mixture of blood and air. If air enters the bloodstream, it may then travel through the pulmonary circulation to the heart and then to other critical organs causing small obstructions to circulation, called **emboli**. These emboli may cause stroke-like signs, myocardial infarction, or even death.

A patient history of exposure to a detonation should make you suspect the possibility of lung injury. Since lung injury occurs more frequently with blasts than other pressure injuries and is usually more serious, assess carefully for signs and symptoms of lung injury in patients with abdominal and ear injuries. Lung injury patients may have progressively worsening crackles, difficulty breathing (**dyspnea**) and, in extreme cases, may cough up blood or blood-tinged sputum (**hemoptysis**). Patients occasionally experience a reduced level of consciousness or small, stroke-like episodes. If there is any reason to suspect lung injury from a blast, transport the victim immediately to the closest trauma centre or other appropriate facility.

If it becomes necessary to ventilate a blast injury patient, do so with caution. The mechanism of injury may have damaged the alveolar-capillary walls and opened small blood vessels to the alveolar space. Positive pressure ventilations may push small air bubbles into the vascular system and create emboli. These emboli may quickly travel to the heart and brain, where they can cause further injury or death. The pressure of the ventilations may also induce **pneumothorax** by pushing air past blast-induced lung defects and into the pleural space. If possible, place the victim in the left lateral recumbent position with the head somewhat down. This positioning will discourage emboli from travelling up the carotid arteries and toward the brain.

Despite the risks associated with ventilating blast injury patients, always provide positive pressure ventilations to any victim with serious dyspnea. Use only the pressure needed to obtain moderate chest rise and respiratory volumes. High-concentration oxygen, as supplied with a reservoir, is also helpful because the bloodstream absorbs small oxygen bubbles more easily than the nitrogen of room air.

Abdomen The blast wave's sudden compression/decompression may also damage the air-filled bowel. Violent movements of the bowel wall cause hemorrhage and possibly wall rupture. Rupture releases bowel contents into the abdominal cavity, leading, over time, to severe infection and irritation (peritonitis).

* **emboli** undissolved solid, liquid, or gaseous matter in the bloodstream that may cause blockage of blood vessels.

* **dyspnea** laboured or difficult breathing.

* **hemoptysis** expectoration of blood from the respiratory tract.

* **pneumothorax** collection of air or gas in the pleural cavity between the chest wall and lung.

Provide careful positive pressure ventilations to any blast injury patient with serious dyspnea.

Blast injuries to the abdomen require no special attention in the early stages of care. The impact of associated injuries—the bowel hemorrhage and spillage of bowel contents—on the patient's overall condition takes time to develop and is not usually apparent at the emergency scene. The only exceptions are when the blast was extremely powerful and the patient was very close to the detonation. In these cases, be alert for signs and symptoms of developing shock, and provide rapid transport and fluid resuscitation as needed.

Ears The ears suffer greatly from blast wave forces associated with ordnance explosion, artillery fire, and even repeated small-arms fire at close range. The structure of the ears explains this. The middle ear is an air-filled cavity containing the organs of hearing (cochlea and stapes) and of positional sense (semicircular canals). The pina (the external portion of the ear) focuses and directs pressure waves (normally, sound waves) through the external auditory canal to the eardrum. The eardrum (tympanic membrane) permits the passage of sound waves but excludes the movement of air into the middle ear. The eustachian tube provides a mechanism for equalizing small and gradual changes in atmospheric pressure between the middle ear and the outside atmosphere. During blast overpressure, however, the eustachian tube cannot equalize the rapid pressure changes. The pressure on the tympanic membrane becomes so great that the membrane stretches or ruptures, resulting in acute hearing loss. The pressure change may be so great as to fracture the delicate bones of hearing, also resulting in acute hearing loss. Hearing losses associated with blasts may be temporary or permanent.

Often, ear injuries, even with as much as a third of the eardrum torn, will improve over time without much attention. Direct your care to supporting the victim and ensuring that the ear canal remains uncontaminated.

Penetrating Wounds Care for penetrating wounds as you would for any serious open wound. Remove as much of the contaminating material as is practical, and cover the site with a sterile dressing. If you encounter a large embedded or impaled object, stabilize the object by securing gauze pads around it or cover it with a non-polystyrene paper cup to prevent movement during transport. Large areas of damaged tissue are prone to infection; keep the wound as clean as possible. Care of penetrating trauma will be discussed at greater length in Chapter 18.

Burns Blasts can also cause extensive burn injuries either from the explosions themselves or from the ignition of other munitions or fuels or of debris or clothing. Care for burn injuries is discussed in detail in Chapter 21.

OTHER TYPES OF BLUNT TRAUMA

Blunt trauma can be caused by still other mechanisms. These include falls, crush injuries, and sports injuries.

Falls

The potential for injury from a fall depends on the height and stopping distance.

In terms of physics, falls are a release of stored gravitational energy. The greater the distance a person falls, the greater the impact velocity, the greater the exchange of energy, and the greater the resultant trauma. As with auto impacts, stopping distance may be more important than the height of the fall. A person may dive pleasurably from a four-metre platform into deep water, but a fall from a second-storey window to a concrete sidewalk results in serious injury. Newton's second law,

$$\text{Force} = \text{Mass} \times \text{Acceleration (or Deceleration)}$$

illustrates that the more rapid the deceleration (the shorter the stopping distance), the greater the force and resultant injury. The nature of the impact surface contour may also affect the nature of the injury. An irregular surface, like building rubble or a stairway, may focus the force of impact, increasing the seriousness of the injury.

Trauma resulting from a fall is dependent on the area of contact and the pathway of energy transmission. If the victim lands feet first, energy is transmitted up the skeletal structure through the calcaneus, tibia, femur, pelvis, and lumbar spine (Figure 17-25). Fractures along this skeletal pathway are common, especially os caleis fractures (heel fractures). The lumbar spine is especially prone to compression injury because it is the only skeletal component supporting the entire upper body. As the victim continues the collision, she may fall forward or backward. In forward falls, an outstretched arm may attempt to break the impact, resulting in shoulder, clavicle, and wrist fractures. Pelvic, thoracic, and head injuries may result from a backward fall. In some cases, the fall will progress with the patient continuing a straight impact. The tongue may be bitten deeply as the weight of the cranium pushes the maxilla against the mandible as it impacts the sternum.

The initial impact may involve other body surfaces with kinetic energy transmitted from the contact point toward the body's centre of mass. In diving injuries, the patient's head hits the lake or pool bottom, while the rest of the body compresses the cervical spine between the head and shoulders. Axial loading crushes the vertebrae, disrupts the spinal cord, and paralyzes the patient. This may result from even a very shallow dive, as from poolside or from within the water.

If the victim falls on outstretched arms, the impact energy is transmitted along the skeletal system from the hand and wrist, to the forearm, elbow, arm, and shoulder. In these cases, the clavicle often fractures because it is the smallest weight-bearing bone along the pathway of impact transmission. With collapse of the upper extremities, the head and neck may experience energy exchange and injury as may the shoulders on collision with the impact surface.

In severe falls, with a person dropping more than three times her own height (six metres for the adult, three metres for the small child), focus your attention on potential internal injuries. Rapid deceleration causes many organs

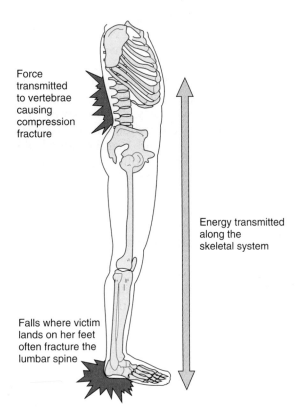

FIGURE 17-25 In falls, energy is transmitted along the skeletal system.

Force transmitted to vertebrae causing compression fracture

Energy transmitted along the skeletal system

Falls where victim lands on her feet often fracture the lumbar spine to be compressed, displaced, and twisted. The heart, for example, is held in the centre of the thorax by the aorta, the vena cavae, and the ligamentum arteriosum. When the victim hits the ground, the heart is pulled downward with such force that it may tear from its aortic attachments, which leads to immediate exsanguination.

In evaluating a fall, determine the point of impact, the fall height or velocity or force of impact, the impact surface, and the transmission pathway of forces along the skeleton. Then anticipate fracture sites and possible internal injuries. During your physical assessment, pay particular attention to the areas where you expect trauma for further signs of injury.

Falls are a common injury mechanism for older or geriatric patients. With increasing age come decreases in coordination, deficits in eyesight and depth perception, and weakening bones. Often, the forces required to break bones are much less in geriatric patients than in younger ones. A brittle bone, like the femur, may actually break during ordinary activities, such as walking down a step, and result in a fall. Assess the circumstances surrounding the fall and the trauma involved, remembering that some fractures in the elderly can occur without the application of serious kinetic forces. Provide careful immobilization and gentle transport for these patients, and ensure that they are comforted and reassured.

Sports Injuries

Sports medicine is a rapidly growing and extensive field, one that certainly cannot be covered completely in this chapter or text. Understanding some basic principles of sports medicine, however, may help you better understand and care for the injured athlete.

Sports injuries are most commonly produced by extreme exertion, fatigue, or direct trauma forces. Injuries can be secondary to acceleration, deceleration, compression, rotation, hyperextension, or hyperflexion. These forces leave behind soft-tissue damage to muscle, connective tissue injury to tendons and ligaments, skeletal trauma to long bones or the spinal column, as well as internal damage to either hollow or solid organs.

When a debilitating sports-related injury occurs, transport the athlete to an emergency department for a complete examination before further participation in the sport is allowed. Injuries that present with minimal pain may be significantly worsened by the stress of further competitive activity. Such stress may cause complete ligament rupture or other soft-tissue injury and increase the potential for permanent disability.

In some contact sports, athletes may experience severe impacts (Figure 17-26). If collision leads to any period of unconsciousness, neurologic deficit, or lowered level of orientation, ensure that the individual is evaluated by emergency department personnel. There is often a strong desire by coaches and players alike for the athlete's return to the game. Until head and cervical spine injuries can be ruled out, however, discourage such action.

Protective gear reduces the chance for and significance of injuries. Gear, however, can sometimes be a contributing factor in sports injuries. In major contact sports, for example, shoes are designed to give maximum traction, using cleats to lock the foot firmly in position. In football, a player might be struck, forcing the body to turn on an immobile foot. Ligaments in the knee may tear, resulting in severe and disabling leg injury. In other cases, protective gear may hinder your complete assessment and patient stabilization.

A newer helmet design for high-school contact sports uses an air-filled bladder to immobilize the head within the device. This fixation may be adequate to immobilize the head within the helmet in cases of suspected spinal injuries. While it is difficult to immobilize a spherical helmet to the flat surface of a spine board, it may be preferable to attempting helmet removal. If your protocols so require,

Sports injuries are most commonly produced by extreme exertion, fatigue, or direct trauma forces.

If a collision leads to any loss of consciousness, neurological deficit, or altered level of consciousness, the athlete should be evaluated by emergency department personnel.

When a debilitating sports-related injury occurs, transport the athlete to an emergency department for a complete examination before further participation in the sport is allowed.

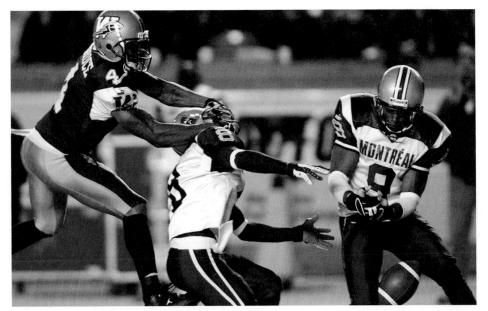

FIGURE 17-26 Contact sports may result in the exchange of great kinetic forces and produce serious injuries.

Source: CP Photo/Winnipeg Free Press—Ken Gigliotti

attempt to immobilize the head and helmet to the long spine board, leaving the shoulder pads in place to help maintain the head and neck in a neutral position.

Crush Injuries

Crush injuries are common types of trauma. They may result from such mechanisms as structural collapse as in an explosion, an industrial or agricultural accident where a limb is caught in machinery, or a traffic accident when a limb is caught under a vehicle. These mechanisms direct great force to soft tissues and bones, compressing surfaces together while stretching semifluid soft tissues laterally. The result may be severe tissue disruption and serious associated hemorrhage.

The injury may be further compounded if the crushing pressure remains in place for an extended period of time. The pressure can disrupt blood flow to and through the limb, causing anaerobic metabolism and some tissue death. This causes a buildup of toxins in the bloodstream. If blood flow returns to the limb, the blood may carry these toxins back to the central circulation. This acidic and toxic blood may then induce cardiac dysrhythmias or seriously damage the kidneys. Another consequence of the release of the crushing pressure is severe and difficult-to-control hemorrhage. The blood vessels within the limb are severely damaged, and bleeding results from many difficult-to-identify locations.

SUMMARY

Blunt trauma accounts for most injury deaths and disabilities. Although vehicle collisions are the most frequent cause of blunt trauma, blast injuries, sports injuries, crush injuries, and falls also account for significant mortality and morbidity. Blunt trauma is difficult to assess accurately, and so you, as the care provider, must look carefully at the mechanism of injury and subtle physical signs to help anticipate serious internal injury. Careful analysis of the mechanism of injury, followed by development of indexes of suspicion for injury, can help you recognize those patients needing rapid entry into the trauma system and those best served by on-scene care and transport to the nearest appropriate care facility.

CHAPTER 18

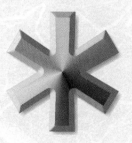

Penetrating Trauma

Objectives

After reading this chapter, you should be able to:

1. Explain the energy exchange process between a penetrating object or projectile and the object it strikes. (pp. 45–49)

2. Determine the effects that profile, yaw, tumble, expansion, and fragmentation have on projectile energy transfer. (pp. 46–49)

3. Describe elements of the ballistic injury process including direct injury, cavitation, temporary cavity, permanent cavity, and zone of injury. (pp. 46–49, 52–54)

4. Identify the relative effects a penetrating object or projectile has when striking various body regions and tissues. (pp. 55–59)

5. Anticipate the injury types and the extent of damage associated with high-velocity/high-energy projectiles, such as rifle bullets; with medium-energy/medium-velocity projectiles, such as handgun and shotgun bullets, slugs, or pellets; and with low-energy/low-velocity penetrating objects, such as knives and arrows. (pp. 49–52)

6. Identify important elements of the scene assessment associated with shootings or stabbings. (pp. 59–61)

7. Identify and explain any special assessment and care considerations for patients with penetrating trauma. (pp. 61–63)

Continued

8. Given several preprogrammed and moulaged penetrating trauma patients, provide the appropriate scene assessment, primary assessment, rapid trauma or focused secondary assessment and history, detailed assessment, and ongoing assessment and provide appropriate patient care and transport. (pp. 45–63)

INTRODUCTION TO PENETRATING TRAUMA

Modern society is experiencing a great increase in the number and severity of penetrating traumas, especially gunshot wounds. About 1300 deaths occur each year in Canada as a result of shootings, compared with approximately 38 000 deaths per year in the United States. In both countries, the number is growing. Many additional mechanisms, including knives, arrows, nails, and pieces of glass or wire, can also cause penetrating trauma. As is the case with auto collisions, physical laws govern the energy exchange process associated with penetrating trauma. Therefore, the types of weapons and projectiles involved and the characteristics of the tissue they strike all affect the severity of injury with penetrating trauma. Understanding the principles of energy exchange and projectile travel will help you anticipate the potential for injuries, recognize the injuries that have occurred, and, ultimately, adequately assess and care for victims of penetrating trauma.

PHYSICS OF PENETRATING TRAUMA

The basic principles of physics that you read about in association with blunt trauma in the last chapter also apply to instances of penetrating trauma. When a projectile strikes a target, it exchanges its energy of motion, more properly called kinetic energy, with the object struck. As you recall, an object's kinetic energy is equal to its mass times the square of its velocity:

$$\text{Kinetic Energy} = \frac{\text{Mass (weight)} \times \text{Velocity (speed)}^2}{2}$$

Thus, the greater the mass of an object, the greater is the energy. If you double the mass of an object, it will have twice the kinetic energy if the speed of the object remains the same. However, the speed (or velocity) of an object has a squared relationship to its kinetic energy. If you double the speed of an object, its kinetic energy increases fourfold. If the speed triples, the energy increases ninefold, and so on (Figure 18-1).

This relationship between mass and velocity explains why very small and relatively light bullets travelling very fast have the potential to do great harm. It also makes clear why different weights of bullets travelling at different velocities cause different amounts of damage. For example, handguns, shotguns, and low-powered rifles are considered to be medium-energy/medium-velocity weapons. They deliver their bullets, slugs, and pellets much faster than low-energy/low-velocity objects, such as knives and arrows, travel but still are slower than bullets delivered by high-energy/high-velocity weapons, such as assault rifles. Thus, a handgun bullet is generally smaller and much slower (250 to 400 metres per second) than a rifle

FIGURE 18-1 The extreme velocity of firearm projectiles gives them great kinetic energy and the potential to do great damage.

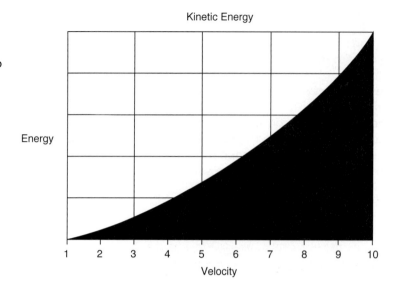

Kinetic Energy

Energy

Velocity

Studies suggest that wounds from rifle bullets are from two to four times more lethal than wounds from handgun bullets.

✳ **ballistics** the study of projectile motion and its interactions with the gun, the air, and the object it contacts.

✳ **trajectory** the path a projectile follows.

✳ **drag** the forces acting on a projectile in motion to slow its progress.

✳ **cavitation** the outward motion of tissue due to a projectile's passage, resulting in a temporary cavity and vacuum.

bullet. A hunting rifle, on the other hand, commonly expels a slightly heavier bullet at speeds of 600 to 1000 metres per second. Hence, the high-energy rifle bullet's kinetic energy is three to nine times greater than the medium-energy handgun bullet's and can be expected to do significantly more damage. Experience in Northern Ireland suggests that rifle bullets are between two and four times as lethal as handgun bullets.

The law of conservation of energy (energy can be neither created nor destroyed) explains why the projectile kinetic energy is transformed into damage as it slows. If a projectile, such as a bullet, remains within the object struck, then all its energy is transferred to the object. If the projectile passes completely through the object, then the energy transferred to the object is equal to the kinetic energy just prior to entry minus the energy remaining in the projectile as it exits.

BALLISTICS

The study of the characteristics of projectiles in motion and their effects on objects they strike is called **ballistics.** The basic physics described above is the starting point for this study. One aspect of ballistics is **trajectory,** or the curved path that a bullet follows once fired from a gun. As it travels through the air, the bullet is constantly pulled downward by gravity. The faster the bullet, the flatter is its curve of travel and the straighter is its trajectory.

A second, more significant, aspect of projectile travel is energy dissipation. Factors that affect energy dissipation include drag, cavitation, profile, stability, expansion, and shape. As a bullet travels through the air, it experiences wind resistance, or **drag.** The faster it travels, the more drag it experiences and the greater is the slowing effect. Since this represents a reduction in bullet speed, it also means, if all else is equal, that the damage caused by a bullet fired at close range will be more severe than from one fired at a distance.

Objects travelling relatively slowly, and without much kinetic energy, such as knives or arrows, will affect only the tissue they contact. High- or medium-velocity projectiles, such as rifle or handgun bullets, however, set a portion of the semifluid body tissue in motion, creating a shock wave and a temporary cavity in the tissue. This stage of the destruction process is known as **cavitation** and is related to the bullet's velocity and how quickly it gives up its energy. The energy exchange rate is related to the size of the projectile's contacting surface, called its profile, and to its shape.

Profile

The **profile** is the portion of the bullet you would see if you looked at it as it travelled toward you. The larger this surface profile, the greater is the energy exchange rate, the more quickly the bullet slows, and the more extensive is the damage to surrounding tissue. For bullets that remain stable during their travel and do not deform, the profile is the bullet's diameter, or **calibre**. To increase the energy exchange rate, bullets are designed to become unstable as they pass from one medium to another or to deform through expansion or fragmentation.

Stability

The location of a bullet's centre of mass affects its stability both during its flight and when it hits a solid or semisolid object. The longer the bullet, the farther the centre of mass is from its leading edge. If the bullet is deflected from straight flight—for example, by the barrel exhaust or by a gust of wind—the lift created by the projectile's tip passing through air at an angle will cause the bullet to tumble. If it continues to tumble, the bullet will slow and the accuracy of the shot will be diminished. To prevent tumbling, bullets are sent spinning through the air by the gun barrel's rifling. This rotation gives a bullet gyroscopic stability like a spinning top. If the spinning bullet is slightly deflected, it will wobble, or **yaw,** then slowly return to straight flight.

When a bullet strikes a dense substance, several things happen. If there is already a yaw, the yaw greatly increases as the bullet begins its penetration. This occurs as the bullet's mass tries to overrun the leading edge. Secondly, the gyroscopic spin designed for stability in air becomes insufficient. A bullet would need to spin at a rate 30 times greater in body tissue than in air to maintain the same stability. The result may be tumbling and a great increase in the bullet's presenting profile. Since a rifle bullet is generally longer than a handgun bullet and has its centre of mass farther back from the leading edge, it is more likely to tumble once it hits body tissue (Figure 18-2). With increased tumbling and a larger presenting profile, a rifle bullet's kinetic energy exchange rate increases, as does its potential for causing damage. In human tissue, a rifle bullet generally rotates 180 degrees and then continues its travel base first.

✱ **profile** the size and shape of a projectile as it contacts a target; it is the energy exchange surface of the contact.

✱ **calibre** the diameter of a bullet expressed in hundredths of an inch (.22 calibre = 0.22 inches); the inside diameter of the barrel of a handgun, shotgun, or rifle.

✱ **yaw** swing or wobble around the axis of a projectile's travel.

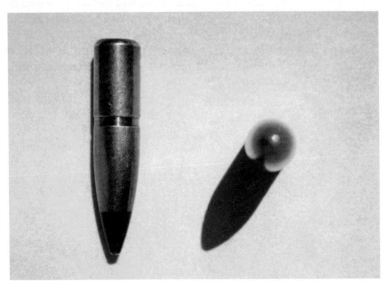

FIGURE 18-2 The presenting surface, or profile, of a bullet changes as it tumbles when it contacts human tissue.

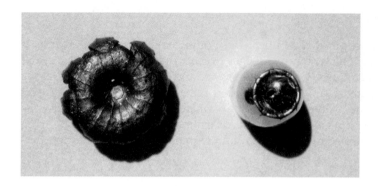

FIGURE 18-3 Some bullets are designed to mushroom on impact, thus increasing their profile, energy exchange rate, and damage potential.

Expansion and Fragmentation

Projectiles also may increase their profile and their energy exchange rate by deforming when they strike a medium denser than air. As the bullet's nose contacts the target, it is compressed by the weight of the rest of the bullet behind it. The nose of the bullet mushrooms outward as the rear of the bullet pushes into it, increasing the projectile's diameter (Figure 18-3). In some cases, the initial impact forces are so great that the bullet separates into several pieces or fragments. This fragmentation increases the energy exchange rate of impact because the total surface area of the fragments is much greater than that of the original bullet profile (Figure 18-4). While handgun bullets are made of relatively soft lead, their velocity, hence their kinetic energy, is generally not sufficient to cause significant deformity. However, some bullets (dum-dums or wad-cutters) are specifically designed to mushroom and/or fragment on impact and thereby increase the damage they cause. Rifle bullets have much greater velocities than do handgun bullets and much more kinetic energy. They are more prone to deform when contacting human tissue, especially bullets used for big-game hunting. Most military ammunition is fully jacketed with impact-resistant metal and seldom deforms solely with soft-tissue collision.

Secondary Impacts

The energy exchange between a projectile and body tissue can also be affected by any object the projectile strikes during its travel. Branches, window glass, or articles of clothing may all deflect a bullet and induce yaw and tumble. They may also cause bullet deformity, and thereby increase the energy exchange rate once the bullet hits the victim.

A special type of secondary impact occurs when the bullet collides with body armour. Kevlar™ and other synthetic fabrics can effectively resist the kinetic en-

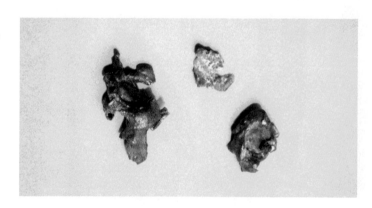

FIGURE 18-4 Some firearm projectiles may break apart, or fragment, on contact, greatly increasing their profile and damage potential.

ergy generated by medium-energy projectiles. This energy is absorbed by the armour and distributed to the victim in much the same way that the recoil of a gun is distributed to the shooter. The impact of the bullet may produce blunt trauma in the person hit (for example, myocardial contusion), but such injuries are generally less damaging than penetration by the bullet would have been. High-energy projectiles may pass through body armour, but in doing so they dissipate some of their energy as blunt trauma, thereby reducing the penetrating kinetic energy as the bullet strikes body tissue. Bullet deformity may increase the rate of energy exchange, but the reduction in kinetic energy reduces the overall injury potential. Ceramic inserts for body armour will stop penetration of most rifle bullets but not without causing significant but less lethal blunt trauma.

Shape

In addition to profile, other aspects of the shape of the bullet affect the energy exchange rate and the resulting damage. Handgun ammunition is rather blunt, is more resistant to travel through human tissue, and releases kinetic energy more quickly. Rifle bullets are more pointed and cut through the tissue more efficiently. However, if the rifle bullet tumbles, it will present a different shape and may exchange energy more rapidly because of both the shape and the increase in profile. If a bullet fragments, the irregular shape of the fragments mean that the projectile will give up its energy more rapidly and through more erratic pathways than will either an intact handgun or rifle bullet.

SPECIFIC WEAPON CHARACTERISTICS

Weapons that commonly cause wounds encountered by paramedics include handguns, domestic rifles, assault rifles, shotguns, and knives and arrows. Each type of weapon has certain characteristics associated with the injuries it produces (Figure 18-5).

Handgun

The handgun is often a small-calibre, short-barrelled, medium-velocity weapon with limited accuracy that is most effective at close range. Because a handgun does not fire a high-velocity, high-energy projectile as a rifle does, its potential for causing damage is limited. The blunter shape of the bullet and, less frequently, its softer composition and associated mushrooming and fragmentation may re-

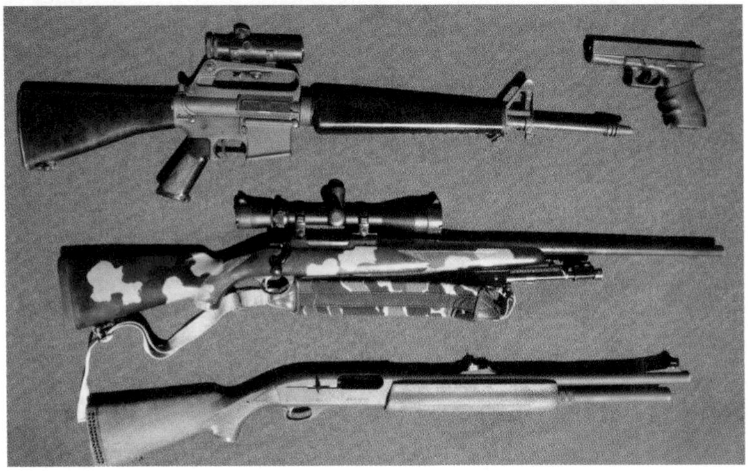

While body armour protects against penetration, impact may result in less lethal but still serious blunt injury.

Content Review

FACTORS AFFECTING ENERGY EXCHANGE BETWEEN A PROJECTILE AND BODY TISSUE

Velocity
Profile
Stability
Expansion and fragmentation
Secondary impacts
Shape

FIGURE 18-5 Firearms include (top to bottom) handguns, assault rifles, domestic rifles, and shotguns.

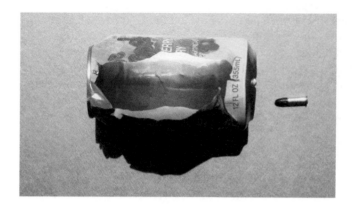

FIGURE 18-6 The energy of the handgun projectile is limited by low projectile weight and its relatively slow velocity.

lease the bullet's energy more rapidly. The damage is still, however, less than that of the higher energy rifle bullet. The severity of injury is usually related to the organs directly damaged by the bullet's passage (Figure 18-6).

Some handguns fire automatically (machine pistols). They continue to discharge bullets until the trigger is released or the magazine empties. While the energy for each projectile remains the same, the damage potential associated with automatic weapons is increased because of the likelihood of multiple impacts or multiple victims.

Rifle

The domestic hunting rifle fires a heavier projectile than does the handgun, through a much longer barrel, and with much greater muzzle velocity. It is either a manually loaded, single-shot weapon with some mechanical loading action to advance the next shell, or a semi-automatic weapon, in which the next shell is fed into the chamber by recoil or exhaust gases. However, no more than one bullet is expelled by each squeeze of the domestic hunting rifle's trigger. The high-energy rifle bullet travels much farther, with greater accuracy, and retains much more of its kinetic energy than does the handgun projectile. Due to the rifle bullet's high speed and energy, it transfers great damaging energy to the target (Figure 18-7). This results in extensive wounds with injuries that extend beyond the projectile's immediate track. Domestic hunting ammunition is especially lethal. It is often designed to expand dramatically on impact, greatly increasing the energy delivery rate and the size of both the temporary cavity and the wound pathway.

The damage caused by high-energy rifle bullets can extend well beyond the actual track of the projectile.

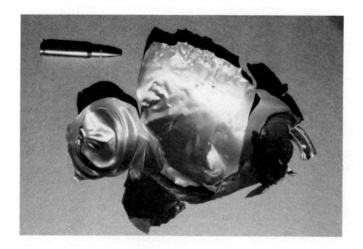

FIGURE 18-7 The energy carried by a rifle bullet is extremely damaging because of its heavier weight and very high velocity.

Assault Rifle

The assault rifle differs from the domestic hunting rifle in that it generally has a larger magazine capacity and will fire in both the semi-automatic and automatic mode. Examples of these weapons include the M16 and the AK47. The resulting injuries are similar to injuries produced by domestic hunting rifles, although multiple wounds and casualties can be expected. Military ammunition is fully jacketed and not designed for expansion and, while still very deadly, the energy delivery is not as severe as with domestic hunting ammunition. Assault weapons in terrorist hands, however, may be loaded with domestic hunting-type ammunition. This greatly increases their injury potential.

Shotgun

The shotgun expels a single projectile (a slug) or numerous spheres (pellets or shot) at medium velocity. The shell is loaded with a particular size of lead shot, varying from 00 (about 8 mm or one-third inch in diameter) to #9 shot (about the size of a pin head). The size of the projectile compartment is approximately the same with various types of loads. This means that the larger the shot, the smaller the number of projectiles. Each projectile shares a portion of the total muzzle energy and adds to the resistance as it moves through air. The shotgun is limited in range and accuracy; however, injuries sustained at close range can be very severe or lethal (Figure 18-8).

Knives and Arrows

In contrast to high- or medium-velocity projectiles, such as rifle or handgun bullets, knives, arrows, and other slow-moving penetrating objects cause low-velocity, low-energy wounds. Because low-velocity objects do not produce either a pressure shock wave or cavitation, damage is usually limited to physical injury caused by direct contact between the blade or object and the victim's tissue. The severity of a low-velocity penetrating wound, however, can often be difficult to assess because the depth and angle of the object's insertion cannot be determined from the visible wound. In addition, an attacker may move the penetrating object about inside the victim, then leave it in place or withdraw it. The penetration can result in serious internal hemorrhage or injury to individual or multiple body organs.

The hunting tips designed for arrows can be especially damaging. These feature three razor-tipped, pointed barbs that are intended to smoothly cut tissue. These tips produce severe internal hemorrhage. Also, any movement of an arrow while it is impaled in the victim increases both the tissue damage and the hemorrhage rate.

The extent of damage is often difficult to assess with wounds caused by low-velocity, low-energy projectiles, such as knives and arrows. Suspect internal hemorrhage and/or injury to body organs.

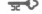

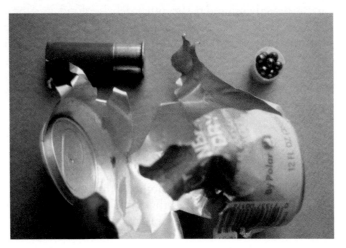

FIGURE 18-8 A shotgun propels small projectiles with limited velocity. However, because of the large number of projectiles, the weapon can be extremely damaging at close range.

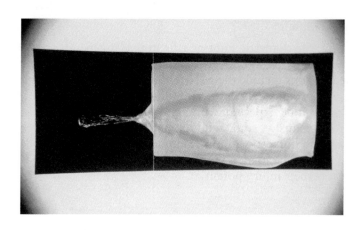

DAMAGE PATHWAY

The damage pathway that a high-velocity projectile inflicts results from three specific factors. They are the direct injury, the pressure shock wave, and cavitation, or the creation of a temporary cavity. These three factors can also create a permanent cavity and a zone of injury (Figure 18-9).

Content Review

FACTORS ASSOCIATED WITH THE DAMAGE PATHWAY OF A PROJECTILE WOUND

Direct injury
Pressure shock wave
Cavitation
　　Temporary cavity
　　Permanent cavity
　　Zone of injury

THE PROJECTILE INJURY PROCESS

The spinning bullet smashes into a semifluid target (such as human tissue) with great speed and kinetic energy. The tip of the bullet strikes tissue, pushing the tissue forward and to the side along the pathway of its travel. This tissue collides with adjacent tissue, ultimately creating a shock wave of pressure moving forward and lateral to the projectile. This shock wave continues to move perpendicular to the bullet's path as it passes. The rapid compression of tissue laterally and the stretching of the tissue as it moves outward from the bullet path crushes and tears the tissue structure. The motion creates a pocket, or cavity, behind the bullet. The pressure within this cavity is reduced, creating suction. This suction draws air and debris into the cavity from the entrance wound and from the exit wound, if one is present. The body tissue's elasticity then draws the sides of the cavity back together, causing the entrance wound, exit wound, and wound pathway to close completely or remain only partially open.

The bullet's exchange of energy with the body leaves various tissues disrupted and injured. Tissue in the direct pathway of the bullet suffers most. It is severely contused and likely to have been torn from its attachments. In addition to the directly injured tissue, other debris, blood, and air are found along the bullet's pathway. The cavitational wave stretches and tears adjacent tissue, damaging cell walls and small blood vessels. The adjacent tissue is injured but will likely regain its normal function slowly. Larger blood vessels torn by the bullet and the cavitational wave release their precious fluid in large quantities into the damaged pathway. Over time, this pathway, because of the disruption in circulation and the introduction of infectious material with the drawing-in of debris, may experience severe infection, which will prolong the healing process.

Direct Injury

Direct injury is the damage done as the projectile strikes tissue, contuses and tears that tissue, and pushes the tissue out of its way. The direct injury pathway is limited to the profile of the bullet as it moves through the body or the profiles of resulting fragments as the bullet breaks apart. Except for magnum rounds (generating particularly high velocities), handgun bullet damage is usually limited to direct injury.

Pressure Shock Wave

When a high-velocity, high-energy projectile strikes human flesh, it creates a pressure shock wave (Figure 18-10). Since most human tissue is semifluid and elastic, the impact of the projectile transmits energy outward very quickly. The tissue cells in front of the bullet are pushed forward and to the side at great speed. They push adjacent cells forward and outward, creating a moving wave of pressure and tissue. The faster and blunter the bullet, the greater is the effect. With high-velocity rifle bullets, pressures are extreme, approaching 100 times the normal atmospheric pressure.

The pressure wave travels very well through fluid, such as blood, and may injure blood vessels distant from the projectile pathway. Air-filled cavities, such as the small air sacs (alveoli) of the lung, compress very easily and absorb the pressure, quickly limiting the shock wave and the resulting temporary cavity. Solid and dense organs, such as the liver and spleen, suffer greatly as the pressure wave moves through them, causing internal hemorrhage and, in extreme cases, fracture.

> *The severity of injury in cases of bullet wounds usually depends on the organs damaged by the bullet's passage.*

Temporary Cavity

The temporary cavity is a space created behind the high-energy bullet as tissue moves rapidly away from the bullet's path. The size of the cavity depends on the amount of energy transferred during the bullet's passage. With rifle bullets, the temporary cavity may be as much as 12 times larger than the projectile's profile. After the bullet's passage, tissue elasticity causes the temporary cavity to close.

Cavitation also produces a subatmospheric pressure within the cavity as it expands. This means that air is drawn in from the entrance wound and the exit wound, if one exists. Debris and contamination enter the cavity with the in-flowing air, adding to the risk of infection.

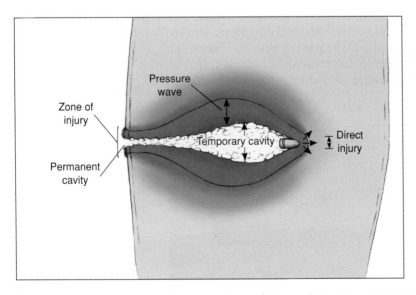

FIGURE 18-10   As a projectile passes through tissue, it creates a pressure wave and a temporary cavity, with results that include direct injury, a permanent cavity, and a zone of injury.

Permanent Cavity

The movement that creates the temporary cavity crushes, stretches, and tears the affected tissues. These processes seriously damage the area in and adjacent to the bullet's path and may also damage the tissue's elasticity. The tissue thus may not return to its normal orientation, resulting in a permanent cavity that in some cases may be larger than the bullet's diameter. This cavity is not a void but is filled with disrupted tissues, some air, fluid, and debris.

Zone of Injury

Associated with most projectile wounds is a zone of injury that extends beyond the permanent cavity. This zone contains contused tissue that does not function normally and may be slow to heal because of cell and tissue damage, disrupted blood flow, and infection.

LOW-VELOCITY WOUNDS

Sharp weapons, such as knives, ice picks, and arrows, or flying objects, such as blast debris or wires thrown by a lawn mower, can cause low-velocity penetrating trauma. In these cases, the relatively slow speed of the object limits the kinetic energy exchange rate as the object enters the victim's body. Consider, for example, the stabbing of a victim by a 70-kilogram attacker who strikes with a knife moving at about three metres per second. Although the mass behind the penetration of the knife blade is significantly greater than a rifle bullet's, the velocity of the knife is vastly lower. This means that injury in such cases is usually restricted to the tissue actually contacted by the penetrating object (Figure 18-11).

While the injury is limited to the penetrating object's pathway, that object may be twisted, moved about, or inserted at an oblique angle. As a result, the entrance wound may not reflect the depth of the object's penetration, the extent of its motion within the body, or the actual organs and tissues it contacts and injures.

Characteristics of the attacker and victim are important to keep in mind when assessing cases of low-velocity penetrating trauma. Knife-wielding males, for example, most often strike with a forward, outward, or crosswise stroke. Females usually strike with an overhand and downward stroke. Victims of these attacks initially attempt to shield themselves with their arms. This means they often receive deep upper-extremity lacerations (commonly called defence wounds). If an attack continues, injuries are often directed to the chest, abdomen, face, neck, or back.

FIGURE 18-11 Damage caused by a low-velocity wounding process, such as that caused by a wire thrown by a lawn mower, is limited to the object's path of travel.

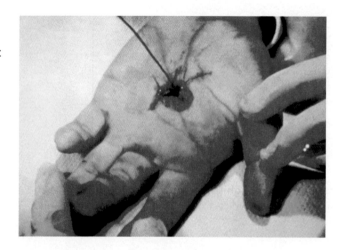

SPECIFIC TISSUE/ORGAN INJURIES

The extent of damage that a penetrating projectile causes within the body varies with the particular type of tissue it encounters. The density of an organ affects how efficiently the projectile's energy is transmitted to surrounding tissues. The tissue's connective strength and elasticity, called **resiliency,** also influence how much tissue damage occurs with the kinetic energy transfer. Structures and tissues within the body that behave differently during projectile passage include connective tissue, solid organs, hollow organs, lungs, and bone.

✳ resiliency the connective strength and elasticity of an object or fabric.

CONNECTIVE TISSUE

Muscles, skin, and other connective tissues are dense, elastic, and held together very well. When exposed to the pressure and stretching of the cavitational wave, these types of tissue characteristically absorb energy while limiting tissue damage. The wound track closes due to the resiliency of the tissue, and serious injury is frequently limited to the projectile's pathway.

ORGANS

Another factor that has profound effects on the victim's potential for survival is the particular organ involved in a penetrating injury. Some organs, such as the heart and brain, are immediately necessary for life functions, and serious injury to them may cause immediate death. When large blood vessels are involved, the hemorrhage can be rapid and severe. A penetrating injury to the urinary bladder, conversely, may not receive surgical intervention for several hours with no threat to the patient's life. When evaluating a wound's seriousness, anticipate the organs injured and the effect their injury is likely to have on the patient's condition and survivability.

Solid Organs

Solid organs, such as the liver, spleen, kidneys, pancreas, and brain, have the density but not the resiliency of muscle and other connective tissues. When struck by the forces of bullet impact, these tissues compress and stretch, resulting in great damage that is more closely associated with the size of the temporary cavity than with the bullet's profile. The tissue returns to its original location, not because of its own elasticity but because of the resiliency of surrounding tissues or the organ capsule. Hemorrhage associated with solid organ projectile damage is often severe.

Be alert to the possibility of severe hemorrhage if you suspect that a projectile has damaged a solid organ.

Hollow Organs

Hollow organs, such as the bowel, stomach, urinary bladder, and heart, are muscular containers holding fluid. The fluid within is noncompressible and rapidly transmits the impact energy outward. If the container is filled and distended with fluid at the time of impact, the energy released can tear the organ apart explosively (Figure 18-12). Slower and smaller projectiles may produce small holes in an organ and permit slow leakage of its contents. If this occurs with the heart, it may produce **pericardial tamponade** (blood filling the pericardial sac, thus limiting heart function) or moderate and slowly life-threatening hemorrhage. If the container is not distended, it is more tolerant of cavitational forces. If a hollow organ, such as the bowel or stomach, holds air, the air compresses with the passage of the pressure wave and somewhat limits the extent of injury. (Large blood vessels respond to projectile passage much like the hollow, fluid-filled, organs.)

✳ pericardial tamponade filling of the pericardial sac with fluid, which in turn limits the filling and function of the heart.

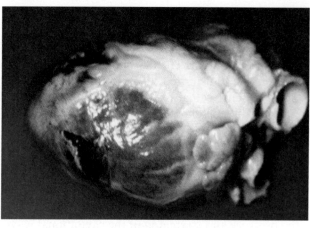

FIGURE 18-12   If a high-velocity bullet strikes the heart during maximum cardiac filling, cardiac rupture and rapid exsanguination may occur.

LUNGS

The lungs consist of millions of small, elastic, air-filled sacs. As the bullet and its associated pressure wave pass, the air is compressed, thereby slowing and limiting the transmission of the cavitational wave. Injury to lung tissue in cases of penetrating trauma is generally less extensive than can be expected with any other body tissue.

A bullet may, however, open the chest wall or disrupt larger airways, thus permitting air to escape into the thorax (pneumothorax) or creating a valve-like defect that results in accumulating pressure within the chest (tension pneumothorax). Bullet wounds only infrequently induce an open pneumothorax (sucking chest wound) because the entrance wound diameter is usually limited to the bullet calibre. Explosive exit wounds of high-powered rifles or close-range shotgun blasts, however, may be large and cause significant disruption of the chest wall integrity. In these cases, a pneumothorax is a more likely outcome.

BONE

In contrast to lung tissue, bone is the densest, most rigid, and nonelastic body tissue of all. When struck by a projectile or its associated pressure wave, bone resists displacement until it fractures, often into numerous pieces. These bone fragments then may distribute the impact energy to surrounding tissue. The projectile's contact with bone may also significantly alter the projectile's path through the body.

GENERAL BODY REGIONS

Several body regions deserve special attention regarding projectile wounds. They include the extremities, abdomen, thorax, neck, and head (Figure 18-13). A projectile's passage also has a special effect on the first and last tissue contacted, the sites of the entrance and the exit wounds.

Extremities

The extremities consist of skin covering muscles and surrounding large long bones. An extremity injury may be debilitating but does not immediately threaten life unless there is severe hemorrhage associated with it. The severity of injury is limited by the resiliency of the skin and muscle, although if the bone is

Injury to lung tissue in cases of penetrating trauma is generally less extensive than can be expected with any other body tissue.

Suspect the possibility of pneumothorax when there has been a significant disruption of chest wall integrity.

Content Review

BODY REGIONS DESERVING SPECIAL ATTENTION WITH PENETRATING TRAUMA
Extremities
Abdomen
Thorax
Neck
Head

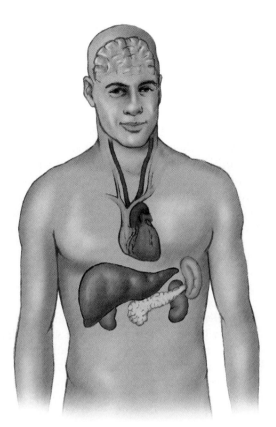

involved, the degree of soft-tissue damage may be increased. In recent military experience, extremity injuries account for between 60 and 80 percent of injuries yet result in less than 10 percent of fatalities. The remaining 20 to 40 percent of penetrating injuries are divided among wounds of the abdomen, thorax, and head and account for more than 90 percent of mortality.

Some 90 percent of penetrating trauma mortality involves the head, thorax, and abdomen.

Abdomen

The abdomen (including the pelvic cavity) is the largest body cavity and contains most of the human organs. The area is not well protected by skeletal structures other than the upper pelvic ring, the lower rib cage border, and the lumbar vertebral column. The passage of a projectile through the abdominal cavity can produce a significant cavitational wave. The major occupant of the cavity, the bowel, is extremely tolerant of compression and stretching, but the liver, spleen, kidneys, and pancreas are highly susceptible to injury and hemorrhage. Since these organs occupy the upper abdominal quadrants, you should consider any penetrating projectile injury to this area to be serious and to have the potential to cause severe internal hemorrhage. Serious consequences should also be anticipated with injuries to the abdominal aorta and inferior vena cava, which are located along the spinal column in the posterior and central abdomen.

Consider any penetrating projectile injury to the abdomen to be serious and to have the potential to cause severe internal hemorrhage.

If a projectile perforates the small or large bowel, those organs may spill their contents into the abdominal cavity. This spillage results in serious peritoneal irritation due to chemical action or infection, although the signs and symptoms take some time to develop. If the injury process disrupts the blood vessels, the free blood will not result in abdominal irritation.

Thorax

Within the chest is a cavity formed by the ribs, spine, sternum, clavicles, and the diaphragm's strong muscle. This thoracic cavity houses the lungs, heart, and major blood vessels as well as the esophagus and part of the trachea. The impact of a bullet with the ribs may induce an explosive energy exchange that injures the surrounding tissue with numerous bony fragments. Lung tissue can absorb much of the cavitational energy while sustaining limited injury itself. However, the heart and great vessels, as fluid-filled containers, may suffer greatly from the energy of the bullet's passage. The damage to these structures and the associated massive hemorrhage may cause almost instant death. Because of the pressure-driven dynamics of respiration, any large chest wound may compromise breathing. Air may pass through a wound instead of the normal airway (pneumothorax) or build up under pressure within the chest wall (tension pneumothorax).

Neck

Monitor the airway closely in any patient with a penetrating wound to the neck.

The neck is an anatomical area traversed by several critical structures. These include the larynx, the trachea, the esophagus, several major blood vessels (the carotid and vertebral arteries and the jugular veins), and the spinal cord. Penetrating trauma in this area is very likely to damage vital structures and lead to airway compromise, severe bleeding, and/or neurological dysfunction. Associated swelling and hematoma formation may compromise circulation and the airway. Additionally, any large penetrating wound may permit air to be drawn into an open external jugular vein and immediately threaten life due to the resulting pulmonary emboli.

Head

Bullet wounds to the head, particularly those that penetrate the skull, are especially lethal.

Suspect the possibility of airway compromise in patients with projectile wounds to the head and face.

The skull is a hollow, strong, and rigid container, housing the brain's delicate semisolid tissue. It is highly susceptible to projectile injury. If a bullet penetrates the skull, its cavitational energy is trapped within the cavity and subjects the brain to extreme pressures. If the released kinetic energy is great enough, the skull may explode outward. In some cases, a bullet may enter the skull and not have enough energy to exit; in such a case, the bullet may continue to travel along the interior of the skull, disrupting more and more brain matter. Bullet wounds to the head, particularly those that penetrate the skull, are especially lethal.

The destructive forces released by a projectile wound to the head may also disrupt the airway and/or the victim's ability to control his own airway. The head and face are also areas with an extensive supply of blood vessels. Penetrating trauma may damage these vessels and result in serious and difficult-to-control hemorrhage.

A frequent occurrence associated with suicide attempts is severe damage to the facial region. As the individual places a shotgun or rifle under the chin and pulls the trigger, the head tilts up and back. This directs the blast entirely to the facial region, but the projectile(s) may not enter the cranium or strike any immediately vital structures. There is, however, serious bleeding. The bleeding and the associated damage can make the airway very hard to control. In these cases, use of an endotracheal tube to secure the airway can be difficult because many airway structures and landmarks are often obliterated by the blast.

Entrance Wound

Entrance wounds are usually the size of the bullet's profile. At this point, cavitational wave energy has not had time to develop and contribute to the wounding process (Figure 18-14). The situation is different, however, with bullets that deform or tumble during flight. With these projectiles, the initial impact can be es-

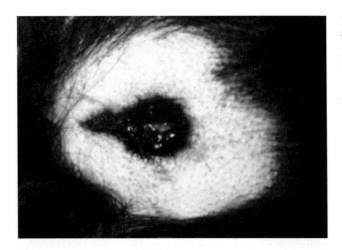

FIGURE 18-14 The entrance wound is often the same size as the projectile's profile and may demonstrate some bruising on the inner border of the wound.

pecially violent, producing a much larger and more disrupted entry wound than the calibre of the bullet alone would suggest.

Bullet entry wounds sustained at close range, a metre or less, display special characteristics. Such wounds may be marked by elements of the barrel exhaust and bullet passage. Tattooing from the propellant residue may form a darkened circle or an oval (if the gun is held at an angle) around the entry wound and contaminate the wound itself. At the wound site, you may notice a small (usually 1 to 2 mm) ridge of discoloration around the entrance caused by the spinning bullet. If the gun barrel is held very close or against the skin as the weapon is fired, it may push the barrel exhaust into the wound, producing subcutaneous emphysema (air within the skin's tissue) and crepitus to the touch. If the barrel is held a few centimetres from the skin, you may notice some burns caused by the hot gases of the barrel exhaust.

Exit Wound

The exit wound is caused by the physical damage both from the passage of the bullet itself and from the cavitational wave. Since the pressure wave is moving forward and outward, the wound may have a "blown outward" appearance. The exit wound may appear as stellate, referring to the tears radiating outward in a star-like fashion (Figure 18-15). Because the cavitational wave has had time to develop, the exit wound may more accurately reflect the potential for damage caused by the bullet's passage than the entrance wound. If the bullet expends all its kinetic energy before it can exit the body, there is no exit wound and the bullet remains within the body. If the bullet does exit, the kinetic energy expended within the body is equal to the kinetic energy before impact minus the energy that remains in the bullet as it leaves the body.

An exit wound may more accurately reflect the potential damage caused by a bullet's passage through the body than an entrance wound.

SPECIAL CONCERNS WITH PENETRATING TRAUMA

SCENE ASSESSMENT

The scene assessment for a shooting or stabbing raises special concerns not associated with most other emergency care situations. The very nature of these injuries should suggest the possibility of danger from further violence and potential injury to you and your crew. Do not approach a shooting or stabbing scene until law-

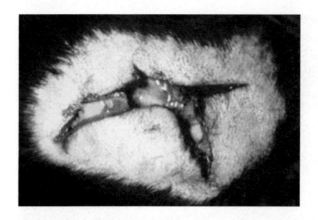

FIGURE 18-15 A bullet's exit wound often has a "blown outward" appearance, with stellate tears.

enforcement personnel arrive and secure it and direct you to enter and provide care. If law-enforcement personnel are not yet on the scene when you arrive, stage your vehicle at least four blocks away and out of sight of the scene. Notify EMS dispatch of your staged location. Do not drive to the scene until requested by law enforcement. On arrival at the scene, if possible, keep the police and their vehicles between you and the shooting or stabbing site. Wait there for the police to indicate that it is safe to approach the patient (Figure 18-16).

As you approach the patient, survey the scene carefully to determine that there are no weapons within the patient's reach. Consider the possibility that the patient may be carrying a knife or other weapon. If you have any doubts, request that the police search the patient for weapons before you begin to provide care.

As you carefully survey the scene of a shooting, try to reconstruct the event. Attempt to determine the patient's original position and his angle to and distance from the shooter. This helps you determine the angle at which the bullet entered the patient (which may not otherwise be revealed by the entrance wound) and whether the wound was received at point blank range or from a distance. Also try to determine the calibre of weapon and its type—handgun, rifle, or shotgun.

If the call involves a knifing injury, attempt to find out the gender and approximate weight of the attacker and the length of the blade. (You probably will not be able to determine the wound depth.) This information will help the emergency department determine the potential severity of the wound.

As you move on to your assessment of the patient, do all that you can to preserve the crime scene while providing any needed patient care. Disturb only those materials around the patient that you must move in order to render care. Cut around any bullet or knife holes in clothing and give the clothing to police for use as evidence. If there is ever any doubt about what to do, however, err on the

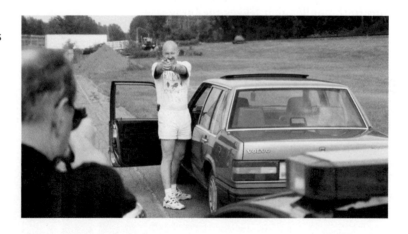

FIGURE 18-16 Ensure that any potentially violent scene is safe and secured by police before entering.

side of providing patient care. (See Chapter 3, the section on "Crime Scene Awareness.") If the victim is obviously dead, employ your jurisdiction's protocols for handling the body, but try to do so without disturbing evidence that may be crucial in determining what happened.

PENETRATING WOUND ASSESSMENT

When assessing the victim of penetrating trauma, try to determine the pathway of the penetrating object and the organs that may have been affected by the wound. Anticipate the impact of potential organ injury, and use this determination in setting priorities for on-scene care or rapid transport of the victim. Remember, however, that a bullet may not travel in a straight line between entrance and exit wounds. Often, a very small shift in a bullet's pathway may mean the difference between tearing open a large blood vessel or missing critical organs completely. The human body is also a dynamic place. The diaphragm moves the kidneys, pancreas, liver, spleen, and heart during respirations; whether or not these organs are injured may be somewhat dependent on the phase of respiration in which the injury occurs.

It is often hard to anticipate the severity of a projectile wound. Injuries to the large blood vessels, heart, and brain may be immediately or rapidly fatal, while injuries to solid organs (liver, pancreas, kidneys, or spleen) may also be deadly but take more time in working their effects. Consequently, always suspect the worst with bullet wounds that involve the head, chest, or abdomen. Provide rapid transport in these cases, and treat shock aggressively.

Provide rapid transport for patients with bullet wounds to the head, chest, or abdomen, and treat aggressively for shock.

PENETRATING WOUND CARE

Certain penetrating wounds need special attention. These include wounds of the face and chest and those involving impaled objects. Their care is described below; care for other penetrating injuries and shock is discussed in later chapters.

Facial Wounds

Some facial gunshot wounds destroy many airway landmarks (Figure 18-17). With wounds like these, endotracheal intubation is extremely difficult. You might find it helpful to visualize the larynx with the laryngoscope while another rescuer gently presses on the chest. Look for any bubbling during the chest compression, and try to pass the endotracheal tube through the bubbling tissue. Then, very carefully ensure that the endotracheal tube is properly placed in the trachea and that lung ventilation is adequate.

If this approach is not effective, two related techniques may restore the airway, at least for long enough to reach more definitive care. These techniques are the

If endotracheal intubation cannot be accomplished in a patient whose airway landmarks have been destroyed by a gunshot wound, emergency cricothyrotomy or cricothyrostomy may be necessary to create a route for ventilations.

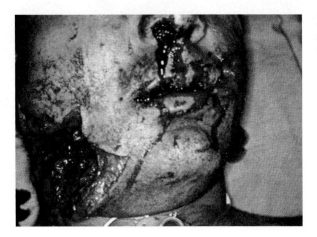

FIGURE 18-17 Facial wounds may distort or destroy airway landmarks.

Anticipate a developing tension pneumothorax if your assessment reveals frothy blood in a patient with a bullet wound to the chest.

cricothyrotomy and the **cricothyrostomy**. These emergency surgical or needle airway procedures perforate the membrane between the thyroid and cricoid cartilages, providing a route for ventilation directly into the lower airway. (These techniques are discussed in detail in Chapter 23, "Head, Facial, and Neck Trauma.")

Chest Wounds

The chest wall is rather thick and resilient. It requires a large wound to create an opening big enough to permit free air movement through the chest wall, an open pheumothorax. Wounds caused by small-calibre handguns usually result in no air movement, while wounds caused by shotgun blasts and exiting high-velocity bullets more commonly cause such injuries. If frothy blood is associated with a chest wound, anticipate a developing tension pneumothorax, in which air builds up under pressure within the thorax. Remember, it takes pressure to push air through the wound and froth the blood. If you completely seal the chest wound, you may stop any outward air flow. This can increase both the speed of development of the tension pneumothorax and its severity. Cover any open chest wound with an occlusive dressing sealed on three sides or an Asherman chest seal (Figure 18-18). If dyspnea is significant, assess for a tension pneumothorax, and if you are an advanced care or critical care paramedic, perform needle decompression as indicated under local protocols. (See Chapter 25, "Thoracic Trauma".)

Always consider the possibility of heart and great vessel damage with a penetrating chest wound. These injuries may lead rapidly to severe internal hemorrhage and death. Another serious complication of penetrating chest trauma is pericardial tamponade. This condition occurs when an object or projectile perforates the heart and permits blood to leak into the pericardial sac. As blood accumulates in the sac, the heart no longer fully fills with blood, and circulation slows. If pericardial tamponade is uncorrected, the **prognosis** for the patient is very poor. However, a needle introduced into the pericardial space, a procedure available at the emergency department, can quickly alleviate the life threat. Therefore, if you suspect this condition, arrange for rapid transport. The assessment of pericardial tamponade is discussed in Chapter 25, "Thoracic Trauma."

Impaled Objects

If an object that causes a low-velocity wound lodges in the body, removal of the object may be dangerous for the patient. If the object became bent as it hit a bone

FIGURE 18-18 Seal open chest wounds with a three-sided dressing or Asherman chest seal, and ensure adequate respirations.

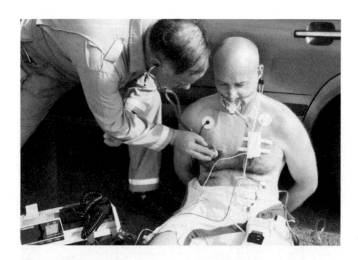

on entry, attempts at removal may cause further injury. If the object is held firmly by soft tissue, it may obstruct blood vessels, thereby restricting blood loss; removal of the object may then increase hemorrhage.

Immobilize impaled objects where and as they are found, and immediately transport the patient. The only impaled objects that you should remove are those lodged in the cheek or trachea that interfere with the airway or those that you must remove to provide CPR, such as those in the back.

Immobilize impaled objects. Only remove those that have lodged in the cheek or those that interfere with the airway or that prevent CPR.

Summary

Penetrating injuries, especially those associated with gunshot wounds, are responsible for a high incidence of prehospital trauma and death. Your understanding of the mechanisms of injury that produce these wounds and an understanding of the types of injuries caused by these mechanisms (index of suspicion) can help you rapidly identify serious life threats and ensure that these patients receive rapid transport to a trauma centre. Special prehospital care techniques, such as sealing an open pneumothorax and managing a difficult airway, can also help you stabilize the patient in the field and help ensure that the patient safely reaches definitive care.

CHAPTER 19

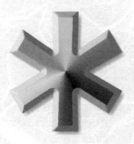

Hemorrhage and Shock

Objectives

After reading this chapter, you should be able to:

1. Describe the epidemiology, including the morbidity/mortality and prevention strategies, for shock and hemorrhage. (pp. 72–74, 82–84)

2. Discuss the anatomy, physiology, and pathophysiology of the cardiovascular system. (see Chapters 12 and 13)

3. Define shock based on aerobic and anaerobic metabolism. (see Chapter 13)

4. Describe the body's physiological response to changes in blood volume, blood pressure, and perfusion. (pp. 83–86)

5. Describe the effects of decreased perfusion at the capillary level. (pp. 83–84)

6. Discuss the cellular ischemic, capillary stagnation, and capillary washout phases related to hemorrhagic shock. (pp. 83–84)

7. Discuss the various types and degrees of shock and hemorrhage. (pp. 72–74, 84–86)

8. Predict shock and hemorrhage based on mechanism of injury. (pp. 74–75 86–87)

9. Identify the need for intervention and transport of the patient with hemorrhage or shock. (pp. 74–79, 86–89)

Continued

10. Discuss the assessment findings and management of internal and external hemorrhage and shock. (pp. 74–79, 86–89)
11. Differentiate between the administration rate and volume of IV fluid in patients with controlled versus uncontrolled hemorrhage. (pp. 89–92)
12. Relate pulse pressure and orthostatic vital sign changes to perfusion status. (pp. 77–78, 88)
13. Define and differentiate between compensated and decompensated hemorrhagic shock. (pp. 84–86)
14. Discuss the pathophysiological changes, assessment findings, and management associated with compensated and decompensated shock. (pp. 84–92)
15. Identify the need for intervention and transport of patients with compensated and decompensated shock. (pp. 86–92)

16. Differentiate among normotensive, hypotensive, and profoundly hypotensive patients. (pp. 86–92)
17. Describe differences in administration of IV fluid in the normotensive, hypotensive, or profoundly hypotensive patients. (pp. 89–91)
18. Discuss the physiological changes associated with application and inflation of the pneumatic antishock garment (PASG). (pp. 91–92)
19. Given several preprogrammed and moulaged hemorrhage and shock patients, provide the appropriate scene assessment, primary assessment, rapid trauma or focused secondary assessment and history, detailed assessment, and ongoing assessment and provide appropriate patient care and transportation. (pp. 65–92)

INTRODUCTION TO HEMORRHAGE AND SHOCK

The loss of the body's most important and dynamic medium, blood, is called **hemorrhage.** Acute and continuing loss of blood robs the body of its ability to provide oxygen and nutrients to and remove carbon dioxide and waste products from the body's elemental building blocks, the cells. In the absence of an adequate volume of circulating blood, the cells and the organs dysfunction and, ultimately, the organism itself dies. The transition between normal function (**homeostasis**) and death is called **shock.** The ability to recognize hemorrhage and shock and the ability to care for them are critical skills for the paramedic and are essential to reducing mortality and morbidity in trauma patients. This chapter provides you with an understanding of the cardiovascular system as it relates to hemorrhage and shock and then describes how to recognize and care for these life-threatening assaults on the human body.

✱ **hemorrhage** an abnormal internal or external discharge of blood.

✱ **homeostasis** the natural tendency of the body to maintain a steady and normal internal environment.

✱ **shock** a state of inadequate tissue perfusion.

The paramedic must be able to recognize hemorrhage and shock in trauma patients in order to reduce mortality and morbidity.

HEMORRHAGE

As noted previously, hemorrhage is loss of blood from the closed vascular system because of injury to the blood vessels. Hemorrhage is usually classified on the basis of the injured vessel from which it flows: capillary, venous, or arterial.

Capillary hemorrhage generally oozes from the wound, normally an abrasion, and clots quickly on its own. The blood is usually bright red because it is well oxygenated.

Venous hemorrhage flows more quickly, though it, too, generally stops in a few minutes. Bleeding associated with venous hemorrhage is generally dark red because the blood has already given up its oxygen as it passed though the capillary beds.

Bleeding associated with arterial hemorrhage flows very rapidly, often spurting from the wound. This blood is well oxygenated and appears bright red as it escapes from the wound. The blood volume lost can be extreme because of the pressure behind arterial bleeding. The spurting nature of arterial hemorrhage results from the variations in the blood pressure driving the blood loss.

While it is convenient to determine the type of hemorrhage, the nature and depth of a wound may make it hard to differentiate between heavy venous and arterial bleeding. Internal hemorrhage cannot be classified by type with the diagnostic techniques available to paramedics providing prehospital care.

CLOTTING

The body's response to local hemorrhage is a complex three-step process called **clotting** (Figure 19-1). As a blood vessel is torn and begins to lose blood, its smooth muscle contracts. This reduces its lumen and the volume and strength of blood flow through it. This is called the **vascular phase.**

At the same time, the vessel's smooth interior lining (the tunica intima) is disrupted, causing a turbulent blood flow. The disturbed blood flow causes frictional damage to the surfaces of the platelets, making them adherent. Platelets then stick to collagen, a protein fibre found in connective tissue, on the vessel's injured inner surface, and to other injured tissue in the area. The blood vessel walls also become adherent. If they are small enough, like capillaries, they may stick together, further occluding blood flow. As platelets adhere to the vessel walls, they **aggregate,** or collect, other platelets. This is the **platelet phase,** the second step of the clotting process. These events occur almost immediately after injury and effectively halt hemorrhage from capillaries and small venous and arterial vessels. While this is a rapid method of hemorrhage control, the resulting clot is unstable.

As time passes, the wound initiates the third and final step of the process, **coagulation.** In this phase, enzymes are released into the bloodstream, initiating a complex sequence of events. These enzymes come from the damaged blood vessel and surrounding tissue (the extrinsic pathway), from the damaged platelets (the intrinsic pathway), or from both. The release of the enzymes triggers a series of chemical reactions that result in the formation of strong protein fibres, or **fibrin.** These fibres entrap red blood cells and form a stronger, more durable clot. This further collection of cells halts all but the most severe hemorrhage. Coagulation normally takes from 7 to 10 minutes. Over time, the cells trapped in the clot protein matrix slowly contract, drawing the wound and the injured vessel together.

The nature of the wound also affects how rapidly and well the clotting mechanisms respond to hemorrhage (Figure 19-2). If the wound lacerates the vessel cleanly in a transverse fashion, the muscles of the vessel wall contract. This retracts the vessel into the tissue, thickening the now shortened tunica media. This thickening further reduces the vessel's lumen, reduces blood flow, and assists the clotting mechanism. If the blood vessel is lacerated longitudinally, rather than transversely, the smooth muscle contraction pulls the vessel open. The vessel does not withdraw,

Content Review

TYPES OF HEMORRHAGE
Capillary
Venous
Arterial

It may be hard to differentiate between heavy venous and arterial bleeding in the field; likewise, paramedics cannot classify internal hemorrhage by type when providing prehospital care.

---

* **clotting** the body's three-step response to stop the loss of blood.

---

* **vascular phase** first step in the clotting process in which smooth blood vessel muscle contracts, reducing the vessel lumen and the flow of blood through it.

Content Review

PHASES OF THE CLOTTING PROCESS
Vascular phase
Platelet phase
Coagulation

---

* **aggregate** to cluster or come together.

---

* **platelet phase** second step in the clotting process in which platelets adhere to blood vessel walls and to each other.

---

* **coagulation** third step in the clotting process, which involves the formation of a protein called fibrin that forms a network around a wound to stop bleeding, ward off infection, and lay a foundation for healing and repair of the wound.

---

* **fibrin** protein fibres that trap red blood cells as part of the clotting process.

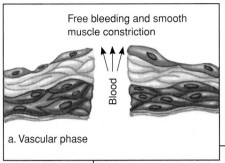

Free bleeding and smooth
muscle constriction

Blood

a. Vascular phase

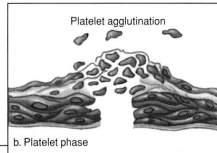

Platelet agglutination

b. Platelet phase

Common pathway

Fibrin

Intrinsic pathway

Extrinsic pathway

Fibrin formation

c. Coagulation phase

FIGURE 19-1   The three steps of the clotting process are the vascular phase, the platelet phase, and coagulation.

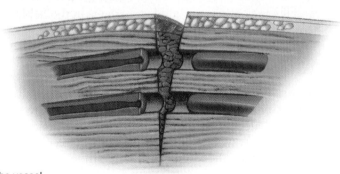

FIGURE 19-2   The type of blood vessel injury often affects the nature of the hemorrhage.

a. A clean lateral cut permits the vessel
to retract and thicken its wall.

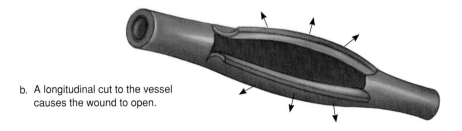

b. A longitudinal cut to the vessel
causes the wound to open.

and the lumen does not constrict. The result is heavy and continued bleeding. Crush trauma often produces this type of damage. The vessels are not torn cleanly and do not withdraw. The actual hemorrhage site is lost in the disrupted tissue, resulting in severe, hard-to-control bleeding from a large wound area.

If a severe hemorrhage continues, frank hypotension reduces the blood pressure at the hemorrhage site. This limits the flow of blood and the dislodging of clots, thus improving the effectiveness of the clotting mechanism.

FACTORS AFFECTING THE CLOTTING PROCESS

The clotting process can be either helped or hindered by a variety of factors. For example, movement at or around the wound site, as in the manipulation of a fracture, may break the developing clot loose and disrupt the forming fibrin strands. For this reason, immediate wound immobilization (splinting) is beneficial.

Aggressive fluid therapy, which is often provided in cases of severe hemorrhage, may adversely change the effectiveness of clotting mechanisms. Aggressive fluid resuscitation may increase blood pressure, which, in turn, increases the pressure pushing against the developing clots. In addition, the water and salts used in fluid therapy dilute the clotting factors, platelets, and red blood cells, further inhibiting the clotting process.

The patient's body temperature also has an effect on the clotting process. As the body temperature begins to fall, as it may in shock states, clot formation is neither as rapid nor as effective as when the body temperature is 37°C (98.6°F). Thus, it is important to keep a patient with severe hemorrhage warm.

Medications may interfere with the body's ability to form a clot and halt both internal and external hemorrhage. Aspirin modifies the enzymes on the surface of platelets that cause them to aggregate after an injury. Ibuprofen and other NSAIDs (nonsteroidal anti-inflammatory drugs) may have a similar but temporary effect. Heparin and warfarin (Coumadin) interfere with the normal generation of protein fibres that produce a stable clot. While these drugs may prevent thrombosis and emboli in patients with heart disease, they may prolong or worsen hemorrhage when that patient is injured. Try to gather information on whether the patient uses such medications when taking the patient history.

HEMORRHAGE CONTROL

Hemorrhage is either internal or external. While there are a number of steps you can take to control external hemorrhage in the field, prehospital care of internal hemorrhage is more limited.

External Hemorrhage

External hemorrhage is easy to identify and care for. It presents with blood oozing, flowing, or spurting from the wound. Bleeding from capillary and venous wounds is easy to halt because the pressure driving it is limited (Figure 19-3). Usually, **direct pressure** on the wound or a combination of direct pressure and elevation work quite well in stopping the bleeding. Bleeding from an arterial wound, however, is powered by the arterial blood pressure, and the blood escapes from the blood vessel with significant force. The normal control and clotting mechanisms help reduce blood loss but do not stop it if the injured vessel is large. To stop bleeding from such a wound, pressure on the bleeding site must exceed the arterial pressure. Direct digital pressure on the site of blood loss, maintained by a dressing and pressure bandage, is most effective. Elevation of the wound area and use of pressure points may also be necessary if the bandage cannot bring about enough pressure directly to the hemorrhage site.

Immediate immobilization (splinting) of the wound site aids the clotting process.

✱ **direct pressure** method of hemorrhage control that relies on the application of pressure to the actual site of the bleeding.

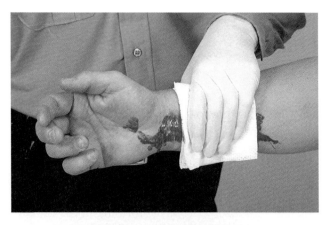

FIGURE 19-3a   Hemorrhage control: Apply direct pressure.

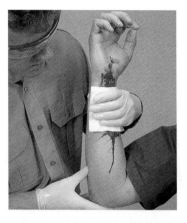

FIGURE 19-3b   Hemorrhage control: Elevate the extremity above the level of the heart.

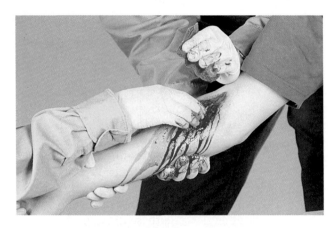

FIGURE 19-3c   Hemorrhage control: If bleeding does not stop, apply direct fingertip pressure.

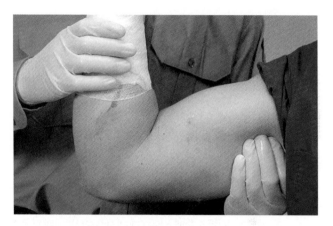

FIGURE 19-3d   Hemorrhage control: If bleeding continues, apply pressure to a pressure point.

Be extremely cautious if you consider using a **tourniquet.** Employ the device *only* to halt persistent, life-threatening hemorrhage. If you apply the tourniquet at a pressure less than the arterial pressure, blood continues to flow into the limb, while the tourniquet restricts venous flow out. The limb's arterial and venous pressures then rise, as does the rate of hemorrhage. If the tourniquet meets its objective and halts all blood flow to the limb, blood loss stops, but so does circulation to the distal extremity. During this absence of perfusion, **lactic acid,** potassium, and other **anaerobic** metabolites accumulate in the stagnant blood. When the tourniquet is released, the resumption of blood flow may transport these toxins into the central circulation with devastating results. Once you apply the tourniquet, therefore, leave it in place until the patient is in the emergency department or some other facility where the negative effects of reperfusion can be addressed. If you must apply a tourniquet, use a wide cravat or belt or a blood pressure cuff (Figure 19-4). A thin or narrow constricting device may damage tissue beneath the tourniquet. Despite these hazards, the tourniquet may be essential in halting life-threatening arterial hemorrhage.

Internal Hemorrhage

Internal hemorrhage is associated with almost all serious blunt and penetrating trauma. As with external hemorrhage, internal hemorrhage can involve capillary, venous, or arterial blood loss. The blood can accumulate in the tissue itself, forming a

＊ **tourniquet** a constrictor used on an extremity to apply circumferential pressure on all arteries to control bleeding.

Use a tourniquet only as a last resort to halt persistent, life-threatening hemorrhage.

＊ **lactic acid** compound produced from pyruvic acid during anaerobic glycolysis.

＊ **anaerobic** able to live without oxygen.

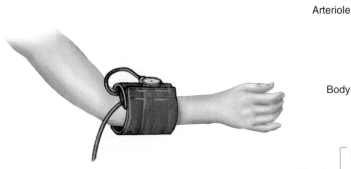

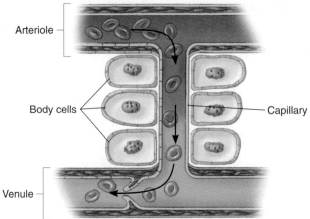

Arteriole

Body cells

Capillary

Venule

a. Blood pressure cuff positioned but not inflated. Normal blood flow.

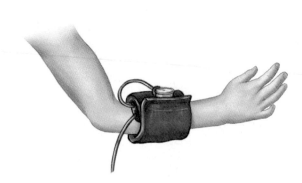

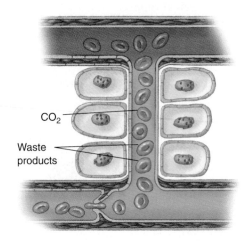

CO_2

Waste products

b. Inflation of BP cuff as a tourniquet cuts off circulation. Blood flow stagnates and metabolic byproducts accumulate.

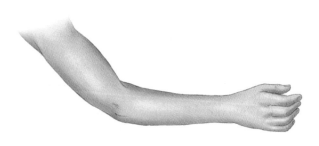

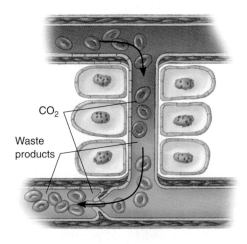

CO_2

Waste products

c. Release of cuff restores circulation. Returning blood flow pushes acidic byproducts back into the central circulation.

FIGURE 19-4   Release of a tourniquet may send accumulated toxins into the central circulation with devastating results for the patient.

visible or hidden contusion, or it can be forced between **fascia** and form a pocket of blood called a **hematoma**. In most of these cases, the hemorrhage is self-limiting because the pressure within the tissue or fascia controls the blood loss. However, large contusions, massive soft-tissue injuries, and large hematomas, especially those affecting large muscle masses, such as the thighs or buttocks, can account for moderate blood and body fluid loss. Fractures of the humerus and tibia/fibula may account for 500 to 750 mL of loss, while femur fractures may account for up to 1500 mL of loss.

In body cavities, such as the chest and the abdominal, pelvic, and retroperitoneal spaces, the resistance to continuing blood loss does not develop. With bleeding in these areas, loss continues unabated until the normal clotting process is effective, the blood pressure drops significantly, or surgical intervention is provided. The best indicators of significant internal hemorrhage are the mechanism of injury (MOI), local signs and symptoms of injury, and the early signs and symptoms of blood loss and shock. If a patient has sustained significant trauma to the chest, abdomen, or pelvis, anticipate significant, continuing, and uncontrolled blood loss. Such a patient requires rapid transport to a trauma centre or hospital for surgical repair of any damaged vessels.

You can assist the natural internal hemorrhage control mechanisms in the extremities by providing a patient with immobilization and elevation. Continued movement of the injury site, especially if it is associated with a long-bone fracture, disrupts the clotting process, causing further soft-tissue, nervous, and vascular damage, and continuing blood loss. If the patient is a victim of serious or multisystem trauma, however, do not spend time on the scene with aggressive skeletal immobilization. Instead, quickly splint the patient to a long spine board and begin transport. Provide splinting of individual limbs, if time permits, during transport.

Internal hemorrhage is often associated with injuries to specific organs and can be related either to trauma or to preexisting medical problems. Internal hemorrhage can also present with external signs of injury or disease in addition to the signs and symptoms of blood loss. These signs can help you identify the nature and location of the blood loss.

The nasal cavity is lined with a rich supply of capillaries to warm and help humidify inspired air. Hypertension, a strong sneeze, or direct trauma may rupture the vessels supplying these capillary beds and produce the moderate to severe hemorrhage called **epistaxis** (Figure 19-5). Prolonged epistaxsis can result in hypovolemia, while blood flowing down the posterior nasal cavity, down the esophagus, and into the stomach may result in nausea, followed by vomiting. Trauma to the oral cavity

* **fascia** a fibrous membrane that covers, supports, and separates muscles and may also unite the skin with underlying tissue.

* **hematoma** collection of blood beneath the skin or trapped within a body compartment.

Provide a patient who has suspected internal bleeding with immobilization and elevation (of extremities) to aid the body's hemorrhage control mechanisms.

* **epistaxis** bleeding from the nose resulting from injury, disease, or environmental factors; a nosebleed.

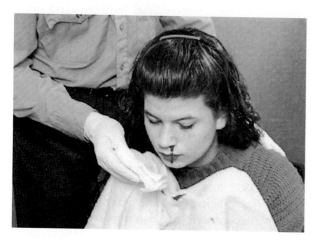

FIGURE 19-5a   To control nosebleed, have the patient sit leaning forward.

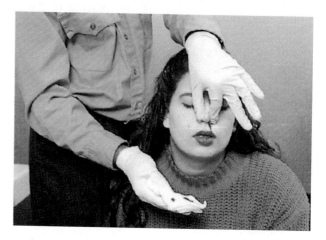

FIGURE 19-5b   Pinch the fleshy part of the patient's nostrils firmly together.

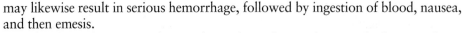

* **esophageal varices** enlarged and tortuous esophageal veins.

* **melena** black, tar-like feces due to gastrointestinal bleeding.

* **anemia** a reduction in the hemoglobin content in the blood to a point below that required to meet the oxygen requirements of the body.

Content Review

STAGES OF HEMORRHAGE

Stage 1—blood loss of up to 15 percent; patient may display some nervousness and marginally cool skin with slight pallor

Stage 2—blood loss of 15 to 25 percent; patient displays thirst, anxiety, restlessness, cool, clammy skin, increased respiratory rate

Stage 3—blood loss between 25 and 35 percent; patient experiences air hunger, dyspnea, severe thirst, anxiety, restlessness; survival unlikely without rapid intervention

Stage 4—blood loss greater than 35 percent; pulse barely palpable, respirations ineffective; patient lethargic, confused, moving toward unresponsiveness; survival unlikely

---

With hemorrhage patients, determine the relative severity of blood loss, the need for aggressive intervention, the length of time since the incident that caused the trauma, the current stage of hemorrhage, and how quickly the patient is moving from one stage to another.

🔑

---

may likewise result in serious hemorrhage, followed by ingestion of blood, nausea, and then emesis.

There are also outward signs that indicate hemorrhage in the lungs and respiratory system. For example, degenerative diseases, such as tuberculosis or cancer, or chest trauma may rupture pulmonary vessels. This leads to the release of blood into the lower airways or alveolar space. The patient may then cough up bright red blood, a sign called hemoptysis.

Trauma, caustic ingestion, degenerative disease (for example, cancer), and rupturing **esophageal varices** may lead to hemorrhage along the esophagus. In these pathologies, blood is likely to travel, via peristalsis, into the stomach, where it collects. Gastric hemorrhage due to ulceration or trauma may also result in the accumulation of blood in the stomach. A significant collection of blood acts as a gastric irritant, inducing vomiting. If the blood is evacuated early, it is bright red in colour. If blood remains in the stomach for some time, emesis resembles coffee grounds in both colour and consistency.

Hemorrhage in the small or large bowel can be associated with trauma, degenerative disease, or diverticulitis (small pouches in the walls of the bowel that collect material, become infected, and may burst). Bowel hemorrhage may present as bleeding from the rectum, or the blood may be digested before release, producing a black and tarry stool called **melena**.

Rectal injury may be caused by pelvic fracture or direct trauma. This presents with bleeding, which may be severe.

Vaginal hemorrhage may be associated with trauma, degenerative disease, menstruation, ectopic pregnancy, placenta previa, and potential or actual miscarriage. Urethral hemorrhage is generally minor and may reflect damage to the prostate or urethra. Blood in the urine reflects bladder injury.

Nontraumatic forms of hemorrhage may be either acute or chronic. Acute hemorrhage moves the victim rapidly toward shock and is quickly recognizable. Chronic hemorrhage is likely to be rather limited in volume, but it does continue over time. The resulting loss depletes the body of red blood cells and leads to **anemia**. This condition reduces the blood's oxygen-carrying capacity, and the patient experiences fatigue and lethargy. Clotting factors may likewise be depleted, which increases the rate of fluid loss and makes any secondary hemorrhage more difficult to control.

STAGES OF HEMORRHAGE

Fluid accounts for about 60 percent of the body's weight and is distributed among the cellular, interstitial, and vascular spaces. The cells contain about 62 percent of the total fluid volume, while the interstitial (nonvascular) space holds 26 percent. Four to five percent of body fluid is found in other spaces, such as the ventricles of the brain and meninges (cerebrospinal fluid). The remaining 7 percent of fluid volume resides in the vascular space. This fluid, called plasma, and the blood cells account for 7 percent of the average adult male's body weight (about 6.5 percent in the female). Fluid in the vascular space is distributed among the heart, arteries, veins, and capillaries and accounts for 5 litres (10 units) of blood volume in the healthy 70-kg adult male.

The effects of hemorrhage can be categorized into four progressive stages as blood volume is lost. These stages relate to the volume of blood lost in acute hemorrhage and that result in "classic" signs and symptoms. Remember, however, that each individual's response to blood loss may vary as may the rate and progress of the loss. Use these categories to help determine the relative severity of the loss and the need for aggressive intervention. It is also important to identify the following: the length of time elapsed since the incident that caused the trauma; the stage of hemorrhage the victim is in when you arrive at her side; and how quickly the patient is moving from one stage to another (Table 19-1).

| Table 19-1 | PATIENT SIGNS ASSOCIATED WITH STAGES OF HEMORRHAGE |

Stage	Blood Loss	Vasoconstriction	Pulse Rate	Pulse (Pressure) Strength	Blood Pressure	Respiratory Rate	Respiratory Volume
1	< 15%	↑	↑	→	→	→	→
2	15–25%	↑↑	↑↑	↓	→	↑	↑
3	25–35%	↑↑↑	↑↑↑	↓↓	↓	↑↑	↓
4	> 35%	↓↓	Variable	↓↓↓	↓↓↓	↓	↓↓

Stage 1 Hemorrhage

Stage 1 hemorrhage is a blood loss of up to 15 percent of the circulating blood volume. In the 70-kg male, that is approximately 500 to 750 mL of blood, about the amount you might donate during a blood drive. The healthy human system can easily compensate for such a blood loss volume by constricting the vascular beds, especially on the venous side. In this stage, the blood pressure remains constant, as do the **pulse pressure**, respiratory rate, and renal output. The central venous pressure may drop slightly, but it returns to normal quickly. The pulse rate elevates slightly, and the patient may display some signs of **catecholamine** (epinephrine and norepinephrine) release, notably nervousness and marginally cool skin with a slight pallor.

✱ **pulse pressure** difference between the systolic and diastolic blood pressures.

Stage 2 Hemorrhage

Stage 2 hemorrhage occurs as 15 to 25 percent (750 to 1250 mL) of the blood volume is lost. The body's first-line compensatory responses can no longer maintain blood pressure, and secondary mechanisms are now employed. Tachycardia becomes clearly evident, and the pulse strength begins to diminish (the pulse pressure is noticeably narrowed). A strong release of catecholamines increases peripheral vascular resistance. This maintains systolic blood pressure but results in peripheral vasoconstriction and cool, clammy skin. Anxiety increases, and the patient may begin to display restlessness and thirst. Thirst occurs as fluid leaves the intracellular and interstitial spaces and the osmotic pressure of the blood changes. Renal output remains normal, but the respiratory rate increases.

✱ **catecholamine** a hormone, such as epinephrine or norepinephrine, that strongly affects the nervous and cardiovascular systems, metabolic rate, temperature, and smooth muscle.

Stage 3 Hemorrhage

Stage 3 hemorrhage occurs when blood loss reaches between 25 and 35 percent of blood volume (1250 to 1750 mL). The body's compensatory mechanisms are unable to cope with the loss, and the classic signs of shock appear. Rapid tachycardia is present as the blood pressure begins to fall. The pulse is barely palpable as the pulse pressure remains very narrow. The patient experiences air hunger and tachypnea. Anxiety, restlessness, and thirst become more severe. The level of responsiveness decreases, and the patient becomes very pale, cool to touch, and diaphoretic. Urinary output declines. Without rapid intervention, this patient's survival is unlikely.

Without rapid intervention, survival of a stage 3 hemorrhage patient is unlikely.

Stage 4 Hemorrhage

Stage 4 hemorrhage occurs with a blood loss of greater than 35 percent of the body's total blood supply. The patient's pulse is barely palpable in the central arteries, if one can be found at all. Respirations are very rapid, shallow, and ineffective. The patient is extremely lethargic and confused, moving rapidly toward unresponsiveness. The skin is very cool, clammy, and extremely pale. Urinary output ceases. Even with aggressive fluid resuscitation and blood transfusions, patient survival is unlikely.

These descriptions of the stages of hemorrhage presume that the patient is a normally healthy adult. Any preexisting condition may affect the volume of blood loss required for movement from one stage to another as well as the speed at which the patient moves through the stages. The patient's state of hydration, from dehydrated to fluid-rich, may also affect how quickly and to what degree compensation takes place.

The rate of the blood loss also has a profound effect on how quickly a patient moves from stage 1 to stage 4. If the blood loss is very rapid, the compensatory mechanisms may not work as effectively. However, a small wound bleeding uncontrollably but very slowly for days may not move the patient from stage 1 to stage 2, even with a loss much greater than 750 mL.

Certain categories of patients—pregnant women, athletes, obese patients, children, and the elderly—react differently to blood loss. The blood volume of a woman in late pregnancy is 50 percent greater than normal. This patient may lose rather large volumes of blood before progressing through the various stages of hemorrhage. Although the mother in this circumstance appears to be somewhat protected from the effects of serious hemorrhage, the fetus is deprived of good circulation early in the blood loss and is more susceptible to harm.

A well-conditioned athlete often has greater fluid and cardiac reserves than a typical patient. This means she may move more slowly through the early stages, with greater percentages of loss needed to advance from one stage to another.

The obese patient, on the other hand, has a blood volume close to 7 percent of ideal body weight but not actual body weight. Thus, the blood volume as a percentage of actual body weight is lower than 7 percent. This means that what appears to be only a small blood loss may have a more serious effect in such a patient.

In infants and young children, blood volumes approximate 8 to 9 percent of body weight, volumes that are proportionally about 20 percent greater than those of adults. However, compensatory mechanisms in infants and children are neither as well developed nor as effective as those in adults. These young patients may not show early signs and symptoms of compensation as clearly as adults. They may instead move quickly into the later stages of shock. Suspect hemorrhage early with child and infant trauma, and treat it aggressively.

The elderly are likewise more adversely affected by blood loss. They have lower volumes of fluid reserves, and their compensatory systems are less responsive to fluid losses. These patients may also be on medications, such as betablockers, that further reduce the body's ability to respond to blood loss and varying blood pressures or on medications, such as aspirin, Coumadin, and heparin, that interfere with the body's natural hemorrhage control system. Often, elderly patients do not experience the tachycardia associated with blood loss, and their blood pressures drop before those of healthy adults. Signs of blood loss and shock may be masked by reduced perceptions of pain in the elderly and by lowered levels of mental acuity due to disease. The elderly also do not tolerate periods of inadequate tissue perfusion well because of chronic cardiovascular inefficiency.

HEMORRHAGE ASSESSMENT

The assessment of various types of trauma patients will be the subject of the next few chapters. In these chapters, only the aspects of assessment that are pertinent to those pathologies will be addressed. Please refer to the patient assessment chapters (Chapter 5, "History Taking"; Chapter 6; "Physical Assessment Techniques"; Chapter 7, "Patient Assessement in the Field"; Chapter 10, "Clinical Decision Making) for a more complete discussion of trauma assessment.

Suspect hemorrhage early in cases of child and infant trauma, and treat it aggressively.

Be aware that signs and symptoms of blood loss in elderly patients may be masked by effects of medications, bodily changes, reduced perception of pain, and the effects of disease.

The assessment of the hemorrhage patient is directed at identifying the source of the hemorrhage and halting any serious and controllable loss of blood. During assessment, you should also examine the circumstances of injury to approximate the volume of blood lost and the rate of past and continuing hemorrhage. This process begins with the scene assessment and continues throughout transport and care.

Scene Assessment

Remember that body substance isolation (BSI) precautions are essential during the assessment of trauma patients. A patient's blood and other body fluids may contain pathogens capable of transmitting HIV, hepatitis, and other diseases to you. Conversely, you may transmit infectious agents to the wounds of the patients you assess and care for. In fact, the risk of your transmitting disease or infection to a patient with open wounds or burns is probably much greater than the risk that she will transmit disease or infection to you. For these reasons, always observe body substance isolation precautions with all trauma patients. These precautions include the use of gloves and a mask when you inspect or palpate any injured area, especially one with open wounds (Figure 19-6). If there is spurting blood, as with arterial hemorrhage, if a patient is combative, or if there is airway trauma with or without bleeding, also wear eye protection and a disposable gown to protect your uniform. Be sure to wash your hands before each ambulance call and do so immediately afterward as well. Scrub vigorously when washing to remove as much of the bacterial load as possible.

If your gloves become contaminated with earth, debris, blood, or body fluids while caring for a patient, change them immediately. If you will be assessing or treating multiple patients, consider double gloving. This means that you put on two or more sets of gloves and remove a set each time you complete assessment of one patient and move on to the next. Place any contaminated gloves, clothing, dressings, or other materials in a biohazard bag, and ensure proper disposal.

The handling of needles presents special problems for prehospital personnel. Once a needle is used, it carries the potential of introducing a patient's blood directly

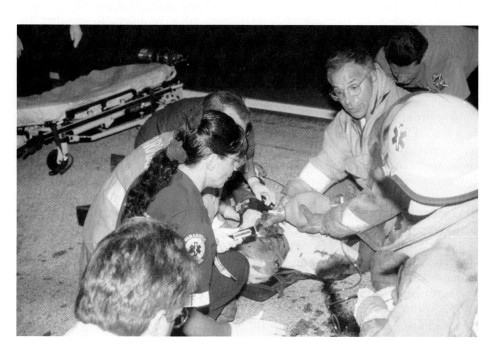

FIGURE 19-6   When caring for a hemorrhaging patient, employ appropriate body substance isolation procedures.

into a caregiver's or bystander's tissues. This greatly increases the likelihood of disease transmission. When dealing with needles, always ensure that they are not recapped but, rather, placed in a properly marked and secure, puncture-resistant sharps container. Should you be pricked by a needle, continue your care, but document the incident immediately on arrival at the emergency department. Wash and cover the wound, then report the incident to your service's infection control officer or other designated officer. There are several prophylactic regimes available that may protect against the transmission of some infectious diseases. Guard against some diseases, such as hepatitis, by obtaining immunizations before you begin your career as a care provider.

Patients may see your gloves and then feel uncomfortable about being treated by someone who is "afraid to touch them." Assure those patients that the gloves and other precautions are for their protection as well as yours.

When appropriate BSI precautions have been taken, continue with the scene assessment. Evaluate the mechanism of injury to anticipate sites of both external and internal hemorrhage. Anticipating external hemorrhage sites focuses your subsequent assessment and care, while anticipating internal hemorrhage affects your decision on whether to provide rapid transport.

When evaluating the mechanism of injury (MOI), also attempt to determine the amount of time that has elapsed between the injury and your evaluation of it. Knowing the length of this time period is very important in determining the amount and rate of blood loss. For example, if you arrive on a scene three minutes after an accident and find a patient losing 150 mL of blood per minute, you can estimate that 450 mL of blood have been lost. You would not expect the patient to display the signs and symptoms of stage 1 hemorrhage. If, however, you arrive 10 minutes after the incident, the same patient, losing blood at the same rate, will have lost 1500 mL of blood and is likely to have reached stage 3. In both cases, the patient is suffering serious, life-threatening hemorrhage. Good assessment and recognition ensures provision of a proper course of care. However, the earlier you arrive at the patient's side, the harder it is to identify serious hemorrhage. For this reason, you must be aware of and appreciate the progressive effects of blood loss and use both the MOI analysis and the time since an incident to increase your suspicions of a problem. Remember, the sooner the signs of later stages of hemorrhage appear, the greater are the rate and volume of blood loss.

The sooner the signs of the later stages of hemorrhage appear, the greater are the rate and volume of blood loss.

Primary Assessment

As you begin the primary assessment, form a general impression of the patient. Be especially alert for any signs and symptoms of internal hemorrhage. These early signs are very subtle and may go unnoticed unless you deliberately look for them. Correct any immediate life threats and provide in-line stabilization if you suspect spinal injury. Assess the patient's initial mental status to determine alertness, orientation, and responsiveness. Be alert for any signs of anxiety, confusion, or combativeness. Any central nervous system deficit may be secondary to hemorrhage, and so be suspicious.

Assess both airway and breathing carefully, noting any tachypnea or air hunger. Administer oxygen via nonrebreather mask at a rate of 15 L/minute. When assessing circulation, pay special attention to the pulse strength (the pulse pressure) and rate. Remember that the pulse pressure narrows well before the systolic pressure begins to drop. The pulse rate, too, may suggest developing shock. A fast—and especially a fast and weak (thready)—pulse may be the first noticeable sign of serious internal blood loss. Note also skin colour and condition. Pale or mottled skin is an early sign of shock, while cool and clammy skin is also an indicator of potential blood loss and shock.

Complete the primary assessment by establishing patient priorities. Decide, on the basis of your findings to this point, whether the patient is to receive a rapid trauma assessment or a focused history and secondary assessment. If any indication, mechanism of injury, sign, or symptom suggests serious internal hemorrhage or uncontrolled external hemorrhage, consider the rapid trauma assessment and then immediate transport of the patient.

Focused History and Secondary Assessment

Your primary assessment findings and the evaluation of the mechanism of injury determine how you will proceed with the focused history and secondary assessment. For trauma patients who have a significant MOI, continue spinal immobilization, and perform a rapid trauma assessment. Then obtain baseline vital signs and a patient history.

For trauma patients who have no significant mechanism of injury and who have revealed no critical findings during primary assessment, perform an assessment focused on the area of injury, then obtain baseline vital signs and a patient history. Finally, provide care as appropriate and transport.

With both types of trauma patients, perform ongoing assessments during transport. If time and the patient's condition permit, you may also perform a detailed secondary assessment. However, you should never delay transport to perform the detailed secondary assessment.

Rapid Trauma Assessment For trauma patients with a significant MOI, you will perform a rapid trauma assessment, inspecting and palpating the patient in an orderly fashion from head to toe. Pay particular attention to areas where critical trauma has occurred and areas where the MOI suggests forces were focused.

Carefully and quickly observe the head for serious bleeding. Internal head injury rarely accounts for the classic signs of shock. However, the scalp bleeds profusely because the vessels there are large and lack the ability to constrict as well as other peripheral vessels. If any external bleeding appears serious, halt it immediately.

Next, examine the neck. The carotid arteries and jugular veins are located close to the skin's surface. Injury to them can produce rapid and fatal exsanguination. An added danger is the aspiration of air directly into an open jugular vein. At times, venous pressure, due to deep inspiration, can be less than atmospheric pressure. Air may then be drawn into the vein, travelling to the heart and forming emboli, which then lodge in the pulmonary circulation. Quickly control any serious hemorrhage from neck wounds with sterile occlusive dressings. If spinal injury is suspected, apply a rigid cervical collar when assessment of the neck is complete, but maintain in-line manual immobilization until the patient is immobilized to a spine board.

Visually sweep the chest and abdomen for any serious external hemorrhage, though such bleeding is infrequent there. You are more likely to note signs of blunt or penetrating trauma, suggesting internal injury and hemorrhage within. Look to the abdomen for signs of soft-tissue injury, contusions, abrasions, rigidity, and guarding and tenderness that suggest internal injury.

Quickly examine the pelvic and groin region. Test the integrity of the pelvic ring by pressing gently on the iliac crest. Remember that pelvic fracture can account for blood loss of more than 2000 mL. Lacerations to the male genitalia may also account for serious external hemorrhage.

Assess the extremities and rule out fractures of the femur, tibia/fibula, or humerus. Keep in mind that femur fracture can account for up to 1500 mL of blood loss, while each tibia/fibula or humerus fracture may contribute an additional 500 to 750 mL of blood loss. Hematomas and large contusions may account for up to 500 mL of blood loss in the larger muscle masses. Quickly check

Content Review

INJURIES THAT CAN CAUSE SIGNIFICANT BLOOD LOSS
Fractured pelvis (2000 mL)
Fractured femur (1500 mL)
Fractured tibia (750 mL)
Fractured humerus (750 mL)
Large contusion (500 mL)

SIGNS AND SYMPTOMS OF INTERNAL HEMORRHAGE

Early
Pain, tenderness, swelling, or discoloration of suspected injury site
Bleeding from mouth, rectum, vagina, or other orifice
Vomiting of bright red blood
Tender, rigid and/or distended abdomen

Late
Anxiety, restlessness, combativeness, or altered mental status
Weakness, faintness, or dizziness
Vomiting of blood the colour of dark coffee grounds
Thirst
Melena
Shallow, rapid breathing
Rapid, weak pulse
Pale, cool, clammy skin
Capillary refill greater than two seconds (most reliable in infants and children under six)
Dropping blood pressure
Dilated pupils sluggish in responding to light
Nausea and vomiting

✱ **hematochezia** passage of stools containing red blood.

✱ **orthostatic hypotension** a decrease in blood pressure that occurs when a person moves from a supine to a sitting or upright position.

✱ **tilt test** drop in the systolic blood pressure of 20 mmHg or an increase in the pulse rate of 20 beats per minute when a patient is moved from a supine to a sitting position; a finding suggestive of a relative hypovolemia.

distal pulse strength and muscle tone in the extremities, comparing findings in the opposing extremities.

Finally, visually sweep the body, including the posterior, for any external hemorrhage that may have gone unnoticed in your examination to this point.

At the end of the rapid trauma assessment, assess the patient's vital signs, obtain a patient history if possible, and inventory the injuries that may contribute to shock. Provide rapid transport for any patient with a MOI or physical findings that meet trauma triage criteria (see Chapter 16, "Trauma and Trauma Systems"). Any patient with injuries likely to induce hemorrhage at the level of stage 2 or greater should likewise receive immediate transport. If travel time to the trauma centre will exceed 20 minutes, consider requesting air medical transport. Be sure to record the results of your assessment carefully. Compare this information with signs and symptoms you discover during the ongoing assessment to identify trends in the patient's condition.

Perform a detailed secondary assessment only when all immediate life threats have been addressed. Normally, this would be when you are en route to the hospital or trauma centre or when transport has been delayed for some reason.

Focused Secondary Assessment Employ the focused trauma assessment for patients without a significant MOI, for example, a patient who has lacerated her finger with a knife. In such cases, the hemorrhage can be controlled on the scene, and the MOI does not suggest additional problems. With such patients, focus your exam on the area injured, inspecting and palpating the area thoroughly, looking for additional injuries beyond the one that prompted the call. Control the hemorrhage, if you have not already done so. Obtain baseline vital signs and a patient history, and prepare and transport the patient.

In some cases, you may want to perform a rapid trauma assessment, even though the patient does not have a significant MOI. This would be the case, for example, if you suspect the patient has more injuries than she has complained of or if her condition suddenly begins to deteriorate. With such patients, it may be necessary to perform a rapid head-to-toe examination, inspecting and palpating all body regions.

Additional Assessment Considerations In the trauma patient with a significant MOI or the medical patient showing signs and symptoms of blood loss and shock, it is important to search for evidence of internal hemorrhage. This evidence may be in the form of blood, or material suggestive of blood, flowing from the body orifices. Bright red blood from the mouth, nose, rectum, or other orifice suggests direct bleeding. The vomiting of material that looks like coffee grounds is associated with partially digested blood in the stomach, suggestive of a long-term and slow hemorrhage. A black, tarry stool called melena suggests blood has remained in the bowel for some time. **Hematochezia** is the passage of stool containing frank blood in it and reflects active bleeding in the colon or rectum.

In the patient with nonspecific complaints—general ill feeling, anxiousness, restlessness—or a lowered level of responsiveness, suspect and look for other signs of internal hemorrhage. Watch for an increasing pulse rate, rising diastolic blood pressure (narrowing blood pressure), and cool and clammy skin.

Also observe for dizziness or syncope when the patient moves from a supine to a sitting or standing position. This condition is called **orthostatic hypotension** and is suggestive of a volume loss, possibly attributable to internal hemorrhage. This phenomenon is the basis of the **tilt test,** which can be employed to determine blood or fluid loss and the body's reduced ability to compensate for normal positional change. Perform this test only on patients who do not already display signs and symptoms of shock. Prepare for the test by obtaining blood pressure and pulse rates from the patient in a supine or seated position. Then have the supine patient move to a seated position or the seated patient stand up and obtain another set of blood pressure and pulse rates. If the systolic blood pressure drops more than 20 mmHg or the pulse rate rises more than 20 beats per minute, the test is considered positive, indicating hypovolemia.

Ongoing Assessment

Once you have rendered all appropriate life-saving care, perform ongoing assessments frequently—at least every five minutes with unstable patients and every 15 minutes with stable ones. Reevaluate your general impression, reassess the patient's mental status, airway, breathing, and circulation, and obtain additional sets of vital signs. Compare each set of findings with earlier ones to determine if the patient's condition is stable, deteriorating, or improving. Pay special attention to the pulse pressure because it is a clear indicator of the body's efforts to compensate for hypovolemia. Also pay particular attention to changes in mental status, noting any increasing anxiety or restlessness.

HEMORRHAGE MANAGEMENT

The management of hemorrhage is an integral part of care for the trauma patient, one that begins during the primary assessment and is shaped by findings of the rapid trauma assessment or the focused secondary assessment.

First, ensure that the airway is patent, that the patient is breathing adequately, and that you have administered high-flow oxygen. If you have not, establish and maintain the airway, and provide the necessary ventilatory support. If you are ACP or CCP certified, be prepared to provide endotracheal intubation if necessary to secure the airway.

Ensure that the patient has a pulse. If not, initiate cardiopulmonary resuscitation (CPR), attach a monitor-defibrillator, and employ advanced cardiac life support measures. Rule out pericardial tamponade and tension pneumothorax as possible causes of cardiac dysfunction. Understand that cardiac arrest in trauma cases due to hypovolemia carries an extremely poor prognosis. When resources are scarce, your efforts may be better utilized caring for other salvageable patients.

During the primary assessment, care for serious (arterial and heavy venous) hemorrhage only after any airway and breathing problems are corrected. Quickly apply a pressure dressing held in place by self-adherent bandage material or a firmly tied cravat. Return to provide better hemorrhage control after you complete the primary and rapid trauma assessments, and set priorities for care of the hemorrhages and other trauma you discover. If the patient displays early signs of shock, consider applying a PASG (pneumatic antishock garment) and initiating fluid therapy; do not, however, delay transport in order to carry out these measures. This must be performed only by a certified ACP or CCP under strict protocols and procedures.

During the initial assessment, care for serious hemorrhage only after any airway and breathing problems are corrected.

Once you have completed the focused history and secondary assessment stage of assessment, begin caring for injuries, including hemorrhage, as you have prioritized them. As you work down your injury priority list and come to a wound, inspect the site to identify the type and exact location of bleeding. This helps you apply pressure—either digitally or with dressings and bandages—most effectively to halt the blood flow. With cases of external hemorrhage, it is important to identify the exact source and type of bleeding and to be sure to look at the wound site.

Document your findings on the prehospital care report. If you document and convey this information clearly to the emergency department staff, you will reduce the need for others to open the wound (thus disrupting the clotting process) to determine and describe its nature.

Direct pressure usually controls all but the most persistent hemorrhage (Figure 19-7). Although systolic blood pressure drives arterial hemorrhage, you can

Direct pressure usually controls all but the most persistent hemorrhage.

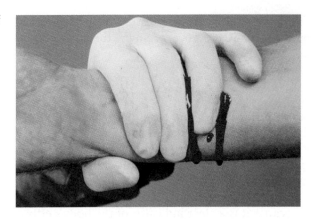

FIGURE 19-7 In most cases of moderate to severe external hemorrhage, direct pressure, maintained by a bandage and dressing, will control bleeding.

stop such a hemorrhage with simple finger pressure properly applied to the source of the bleeding. If a wound looks as though it may pose a problem, insert a wad of dressing material over the site of the heaviest bleeding and apply a bandage over the dressing. This focuses pressure on the site and away from the surrounding area. If bleeding saturates the dressing, cover it with another dressing, and apply another bandage to keep pressure on the wound. Removing the soaked bandage and dressing disrupts the clotting process and prolongs the hemorrhage. If, however, the wound continues to bleed through your layers of dressings and bandages, consider removing the dressing materials you have applied, directly visualizing the exact site of bleeding, and then reapplying a wad of dressing and firm direct pressure to the precise hemorrhage site.

If direct pressure alone does not halt the blood flow to an extremity, consider elevation. Elevation reduces the systolic blood pressure because the heart has to push the blood against gravity and up the limb. Employ elevation only when there is an isolated bleeding wound on a limb and movement will not aggravate any other injuries.

If bleeding still persists, find an arterial pulse point proximal to the wound, and apply firm pressure there (Figure 19-8). This further reduces the blood pressure within the limb and should reduce the hemorrhaging.

Other techniques that can aid in hemorrhage control include limb splinting and the use of pneumatic splints. Splinting helps maintain the stability of the wound site, thus assisting the mechanisms by which clots develop. Splinting may also protect the site from injuries that might occur if the patient is jostled during extrication and transport or as you assess and care for other wounds. Pneumatic splints can also prevent movement of an injured limb. They may also be helpful in holding dressings in place and in applying direct pressure to a limb circumferentially.

Consider using a tourniquet only as a last resort when hemorrhage is prolonged and persistent. As mentioned earlier, there are hazards associated with tourniquet use. Apply a blood pressure cuff just proximal to the hemorrhage site and inflate it to apply a pressure about 30 mmHg greater than the systolic blood pressure. Ensure there is no continued bleeding after you apply the tourniquet, and mark the patient's forehead with the letters "TQ" and the time of application.

Specific Wound Considerations

There are several types of wounds that require special attention for hemorrhage control. They include head wounds, neck wounds, large gaping wounds, and crush injuries.

Head injuries raise some special concerns regarding hemorrhage control. Head wounds may be associated with both severe hemorrhage and the loss of

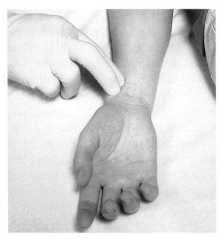

a. Radial artery for hand

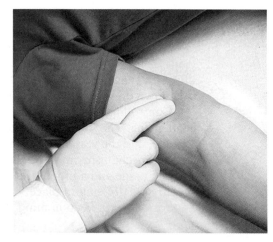

b. Brachial artery for forearm

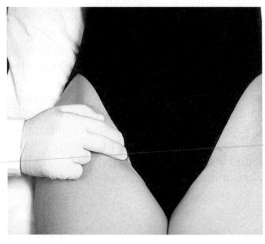

c. Femoral artery for thigh

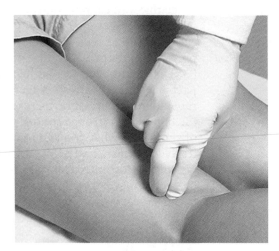

d. Popliteal artery for leg and foot

FIGURE 19-8   Common pressure points for hemorrhage control.

skull integrity (fracture). Control bleeding with such wounds very carefully, using gentle direct pressure around the wound site and against the stable skull. Fluid drainage from the ears and nose may be secondary to skull fracture. Cerebrospinal fluid, as it escapes the cranial vault, relieves the building intracranial pressure. Halting the flow of fluid would end this relief mechanism and compound the increase in pressure. In addition, stopping the flow may provide a pathway for pathogens to enter the meninges and cause serious infection (meningitis). Cerebrospinal fluid quickly regenerates as the injury heals. Thus, if there is hemorrhage from either the nose or ear canal, simply cover the area with a soft, porous dressing, and bandage it loosely.

Neck wounds carry the risk of air being drawn into the venous circulation with life-threatening results. Cover any open neck wound with an occlusive dressing held firmly in place. Do not employ circumferential bandages to create direct pressure with neck wounds. Digital pressure controls most, if not all, neck bleeding. It may, however, be necessary to apply and maintain this manual pressure continuously during the patient's prehospital care.

With head injury patients, do not attempt to stop the flow of blood or fluid from the nose or ear canal, but cover the area with porous dressing to collect the material, and bandage loosely.

Cover any open neck wound with an occlusive dressing held firmly in place.

Gaping wounds often present hemorrhage control problems. With such wounds, bleeding originates from many sites and the open nature of these wounds prevents application of uniform direct pressure. To manage bleeding from such a wound, create a mass of dressing material approximating the volume and shape of the wound. Place the material with the sterile, nonadherent side down on the wound and bandage it firmly in place.

Controlling hemorrhage associated with crush injuries can be particularly challenging. The source of hemorrhage in such cases is frequently difficult to determine, and the vessels are damaged in such a way that the normal hemorrhage control mechanisms may be ineffective. Place a dressing around and over the crushed tissue and a blood pressure cuff over that, and inflate to apply pressure, holding the dressing in place. If bleeding is heavy and persistent, consider using a tourniquet, but keep in mind the precautions discussed previously.

Transport Considerations

Consider rapid transport for any patient who experiences serious external hemorrhage that you cannot control and for any patient with suspected serious internal hemorrhage.

Consider rapid transport for any patient who experiences serious external hemorrhage that you cannot control and for any patient with suspected serious internal hemorrhage. Be vigilant for any signs of compensation for blood loss and for the early signs of shock. Monitor your patient's mental status, pulse rate, and blood pressure (for narrowing pulse pressure). When in doubt, transport immediately.

Understand that serious hemorrhage can have a significant psychological impact on patients. Stress triggers the "fight-or-flight" response, increases heart rate and blood pressure, increases the body's metabolic demands, works against the body's hemorrhage control mechanisms, and contributes to the development of shock. Do what you can to ease the anxieties of such patients. Communicate freely with them, and explain what care measures you are taking and why. Be especially alert to their comfort needs, and address them as appropriate. If possible, keep these patients from seeing their injuries or the serious injuries affecting friends and other accident victims.

SHOCK

Shock is the underlying killer of all trauma patients and often presents with only subtle signs and symptoms.

A simple medical definition of shock is "a state of inadequate tissue perfusion." Beyond that simple definition, however, shock is the transitional stage between normal life, called homeostasis, and death. It is the underlying killer of all trauma patients and often presents with only subtle signs and symptoms until the body can no longer compensate. Then the victim moves quickly, and often irreversibly, toward death. Because of this, you, as a paramedic, must understand the process of shock and recognize its earliest signs and symptoms.

Cells are the microscopic building blocks of the human body. When cells cease to function—and if the process is not reversed—the result is cell death, which leads to tissue death, then to organ failure, and ultimately to the death of the organism. In order for cells to function, they must be continually perfused by blood, carried through the capillaries, in order to receive a constant supply of oxygen and other nutrients and to eliminate waste products.

Shock is a tissue perfusion problem affecting the individual body cells. There are many causes of shock, though all are commonly manifested by signs and symptoms of cardiovascular system compensation, followed by decompensation and, ultimately, collapse. The best way to understand shock and how body systems compensate for it is to look at the cell and its functions and then to examine how the body provides for the cells' metabolic needs and how this process can fail. Normal cell **metabolism** is discussed in Chapter 12, while the pathophysiology of shock is discussed in Chapter 13.

✱ **metabolism** the total changes that take place in an organism during physiological processes.

THE BODY'S RESPONSE TO BLOOD LOSS

The sympathetic nervous system and the hormones it releases begin progressive responses as hemorrhage causes blood to leave the cardiovascular system. As the draw-down of the vascular volume reaches the heart, the right atrium does not completely fill. This means the atrium's output does not engorge the ventricle. Cardiac contractility therefore suffers as the ventricular myocardium does not stretch. The stroke volume drops, and there is an immediate drop in the systolic blood pressure. This decreased pressure reduces the cardiovascular system's ability to drive blood through the capillary beds. The baroreceptors in the neck recognize this decrease in blood pressure and signal to the medulla oblongata. The vasomotor centre increases the peripheral vascular resistance and increases venous tone, while the cardioacceleratory centre increases heart rate and contractile strength. With the reduced venous capacitance and a slight increase in heart rate and peripheral vascular resistance, the blood pressure returns to normal, as does tissue perfusion. These actions normally compensate for small blood losses. If the blood loss stops, the body reconstitutes the blood from the interstitial fluid and replaces the lost red blood cells gradually, without noticeable or ill effects.

Cellular Ischemia

If blood loss continues, the venous system constricts to its limits in order to maintain cardiac preload. However, it becomes more and more difficult for the venous system to compensate because its limited musculature begins to tire. Peripheral vascular resistance also continues to increase to maintain the systolic blood pressure. As it does, the diastolic blood pressure rises, the pulse pressure narrows, and the pulse weakens. The constriction of arterioles means that less and less blood is directed to the noncritical organs, and those organs' supply of oxygen is reduced. The skin, the largest of the noncritical organs, receives reduced circulation and becomes cool, pale, and moist. If the hemorrhage continues, some noncritical organ cells begin to starve for oxygen. Anaerobic metabolism is their only energy source, and carbon dioxide and lactic and other acids begin to accumulate. Cellular hypoxia begins, followed by **ischemia.** The heart rate increases but only slowly because the other compensatory mechanisms are still effectively maintaining preload.

* **ischemia** a blockage in the delivery of oxygenated blood to the cells.

As the blood loss increases, more and more body cells are deprived of their oxygen and nutrient supplies, and more and more waste products accumulate. The bloodstream becomes acidic, and the body's chemoreceptors stimulate an increase in depth and rate of respirations. Circulating catecholamines and increasing acidosis cause alterations in the level of orientation, and the patient becomes anxious, restless, and possibly combative. Ischemia now affects not only noncritical organs but also the arterioles. These vessels, which also require oxygen, become hypoxic and begin to fatigue. Meanwhile, the coronary arteries are providing a decreasing amount of oxygenated blood to the labouring heart.

If the blood loss stops, the blood draws fluid from within the interstitial space, at a rate of up to one litre per hour, to restore its volume, and erythropoietin accelerates the production of red blood cells. The kidneys reduce urine output to conserve water and electrolytes, and a period of thirst provides the stimulus for the patient to drink liquids and replace the lost volume on a more permanent basis. Transfusion with whole blood may be required at this point. While some signs of circulatory compromise and fatigue are present, the patient's recovery is probable with a period of rest.

Capillary Microcirculation

If blood loss continues, sympathetic stimulation and reduced perfusion to the kidneys, pancreas, and liver cause release of hormones. Angiotensin II further increases peripheral vascular resistance and reduces the blood flow to more of the body's tissues. If the blood loss continues, circulation is further limited to only those organs most critical to life. This further decrease in circulation leads to an increase in cellular hypoxia in noncritical tissues, and more cells begin to use anaerobic metabolism for energy in a desperate attempt to survive. The buildup of lactic acid and carbon dioxide relaxes the precapillary sphincters. The circulating blood volume is diminished both by the continued hemorrhage and by fluid loss as the capillary beds engorge. Postcapillary sphincters remain closed, forcing fluids into the interstitial spaces by **hydrostatic pressure.** The circulatory crisis worsens as the compensatory mechanisms begin to fail. Interstitial edema reduces the ability of the capillaries to provide oxygen and nutrients to and remove carbon dioxide and other waste products from the cells. The capillary and cell membranes also begin to break down. Red blood cells begin to clump together, or agglutinate, in the hypoxic and stagnant capillaries forming columns of coagulated cells called **rouleaux.**

* **hydrostatic pressure** the pressure of liquids in equilibrium; the pressure exerted by or within liquids.

* **rouleaux** group of red blood cells that are stuck together.

Capillary Washout

The building acidosis from the accumulating lactic acid and carbon dioxide (carbonic acid) finally causes relaxation of the postcapillary sphincters. With relaxation, those byproducts along with potassium (released by the cells to maintain a neutral environment in the presence of building acidosis) and the columns of coagulated red blood cells are dumped into the venous circulation. This **washout** causes profound metabolic acidosis and releases microscopic emboli. Cardiac output drops toward zero; peripheral vascular resistance drops toward zero; blood pressure drops toward zero; cellular perfusion, even to the most critical organs, drops toward zero. The body moves quickly and then irreversibly toward death.

* **washout** release of accumulated lactic acid, carbon dioxide (carbonic acid), potassium, and rouleaux into the venous circulation.

STAGES OF SHOCK

The shock process, as described above, can be divided into three stages based on presenting signs and symptoms. The stages are progressively more serious and include compensated, decompensated, and irreversible shock (Table 19-2).

Compensated Shock

Compensated shock is the initial shock state. In this stage, the body is still capable of meeting its critical metabolic needs through a series of progressive compensating actions (Figure 19-9). These progressive compensations create a series of signs and symptoms that range from the subtle to the obvious. The compensated shock stage ends with the precipitous drop in blood pressure. Compensated shock is the shock stage in which prehospital interventions and rapid transport are most likely to meet with success.

The body's first recognizable response to serious blood loss is probably an increase in pulse rate. However, a rate increase due to blood loss may be difficult to differentiate from tachycardia due to excitement and the "fight-or-flight" response. The first sign usually attributable to shock is a narrowing pulse pressure and weakening pulse strength (weak and rapid pulse). As the condition becomes more serious, vasoconstriction causes the victim's skin to become pale, cyanotic, or ashen as blood is directed away from the skin and toward the more critical organs. The skin becomes cool and moist (clammy), and capillary refill times begin to exceed three

* **compensated shock** hemodynamic insult to the body in which the body responds effectively. Signs and symptoms are limited, and the human system functions normally.

Compensated shock is the shock stage in which prehospital interventions and rapid transport are most likely to meet with success.

Content Review

STAGES OF SHOCK
Compensated
Decompensated
Irreversible

Table 19-2   THE STAGES OF SHOCK

Compensated Shock

Initial stage of shock in which the body progressively compensates for continuing blood loss.

- Pulse rate increases
- Pulse strength decreases
- Skin becomes cool and clammy
- Progressing anxiety, restlessness, combativeness
- Thirst, weakness, eventual air hunger

Decompensated Shock

Begins when the body's compensatory mechanisms can no longer maintain preload.

- Pulse becomes unpalpable
- Blood pressure drops precipitously
- Patient becomes unconscious
- Respirations slow or cease

Irreversible Shock

Shortly after the patient enters decompensated shock, the lack of circulation begins to have profound effects on body cells. As they are irreversibly damaged, the cells die, tissues dysfunction, organs dysfunction, and the patient dies.

seconds. As compensation becomes more acute, the victim becomes anxious, restless, or combative and complains of thirst and weakness. Near the end of the compensated shock stage, the patient may experience air hunger and tachypnea.

Decompensated Shock

Decompensated shock begins as the body's compensatory mechanisms can no longer respond to a continuing blood loss. Mechanisms that initially compensated for blood loss now fail, and the body moves quickly toward complete

✱ **decompensated shock** continuing hemodynamic insult to the body in which the compensatory mechanisms break down. The signs and symptoms become very pronounced, and the patient moves rapidly toward death.

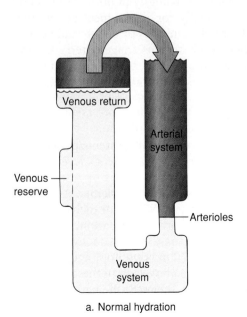
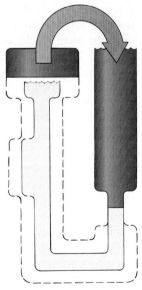

a. Normal hydration

b. Hypovolemia and venous compensation

FIGURE 19-9   In compensated shock, the body reduces venous capacitance in response to blood loss.

collapse. Entry into decompensated shock is indicated by a precipitous drop in systolic blood pressure. Despite all compensatory mechanisms, venous return is inadequate, and the heart no longer has enough blood volume to pump. Even extreme tachycardia produces little cardiac output. No amount of vascular resistance can maintain blood pressure and circulation. Even the most critical organs of the body are hypoperfused. The heart, already hypoxic because of poor perfusion and the increased oxygen demands created by tachycardia, begins to fail. This state may be indicated by the presence of a bradycardia. In this stage, the brain is extremely hypoxic. This means that the patient displays a rapidly dropping level of responsiveness. The brain's control over bodily functions, including respiration, ceases, and the body takes on a death-like appearance.

Irreversible Shock

Irreversible shock exists when the body's cells are badly injured and die in such quantities that the organs cannot carry out their normal functions. While aggressive resuscitation may restore blood pressure and pulse, organ failure ultimately results in organism failure. The transition to irreversible shock is very difficult to identify in the field. Clearly, the longer a patient is in decompensated shock, the more likely it is that she has moved to irreversible shock.

SHOCK ASSESSMENT

You must be able to recognize shock as early as possible in your patient assessment and begin to provide care just as promptly. You must search out the signs and symptoms of shock in each phase of the assessment process: the scene assessment, the primary assessment, the rapid trauma assessment or focused history and secondary assessment, and—when appropriate—the detailed secondary assessment. Further, you must carefully monitor for the development or progression of shock with frequent ongoing assessments during care and transport of the trauma patient.

Scene Assessment

Anticipate shock during the scene assessment. Analyze the forces that caused the trauma and their impacts on your patient for the possibility of both external and internal injuries and hemorrhage. Look especially for injury mechanisms that might result in internal chest, abdominal, or pelvic injuries or in external hemorrhage from the head, neck, and extremities. Apply trauma triage criteria as early as practical to identify the patients who are most likely to require immediate transport to the trauma centre and access to air medical transport if appropriate.

Primary Assessment

The primary assessment directs your attention to the body systems/patient priorities that present the early signs of shock. Determine the patient's level of consciousness, responsiveness, and orientation. Any mental deficit or restlessness, anxiety, or combativeness may be due to blood loss and hypovolemia. As you assess the airway and breathing, apply high-flow oxygen. Watch for tachypnea and air hunger, which are late signs of shock. When assessing circulation, recall that tachycardia suggests hypovolemia. Baseline rates suggestive of tachycardia are about 160 in the infant, 140 in the preschooler, 120 in the school-age child and 100 in the adult. An increase of 20 beats per minute above any of these rates suggests a significant blood loss. The weaker the pulse, the more the patient is compensating for blood loss.

Carefully observe the patient's body surface, and be quick to anticipate potential shock, either as a cause of or a contributing factor to the patient's condition. Look also to the general condition of the skin. It should be warm, pink, and dry. If it is cyanotic, grey, ashen, pale, and cool and moist (clammy), suspect peripheral vasoconstriction, an early sign of shock.

Watch the pulse oximeter for the saturation value, and keep it above 95 percent if possible. As compensation increases and the pulse strength diminishes, the pulse oximeter readings will become more and more unreliable. If you note erratic or intermittent readings on the device, suspect increasing cardiovascular compensation and progressing shock as the reason.

Conclude the primary assessment by establishing patient priorities. If any indication, MOI, sign, or symptom suggests serious internal hemorrhage or uncontrolled external hemorrhage, consider rapid trauma assessment. If the patient has minor and isolated injuries, move to the focused history and secondary assessment.

Focused History and Secondary Assessment

As noted earlier, the order in which the steps of the focused history and secondary assessment are performed vary with the patient's MOI. For trauma patients who have no significant mechanism, perform an assessment focused on the area of injury, obtain baseline vital signs, and gather a patient history. For trauma patients who have a significant MOI, continue spinal immobilization, perform a rapid trauma assessment, and then obtain baseline vital signs and a patient history. Remember that trauma patients with significant mechanisms of injury are the most likely to suffer from shock.

The rapid trauma assessment is performed on a patient with a significant MOI or signs of shock or serious injury.

Rapid Trauma Assessment When you have a trauma patient with a significant MOI, perform a rapid trauma assessment, inspecting and palpating the patient from head to toe (Figure 19-10). Immediately control any significant hemorrhage. Put a dressing and bandage over the wound, and apply direct pressure. Provide more complete hemorrhage control once you attend to the other priorities.

The focused secondary assessment is performed on a trauma patient with an expected, isolated, nonserious injury.

Be sure to examine areas of the body where you expect to find serious injury, as suggested by your scene assessment. Pay special attention to the areas most likely to suffer serious, life-threatening injuries: the head, neck, chest, abdomen, and pelvis. Minor reddening may be the only sign of a developing contusion and serious internal injury. Also examine the neck veins. In the supine, normovolemic patient, they should be full. If they are flat, suspect hypovolemia.

During your rapid trauma assessment, rule out the possibility of obstructive shock. Assess the chest to identify any tension pneumothorax. Look for dyspnea,

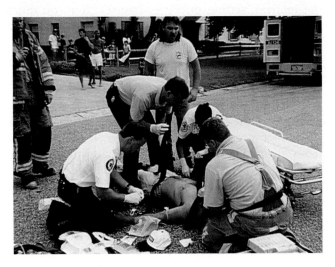

FIGURE 19-10 The rapid trauma assessment focuses on potential shock-inducing injuries to the head, neck, and torso.

a hyperinflated chest, distended jugular veins, resonant percussion, diminished or absent breath sounds on the affected side, lower tracheal shift to the opposite side, and any subcutaneous emphysema. Also suspect and search for pericardial tamponade. Look for penetrating injury, distended jugular veins, muffled or distant heart tones, tachycardia, and progressive and extreme hypotension. Pericardial tamponade requires immediate and rapid transport to a trauma centre. If the patient received significant anterior chest trauma, suspect myocardial contusion. Apply an electrocardiogram (ECG) monitor, and analyze the cardiac rhythm.

During the assessment, be alert to the possibility that hemorrhagic shock is not the problem or is not the only problem affecting your patient. Such conditions as stroke, epilepsy, or heart attack can lead to auto collisions and other traumatic events. Be careful to rule out cardiogenic shock by questioning the patient about crushing substernal chest discomfort and looking for pulmonary edema, jugular vein distention, and cardiac dysrhythmias (see Chapter 28, "Cardiology"). Also suspect and check for neurogenic shock (see Chapter 24, "Spinal Trauma"). Look for the presence of pink and warm skin below the point of nervous system injury, while the skin above the injury is pale, cool, and clammy. Other shock states, such as anaphylactic, septic, and diabetic shock are not likely unless the patient history suggests them.

Quickly take a set of vital signs, concentrating on both the pulse rate and the pulse pressure. If the pulse is weak, its rate is elevated, or the pulse pressure is diminished, suspect serious hemorrhage. Gauge your findings against the MOI and the time from the injury to your assessment. The shorter the time and the more pronounced the signs and symptoms, the more rapidly the patient is moving toward decompensation and then irreversible shock.

Complete this step of the assessment process by gathering a patient history. Listen to any patient complaints of weakness, thirst, or nausea, which may be further signs of shock. Be especially alert for patient complaints suggestive of a myocardial infarction. Be prepared to monitor the heart for dysrhythmias.

At the end of the rapid trauma assessment or the focused history and secondary assessment, inventory your findings. Set the patient's priority for transport, and set priorities for the order in which you will care for injuries. Again, if any indication, MOI, sign, or symptom suggests serious internal hemorrhage or uncontrolled external hemorrhage, consider rapid transport of the patient. Approximate the probable volume of blood lost to fractures, large contusions, and hematomas. Also note the probable locations of internal hemorrhage, and attempt to estimate the blood loss from them. Identify all significant injuries, and assign each a priority for care. While you may not complete the care for all the injuries, setting priorities ensures that you quickly address those injuries most likely to contribute to the patient's hypovolemia and shock.

Detailed Secondary Assessment

Consider performing a detailed secondary assessment on a potential shock patient only after all priorities have been addressed and the patient is either en route to the trauma centre or if such circumstances as a prolonged extrication prevent immediate transport. If you have the time, assess the patient from head to toe and look for any additional signs of injury. You should remove all of the patient's clothing, being careful not to cut the patient in the process. This will allow you to visualize the entire body for injuries.

Remember that your early arrival at the patient's side may mean that the ecchymosis (black-and-blue discoloration) associated with injuries has not had time to develop. So, be very careful to look for reddening (erythema) and areas of local warmth, suggestive of trauma.

During assessment, be alert to the possibility that hemorrhagic shock is not the problem or is not the only problem affecting your patient.

Ongoing Assessment

After completing the primary assessment and the rapid trauma assessment or focused history and secondary assessment, perform serial ongoing assessments. Reassess mental status, airway, breathing, and circulation. Reestablish patient priorities, and reassess and record the vital signs. This ongoing assessment allows you to identify any trends in the patient's condition. Pay particular attention to the pulse rate and pulse pressure. If the pulse rate is increasing and the difference between the diastolic and systolic pressures is decreasing, suspect increasing compensation and worsening shock. Perform a focused assessment for any changes in symptoms the patient reports. Also, check the adequacy and effectiveness of any interventions you have performed. Provide this ongoing assessment every five minutes for the seriously injured patient or for any patient who displays any of the signs or symptoms of shock.

SHOCK MANAGEMENT

Airway and Breathing Management

Management of the shock patient begins with corrective actions taken during the primary assessment. One of the primary principles of shock care is to ensure the best possible chance for tissue oxygenation and carbon dioxide offload. Accomplish this by ensuring or providing good ventilations with supplemental high-flow oxygen (12–15 L/min via nonrebreather mask). If the patient is moving air ineffectively (at a breathing rate less than 12/min or with inadequate respiratory volume), provide positive pressure ventilations (PPV).

Positive pressure ventilation to the breathing patient, called **overdrive respiration,** is coordinated with the patient's breathing attempts if possible (Figure 19-11). However, ensure that the ventilations provide both a good respiratory volume (at least 800 mL) and an adequate respiratory rate (at least 12 to 16 per minute). Overdrive respiration may be indicated in patients with rib fractures, flail chest, spinal injury with diaphragmatic respirations, head injury, or any condition in which the patient, because of bellows system or respiratory control failure, is not breathing adequately on her own.

If the patient is unconscious or semiconscious and unable to protect her airway, be aggressive in your care. Intubation may be required. Shock patients frequently vomit, and gastric aspiration presents a serious, possibly fatal, consequence. If there are any signs of a tension pneumothorax presenting with decreased or absent breath sounds on the affected side, tracheal deviation, and hypotension, provide needle decompression. Needle decompression should be performed either at the second intercostal space, midclavicular line or at the fifth intercostal space, midaxillary line (see Chapter 25, "Thoracic Trauma"). Continue to monitor the patient en route to the hospital, ensuring adequate oxygenation and perfusion.

Hemorrhage Control

Provide rapid control of any significant external hemorrhage. Use direct pressure and elevation where practical, and pressure points as needed.

Fluid Resuscitation

The field treatment of choice for fluid resuscitation in trauma cases is blood. Blood, however, must be refrigerated, typed, and cross-matched. (O-negative blood may be given in emergency circumstances.) Blood also has a short shelf life and is costly for field use. The most practical fluid for prehospital administration, then, is Ringer's Lactate solution. Ringer's Lactate best matches the electrolyte concentration of plasma and does not produce the hyperchloremic acidosis associated with

A primary principle of shock care is to ensure the best possible chance for tissue oxygenation and carbon dioxide offload; do this by providing supplemental high-flow oxygen or positive pressure ventilation.

* **overdrive respiration** positive pressure ventilation supplied to a breathing patient.

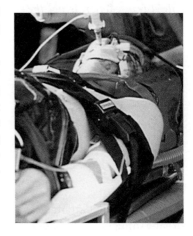

FIGURE 19-11   Ensure that the potential shock patient receives adequate ventilation, using overdrive respiration if necessary.

The most practical choice for prehospital fluid resuscitation is Ringer's Lactate solution.

the infusion of large volumes of normal saline. However, normal saline is an acceptable second choice and has few drug and fluid incompatability problems.

Some hypertonic and synthetic solutions show promise for fluid resuscitation. None of these, however, has been identified as superior to isotonic electrolyte solutions for prehospital use. Hypertonic solutions can mobilize the interstitial and cellular fluid volumes to replace lost blood volume, but they cannot carry either the oxygen or the clotting factors essential for hemorrhage control. Synthetic agents are now available that can carry oxygen and may, in the future, assist the clotting process. These agents, however, are expensive, have short shelf lives, and pose some patient compatibility problems.

When administering fluids to a trauma patient or to any patient who may need large fluid volumes, consider the internal lumen size of both the catheter and the administration set. Fluid flow is proportional to the fourth power of the internal diameter. This means that if you double the lumen's diameter, the same fluid under the same pressure will flow 16 times more quickly. Hence, use the largest catheter you can introduce into the patient's vein and use a large-bore trauma or blood administration set (Figure 19-12).

Catheter length and fluid pressure also influence fluid flow. The longer the catheter, the greater is the resistance to flow. The ideal catheter for the shock patient is relatively short, 3.75 cm or shorter. An increase in pressure increases fluid flow. This means that the higher you position the bag or the greater the pressure differential between the solution and the venous system, the faster will be the fluid flow. If you cannot elevate the fluid bag, position it under the patient, or place it in a pressure infuser or a blood-pressure cuff inflated to 100 or 200 mmHg.

Electrolyte administration is indicated for patients with the classic signs and symptoms of shock. When you have controlled external hemorrhage and there is no reason to suspect serious internal hemorrhage, employ aggressive fluid resuscitation. Moderate fluid resuscitation is also prudent for patients with blunt trauma to the chest or abdomen. Administer 1 L of Ringer's Lactate solution rapidly via IV (Figure 19-13). Use trauma or blood tubing to ensure unimpeded flow, and initiate the IV with a large-bore (14- or 16-gauge) catheter. In children, infuse 20 mL/kg of body weight rapidly when you see any signs and symptoms of shock. Administer a second fluid bolus if the vital signs do not improve after the first bolus or if, at some later time, the patient again begins to deteriorate. The objective of fluid resuscitation in the field is not the return of normal vital signs but the stabilization of vital signs until the patient reaches the trauma centre.

If there is penetrating trauma to the chest and/or you cannot control other hemorrhages, be more conservative with fluid administration. Cautiously control fluid volume, remembering that your goal is maintaining vital signs, not improving them. Increases in blood pressure can dislodge developing clots and disrupt the normal clotting processes. The result may be further hemorrhage with further

The objective of prehospital fluid resuscitation is not the return of normal vital signs but the stabilization of vital signs until the patient reaches the trauma centre.

FIGURE 19-12 Catheter size greatly influences fluid flow. Shown here are 22-, 18-, 14-, and 8-gauge catheters.

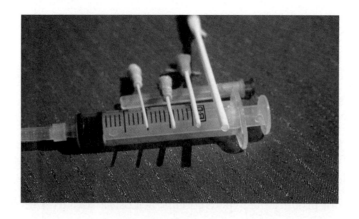

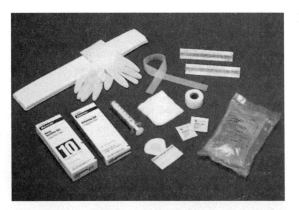

FIGURE 19-13   Supplies for initiating IV therapy.

dilution of the clotting factors and hemoglobin. Closely monitor your patient's vital signs, and administer Ringer's Lactate solution to keep the patient's mental status and pulse pressure at a steady level. Maintain the blood pressure at a steady level, even if it has dropped below 100 mmHg. Studies suggest that a blood pressure of 90 mmHg may be optimal for the patient with continuing internal hemorrhage. Do not, however, let the pressure drop below 50 mmHg.

Temperature Control

Trauma and blood loss deal serious blows to the mechanisms that normally adjust the body's core temperature. Reduced body activity reduces heat production to subnormal levels. Cutaneous vasoconstriction decreases the skin's ability to act as part of the body's temperature control system. The result is a patient highly susceptible to fluctuations in body temperature. In cases of trauma, patients commonly lose heat more rapidly than normal. At the same time, the heat-generating reflexes, like shivering, are ineffective and, in fact, are counterproductive to the shock care process.

In all except the warmest environments, help conserve body temperature by covering the patient with a blanket and keeping the patient compartment of the ambulance very warm. If you infuse fluids, ensure that they are well above room temperature—ideally at body temperature or slightly above (no more than 40°C). Use fluid warmers, or keep IV solutions in a compartment that is warmer than the rest of the ambulance. Be very sensitive to any patient complaints about being cold, and provide whatever assistance you can to ensure that heat loss is limited.

In all but the warmest environments, cover the hemorrhage or shock patient with a blanket, and keep the patient compartment of the ambulance very warm.

Pneumatic Antishock Garment

The **pneumatic antishock garment (PASG)**, sometimes referred to as the medical antishock trouser (MAST), is a device designed to apply firm circumferential pressure around the lower extremities, pelvis, and lower abdomen. The device is intended to compress the vascular space, thereby accomplishing four objectives:

* To increase peripheral vascular resistance by pressurizing the arteries of the lower abdomen and extremities
* To reduce the vascular volume by compressing venous vessels
* To increase the central circulating blood volume with blood returned from areas under the garment
* To immobilize the lower extremities and the pelvic region

Research has revealed potential problems with PASG use. The abdominal component of the PASG pressurizes the abdominal cavity, increasing the work

✱ pneumatic antishock garment (PASG) garment designed to produce uniform pressure on the lower extremities and abdomen; used with shock and hemorrhage patients in some EMS systems.

FIGURE 19-14 Emotional support for the seriously injured trauma patient is an important part of shock patient care.

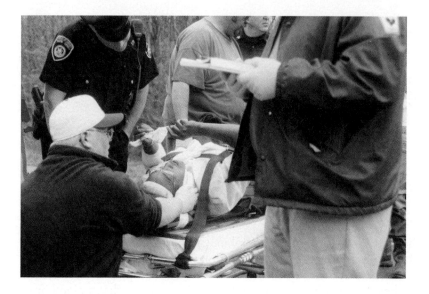

associated with breathing and, in some cases, reducing chest excursion. Application of the garment also increases mortality when used in cases of penetrating chest trauma. In light of this information, it is imperative that you understand the limitations of the device and comply with your local protocols and medical direction when considering use of the PASG.

Pharmacological Intervention

In shock, pharmacological interventions are generally limited, especially in hypovolemic patients. The sympathetic nervous system efficiently compensates for low volume, and no agent, other than intravenous fluid and, in some cases, blood and blood products, has been shown to be effective in the prehospital setting. For cardiogenic shock, fluid challenge, vasopressors (e.g., dopamine), and the other cardiac drugs are indicated (see Chapter 28, "Cardiology"). For spinal and obstructive shock, consider intravenous fluids, such as normal saline and Ringer's Lactate solution. For distributive shock, consider IV fluids, dopamine, and use of the PASG.

The patient who has experienced trauma sufficient to induce hemorrhage and hypovolemia will be anxious and bewildered. As the care provider at the patient's side, it is your responsibility to be calm and reassuring, thus counteracting the natural "fight-or-flight" response (Figure 19-14). By acting in this manner, you not only help your patient deal with the event's emotional trauma but also combat some of the negative effects of sympathetic stimulation.

SUMMARY

Significant hemorrhage and its serious consequence, shock, are genuine threats to the trauma patient's life. The signs of these threats are often subtle or hidden, especially if bleeding is internal. Only through careful analysis of the mechanism of injury during the scene assessment and careful evaluation of the patient during the assessment process can you recognize and then treat these life-threatening problems. Treatment often involves rapidly bringing the patient to the services of a trauma centre and, while doing so, providing aggressive care—supplemental oxygen, positive pressure ventilations, and fluid resuscitation, aimed at maintaining vital signs, not necessarily improving them. With this approach, you afford your patient the best chance for survival.

CHAPTER 20

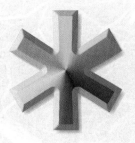

Soft-Tissue Trauma

Objectives

After reading this chapter, you should be able to:

1. Describe the incidence, morbidity, and mortality of soft-tissue injuries. (p. 95)
2. Describe the anatomy and physiology of the integumentary system, including epidermis, dermis, and subcutaneous tissue. (see Chapter 12)
3. Identify the skin tension lines of the body. (pp. 98–99)
4. Predict soft-tissue injuries based on mechanism of injury. (pp. 113–117)
5. Discuss blunt and penetrating trauma. (pp. 95–101)
6. Discuss the pathophysiology of soft-tissue injuries. (pp. 95–111)
7. Differentiate among the following types of soft-tissue injuries:

a. Closed (pp. 96–97)
   i. Contusion
   ii. Hematoma
   iii. Crush injuries
b. Open (pp. 97–101)
   i. Abrasions
   ii. Lacerations
   iii. Incisions
   iv. Punctures
   v. Impaled objects
   vi. Avulsions
   vii. Amputations

8. Discuss the assessment and management of open and closed soft-tissue injuries. (pp. 113–133)
9. Discuss the incidence, morbidity, and mortality of crush injuries. (pp. 97, 128–130)

Continued

10. Define the following conditions:
    a. Crush injury (pp. 97, 109–110, 128–130)
    b. Crush syndrome (pp. 97, 110, 128–130)
    c. Compartment syndrome (pp. 130–131)
11. Discuss the mechanisms of injury, assessment findings, and management of crush injuries. (pp. 97, 109–110, 128–130)
12. Discuss the effects of reperfusion and rhabdomyolysis on the body. (pp. 110, 130)
13. Discuss the pathophysiology, assessment, and care of hemorrhage associated with soft-tissue injuries, including:
    a. Capillary bleeding (pp. 102, 120)
    b. Venous bleeding (pp. 102, 120)
    c. Arterial bleeding (pp. 102, 120–122)
14. Describe and identify the indications for and application of the following dressings and bandages: (pp. 111–113)
    a. Sterile/nonsterile dressing
    b. Occlusive/nonocclusive dressing
    c. Adherent/nonadherent dressing
    d. Absorbent/nonabsorbent dressing
    e. Wet/dry dressing
    f. Self-adherent roller bandage
    g. Gauze bandage
    h. Adhesive bandage
    i. Elastic bandage
    j. Triangular bandage

15. Predict the possible complications of an improperly applied dressing or bandage. (pp. 111–113, 125)
16. Discuss the process of wound healing, including the following:
    a. Hemostasis (pp. 102–104)
    b. Inflammation (p. 104)
    c. Epithelialization (p. 104)
    d. Neovascularization (pp. 104–105)
    e. Collagen synthesis (p. 105)
17. Discuss the assessment and management of wound healing. (pp. 102–111)
18. Discuss the pathophysiology, assessment, and management of wound infection. (pp. 105–107)
19. Formulate treatment priorities for patients with soft-tissue injuries in conjunction with the following:
    a. Airway/face/neck trauma (p. 131)
    b. Thoracic trauma (open/closed) (pp. 131–132)
    c. Abdominal trauma (p. 132)
20. Given several preprogrammed and moulaged soft-tissue trauma patients, provide the appropriate scene assessment, primary assessment, rapid trauma or focused secondary assessment and history, detailed assessment, and ongoing assessment and provide appropriate patient care and transportation. (pp. 113–133)

INTRODUCTION TO SOFT-TISSUE INJURIES

The skin is one of the largest, most important organs of the human body, comprising 16 percent of total body weight. It provides a protective envelope that keeps invading pathogens out while containing body substances and fluids. It is also a key organ of sensation as well as a radiator of excess body heat in warm weather and a conservator of heat in cold conditions. Even as it accomplishes these various functions, the skin remains a durable, pliable, and accommodating tissue, and one that is highly capable of repairing itself.

Known collectively as the **integumentary system,** the skin is the first tissue of the human body to experience the effects of trauma. Because skin covers the entire body surface, any penetrating injury or the kinetic forces of blunt injury must pass through it before affecting other vital organs. Often, the signs of this energy transmission can only be observed with very careful examination of the skin. Therefore, the skin is of great significance at all stages of the patient assessment process.

Trauma to the skin may present as open injuries—abrasions, lacerations, incisions, punctures, avulsions, and amputations—or as closed injuries—contusions, hematomas, and crush injuries. Such injuries infrequently threaten life but may endanger blood vessels, nerves, connective tissue, and other important internal structures. Uncontrolled blood loss may lead to hypovolemia and shock, while the wound may provide a pathway for infection.

> ✳ **integumentary system** skin, consisting of the epidermis, dermis, and subcutaneous layers.

EPIDEMIOLOGY

Soft-tissue injuries are, by far, the most common form of trauma. Most, but not all, open wounds require only simple care and limited suturing. A significant minority, however, damage arteries, nerves, or tendons and can lead to permanent disability. Uncontrolled external hemorrhage of an otherwise uncomplicated open wound is a very rare but completely preventable situation that sometimes occurs with this type of injury and can result in death. Of the open wounds presenting to emergency departments, up to 6.5 percent will eventually become infected, resulting in significant morbidity.

> *Soft-tissue injuries are the most common type of trauma.*
>

Closed wounds share a similar epidemiology, except that they are probably even more common than open injuries. Most minor "bumps and bruises" never reach the paramedic, as most patients elect to self-treat all but the most serious cases. Despite their frequency and usually minor nature, closed injuries *can* result in significant pain, suffering, and morbidity. Infection, however, is not usually a complication with closed wounds. Risk factors for soft-tissue wounds include age (especially school-age children and the elderly), alcohol or drug abuse, and occupation. Labourers, machine operators, and others whose hands and body parts are exposed to heavy objects, machines, or tools are at great risk.

Simple measures can reduce risks and prevent soft-tissue injuries. For example, locating playgrounds on grass, sand, gravel, or other forgiving surfaces and padding the equipment in them can cut injury rates among children. In factories, machine guards, fail-safe switches, and similar engineering controls can reduce injuries. Protective clothing, such as steel-toed boots and leather gloves, also provide simple methods of reducing the incidence and severity of soft-tissue injuries.

PATHOPHYSIOLOGY OF SOFT-TISSUE INJURY

Although we often take the skin's functions for granted, soft-tissue injury can seriously affect health, causing severe blood and fluid loss, infection, hypothermia, and other problems.

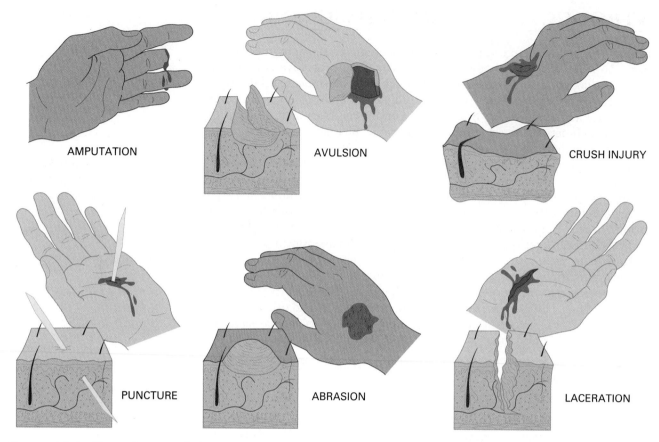

AMPUTATION   AVULSION   CRUSH INJURY

PUNCTURE   ABRASION   LACERATION

FIGURE 20-1   Types of open soft-tissue injuries.

Trauma is a violent transfer of energy that produces an open or closed wound to the skin and possible injury to the structures underneath. Wounds can be either blunt or penetrating (Figure 20-1). While all penetrating wounds are open, blunt trauma can, on occasion, create open wounds. Common soft-tissue injuries include closed wounds (contusions, hematomas, and crush injuries) and open wounds (abrasions, lacerations, incisions, punctures, avulsions, and amputations). Each type of wound is different and deserves special consideration.

CLOSED WOUNDS

Contusions

Contusions are blunt, nonpenetrating injuries that crush and damage small blood vessels (Figure 20-2). Blood is drawn to the inflamed tissue, causing a reddening called **erythema**. Blood also leaks into the surrounding interstitial spaces through damaged vessels. As the hemoglobin within the free blood loses its oxygen, it becomes dark red and then blue, resulting in the black-and-blue discoloration called **ecchymosis**. Because the development of ecchymosis is a progressive process, the discoloration may not be evident during prehospital care.

Contusions are more pronounced in areas where the mechanism causing the injury (for example, a steering wheel) and skeletal structures (such as the ribs or skull) trap the skin. Occasionally, a chest injury displays an erythematous or ecchymotic outline of the ribs and sternum, reflecting an impact with the auto dashboard or some other blunt object. Early signs of such an injury may be difficult to identify, but they will become more evident as time passes and discoloration increases.

✱ **contusion** closed wound in which the skin is unbroken, although damage has occurred to the tissue immediately beneath.

✱ **erythema** general reddening of the skin due to dilation of the superficial capillaries.

✱ **ecchymosis** blue-black discoloration of the skin due to leakage of blood into the tissues.

Hematomas

Soft-tissue bleeding can occur within the tissue and at times can be quite significant. When the injury involves a larger blood vessel, most commonly an artery, the blood can actually separate tissue and pool in a pocket called a **hematoma**. These injuries are very visible in cases of head trauma because of the unyielding skull underneath. Hematomas tend to be less pronounced in other body areas, even though they can contain significant hemorrhage. Severe hematomas to the thigh, leg, or arm may contribute significantly to hypovolemia. A hematoma in the thigh, for example, can contain mote than a litre of blood before swelling becomes noticeable.

Crush Injury

The term **crush injury** describes a collection of traumatic insults that include crush injury and crush syndrome. A body part that is crushed, possibly by a heavy object, sustains deep injury to the muscles, blood vessels, bones, and other internal structures (Figure 20-3). Damage can be massive, despite minimal signs displayed on the skin itself. **Crush syndrome** is the term used to describe the systemic effects of a crush injury. If the pressure that causes a crush injury remains in place for several hours, the resulting destruction of skeletal muscle cells leads to the accumulation of large quantities of myoglobin (a cell protein), potassium, lactic acid, uric acid, and other toxins. When the pressure is released, these products enter the bloodstream. They circulate, causing a severe metabolic acidosis. These materials are also toxic to the kidneys and heart. Crush syndrome is thus a potentially life-threatening trauma event. It will be discussed in more detail later in this chapter.

OPEN WOUNDS

Abrasions

Abrasions are typically the most minor of injuries that violate the protective envelope of the skin. They involve a scraping or abrasive action that removes layers of the epidermis and the upper reaches of the dermis (Figure 20-4). Bleeding can be persistent but is usually limited because the injury involves only superficial capillaries. If the injury compromises a large area of the epidermis, it carries the danger of serious infection.

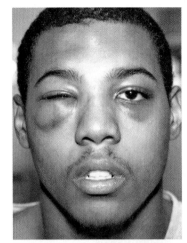

FIGURE 20-2   A contusion. Note that the discoloration of a contusion is a delayed sign.

✱ **hematoma** collection of blood beneath the skin or trapped within a body compartment.

✱ **crush injury** mechanism of injury in which tissue is locally compressed by high pressure forces.

✱ **crush syndrome** systemic disorder of severe metabolic disturbances resulting from the crush of a limb or other body part.

✱ **abrasion** scraping or abrading away of the superficial layers of the skin; an open soft-tissue injury.

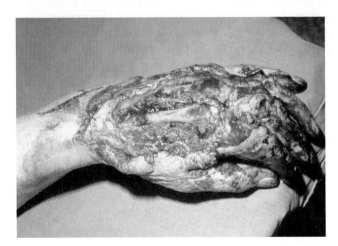

FIGURE 20-3   A crush injury.

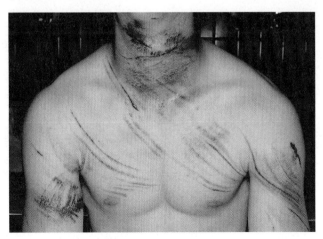

FIGURE 20-4   Abrasions.

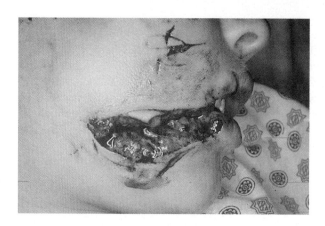

FIGURE 20-5 Lacerations (secondary to animal bite).

✳ **laceration** an open wound, normally a tear with jagged borders.

✳ **tension lines** natural patterns in the surface of the skin revealing tensions within.

✳ **incision** very smooth or surgical laceration, frequently caused by a knife, scalpel, razor blade, or piece of glass.

✳ **puncture** specific soft-tissue injury involving a deep, narrow wound to the skin and underlying organs that carries an increased danger of infection.

Lacerations

A **laceration** is an open wound that penetrates more deeply into the dermis than an abrasion does (Figure 20-5). A laceration tends to involve a smaller surface area, being limited to the tissue immediately surrounding the penetration. It endangers the deeper and more significant vasculature—arteries, arterioles, venules, and veins—as well as nerves, muscles, tendons, ligaments, and perhaps some underlying organs. As with an abrasion, the injury breaks the skin's protective barrier and provides a pathway for infection.

Note that the skin does not merely hang on the flesh but, rather, is spread over the body and attached to fit the contours of the underlying structures. This creates natural stretch or tension in the skin. The orientation of tension in the skin is revealed in characteristic patterns called **tension lines** (Figure 20-6). The effects of tension on the skin become evident when the skin is transected, as with a laceration. Lacerations cutting across the tension lines have a tendency to be pulled apart and thus spread widely or gape. Lacerations parallel to the tension lines tend to gape very little. Wounds that spread widely tend to bleed more than those with minimal gaping. Large gaping wounds heal more slowly and are more likely to leave noticeable scars than are wounds that spread less.

The tension represented by skin tension lines can be either static or dynamic. Static tension is noted in areas with limited movement of the tissue and structures beneath, as in the anterior abdomen or between the joints in the extremities. Dynamic tension lines occur in areas subject to great movement, as in the skin over such joints as the elbow, wrist, or knee. The increased motion in areas with dynamic skin tension lines means that the clotting and tissue mending processes in these areas are more frequently interrupted, disrupting and complicating skin repair.

You should note the laceration's orientation to the skin tension lines during your assessment of the patient. Remember that if the orientation parallels those lines, the wound may remain closed. If it is perpendicular to them, the wound may gape open.

Incisions

An **incision** is a surgically smooth laceration, often caused by a sharp instrument such as a knife, straight razor, or piece of glass. Such a wound tends to bleed freely. In all other ways, it is a laceration.

Punctures

Another special type of laceration is the **puncture**. It involves a small entrance wound with damage that extends into the body's interior (Figure 20-7). The

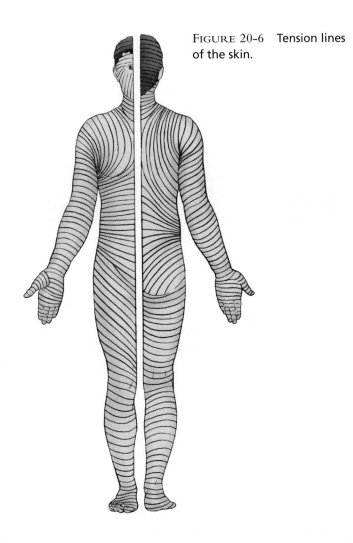

FIGURE 20-6 Tension lines of the skin.

wound normally seals itself and presents in a way that does not reflect the actual extent of injury. If the puncture penetrates deeply, it may involve not just the skin but also the underlying muscles, nerves, bones, and organs. A puncture additionally carries an increased danger of infection. A penetrating object introduces bacteria and other pathogens deep into a wound. There, the disrupted tissue and blood vessels, along with a reduced oxygen level, create a warm and moist environment that is ideal for the colonization of bacteria.

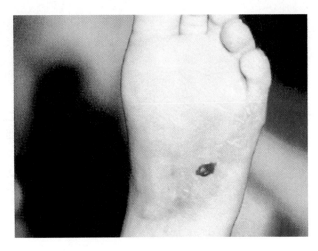

FIGURE 20-7 A puncture wound.

FIGURE 20-8   An impaled object.

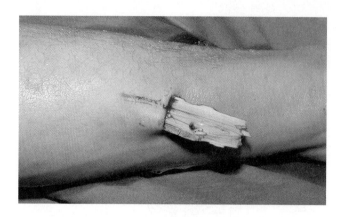

Impaled Objects

✱ **impaled object** foreign body embedded in a wound.

An **impaled object** is not a wound itself but, rather, a wound complication often associated with a puncture or laceration. Impaled objects are important for the damage they may cause if withdrawn. Frequently, embedded objects are irregular in shape and become entangled in important structures, such as arteries, nerves, or tendons (Figure 20-8). Their removal in the field can result in further damage. Perhaps more critically, the embedded object may have lacerated a large blood vessel and the object's presence temporarily blocks, or tamponades, blood loss. Removal of the object may cause an uncheckable flow of blood. This situation is particularly dangerous when the object is impaled in the neck or trunk, where the application of effective direct pressure is difficult or impossible.

Avulsions

✱ **avulsion** forceful tearing away or separation of body tissue; an avulsion may be partial or complete.

✱ **degloving injury** avulsion in which the mechanism of injury tears the skin off the underlying muscle, tissue, blood vessels, and bone.

Avulsion occurs when a flap of skin, although torn or cut, is not torn completely loose from the body (Figure 20-9). Avulsion is frequently seen with blunt trauma to the skull, where the scalp is torn and folds back. It may also occur with animal bites and machinery accidents. The seriousness of the avulsion depends on the area involved, the condition of the circulation to (and distal to) the injury site, and the degree of contamination.

A special type of avulsion is the **degloving injury.** In this wound, the mechanism of injury tears the skin off the underlying muscle, connective tissue, blood vessels, and bone. It is a particularly gruesome injury, occurring occasionally with farm and industrial machinery. The device pulls the skin off with great force

FIGURE 20-9   An avulsion.

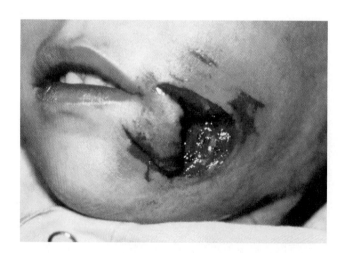

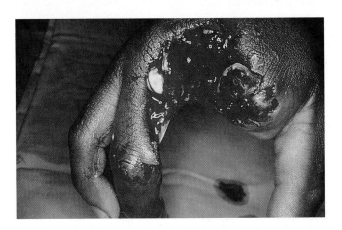

FIGURE 20-10   A ring-type degloving injury.

as the skeletal tissue underneath is held stationary. The wound exposes a large area of tissue and is often severely contaminated. This type of injury carries a poor prognosis. If, however, the vasculature and innervation remain intact, there may be some hope for future use of the digit or extremity.

A variation of the degloving process is the ring injury (Figure 20-10). As a person jumps or falls, the ring is caught, pulling the skin of the finger against the weight of the victim. The force may tear the upper layers of tissue away from the phalanges, exposing the tendons, nerves, and blood vessels. Although the ring injury involves a smaller area, it is otherwise a degloving injury.

Amputations

The partial or complete severance of a digit or limb is an **amputation** (Figure 20-11). It often results in the complete loss of the limb at the site of severance. The hemorrhage associated with the amputation may be limited if the limb or digit is cut cleanly or may be severe and continuing if the wound is a jagged or crushing one. The surgeon may attempt to reattach the amputated part or use its skin for grafting as he repairs the remaining limb. If this skin is unavailable, the surgeon may have to cut the bone and musculature back further to close the wound. This reduces the length of the limb as well as its future usefulness.

✱ **amputation** severance, removal, or detachment, either partial or complete, of a body part.

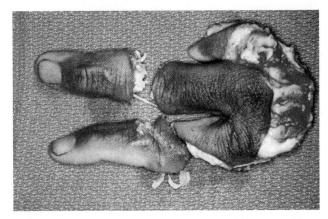

FIGURE 20-11   An amputation of the first two fingers.

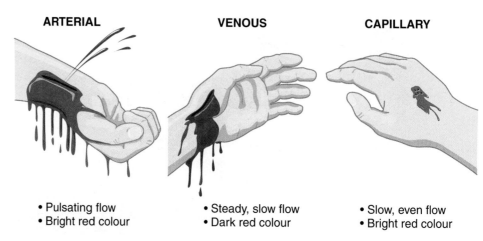

ARTERIAL	VENOUS	CAPILLARY
• Pulsating flow • Bright red colour	• Steady, slow flow • Dark red colour	• Slow, even flow • Bright red colour

FIGURE 20-12 Hemorrhage. Arterial hemorrhage is bright red and flows rapidly from a wound. Venous hemorrhage is darker red and flows slowly. Capillary hemorrhage is also bright red and flows slowly.

HEMORRHAGE

Soft-tissue injuries frequently cause blood loss, ranging from inconsequential to life threatening. The loss can be arterial, venous, or capillary (Figure 20-12). Bleeding can be easy or almost impossible to control. Hemorrhage is usually dark red with venous injury, red with capillary injury, and bright red with arterial injury. The rate of hemorrhage also varies from oozing capillary, to flowing venous, to pulsing arterial bleeding. In practice, it may be hard to differentiate among the types and origins of hemorrhage. It is important, however, to determine the rate and quantity of blood loss. This information helps you decide on the most effective means of stopping the blood flow and to prioritize the patient for care and transport.

Often, the nature of the soft-tissue wound may be more important than the size or type of vessel involved in determining the severity of the blood vessel injury. If a moderately sized vein or artery is cut cleanly, the muscles in its walls contract. This constricts the vessel's lumen and retracts the severed vessel into the tissue. As the muscle is drawn back from the wound, it thickens and further restricts the lumen. This restricts blood flow, reduces the rate of loss, and assists the clotting mechanisms. Therefore, clean lacerations and amputations generally do not bleed profusely. If, on the other hand, the vessel is not severed cleanly but is laid open instead, muscle contraction opens the wound, thereby increasing and prolonging blood loss.

WOUND HEALING

Wound healing is a complex process that begins immediately following injury and can take many months to complete. Wound healing is an essential component of homeostasis, the process whereby the body maintains a uniform environment for itself. Although it is useful to divide the wound healing process into stages or parts, it is important to note that these phases overlap considerably and are intertwined physiologically (Figure 20-13).

Hemostasis

Arguably the most important aspect of wound healing is the body's ability to stop most bleeding on its own. This process is called **hemostasis.** Without hemostasis, even the most trivial nicks and scratches would continue to bleed, leading to life-

---

During assessment, it is important to determine the rate and quantity of hemorrhage.

Content Review

STAGES OF WOUND HEALING
Hemostasis
Inflammation
Epithelialization
Neovascularization
Collagen synthesis

✱ **hemostasis** the body's natural ability to stop bleeding, the ability to clot blood.

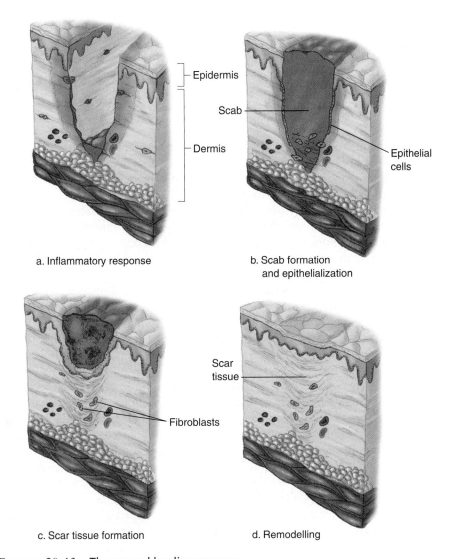

a. Inflammatory response

b. Scab formation
and epithelialization

c. Scar tissue formation

d. Remodelling

Epidermis

Dermis

Scab

Epithelial
cells

Fibroblasts

Scar
tissue

FIGURE 20-13   The wound healing process.

threatening hemorrhage. Hemostasis has three major components related to the vasculature, the platelets, and the clotting cascade.

Hemostasis begins almost immediately following injury. Arteries, arterioles, and some veins are endowed with a muscular layer that reflexively constricts the vessel in response to local injury. The longitudinal muscles, too, play a role by retracting the cut ends of larger vessels back into the contracted muscle, thus reducing flow. This immediate response usually reduces but does not entirely stop bleeding. Capillaries, which do not have a muscle layer, cannot contract and thus continue to bleed. This explains the continuing but minor bleeding associated with capillary wounds, such as paper cuts and minor abrasions.

Platelets begin the clotting process. The damaged vessel wall becomes "sticky," as do the platelets in the turbulent flow of the disrupted vessel. Platelets stick to the vessel wall and to one another. This forms a platelet plug, reducing blood flow or, in small vessels, stopping it altogether.

When a blood vessel is injured, the disrupted tunica intima exposes collagen and other structural proteins to the blood. These proteins activate a complicated series of enzyme reactions that change certain blood proteins into long fibrin strands. These strands then entrap erythrocytes and produce a gelatinous mass that further occludes the bleeding vessel. This complex process, called coagulation, stops all but the most severe and persistent hemorrhage. With time, the clot shrinks or contracts, bringing the wound margins closer together, further facilitating wound healing. When the clot is no longer needed, it is reabsorbed by the body and any superficial scab merely drops off.

Inflammation

Shortly after hemostasis begins, the body sets in motion a very complex process of healing called **inflammation.** The inflammatory process involves a host of elements including various kinds of white blood cells, proteins involved in immunity, and hormone-like chemicals that signal other cells to mobilize.

Cells damaged by direct trauma or by invading pathogens release a number of proteins and chemicals into the surrounding tissue and blood. These agents, called **chemotactic factors,** recruit cells responsible for consuming cellular debris, invading bacteria, or other foreign or damaged cells and for beginning the inflammatory process. The first cells to arrive are specialized white blood cells called **granulocytes** and **macrophages.** These cells (also called phagocytes) are capable of engulfing bacteria, debris, and foreign material, digesting them, and then releasing the byproducts in a process called **phagocytosis.** Other white blood cells called lymphocytes, in combination with immunoglobulins or immune proteins, are also mobilized. Lymphocytes attack invading pathogens directly or through an antibody response.

The injury process, the material released from injured cells, and the debris released as the phagocytes destroy invading cells cause mast cells to release histamine. Histamine dilates precapillary blood vessels, increases capillary permeability, and increases blood flow into and through the injured or infected tissue. This brings much-needed oxygen and more phagocytes to the injured area and draws away the byproducts of cell destruction and repair. The increasing blood flow and local tissue metabolism also increase tissue temperature, which may, in turn, denature pathogen membranes. This response produces a swollen (edematous), reddened (erythematous), and warm region, characteristic of inflammation in response to local infection or injury. The result of the inflammation stage is the clearing away of dead and dying tissue, removal of bacteria and other foreign substances, and the preparation of the damaged area for rebuilding.

Epithelialization

Epithelialization is an early stage in wound healing in which epithelial cells migrate over the surface of the wound. The stratum germinativum cells rapidly divide and regenerate, thus restoring a uniform layer of skin cells along the edges of the healing wound. In clean, surgically prepared wounds, complete epithelialization may take place in as little as 48 hours. Except in minor, superficial wounds, the new epithelial layer is not a perfect facsimile of the original, undamaged skin. Instead, the new skin layer may be thinner, pigmented differently, and devoid of normal hair follicles. However, the new skin is usually quite functional and cosmetically similar to the original. If the wound is very large, epithelialization may be incomplete, and collagen will show through as a shiny, pinkish line of tissue called a scar.

Neovascularization

In order for healing to take place, new tissue must grow and regenerate. That requires blood rich in oxygen and nutrients. The body responds to this increased

---

* **inflammation** complex process of local cellular and biochemical changes as a consequence of injury or infection; an early stage of healing.

* **chemotactic factors** chemicals released by white blood cells that attract more white blood cells to an area of inflammation.

* **granulocytes** white blood cells charged with the primary purpose of neutralizing foreign bacteria.

* **macrophage** immune system cell that has the ability to recognize and ingest foreign pathogens.

* **phagocytosis** process in which a cell surrounds and absorbs a bacterium or other particle.

* **epithelialization** early stage of wound healing in which epithelial cells migrate over the surface of the wound.

demand by generating new blood vessels in a process called **neovascularization.** These vessels bud from undamaged capillaries in the wound margins and then grow into the healing tissue. Neovascularized tissue is very fragile and has a tendency to bleed easily. It takes weeks to months for the newly formed blood vessels to become fully resistant to injury and for the surrounding tissue to strengthen enough to protect the new and delicate circulation.

Collagen Synthesis

Collagen is the body's main structural protein. It is a strong, tough fibre forming part of hair, bones, and connective tissue. Scar tissue, cartilage, and tendons are almost entirely collagen. Specialized cells called **fibroblasts** are brought to the wound area and synthesize collagen as an important step in rebuilding damaged tissues. Collagen binds the wound margins together and strengthens the healing wound. It is important to note that as the wound heals, it is not "as good as new." Regenerated skin has only about 60 percent of the tensile strength of undamaged skin at four months, when the scar is fully mature. This accounts for the occasional reinjury and reopening of wounds weeks or months after healing. The fibroblasts continue to reshape the scar tissue and shrink the wound for months after the scab falls off. This **remodelling** involves reorganizing collagen fibres into neat, parallel bands, strengthening the healing tissue still more. Remodelling can continue for up to 6 to 12 months after the initial injury, and so the final cosmetic outcome of the healing process may not be evident until then.

INFECTION

Infection is the most common and, next to hemorrhage, the most serious complication of open wounds. Approximately 1 in 15 wounds seen at the emergency department results in a wound infection. These infections delay healing. They may also spread to adjacent tissues and endanger cosmetic appearances. Occasionally, they cause widespread or systemic infection, called sepsis.

The most common causes of skin and soft-tissue infections are the *Staphylococcus* and *Streptococcus* bacterial families. These bacteria are gram positive (gram staining is a procedure to differentiate between types of bacteria), aerobic, and very common in the environment. *Staphylococcus* bacteria frequently colonize on the surface of normal skin, and so it is not surprising to find them driven into wounds by the forces of trauma. Less commonly, wound infections are caused by other bacteria, such as gram-negative rods, including *Pseudomonas aeruginosa* (diabetics and foot puncture wounds) and *Pasteurella multocida* (cat and dog bites).

It takes bacteria a few days to grow into numbers sufficient to cause noticeable signs or symptoms of infection. Infections appear at least two to three days following the initial wound and commonly present with pain, tenderness, erythema, and warmth. Infection earlier than that is very unusual. Pus, a collection of white blood cells, cellular debris, and dead bacteria, may be visible draining from the wound. The pus is usually thick, pale yellowish-to-greenish in colour, and has a foul smell. Visible red streaks, or **lymphangitis,** may extend from the wound margins up the affected extremity proximally. These streaks represent inflammation of the lymph channels as a result of the infection. The patient may also complain of fever and malaise, especially if the infection has begun to spread systemically.

* **neovascularization** new growth of capillaries in response to healing.

* **collagen** tough, strong protein that makes up most of the body's connective tissue.

* **fibroblasts** specialized cells that form collagen.

* **remodelling** stage in the wound healing process in which collagen is broken down and relaid in an orderly fashion.

Infection is the most common complication of open wounds.

* **lymphangitis** inflammation of the lymph channels, usually as a result of a distal infection.

Infection Risk Factors

Risk factors for wound infections are related to the host's health, the type and location of the wound, any associated contamination, and the treatment provided. Diabetics, the infirm, the elderly, and individuals with serious chronic diseases, such as chronic obstructive pulmonary disease (COPD), are at greater risk for infection and heal more slowly and less efficiently than healthy individuals. Patients with any significant disease or preexisting medical problem, such as cancer, anemia, hepatic failure, or cardiovascular disease, have difficulty mobilizing the immune and tissue-repair response necessary for good wound healing. Human immunodeficiency virus (HIV) causes acquired immune deficiency syndrome (AIDS), attacks the body's immune system, and seriously impairs its ability to ward off infection, increasing risk significantly. Smoking constricts blood vessels and robs healing tissues of needed oxygen and nutrients, also increasing infection risk.

Several drugs detract from the body's ability to fight infection. Persons on immunosuppressant medications, such as prednisone or cortisone (corticosteroids), and nonsteroidal anti-inflammatory drugs (NSAIDs), such as ibuprofen, are also at increased risk for serious infection. Colchicine, a drug used to treat gout, also reduces the body's inflammation response. Neoplastic agents, which are used to combat rapidly reproducing cancer cells, also disrupt cell regeneration at an injury site.

The type of wound—for example, a puncture or an extensive crush injury—may influence the likelihood of infection.

The wound type strongly affects the likelihood of a wound infection. A puncture wound traps contamination deep within tissue where there is a perfect environment for bacterial growth. Avulsion tears away blood vessels and supporting structures, robbing the damaged tissue of its blood supply, a critical factor in preventing or reducing infection. Crush injuries and other wounds that produce large areas of injured or dead (devitalized) tissue provide an excellent environment for bacterial growth and are at great risk for wound infection.

In a similar fashion, wound location influences infection risk. Well-vascularized areas, such as the face and scalp, are highly resistant to infection. Distal extremities, the feet in particular, are at greater risk.

Clean objects, such as uncontaminated sheet metal or a clean knife, usually leave only small amounts of bacteria in a wound and, consequently, do not often cause infections. However, objects contaminated with organic matter and bacteria, such as a nail on a barnyard floor, a knife used to clean raw meat, or a piece of wood, pose much greater risks of infection. The infection risk associated with bites caused by mammals, carnivores in particular, is very great. Bites by humans, cats, and dogs are among the most common and most serious types of bites.

The type of treatment provided for a wound affects the risk of infection. Use of sterile dressings and clean examination gloves minimizes wound contamination during prehospital treatment. Gloves protect not only the rescuer but also the patient from contaminants on the rescuer's hands. Irrigation of wounds with sterile saline using a pressurized stream device has been shown to reduce bacterial loads and reduce infection rates. Closing wounds (with sutures or staples, for example) increases infection risks compared with leaving wounds open. However, the risks associated with wound closure are frequently accepted in order to achieve the best possible cosmetic outcome and more rapid healing.

In most cases, routine use of antibiotics with wounds does not help reduce infection rates and, in fact, may increase the likelihood of infection with antibiotic-resistant microorganisms. Antibiotics may be helpful if given within the first hour or so after occurrence of deep major wounds, such as those from gunshots or stabbings, puncture wounds to the feet, and wounds where retention of a foreign body is suspected.

Infection Management

Despite the potential problems noted above, the mainstay in treatment for infections is the use of chemical bactericidals, also know as antibiotics. Antibiotics for the treatment of gram-positive infections include the antistaphylococcal penicillin, cephalosporin, and erythromycin in patients allergic to penicillin. The pharmalogical approach against pseudomonas often requires the use of two drugs, while pasteurella is adequately treated with penicillin.

On occasion, a wound forms a collection of pus called an abscess and requires a minor incision and drainage to correct. Surgical removal of this material helps the body return to normal more quickly.

Gangrene One of the rarest and most feared wound complications is **gangrene**. Gangrene is a deep space infection usually caused by the anaerobic bacterium *Clostridium perfringens*. These bacteria characteristically produce a gas deep within a wound, causing subcutaneous emphysema and a foul smell whenever the gas escapes. Once they have become established, the bacteria are particularly prolific and can rapidly involve an entire extremity. Left unchecked, gangrene frequently leads to sepsis and death. In the days before antibiotics, amputation was frequently necessary to stop the spread of the infection. Modern treatment with a combination of antibiotics, surgery, and hyperbaric oxygenation effectively arrests most cases of gangrene early in their course.

✳ gangrene deep space infection usually caused by the anaerobic bacterium *Clostridium perfringens*.

Tetanus Another highly feared but, fortunately, rare complication of wound infections is tetanus, or lockjaw. Tetanus is caused by the bacterium *Clostridium tetani*, and like its cousin *Clostridium perfringens*, it is anaerobic. Tetanus presents with few signs or symptoms at the local wound site, but the bacteria produce a potent toxin that causes widespread, painful, involuntary muscle contractions. Early observers noted mandibular trismus, or jaw-clenching ("lockjaw"). There is an antidote for the tetanus toxin, but it only neutralizes circulating toxin molecules, not those already bound to the motor endplates. Thus, treatment is slow and recovery prolonged.

Fortunately, tetanus is preventable through immunization. Widespread immunization has reduced its incidence to a very few cases. The standard immunization is a series of three shots in childhood, with boosters every 10 years thereafter.

OTHER WOUND COMPLICATIONS

Several circumstances or conditions can interfere with normal wound healing processes. These conditions include impaired hemostasis, rebleeding, and delayed healing.

Impaired Hemostasis

Several medications can interfere with hemostasis and the clotting process. Aspirin is a powerful inhibitor of platelet aggregation, and it is used clinically to help prevent clot formation in the coronary and cerebral arteries of patients at risk for myocardial infarction or cerebrovascular accident (stroke). Thus, a side effect of aspirin use is a prolongation of clotting time, an important consideration in a patient who has sustained significant trauma or is undergoing major surgery. Likewise, anticoagulants, such as Coumadin (warfarin) and heparin, and thrombolitics, such as TPA (tissue plasminogen activator) and streptokinase, interfere with or break down the protein fibres that form clots and are used to prevent or destroy obstructions at critical locations. They also adversely affect clot development in soft-tissue wounds. Penicillins may increase clotting times and interfere with blood cell production. Additionally,

Some medications, such as aspirin, warfarin, and heparin, can interfere with the clotting process.

abnormalities in proteins involved in the fibrin formation cascade may result in delayed clotting, as is the case in hemophiliacs.

Rebleeding

Despite treatment that provides adequate initial control of bleeding, rebleeding is possible from any wound. Movement of underlying structures, such as muscles or bones, or of the bandage or dressing material may dislodge clots and re-institute hemorrhage.

Also, hemorrhage that appears to have been stopped may actually be bleeding into an oversized dressing until it saturates the dressing and pushes through it. Monitor your dressings and bandages frequently to ensure that blood loss is not continuing.

Partially healed wounds are also at risk for rebleeding. Postoperative wounds in particular can start bleeding again with life-threatening results. Because patients are discharged from hospitals more quickly these days than in the past and return home sooner after surgery, anticipate this potential complication.

Delayed Healing

* **serous fluid** a cellular component of blood, similar to plasma.

In some patients, the wound repair process may be delayed or even arrested, resulting in incomplete wound healing. Persons at greatest risk for this complication are diabetics, the elderly, the chronically ill, and the malnourished. Seriously or chronically infected wounds and those in locations with limited blood flow (distal extremities) are also at risk for incomplete healing. Incompletely healed wounds remain tender and are easily reinjured. A pale yellow or blood-tinged **serous fluid** may drain from them. Out-of-hospital treatment of incompletely healed wounds includes frequent changes of sterile, nonadherent dressings and protection of the wound.

Compartment Syndrome

* **compartment syndrome** muscle ischemia that is caused by rising pressures within an anatomical fascial space.

Compartment syndrome is a complication of closed and, occasionally, open wounds. In compartment syndrome, an extremity injury causes significant edema and swelling in the deep tissues. Because the extremity muscles are encapsulated in tough, inflexible fasciae, the swollen tissue has "nowhere to go," and the pressure in the compartment rises (Figure 20-14). When the pressure rises above 45 to 60 mmHg, the blood flow to that muscle group or compartment is compromised and ischemia ensues. If the condition continues for more than a few hours, irreversible damage and permanent disability may result. The muscle mass may die, and its contribution to limb function may be lost. Frequently, the resulting scar tissue shortens the length of the muscle strand and produces what is called Volkmann's contracture, thus further reducing the usefulness of the limb after compartment syndrome. All extremities may experience compartment syndrome, but the lower extremities, especially the calf, are at greatest risk because of their bulk and fascial anatomy.

Abnormal Scar Formation

* **keloid** a formation resulting from overproduction of scar tissue.

During the healing process, scar tissue sometimes develops abnormally. A **keloid** is excessive scar tissue that extends beyond the boundaries of a wound. It develops most commonly in darkly pigmented individuals and develops on the sternum, lower abdomen, upper extremities, and ears. Another healing abnormality

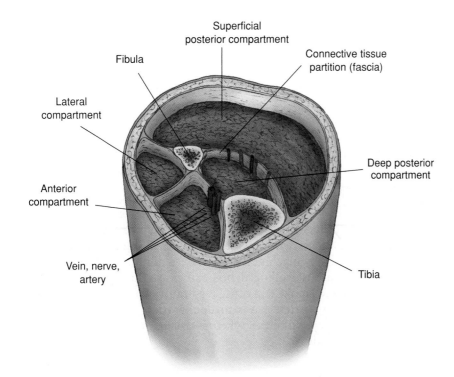

Superficial
posterior compartment

Fibula

Connective tissue
partition (fascia)

Lateral
compartment

Deep posterior
compartment

Anterior
compartment

Vein, nerve,
artery

Tibia

FIGURE 20-14   Musculoskeletal compartments segregated by fascia.

is hypertrophic scar formation. This is an excessive accumulation of scar tissue, usually within the injury border, that is often associated with dynamic skin tension lines, like those at flexion joints.

Pressure Injuries

A special type of soft-tissue injury is the pressure injury, which is caused by prolonged compression of the skin and tissues beneath. This may occur in the chronically ill (bed-ridden) patient, the patient who falls and remains unconscious for hours (due to alcohol intoxication, stroke, or drug overdose), or the patient who is entrapped with no crushing mechanism. The patient's weight against the ground or other surface compresses tissue and induces hypoxic injury. The injury is similar to a crush injury, although the mechanism is more passive and more likely to go unnoticed. Pressure injury may also occur when a long spine board, air splint, or rigid splint remains on a patient for an extended time.

Pressure injuries may occur if a long spine board or splint is left on a patient for an extended period.

CRUSH INJURY

Crush injury involves a trauma pattern in which body tissues are subjected to severe compressive forces. A crush injury can be relatively minor (for example, one that involves only a finger or part of an extremity) or it can be massive (one that affects much or all of the body). The mechanisms of injury can be varied. A packing machine might compress a worker's finger or extremity; a collapsed jack might trap a mechanic's leg under a car wheel; the seat and steering column might compress a driver's chest between them in an auto collision; or debris from a building collapse or trench cave-in might bury a construction worker.

A crush injury disrupts the body's tissues—muscles, blood vessels, bone, and, in some cases, internal organs. With such injuries, the skin may remain intact and the limb may appear normal in shape, or the skin may be severely cut and bruised and the extremity mangled and deformed. In both cases, however, the damage within is extensive. The injury often results in a large area of destruction with limited effective circulation, thus creating an excellent growth medium for bacteria. Hemorrhage with crush injuries may be difficult to control for several reasons: The actual source of the bleeding may be hard to identify; several large vessels may be damaged; and the general condition of the limb does not support effective application of direct pressure. The resulting tissue hypoxia and acidosis may result in muscle rigor, with muscles that may feel very hard and "wood-like" on palpation.

Associated Injury

When patients have been subjected to mechanisms that cause crush injuries, those mechanisms or others associated with them often result in additional injuries. For example, patients who have received crush injuries in building collapses or when entrapped by machinery may suffer additional fractures and open or closed soft-tissue injuries. Falling debris can cause direct injury, both blunt and penetrating. Dust and smoke can cause respiratory and eye injuries. Also, entrapment for any length of time leads to dehydration and hypothermia. You should consider all these possibilities when assessing and providing emergency care to victims of crush injury.

CRUSH SYNDROME

necrosis tissue death, usually from ischemia.

rhabdomyolysis acute disease that involves the destruction of skeletal muscle.

Crush syndrome occurs when body parts are entrapped for four hours or longer. Shorter periods of entrapment may result in direct body part damage, but they usually do not cause the broad, systemic complications of crush syndrome. The crushed skeletal muscle tissue undergoes **necrosis** and cellular changes with resultant release of metabolic byproducts. This degenerative process, called traumatic **rhabdomyolysis** (skeletal muscle disintegration), releases many toxins. Chief among these byproducts of cellular destruction are myoglobin (a muscle protein), phosphate and potassium (from cellular death), lactic acid (from anaerobic metabolism), and uric acid (from protein breakdown). These byproducts accumulate in the crushed body part but, because of the entrapment and the resulting minimal circulation through the injured tissue, do not reach the systemic circulation. Once the limb or victim is extricated and the pressure is released, however, the accumulated byproducts and toxins flood the central circulation.

High levels of myoglobin can lodge in the filtering tubules of the kidney, especially with patients who are in hypovolemic (shock) states, leading to renal failure, a leading cause of delayed death in crush syndrome. More immediate problems include hypovolemia and shock from the flow of sodium, chloride, and water into the damaged tissue. Increased blood potassium (hyperkalemia) can reduce the cardiac muscle's response to electrical stimuli, induce cardiac dysrhythmias, and lead to sudden death. Rising phosphate levels (hyperphosphatemia) can lead to abnormal calcifications in the vasculature and nervous system, compounding problems for the patient. In addition, as oxygenated circulation returns to the cells, the aerobic process by which uric acid is produced can operate again, thus increasing cellular acidity and injury.

INJECTION INJURY

A unique type of soft-tissue injury is the injection injury. A bursting high-pressure line, most commonly a hydraulic line, may inject fluid through a patient's skin and into the subcutaneous tissues. If the pressure is strong enough, the fluid may push between tissue layers and travel along the limb (Figure 20-15). The fluid thus

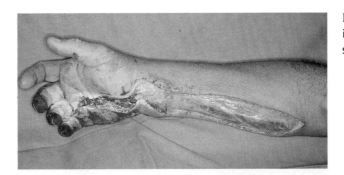

injected—for example, a petroleum-based hydraulic fluid—may then chemically damage the surrounding tissue. The body's repair mechanisms are unprepared to remove the great quantities of injected material, and the resulting damage is severe. A limb may be lost due to the direct physical damage from the injection process, the chemical damage done by the injected material, or the infection that develops after the injection.

DRESSING AND BANDAGE MATERIALS

There are several types of dressings and bandages that are effective in prehospital care. A dressing is the material placed directly on the wound to control bleeding and maintain wound cleanliness (Figure 20-16). A bandage is the material used to hold a dressing in place and to apply direct pressure to control hemorrhage (Figure 20-17). Dressings and bandages have various designs and are used for a variety of purposes in emergency care.

Sterile/Nonsterile Dressings

Sterile dressings are cotton or other fibre pads that have been specially prepared to be free of microorganisms. They are usually packaged individually and remain sterile for as long as the package is intact. Once the packaging is opened, sterile dressings become contaminated by airborne dust and particles that harbour

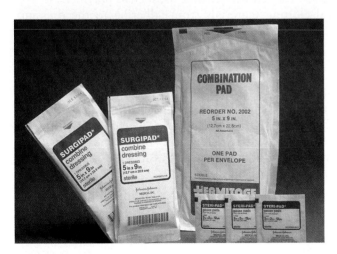

a. A variety of sterile dressings

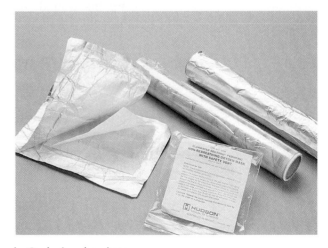

b. Occlusive dressings

FIGURE 20-16 Assorted dressings used in the care of soft-tissue injuries.

FIGURE 20-17   Kerlix, a type of self-adherent roller bandage.

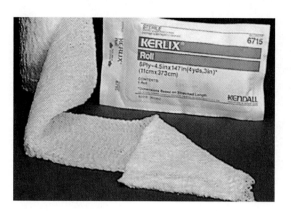

Content Review

TYPES OF BANDAGING AND DRESSING MATERIALS

Dressings
  Sterile/nonsterile
  Occlusive/nonocclusive
  Adherent/nonadherent
  Absorbent/nonabsorbent
  Wet/dry
Bandages
  Roller
  Gauze
  Adhesive
  Elastic
  Triangular

bacteria and other microorganisms. Sterile dressings are designed to be used in direct contact with wounds.

Nonsterile dressings are clean—that is, free of gross contamination—but are not free of microscopic contamination and microorganisms. Nonsterile dressings are not intended to be applied directly to a wound but, rather, to be placed over a sterile dressing to add bulk or absorptive power.

Occlusive/Nonocclusive Dressings

Some dressings, such as sterilized plastic wrap and petroleum-impregnated gauze, are designed to prevent the movement of fluid and air through them. These dressings are called occlusive and are helpful in preventing air aspiration into chest wounds (open pneumothorax) and open neck wounds (air emboli into the jugular vein). Most dressing material is nonocclusive.

Adherent/Nonadherent Dressings

Adherent dressings are untreated cotton or other fibre pads that will stick to drying blood and fluid that has leaked from open wounds. Adherent dressings have the advantage of promoting clot formation and thus reducing hemorrhage, but their removal from wounds can be quite painful. Removal or disturbance of an adherent dressing is also likely to break the clot and cause rebleeding. Nonadherent dressings are specially treated with chemicals, such as polymers, to prevent the wound fluids and clotting materials from adhering to the dressing. Nonadherent dressings are preferred for most uncomplicated wounds.

Absorbent/Nonabsorbent Dressings

Absorbent dressings readily soak up blood and other fluids, much as a sponge soaks up water. This property is helpful in many bleeding situations. Nonabsorbent dressings absorb little or no fluid and are used when a barrier to leaking is desired. The clear membrane dressings frequently placed over intravenous puncture sites are good examples of nonabsorbent dressings. Most other dressings used in prehospital care are absorbent dressings.

Wet/Dry Dressings

Wet dressings are sometimes applied to special types of wounds, such as burns. They are also used in the hospital to effect healing in some complicated postoperative wounds. Sterile normal saline is the usual fluid used to wet dressings. Wet dressings provide a medium for the movement of infectious material into wounds, however, and are not commonly used in prehospital care, except with such injuries as abdominal eviscerations or burns involving only a limited body surface area. Dry dressings are the type most often employed for wounds in prehospital care.

Self-adherent Roller Bandages

The most common and convenient bandage material is the soft, self-adherent, roller bandage (Kling or Kerlix). It has limited stretch and resists unravelling as it is rolled over itself. It conforms well to body contours and is quick and easy to use. This bandage is most appropriate for injuries located where it can be wrapped circumferentially. It comes in rolls from 2.5 to 15.25 cm wide.

Gauze Bandages

Like soft, self-adherent bandages, gauze bandages are a convenient material for securing dressings. They do not stretch, however, and thus do not conform as well to body contours as the self-adherent material, but they are otherwise functional for bandaging. Since gauze bandages do not stretch, they may increase the pressure associated with tissue swelling at injury sites. Gauze usually comes in rolls from 1.25 to 5 cm wide.

Adhesive Bandages

An adhesive bandage (or adhesive tape) is a strong plastic, paper, or fabric material with adhesive applied to one side. It can effectively secure a small dressing to a location where circumferential wrapping is impractical. When used circumferentially, an adhesive bandage does not allow for any swelling and permits pressure to accumulate in the tissues beneath it. Adhesive bandages usually come in widths that range from 0.6 to 7.6 cm.

Elastic (or Ace) Bandages

Elastic bandages stretch easily and conform to the body contours. Elastic bandages provide stability and support for minor musculoskeletal injuries, but they are not commonly used in prehospital care. When you do use these bandages, however, remember that it is very easy to apply too much pressure with them. Each consecutive wrap applied will contain and add to pressure on the wound site. Swelling associated with the wound may increase the pressure until blood flow through and out of the affected limb is reduced or stopped.

Triangular Bandages

Triangular bandages, or cravats, are large triangles of cotton fabric. They are strong, nonelastic bandages commonly used to make slings and swathes and, in some cases, to affix splints. They can also be used to hold dressings in place, but they do not conform as well to body contours as soft, self-adherent bandages and do not maintain pressure or immobilize wound dressings very well.

ASSESSMENT OF SOFT-TISSUE INJURIES

Proper evaluation of the skin can tell you more about the body's condition after trauma than any other aspect of patient assessment. Not only is the skin the first body organ to experience the effects of trauma, it is the first and often the only organ to display them. Therefore, assessment of the skin and its injury must be deliberate, careful, and complete. While the processes that cause soft-tissue

Wound assessment must be comprehensive to ensure that care of each injury can be assigned an appropriate priority.

injuries and the manifestations of those injuries vary, prehospital assessment is a simple, well-structured process. Follow the assessment process carefully and completely to ensure that you establish the nature and extent of each injury. Doing so enables you to assign soft-tissue injuries, and other injuries associated with them, the appropriate priorities for care.

Assessment of patients with soft-tissue wounds follows the same general progression as the assessment of other trauma patients. First, assess the scene, ruling out potential hazards, identifying the mechanism of injury, and determining the need for additional medical and rescue resources. Next, perform a quick primary assessment and identify and care for any immediately life-threatening injuries. For the patient with a mechanism of injury or signs and symptoms that suggest serious trauma, you will perform a rapid trauma assessment and use trauma triage criteria to determine the need for rapid transport. For a patient with no significant mechanism of injury and no indication from the primary assessment of a serious injury or life threat, perform a focused trauma assessment and gather vital signs and patient history at the scene. Perform a detailed secondary assessment only if conditions warrant and time permits. Provide serial ongoing assessments to track your patient's response to his injuries and your care.

SCENE ASSESSMENT

During the scene assessment, look for evidence that will help you determine the mechanism of injury and anticipate the likely injuries and their severity. While soft-tissue injuries are not usually life threatening, they can suggest other, serious life threats. Remember: No injury mechanism can affect the human body without first travelling through the skin. Identify where injury is likely, and be prepared to carefully examine the skin for evidence that suggests internal injury. Consider mechanisms of injury that could cause entrapment and either crush injury or crush syndrome.

No mechanism of injury can affect the human body without first passing through the skin.

Be alert to the fact that the mechanisms that injured the patient may still be present and pose threats to you and other rescuers. Rule out or eliminate any threats to yourself or fellow care providers before entering the scene (Figure 20-18).

Because trauma and injuries that penetrate the skin are likely to expose you to the hazards of contact with a patient's body fluids, don sterile gloves, and observe other body substance isolation procedures as you approach the patient. Recognize that arterial bleeding and hemorrhage associated with the airway can cause blood to splatter at the scene. If you suspect these injuries, don splash protection-wear for your eyes and clothing.

FIGURE 20-18 During the scene assessment, rule out hazards, utilize PPE, and analyze the mechanism of injury.

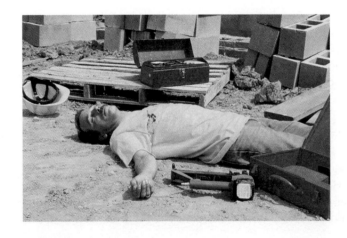

PRIMARY ASSESSMENT

Begin your primary assessment by establishing manual cervical in-line immobilization if you suspect significant head or spine injury and by forming a general impression of the patient. Determine the patient's level of consciousness, and assess the airway, breathing, and circulation. Assess perfusion by noting skin colour, temperature, and condition and by assessing capillary refill.

During this assessment, pay particular attention to the location and types of visible wounds to gain further understanding of the mechanism of injury and whether it produced blunt or penetrating trauma. If responsive, the patient may be able to give you critical information about how the wound occurred. If the patient is unable to speak, emergency medical responders or bystanders may be able to provide this information. Deal with any immediate threats to the patient's life as you discover them.

FOCUSED HISTORY AND SECONDARY ASSESSMENT

Use the information you have gathered through the primary assessment to determine how to proceed in the assessment process. Patients with serious trauma, suggested by a significant mechanism of injury or the findings of the primary assessment, will receive a rapid trauma assessment. All other patients will receive a focused trauma assessment.

Significant Mechanism of Injury—Rapid Trauma Assessment

In the rapid trauma assessment, you will perform a swift evaluation of the patient's head, neck, chest, abdomen, pelvis, extremities, and posterior body. Examine these areas for signs of internal or life-endangering injuries. Quickly investigate any discolorations, deformities, temperature variations, abnormal muscle tone, or open wounds.

Ensure that any wounds you discover or the injuries suggested beneath them do not involve or endanger the airway or breathing or contribute significantly to blood loss. Focus your immediate care during the rapid trauma assessment on continuing to ensure the patient's airway and breathing and then on controlling severe blood loss.

Inspect and palpate areas where the mechanism of injury suggests serious injuries may exist. Again, look for discoloration, temperature variation, abnormal muscle tone, and deformity suggestive of trauma (Figure 20-19). If the mechanism of injury suggests open wounds, sweep body areas hidden from sight with gloved

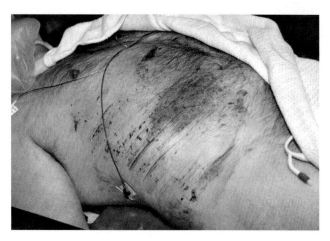

FIGURE 20-19   Often, the only signs of serious internal injury are external soft-tissue injuries.

hands; this will rule out the possibility of unseen blood loss and pooling. Control moderate to severe hemorrhage immediately. Hemorrhage control need not be definitive but should stop continuing significant blood loss. Once more serious injuries are cared for, you can return and dress and bandage wounds more carefully.

Survey bleeding wounds to determine the type of hemorrhage—arterial, venous, or capillary. Attempt to approximate the volume of blood lost since the time of the accident, which suggests the rate of blood loss.

Carry out your exam using the methods described in "Assessment Techniques" later in this chapter. Apply a cervical spinal immobilization collar once you have completed the rapid assessment of the head and neck. Continue to provide manual immobilization, however, until the patient is fully immobilized to a backboard.

When the rapid trauma assessment is complete, obtain a set of baseline vital signs and a patient history. Be sure to maintain manual in-line immobilization while the signs and history are being gathered. If you have enough personnel, the vital signs and history may be obtained simultaneously as the rapid trauma assessment is performed.

When obtaining the history, be sure to question the patient about medications, especially those that may have some direct relevance to soft-tissue injuries. For example, the patient's tetanus history is important with any penetrating trauma. Determine if the patient has had a tetanus booster and how long ago it was given. Note that a patient's routine use of aspirin or blood thinners—for example, heparin or warfarin for stroke or MI risk—may affect the body's ability to halt even minimal hemorrhage. Ask about use of anti-inflammatory medications, such as prednisone, because those medications reduce the inflammatory response and slow the normal healing process. Question the patient about any preexisting diseases. Note that certain diseases, especially HIV, AIDS, or anemia, increase the risks of infection and the problems of hemorrhage control.

At the conclusion of the rapid trauma assessment, confirm the decision either to transport the patient immediately with further care provided en route to the hospital or to remain at the scene and complete treatment of non-life-threatening injuries. Consider the rate and volume of any blood loss and any uncontrollable bleeding in this decision.

If your patient's condition merits care at the scene, prioritize the soft-tissue wounds you have identified to establish an order of care to follow. The few moments taken to sort out injuries and to plan the management process saves valuable time in the field. This also ensures that you provide early care for injuries with the highest priority.

No Significant Mechanism of Injury— Focused Trauma Assessment

When a patient has a soft-tissue injury but neither a significant mechanism of injury nor an indication of a serious problem from the primary assessment—for example, a cut finger or a knee abrasion from a fall—the sequence of assessment steps is different from that for a patient with a significant injury mechanism. Begin this phase of the assessment with a focused trauma assessment, which is an exam directed at the injury site—the finger or the knee in the examples noted above. A full head-to-toe rapid trauma assessment is not necessary in most such cases, but a primary assessment should be completed on every patient eventually.

Direct the focused assessment at the site of the chief complaint and any area of injury suggested by the mechanism of injury. Use the examination techniques of inquiry, inspection, and palpation (described below) to evaluate the injury and the surrounding area. In the case of a wound to an extremity, be sure to check the distal extremity for pulses, capillary refill, colour, and temperature. Then, obtain a set of baseline vital signs and a history from the patient. If any of your findings suggest the patient has more serious injuries, perform a rapid trauma assessment, and consider rapid transport.

DETAILED SECONDARY ASSESSMENT

Once the rapid or focused trauma assessment has been completed, vital signs and history gathered, and necessary emergency care steps have been taken, you may perform a detailed secondary assessment. Like the rapid trauma assessment, this head-to-toe evaluation of the skin (and the rest of the body) involves the techniques of inquiry, observation, and palpation. The detailed assessment should follow a planned and comprehensive process, ideally progressing from head to toe, although the order is not critical. The main purpose of the detailed assessment is to pick up any additional information regarding the patient's condition and to search for any unsuspected or subtle injuries. Manage any additional injuries you discover during the examination. The detailed secondary assessment is usually performed during transport, or on scene if transport has been delayed. Never delay transport to perform it, and only perform it if the patient's condition permits.

The detailed head-to-toe assessment should be performed at the scene only if significant and life-threatening bleeding can be ruled out.

ASSESSMENT TECHNIQUES

The assessment techniques described below can be used during both the rapid trauma assessment and the detailed secondary assessment.

Inquiry

Question the patient about the mechanism of injury, any pain, pain on touch or movement, and any loss of function or sensation specific to an area. Additionally, attempt to determine the exact nature of the pain or sensory or motor loss by using elements of the OPQRST mnemonic (see Chapter 7, "Patient Assessment in the Field"). Question the patient about signs and symptoms before touching an area.

Inspection

Continue the assessment by carefully observing a particular body region. Identify any discolorations, deformities, or open wounds in those regions.

Determine if any discoloration is local, distal, or systemic, reflecting local injury, circulation compromise, or systemic complications, such as shock. Contusions, blood vessel injuries, dislocations, and fractures may cause local discoloration, including erythema or ecchymosis. Distal discoloration may present as a pale, cyanotic, or ashen-coloured limb distal to the point of circulation loss. You may also notice systemic discoloration, such as pale, ashen, or greyish skin in all limbs, suggestive of hypovolemia and shock.

Examine any deformities you find to determine their cause. Is the deformity due to a developing hematoma, the normal swelling associated with the inflammatory process, or underlying injuries?

Inspect in detail any wounds you discover. Study the wound to determine its depth and evaluate its potential for damage to underlying muscles, nerves, blood vessels, organs, or bones. If possible, identify the object that caused the wound, and determine the amount of force transmitted by it to the body's interior. Ascertain if there are any foreign bodies, contamination, or impaled objects in the wound. Finally, identify the nature and location of any hemorrhage.

Observe each wound carefully so that you can describe it to the attending physician after you dress and bandage the injury. This information will help the emergency department staff prioritize the patient's injuries. Careful observation

The wound should be observed in such a way that it can later be described to the attending physician.

will also aid you in preparation of your prehospital care report. Adequate lighting is crucial for evaluating wounds. If necessary, defer this portion of the detailed secondary assessment until better lighting is available, as in the back of the ambulance.

If a patient's limb or digit has been amputated, have other rescuers conduct a brief but thorough search for the amputated part. If the part cannot be located immediately or remains entrapped, do not delay patient transport. Instead, leave someone at the scene to continue the search. Ensure that once the body part is retrieved, it is properly handled, packaged, and brought to the same hospital as the patient.

Palpation

In addition to questioning the patient and inspecting the body regions, you should palpate the body's entire surface. Be alert for any deformity, asymmetry, temperature variation, unexpected mass, or localized loss of skin or muscle tone. Gently palpate all apparent closed wounds for evidence of tenderness, swelling, crepitus, and subcutaneous emphysema. Avoid palpating the interior of open wounds, which may introduce contamination and disturb the clotting process. Ascertain the presence or absence of distal pulses and capillary refill time with any extremity injury. Also, check motor and sensory functions distal to any extremity wound and compare the findings with those from the opposite limb.

ONGOING ASSESSMENT

During transport, provide an ongoing assessment, reassessing the patient's mental status, airway, breathing, and circulation, gathering additional sets of vital signs, and evaluating the sites of the patient's injuries. Also, inspect any interventions you have performed. Provide an ongoing assessment at least every five minutes with unstable patients and every 15 minutes with stable patients. If you note any change in the patient's condition, modify your priorities for transport and care accordingly.

MANAGEMENT OF SOFT-TISSUE INJURY

The management of minor wounds is a late priority in the care of the trauma patient unless extensive bleeding is noted.

Once you complete your patient assessment, take steps to manage the soft-tissue injury, either in the field or en route to the hospital. Control of blood loss, prevention of shock, and decontamination of affected areas take priority. The following sections describe some of the most important of these care steps.

Unless you note extensive bleeding, wound management by dressing and bandaging is a late priority in the care of trauma patients. Dress and bandage wounds whose bleeding does not represent a life threat only after you stabilize your patient by caring for higher priority injuries.

OBJECTIVES OF WOUND DRESSING AND BANDAGING

The three objectives of bandaging are to control hemorrhage, keep the wound clean, and immobilize the wound site.

The dressing and bandaging of a wound has three basic objectives. These are to control all hemorrhaging, keep the wound as clean as possible, and immobilize the wound (Procedure 20-1). The appearance of the final dressing and bandage is not as critical as achievement of these three objectives.

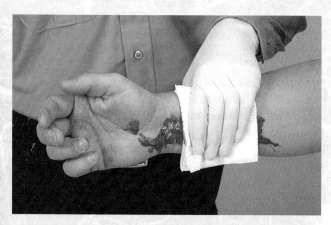

20-1a   Apply direct pressure with a dressing to the site of hemorrhage.

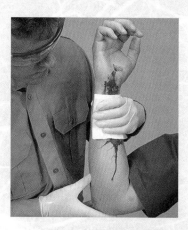

20-1b   Elevate the hemorrhage site if there is no serious musculoskeletal injury.

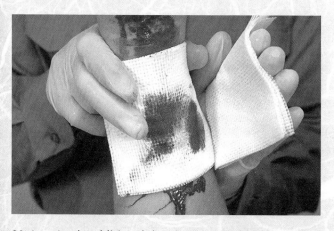

20-1c   Apply additional dressings as needed.

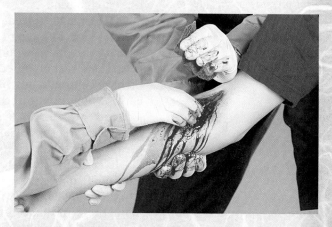

20-1d   If serious hemorrhage persists, expose the wound, and place digital pressure with a gloved hand on the site of bleeding.

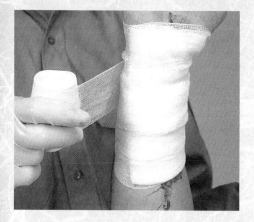

20-1e   Bandage the dressing in place, maintaining pressure on the wound.

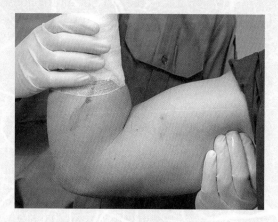

20-1f   Apply digital pressure to a proximal artery if the hemorrhage persists.

Hemorrhage Control

The primary method—and the most effective one—of controlling hemorrhage associated with soft-tissue injury is direct pressure. In cases of serious hemorrhage flowing from a wound with some force, place a small dressing directly over the site of the bleeding, and apply pressure directly to it with a finger. When the bleeding is the more commonly encountered slow-to-moderate type, use a dressing that has been sized to cover and pad the wound. Then, simply wrap the dressing with a soft, self-adherent bandage using moderate pressure to halt the blood loss. Monitor the wound frequently to ensure bleeding has stopped.

Elevation can assist in the control of hemorrhage, although it is generally not as effective as direct pressure. Elevation reduces arterial pressure in the extremity and increases venous return. Elevation can thus reduce edema and increase blood flow through the wound and injured extremity. This promotes good oxygenation and wound healing. Do not elevate a limb, however, if doing so will cause any further harm as would be the case if the patient has a suspected spinal or associated musculoskeletal injury or if there is an object impaled in the limb.

Use pressure points to assist with bleeding control and the clotting process when direct pressure and elevation together do not control it. Locate a pulse point immediately proximal to the wound and above a bony prominence. Apply firm pressure and maintain it for at least 10 minutes. Ensure that the hemorrhage does not continue.

Occasionally, bleeding from a soft-tissue injury can be difficult to control. If the bleeding continues despite the use of direct pressure, elevation, and pressure points, reassess the wound to be sure you have determined the exact site of blood loss. Then, reapply direct digital pressure to that precise point. Too often, hemorrhage continues because the bandaging technique distributes pressure over the entire wound site, rather than focusing it directly on the source of the bleeding. The force driving the hemorrhage is no greater than the patient's systolic blood pressure, and properly applied digital pressure can thus easily provide a pressure greater than this to compress the vessel and halt any blood loss.

In certain circumstances, the use of direct pressure, elevation, and a pressure point may not control hemorrhage. Crush injuries and amputations are situations in which normal bleeding control measures are often ineffective. With these traumatic injuries, several blood vessels are jaggedly torn, confounding the body's normal hemorrhage control mechanisms and making it difficult to pinpoint the source of bleeding. Even if the source of bleeding can be found, applying firm direct pressure to it may be difficult. In such cases, the application of a tourniquet may be useful. The tourniquet should be considered the last option for controlling hemorrhage. If properly applied, the tourniquet will stop the flow of blood; however, its use has serious associated risks. Keep the following precautions in mind whenever you consider using a tourniquet.

1. If the pressure applied is insufficient, the tourniquet may halt venous return while permitting continued arterial blood flow into the extremity, increasing the rate and volume of blood loss.

2. When the tourniquet is applied properly, the entire limb distal to the device is without circulation. Hypoxia, ischemia, and necrosis may permanently damage the tissue distal to the tourniquet.

3. When circulation is restored, the blood flows and pools in the extremity, adding to any hypovolemia. In addition, any blood that returns to the central circulation is highly hypoxic, acidic, and toxic. This blood can cause shock, lethal dysrhythmias, renal failure, and death. The return of circulation may also restart hemorrhage and introduce emboli into the central circulation.

A combination of techniques for hemorrhage control may be effective when bleeding is resistant to direct pressure.

To halt hemorrhage, apply firm pressure to the site for at least 10 minutes.

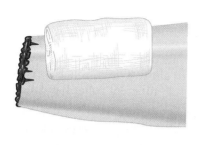

a. Place a bulky dressing over the distal artery.

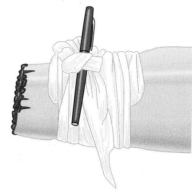

b. Apply a pressure exceeding the systolic pressure.

FIGURE 20-20 The steps of tourniquet application.

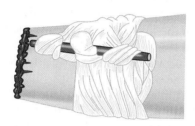

c. Secure the tourniquet, and monitor the wound site for continuing hemorrhage.

Do not use a tourniquet unless you cannot control severe bleeding by any other means. Place it just proximal to the wound site, but stay away from the elbow or knee joints (Figure 20-20). Apply the tourniquet in a way that will not injure the tissue beneath. For example, do not use very narrow material, like rope or wire, for a tourniquet; applying great pressure to a limb with such material may cause serious injury in the compressed tissue. Instead, select a two-inch or wider band for compression.

A readily available, effective, and easily controllable tourniquet is the sphygmomanometer (regular for the upper extremity and thigh for the lower). It is wide, simple to apply, rapid to inflate, and easy to monitor. Inflate it to a pressure 30 mmHg above the patient's systolic blood pressure and beyond the pressure at which the patient's hemorrhage ceases.

Once you apply a tourniquet, leave it in place until the patient arrives at the emergency department. Monitor the tourniquet during transport to ensure that it does not lose pressure, and watch for signs of renewed bleeding. If bleeding starts again, increase the tourniquet pressure. Alert the hospital staff to your use of the tourniquet during transport as well as upon arrival. Mark the patient's forehead clearly with the letters "TQ," and note the time the tourniquet was applied.

Do not release a tourniquet in the field, except under exceptional circumstances and then only during consultation with medical direction. Be prepared to provide vigorous fluid resuscitation, ECG monitoring, dysrhythmia treatment, and rapid transport if a tourniquet release is attempted.

Do not use a tourniquet unless you cannot control bleeding by any other means.

Once applied, a tourniquet should be left in place until the patient arrives at the emergency department.

Sterility

Once you halt severe bleeding, keep the wound as sterile as possible. Under field conditions, this may simply mean keeping the wound as clean as reasonably possible. With very small open wounds, like an IV start or a small laceration, you may consider the application of an antibacterial ointment to help with infection control. However, the effectiveness of such ointments on larger wounds is limited, and ointments are not generally applied to these wounds.

Under normal conditions, you need not cleanse the wound. If a wound is grossly contaminated, however, irrigate it with normal saline or Ringer's Lactate solution. A 1000-mL bag of saline, connected to a macrodrip administration set and pressurized by squeezing the bag under your arm, may allow rapid and gentle wound cleansing. Try to move any contamination from the centre of the wound outward. You may also carefully remove larger particles—glass, gravel, debris, and so forth—if you can do this swiftly and without inducing further injury.

Apply a bandage to make the dressing appear as neat as time and the conditions under which you are working will allow. Often, this is as easy as covering the entire dressing with wraps of soft, self-adherent roller bandage. The neat appearance calms and reassures the patient, while the bandaging reduces contamination and the chances of posttrauma infection.

Immobilization

Immobilization is an important, but frequently overlooked, component of hemorrhage control.

The last objective of bandaging is immobilization. The stability of the wound site helps the natural clotting mechanisms operate and reduces the patient's discomfort. Maintaining gentle pressure with the bandage may reduce pain and local swelling. Immobilize the limb with bandaging material to the patient's body or to a rigid surface, such as a padded board or ladder splint.

When immobilizing a limb, do not use elastic bandaging material or apply the bandage too tightly. The edema that develops rapidly with an injury puts increasing pressure on underlying tissue. This pressure may quickly reduce or halt circulation.

Frequently monitor any limb that you bandage circumferentially to ensure that the distal pulse remains strong and that the distal extremity maintains good colour and does not swell. If you cannot locate the distal pulse, monitor capillary refill, skin colour, and temperature. If signs or symptoms suggest that the distal circulation is compromised, elevate the extremity, if possible, and check and consider loosening the bandage.

Pain and Edema Control

Treat painful soft-tissue injuries or those likely to cause large debilitating edema with the application of cold packs and moderate-pressure bandages. Cold reduces inflammatory response and local edema. It also dulls the pain associated with serious soft-tissue trauma. Use a commercial cold pack or ice in a plastic bag wrapped in a dry towel and apply it to the wound. Do not use a cold pack directly against the skin as it cools beyond any therapeutic value. Direct application of a cold pack may also cause tissue freezing, especially in areas with reduced circulation.

Some moderate pressure over the wound area may also help reduce pain and wound edema. In cases where the patient reports severe pain, consider use of morphine sulphate or other analgesics for patient comfort. Administer morphine in 2-mg increments titrated to pain relief every five minutes (up to a total of 10 mg).

ANATOMICAL CONSIDERATIONS FOR BANDAGING

Each area of the body has specific anatomical characteristics. Your application of bandages and dressings should take these characteristics into account to provide effective prehospital wound care (Figure 20-21).

Scalp

The scalp has a rich supply of vessels that can bleed heavily when injured. It is commonly said that head wounds rarely account for shock, but scalp hemorrhage can be severe, difficult to control, and lead to the loss of moderate to large volumes of blood.

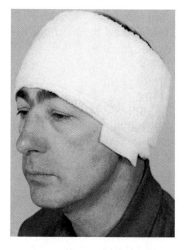

a. Head and/or ear bandage

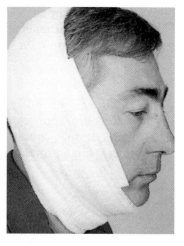

b. Cheek and ear bandage
(be sure mouth will open)

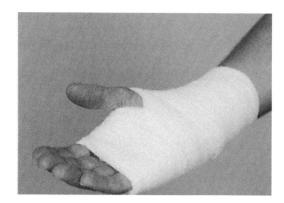

c. Hand bandage

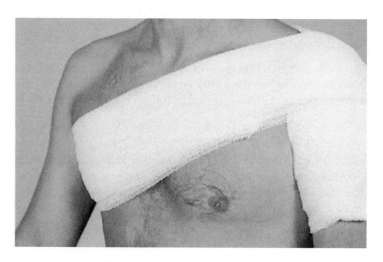

d. Shoulder bandage

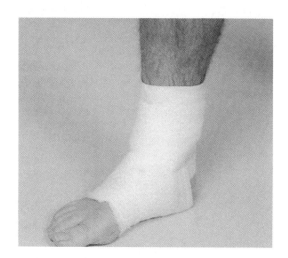

e. Foot and/or ankle bandage

FIGURE 20-21   Good bandaging uses the natural body curves and the self-adherent characteristics of bandages to hold dressings firmly in place.

In scalp hemorrhage uncomplicated by skull fracture, direct pressure against the skull is effective in the control of bleeding. To hold a dressing in place and maintain pressure, wrap a bandage around the head, capturing the occiput or brow or, in some cases, passing the bandage under the chin (while still allowing for jaw movement).

If a head wound is complicated by fracture, be very careful in your application of pressure. Apply gentle digital pressure around the wound and attempt to locate the small scalp arteries that feed it to use as pressure points. Then, simply hold a dressing on the wound without much pressure.

Face

Facial wounds are frequently gruesome and bleed heavily. Gentle direct pressure to these wounds can effectively control hemorrhage. You can maintain this pressure by wrapping a bandage around the head. Be careful to ensure a clear airway, and use your bandaging to splint any facial instability.

Remember, blood is a gastric irritant and swallowed blood may induce emesis. Be ready to provide suctioning in patients with oral or nasal hemorrhage because unexpected emesis may compromise the airway.

Ear or Mastoid

Wounds to the ear region can be easily bandaged by wrapping the head circumferentially. Use open gauze to collect, not stop, any bleeding or fluids flowing from the ear canal. These materials may contain cerebrospinal fluid, and halting their flow may add to any increasing intracranial pressure.

Neck

Minor neck wounds may be lightly wrapped circumferentially with bandages or taped to hold dressings in place. If bleeding is moderate to severe, however, direct manual pressure may be necessary because the amount of pressure applied by circumferential wrapping may compromise both the airway and circulation to and from the head. In cases of large wounds or moderate to severe bleeding, also consider using an occlusive dressing to prevent aspiration of air into a jugular vein.

Shoulder

The shoulder is an easy area to bandage as soft, self-adherent roller bandages readily conform to body contours. Use the axilla, arm, and neck as points of fixation, but be careful not to put pressure on the anterior neck and trachea.

Trunk

For minor trunk wounds, adhesive tape may be sufficient to hold dressings in place. With larger wounds, bandaging can be more difficult because you must wrap the patient's body circumferentially to apply direct pressure to a wound. Applying a bandage in this way may require moving the patient unnecessarily and risk causing or worsening an injury.

Groin and Hip

The groin and the hip are easy places to affix a dressing. Bandage by following the contours of the upper thighs and waist, similar to the technique of bandaging a shoulder. Be careful here, though. Any movement of the patient is likely to affect the tightness of the bandage and the amount of pressure over the dressing. With these injuries, therefore, apply the bandage after the patient is in final position for transport.

Elbow and Knee

Joints, especially the elbow and knee, are difficult to bandage. Bandage using circumferential wraps, and then splint the area to ensure that the bandage does not loosen with movement. If possible, place the joint in a position halfway between flexion and extension. This position, called the position of function, relaxes the muscles controlling the joint and the skin tension lines and is most comfortable for the patient during long transports or periods of immobilization.

Hand and Finger

Hand and finger injuries are easy to bandage by simple circumferential wrapping. Again, consider placing the hand or digit in the position of function, halfway between flexion and extension. Accomplish this by placing a large, bulky dressing in the palm of the patient's hand and then wrapping around it. You may use a malleable finger splint to obtain the position of function and then wrap circumferentially to splint the finger.

Ankle and Foot

Ankle and foot wounds are also easy to bandage by wrapping circumferentially and by using the natural body contours. If strong direct pressure is needed to maintain hemorrhage control, start your wrapping from the toes, and work proximally. This ensures that the pressure of bandaging does not form a venous tourniquet and compromise circulation to this very distal injury.

COMPLICATIONS OF BANDAGING

Bandaging can lead to some complications, although such occurrences are infrequent. If a bandage—particularly a circumferential bandage—is too tight, the area beneath it may continue to swell, increasing pressure in the area of the wound. This can lead to decreased blood flow and ischemia distal to the bandage. Pressure can build to such an extreme that the bandage acts like a tourniquet. Pain, pallor, tingling, loss of pulses, and prolonged capillary refill time are typical signs of developing pressure and ischemia. Avoid this complication by making bandages snug but not too tight. A useful technique is to wrap a bandage only so tight that one finger can still be easily slipped beneath it.

Bandages and dressings left on too long can become soaked with blood and body fluids and then serve as incubators for infection. This problem usually takes at least two to three days to develop and is not a common concern in most prehospital settings.

The size of the dressing is an important consideration in bandaging. An unnecessarily large and bulky dressing can prevent proper inspection of a wound and hide contamination and continued serious bleeding. Too small a dressing can become lost in a wound and become, in effect, a foreign body. This is most frequently a problem with large, gaping wounds and deep wounds that penetrate the thoracic or abdominal cavities. When dressing a wound, choose a dressing just larger than the wound but not so small as to become lost in it.

Frequently check the pressure beneath a bandage to ensure good distal circulation.

CARE OF SPECIFIC WOUNDS

Some circumstances—amputations, impalements, and crush syndrome cases—deserve special attention during the patient management process. These injuries can challenge even the seasoned paramedic to provide the most appropriate care.

Amputations

Amputations may bleed either heavily or minimally. Attempt to control hemorrhage with direct pressure by applying a large, bulky dressing to the wound. If this fails to control hemorrhage, consider using a tourniquet just above the point of severance. If there is a crush wound associated with the limb loss, apply the tourniquet just above the crushed area. Do not delay patient transport while locating or extricating the amputated body part. Transport the patient immediately, and then have other personnel transport the part once it is located or released from entrapment.

Current recommendations for managing separated body parts include dry cooling and rapid transport. Place the amputated part in a plastic bag, and immerse the bag in cold water (Figure 20-22). The water may have a few ice cubes

Current recommendations for managing amputated body parts include dry cooling and rapid transport.

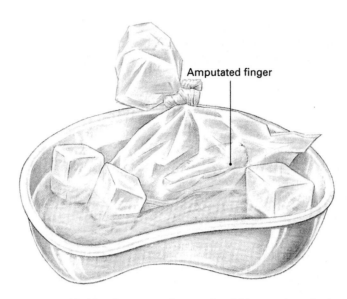

FIGURE 20-22   Amputated parts should be put in a dry bag, sealed, and placed in cool water that contains a few ice cubes.

in it, but avoid direct contact between the ice and the injured part. Even if the amputated part cannot be totally reattached, skin from it may be used to cover the limb end (Figure 20-23).

Impaled Objects

Do not remove impaled objects because of the risk of serious, uncontrollable bleeding.

When possible, immobilize all impaled objects in place (Figure 20-24). Position bulky dressings around the object to stabilize it, and tape over the dressings to hold them in place. Try to make movement of the patient to the ambulance and transport to the emergency department as smooth and nonjarring as possible. Remember that any movement of the impaled object is likely to cause continued internal bleeding and additional tissue damage.

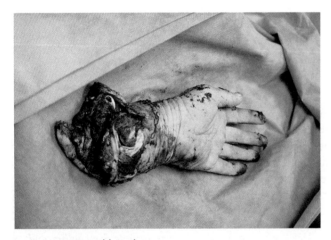

a. An amputated hand

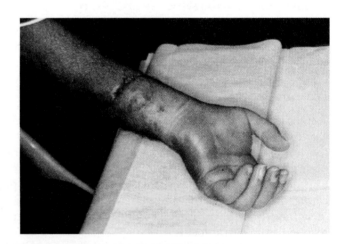

b. A successfully reimplanted hand

FIGURE 20-23   Amputated parts should be located and transported with the patient to the hospital for possible reattachment.

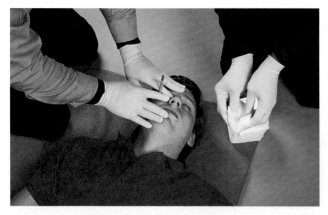

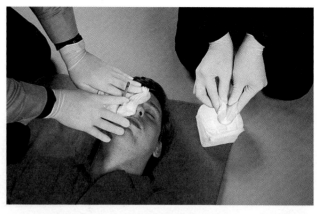

a. Manually stabilize any impaled object.

b. Use bulky padding or dressing to immobilize the object.

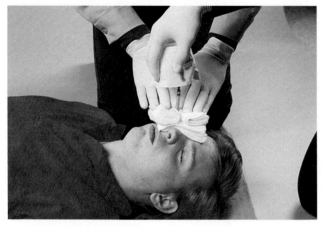

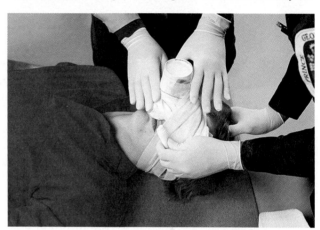

c. If the object protrudes, cover it with a paper cup.

d. Bandage the cup and padding securely in place.

FIGURE 20-24　Stabilization of an impaled object.

If the impaled object is too large to transport or is affixed to something that cannot be moved, such as a reinforcing rod set in concrete, consider cutting it. Use appropriate techniques and tools depending on the circumstances of the impalement. A hand or power saw, an acetylene torch, or bolt cutters might be employed. Whatever tools and techniques are used, be sure to take steps to limit the heat, vibration, or jolting transmitted to the patient. Provide the best possible support for both the object and the patient during the cutting procedure.

There are some special circumstances in which you *should* remove an impaled object. For example, you may remove an object impaled in the cheek if the removal is necessary to maintain a patent airway (Figure 20-25). In this case, be prepared to apply direct pressure to the wound both from inside the cheek (intraorally) and externally.

Another object that would require removal is one impaled in the central chest or back of a patient who needs cardiopulmonary resusatation (CPR). In such a circumstance, the risk associated with not performing resuscitation outweighs the risk of removing the object. Be aware, however, that a trauma patient who needs CPR has a very poor prognosis.

Another complication associated with an impaled object occurs when a patient is impaled on an object that cannot be cut or moved. In such a case, contact medical direction for advice and guidance. If the object is impaled in a limb, bleeding may be controllable. If it has entered the head, neck, chest, or abdomen, it may not be.

Only remove impaled objects that obstruct the airway or prevent CPR.

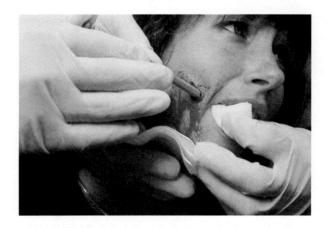

FIGURE 20-25 Objects impaled in the cheek may be removed because the sites of hemorrhage can be controlled and the object may interfere with airway control.

Crush Syndrome

The key to successful prehospital management of a crush syndrome patient is anticipation of the problem and prevention of its effects. Since, by definition, all crush syndrome patients are victims of prolonged entrapment, cases can be identified before extrication is complete. The focus of prehospital crush injury care is on rapid transport, adequate fluid resuscitation, diuresis, and—possibly—systemic alkalinization.

The prehospital approach to crush syndrome is similar to that with other trauma patients. Ensuring scene safety is particularly important in these cases. Crush syndrome victims are often buried in heavy rubble or other large debris, and access may be difficult (Figure 20-26). You may need to request the assistance of specialized personnel and their equipment—urban search and rescue teams, or trench, heavy, or confined space rescue teams. Never place yourself or other rescuers in unreasonable danger when providing care or attempting a rescue.

Once the scene is safe and you can reach the patient, conduct a primary assessment. Remove debris from around the head, neck, and thorax to minimize airway obstruction and restriction of ventilation. Control any reachable and obvious bleeding. Perform as much of the initial and rapid trauma assessment as possible, keeping in mind that portions of the patient's body will be inaccessible as a result of the entrapment. The dark, dusty, and cramped conditions of many confined spaces may force you to improvise. Be alert for signs and symptoms of associated injuries, such as dust inhalation, dehydration, and hypothermia.

Remember that the greater the body area compressed and the longer the time of entrapment, the greater is the risk of crush syndrome. Initially, a trapped pa-

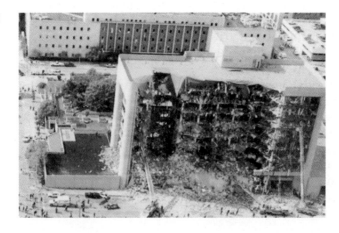

FIGURE 20-26 Explosion and structural collapse frequently produce crush injury and crush syndrome.

tient will usually complain only of entrapment symptoms: pain, lack of motor function, tingling, or loss of sensation in the affected limb. The patient may also experience flaccid paralysis and sensory loss in the limb unrelated to the normal distribution of peripheral nerve control and sensation.

As long as the body part is still trapped and the metabolic byproducts of the crush injury are confined to the entrapped part, the patient will not experience the full effects of crush syndrome. With extrication, however, toxic byproducts are released into the circulation, and the patient may rapidly develop shock and die. If the patient survives the initial release of the byproducts, he remains at great risk of developing renal failure with serious morbidity or delayed death. Note, too, that a crush injury may also induce compartment syndrome (explained below), especially with prolonged entrapment.

Once you have ensured the patient's ABCs, turn your attention to obtaining IV access. Intravenous fluids and selected medications are important in treating crush syndrome. Initiate two large-bore IVs if possible. Because of the entrapment, it may be necessary to consider alternative IV sites, such as the external jugular vein or the veins of a lower extremity. Avoid any site distal to a crush injury.

When you encounter crush syndrome, it is unlikely that your protocols will address it fully. Contact the trauma centre for medical direction and communicate, online, with the emergency physician. Expect to provide frequent vital sign and patient updates, and be prepared to administer large fluid volumes and, possibly, alkalizing agents.

Base hospital physicians may order an infusion of 1000 to 1500 mL (20–30 mL/kg) of normal saline or, more ideally, 5 percent dextrose in 0.5 normal saline, even in a patient not yet showing signs of shock. Avoid Ringer's Lactate or other solutions containing potassium. Then, infuse solution at a rate of 1000 mL/h (20 mL/kg/h) for as long as the patient remains trapped (up to 12 litres in 24 hours). Continue this infusion rate until the patient reaches the hospital. As with all patients receiving large volumes of crystalloids, periodically query the patient for symptoms of shortness of breath, and auscultate the lungs for evidence of pulmonary edema (e.g., crackles). Stop or reduce the fluid flow rate if you suspect pulmonary edema. In young, healthy adults and children, this rarely occurs at the fluid flow rates described here.

Alkalinization of the blood and urine is a consideration for preventing and treating crush syndrome. In combination with fluid resuscitation, alkalinization can correct acidosis, help prevent renal failure, and help correct hyperkalemia. Sodium bicarbonate 1 mEq/kg initially, followed by 0.25 mEq/kg/h thereafter, may be administered according to protocol. It is preferable to add the bicarbonate to the normal saline bag, rather than administering it as a bolus or IV push.

Diuretics may help keep the kidneys well perfused and more resistant to failure during crush syndrome. Mannitol, an osmotic diuretic, is the drug of choice as it draws interstitial fluid into the vascular space and eliminates it as mannitol is excreted by the kidneys. Furosemide, a loop diuretic, inhibits the reabsorption of both sodium and chloride. Its use is not advisable in hypovolemic states because it may add to the electrolyte imbalance. These treatments will reflect critical care or advanced care paramedic status.

Consider applying a tourniquet before the entrapping pressure is released if you have been unable to medicate the patient and provide fluid resuscitation. The tourniquet will sequester the toxins and prevent reperfusion injury. Tourniquet use, however, will continue the development of crush syndrome and worsen its effects.

In cases where the entrapping object may not be moved for many hours or days, medical direction may consider field amputation. This operation is mostly performed by a physician responding to the scene.

Cardiac (ECG) monitoring is important with all crush syndrome patients. Dysrhythmias may develop at any time but are most likely to occur immediately

Note: The milliequivalent (mEq) is a means of measuring electrolytes in a standard solution and is based on the molecular weight of the electrolyte in question.

following the release of pressure on patient extrication. Sudden cardiac arrest should be treated in the usual fashion with defibrillation. As the critical care paramedic, consider 500 mg calcium chloride IV push (in addition to the sodium bicarbonate) to counter life-threatening dysrhythmias induced by hyperkalemia. Watch for the tenting, or peaking, of the T-wave, a prolonged P-R interval, and S-T segment depression. Be sure to flush the IV line between infusions or to use fresh lines because calcium chloride and sodium bicarbonate tend to precipitate.

Once the patient is freed from entrapment, be prepared to treat rapidly progressing shock. Continue the normal saline infusions at 20 mL/kg/h. Rapidly transport the patient to an appropriate hospital (usually a trauma centre) in all cases of suspected crush syndrome.

Prehospital care of the crushed limb or body parts requires no special techniques. Cover open wounds, and splint fractures, keeping in mind that progressive swelling will necessitate ongoing reassessment, with monitoring of distal circulation and the tightness of bandages, straps, and splints. Handle all crushed limbs gently because the ischemic tissue is prone to injury. Elevation of severely crushed extremities is not indicated in the prehospital setting.

Care at the hospital for crush injury is aggressive and may use such techniques as débridement and hyperbaric oxygenation. During hyperbaric oxygenation, the patient is placed in a chamber containing artificially high concentrations of oxygen under several atmospheres of pressure. This pressure drives oxygen into poorly oxygenated tissue to help with the destruction of anaerobic bacteria and to increase tissue oxygenation for repair and regeneration, ultimately reducing tissue necrosis and edema. Hyperbaric oxygenation is most effective when provided early in the course of care.

Hospital care for crush injuries also includes administration of several medications as well as hemodialysis to help salvage the kidneys from the ravages of myoglobin and other toxic agents. Allopurinol, a xanthine oxidase inhibitor, interferes with the production of uric acid, a byproduct of skeletal muscle destruction, and may help reperfusion of both the kidneys and the skeletal muscles. It is most effective if administered immediately before release of the compression. Amiloride hydrochloride is a potassium-sparing diuretic that inhibits the sodium/calcium exchange. Mannitol, tetanus toxoid, and prophylactic antibiotics may also be administered in the hospital to treat crush syndrome.

Compartment Syndrome

The most prominent symptom of compartment syndrome is severe pain, often disproportionate to the physical findings. Other signs are often subtle or absent, or they may be overshadowed by the original injury, such as a fracture or contusion. Some people suggest using the six Ps—pain, paresthesia, pallor, pressure, paralysis, pulselessness—to identify compartment syndrome, but many of these signs are not dependable, or they appear very late in the course of the injury. Motor and sensory functions are usually normal with compartment syndrome, as are distal pulses. Even capillary refill shows little change. It is important to note that compartment syndrome rarely occurs within the first four hours after an acute injury. It is more likely to appear six to eight hours (or as much as a day or more) after the initial injury. Recognition of compartment syndrome can be challenging and requires a healthy suspicion of the problem.

The first step in prehospital treatment for compartment syndrome is care of the underlying injury. Splint and immobilize all suspected fractures, and use traction as appropriate for femur fractures. Apply cold packs to severe contusions. Elevation of the affected extremity is the single most effective prehospital treatment for compartment syndrome. This reduces edema, increases venous return,

Once the crush injury patient is freed from entrapment, anticipate the rapid development of shock.

The most prominent symptom of compartment syndrome is pain disproportionate to the physical findings.

lowers compartment pressure, and helps prevent ischemia. In the hospital, compartment syndrome is treated surgically, through fasciectomy, a procedure that incises the restrictive fascia.

SPECIAL ANATOMICAL SITES

Several anatomical sites pose challenges to care of soft-tissue injuries. These include the face and neck, the thorax, and the abdomen.

Face and Neck

Soft-tissue injuries to the face and neck present potential challenges owing to the anatomical relationships of the airway and great vessels. Injuries to the face may result in blood and tissue debris in the airway, posing risks of airway obstruction, asphyxia, and aspiration (Figure 20-27). Pooled secretions and tissue edema may add to airway problems. Trauma to the face or neck may also distort the anatomical structures of the upper airway, leading to airway compromise and complicating attempts at endotracheal intubation.

Emergency treatment of face and neck injuries can be challenging and may tax your skills. First, gain control of the airway. Open the airway using manual manoeuvres. If you suspect the possibility of spinal injury, use the jaw-thrust manoeuvre in conjunction with in-line manual immobilization. Aggressively suction blood, saliva, and debris from the pharynx, but avoid stimulating the gag reflex in the patient or inducing emesis. Insert an oro- or nasopharyngeal airway as needed.

Visualized endotracheal intubation is the gold standard for securing the airway, but achieving it is fraught with complications in cases of face and neck trauma. Secretions and blood may prevent adequate visualization, even with aggressive suctioning. Airway edema can distort the anatomy beyond recognition and even prevent passage of the endotracheal tube. In all cases, meticulous and absolute ascertainment of tube placement is mandatory to avoid fatal hypoxia.

Although not routinely used by paramedics in Canada, in desperate circumstances, needle cricothyrostomy or surgical cricothyrotomy may be life saving. Avoid placing the needle or making the incision through neck hematomas to avoid life-threatening bleeding.

Once you have secured the airway, focus your attention on any serious bleeding from the face or neck. Direct pressure is usually successful for bleeding control, but be certain to avoid compressing or occluding the airway. Pressure points and tourniquets should not be used because of the risks of cerebral ischemia and strangulation. Open neck wounds also carry the danger of air aspiration and emboli. Cover any open neck wound with an occlusive dressing, which should then be held or bandaged firmly in place. Because of the neck's anatomy, you may have to maintain digital pressure throughout the course of prehospital care to ensure effective bleeding control.

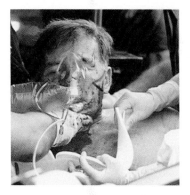

FIGURE 20-27 Severe facial soft-tissue injuries may interfere with airway control and distort landmarks used for intubation.

Thorax

Superficial soft-tissue injury to the thorax may suggest more serious intrathoracic injuries. The pleural space extends superiorly to the supraclavicular fossa and inferiorly to include the entire rib cage both anteriorly and posteriorly. Trauma to this area is likely to injure both the pleura and lungs. Small "lacerations" may actually be deep, penetrating stab or gunshot wounds with resultant hemothorax, pneumothorax, pericardial tamponade, penetrating trauma to the heart, or injury to the great vessels, esophagus, bronchi, or diaphragm. A seemingly minor "rib bruise" may be the only visible sign of serious lung or cardiac contusions beneath.

Perform a thorough secondary assessment to detect any signs of internal bleeding, pulmonary edema, dysrhythmias, or shock. However, never explore a thoracic wound beyond the skin edges. Probing deeper can convert a minor wound to a pneumothorax or a bleeding disaster. Consider all thoracic wounds to be potentially life threatening until evidence proves otherwise. See Chapter 25, "Thoracic Trauma," for detailed care procedures.

Dress all open thoracic wounds with sterile dressings in the usual fashion. Be alert, however, for the presence of air bubbling, subcutaneous emphysema, crepitus, or other hints of open pneumothorax. Be extremely cautious about making an airtight seal on any thoracic wound because doing so can rapidly lead to tension pneumothorax and death. Instead, use an occlusive dressing sealed on three sides or an Asherman chest seal, and be prepared to assist ventilations. Auscultate the chest, and monitor respirations frequently. Watch the occlusive dressing so that it does not seal with blood against the chest wall and convert a simple pneumothorax into a tension pneumothorax.

Abdomen

The peritoneal cavity extends approximately from the symphysis pubis inferiorly to the diaphragm superiorly. As the diaphragm rises and falls with respiration, so, too, does the border between the abdominal and thoracic cavities. You cannot know the exact position of the diaphragm at the time the injury occurred, and so suspect associated injuries to both abdominal and thoracic organs if the soft-tissue injury involves the region between the rib margin and the fifth rib anteriorly, the seventh rib laterally, and the ninth rib posteriorly.

Blunt or penetrating trauma to the abdomen can injure both hollow and solid organs, penetrate or rupture the diaphragm, and cause serious internal bleeding. Anteriorly and just underlying the rib margin are the liver on the right and the spleen on the left. Posteriorly, the kidneys (not true abdominal organs since they lie retroperitoneally) are located in the costovertebral angle region. Hollow organs—bowel, stomach, and urinary bladder—may rupture. In addition to bleeding copiously, these organs may release their contents and cause inflammation of the peritoneum.

Consider any soft-tissue wound in the abdominal region as potentially damaging to the underlying organs. Signs and symptoms of internal damage can be subtle, particularly early on. Eviscerations and other massive injuries are obvious, but other internal injuries that are just as serious may not be apparent. Prehospital treatment is primarily supportive and includes ensuring adequate oxygenation, preventing shock, and dressing open wounds (see Chapter 26, "Abdominal Trauma").

WOUNDS REQUIRING TRANSPORT

Transport any patient with a wound that involves a structure beneath the integument for emergency department evaluation. This includes wounds involving, or possibly involving, nerves, blood vessels, ligaments, tendons, or muscles. Transport any patient with a significantly contaminated wound, a wound involving an impaled object, or a wound that was received in a particularly unclean environment. Also, transport any patient with a wound with likely cosmetic implications, such as facial wounds or large gaping wounds.

SOFT-TISSUE TREATMENT AND REFERRAL/RELEASE

In some EMS systems, paramedics are permitted to treat and release patients with minor and superficial soft-tissue injuries or treat and then refer them to their personal physicians. This generally occurs under online medical direction or according to strict protocols.

In such circumstances, you must evaluate and dress the wound. Then, explain to the patient the steps to follow for continuing care of the injury. Tell the patient of the need to change the dressing and to monitor the injury site for further hemorrhage or developing infection. Provide the patient with simple written instructions (approved and/or published by medical direction) explaining wound care, monitoring, protection, dressing change, cleansing, and the signs of such problems as infection or hemorrhage.

Instruct the patient to contact a physician if certain signs and symptoms appear, and describe those signs and symptoms thoroughly. Ensure that the patient has the means to obtain followup by a physician or health-care provider, and again stress the circumstances in which such followup care should be sought. During any referral or release, if the patient's tetanus immunization history is unclear or it has been longer than five years since the last immunization, instruct the patient to obtain a tetanus booster immediately.

Document all referral/release incidents carefully in the prehospital care report. The report should include a description of the nature and extent of the wound and of the care provided for it. Note in the report all instructions and materials provided to the patient and any medical direction you received.

SUMMARY

Soft-tissue injury may compromise the skin—the envelope that protects and contains the human body. Any trauma must penetrate the skin before it can harm the interior organs and threaten life. Any damage to the skin may interfere with its ability to contain fluids and blood and to prevent damaging agents from entering the body. For these reasons, the assessment and care of soft-tissue injuries are important parts of prehospital care.

Assess wounds carefully, since they may provide the only overt signs of serious internal injury. Realize that discoloration and swelling take time to develop and may not be as apparent in the field as when you present the patient at the emergency department. Look carefully for the early signs of wounds, and use the mechanism of injury to locate potential trauma sites. When caring for soft-tissue injuries, keep in mind the basic goals: controlling hemorrhage, keeping the wound as clean as possible, and immobilizing the injury site.

CHAPTER 21

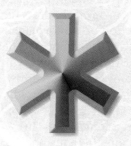

Burns

Objectives

After reading this chapter, you should be able to:

1. Describe the anatomy and physiology of the skin and remaining human anatomy as they pertain to thermal burn injuries. (see Chapter 12)

2. Describe the epidemiology, including incidence, mortality, morbidity, and risk factors, of burn injuries as well as strategies to prevent such injuries. (p. 136)

3. Describe the local and systemic complications of a thermal burn injury. (pp. 136–138, 148–151)

4. Identify and describe the depth classi-fications of burn injuries, including superficial burns, partial thickness

burns, and full thickness burns. (pp. 146–147)

5. Describe and apply the "rule of nines" and the "rule of palms" methods for determining body surface area percentage of a burn injury. (pp. 147–148)

6. Identify and describe the severity of a burn, including a minor burn, a moderate burn, and a critical burn. (pp. 153–156)

7. Describe the effects age and pre-existing conditions have on burn severity and a patient's prognosis. (pp. 150, 155)

Continued

8. Discuss complications of burn injuries caused by trauma, blast injuries, airway compromise, respiratory compromise, and child abuse. (pp. 144–146, 151–153, 159)

9. Describe thermal burn management, including considerations for airway and ventilation, circulation, pharmacological and nonpharmacological measures, transport decisions, and psychological support/communication strategies. (pp. 151–159)

10. Describe special considerations for a pediatric patient with a burn injury and describe the criteria for determining burn severity. (pp. 147–148, 150, 155)

11. Describe the specific epidemiologies, mechanisms of injury, pathophysiologies, and severity assessments for inhalation, chemical, and electrical burn injuries and for radiation exposure. (pp. 159–166)

12. Discuss special considerations that affect the assessment, management, and prognosis of patients with inhalation, chemical, and electrical burn injuries and with exposure to radiation. (pp. 159–166)

13. Differentiate between supraglottic and subglottic inhalation burn injuries. (pp. 144–146)

14. Describe the special considerations for a chemical burn injury to the eye. (pp. 163–164)

15. Given several preprogrammed, simulated thermal, inhalation, electrical, and chemical burn injury and radiation exposure patients, provide the appropriate scene assessment, primary assessment, rapid trauma or focused secondary assessment and history, detailed assessment, and ongoing assessment and provide appropriate patient care and transportation. (pp. 151–166)

INTRODUCTION TO BURN INJURIES

The incidence of burn injuries in Canada and other developed countries has been declining for several decades. According to the Firefighters Burn Treatment Society, more than 200 000 (about 1 percent) Canadians are seen each year for burn injuries.

Burn injuries are second only to motor-vehicle collisions as the overall leading cause of death. According to the University of Toronto, smoke inhalation is the most common cause of death (30 percent) among those who suffer major burns. Some 3 to 5 percent of these burns are considered life threatening. Persons at greatest risk for serious burns include the very young and the very old, the infirm, and certain workers, such as firefighters, metal smelters, and chemical workers. Burn injuries remain the second leading cause of death in children under 12 years of age and the fourth overall cause of trauma death.

Much of the national decline in burn mortality is attributed to improved building codes, safer construction techniques, and the use of smoke detectors. Smaller but still important effects are attributed to educational campaigns aimed primarily at school children. Other simple and inexpensive measures that have helped prevent burns include keeping cigarette lighters and matches away from children and reducing household hot-water temperatures to below scalding levels.

Burns are a specific subset of soft-tissue injuries with a specific pathological process. While the term "burn" suggests combustion, the actual process that produces burn injuries is much different. The human body is predominantly water and does not support combustion. Instead, body tissues change chemically, evaporating water and denaturing the proteins that make up cell membranes. The result can be widespread damage to the skin, or integumentary system.

Although the skin and its functions are often taken for granted, burn injury to this organ can subject a patient to severe fluid loss, infection, hypothermia, and other injuries.

PATHOPHYSIOLOGY OF BURNS

Burns result from the disruption of proteins in the cell membranes. Burns can be caused by several different mechanisms including thermal, electrical, chemical, and radiation energies. Being able to understand the mechanism of a burn and to determine the degree and area of burn helps you assess the seriousness of the burn and thus guide your care.

TYPES OF BURNS

Soft-tissue burns occur secondary to thermal (heat), electrical, chemical, or radiation insults to the body. While the resulting burns are much the same, the damage process differs with the various mechanisms. The following sections describe each of these four types of burns.

Thermal Burns

A thermal burn causes damage by increasing the rate at which the molecules within an object move and collide with each other. We measure the energy of this molecular motion as temperature. At a temperature greater than absolute zero, the molecules of any object move about. As the object's temperature increases, so does the speed of the molecules and the incidences of their collisions with other molecules. These changes in internal energy cause many substances—for example, steel—to expand with increasing temperature. Heat energy may also cause chemical changes. As temperature increases, such substances as gasoline may

Content Review

BASIC TYPES OF BURNS
Thermal
Electrical
Chemical
Radiation

combine with oxygen. The nature of matter may change as well. Water, for example, may change into ice (with decreasing heat energy) or steam (with increasing heat energy). An egg changes its nature as the proteins break down, or **denature,** in a hot frying pan. This is why cooked eggs have a rubbery consistency.

Similar changes also take place in burned tissue. As molecular speed increases, the cell components, especially membranes and proteins, begin to break down as in the case of the egg in a frying pan. The result of exposure to extreme heat is progressive injury and cell death.

The extent of burn injury relates to the amount of heat energy transferred to the patient's skin. The amount of that heat energy, in turn, depends on three components of the burning agent: its temperature, the concentration of heat energy it possesses, and the length of its contact time with the patient's skin.

Obviously, the greater the temperature of an agent, the greater is the potential for damage. However, it is also important to consider the amount of heat energy possessed by the object or substance. Receiving a blast of heated air from an oven at 177°C is much less damaging than contact with hot cooking oil at the same temperature. In general, water, oils, and other liquids have a fairly high heat energy content. This content is roughly related to the density of the material. In a similar fashion, solids also usually have a high heat content. Gases, on the other hand, usually have less capacity to hold heat owing to their less dense nature.

Duration of exposure to the heat source is also obviously important in determining the severity of a burn. A patient's momentary contact with hot oil would result in less damage than if the oil were poured onto her shoe.

A burn is a progressive process, and the greater the heat energy transmitted to the body, the deeper is the wound. Initially, the burn damages the epidermis by the increase in temperature. As contact with the substance continues, heat energy penetrates farther and deeper into the body tissue. Thus, a burn may involve the epidermis, dermis, and subcutaneous tissue as well as muscles, bone, and other internal tissue.

At the level of local tissues, thermal burns cause a number of effects collectively termed **Jackson's theory of thermal wounds.** This theory helps us understand the physical effects of high heat and helps explain a number of clinical effects (Figure 21-1).

With a burn, the skin nearest the heat source suffers the most profound changes. Cell membranes rupture and are destroyed, blood coagulates, and structural proteins denature. This most damaged area is the **zone of coagulation.** If the zone of coagulation penetrates the dermis, the resulting injury is termed a full-thickness or third-degree burn. Adjacent to this area is the **zone of stasis,** a less damaged yet still inflamed region where blood flow decreases. More distant from the burn source is a broader area where inflammation and changes in blood flow are limited. This is the **zone of hyperemia;** this zone accounts for the erythema (redness) associated with some burns.

Large burns have profound pathological effects on the body as a whole. In general, these effects are important in any burn that covers more than 15 to 20 percent of the patient's body surface area. To understand these effects and the resulting burn shock, you must first learn a little about the progression of burns.

The body's response to burns occurs over time and can usefully be classified into four stages. The first stage occurs immediately following the burn and is called the **emergent phase.** This is the body's initial reaction to the burn. This phase includes a pain response as well as the outpouring of catecholamines in response to the pain and the physical and emotional stress. During this stage, the patient displays tachycardia, tachypnea, mild hypertension, and mild anxiety.

* **denature** alter the usual substance of something.

* **Jackson's theory of thermal wounds** explanation of the physical effects of thermal burns.

Content Review

EFFECTS OF HEAT ACCORDING TO JACKSON'S THEORY OF THERMAL WOUNDS

Zone of coagulation—most damaged area nearest heat source; cell membranes rupture and are destroyed, blood coagulates, structural proteins denature

Zone of stasis—adjacent to most damaged region; inflammation present, blood flow decreased

Zone of hyperemia—area farthest from heat source; limited inflammation and changes in blood flow

* **zone of coagulation** area in a burn nearest the heat source that suffers the most damage and is characterized by clotted blood and thrombosed blood vessels.

* **zone of stasis** area in a burn surrounding the zone of coagulation and that is characterized by decreased blood flow.

* **zone of hyperemia** area peripheral to a burn that is characterized by increased blood flow.

* **emergent phase** first stage of the burn process that is characterized by a catecholamine release and pain-mediated reaction.

✱ fluid shift phase stage of the burn process in which there is a massive shift of fluid from the intravascular to the extravascular space.

✱ intravascular space the volume contained by all the arteries, veins, capillaries, and other components of the circulatory system.

✱ extravascular space the volume contained by all the cells (intracellular space) and the spaces between the cells (interstitial space).

✱ hypermetabolic phase stage of the burn process in which there is increased body metabolism in an attempt by the body to heal the burn.

✱ resolution phase final stage of the burn process in which scar tissue is laid down and the healing process is completed.

✱ voltage the difference of electric potential between two points with different concentrations of electrons.

✱ current the rate of flow of an electric charge.

✱ ampere basic unit for measuring the strength of an electric current.

✱ resistance property of a conductor that opposes the passage of an electric current.

✱ ohm basic unit for measuring the strength of electrical resistance.

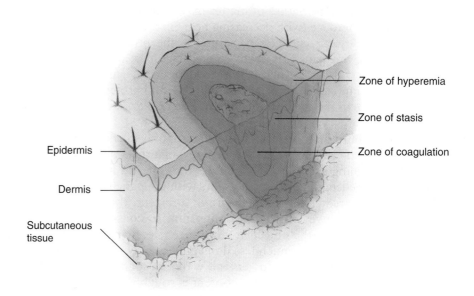

FIGURE 21-1   The zones of injury commonly caused by a thermal burn.

The **fluid shift phase** follows the initial phase and can last for up to 18 to 24 hours. The fluid shift phase begins shortly after the burn and reaches its peak in six to eight hours. You are therefore likely to see it in the prehospital setting. In this phase, damaged cells release agents that initiate an inflammatory response in the body. This increases blood flow to the capillaries surrounding the burn and increases the permeability of the capillaries to fluid. The response results in a large shift of fluid away from the **intravascular space** into the **extravascular space** (massive edema). Note that the capillaries leak fluid (water, electrolytes, and some dissolved proteins) and not blood cells. Blood loss from burns uncomplicated by other trauma is usually minimal.

After the fluid shift phase comes the **hypermetabolic phase,** which may last for many days or weeks depending on the burn severity. This phase is characterized by a large increase in the body's demands for nutrients as it begins the long process of repairing damaged tissue. Gradually, this phase evolves into the **resolution phase,** in which scar tissue is laid down and remodelled, and the burn patient begins to rehabilitate and return to normal function.

Electrical Burns

Electricity's power is the result of an electron flow from a point of high concentration to one of low concentration. The difference between the two concentrations is called the **voltage.** It is helpful to envision voltage as the "pressure" of the electric flow. The rate or the amount of flow in a given time is termed the **current** and is measured in **amperes.**

Another factor that affects the flow of electricity is **resistance.** Resistance is measured in **ohms.** Copper electrical wire has very little resistance and allows a free flow of electrons. Tungsten (the filament in a light bulb) is moderately resistant and heats, glows, and emits light as more and more current is applied to it.

The relationship between current (*I*), resistance (*R*), and voltage (*V*) is well known as **Ohm's law:**

$$V = IR \text{ or } I = V/R$$

Like tungsten, the internal parts of the human body are moderately resistant to the flow of electricity. The skin, however, is highly resistant to electrical flow. Moisture or sweat on the skin lowers this resistance. If the human body is subjected to voltage, the body initially resists the flow. If the voltage is strong enough, the current begins to pass into and through the body. As it does, heat energy is created. The heat produced is proportional to the square of the current flow and is related to power, *P*, as expressed in **Joule's law:**

$$P = I^2R$$

The highest heat occurs at the points of greatest resistance, often at the skin. This accounts for the severe "entry" and "exit" wounds sometimes seen in electrical injuries. Dry, callused skin can have enormous resistance values, ranging from 500 000 to 1 000 000 ohms/cm. Wet skin, particularly the thin skin on the palm side of the arm or on the inner thigh, can have values as low as 300 to 10 000 ohms/cm. Mucous membranes have very low resistance (100 ohms/cm) and allow even small currents to pass. This accounts for the relative ease with which household current can cause lip and oral burns in children who accidentally bite electrical cords (Figure 21-2).

With low currents, the heat energy produced is of little consequence. But if the voltage or current is high, profound body damage can occur. The longer the duration of contact, the greater is the potential for injury. Electrical burns can be particularly damaging because the burn heats the victim from the inside out, causing great damage to internal organs and structures while possibly leaving little visible damage on the surface, save for the entry and exit wounds (Figure 21-3).

Thermal injury due to electrical current occurs as energy travels from the point of contact to the point of exit. At both these points, the concentration of electricity is great, as is the degree of damage you might expect. The smaller the area of contact, the greater is the concentration of current flow and the greater is the injury. Between the entrance and exit points, the energy spreads out over a larger cross-sectional area and generally causes less injury. Electrical current may follow blood vessels and nerves because they offer less resistance than muscle and

* **Ohm's law** the physical law identifying that the current in an electrical circuit is directly proportional to the voltage and inversely proportional to the resistance.

* **Joule's law** the physical law identifying that the rate of heat production is directly proportional to the resistance of the circuit and to the square of the current.

Electrical burns can be particularly damaging because the current burns the victim from the inside out.

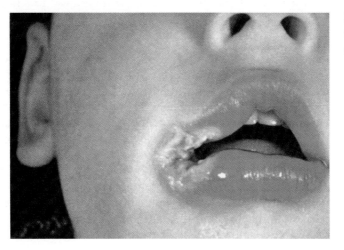

FIGURE 21-2 Electrical burns to a child's mouth caused by chewing on an electrical cord.

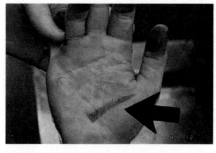

a. Entrance wound   b. Exit wound

FIGURE 21-3   Injuries due to electrical shock.

bone. This may lead to serious vascular and nervous injuries deep within the involved limbs or body cavity.

Electrical contact also interferes with control of muscle tissue. The passage of current, especially alternating current, severely disrupts the complicated electrochemical reactions that control muscles. If contact with a current as low as 20 to 50 milliamperes (mA) is maintained for a period of time, the muscles of respiration may be immobilized. The result is prolonged respiratory arrest, anoxia, hypoxemia, and—eventually—death. Electrical currents greater than 50 mA may also disrupt the heart's electrical system, causing ventricular fibrillation accompanied by ineffective pumping action. Alternating electrical current, such as that found in household current, can also cause tetanic convulsions or uncontrolled contractions of muscles. If the victim is holding a wire at such a time, the victim may be unable to let go, thereby prolonging the exposure and increasing the severity of injury. This can occur with as little as 9 mA of current.

Electrical injury may also disrupt muscular and other tissue, leading to its degeneration. As the tissue dies, it releases materials toxic to the human body. These materials may damage the liver and kidneys, leading to their failure.

At times, electrical energy may cause flash burns secondary to the heat of current passing through adjacent air. Air is very resistant to the passage of electrical current. If the current is strong enough and the space through which it passes is small, the electricity arcs, producing tremendous heat. If the patient's skin is close by, the heat may severely burn or vaporize tissue. In addition, the heat may ignite articles of clothing or other combustibles and produce thermal burns.

Chemical Burns

Chemical burns denature the biochemical makeup of cell membranes and destroy the cells. Such injuries are not transmitted through the tissue as are thermal injuries. Instead, a chemical burn must destroy the tissue before it can chemically burn any deeper. This fact generally limits the "burn" process unless very strong chemicals are involved (Figure 21-4). Agents that can cause chemical burns are too numerous to mention. However, the most common causes of these burns are either strong acids or bases (alkalis).

Both acids and alkalis burn by disrupting cell membranes and damaging tissues on contact. As they cause damage, acids usually form a thick, insoluble mass, or coagulum, at the point of contact. This process is called **coagulation necrosis** and helps limit the depth of acid burns. Alkalis, however, do not form a protective coagulum. Instead, the alkali continues to destroy cell membranes, re-

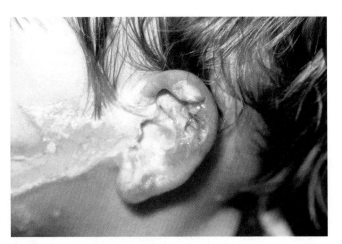

FIGURE 21-4 A chemical burn to the ear.

leasing the intercellular and interstitial fluid, destroying tissue in a process called **liquefaction necrosis.** This process allows the alkali to rapidly penetrate the underlying tissue, causing progressively deeper burns. For this reason, alkali burns can be quite serious.

Radiation Injury

Nuclear radiation has bombarded Earth since long before recorded time. It is a daily, natural phenomenon. Radiation becomes a danger when people are exposed to synthetic sources that greatly increase the intensity of radiation. Medicine and industry use radioactive materials for diagnostic testing and treatment and for energy production. Deaths from exposure to radiation are extremely rare as are serious injuries because of the safety measures commonly used with the handling of nuclear materials. The risk of injury comes from accidents associated with improper handling, either in the on-site environment or during transport. In addition, the possibility of large-scale exposure to radiation from terrorist acts is considered to be increasing.

Nuclear radiation causes damage through a process known as **ionization.** A radioactive energy particle travels into a substance and changes an internal atom (Figure 21-5). In the human body, the affected cell either repairs the damage, dies, or goes on to produce damaged cells (cancer). The cells most sensitive to radiation injury are the cells that reproduce most quickly, like those responsible for erythrocyte, leukocyte, and platelet production (bone marrow), cells lining the intestinal tract, and cells involved in human reproduction.

We commonly encounter four types of radiation:

- *Alpha Radiation* The nucleus of an atom releases **alpha radiation** in the form of a small helium nucleus. Alpha radiation is a very weak energy source and can travel only centimetres through the air. Paper or clothing can easily stop alpha radiation. This radiation also cannot penetrate the epidermis. On the subatomic scale, however, alpha particles are massive and can cause great damage over the short distance they travel. Alpha radiation is only a significant hazard if the patient inhales or ingests contaminated material, thus bringing the source in close proximity to sensitive respiratory and digestive tract tissues.

✱ **liquefaction necrosis** the process in which an alkali dissolves and liquefies tissue.

✱ **ionization** the process of changing a substance into separate charged particles (ions).

✱ **alpha radiation** low-level form of nuclear radiation; a weak source of energy that is stopped by clothing or the first layers of skin.

Content Review

TYPES OF RADIATION
Alpha—very weak, stopped by paper, clothing, or the epidermis

Beta—more powerful than alpha; can travel two to three metres through air; can penetrate some clothing and the first few millimetres of skin

Gamma—most powerful ionizing radiation; great penetrating power; protection requires thick concrete or lead shielding

Neutron—great penetrating power but uncommon outside nuclear reactors and bombs

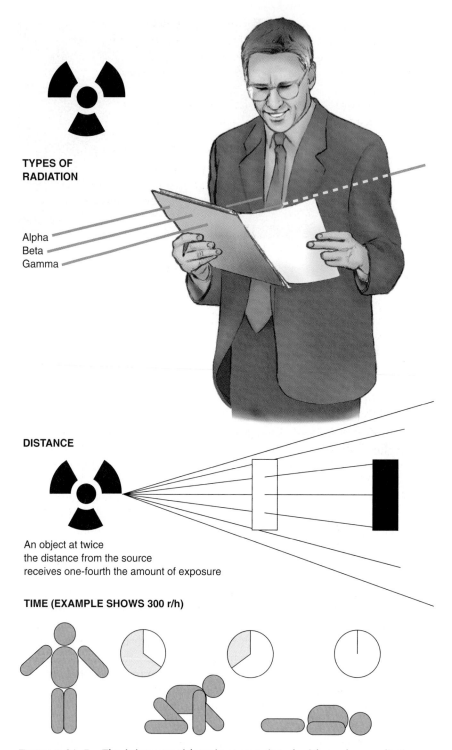

Alpha
Beta
Gamma

DISTANCE

An object at twice
the distance from the source
receives one-fourth the amount of exposure

TIME (EXAMPLE SHOWS 300 r/h)

FIGURE 21-5   The injury considerations associated with nuclear radiation.

✱ beta radiation medium-
strength radiation that is
stopped with light clothing or
the uppermost layers of skin.

- *Beta Radiation* A second type of radiological particle produces **beta
radiation.** Its energy is greater than that of alpha radiation.
However, the beta particle is relatively lightweight, with the mass of
an electron. Beta radiation can travel two to three metres through
air and can penetrate a few layers of clothing. Beta particles can
invade the first few millimetres of skin and thus have the potential
for causing external as well as internal injury.

- *Gamma Radiation* **Gamma radiation,** also known as x-rays, is the most powerful type of ionizing radiation. It has the ability to travel through the entire body or ionize any atom within. Its lack of mass or charge (it is pure electromagnetic energy) helps give it great penetrating power. Gamma radiation evokes the greatest concern for external exposure. It is the most dangerous and most feared type of radiation because it is difficult to protect against. Many metres of concrete or many centimetres of lead are needed to protect against the highest-energy gamma rays. Fortunately, exposure to high-energy gamma rays is rare; it occurs only in individuals who are exposed to nuclear blasts, are near the cores of nuclear reactors, or are very close to highly radioactive materials. More modest amounts of concrete, steel, or lead can provide shielding from the more common and lower-energy x-rays and gamma rays.

- *Neutron Radiation* Neutrons are small, yet moderately massive sub-atomic particles with no charge. Their small size and lack of charge account for their great penetrating power. Fortunately, strong **neutron radiation** is uncommon outside nuclear reactors and bombs.

* **gamma radiation** powerful electromagnetic radiation emitted by radioactive substances with powerful penetrating properties; it is stronger than alpha and beta radiation.

* **neutron radiation** powerful radiation with penetrating properties between that of beta and gamma radiation.

Exposure to radiation and the effects of ionization can occur through two mechanisms. In the first, an unshielded person is directly exposed to a strong radioactive source, for example, an unstable material, such as uranium. The second mechanism of exposure is contamination by dust, debris, or fluids that contain very small particles of radioactive material. These contaminants give off weaker radiation than a direct radioactive source, such as uranium. However, the close proximity of these contaminants to the body and their longer contact times with it may result in greater exposure and contamination. Note that most substances, including human tissue, do not give off radiation. The patient himself is not the danger in a radiation exposure incident. Any danger comes from the radioactive source, such as the contaminated material on the patient.

Three factors are important to keep in mind whenever you are called to incidents of radiation exposure: the duration of exposure; the distance from the radioactive source; and the shielding between you, the patient, and the source. Knowledge of these three factors can minimize your own exposure and potential for injury.

- *Duration.* Radiation exposure is an accumulative danger. The longer you or the patient remain exposed to the source, the greater is the potential for injury.

- *Distance.* Radiation strength diminishes quickly as you move farther from the source. The effect is similar to that of a light bulb's brightness. At one metre, you can easily read by it, while at a hundred metres the light barely casts a shadow. Mathematically, the relationship is inverse and squared. As you double your distance from the radioactive source, its strength drops to one-fourth. As you triple the distance, its strength diminishes to one-ninth, and so on.

- *Shielding.* The more the material between you and the source, the less radioactive exposure you experience. With alpha and beta radiation, shielding is very easy to provide and reasonably effective. With gamma and neutron sources, dense objects, such as earth, concrete, metal, and lead, are needed to provide any real protection.

Content Review

FACTORS AFFECTING EXPOSURE TO RADIATION
Duration of exposure
Distance from the source
Shielding from the source

* **rad** basic unit of absorbed radiation dose.

* **Gray** a unit of absorbed radiation dose equal to 100 rads.

Radiation exposure is measured with a Geiger counter, while cumulative exposure is recorded by a device called a dosimeter. They record units of radiation expressed as either the **rad** or the **Gray** (Gy), 1 Gray being equal to 100 rads.

Different tissues are sensitive to different levels of absorbed radiation. As little as 0.2 Gy can cause cataracts in exposed eyes and damage the blood-cell-producing bone marrow (also called hematopoietic) tissue. The radiation dose that is lethal to about 50 percent of exposed individuals is approximately 4.5 Gy.

With whole body exposure, and as the radiation dose increases, the signs and symptoms of exposure appear earlier and become more severe. The first signs of serious exposure are slight nausea and fatigue, occurring between 4 and 24 hours after exposure. As the radiation dose moves into the lethal range, the severity of the nausea increases and is joined by anorexia, vomiting, diarrhea, and malaise. Erythema of the skin may be present, and fatigue becomes more intense. These signs appear within two to six hours. With exposure to even higher, fatal doses, the patient displays all the signs of radiation exposure almost immediately and soon thereafter experiences confusion, watery diarrhea, and physical collapse. Note that the signs and symptoms of radiation exposure and the injuries associated with it vary because individual sensitivity to radiation exposure varies greatly.

Prolonged exposure to even small amounts of radiation may produce long-term and delayed problems. Infertility is a potential injury because the cells producing eggs and sperm are highly susceptible to ionization damage. Cancer is another delayed and severe side effect. It may occur years or even decades after a radiation exposure.

Inhalation Injury

Inhalation injury may be associated with burns, especially if the injury occurred in an enclosed space.

The burn environment frequently produces inhalation injury. This is especially true if the patient is in a closed space or is unconscious. A patient who is unconscious or trapped in a smoke-filled area eventually inhales gases, heated air, flames, or steam. The inhalation results in airway and respiratory injuries.

You can expect to find the following inhalation conditions in a burn environment (Figure 21-6). Keep them in mind as you survey the scene and take the necessary protective measures.

Toxic Inhalation Modern residential and commercial construction uses synthetic resins and plastics that release toxic gases as they burn. Combustion of these materials can form such toxic agents as compounds of cyanide and hydrogen sulphide. If a patient inhales these gases, the gases react with the lung tissue, causing internal chemical burns, or they diffuse across the alveolar–capillary membrane and enter the bloodstream, causing systemic poisoning. The signs and symptoms of these injuries may present immediately following exposure, or their onset may be delayed for an hour or two after inhalation. Toxic inhalation injury occurs more frequently than thermal inhalation burns.

Suspect carbon monoxide poisoning in any patient who was in an enclosed space during combustion.

Carbon Monoxide Poisoning An additional concern associated with the burn environment is carbon monoxide (CO) poisoning. Suspect it in any patient who has been within an enclosed space during combustion. Carbon monoxide is created during incomplete combustion, like that that may occur with a faulty heating unit or when someone tries to heat a room with an unvented device, such as a barbecue grill. Poisoning occurs because carbon monoxide has an affinity for hemoglobin more than 200 times greater than does oxygen. If your patient has inhaled carbon monoxide, even in the smallest quantities, the carbon monoxide displaces oxygen in the hemoglobin and remains there for hours. The result is hypoxemia. Hypoxemia, which is difficult to detect, subtly compromises the delivery of oxygen to the patient's vital organs. If carbon monoxide inhalation is associated with airway burns, the respiratory compromise will be further compounded.

Airway Thermal Burn Another, though less frequent, injury is the airway thermal burn. Very moist mucosa lines the airway and helps insulate it against heat damage.

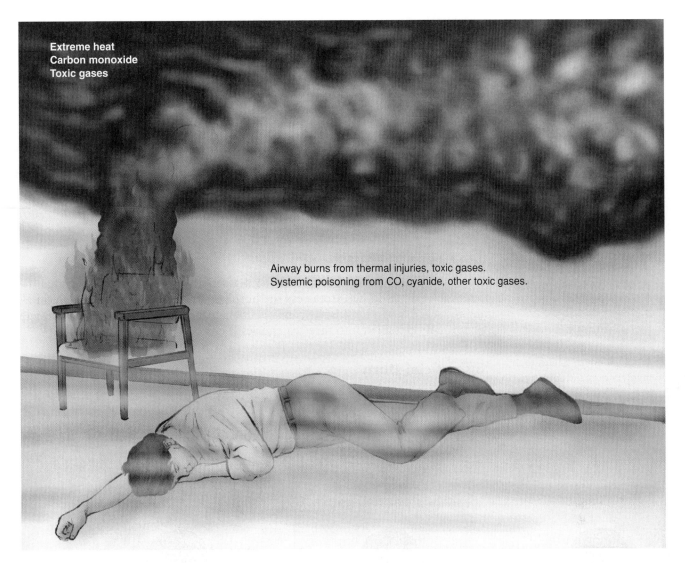

Extreme heat
Carbon monoxide
Toxic gases

Airway burns from thermal injuries, toxic gases.
Systemic poisoning from CO, cyanide, other toxic gases.

FIGURE 21-6   Hazards of fire in an enclosed environment.

Because of this mucosa, **supraglottic,** or upper airway, structures may absorb the heat and prevent lower airway burns. High levels of thermal energy are required to evaporate the fluid and injure the cells. Inspiration of hot air or flame rarely produces enough heat to cause significant thermal burns to the lower airway.

Superheated steam has greater heat content than hot, dry air and can cause **subglottic,** or lower airway, burns. Superheated steam is created under great pressure and can have a temperature well above 100°C (212°F). A common hazard to firefighters, superheated steam develops when a stream of water strikes a hot spot and vaporizes explosively. The blast can dislodge the mask of a firefighter's self-contained breathing apparatus (SCBA), exposing her to superheated steam inhalation. The steam contains enough heat energy to severely burn the upper airway. It also may damage the lower respiratory tract, although this happens less frequently.

Risk factors for inhalation injuries associated with burns include standing in the burn environment (hot gases rise), screaming or yelling there (the open glottis allows toxic gases to enter the lower airway), and being trapped in a closed burn environment.

✱ **supraglottic** referring to the upper airway.

✱ **subglottic** referring to the lower airway.

Superheated steam is a common cause of airway burns.

With any thermal or smoke-related chemical burn injury to the respiratory tract, there is the danger of airway restriction, severe dyspnea, and possible respiratory arrest. The airway is a narrow tube, lined with extremely vascular tissue. If damaged, this tissue swells rapidly, seriously reducing the size of the airway lumen. The patient presents with minor hoarseness, followed precipitously by dyspnea. Stridor, high-pitched "crowing" sounds on inspiration, is an ominous sign of impending airway obstruction. Other clues leading you to suspect potential airway burns include singed facial and nasal hair, black-tinged (carbonaceous) sputum, and facial burns. The airway injury may be so extensive as to induce complete respiratory obstruction and arrest. Accurate assessment is important because 20 to 35 percent of patients admitted to burn centres and some 60 to 70 percent of burn patients who die have an associated inhalation injury.

DEPTH OF BURN

After you determine the burn source and assess the possibility of associated inhalation injury, you need to assess the burn's severity. One element in determining the severity of a burn is the depth of damage it causes. Depth of burn damage is normally classified into three categories (Figure 21-7).

Superficial Burn

The **superficial burn**, also termed a first-degree burn, involves only the epidermis. It is an irritation of the living cells in this region and results in some pain, minor edema, and erythema. It normally heals without complication.

✱ **superficial burn** a burn that involves only the epidermis; characterized by reddening of the skin; also called a first-degree burn.

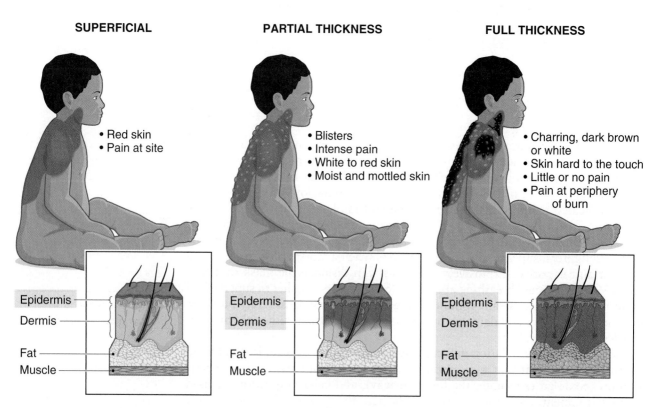

SUPERFICIAL

- Red skin
- Pain at site

Epidermis
Dermis
Fat
Muscle

PARTIAL THICKNESS

- Blisters
- Intense pain
- White to red skin
- Moist and mottled skin

Epidermis
Dermis
Fat
Muscle

FULL THICKNESS

- Charring, dark brown or white
- Skin hard to the touch
- Little or no pain
- Pain at periphery of burn

Epidermis
Dermis
Fat
Muscle

FIGURE 21-7   Classification of burns by depth.

Partial Thickness Burn

The **partial thickness burn,** also termed a second-degree burn, penetrates slightly deeper than a superficial burn and produces blisters. Heat energy travels into the dermis, involving more of the tissue and resulting in greater destruction. The partial thickness burn is similar to a superficial burn in that it is reddened, painful, and edematous. You can differentiate it from the superficial burn only after blisters form. Because there are many nerve endings in the dermis, both superficial and partial thickness burns are often very painful. With both superficial and partial thickness burns, the dermis is still intact and complete skin regeneration is very likely.

The sunburn is a common, but specialized, type of burn. Ultraviolet radiation causes the burn, rather than normal thermal processes. The radiation penetrates superficially and damages the uppermost layers of the dermis. Sunburn can present as either a superficial or a partial thickness burn.

Another similar type of burn occurs as someone watches an arc welder without proper eye protection. The lens of the eye focuses the high-intensity ultraviolet light on the retina, where it burns the tissue. This results in delayed eye pain and, possibly, transient blindness.

Full Thickness Burn

The **full thickness,** or third-degree, **burn,** penetrates both the epidermis and the dermis and extends into the subcutaneous layers or even deeper, into muscles, bones, and internal organs. These burns destroy the tissue's regenerative properties and the peripheral nerve endings. The injury is painless because of the nerve destruction, but the margins of the full thickness burn are frequently partial thickness burns, which can be quite painful. The full thickness burn takes on various colorations, depending on the nature of the burning agent and the damaged, dying, or dead tissue. They can be white, brown, or a charred colour and typically have a dry, leather-like appearance. Because the burn destroys the entire dermis, healing is difficult unless the wound is small or skin grafting is possible.

BODY SURFACE AREA

Another factor affecting burn severity is how much of a person's **body surface area (BSA)** the burn involves. There are two approaches to estimating the BSA involved in a burn. The first, the rule of nines, is useful in estimating large burn areas. The second method, the rule of palms, is helpful in assessing smaller wounds more accurately.

Rule of Nines

The **rule of nines** identifies 11 topographical adult body regions, each of which approximates 9 percent of the patient's BSA (Figure 21-8). These regions are the entire head and neck; the anterior chest; the anterior abdomen; the posterior chest; the lower back (the posterior abdomen); the anterior surface of each lower extremity; the posterior surface of each lower extremity; and each upper extremity. The genitalia make up the remaining 1 percent of BSA.

Because infant or child anatomy differs significantly from that of adults, you have to modify the rule of nines to maintain an accurate approximation of BSA. Divide the head and neck area into the anterior and posterior surface and award 9 percent for each. Reduce the surface area of each lower extremity by 4.5 percent to ensure that the total body surface area remains at 100 percent. The rule of nines is, at best, an approximation of the area burned. It is, however, an expedient and useful tool to help measure the burn's extent.

✱ **partial thickness burn** burn in which the epidermis is burned through and the dermis is damaged; characterized by redness and blistering; also called a second-degree burn.

Content Review

DEPTH OF BURN

Superficial (first-degree)—involves only the epidermis; produces pain, minor edema, and erythema (redness)

Partial thickness (second-degree)—involves epidermis and dermis; produces pain, edema, erythema, blisters

Full thickness (third-degree)—involves all skin layers and possibly structures beneath; painless, but tissue is destroyed; white, brown, or charred, leather-like appearance

---

✱ **full thickness burn** burn that damages all layers of the skin; characterized by areas that are white and dry; also called third-degree burn.

✱ **body surface area (BSA)** amount of a patient's body affected by a burn.

✱ **rule of nines** method of estimating amount of body surface area burned by a division of the body into regions, each of which represents approximately 9 percent of total BSA (plus 1 percent for the genital region).

THE RULE OF NINES

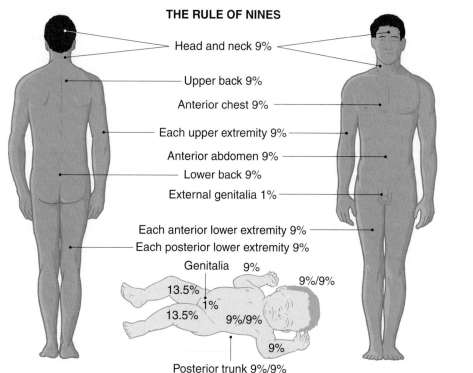

Head and neck 9%

Upper back 9%

Anterior chest 9%

Each upper extremity 9%

Anterior abdomen 9%

Lower back 9%

External genitalia 1%

Each anterior lower extremity 9%

Each posterior lower extremity 9%

Genitalia   9%

13.5%   9%/9%

1%

13.5%   9%/9%

9%

Posterior trunk 9%/9%

FIGURE 21-8   The rule of nines.

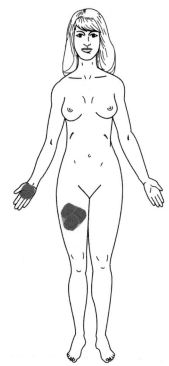

FIGURE 21-9   Using the rule of palms, the surface of the patient's palm represents approximately 1 percent of BSA and is helpful in estimating the area of small burns.

Rule of Palms

* **rule of palms** method of estimating amount of body surface area burned that sizes the area burned in comparison with the patient's palmar surface.

The **rule of palms,** an alternative system for approximating the extent of a burn, uses the palmar surface as a point of comparison in gauging the size of the affected body area (Figure 21-9). The patient's palm (the hand less the fingers) represents about 1 percent of the BSA, whether the patient is an adult, a child, or an infant. If you can visualize the palmar surface area and apply it to the burn area mentally, you can then obtain an estimate of the total BSA affected.

The rule of palms is easier to use for local burns of up to about 10 percent BSA, while the rule of nines is simpler and more appropriate for larger burns. There are many other burn approximation techniques that are both more specific to age and, in general, more accurate. However, these techniques are more complicated and time consuming to use. Both the rule of nines and the rule of palms provide reasonable approximations of BSA when used properly in the field.

SYSTEMIC COMPLICATIONS

Burns cause several systemic complications. These can affect the overall severity of a burn. Typical complications include hypothermia, hypovolemia, eschar formation, and infection.

Hypothermia

A burn may disrupt the body's ability to regulate its core temperature. Tissue destruction reduces or eliminates the skin's ability to contain the fluid within. The burn process releases plasma and other fluids, which seep into the wound. There they evaporate and rapidly remove heat energy. If the burn is extensive, uncontrolled body heat loss induces rapid and severe hypothermia.

Hypovolemia

Hypovolemia also may complicate the severe burn. The inability of damaged blood vessels to contain plasma causes a shift of proteins, fluid, and electrolytes into the burned tissue. Additionally, the loss of plasma protein reduces the blood's ability, through osmosis, to draw fluids from the uninjured tissues. This, in turn, compromises the body's natural response to fluid loss and may produce a profound hypovolemia. Although this is a serious complication of the extensive burn, it takes hours to develop. Modern aggressive fluid resuscitation can effectively counteract this aspect of the burn process.

A related complication is electrolyte imbalance. With the massive shift of fluid to the interstitial space, the body's ability to regulate sodium, potassium, and other electrolytes becomes overwhelmed. In addition, large thermal and electrical burns can lead to massive tissue destruction with a resultant release of breakdown products into the bloodstream. Potassium is one such breakdown product, and its oversupply, or hyperkalemia, can lead to life-threatening cardiac dysrhythmias. Careful electrocardiographic (ECG) monitoring and appropriate fluid resuscitation can help prevent hyperkalemic complications.

Eschar

Skin denaturing further complicates full thickness thermal burns. As the burn destroys the dermal cells, they become hard and leathery, producing what is known as an **eschar.** The skin as a whole constricts over the wound site, increasing the pressure of any edema beneath and restricting the flow of blood (Figure 21-10). If the extremity burn is circumferential, the constriction may be severe enough to occlude all blood flow into the distal extremity. In the case of a thoracic burn, eschar may drastically reduce chest excursion and respiratory tidal volume.

✳ **eschar** hard, leathery product of a deep full thickness burn; it consists of dead and denatured skin.

Infection

Although infection is the most persistent killer of burn victims, its effects do not appear for several days following the acute injury. Pathogens invade the wound shortly after the burn occurs and continue to do so until the wound heals. These pathogens pose a hazard to life when they grow to massive numbers, a process that takes days or weeks. To reduce the patient's exposure to infectious pathogens, carefully employ body substance isolation, use sterile dressings and clean equipment, and avoid gross contamination of the burn.

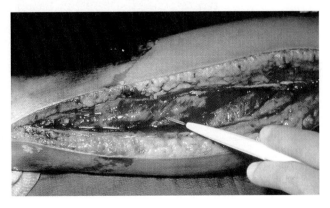

FIGURE 21-10 The constriction created by an eschar can limit chest excursion or cut off blood flow to and from a limb.

Organ Failure

As noted above, the burn process releases material from damaged or dying body cells into the bloodstream. Myoglobin from the muscles clogs the tubules of the kidneys and, with hypovolemia, may cause kidney failure. Hypovolemia and the circulating byproducts of cellular destruction may also induce liver failure. In addition, the release of cellular potassium into the bloodstream affects the heart's electrical system, causing dysrhythmias and possible death.

Special Factors

Consider any patient with a preexisting illness or disease or any pediatric or geriatric patient as having a more serious burn injury.

Certain factors involving the burn patient's overall health and age will also affect the patient's response to a burn and should influence your field decisions regarding treatment and transport. Geriatric and pediatric patients and those who are already ill or otherwise injured have greater difficulty coping with burn injuries than have healthy individuals. The pediatric patient has a high body surface area to body weight ratio, which means the fluid reserves needed for dealing with the effects of a burn are low. Geriatric patients have reduced mechanisms for fluid retention and lower fluid reserves. They are also less able to combat infection and more apt to have underlying diseases. Those who are ill are already using the energy of their bodies to fight their diseases; with burns, these patients have additional medical stresses to combat. The fluid loss that accompanies a burn also compounds the effects of blood loss in a trauma patient. This patient now must recover from two injuries.

Physical Abuse

When assessing any burn, particularly in a child or an elderly and infirm adult, be alert for any signs of potential physical abuse. Look for mechanisms of injury that do not make sense, such as stove burns on an infant who cannot yet stand or walk. Certain burn patterns should also give rise to suspicion. Multiple circular burns each about a centimetre in diameter may mean intentional cigarette burns. Infants who have been dipped in scalding hot water will have characteristic circumferential burns to their buttocks as they raise their feet and legs in an attempt to avoid the burning water (Figure 21-11). Branding is an unusual form of abuse and is sometimes seen in ritualistic or hazing ceremonies in some groups. In all cases of

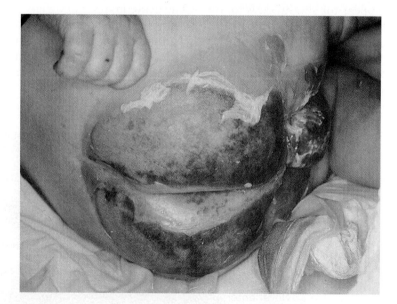

FIGURE 21-11   Burn injury from placing a child's buttocks in hot water as punishment.

suspected abuse, document your findings objectively and accurately, report them to the person assuming patient care in the emergency department, and notify the proper authorities as provincial or territorial and local laws require.

ASSESSMENT OF THERMAL BURNS

Skin evaluation tells more about the body's condition than any other aspect of patient assessment. Not only is the skin the first body organ to experience the effects of burns, but it is also the first and often the only organ to display them. Therefore, assessment of the skin and the associated burns must be deliberate, careful, and complete.

Although the burn process varies, assessment is simple and well structured. Assess burn patients carefully and completely to ensure that you establish the nature and extent of each injury. This helps you assign burns the appropriate priority for care.

The assessment of thermal burns follows established procedures for performing the scene assessment, the primary assessment, the rapid trauma assessment or focused history and secondary assessment, the detailed secondary assessment, and the ongoing assessment.

SCENE ASSESSMENT

The safety of your patients, fellow rescuers, and yourself depends on a complete and thorough scene assessment. Look around carefully as you arrive at the scene to ensure there is no continuing danger to you or your patient. Examine the scene to ensure it is safe for you to enter. If there is any doubt, do not enter until the scene is made safe by appropriate emergency personnel (Figure 21-12).

On calls involving burn patients, be wary of entering enclosed spaces, such as a bedroom or a garage, if there is recent evidence of a fire. Even small fires can cause intense heat in small, enclosed spaces. This can rapidly lead to a near-explosive process (called flashover) in which the temperature of the contents of a room rise to the point of rapid ignition. Flashover is frequently fatal to victims caught in the immediate area.

Another significant hazard at fire-ground scenes is the buildup of toxic gases. Carbon monoxide, cyanide, and hydrogen sulphide are common byproducts of

> *Be wary of entering any enclosed space associated with a fire because of the dangers of flashover and toxic gases.*
>

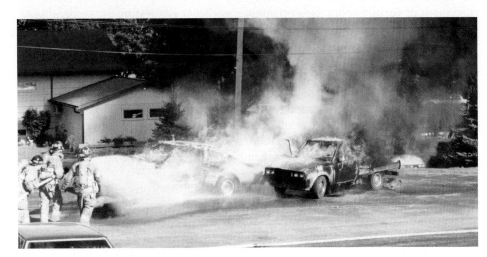

FIGURE 21-12   Never enter a fire scene until it has been safely contained by appropriately trained personnel.

combustion and can be produced in large quantities in some fires. Cyanide, in particular, can kill after as little as 15 seconds of exposure, a time short enough to fell any would-be rescuer without proper protection.

Never enter any potentially hazardous scene. Instead, ensure that the fire is thoroughly extinguished or that the patient is brought to you by persons skilled in working in hazardous environments who are using proper personal protective equipment. Ensure that the area where you will be caring for the patient is free from such dangers as structural collapse, contamination, electricity, and any other hazards.

Once at the burn patient's side, stop the burning process so it no longer threatens you or the patient. Extinguish any overt flame using copious irrigation, if water is available. Alternatively, a heavy wool or cotton blanket (avoid most synthetics, such as nylon or polyester) will smother flames.

Quickly survey the patient for other materials she is wearing that may continue the burn process. Remember that burn patients may be an actual hazard both to themselves and to you. Leather articles, such as shoes, belts, or watchbands, can smoulder for hours and continue to induce thermal injury. Watches, rings, and other jewellery may also hold and transmit heat or may restrict swelling tissue and occlude distal circulation. Synthetics (such as a nylon windbreaker) produce great heat as they burn and leave a hot, smouldering residue once the overt flames are out. Remove materials such as those described above as soon as possible. Be careful as you check for and remove these items. They may still be hot enough to burn you.

Once the scene is safe and there are no further dangers to you or others, consider the burn mechanism. Ask yourself: "Is there any possibility that the patient was unconscious during the fire or trapped within the building?" If so, be ready to place a special emphasis on your assessment and management of the patient's airway and breathing. Watch for any signs of airway restriction, and be alert to possible poisoning from carbon monoxide or other toxic gases.

Also, consider and examine for other mechanisms of injury associated with the burn. Remember that the victim, in attempting to escape the flames, may have fallen down a flight of stairs or jumped from a second- or third-storey window. Anticipate skeletal and internal injuries. In cases of electrical burns, consider the possibility that muscle spasms caused by contact with high voltage may also have caused skeletal fractures. Be aware that trauma injuries will increase the severity of the burn's impact on your patient.

Conclude the scene assessment by considering the need for other resources to manage the scene and treat the patient. Request additional EMS, police, and fire personnel and equipment as necessary. If you suspect serious airway involvement or carbon monoxide poisoning, consider requesting air medical service to reduce transport time to the hospital or burn/trauma centre.

PRIMARY ASSESSMENT

Start your primary assessment by forming a general impression of the patient. Rule out any danger of associated trauma or the possibility of head and spine injury. Evaluate the patient's level of consciousness, and if the patient displays an altered state of consciousness, consider toxic inhalation as a cause. Protect the patient from further cervical injury if indicated by the suspected mechanism of injury or by the patient's symptoms.

Next, ensure that the airway is patent. If it is not, protect it. You must give the airway of a burn patient special consideration. Look for the signs of any thermal or inhalation injury during your initial airway exam (Figure 21-13). Look carefully at the facial and nasal hairs to see if they have been singed. Examine any sputum and the areas around the mouth and nose for carbonaceous residue or any other evidence of inhalation. Listen for airway sounds, such as stridor, hoarseness, or coughing, that indicate irritation or inflammation of the

Look for and extinguish smouldering shoes, belts, or watchbands early in the assessment of burn patients.

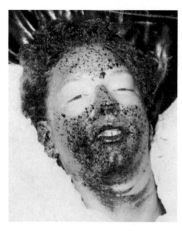

FIGURE 21-13 Facial burns or carbonaceous material around the mouth and nose suggest the possibility of chemical and thermal burns to the airway.

mucosa. Such sounds should alert you to the possibility that the airway has been injured and that progressive swelling of the airway is likely. Stridor, in particular, is a serious finding. Consider a patient with any signs of respiratory involvement as a potential acute emergency, and provide immediate care and transport.

With patients in whom respiratory involvement is suspected, provide humidified high-flow, high-concentration oxygen, and prepare the equipment for assisting ventilations. High-concentration oxygen (at levels approaching 100 percent) is especially important for burn patients because they may be suffering from carbon monoxide poisoning. Very high oxygen percentages more effectively provide oxygen to body cells and may reduce the half-life of the carbon monoxide by up to two-thirds.

Burn patients may progress rapidly from mild dyspnea to total respiratory arrest. While the intubation of a respiratory burn patient may be difficult in the field, there are distinct advantages to performing it early. The edema is progressive and gradually reduces the airway lumen. If intubation is delayed until the patient becomes extremely dyspneic or goes into respiratory arrest, the airway may be so edematous that it will be difficult, if not impossible, to intubate.

If you elect field intubation for the burn patient (and medical direction approves as you are an advanced care or critical care paramedic), perform it quickly and carefully. The airway is already narrowing, and the normal trauma associated with intubation could make matters worse. Intubation can be more complicated if the patient is conscious and resists the process (see Chapter 23). You may also find nasotracheal intubation useful. In any case, select the crew member with the most experience to ensure that intubation is completed quickly and with the least amount of associated airway trauma.

As with all intubation, it is best to maintain an airway using the largest endotracheal tube possible. Be sure, however, to have at hand several tubes smaller than you would normally use because edema may have reduced the size of the airway. Select the largest tube that you think will easily pass through the cords.

Ensure that the patient's breathing is adequate in both volume and rate. Carefully assess tidal volume if there are circumferential burns of the chest because the developing eschar may restrict chest excursion. Ventilate as necessary via bag-valve mask using the reservoir and high-flow oxygen.

In cases of severe airway burns, intubate early. If intubation is delayed until the patient arrives at the emergency department, the airway may be so edematous that it may be difficult or impossible to intubate.

FOCUSED AND RAPID TRAUMA ASSESSMENT

The focused history and secondary assessment for the burn patient are much the same as for any other trauma patient, beginning with a rapid trauma assessment or a focused secondary assessment and proceeding to the taking of baseline vital signs and a patient history. With a burn patient, however, you must also accurately approximate the area of the burn and its depth. This approximation guides your care and helps emergency department personnel prepare for patient arrival.

Except in cases of clearly localized burns, examine the patient's entire body surface, both anterior and posterior. Remove any clothing that was or could have been involved in the burn. If any of the clothing adheres to the burn or resists removal, cut around it as necessary.

Apply the rule of nines to determine the total body surface area (BSA) burned. Add 9 percent if the burn involves an entire "rule of nines" region. If it only involves a portion, add that proportion of 9 percent. For example, if one-third of the upper extremity is burned, the surface area approximation is 3 percent (one-third of 9 percent = 3 percent). For small burns, use the rule of palms to approximate the affected BSA.

The depth of a burn injury is also an important consideration. Identify areas of painful sensation as partial thickness burns (Figure 21-14). Consider those that present with limited or absent pain as probable full thickness burns

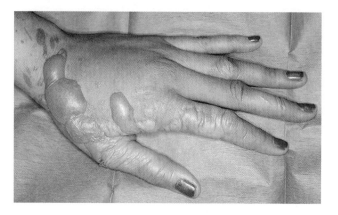

FIGURE 21-14   A partial thickness burn.

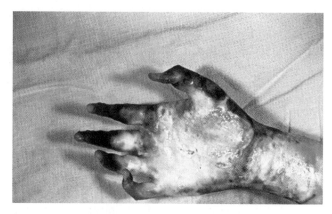

FIGURE 21-15   A deep full thickness burn.

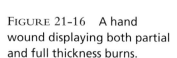

Burns to the face, hands, feet, joints, genitalia, and circumferential burns are of special concern.

(Figure 21-15). This differentiation is difficult because partial thickness injury and its associated pain commonly surrounds the full thickness burn (Figure 21-16). See Table 21-1 for the characteristics of the different types of burns.

A third consideration in determining the severity of a burn is the area of the body affected. The face, hands, feet, joints, genitalia, and circumferential burns deserve particular consideration. Each presents with special problems to patients and their recovery.

You have already assessed the face for burns to eliminate respiratory involvement. But this area also needs special consideration for aesthetic reasons. Facial damage and scarring may be more socially debilitating than a joint or limb burn. Carefully assess and give a high priority to these injuries, even if you do rule out respiratory involvement.

Consider burns involving the feet or the hands as serious. These areas are critical for much of the patient's daily activities. Serious burns and the associated scar tissue make thermal hand or foot injuries extremely debilitating. Assess these areas and communicate the precise location of the injury and the degree of the burn to the receiving physician. Joint burns can likewise be debilitating for patients. Scar tissue replaces skin, leading to loss of joint flexibility and mobility. Give any burn assessed as full thickness that involves the hands, feet, or joints a higher priority than a burn of equal surface area and depth elsewhere.

Also, pay particular attention to burns that completely ring an extremity, the thorax, the abdomen, or the neck. Due to the nature of a full thickness burn, the area underneath the burn may be drastically compressed as an eschar forms. The resulting constriction may hinder respirations, restrict distal blood flow, or cause hypoxia of the tissues beneath. Carefully assess any burn encircling a part of the

FIGURE 21-16   A hand wound displaying both partial and full thickness burns.

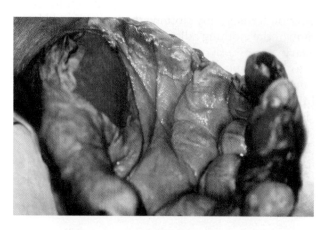

Table 21-1 CHARACTERISTICS OF VARIOUS DEPTHS OF BURNS

	Superficial (First-Degree)	Partial Thickness (Second-Degree)	Full Thickness (Third-Degree)
Cause	Sun or minor flame	Hot liquids, flame	Chemicals, electricity, hot metals, flame
Skin colour	Red	Mottled red	Pearly white and/or charred, translucent, and parchment-like
Skin	Dry with no blister	Blisters with weeping	Dry with thrombosed blood vessels
Sensation	Painful	Painful	Anesthetic
Healing	3–6 days	2–4 weeks	May require skin grafting

body for distal circulation or other signs of vascular compromise. Once you note such an injury, perform ongoing assessments to monitor distal circulatory status.

Finally, assign a higher priority to any burns affecting pediatric or geriatric patients or patients who are ill or otherwise injured. Serious burns cause great stress for these patients. The massive fluid and heat loss as well as the infection often associated with burns challenge the ability of body systems to perform adequately. Consider a burn more serious whenever it is accompanied by any other serious patient problem.

Once you determine the depth, extent, and other factors that contribute to burn severity, categorize the patient as having either minor, moderate, or severe burns. Use the criteria in Table 21-2 as a guide.

The severity of a burn should be increased one level with pediatric and geriatric patients and patients suffering from other trauma or acute medical problems. Also consider burns as critical with a patient who shows any signs or symptoms of respiratory involvement. Such patients require immediate transport to a burn (or trauma) centre, if possible (Table 21-3).

The burn centre is a hospital with a commitment to providing specialty treatment to burn patients. That commitment includes measures necessary to reduce

The head-to-toe examination should continue at the scene only if significant and life-threatening burns can be ruled out.

Table 21-2 BURN SEVERITY

Minor

Superficial: BSA < 50 percent (sunburns, etc.)

Partial thickness: BSA < 15 percent

Full thickness: BSA < 2 percent

Moderate

Superficial: BSA > 50 percent

Partial thickness: BSA < 30 percent

Full thickness: BSA < 10 percent

Critical

Partial thickness burns: BSA > 30 percent in an adult, > 20 percent in a child

Full thickness burns: BSA > 10 percent in an adult, any amount in a child

Any burns to face, hands, or perineum

Burns complicated by respiratory tract injuries, other major injuries or fractures, or electrocution

Any burns in high-risk patients, such as the elderly, debilitated, or immuno-compromised

Source: American Burn Association.

Table 21-3	INJURIES THAT BENEFIT FROM BURN CENTRE CARE
	Partial thickness (second-degree) burn greater than 15 percent of BSA
	Full thickness (third-degree) burn greater than 5 percent BSA
	Significant burns to the face, feet, hands, or perineal area
	High-voltage electrical injuries
	Inhalation injuries
	Chemical burns causing progressive tissue destruction
	Associated significant injuries

Source: American Burn Association.

the risk of infection presented by serious burns. The centre must also have the resources to perform delicate skin grafts necessary to replace destroyed skin. Because serious burns leave scar tissue that covers joints and other important areas and affects movement, the centre can provide rehabilitation programs requiring prolonged patient stays and intensive nursing care. While immediate transport to a burn centre is not as critically time dependent as transport for other seriously injured patients to a trauma centre, the burn centre's resources can optimize a patient's recovery prospects.

Conclude the focused history and secondary assessment by prioritizing the patient for transport. Rapidly transport any patient with full thickness burns over a large portion of the BSA. Patients with associated injuries to the face, joints, hands, feet, or genitalia are also candidates for immediate transport. Other cases needing rapid transport include patients who have experienced smoke, steam, or flame inhalation, or any geriatric, pediatric, otherwise ill, or trauma patient. Direct these patients to the nearest burn centre as described by your local protocols or by online medical direction.

ONGOING ASSESSMENT

Conduct ongoing assessments for all burn patients, every 15 minutes for minor burns and every five minutes for moderate or critical burns. Although the burn injury mechanism has been halted, the nature of the burn will continue to affect the patient. In addition to monitoring vital signs, watch for early signs of hypovolemia and airway problems. Also, be cautious about aggressive fluid therapy. Monitor for lung sounds and respiratory effort suggestive of pulmonary edema, and slow the fluid resuscitation if any signs develop. Also, carefully monitor distal circulation and sensation with any circumferential burn. Finally, monitor the ECG to identify any abnormalities, which may be caused by electrolyte imbalances secondary to fluid movement and tissue destruction.

MANAGEMENT OF THERMAL BURNS

Once you complete your burn patient assessment and correct or address any immediate life threats, you can begin certain burn management steps, either in the field or en route to the hospital. These include the prevention of shock, hypothermia, and any further wound contamination.

Thermal burn management can be divided into two categories: that for local and minor burns and that for moderate to severe burns.

LOCAL AND MINOR BURNS

Use local cooling to treat minor soft-tissue burns involving only a small proportion of the body surface area at a partial thickness. Provide this care only for partial thickness burns that involve less than 15 percent of the BSA or very small full thickness burns (less than 2 percent BSA). Cooling of larger surface areas may subject the patient to the risk of hypothermia. Cold or cool water immersion has some effect in reducing pain and may limit the depth of the burning process if applied immediately (within one or two minutes) after the burn.

If you have not already done so, remove any article of clothing or jewellery that might possibly act to constrain edema. As body fluids accumulate at the injury site, the site begins to swell. If the swelling encounters any constriction, it increases pressure on other tissue and may, in effect, serve as a tourniquet. This pressure may result in the loss of pulse and circulation distal to the injury. Evaluate distal circulation and sensation frequently during care and transport.

Also, provide the burn patient with comfort and support. Even rather minor burns can be very painful. Calm and reassure the patient. In severe cases, consider morphine sulphate or fentanyl analgesia if an ACP/CCP is transporting the patient.

Standard in-hospital treatment for minor burns includes the application of topical (not systemic) antibiotic ointments, such as silver sulphadiazine, and bulky sterile dressings. Encourage the patient, as much as possible, to keep the burn area elevated. Provide analgesia in either oral or parenteral form, as burns can be quite painful. Full thickness burns are open wounds, and so any patient without an up-to-date tetanus immunization status is given a booster of tetanus-diphtheria toxoid.

MODERATE TO SEVERE BURNS

Use dry, sterile dressings to cover partial thickness burns that involve more than 15 percent BSA or full thickness burns involving more than 5 percent of the BSA. Dressings keep air movement past the sensitive partial thickness burn to a minimum and thereby reduce pain. Bulky sterile dressings also provide padding against minor bumping and other trauma. In full thickness burns, they provide a barrier to possible contamination.

Keep the patient warm. When burns involve large surface areas, the patient loses the ability to effectively control body temperature. If the burn begins to seep fluid, as in a full thickness burn, evaporative heat loss can be extreme. Cover such an area with dry sterile dressings, cover the patient with a blanket, and maintain a warm environment. If transport time is less than 20 minutes and the risk of hypothermia is low, damp dressings may be applied to the patient's burns.

When treating full thickness burns to the fingers, toes, or other locations where burned surfaces may contact each other, place soft, nonadherent bandages between the burned skin areas (Figure 21-17). Without this precaution, the disrupted and wet wounds would stick together and cause further damage when pulled apart for care at the emergency department.

Cool water immersion of minor localized burns may be effective if accomplished in the first few minutes after a burn.

Cover extensive partial and full thickness burns with dry sterile dressing, keep the patient warm, and initiate fluid resuscitation.

Use soft, nonadherent dressings between areas of full thickness burns, as between the fingers and toes, to prevent adhesion.

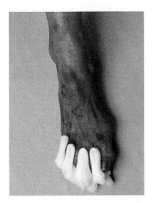 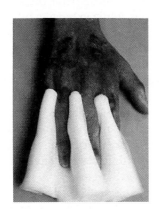 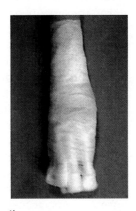

FIGURE 21-17 Separate burned toes and fingers with dry sterile gauze.

If the surface area of the burn is great and the transporting unit is an ACP/CCP, medical direction may ask you to provide aggressive fluid therapy during prehospital care. While hypovolemia is not an early development after a burn, fluid migration into the wound later during the burn cycle eventually leads to serious fluid loss. Early and aggressive fluid therapy can effectively reduce the impact of this fluid loss.

If burns cover all the normal IV access sites, you may place the catheter through tissue with partial thickness burns, proximal to any more serious injury. (Full thickness burns usually damage the blood vessels or coagulate the blood, making intravenous cannulation difficult and possibly impeding effective fluid flow.) Be careful with insertion. The skin may be leathery, but the tissue underneath is very delicate.

Establish intravenous routes in any patient with moderate to severe burns. Introduce two large-bore catheters, and hang 1000-mL bags of either normal saline (preferred) or Ringer's Lactate solution. Current fluid resuscitation formulas recommend 4 mL of fluid for every kilogram of patient weight multiplied by the percentage of body surface area burned:

$$4 \text{ mL} \times \text{Patient weight in kg} \times \text{BSA burned} = \text{Amount of fluid}$$

Thus for a 70-kg patient with 30 percent BSA burned, the calculation is

$$4 \times 70 \times 30 = 8400 \text{ mL}$$

The patient needs half this amount of fluid in the first eight hours after the burn. This particular fluid resuscitation protocol is known as the Parkland formula. Other variations exist and may be in use in your local area. In most prehospital situations where transport time is short (less than one hour), an initial fluid bolus of 0.5 mL of fluid for every kilogram of patient weight multiplied by the percentage of BSA burned is reasonable:

$$0.5 \text{ mL} \times \text{Patient weight in kg} \times \text{BSA burned} = \text{Amount of fluid}$$

Thus, for an 80-kg patient with 20 percent BSA burned, the calculation is

$$0.5 \times 80 \times 20 = 800 \text{ mL}$$

You may repeat this infusion once or twice during the first hour or so of care.

Be cautious and conservative when administering fluids to the burn patient if there is any possibility of airway or lung injury. Rapid fluid administration may worsen airway swelling or the edema that accompanies toxic inhalation. Whenever you administer fluid to a burn patient, carefully monitor the airway, and auscultate for breath sounds frequently.

Burns are quite painful, and yet the pain is often paradoxical to the burn severity. Less severe superficial and partial thickness (first- and second-degree) burns are very uncomfortable, while extensive full thickness (third-degree) burns are often almost without pain. Provide patients in severe pain with narcotic analgesia if within your scope of practice. Consider morphine in 2 mg IV increments every five minutes until suffering is relieved. Use morphine with caution, as it may depress the respiratory drive and increase any existing hypovolemia. Fentanyl 50 μg (micrograms) may also be administered as an alternative.

Infection is another typical and deadly problem associated with extensive soft-tissue burns. This life-threatening condition does not develop until well after prehospital care is concluded. However, proper field care can significantly reduce mortality and morbidity. Providing a clean environment and sterile dressings can lessen the bacterial load for the patient.

Emergency department personnel will continue fluid resuscitation for serious burn patients, according to the Parkland or another suitable formula. They will

Be cautious and conservative when administering fluids to the burn patient with inhalation injury.

perform arterial blood gas evaluation to determine oxygen tension, carbon monoxide concentration, and cyanide poisoning levels. Urine output and cardiac monitoring are instituted as well. The staff will ensure adequate administration of parenteral narcotic analgesia and provide tetanus immunization if necessary. They will closely evaluate severe circumferential burns for eschar development. If the blood flow in an extremity or respirations are impaired, the physician may perform an escharotomy.

INHALATION INJURY

If you suspect thermal (or chemical) airway burns and airway compromise is imminent, intubation can be life saving. Once you ensure the patient's airway, provide high-flow oxygen by nonrebreather mask at 15 litres per minute (Lpm). Oxygen not only counters hypoxia but is also therapeutic in carbon monoxide and cyanide poisoning. A centre capable of providing hyperbaric oxygen therapy for patients with suspected carbon monoxide poisoning may be useful. The hyperbaric chamber provides oxygen under the pressure of two or more atmospheres. This pushes oxygen into the patient's bloodstream, carrying it directly to the body's cells. Hyperbaric oxygenation also drives carbon monoxide from the hemoglobin, shortening the time to recovery. If hyperbaric oxygen therapy is available in your area, any patient suffering from smoke inhalation or suspected carbon monoxide poisoning could be considered for treatment at the facility.

Early intubation can be life saving for the inhalation injury patient.

Suspect cyanide toxicity in patients with severe symptoms, such as dyspnea, chest pain, altered mental status, seizures, and unconsciousness. To be effective, antidotal treatment of serious cyanide poisoning must be started early. Vapour exposures are likely to result in severe respiratory distress or apnea in addition to unconsciousness. Rapid airway intervention with endotracheal intubation and ventilatory support with a bag-valve mask are initial priorities. However, a rapid shift to antidotal therapy is essential to save the patient.

Administration of the antidote for cyanide in the hospital is a two-stage process, first using a nitrite compound, followed by a sulphur-containing compound (Figure 21-18). The nitrite acts by converting the hemoglobin (the primary oxygen-carrying protein in the blood) to methemoglobin. Methemoglobin then binds the cyanide, removing it from the cytochrome$_{a3}$ (an enzyme necessary for oxygen processing by cells). The sulphur-containing antidote then removes the cyanide by forming a nontoxic compound, which is excreted in the urine.

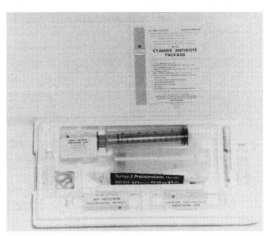

FIGURE 21-18   A cyanide antidote kit.

ASSESSMENT AND MANAGEMENT OF ELECTRICAL, CHEMICAL, AND RADIATION BURNS

ELECTRICAL INJURIES

Until the power is turned off, no one should be allowed to approach the electrical burn patient.

Be certain that the power has been turned off before you approach the scene of a suspected electrical injury. Until it is done, do not allow anyone to approach the patient or the proximity of the electrical source. Remember that an energized power line need not spark or whip around to be deadly; a power line simply lying on the ground can still present a significant danger. Note also that some utility lines have breakers that will try to reestablish power periodically. Establish a safety zone if there is any question about the status of lines that are down. Keep vehicles and personnel at a distance from downed lines or the source pole that is greater than the distance between the power poles. Also be aware that downed power lines may energize metal structures, such as buildings, vehicles, or fences.

Once the scene is secure, assess the patient and prepare her for transport. Search for entrance and exit wounds. Look specifically for possible contact points with both the ground and the electrical source. In some circumstances, multiple entrance and exit wounds are present. Remember that electrical current passes through the body and therefore may cause significant internal burns, especially to blood vessels and nerves, whereas the assessment reveals only minimal superficial findings. Rapidly progressive cardiovascular collapse can follow contact with an electrical source. Also, examine the patient for any fractures resulting from forceful muscle contractions caused by the current's passage.

As with thermal burns, look for smouldering shoes, belts, or other items of clothing. Such items may continue the burning process well after the current is turned off. Also remove rings, watches, and any other constrictive items from the fingers, limbs, and the neck.

Monitor the electrical burn patient for abnormalities in the ECG.

Perform ECG monitoring for possible cardiac disturbances in victims of electrical burns. Electrical current may induce dysrhythmias, including bradycardias, tachycardias, ventricular fibrillation, and asystole. Ensure that emergency department personnel examine any patient who has sustained a significant electrical shock. The damage the current causes may be internal and not apparent to you or your patient during assessment. Consider a patient with any significant electrical burn or exposure as a high priority for immediate transport.

Lightning strikes on humans occur rarely, but in Canada, they result in 16 deaths per year on average. Strikes on people riding tractors, on open water, on golf courses, and under trees are most common, and men are the victims of 75 percent of all strikes. A lightning strike is a high-voltage (up to 100 000 volts), high-current (10 000 amperes), and high-temperature (> 27 000°C) event that lasts only a fraction of a second. A direct strike will impart this energy to the patient (Figure 21-19). However, the lightning will often strike a nearby object with some voltage travelling sideways (sideflash), or the voltage may radiate outward in alternate pathways from the strike point, thus diminishing the voltage (step voltage).

By the time anyone reaches the victim of a lightning strike, the electricity has long since dissipated. (There will be, however, a continued risk of further strikes as long as the storm remains nearby.) There is no danger of electrical shock from touching the victim of a lightning strike. The victim's clothing, however, may continue to smoulder; so, remove it as necessary. Among other serious effects, lightning can produce a sudden cessation of breathing. Despite being apneic and perhaps even pulseless, these patients frequently survive with prompt prehospital intervention.

Treat visible burns ("entrance" and "exit" wounds), just as any thermal burn, with cooling if necessary, followed by the application of dry sterile dressings. Do

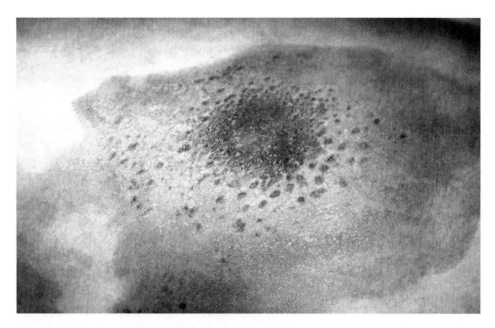

FIGURE 21-19   A typical lightning strike injury.

not focus too much on the visible burns, but recognize that the electricity has passed through the body, possibly causing widespread internal effects.

Treat cardiac or respiratory arrest in electrical burn patients with aggressive airway, ventilatory, and circulatory management. Patients in cardiac arrest because of contact with electrical current have a high survival rate if prehospital intervention is prompt. Check immediately for ventricular fibrillation, and defibrillate if necessary. Secure the airway with an oropharyngeal airway (OPA); if ACP/CCP, use an endotracheal tube; and begin ventilations and chest compressions. The usual resuscitative procedures for cases of cardiac arrest apply equally when the cause of the arrest is electrical injury; they might include the use of epinephrine, lidocaine, or atropine.

For serious electrical burn injuries, initiate at least two large-bore IVs and give an initial 20 mL/kg fluid bolus. If the electrical burn is severe, provide additional fluid using the Parkland or another formula.

CHEMICAL BURNS

As you perform the scene assessment, identify the nature of the chemical spill/contamination, and if possible, approach from upwind. Identify the location of the chemical, and ensure that it poses no hazard to you, other rescuers, or the public through communication with dispatch and CANUTEC. Be wary of toxic fumes and cross-contamination from the patient and the surrounding environment. If necessary, have hazardous material team members evacuate and decontaminate the victim before you begin assessment and care. Seek out personnel on the scene who are familiar with the agent, and consult with them regarding dangers posed by the agent and any specific medical care and patient handling procedures required with it.

During your assessment and care, always wear medical examination gloves, but never presume that they will protect you from the chemical agent. Take appropriate protective action against airborne dust, toxic fumes, and splash exposure for both you and the patient (goggles and mask as needed). Wear a disposable gown if there is danger of the agent contacting your clothing. Make certain the

In dealing with a chemical burn, take all precautions to ensure that no one else becomes contaminated.

agent is isolated and no longer a danger to the patient or others. Remove any of the patient's clothing that you suspect may be contaminated, and isolate it from accidental contact. Save the clothing, and ensure that it is disposed of properly. Identify the type of agent, its exact chemical name, the length of the patient's contact time with it, and the precise areas of the patient's body affected by it.

As you begin your primary assessment, ensure that the patient is alert and fully oriented and that airway and breathing are unaffected by the contact. If there is any airway restriction or respiratory involvement, consider early management. As airway tissue swells, the obstruction worsens and airway management may become more difficult. Monitor the patient's heart rate, and consider ECG monitoring because many chemicals (for example, organophosphates) may affect the heart. If the patient is stable, begin the rapid trauma assessment.

Examine any chemical burn carefully to establish the depth, extent, and nature of the injury. If you suspect the involvement of phenol, dry lime, sodium, or riot control agents, treat as indicated below.

- *Phenol* A gelatinous caustic called phenol is used as a powerful industrial cleaner. Phenol is very difficult to remove because it is sticky and insoluble in water. Alcohol, which dissolves it, is frequently available in places where phenol is regularly used. You can use the alcohol to remove the phenol and follow with irrigation using large volumes of cool water.

- *Dry Lime* Dry lime is a strong corrosive that reacts with water. It produces heat and subsequent chemical and thermal injuries. Brush dry lime off the patient gently but as completely as possible. Then, rinse the contaminated area with large volumes of cool to cold water. While the water reacts with any remaining lime, it cools the contact area and removes the rest of the chemical. By rinsing with water, you ensure that the lime reacts with that water, rather than with the water contained within the patient's soft tissues.

- *Sodium* Sodium is an unstable metal that reacts destructively with many substances, including human tissue. It reacts vigorously with water, creating extreme heat, explosive hydrogen gas, and possible ignition. Sodium is normally stored submerged in oil because the metal reacts with oxygen in the air. If a patient is contaminated with sodium, decontaminate her quickly by gentle brushing. Then, cover the wound with oil used to store the substance.

- *Riot Control Agents* These agents, which include tear gas (chlorbenzlidene malonitrile, CS), chloracetophenon (CN, mace), and oleoresin capsicum (OC, pepper spray), deserve special mention because people are the targets of their intended use and because that use is frequent. These agents cause intense irritation of the eyes, mucous membranes, and respiratory tract. In general, they do not cause permanent damage when properly deployed. Patients who have come in contact with them typically present with eye pain, tearing, and temporary "blindness." Coughing, gagging, and vomiting are not uncommon. Treatment is supportive, and most patients recover spontaneously within 10 to 20 minutes of exposure to fresh air. If necessary, irrigate the patient's eyes with normal saline if you suspect that any riot agent particles remain.

Irrigation with copious amounts of cool water is indicated for burns from an unknown chemical agent.

If it has not been done earlier, decontaminate the patient who has come in contact with any other chemical capable of causing tissue damage. Stop the damage by irrigating the site with large volumes of water (Figure 21-20). Water rinses

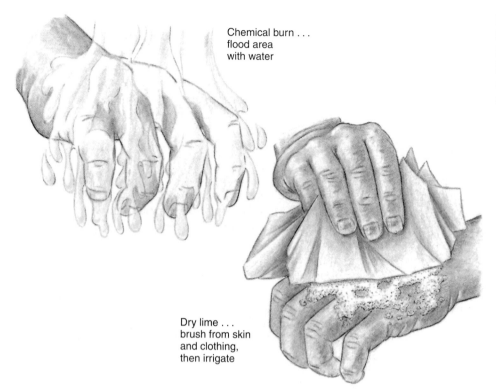

Chemical burn . . .
flood area
with water

Dry lime . . .
brush from skin
and clothing,
then irrigate

FIGURE 21-20   Chemical burns should be flushed with large quantities of water. Dry lime should be first brushed away before applying cool water.

away the offending material and dilutes any water-soluble agents. Water also reduces the heat and rate of the chemical reaction and, ultimately, the chemical's effects on the patient's skin. If the contamination is widespread, douse the patient with large volumes of water. Use a garden hose or low-pressure water from a fire truck. Ensure that the water is neither too warm nor too cold.

When the patient has been thoroughly rinsed for a few minutes, remove any remaining clothing. Take care that the process does not contaminate rescuers. If the agent is dangerous, save all clothing, and contain the rinse water for proper disposal at a later time. Next, gently wash the burn with a mild soap (such as ordinary dish soap) and a soft brush or sponge. Be careful not to cause further soft-tissue damage. After washing, gently irrigate the wound with a constant flow of water. While the pain and the burning process may appear to subside, it is important to continue the irrigation until the patient arrives at the emergency department. If practical, transport the label from the corrosive's container or a sample of the agent (safely contained and marked) along with the patient. On arrival at the hospital, be sure to describe to emergency department personnel, and enter in your prehospital care report, any first aid given prior to your arrival.

With chemical burns, pay particular attention to the patient's eyes. Eyes are very sensitive to chemicals and can easily be damaged even by weak agents. Prompt treatment of chemical eye injury is critical and can reduce damage to and preserve eyesight. Ask the patient about the chemical that came in contact with the eyes, eye pain, vision changes, and contact lens use. Examine the eyes for eyelid spasm (**blepharospasm**), conjunctival erythema, discoloration, tearing, and other evidence of burns or irritation.

If there were chemical splashes, irrigate the eye with large volumes of water. Alkali burns are especially damaging, and in such cases, you should flush the eye for at least 15 minutes. Irrigate acid burns for at least five minutes. Flush injury by splashes of an unknown agent for up to 20 minutes. Do not, however, delay transport while irrigating.

Do not use any antidote or any neutralizing agent on chemical burns.

* **blepharospasm** twitching of the eyelids.

Irrigate all alkali burns to the eye for at least 15 minutes.

A useful technique for irrigation is to set up a bag of normal saline (Ringer's Lactate is an acceptable substitute) and use the flow regulator to control the flow of fluid into the nasal corner of the eye. Turn the patient's head to the side to facilitate drainage and avoid cross-contaminating the other eye with the waste fluid. Be alert for contact lenses in cases where chemicals are splashed into the eyes. Chemicals may become trapped under the lenses, preventing adequate irrigation. Gently remove the lenses while continuing irrigation.

RADIATION BURNS

An incident involving potential radiation exposure or burns must be a concern during both dispatch and response phases of the emergency call. Because radiation can be neither seen nor felt, it can endanger EMS personnel unless the hazard has been anticipated and proper precautions taken. If you suspect radiation exposure, approach the scene very carefully (Figure 21-21). If the incident occurs at a power generation plant or in an industrial or a medical facility, seek out personnel knowledgeable about the radioactive substance being used. Such persons are always on staff, and frequently on site, at these facilities. Stay a good distance from the scene, and ensure that bystanders, rescuers, and patients remain far from the source of the exposure. Remember that distance and the nature of the materials, like concrete or earth, between you and the radiation source reduce potential exposure. If the exposure could be from dust or fire, approach from and remain upwind of the radiation source.

In radiation exposure incidents, ensure that personnel trained in radiation hazards isolate the source, contain it, and test the scene for safety. If this is impossible, move the patient to a site remote from the radioactivity source where you can give care without danger to either you or the patient. Plan the removal carefully. Use as much shielding as possible and keep exposure times to a minimum. Remember, the dose of radiation received is related to three primary factors: duration, distance, and shielding.

If there is a risk that patients are contaminated, ensure that they are properly decontaminated before you begin assessment and care. If available for this task, use persons knowledgeable in decontamination and monitoring techniques and who have the appropriate protective gear. If this is not possible, don goggles, a mask, gloves, and a disposable gown. Direct the evacuation team to place the patients in a decontamination area remote from your vehicle and other personnel and where any contamination can be contained. Have the patients disrobe or carefully disrobe them, rinse them with large volumes of water, and then wash them with a

Because radiation can be neither seen nor felt, it can endanger EMS personnel unless proper precautions are taken.

Duration, distance, and shielding are important factors in determining radiation dose exposure.

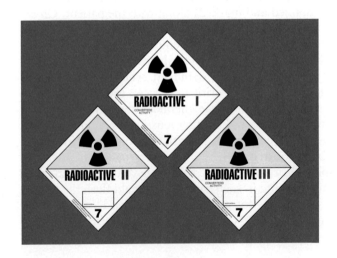

FIGURE 21-21 Warning labels may indicate the presence of radioactive materials.

soft brush and rinse again. Ordinary dish soap is effective as a cleansing agent. As in incidents of chemical contamination, save all clothing and decontamination water, and dispose of them safely. Perform decontamination before moving the patients to the ambulance.

Carefully document the circumstances of the radioactive exposure. If possible, identify the source and strength of the agent. Determine the patient's proximity to the source during the exposure as well as the length of exposure.

Once decontaminated, treat a radiation exposure patient as you would any other patient. Because the human body by itself cannot be a source of ionizing radiation, the decontaminated patient poses no threat to you or your crew. Remember, however, that any contaminated material remaining on the patient or any contamination transferred to you does provide a source of radiation exposure and may contaminate you and your vehicle.

Once properly decontaminated, the radiation injury patient presents no radiation danger to caregivers.

The actual assessment of a patient exposed to radiation is quite simple and usually reveals minimal signs or symptoms of injury. Only extreme exposures result in the classical presentation of nausea, vomiting, and malaise. Burns are extremely rare, although they may occur if the exposure is extremely intense. Even though a patient seems well, the delayed consequences of high-dose radiation exposure can be devastating. If you note any early patient complaints, record the findings in the patient's own words and include the time the complaint first was made. This information is helpful in determining the patient's degree of radiation exposure (Table 21-4).

Treat the symptoms of the radiation injury patient, make the patient as comfortable as possible, and offer psychological support. Cover any burns with sterile dressing and, if general symptoms are noticeable, provide oxygen, and initiate an IV. Maintain the patient's body temperature, and provide transport to the emergency department.

Table 21-4 DOSE–EFFECT RELATIONSHIPS TO IONIZING RADIATION

Whole Body Exposure Dose (RAD)	Effect
5–25	Asymptomatic. Blood studies are normal.
50–75	Asymptomatic. Minor depressions of white blood cells and platelets in a few patients.
75–125	May produce anorexia, nausea, and vomiting, and fatigue in approximately 10–20 percent of patients within two days.
125–200	Possible nausea and vomiting. Diarrhea, anxiety, tachycardia. Fatal to less than 5 percent of patients.
200–600	Nausea and vomiting. Diarrhea in the first several hours. Weakness, fatigue. Fatal to approximately 50 percent of patients within six weeks without prompt medical attention.
600–1 000	"Burning sensation" within minutes. Nausea and vomiting within 10 minutes. Confusion, ataxia, and collapse within one hour. Watery diarrhea within one to two hours. Fatal to 100 percent within short time without prompt medical attention.

Localized Exposure Dose (RAD)	Effect
50	Asymptomatic.
500	Asymptomatic (usually). May have risk of altered function of exposed area.
2 500	Atrophy, vascular lesion, and altered pigmentation.
5 000	Chronic ulcer, risk of carcinogenesis.
50 000	Permanent destruction of exposed tissue.

ONGOING ASSESSMENT

Monitor patients with inhalation, chemical, and electrical burns and radiation exposure patients for signs of increasing complications associated with their burn mechanisms. Also, monitor blood pressure, pulse, and respirations, and note down any trends. Perform these evaluations every 15 minutes in stable patients and every five minutes in unstable patients.

SUMMARY

Burn injuries may compromise the skin—the protective envelope that protects and contains the human body. Burn damage to the skin may interfere with its ability to contain water within the body and to prevent damaging agents from entering. For these reasons, assessment and care of these soft-tissue injuries are important.

Assess the burn to determine its depth and the extent of the body surface area it involves. Be sensitive to any respiratory, joint, hand, foot, or circumferential regions affected by the burn. Give special consideration to pediatric and geriatric burn patients and to burn patients who are also ill or otherwise injured. Consider all these factors in determining the overall severity of a burn. If the patient's condition warrants, institute aggressive care. Anticipate airway compromise and fluid loss. Secure the airway very early in prehospital care. Initiate IV access, and begin fluid administration.

Electrical, chemical, or radiation burns require special care and assessment. An electrical burn requires careful assessment to determine the area and depth of burn involvement and should be followed by wound site dressing and cardiac monitoring. Chemical burns need rapid and effective decontamination. Radiation burns call for extreme care in removing the patient from the radiation source and in providing decontamination and supportive care.

CHAPTER 22

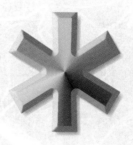

Musculoskeletal Trauma

Objectives

After reading this chapter, you should be able to:

1. Describe the incidence, morbidity, and mortality related to musculo-skeletal injuries. (pp. 168–169)
2. Discuss the anatomy and physiology of the muscular and skeletal systems. (see Chapter 12)
3. Predict injuries based on the mechanism of injury: (pp. 169–175)
   - Direct
   - Indirect
   - Pathological
4. Discuss the types of musculoskeletal injuries:
   - Fractures (open and closed) (pp. 172–174)
   - Dislocations/fractures (pp. 171–172)
   - Sprains (p. 171)
   - Strains (p. 171)
5. Describe the six Ps of musculoskeletal injury assessment. (p. 180)
6. List the primary signs and symptoms of extremity trauma. (pp. 177–182)

Continued

7. List other signs and symptoms that can indicate a less obvious extremity injury. (pp. 180–182)
8. Discuss the need for assessment of pulses, motor function, and sensation before and after splinting. (p. 185)
9. Identify the circumstances requiring rapid intervention and transport when dealing with musculoskeletal injuries. (pp. 178–179)
10. Discuss the general guidelines for splinting. (pp. 184–189)
11. Explain the benefits of the application of cold and heat for musculoskeletal injuries. (p. 190)
12. Describe age-associated changes in bones. (p. 175)
13. Discuss the pathophysiology, assessment findings, and management of open and closed fractures. (pp. 173–174, 191–194)
14. Discuss the relationship between the volume of hemorrhage and open or closed fractures. (pp. 179, 191, 192)
15. Describe the special considerations involved in femur fracture management. (pp. 191–192)
16. Discuss the pathophysiology, assessment findings, and management of dislocations. (pp. 171–172, 195–199)

17. Discuss the prehospital management of dislocations/fractures, including splinting and realignment. (pp. 191–199)
18. Explain the importance of manipulating a knee dislocation/fracture with an absent distal pulse. (pp. 195–196)
19. Describe the procedure for reduction of a shoulder, finger, or ankle dislocation/fracture. (pp. 196–199)
20. Discuss the pathophysiology, assessment findings, and management of sprains, strains, and tendon injuries. (pp. 171, 199)
21. Differentiate among musculoskeletal injuries on the basis of the assessment findings and history. (pp. 177–183)
22. Given several preprogrammed and moulaged musculoskeletal trauma patients, provide the appropriate scene assessment, primary assessment, rapid trauma or focused secondary assessment and history, detailed assessment, and ongoing assessment and provide appropriate patient care and transport. (pp. 177–203)

INTRODUCTION TO MUSCULOSKELETAL TRAUMA

Incidences of musculoskeletal injury are second in frequency only to soft-tissue injuries in trauma.

In trauma, incidence of musculoskeletal injuries are second in frequency only to soft-tissue injuries. They usually result from application of significant direct or transmitted blunt kinetic forces. Skeletal or muscular injuries may also occasionally result from penetrating mechanisms of injury. Thousands of Canadians sustain musculoskeletal injuries each year from a variety of sources, including sports injuries, motor vehicle crashes, falls, and acts of violence. These incidents can cause a variety of injuries to the body's bones, cartilage, ligaments, muscles, or tendons. While injuries to the upper extremities can be painful and sometimes debilitating, they rarely threaten life. Lower extremity injuries, on the other hand, are generally associated with a greater magnitude of force and greater secondary blood loss and, thus, more often constitute threats to life or limb. In addition, the same forces responsible for a musculoskeletal injury may damage internal organs, nerves, and blood vessels, causing serious problems throughout the body. In fact, most patients (up to 80 percent) who suffer multisystem trauma experience significant musculoskeletal injuries.

Up to 80 percent of patients who suffer multisystem trauma experience significant musculoskeletal injuries.

PREVENTION STRATEGIES

Stopping injury before it occurs—injury prevention—is the optimal way to reduce musculoskeletal injuries. Strategies for preventing musculoskeletal injuries include application of modern vehicle and highway designs and safe driving practices, including the use of restraint systems. Auto collisions are the greatest single cause of musculoskeletal injuries, and improved vehicle safety has done much to reduce injury incidence and severity. Workplace safety standards have done much to reduce on-the-job injuries. These standards include criteria for proper footwear, scaffolding, fall protection devices, and the like. Sports injuries, which most commonly affect the musculature, joints, and long bones, account for a significant number of traumas. While protective gear, improved equipment design, and better conditioning of athletes have reduced injuries, the very nature of contact sports means that these activities remain a significant cause of injury. Household accidents and falls also account for many musculoskeletal injuries. Use of good safety practices—for example, proper footwear, well-designed railings, proper use of step ladders—can reduce injury incidence at home.

PATHOPHYSIOLOGY OF THE MUSCULOSKELETAL SYSTEM

The musculoskeletal injury process is a complicated one, resulting in much more damage than does the disruption of an inert structural element of the body. Bone is living tissue and requires a continuous supply of oxygenated circulation. Bone lies deep within muscle tissue, and major nerves and blood vessels parallel it as they travel to the distal extremity. At points of articulation, there is a complex arrangement of ligaments, cartilage, and synovial fluid that holds the joint together while permitting a wide range of movement. Finally, the muscles attach and direct skeletal movement through the collections of fibres, fasciculi, and muscle bodies connected to the skeletal system by tendons. This complex arrangement of connective, skeletal, vascular, nervous, and muscular tissue is endangered whenever significant kinetic forces are applied to the extremities. If the forces are severe enough, they are likely to cause muscular, joint, or skeletal injury.

Bone is living tissue and requires a constant supply of oxygenated circulation.

MUSCULAR INJURY

Muscular injuries may result from direct blunt or penetrating trauma, overexertion, or problems with oxygen supply during exertion. These injuries include contusions, penetrating injuries, fatigue, cramps, spasms, and strains. Muscular problems usually do not contribute significantly to hypovolemia and shock, with the exceptions of severe contusions with large associated hematomas and penetrating injuries with extensive hemorrhage.

Content Review
TYPES OF MUSCULAR INJURIES
Contusion
Compartment syndrome
Penetrating injury
Muscle fatigue
Muscle cramp
Muscle spasm
Muscle strain

Contusion

Severe trauma frequently crushes muscles between a blunt force and the skeletal structure beneath. This damages both the muscle cells and the blood vessels that supply them. Small blood vessels rupture, leaking blood into the interstitial spaces and causing pain, erythema, and then ecchymosis. Blood in the interstitial spaces and muscle cell damage set off the body's inflammatory response. Capillary beds engorge with blood, and fluid shifts to the interstitial space, leading to tissue edema. The injury may also cause blood to pool beneath tissue layers in a hematoma. In more massive body muscles, like those of the thigh, buttocks, calf, or arm, large volumes of blood may accumulate, contributing significantly to hypovolemia. A large hematoma or significant muscular edema will increase the diameter of the injured limb, especially compared with the opposing uninjured limb. For the most part, however, signs of muscle injury remain hidden beneath the skin.

Compartment Syndrome

Contusion, crush injury, and fracture may damage the soft tissue of the extremity and cause both internal hemorrhage and swelling. As the swelling and pooling of blood increase, pressure may build within the fascial compartment that contains them. This pressure first restricts capillary blood flow and compresses and damages nerves. If the pressure continues to build, it restricts and then halts venous return through the limb and ultimately stops arterial circulation. The first signs of this developing injury are tension (a feeling like a contracted muscle) within the limb and some loss of distal sensation, especially in the webs of the fingers or toes. The patient may complain of pain and appear more seriously injured than the mechanism of injury or outward signs might suggest. In addition, your moving of the patient's limb (passive extension) may elicit increased pain. Pulse deficit is a late sign of compartment syndrome.

Penetrating Injury

Deep lacerations may penetrate skin and subcutaneous tissues, thus affecting the muscle masses and tendons below. Massive wounds involving a large percentage of a muscle body or those injuring or severing a tendon may reduce the distal limb's strength or render muscular control ineffective. When a tendon or muscle is cut, contraction of the opposing muscle moves the limb, while the injured muscle/tendon is unable to return the limb toward the neutral position. Such injuries call for surgical intervention to identify and rejoin the damaged tendon or muscle body. These wounds may also introduce infectious agents, damage muscle tissue, and affect the muscle's blood supply. The resulting infection, ischemia, or a combination of the two may result in further tissue injury and poor healing.

Fatigue

* **fatigue** condition in which a muscle's ability to respond to stimulation is lost or reduced through overactivity.

Muscle **fatigue** occurs as the muscles reach their limit of performance. Exercise draws down the muscle's oxygen and energy reserves and causes accumulation of metabolic byproducts. The cell environment becomes hypoxic, toxic, and energy deprived. Fewer and fewer muscle fibres are able to contract. The strength of the muscle mass diminishes, and further exertion becomes painful. Until adequate circulation restores oxygen and the muscle cells can replenish energy sources, the muscle fibres and muscle body remain weakened.

Muscle Cramp

* **cramping** muscle pain resulting from overactivity, lack of oxygen, and accumulation of waste products.

Cramping is not really an injury but an "angina" of the muscle tissue. Muscle pain results when exercise consumes the available oxygen and energy sources and the circulatory system fails to remove metabolic waste products. The pain begins during or immediately after vigorous exercise or after the limb has been left in an unusual position for a period of time (obstructing circulatory flow). Cramping is usually associated with continuous muscle contraction (spasm). Changing the limb's position or massaging it may help return the circulation and reduce the pain. Once rest and adequate circulation restore the metabolic balance, the pain of muscle cramp usually subsides.

Muscle Spasm

In muscle **spasm,** the affected muscle goes into an intermittent (clonic) or continuous (tonic) contraction. The spasm may be firm enough to feel like the deformity associated with a fracture and can confound assessment. (The extreme of muscle spasm is rigor mortis, an anoxic, rigid, whole-body muscle spasm that occurs after death.) As with the cramp, the spasm usually subsides uneventfully with the restoration of circulation.

* **spasm** intermittent or continuous contraction of a muscle.

Strain

A **strain** occurs when muscle fibres are overstretched by forces that exceed the strength of the fibres. The muscle fibres then stretch and tear, causing pain that increases with any use of the muscle. The injury may occur with extreme muscle stress, as during heavy lifting or sprinting, or at times of fatigue, when only a limited number of fibres are in contraction. With a strain, the fibres are damaged without internal bleeding, edema, or discoloration. The site of injury is generally painful to palpation, and patients normally report pain that limits use of the affected muscle.

* **strain** injury resulting from overstretching of muscle fibres.

JOINT INJURY

Joint injuries include sprains, subluxations, and dislocations. The following sections detail the pathologies behind each of these injuries.

Sprain

A **sprain** is a tearing of a joint capsule's connective tissues, specifically a ligament or ligaments. This injury causes acute pain at its site, followed shortly by inflammation and swelling. Ecchymotic discoloration occurs over time but not usually during prehospital care. The tearing of ligaments weakens the joint. Continued use of the joint may lead to its complete failure. Sprains are classified, or graded, according to their severity, using the following criteria:

- *Grade I* Minor and incomplete tear. The ligament is painful, and swelling is usually minimal. The joint is stable.
- *Grade II* Significant but incomplete tear. Swelling and pain range from moderate to severe. The joint is intact but unstable.
- *Grade III* Complete tear of the ligament. Due to severe pain and spasm, the sprain may present as a fracture. The joint is unstable.

* **sprain** tearing of a joint capsule's connective tissues.

* **subluxation** partial displacement of a bone end from its position in a joint capsule.

Subluxation

A **subluxation** is a partial displacement of a bone end from its position within a joint capsule. It occurs as the joint separates under stress, stretching the ligaments. The subluxation differs from the sprain in that it more significantly reduces the joint's integrity. The injured joint is painful and swells quickly, its range

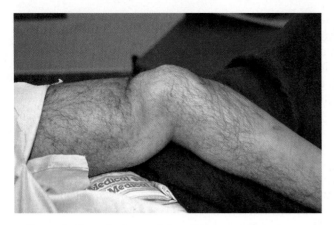

a. Presentation of a knee dislocation

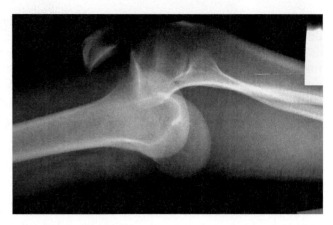

b. X-ray of the dislocation

FIGURE 22-1   Knee dislocation.

of motion is limited, and the joint is unstable. Hyperflexion, hyperextension, lateral rotation beyond the normal range of motion, or application of extreme axial force are common causes of subluxations.

Dislocation

 dislocation complete displacement of a bone end from its position in a joint capsule.

A **dislocation** is a complete displacement of a bone end from its normal joint position (Figure 22-1). The joint then fixes in an abnormal position with noticeable deformity. The site is painful, swollen, and immobile. This type of injury carries with it the danger of entrapping, compressing, or tearing blood vessels and nerves. Dislocation occurs when the joint moves beyond its normal range of motion with great force. By its nature, a dislocation has serious associated ligament damage and may involve injury to the joint capsule and articular cartilage.

BONE INJURY

The fracture is an involved process that ultimately disrupts the continuity of the bone. When extreme compressional forces or significant lateral forces exceed the tensile strength of a bone, the bone fractures.

A fracture may be caused by direct injury—for example, an auto bumper strikes a patient's femur or a high-powered rifle bullet slams into a patient's thigh and then femur. The cause of the fracture may also be indirect. This might occur when a bike rider is thrown over the handlebars and braces the fall with an outstretched arm. In this case, the energy of impact is transmitted from the hand to the wrist, to the forearm, to the upper arm, to the shoulder, to the clavicle. The transmitted force fractures the clavicle and may cause internal injury to blood vessels and the upper reaches of the lung. For this reason, always analyze the mechanism of injury carefully, recognizing that kinetic forces may be transmitted and cause injury far from the point of impact. Remember, 80 percent of multisystem trauma cases have associated serious musculoskeletal injury.

Recognize that kinetic forces may be transmitted through the skeletal system and cause injury remote from the impact site.

As kinetic energy is transmitted to the bone and the bone fractures, the collagen, osteocytes, salt crystals, blood vessels, nerves, and medullary canal of the bone, as well as its periosteum and endosteum (the inner lining of the medullary canal) are disrupted. If the broken bone ends displace, they may further injure surrounding muscles, tendons, ligaments, veins, and arteries. The result is a serious insult to the limb structure.

Vascular damage may restrict blood flow to the distal limb, increasing capillary refill time, diminishing pulse strength and limb temperature, and causing discoloration and paresthesia (a "pins-and-needles" sensation). Nerve injury may result in distal paresthesia, anesthesia (loss of sensation), paresis (weakness), and paralysis (loss of muscle control). Muscle or tendon damage may interfere with the victim's ability to move the limb. If muscle tissue is badly damaged where fasciae firmly contain it, compartment syndrome may develop.

If the bone does not seriously displace and the forces causing fracture do not penetrate, the surrounding skin remains intact, and the resulting injury is termed a **closed fracture.** If the sharp bone ends displaced by the forces causing the fracture or other subsequent motion of the limb lacerate through the muscle, subcutaneous tissue, and skin, the result is termed an **open fracture** (Figure 22-2). An open fracture may also occur when a bullet travels through the limb and fractures the bone. Open fractures carry the risk of associated infection within the disrupted soft, bone, and medullary tissues. Such an infection may seriously reduce the bone's ability to heal. Where bones are located very close to the skin, as with the tibia (the shin), an open fracture can occur with relatively minimal bone displacement.

Surprisingly, some fractures may be relatively stable (Figure 22-3). When the bone suffers a small crack that does not disrupt its total structure, the injury is termed a **hairline fracture.** This type of injury weakens the bone and is painful, but the bone remains in position, retaining some of its strength. Another type of relatively stable bone injury is the **impacted fracture.** In some cases of compression, the bone impacts on itself, resulting in a compressed but aligned bone. As in a hairline fracture, the bone in an impacted fracture remains in position and retains some of its original strength. The danger with both hairline and impacted fractures is that further stress and movement may fracture the remaining bone and displace the bone ends, increasing both the severity of the injury and its healing time.

✱ **closed fracture** a broken bone in which the bone ends or the forces that caused the break do not penetrate the skin.

✱ **open fracture** a broken bone in which the bone ends or the forces that caused the break penetrate the surrounding skin.

✱ **hairline fracture** small crack in a bone that does not disrupt its total structure.

✱ **impacted fracture** break in a bone in which the bone is compressed on itself.

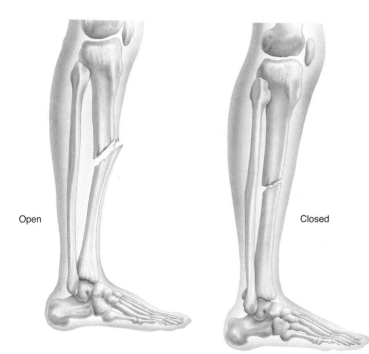

Open   Closed

FIGURE 22-2 Open and closed fractures.

FIGURE 22-3 Some types of fractures.

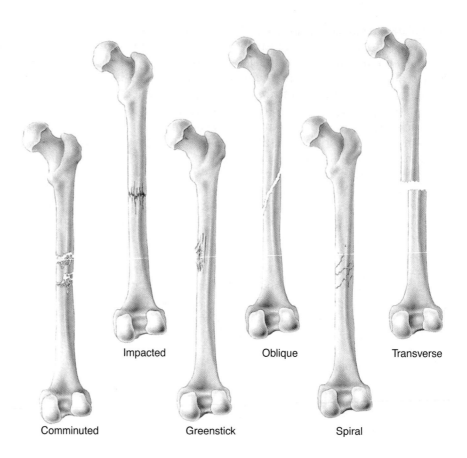

Impacted

Oblique

Transverse

Comminuted

Greenstick

Spiral

✱ **transverse fracture** a break that runs across a bone perpendicular to the bone's orientation.

✱ **oblique fracture** break in a bone running across it at an angle other than 90 degrees.

✱ **comminuted fracture** fracture in which a bone is broken into several pieces.

✱ **spiral fracture** a curving break in a bone as may be caused by rotational forces.

✱ **fatigue fracture** break in a bone associated with prolonged or repeated stress.

There are several fracture types whose physical characteristics can be revealed only by x-rays. For example, the **transverse fracture** is a complete break in the bone that runs straight across it at about a 90-degree angle. A fracture that runs at an angle across the bone is considered an **oblique fracture**. A fracture in which the bone has splintered into several smaller fragments is a **comminuted fracture**; this type of fracture is often associated with crushing injuries or the impact of a high-velocity bullet. Fractures involving a twisting motion may result in a curved break around the bone shaft known as a **spiral fracture**. Spiral fractures can occur with twisting motions, as when a child's arm is rotated by an adult or when an adult's limb is pulled into machinery, such as an auger.

The **fatigue fracture** is associated with prolonged or repeated stress, such as walking. The bone generally weakens and fractures without the application of great kinetic force. An example is the metatarsal fatigue fracture, also known as a march fracture.

A rare but serious complication of fracture is fat embolism. The bone's disruption may damage adjacent blood vessels and the medullary canal. The injury may then release fat, stored in a semiliquid form, into the wound site where it enters the venous system and travels to the heart. The heart distributes the fat to the pulmonary circulation where it becomes pulmonary emboli. Fat embolism is usually associated with severe or crush injuries or postinjury manipulation of larger long bone fractures.

Pediatric Considerations

The bones of infants, young children, and, to a degree, older children contain a greater percentage of cartilage than those of adults and are still growing from the epiphyseal plate. Pediatric patients, thus, often sustain different types of fractures from those of adults.

The flexible nature of pediatric bones is responsible for the **greenstick fracture**, a type of partial fracture. The injury disrupts only one side of the long bone and remains angulated, resisting alignment due to the disrupted bone fibres on the fracture side. During the bone repair process, the injured side experiences more rapid growth than the other side. This results in increasing angulation of the bone as it heals. Surgeons often complete a greenstick fracture by breaking the bone fully, thereby ensuring proper healing.

A child's bone grows at the epiphyseal plate, which forms a weak spot in the diaphysis. In pediatric trauma, this is a common site of the long bone disruption, called an **epiphyseal fracture**. If the growth plate is disrupted, the disruption may lead to a reduction or halt in bone growth, a condition most commonly involving the proximal tibia.

✱ greenstick fracture partial fracture of a child's bone.

✱ epiphyseal fracture disruption in the epiphyseal plate of a child's bone.

Geriatric Considerations

The aging process causes several changes to the musculoskeletal system. A gradual, progressive decrease in bone mass and collagen structure begins at about the age of 40 and results in bones that are less flexible, more brittle, and more easily fractured. The bones also heal more slowly. The aging adult loses some muscle strength and coordination, increasing the likelihood of skeletal injury. Fractures of the lumbar spine and femoral neck occur because of stress, often without history of significant trauma.

Another age-related and more significant problem secondary to poor bone remodelling is called **osteoporosis**. Osteoporosis is an accelerated degeneration of bone tissue due to loss of bone minerals, principally calcium. It typically affects women more than men and becomes most serious after menopause. The condition leads to increases in bone structure degeneration, spinal curvature, and incidences of fractures.

✱ osteoporosis weakening of bone tissue due to loss of essential minerals, especially calcium.

Pathological Fractures

Pathological fractures result from disease pathologies that affect bone development or maintenance. Such problems may be caused by tumours of the bone, periosteum, or articular cartilage or by diseases that release agents that increase osteoclast activity and osteoporosis. Other diseases and infections can have the same impact on bone tissue and cause fractures, especially in older patients. Radiation treatment may also kill bone cells, resulting in localized bone degeneration, weakened bones, and fractures. These fractures are not likely to heal well, if they heal at all.

GENERAL CONSIDERATIONS WITH MUSCULOSKELETAL INJURIES

The potential effects of trauma can be better anticipated when the skeletal structure and the musculature are examined together. It is important to note that long bones are smallest through the diaphysis and largest at the epiphyseal area, or joint. The external extremity diameter is greatest surrounding the midshaft due to the placement of skeletal muscle. This anatomical relationship is significant when looking at the potential for nervous or vascular injury.

Since there is limited soft tissue surrounding joints, joint fractures, dislocations, and—to a lesser degree—subluxations and sprains may cause severe problems beyond the direct injury. Any swelling, deformity, or displacement may

Because there is limited soft tissue surrounding joints, injuries there may cause severe problems beyond the direct injury because blood vessels and nerves may be affected.

compromise the nerve and vascular supply to the distal extremity. Fractures near a joint are more likely to compress or sever blood vessels or nerves. With shaft fractures, neurovascular injury is less likely, although manipulation of the fracture site or gross deformity may still endanger vessels and nerves running along the bone.

Areas around the joints are further endangered because blood vessels supplying the epiphysis enter the long bone through the diaphysis. If a fracture close to the epiphysis displaces the bone ends, it may compromise this blood supply with devastating results. The distal bone tissue may die without adequate circulation, destroying the joint and its function.

Once injury occurs, the stability of the extremity is reduced. Any additional movement can increase pain, damage to soft tissues, and the possibility of vascular or nerve involvement. Even slight manipulation can cause internal trauma. For example, a fractured femur has bone ends that are about the size of a broken broom handle. If, during extrication, splinting, and patient transport, the bone ends move about within the soft tissue, the resulting damage may be much more severe than that which initially occurred with the fracture. Manipulation of the injury site may also increase the likelihood of introducing bone fragments or fat emboli into the venous system, causing pulmonary embolism.

Another complication associated with long bone fracture is muscle spasm induced by pain. In a long bone fracture, pain causes the surrounding muscles to contract. This contraction forces the broken bone ends to override the fracture site. The result, in the case of the femur, is two broom-handle-sized bones driven into the muscles of the thigh, causing a cycle of more pain, more spasm, and more damage.

Bone Repair Cycle

The bone repair cycle is a complex process that results in almost complete healing. When trauma fractures a bone, the periosteum tears, as do local blood vessels, soft tissues, and the endosteum. Blood fills the injured area and congeals, establishing a red blood cell and collagen clot. This hemorrhagic clot is not very stable but does begin the bone repair process. Osteocytes from the bone ends begin to multiply rapidly and produce osteoblasts. These osteoblasts lay down salt crystals within the collagen clot fibres. This establishes lengthening and widening regions of skeletal tissue from each disrupted bone end. Over time, the two growing ends join and form a large knob of cancellous bone, called the **callus**, that encapsulates the fracture site.

As the process continues, the deposition of salts and the increasing collagen fibre matrix strengthen the callus and stabilize the bone to near-normal strength. Then, osteoclasts dissolve salt crystals and collagen in areas where stress is minimal, while osteoblasts lay down new collagen and salts in high-stress areas. Through this process, the bone is remodelled until it looks very much like it did before the injury. If a fracture occurs when a patient is young and the bone ends are well aligned, there may be little evidence to suggest an injury ever occurred. If the bone ends are misaligned or if the bone experiences stress, infection, or movement before it has a chance to heal properly, the injury site may never return to normal and may leave the person with some disability.

Inflammatory and Degenerative Conditions

Patients suffering from inflammatory and degenerative conditions may complain of joint pain, tenderness, and fatigue. These patients may also have difficulty walking and moving, may require additional assistance with their normal daily activities, and be prone to musculoskeletal injuries. Common inflammatory diseases of the musculoskeletal system include bursitis, tendinitis, and arthritis.

* **callus** thickened area that forms at the site of a fracture as part of the repair process.

Bursitis

Bursitis is an acute or chronic inflammation of the bursae, the small synovial sacs that reduce friction and cushion the ligaments and tendons from trauma. Bursitis may result from repeated trauma, gout, infection, and, in some cases, unknown etiologies. A patient with bursitis experiences localized pain, swelling, and tenderness at or near a joint. Commonly affected locations include the olecranon (elbow), the area just above the patella, and the shoulder.

Tendinitis

Tendinitis is characterized by inflammation of a tendon and its protective sheath and has a presentation similar to that of bursitis. Repeated trauma to a particular muscle group is a common cause of the condition, which usually affects the major tendons of the upper and lower extremities.

Arthritis

Arthritis is literally an inflammation of a joint. Three of the most common types of arthritis are osteoarthritis, rheumatoid arthritis, and gout (more formally known as gouty arthritis).

Osteoarthritis, which is also known as degenerative joint disease, is the most common type of connective tissue disorder. It is characterized by a general degeneration, or "wear-and-tear," of articular cartilage that results in irregular bony overgrowths. Signs and symptoms include pain, stiffness, and diminished movement in the joints. Joint enlargement may be visible, especially in the fingers. Predisposing factors for osteoarthritis include trauma, obesity, and aging.

Rheumatoid arthritis is a chronic, systemic, progressive, and debilitating disease resulting in deterioration of peripheral joint connective tissue. It is characterized by inflammation of the synovial joints, which causes immobility, pain, increased pain on movement, and fatigue. The disease occurs two to three times more frequently in women than in men. In extreme cases, flexion contractures may develop due to muscle spasms induced by inflammation.

Gout is an inflammation in joints and connective tissue produced by an accumulation of uric acid crystals. It occurs most frequently in males who often have high concentrations of uric acid in the blood. Uric acid is a metabolism end-product that is not easily dissolved. Signs and symptoms of gout include peripheral joint pain, swelling, and possible deformity.

MUSCULOSKELETAL INJURY ASSESSMENT

With the majority of patients, fractures, dislocations, or muscular injuries only infrequently threaten life or seriously contribute to the development of shock. In most circumstances, a patient with an isolated fracture, dislocation, or trauma to muscular or connective tissue will receive complete assessment and management at the scene.

However, serious musculoskeletal injury is common in a patient who presents with other serious injuries. As you read earlier, energy is often transmitted from the point of impact along the skeletal system to the internal organs. Thus, when you discover a skeletal injury, always look for indications of the severity of the trauma forces and the possibility that the forces also caused internal injuries.

As with any trauma patient, the assessment process progresses through the scene assessment, the primary assessment, either the rapid trauma assessment or focused secondary assessment and history, the detailed secondary assessment

---

* **bursitis** acute or chronic inflammation of the small synovial sacs.

* **tendinitis** inflammation of a tendon and/or its protective sheath.

* **arthritis** inflammation of a joint.

* **osteoarthritis** inflammation of a joint resulting from wearing down of the articular cartilage.

* **rheumatoid arthritis** chronic disease that causes deterioration of peripheral joint connective tissue.

* **gout** inflammation of joints and connective tissue due to buildup of uric acid crystals.

When you discover a skeletal injury, always look for indications of the severity of the trauma forces and the possibility that the forces also caused internal injuries.

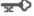

when appropriate, and serial ongoing assessments. You will usually focus your attention on musculoskeletal injuries during the rapid trauma assessment or focused assessment and history and then as part of the detailed secondary assessment.

SCENE ASSESSMENT

Remember to ensure scene safety, and don the appropriate personal protective equipment before approaching any scene. Gloves are mandatory when dealing with open musculoskeletal wounds, but those wounds, by themselves, do not usually suggest the need for protective eyewear, mask, or gown. Since most musculoskeletal injuries result from trauma, analyze the mechanism of injury to anticipate the nature and severity of those injuries. Enhance your analysis of the mechanism of injury by talking with the patient, family members, and bystanders to identify what happened and how.

PRIMARY ASSESSMENT

It is imperative that assessment of the trauma patient begin with an evaluation of the patient's mental status and ABCs (airway, breathing, circulation). During this primary assessment, you must also identify the potential for spinal injury and the need for spinal precautions. Remember, any serious musculoskeletal injury suggests kinetic energy forces sufficient to cause spinal injury, and so always take spinal precautions with such an injury. Proceed with the primary assessment and ensure that any life-threatening injuries are addressed before moving on in the assessment process. Never let the gruesome nature of a musculoskeletal injury distract you from performing a proper primary assessment and identifying and caring for life-threatening injuries first (Figure 22-4).

Patients with musculoskeletal injuries are classified into four categories:

1. Patients with life- and limb-threatening injuries
2. Patients with life-threatening injuries and minor musculoskeletal injuries
3. Patients with non-life-threatening injuries but serious limb-threatening musculoskeletal injuries
4. Patients with non-life-threatening injuries and only isolated minor musculoskeletal injuries

Perform a rapid trauma assessment for those patients with possible life- or limb-threatening injuries. A patient without life threat but with serious musculoskeletal injury may receive the rapid trauma assessment or the focused secondary assessment and history, depending on the mechanism of injury and the information you discover during the primary assessment. Provide patients who have isolated and simple musculoskeletal injuries with a focused secondary assessment and history, though you must remain watchful for any sign or symptom of more seri-

Any serious musculoskeletal injury suggests kinetic energy forces sufficient to cause spinal injury, and so always take spinal precautions.

Never let the gruesome nature of a musculoskeletal injury distract you from identifying and caring for the more subtle but life-threatening injuries first.

Content Review

CLASSIFICATION OF PATIENTS WITH MUSCULOSKELETAL INJURIES

Life- and limb-threatening injuries
Life-threatening injuries, minor musculoskeletal injuries
Non-life-threatening injuries, serious limb-threatening injuries
Non-life-threatening injuries, isolated minor musculoskeletal injuries

FIGURE 22-4 As you begin assessment, examine the patient quickly for musculoskeletal injuries, but remember that they are not often life threatening.

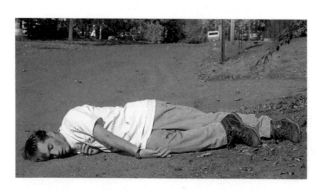

ous injury and the need for both a rapid trauma assessment and rapid patient transport to a trauma centre.

RAPID TRAUMA ASSESSMENT

The rapid trauma assessment is performed on any patient with any sign, symptom, or mechanism of injury that suggests serious injury. While musculoskeletal injuries do not often cause life-threatening hemorrhage, remember that 80 percent of patients with serious multisystem trauma have associated musculoskeletal injury. When you have evidence of serious musculoskeletal injury, maintain a high index of suspicion for serious internal injury.

Perform the rapid trauma assessment in a carefully ordered way, progressing through an evaluation of the head, neck, chest, and abdomen, and arriving at the pelvis. Pay particular attention to the possibility of pelvic fracture because such an injury may account for hemorrhage of more than two litres. Check the stability of the pelvic ring by directing firm pressure downward, inward pressure on the iliac crests, and then directing downward pressure on the symphysis pubis. If the pressure reveals any instability or crepitus or elicits a response of pain from the patient, suspect pelvic fracture. Crepitus is a grating sensation felt as bone ends rub against one another. If you feel crepitus once, presume that bone injury exists, and do not attempt to re-create the sensation.

A pelvic fracture may account for hemorrhage of more than two litres.

In assessing the thighs, look for signs of tissue swelling and femur fracture. Each femur fracture may account for as much as 1500 mL of blood loss. Evidence of this loss may be hidden within the tissue and muscle mass of the thigh, and so compare one thigh with the other to evaluate swelling. Monitor for the signs that the patient is compensating for blood loss, and consider both fluid resuscitation and rapid transport without delay.

A femur fracture may account for as much as 1500 mL of blood loss.

While fractures and muscular injuries of the extremities may not by themselves produce shock, they may significantly contribute to hypovolemia. Consider the effects of these injuries in your decision on whether to provide rapid transport or on-scene care. Further, fractures and dislocations may entrap or damage blood vessels or nerves, thus seriously threatening the future use of a limb. Quickly survey each limb, and check the distal pulses, temperature, sensation (if the patient is conscious), motor function, and muscle tone.

Complete the rapid trauma assessment by gathering a patient history and a baseline set of vital signs (which may be done at the same time the secondary assessment is being performed). If the rapid trauma assessment reveals a serious threat to life or limb, rapidly transport the patient to the nearest appropriate facility.

FOCUSED HISTORY AND SECONDARY ASSESSMENT

The focused history and secondary assessment directs your attention to the injuries found or suggested during the primary assessment by the mechanism of injury and the patient's signs and symptoms. This step of the assessment process is performed for patients without life-threatening injuries and permits both assessment and care focused on isolated injuries.

Begin the focused secondary assessment by observing and inquiring carefully for signs and symptoms of fracture, dislocation, or other musculoskeletal injury in each limb with suspected injury (Figure 22-5). Expose and visualize the entire limb by removing any restrictive clothing or cutting it away carefully. In doing so, avoid manipulation of any potential injury site. Inspect the injury site carefully to locate any deformities (angulation or swelling), discolorations (unlikely in the first minutes after the incident), and indications of soft-tissue wounds that suggest injury beneath. Any unusual limb placement, asymmetry, or inequality in limb length

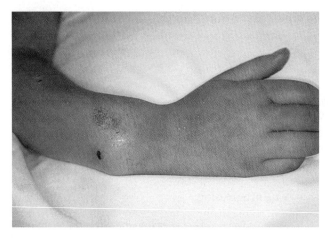

a. A fracture will often present with deformity.

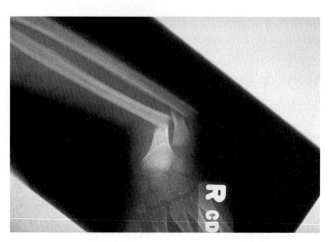

b. An x-ray of the fracture.

FIGURE 22-5   Presentation of a forearm fracture.

(when compared with the opposing limb) should also arouse suspicion of musculo-skeletal injury. Consider the possibility that any open wounds communicate with an associated fracture or dislocation. Observe for any contamination or sign of the bone protruding. Question the patient about pain, pain with attempted movement, discomfort, or unusual feeling or sensation. Also, inquire about weakness, paralysis, paresthesia, or anesthesia. It may be helpful to think of the six Ps as a way to remember the key elements to be alert for when evaluating an extremity:

- *Pain.* The patient may report this upon palpation (tenderness) or movement.
- *Pallor.* The patient's skin may be pale or flushed, and capillary refill may be delayed.
- *Paralysis.* The patient may be unable to move, or have difficulty in moving, an extremity.
- *Paresthesia.* The patient may report numbness or tingling in the affected extremity.
- *Pressure.* The patient reports a feeling of tension within the extremity.
- *Pulses.* These may be diminished or absent in the extremity.

If you do not identify a specific injury, palpate the extremity for instability, deformity (swelling or angulation), crepitus, unusual motion (joint-like motion where a joint does not exist), muscle tone (normal, flaccid, or spasmodic), or any regions of unusual warmth or coolness. Palpate the entire anterior and posterior surfaces, then the lateral and medial surfaces. Your assessment must be gentle, yet complete. Record any abnormal signs. When assessing the feet, carefully evaluate the distal circulation. Assess pulses for presence and relative strength, and then compare bilaterally. Test the skin for humidity and warmth. Suspect circulatory compromise if capillary refill time is prolonged compared with the uninjured limb. Observe the skin for discoloration, noting any erythema, ecchymosis, or any abnormal hue (pale, ashen, or cyanotic). Approximate the level at which any deficit begins, and note any relation to possible extremity injury.

In a conscious and responsive patient, evaluate sensation and muscle strength distal to the injury (Figure 22-6). Check tactile (touch) response by touching or stroking the bottom of the foot with the blunt end of a bandage scis-

Content Review

THE SIX Ps IN
EVALUATING LIMB INJURY

Pain
Pallor
Paralysis
Paresthesia
Pressure
Pulses

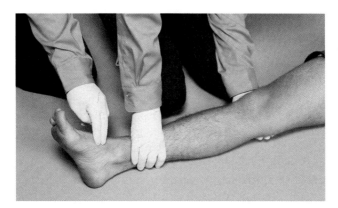

FIGURE 22-6 Evaluate the distal extremity for pulse, temperature, colour, sensation, and capillary refill.

sors or other similar instrument. Ask the patient to describe the feeling. If the patient is responsive and if there is no indication that the limb is injured, ask the patient to push down with the balls of both feet (plantar flexion) against your hands. Then, ask the patient to pull upward with the top of the feet (dorsiflexion), again against your hands. If you feel any unilateral or bilateral weakness or the patient reports any pain, document the finding on the prehospital care report, and look for the cause. Check abnormal sensation and the patient's ability to wiggle the toes or fingers.

Assess for potential upper extremity injury in a manner similar to your assessment of the lower extremity. Expose, observe, question about, and then palpate the limb as described above. Determine tactile response by using the back of the patient's hand. Test muscular strength by having the patient squeeze two of your fingers. Compare strength and sensation bilaterally, identify any deficit, and attempt to locate the cause. Evaluate the upper extremity, and ensure it is uninjured before you use it for blood pressure determination.

When the assessment of an extremity suggests injury, treat the limb as though a fracture or dislocation exists because the only definitive way to rule out these injuries is by x-ray examination. Also, note that splinting protects strains, sprains, and subluxations as well as fractures and dislocations from further injury. Treating a soft-tissue or muscular injury as a fracture or dislocation produces nothing more harmful than slight discomfort for the patient. Failure to immobilize an injury properly, however, may lead to additional soft-, skeletal, connective, vascular, or nervous tissue damage and possibly cause permanent harm.

If possible, find the exact site of injury and determine if it involves a joint area or a long bone shaft. Form a clear visual image of the injury site in your mind so that you can describe the injury in the patient care report and to the receiving physician. Remember that the splinting device may hide the site from view, leaving the attending physician unable to determine what exists beneath it. A good description of the wound may delay the need to remove the splint to view the injury.

One complication of musculoskeletal injury to the extremities is compartment syndrome. This condition results from bleeding into, or edema within, a muscle mass surrounded by fasciae that do not stretch. The buildup of pressure then compresses capillaries and nerves, leading to local tissue ischemia and then necrosis, with some loss of distal sensation. A pulse deficit may be a very late finding in compartment syndrome. Suspect compartment syndrome in any patient who has any paraesthesia, especially in the webs between the medial toes or fingers, who has an extremity injury with a firm mass or increased skin tension at the injury site, or who has pain out of proportion to the nature of the injury or pain that increases when you move the limb. Also suspect compartment syndrome in any unconscious patient with a swollen limb. Compartment syndrome most often occurs in the forearm or leg.

When the assessment of an extremity suggests injury, treat the limb as though a fracture or dislocation exists.

Form a clear mental picture of the injury site, and be able to describe it to the emergency physician.

Content Review

EARLY INDICATORS OF COMPARTMENT SYNDROME
Feeling of tension within limb
Loss of distal sensation (especially in webs of fingers and toes)
Complaints of pain
Condition more severe than mechanism of injury would indicate
Pain on passive extension of extremity
Pulse deficit (late sign)

During the secondary assessment, question the patient about the symptoms of injury. Ensure that your verbal investigation is detailed and complete. Determine the nature and location of pain and tenderness or dysfunction. The patient's description of the fracture or dislocation event may also be helpful. The patient may state that he felt the bone "snap" or the joint "pop out." Determine whether the bone snapping caused the fall or the fall caused the fracture. Evaluate the amount of pain and discomfort the patient is experiencing with the injury. For example, an elderly patient may present with a fractured hip and limited pain, a presentation usually related to a degenerative disease and secondary fracture. These findings may suggest that you adopt a less aggressive approach to care for this patient, focusing on the patient's comfort, rather than on traction splinting and shock care. Also, identify the signs and symptoms of injury as well as pertinent allergies, medications, past medical history, last oral intake, and events leading up to the incident.

Compare the findings of your assessment with the index of suspicion for injury you developed during the scene assessment. If you have found less significant injury than you suspected, consider reevaluating the patient to ensure that no injury has been overlooked. If you find a more significant injury, suspect other severe injury may have occurred elsewhere and expand your focused assessment.

As you conclude the focused history and secondary assessment, identify all injuries found, prioritize them, and establish the order of care for them. Identify the extent to which each injury may contribute to hemorrhage and shock. Then, prioritize the patient for transport. Taking these few moments to sort out what is wrong with the patient and to plan care steps will increase the efficiency of your patient care, reduce on-scene time, and ensure that the patient receives the proper care at the right time.

At the conclusion of the rapid trauma assessment or the focused assessment, identify all injuries and prioritize them for care.

DETAILED SECONDARY ASSESSMENT

After you have ruled out or addressed potential threats to the patient's life or limbs, attended to any serious problems, and assessed any suspected injuries, you may perform a detailed secondary assessment. You will most likely perform the detailed secondary assessment on the patient who is unconscious or has a lowered level of consciousness. The assessment may be performed at the scene or, more likely, en route to the hospital. The detailed secondary assessment is a search for the signs and symptoms of further injury. It is performed as a head-to-toe evaluation, looking specifically where you have not looked before and with enough care to identify any subtle indications of injury. Be alert for the signs and symptoms of internal or external injury or hemorrhage. Use the same assessment techniques for evaluating musculoskeletal injuries during the detailed secondary assessment that you employed during the rapid trauma assessment and focused history and secondary assessment.

ONGOING ASSESSMENT

The ongoing assessment focuses on serial measurement of the patient's vital signs and level of consciousness, and the signs and symptoms of the major trauma affecting the patient. For patients with musculoskeletal injuries, monitor distal sensation and pulses frequently. Remember to ask about the patient's complaints and description of the musculoskeletal injury, watching for any changes in the responses. As time passes and the effects of the "fight-or-flight" response wear off, the patient may display more significant and specific symptoms of injury. The patient may also begin to complain of other injuries masked earlier by the chief complaint and of other major pain or discomfort. If this occurs, provide a focused assessment on the area of complaint, and modify your patient priorities as additional injuries are found.

During the ongoing assessment, be sure to ask about the patient's complaints and description of the musculoskeletal injury because over time, the patient may display more significant and specific symptoms of injury and complain of other injuries masked earlier by the chief complaint.

SPORTS INJURY CONSIDERATIONS

Many of the musculoskeletal injuries you encounter as a paramedic are associated with sports activities. Such activities as football, basketball, soccer, baseball, in-line skating, skiing, snowboarding, bicycling, wrestling, hiking, and hockey often lead to injuries in participants. When you are called to the scene of a sports injury, assess the mechanism of injury and determine whether there was a major kinetic force involved and whether it is a hyperextension or flexion injury or a fatigue-type injury. Athletic injuries often affect major body joints, such as the shoulder, elbow, wrist, knee, and ankle. Injuries in these areas are especially troubling for patients because serious ligament damage might preclude future participation in sports and limit limb usefulness. It is imperative that any potentially significant sports injury be attended to by an emergency department physician. The competitive natures of players, teammates, coaches, and athletic trainers may lead them to downplay injuries in order to keep an injured athlete in competition. Allowing an injured athlete to keep playing, however, places additional stress on the injury and may result in further, and more debilitating, damage.

Any potentially significant sports injury should be attended to by an emergency department physician.

MUSCULOSKELETAL INJURY MANAGEMENT

Management of musculoskeletal injuries is not normally a high priority in trauma patient care. It usually does not occur until after you have completed the primary assessment, stabilized the airway, breathing, and circulation, and finished the rapid trauma assessment. While the focus of care for the serious trauma patient is the current life threats, some protection for serious musculoskeletal injuries is provided by moving the patient as a unit (with axial alignment) and by packaging the patient for transport using the long spine board (see Chapter 24, "Spinal Trauma"). These techniques help you reduce the risks of aggravating musculoskeletal injuries, increasing hemorrhage, and worsening shock and patient outcome.

Fractures of the pelvis and, to a lesser degree, the femur can significantly contribute to hypovolemia and shock. These injuries deserve a high priority in patient care. Other musculoskeletal injuries that merit a priority for care include those that threaten a limb, such as injuries with loss of distal circulation or sensation (most commonly joint injuries), and those that cause compartment syndrome (most likely leg or forearm injuries). You may prioritize other injuries by the relative size of the bone fractured or the body area involved and by the energy that was required to cause injury. Prioritize the patient's musculoskeletal injuries for care, then proceed with splinting and transport.

GENERAL PRINCIPLES OF MUSCULOSKELETAL INJURY MANAGEMENT

The objectives of musculoskeletal injury care are to reduce the possibility of any further injury during patient care and transport and to reduce the patient's discomfort. Accomplish these goals by protecting open wounds, positioning the extremity properly, immobilizing the injured extremity, and monitoring neurovascular function in the distal limb. In some cases, care involves manipulating the injury to reestablish distal circulation and sensation or simply to restore normal anatomical position for the patient in the event of prolonged extrication or transport. In most cases, care for musculoskeletal injuries will also include application of a splinting device.

As you begin to care for a patient with musculoskeletal injuries, talk to him and explain what you are doing, why, and what impact it will have on the patient. Alignment and splinting will likely first cause an increase in pain followed by a significant reduction in it. By telling the patient of this in advance, you will increase confidence in both your intent to help and your ability to provide care.

Protecting Open Wounds

If there is any open wound in close proximity to the fracture or dislocation, consider the fracture or dislocation to be an open one. Carefully observe the wound and note any signs of muscle, tendon, ligament, or vascular injury, and be prepared to describe the wound in your report and at the emergency department. Cover the wound with a sterile dressing held in place with bandaging or a splint. Frequently, the attempts to align a limb, the splinting process, or the application of traction will draw protruding bones back into the wound. This is an expected consequence of proper care but must be brought to the attention of the attending emergency department physician.

Positioning the Limb

Proper limb positioning is essential to ensure patient comfort, to reduce the chances of further limb injury, and to encourage venous drainage. Proper positioning is different with fractures and dislocations, although splinting with the limb in a normal anatomical position, the position of function, is beneficial for both.

Limb alignment is appropriate for any fractures of the midshaft femur, tibia/fibula, humerus, or radius/ulna. Alignment can be maintained by using the speed, malleable, or traction splint. Proper alignment of a fracture enhances circulation and reduces the potential for further injury to surrounding tissue. It is also very difficult to immobilize a limb with a fracture in an unaligned, angulated position because the fracture segments are short and buried in soft tissue. Perform any limb alignment with great care so as to avoid damaging the tissue surrounding the fracture site. During the process, the proximal limb should remain in position while you bring the distal limb to the position of alignment using gentle axial traction. Stop the process when you detect any resistance to movement or when the patient reports any significant increase in pain.

Generally, you should not attempt alignment of dislocations and serious injuries within 7 cm of a joint. Only attempt to manipulate such injury sites if the distal circulation is compromised. In such a case, try to move the joint, while another care provider palpates the distal pulse. If the pulse is restored, if you meet significant resistance to movement, or if the patient complains of greatly increased pain, stop the manipulation and splint the injured limb as it is. Be sure to transport the patient quickly because a loss of circulation can endanger the future usefulness of the limb.

Proper positioning of injured limbs is important for maintaining distal circulation and sensation and increasing patient comfort. Deformities and extremes of flexion or extension put pressure on the soft tissues and may compress nerves and blood vessels. These positions also fatigue the surrounding muscles and increase the pain associated with the injury. By placing the uninjured joints of the limb halfway between flexion and extension in what is called the position of function, you place the least stress on the joint ligaments and the muscles and tendons surrounding the injury. Place the limb in the position of function whenever possible (Figure 22-7). Note, however, that some injuries and some splinting devices commonly used for musculoskeletal injuries may preclude this positioning.

When practical, elevate the injured limb. This will assist with venous drainage and reduce the edema associated with musculoskeletal injury.

Stop realignment attempts when you detect any resistance to movement or when the patient reports any significant increase in pain.

Do not attempt alignment of dislocations and serious injuries within 7 cm of a joint.

When possible, place injured limbs in the position of function or a neutral position.

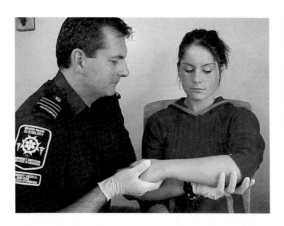

FIGURE 22-7 Gently position the limb in the position of function, unless your attempts meet with resistance or a significant increase in pain or the injury is within 7 cm of a joint.

Immobilizing the Injury

The aim in immobilizing musculoskeletal injuries is to prevent further injury caused by the movement of broken bone ends and bone ends dislodged from a joint and by further stress placed on muscles, ligaments, or tendons already injured by a strain, sprain, subluxation, dislocation, or fracture. This immobilization is usually accomplished through the use of a splinting device.

Since most long bones lie buried deep within the musculature of the extremities, it is very difficult to immobilize them directly. Hence, we immobilize the joint above and the joint below the injury, regardless of whether the injury occurs at a joint or midshaft in a long bone. This ensures that no motion is transmitted through the injury site as might occur, for example, with the rotation (supination/pronation) of the radius against the ulna at the elbow when the wrist turns.

Wrap any splinting device or associated bandage from a distal point to a proximal one. This ensures that the pressure of bandaging moves any blood into the systemic circulation and does not trap it in the distal limb. This method of wrapping thus assists venous drainage and the healing process. Apply firm pressure when wrapping, but be sure you can easily push a finger beneath the wrapping.

Checking Neurovascular Function

It is imperative that you identify the status of the circulation, motor function, and sensation distal to the injury site before, during, and after splinting of all musculoskeletal injuries. The check before splinting identifies a baseline condition and establishes that the initial injury has not disrupted circulation. The check during splinting ensures that inadvertent limb movement or circumferential pressure does not compromise distal circulation. The check after splinting identifies any restriction caused by progressive swelling of the injured area against the splinting device. Clearly identify and document these evaluations whenever you apply a splint.

To perform this evaluation, first palpate for a pulse, and ensure that it is equal in strength to that of the opposing limb. If the pulse cannot be located or is weak, check capillary refill and skin temperature, colour, and condition. Again, compare your findings with those for the opposing limb. Ask the patient to describe the sensation when you rub or pinch the bottom of the foot or back of the hand, and ask him to move the fingers or toes. The patient response establishes your baseline circulation, sensory, and motor findings. Reevaluate pulse, motor function, and sensation frequently during the remaining care and transport. If a care provider is holding the limb while you apply the splint, have him monitor both pulse and skin temperature. That care provider can then immediately note any compromise in circulation.

Always check pulses, motor function, and sensation in the distal extremity before, during, and after splinting.

Splinting Devices

An essential part of managing any musculoskeletal system injury is the use of devices to immobilize a limb and permit patient transport without causing further injury. These devices, called splints, are designed to help you reduce or eliminate any movement of the injured extremity. Splints come in several forms that can assist in immobilizing common fractures and dislocations associated with musculoskeletal trauma (Figure 22-8). They include rigid, formable, soft, traction, and other splints.

Rigid Splints

Rigid splints, as the name implies, are firm and durable supports for the injured limb. They can be constructed of cardboard, plastic, metal, synthetic products, or wood. Such devices very effectively immobilize injury sites but require adequate padding to lessen patient discomfort. This padding may be built into the splint or may simply be a bulky dressing affixed to the splint with soft bandaging. Several types of commercially available rigid splints are used in prehospital care. They are usually flat and rigid devices and are about 7 cm wide and from 40 to 120 cm long. The injured limb that is in alignment is immobilized to the splint by circumferential wrapping, while an angulated limb may be held in position by cross-wrapping at two locations.

A special form of rigid splint is the pre-formed splint. It is usually a stamped metal or pre-formed plastic or fibreglass device shaped to the contours of the distal limbs. These splints are usually available for the ankles and hands.

Formable Splints

Another type of rigid splint is the formable, or malleable, splint. It is made up of a material that you can easily shape to match the angulation of a limb. You then affix the formed splint to the limb with circumferential bandaging. Formable splints include both the ladder splint, which is a matrix of soft metal wires soldered together, and the metal sheet splint, which is made up of thin aluminum or another easily shaped metal.

Soft Splints

Soft splints use padding or air pressure to immobilize an injured limb. Among the varieties of soft splints are air splints, which include pillow splints.

The air splint provides immobilization as air pressure fills the splint and compresses the limb. Since the splint is a formed cylinder and may include shaping

FIGURE 22-8   A variety of splints are available for musculoskeletal injuries.

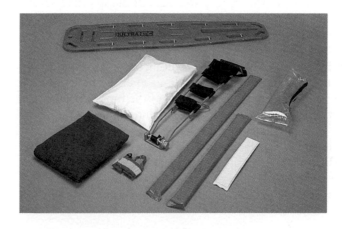

for the foot, it immobilizes the limb in an aligned position. Air splints should not be used with long-bone injuries at or above the knee or elbow because they cannot prevent movement of hip or shoulder joints and are thus unable to immobilize the proximal joints of the limb. Air splints also apply a pressure that may be helpful in controlling both external and internal hemorrhage. While these devices may limit assessment of the distal extremity, they do permit observation because they are transparent.

Monitor pressure within the air splint as it may change with changes in altitude or temperature.

Monitor air splints carefully with any changes in temperature or atmospheric pressure. Increases in ambient heat or decreases in pressure, as during an ascent in a helicopter, will increase the pressure within the splint. Conversely, decreases in temperature or a descent in a helicopter will decrease pressure in the splint. Constantly monitor the pressure in the air splint to ensure it does not rise or fall during your care.

The pillow splint is a comfortable splint for ankle and foot injuries. The foot is simply placed on the pillow, and the outer fabric is drawn around the foot and pillow. The outer fabric is pinned together or wrapped circumferentially with bandage material around the injury site. This device applies gentle and uniform pressure to effectively immobilize the distal extremity. Using a bulky blanket or two and wrapping them firmly may also provide the same type of immobilization.

Traction Splints

The traction splint was developed during World War I and used extensively during World War II. This splint dramatically reduced both mortality and limb loss from femur fractures caused by projectile wounds, blast injuries, and other traumas. Today, the traction splint is the mainstay of prehospital care for the isolated traumatic femur fracture.

The traction splint is a frame that applies a pull (traction) on the injured extremity and against the trunk. The application of traction is useful when splinting the femur, which is surrounded by very heavy musculature. Frequently, the pain of fracture initiates muscle spasm that causes the bone ends to override each other causing further pain and muscle spasm and aggravating the original injury. The traction splint prevents overriding of the bone ends, lessens patient pain, and may help relax any muscle spasm.

There are basically two styles of traction splint: the bipolar frame device and the unipolar device (Figure 22-9). The bipolar (Hare or Thomas) traction splint has a half-ring that fits up and against the ischial tuberosity of the pelvis. A distal ratchet connects to a foot harness and pulls traction from the foot and against the pelvis. The frame lifts and supports the limb, and a foot stand suspends the injured limb above the ground. This construction helps prevent movement of the limb during transport of the patient, while the elevation supplied by the stand enhances venous drainage. The unipolar (Sager) traction splint uses a single lengthening shaft to pull a foot harness against pressure applied to the pubic bone. The cravats provided stabilize the extremity, and so you must observe greater care whenever you move the patient. The unipolar splint can be utilized for patients with bilateral fractures.

Other Splinting Aids

Vacuum splints can conform to the exact shape of a limb (Figure 22-10). An injured limb is placed on a bag containing small plastic particles. The splint is shaped around the limb, and then the air is withdrawn from the device. The suction locks the particles in position, immobilizing the splint to the contours of the limb. The only disadvantage to vacuum splinting is that during air evacuation there is a small amount of shrinkage and a reduction in the splinting effect.

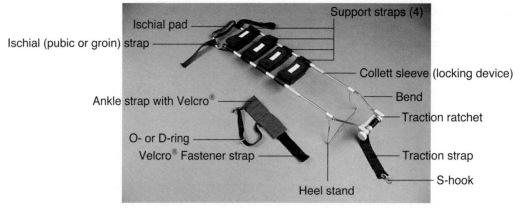

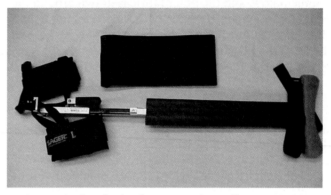

Ischial pad

Ischial (pubic or groin) strap

Support straps (4)

Collett sleeve (locking device)

Ankle strap with Velcro®

Bend

Traction ratchet

O- or D-ring

Velcro® Fastener strap

Traction strap

S-hook

Heel stand

a. A bipolar frame traction splint

b. A unipolar frame traction splint

Figure 22-9   Traction splints.

Cravats or Velcro® straps can augment the effectiveness of rigid splints. You can secure the lower extremities, one to the other, to help the patient control the musculoskeletal injury site, or you can use a sling and swathe to help immobilize a splinted upper extremity to the chest. Fractures of the humerus are difficult to immobilize because the shoulder is such a large and mobile part of the body. A sling may hold the elbow at a fixed angle, while a swathe secures the limb against the body to limit further shoulder movement. By holding a thumb in the fold of the elbow, the patient can easily reduce any movement of the limb and complement the splinting process.

Figure 22-10   Suction the air out of a vacuum splint until the device is rigid. Reassess pulse, motor function, and sensation in the extremity after application.

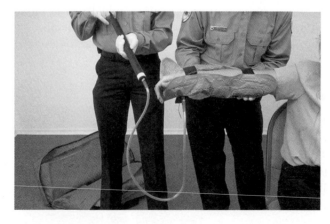

In some cases of serious musculoskeletal injury, other injuries preclude the splinting of individual fractures and dislocations. In such cases, you may splint the limbs to the body with cravats or bandage material and immobilize the patient to the long spine board. Simply strap the body and limbs to the board, and transport the patient as a unit. While this is not definitive splinting, it will provide reasonable protection for musculoskeletal injuries.

FRACTURE CARE

For prehospital care purposes, consider a joint injury to be any muscular or connective tissue injury or dislocation or fracture within 7 cm of a joint. Fractures are then defined as shaft injuries at least 7 cm away from the joint. These definitions are essential because an injury near the joint carries a higher incidence of blood vessel and nerve involvement and requires a different approach to positioning and splinting.

Consider any injury within 7 cm of a joint to be a joint injury.

Begin fracture care by ensuring distal pulses, sensation, and motor function. Then, align the limb for splinting. Quickly recheck the circulation and motor and sensory functions below the injury. If you identify any neurovascular deficit, attempt to correct the problem by gentle repositioning, even if the limb is relatively aligned. If the limb is angulated, proceed with realignment. Remember that most splinting devices are designed to immobilize aligned limbs and that alignment provides the best chance for ensuring good neurovascular function distal to the injury.

To move an injured limb from an angulated position into alignment, use gentle distal traction applied manually. Have an assisting paramedic immobilize the proximal limb in the position found. Grasp the distal limb firmly, and apply traction along the limb's axis, gently moving it from the angulated to an aligned position. Should you feel any resistance to movement or notice a great increase in patient discomfort, stop the alignment attempt, and splint the limb as it lies. Once you complete the alignment, recheck the distal neurovascular function. If it is adequate, proceed with splinting. If function is inadequate, move the limb around slightly, while another care provider monitors for a pulse. If one attempt at gentle manipulation does not reestablish a pulse, splint and transport the patient quickly.

Proceed with splinting by selecting an appropriate device, and secure the limb to it in a way that ensures you immobilize both the fracture site and the adjacent joints. Have the care provider who is holding the limb apply a gentle traction to stabilize the limb (and monitor the distal pulse) during splinting. If you apply your splint properly, the device may maintain this traction and provide greater stabilization of the limb and greater patient comfort. Secure the limb to the body (upper extremity) or to the opposite limb (lower extremity) to protect it and to give the patient some control over the limb.

JOINT CARE

Joint care, too, begins with assessment for distal neurovascular function. If you find the pulse, sensation, and motor functions to be adequate, immobilize the joint in the position found. Use a ladder or other malleable splint, shaped to the limb's angle, or cross-wrap with a padded rigid splint to immobilize the joint in place. Ensure that your splinting immobilizes the injured joint and both the joint above and the joint below the injury. If not, secure the limb firmly to the body to immobilize these joints.

Unless you identify a neurovascular deficit, immobilize joint injuries as you find them.

If circulation or motor or sensory function is lost below the joint injury, consider moving the limb to reestablish it. While you gently move the limb, have another care provider monitor the circulation and sensation. If you can reestablish neurovascular function quickly, splint the limb in the new position. If not, splint the limb, and provide quick transport to the patient.

With some joint injuries, you may attempt to return the displaced bone ends to their normal anatomical position. This process is called **reduction** and has both benefits and hazards. An early return to normal position reduces stress on the ligaments and basic joint structure and facilitates better distal circulation and sensation. However, the process creates the risk of trapping blood vessels or nerves as the bone ends return to their normal anatomical positions. Attempt reduction of a dislocation only when you are sure the injury *is* a dislocation, when you expect the patient's arrival at the emergency department to be delayed (prolonged extrication or long transport time), or when there is a significant neurovascular deficit. Do not attempt a reduction if the dislocation is associated with other serious injuries. Consult your protocols and medical direction to determine the criteria used in your system for attempting dislocation reduction.

When performing a joint reduction, you attempt to protect the articular surface while directing the bones back to their normal anatomical position. Begin the process by providing the patient with analgesic therapy to reduce pain associated with the injury and the reduction itself. Then, have an assisting care provider hold the proximal extremity in position and provide a countertraction during the reduction. You then apply traction to pull the bone surfaces apart, reducing the pressure between the nonarticular surfaces. Slowly increase traction, and direct the displaced limb toward its normal anatomical position. Successful relocation is indicated when you feel the joint "pop" back into position, the patient experiences a lessening of pain, and the joint becomes mobile within at least a few minutes of the procedure. Carefully evaluate the distal circulation, sensation, and motor function after the reduction. If the procedure does not meet with success within a few minutes, splint the limb as it is, and provide rapid transport for the patient. If the reduction is successful, splint the limb in the position of function, and transport the patient.

MUSCULAR AND CONNECTIVE TISSUE CARE

Injuries to the soft tissues of the musculoskeletal system deserve special care. While such injuries are not usually life threatening, they can be very painful and, in some cases, threaten limbs. For example, compartment syndrome can restrict capillary blood flow, venous blood return, and nerve function beyond the site of the injury. If such an injury is not discovered and relieved, it may produce severe disability. Deep contusions and especially large hematomas can also contribute to blood loss and hypovolemia. Once you have provided care for life threats, fractures, joint injuries, and other limb threats, give your attention to injuries to muscular and connective tissues.

To manage these muscle, tendon, and ligament injuries, immobilize the region surrounding them. Doing so will reduce the associated internal hemorrhage and pain. Provide gentle circumferential bandaging (loose enough to let you slide a finger underneath) to further reduce hemorrhage, edema, and pain, but be sure to monitor distal circulation. Loosen the bandage further if there are any signs of neurovascular deficit. Application of local cooling will reduce both edema and patient discomfort. Be careful to wrap any cold or ice pack in a dressing to prevent too drastic a cooling and any consequent injury. You may apply heat to the wound after 48 hours to enhance both circulation and healing. If possible, place the limb in the position of function, and elevate the extremity to ensure good venous return, limit swelling, and reduce patient discomfort. Monitor distal neurovascular function to ensure that your actions do not compromise circulation, sensation, or motor function.

CARE FOR SPECIFIC FRACTURES

Pelvis

Pelvic fractures involve either the iliac crest or the pelvic ring. While iliac crest fractures may reflect serious trauma, they do not represent a life threat as in ring fractures. Iliac crest fractures are often isolated and stable injuries that you can care for by simple patient immobilization.

Pelvic ring fractures, conversely, are often serious, life-threatening events. The ring shape of the pelvis provides strength to the structure, but when it breaks, two fracture sites usually result. The kinetic forces necessary to fracture the pelvic ring are significant and are likely to produce fractures and internal injuries elsewhere. In addition, the pelvis is actively involved in blood cell production, has a rich blood supply, and its interior surface is adjacent to major blood vessels serving the lower extremities. Injury to the pelvic ring, therefore, can result in heavy hemorrhage that is likely to empty into the pelvic and retroperitoneal spaces and account for blood loss in excess of two litres. Such injury may result in circulation loss to one or both lower extremities. Pelvic fractures may also be associated with hip dislocations and injuries to the bladder, female reproductive organs, the urethra, the prostate in the male, and the end of the alimentary canal (anus and rectum). Clearly, pelvic ring fractures are very serious injuries.

The objectives of pelvic injury care are to stabilize the fractured pelvis, support the patient hemodynamically, and provide rapid transport to a trauma centre.

Always consider a pelvic fracture patient to be a candidate for rapid transport.

Femur

Femur fractures may be traumatic, resulting from the application of very strong and violent forces, or atraumatic, resulting from degenerative diseases. Patients with disease-induced fractures usually are of advancing age and present with a history of a degenerative disease, a clouded or limited history of trauma, and only moderate discomfort. Care for such patients by immobilizing them as found and then providing gentle transport. Generally, you can provide effective splinting by placing the patient on a long spine board and padding with pillows and blankets for patient comfort. Use of a traction splint is not essential if pain is not inducing the spasms that cause broken bone ends to override.

A patient who has suffered a traumatic femur fracture usually experiences extreme discomfort, often writhing in pain. In such a case, providing distal traction immobilizes both bone ends, relieves muscle spasms, and reduces the associated pain. Traction splinting is the best avenue for care of the hemodynamically stable patient with a femur fracture. However, the traction splint is not indicated if the patient has concurrent serious knee, tibia, or foot injuries.

Proximal fractures (surgical neck and intertrochanteric fractures) are frequently caused by hip injuries, transmitted forces, or the degenerative effects of aging. Mid-shaft fractures often result from high-energy, lateral traumas and are associated with significant blood loss. Injuries to the distal femur (condylar and epicondylar fractures) can be extensive and are likely to involve blood vessels, nerves, and connective tissue. The energy necessary to fracture the femur may be sufficient to dislocate the hip and cause serious internal injuries elsewhere in the body.

You may find it difficult to differentiate between proximal fractures of the femur (hip fractures) and anterior hip dislocations. Generally, a femur fracture presents with the foot externally rotated (turned outward) and the injured limb shortened when compared with the other. This difference may be slight and may be unnoticeable if the patient's legs are not straight and parallel. An anterior

Atraumatic femur fractures may be splinted by gently placing the patient on a long spine board.

dislocation presents similarly to the femur fracture, but with the head of the femur protruding in the inguinal region. When in doubt, treat it as a dislocation.

If you suspect femur fracture, align the limb, determine the status of circulation and sensory and motor function, and apply the traction splint (Figure 22-11). (If you use manual traction to align the femur, maintain it until the splint is applied and continues the traction.) Adjust the length of the splint to the injured extremity, position the device against the pelvis, and secure it in position with the inguinal strap. With a bipolar splint, apply the ankle hitch, provide gentle traction, and elevate the distal limb to place the splint's ring against the ischial tuberosity. With a unipolar splint, position the T-shaped support against the pubic bone and simply apply the ankle hitch. Ensure that hitch and splint hold the foot and limb in an anatomical position as you apply firm traction. Position and secure the limb to the splint with straps, then gently move the patient and splint to the long spine board. Firmly secure the patient and limb for transport.

Guide your application of traction by the patient's response. Ask the patient how the limb feels as you initiate and increase the amount of traction. Stop the application of traction when the limb is immobilized and patient discomfort decreases. Remember, as the traction splint prevents the overriding of bone ends, the pain of injury decreases. This reduces the strength of muscle spasm and lets the limb return to its initial length. This, in turn, reduces the traction provided by the splint, which means that the bone ends will no longer be as well immobilized. Do not use traction splints on a suspected pelvic fracture.

When the need for rapid transport or other patient injuries preclude the use of the traction splint, consider using the long spine board for immobilizing and transporting the femur fracture patient. Use long padded rigid splints, one medial and one lateral, to quickly splint the injured limb, and then tie that limb to the uninjured one. Use a scoop stretcher or another device or movement technique to transfer the patient to a long spine board, and secure the patient firmly on it.

Tibia/Fibula

Fibular fractures are relatively stable, while tibial fractures are not.

Fractures of the leg bones, the tibia and the fibula, can occur separately or together. The tibia is the most commonly fractured leg bone and may be broken by direct force, crushing injury, or twisting forces. Tibial fracture is likely to cause an open wound. Fibular fractures are often associated with damage to the knee or ankle. If the tibia is fractured and the fibula is intact, the extremity may not

FIGURE 22-11 The traction splint effectively immobilizes femur fractures.

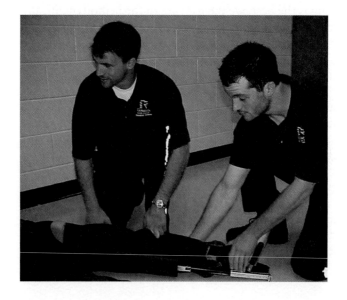

angulate, but it cannot bear weight. If only the fibula is broken, the limb may be relatively stable. Injuries to either bone may result in compartment syndrome. Direct trauma suffered during an auto collision or athletic impact frequently causes these tibia and fibula injuries.

Align the injured limb, assess circulation, sensation, and motor function, and then immobilize the limb with gentle traction. A full-leg air splint (one that accommodates the foot) or lateral and medial padded rigid splints will provide effective immobilization (Figure 22-12). You may also use a speed splint as long as it accommodates the full limb and is rigid enough to maintain immobilization. After you splint the injured limb, secure it to the uninjured leg. This affords some protection against uncontrolled movement and may reassure the patient that he still has some control over the extremity.

Clavicle

The clavicle is the most frequently fractured bone in the human body. Fractures to it usually result from transmitted forces directed along the upper extremity that cause relatively minor skeletal injury. The clavicle, however, is located adjacent to both the upper reaches of the lung and the vasculature that serves the upper extremity and head. Hence, an injury to the clavicle has the potential to cause serious internal injury, especially if powerful mechanisms of injury are involved. The clavicular fracture patient often presents with pain and the shoulder shifted forward with palpable deformity along the clavicle. Accomplish splinting either by immobilizing the affected limb in a sling and swathe or by wrapping a figure-eight bandage around the shoulders, drawing the shoulders back, and then securing the bandage tension. Monitor the patient carefully for any sign of internal hemorrhage or respiratory compromise.

Humerus

A fractured humerus is very difficult to immobilize at its proximal end. The proximal humerus is buried within the shoulder muscles, and the shoulder joint is highly mobile atop the thoracic cage. The axillary artery runs through the axilla, making it difficult to apply any mechanical traction to the limb without compromising circulation. Hence, the most effective techniques for splinting this fracture are to apply a sling and swathe to immobilize the bent limb against the chest or to tie the extended and splinted limb to the body.

The preferred technique is to use the sling and swathe. Apply a short padded rigid splint to the lateral surface of the arm to distribute the pressure of the swathing and better immobilize the arm. Sling the forearm with a cravat, catching

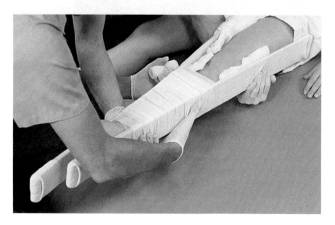

FIGURE 22-12 Placement of long padded board splints laterally and medially can effectively splint tibia/fibula fractures.

just the wrist region and not the elbow. This permits some gravitational traction in the seated patient and prevents inadvertent application of pressure by the sling, which could push the limb together. Then, use several cravats to gently swathe the arm and forearm to the chest. If the patient is conscious, have him place the thumb of the uninjured extremity in the fold of the elbow to help control the injured limb's motion. This gives the patient control over the limb, decreases limb movement, and increases comfort.

You may also immobilize the limb by using a long padded rigid splint affixed to the extended limb. Place the splint along the medial aspect of the upper extremity, and ensure that it does not apply pressure to the axilla. Such pressure disrupts axillary artery blood flow to the limb and is uncomfortable for the patient. Secure the splint firmly to the limb, wrapping from the distal end toward the proximal end. Then, secure the splint to the supine patient's body, and move the patient and splint to a long spine board.

Radius/Ulna

The forearm may fracture anywhere along its length, and the fracture may involve the radius, the ulna, or both. Most commonly, fracture occurs at the distal end of the radius, just above the articular surface. This is known as a Colles' fracture, and it presents with the wrist turned up at an unusual angle. Another term for this injury is the "silver fork deformity" because it is contoured like a fork and the distal limb often becomes ashen. As with most joint fractures, the major concern here is for distal circulation and innervation. If you find a neurovascular injury, use only slight adjustments to restore nervous or circulatory function because movement in this area is likely to cause further injury.

When possible, leave a distal digit exposed to evaluate capillary refill and skin colour and temperature.

Splint forearm fractures with a short, padded rigid splint affixed to the forearm and hand. Secure the hand in the position of function by placing a large wad of dressing material in the palm to maintain a position like that of holding a large ball. Place the rigid splint along the medial forearm surface and wrap circumferentially from the fingers to the elbow. Leave at least one digit exposed to permit checking for capillary refill. Bend the elbow across the chest and use a sling and swathe to hold the limb in position. This provides relative elevation and improved venous drainage in both seated and supine patients.

The air splint or long padded rigid splint, tied firmly to the body, may also adequately immobilize forearm fractures (Figure 22-13). When using these devices, remember to place the hand in the position of function to increase patient comfort.

FIGURE 22-13 A malleable splint can effectively splint fractures of the radius and/or ulna.

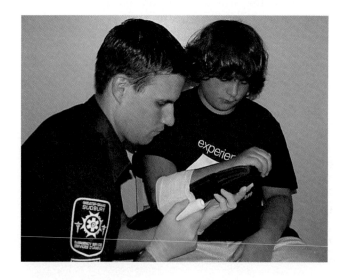

CARE FOR SPECIFIC JOINT INJURIES

Hip

The hip may dislocate in two directions, anteriorly and posteriorly. The anterior dislocation presents with the foot turned outward and the head of the femur palpable in the inguinal area. The posterior dislocation is most common and presents with the knee flexed and the foot rotated internally. The displaced head of the femur is buried in the muscle of the buttocks. Immobilize a patient with either type of dislocation on a long spine board using pillows and blankets as padding to maintain the patient's position and provide comfort. If distal circulation, sensation, or motor function is severely compromised, consider one attempt at reduction of a posterior dislocation. (Consult local protocols and medical direction to identify criteria for reduction attempts.) However, do not attempt reduction if there are other serious injuries, like a pelvic fracture, associated with the hip dislocation. Anterior dislocations, in general, cannot be managed by reduction in the prehospital setting.

For reduction of a posterior hip dislocation, have a care provider hold the pelvis firmly against the long spine board or other firm surface by placing downward pressure on the iliac crests. Flex the patient's hip and knee at 90 degrees, and apply a firm, slowly increasing traction along the axis of the femur. Gently rotate the femur externally. It takes some time for the muscles to relax, but when they do, the head of the femur will "pop" back into position. If you feel this "pop" or if the patient reports a sudden relief of pain and is able to extend the leg easily, the reduction has likely been a success. Immobilize the patient in a comfortable position, either in flexion (not to exceed 90 degrees) or fully supine with the hip and leg in full extension. Reevaluate sensation, motor function, and circulation. If the femur head does not move into the acetabulum after a few minutes of your attempted reduction, immobilize the patient as found, and provide rapid transport.

Knee

Knee injuries may include fractures of the femur, the tibia, or both, patellar dislocations, or frank dislocations of the knee. Because the knee is such a large joint and bears such a great amount of weight, an injury to it is serious and threatens the patient's future ability to walk. Another concern with knee injury is possible injury to the major blood vessel traversing the area, the popliteal artery. This artery is less mobile than blood vessels in other joints, which leaves it more subject to injury and distal vascular compromise.

Immobilize knee joint fractures and patellar dislocations in the position found unless distal circulation, sensation, or motor function is disrupted. If the limb is flexed, splint it with two medium rigid splints, placing one medially and one laterally (Figure 22-14). Cross-wrap with bandage material to secure the limb in position. You may also use ladder or malleable splints, conformed to the angle of the limb and placed anteriorly and posteriorly, or a vacuum splint to immobilize the knee. If the limb is extended, simply apply two padded rigid splints or a full-leg air splint.

Dislocation of the patella is more common than dislocation of the knee joint and usually leaves the knee in a flexed position with a lateral displacement of the patella. The injured knee appears significantly deformed, though patellar dislocation has a lower incidence of associated vascular injury than does knee dislocation.

Anterior dislocations of the knee produce an extended limb contour that lifts at the knee (moving from proximal to distal), while posterior dislocations produce a limb that drops at the knee. (Ensure that the injury is not a patellar dislocation.) If there is neurovascular compromise, have another care provider

> *Immobilize knee injuries in the position found unless you discover significant distal circulation, sensation, or motor deficit.*

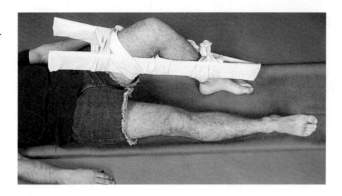

FIGURE 22-14 Angulated knee dislocations can be immobilized with two padded rigid splints.

immobilize the femur. You should then grasp the limb just above the ankle and at the calf muscle and apply a firm and progressive traction, first along the axis of the tibia and then pulling the limb toward alignment with the femur. With posterior dislocations, a third care provider may provide moderate downward pressure on the distal femur and upward pressure on the proximal tibia to facilitate the reduction. As with most dislocations, success is measured by feeling the bone end "pop" back into place, the patient reporting a dramatic reduction in pain, and noting a freer movement of the limb at the knee joint. Once you reduce the knee dislocation, immobilize the joint in the position of function, and transport the patient. If you cannot reduce the dislocation with a few minutes of distal traction, immobilize the extremity in the position found, and transport the patient quickly. Perform a knee dislocation reduction, even if the patient has good distal circulation and nervous function, when the time to definitive care is likely to exceed two hours.

Ankle

Ankle injuries often produce a distal lower limb that is grossly deformed, due to malleolar fracture, dislocation, or both. Sprains are also injuries of concern, although with them the limb remains in anatomical position. Splint sprains or nondisplaced fractures with an air splint (shaped to accommodate the foot) speed splint or other rigid splints, padded liberally and wrapped firmly. You may also use a pillow splint, especially if there is any ankle deformity (Figure 22-15). Apply local cooling to ease the pain and reduce swelling.

Ankle dislocation may occur in any of three directions: anteriorly, posteriorly, and laterally. The anterior dislocation presents with a dorsiflexed (upward pointing) foot that appears shortened. The posterior dislocation appears to

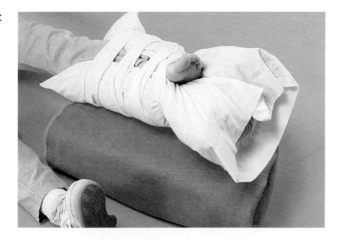

FIGURE 22-15 A pillow splint can be used for injuries to the ankles and feet.

lengthen the plantar flexed (downward pointing) foot. The lateral dislocation is the most common and presents with a foot turned outward with respect to the ankle. If distal neurovascular compromise indicates the need for reduction, have a care provider grasp the calf, hold it in position, and pull against the traction you apply. You should then grasp the heel with one hand and the metatarsal arch with the other. Pull a distal traction to disengage the bone ends and protect the articular cartilage during the relocation. For anterior dislocations, move the foot posteriorly with respect to the ankle; with lateral dislocations, rotate the foot medially; with posterior dislocations, pull the heel toward you and the foot toward you, then away. The joint should return to normal position with a "pop," and there should be a reduction in patient pain and an increase in the mobility of the joint. Apply local cooling, and immobilize the limb. If the procedure does not result in joint reduction within a few minutes, splint the joint as found, and provide rapid patient transport.

Foot

Injuries to the foot include dislocations and fractures to the calcanei (heel bones), metatarsals, and phalanges. Injuries to the calcanei generally result from falls and can cause significant pain and swelling. Injuries to the metatarsals and phalanges can result from penetrating or blunt trauma or the typical "stubbing" of a toe. Fatigue fractures of the metatarsal bones, or "march fractures," are relatively common. These injuries are reasonably stable, even though the extremity cannot bear weight. When foot or ankle injury is suspected, anticipate both bilateral foot injuries and lumbar spinal injury.

Immobilize foot injuries in much the same way as you do with ankle injuries. Use pillow, vacuum, rigid, or air splints (with foot accommodation). If possible, leave some portion of the foot accessible so that you can monitor distal capillary refill or, at least, skin temperature and colour.

Shoulder

Fractures to the shoulder most commonly involve the proximal humerus, lateral scapula, and distal clavicle. Dislocations can include anterior, posterior, or inferior displacement of the humoral head. Anterior dislocations displace the humoral head forward, resulting in a shoulder that appears "hollow" or "squared off," with the patient holding the arm close to the chest and forward of the mid-axillary line. Posterior dislocations rotate the arm internally, and the patient presents with the elbow and forearm held away from the chest. Inferior dislocations displace the humoral head downward, with the result that the patient's arm is often locked above the head.

You should immobilize shoulder injuries, like all joint injuries, as found, unless pulse, sensation, or motor function distal to the injury is absent. Immobilize anterior and posterior dislocations with a sling and swathe, and if needed, place a pillow under the arm and forearm. Immobilization of any inferior dislocation (with the upper extremity fixed above the head) will call for ingenuity on your part in splinting. In such cases, immobilize the extended arm in the position found. Using cravats, tie a long, padded splint to the torso, shoulder girdle, arm, and forearm to immobilize the arm above the head. Gently move the patient to the long spine board, and secure both splint and patient to the spine board.

Begin reduction of anterior and posterior shoulder dislocations by placing a strap across the patient's chest, under the affected shoulder (past the axilla) and across the back. Have a care provider be prepared to pull countertraction across the chest and superiorly using the strap. You, meanwhile, should flex the patient's elbow, drawing the arm somewhat away from the body (abduction) and pull firm traction along the axis of the humerus. Some slight internal and external rotation of the humerus may facilitate reduction. For reduction of inferior dislocations, have another care provider hold the thorax while you flex the elbow. Gradually apply firm traction along the axis of the humerus, and gently rotate the arm externally. If the joint does not relocate in a few minutes, immobilize it as it lies, and transport the patient. If reduction is successful, immobilize the upper extremity in the normal anatomical position with a sling and swathe.

Elbow

Elbow dislocations should not be reduced in the prehospital setting.

Elbow injuries display a high incidence of nervous and vascular involvement, especially in children. As in the knee, the blood vessels running through the elbow region are held firmly in place. The probability is high, therefore, that any fracture or dislocation will involve the brachial artery and the medial, ulnar, and radial nerves. Assess the distal neurovascular function, and if you detect a deficit, move the joint very carefully and minimally to restore distal circulation. Then, splint the elbow with a single padded rigid splint, providing cross-strapping as necessary, or use a ladder splint bent to conform to the angle of the limb (Figure 22-16). Keeping the wrist slightly elevated above the elbow, secure the limb to the chest using a sling and swathe. This position increases venous return and reduces the swelling and pain associated with the injury.

Wrist/Hand

When splinting the distal upper extremity, place padding in the palm of the hand to maintain the position of function.

Fractures of the hand and wrist are commonly associated with direct trauma. They present with very noticeable deformity and significant pain reported by the patient. These fractures are of serious concern to the patient. Since the hand and wrist bones are small, any fracture is in close proximity to a joint. Exercise concern when you care for these injuries because of the possibility of vascular and neural involvement.

You can effectively immobilize musculoskeletal injuries of the forearm, wrist, hand, or fingers with a padded rigid or malleable splint. Place a roll of bandaging, a wad of dressing material, or some similar object in the patient's hand to maintain the position of function. Then, secure the extremity to the padded board or malleable splint. Be sure to leave some portion of the distal extremity accessible so that you can monitor the adequacy of perfusion and sensation. Place the wrist above the elbow to assist venous return and reduce distal swelling.

Hand and wrist injuries are very common, particularly among athletes and children. A particular type of wrist fracture is the Colles' fracture, in which the wrist has a "silver fork" appearance. Fortunately, such injuries are seldom serious and can be managed in the prehospital setting quite easily.

Finger

Forces may displace the phalanges from their joints, resulting in deformity and pain. Displacement usually occurs between the phalanges or between the proximal phalanx and the metacarpal and causes the bone to be moved either anteriorly or posteriorly. (Amputations are multisystem injuries that severely damage the musculoskeletal system. They are addressed in depth in Chapter 20, "Soft-Tissue Trauma.")

Splint finger fractures using tongue blades or small, malleable splints designed to be shaped to the contour of the injured finger. The finger may also be taped to the adjoining fingers to limit additional movement. The hand is then placed in the position of function and further immobilized.

Finger dislocations usually involve the proximal joint (and sometimes the distal joint) with the digit commonly displacing posteriorly. If reduction is indicated,

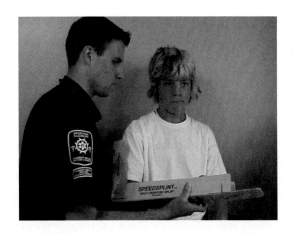

FIGURE 22-16 Use a corrugated board splint such as a Speedsplint to immobilize angulated fractures or dislocations of the elbow.

grasp the distal finger, and apply a firm distal traction. Then, direct the digit toward the normal anatomical position by moving its proximal end. You should feel the finger "pop" into place, and the digit should resume its normal alignment when compared with the uninjured finger on the other hand. Splint the finger with a slight bend (10 to 15 degrees), and immobilize the hand in the position of function.

SOFT AND CONNECTIVE TISSUE INJURIES

Tendon, ligament, and muscle injuries are rarely, if ever, life threatening. Massive muscular contusions and hematomas can, however, contribute to hypovolemia, while ligament and tendon injuries can endanger the future functioning of a limb. Be careful about permitting the patient to put further stress on a limb, especially with higher grades of sprains. The weakened ligaments may fail completely, resulting in dislocation or complete joint instability. For the purpose of care, treat these injuries as you would dislocations, and immobilize the adjacent joints. Monitor distal neurovascular function because tissue swelling within the circumferential wrapping of a splint may compress blood vessels and nerves. Care for muscular injuries with immobilization, gentle compression with snug (but not overly tight) dressings, and local cooling to suppress edema and pain using cold packs or ice wrapped in dressing material. Be watchful for signs of compartment syndrome, especially in the calf and forearm regions.

Open wounds involving the muscles, tendons, and ligaments can be severe and debilitating. Carefully evaluate such wounds for signs of connective tissue involvement. Be especially watchful in the case of deep open injuries close to the joints. With such wounds, the likelihood of tendon and ligament disruptions is great and may affect the use of the joint, the muscles controlling the joint, or the muscles controlling joint movement distal to the injury. Carefully evaluate for circulation, sensation, and motor function below these injuries.

Injury to a muscle or tendon may limit its ability to either extend or flex the limb. The opposing muscle moves the limb, while the injured muscle cannot return it to the normal position. With limb injuries, note any unusual limb position, especially if the patient is unable to return the limb to a neutral position. At any sign of pain or dysfunction, splint the limb.

MEDICATIONS

Medications are frequently administered to the patient who has musculoskeletal injury to relieve pain and to premedicate before correction of a dislocation. Medications used include nitrous oxide, diazepam, midazolam, morphine, fentanyl, and meperidine.

Tendon, ligament, and muscle injuries are rarely life threatening.

Care for muscular injuries with immobilization, gentle compression with snug dressings, and local cooling to suppress edema and pain.

Sedatives/Analgesics

Nitrous Oxide Nitrous oxide (Nitronox®) is a nitrogen and oxygen compound in a gaseous state. It is administered in the prehospital setting for its anesthetic properties, specifically to reduce the perception of pain in cases of musculoskeletal injuries. For prehospital care, it is administered in a 50-percent nitrous oxide and 50-percent oxygen mixture via a special regulator and a self-administration mask. Self-administration of nitrous oxide prevents overmedication because the patient will drop the mask when too heavily sedated.

Nitrous oxide is nonexplosive, and its analgesic effects dissipate within two to five minutes of discontinuing administration. High concentrations of nitrous oxide may lead to hypoxia and may cause respiratory depression and vomiting. These side effects are minimized, however, because the gas is premixed with oxygen by the administration set during prehospital delivery.

The chief concern with the use of nitrous oxide is that is diffuses easily into air-filled spaces in the body, increasing the pressure within them. This diffusion is especially dangerous in patients with pneumothorax or tension pneumothorax, bowel obstruction, and middle ear obstruction. Rule out COPD (chronic obstructive pulmonary disease) and these pathologies before you administer nitrous oxide in the prehospital setting.

The nitrous oxide administration device consists of two cylinders of equal size, one holding oxygen (green) and the other, nitrous oxide (blue). The gases are mixed in a special blender/regulator and provided to the patient when his inspiration generates a less-than-atmospheric pressure. The patient must hold the administration mask firmly to the face to trigger administration, which prevents administration in a patient who is heavily sedated. Nitrous oxide is a controlled substance, and its use is carefully monitored for provider abuse.

Diazepam Diazepam (Valium®) is a benzodiazepine with both anti-anxiety and skeletal muscle relaxant qualities. The drug reduces the patient's perception and memory of pain. It is used for musculoskeletal injuries and to medicate patients before painful procedures, such as cardioversion and dislocation reduction. It is administered in a slow IV bolus of 5 to 15 mg, not to exceed 5 mg/min, into a large vein. Diazepam is rather fast acting, with IV effects occurring almost immediately and reaching peak effectiveness in 15 minutes. Its duration of effectiveness is from 15 to 60 minutes. Do not mix diazepam with any other drugs, and flush the IV line before and after administration. Administer diazepam as close to the IV catheter as possible, and do not inject it into a plastic IV bag. Diazepam is readily absorbed by plastic, which quickly reduces its concentration.

Diazepam is usually supplied in single-use vials or preloaded syringes containing 2 mL of a 5-mg/mL solution (10 mg). Administer 5 to 15 mg IV, and repeat in 10 to 15 minutes if necessary.

The effects of diazepam may be reversed by the administration of flumazenil. Usually, 2 mL of a 0.1-mg/mL solution is given IV (over 15 seconds), with a second dose repeated at 60 seconds.

Midazolam Midazolam (Versed®), a potent but short-acting benzodiazepine with strong hypnotic and amnestic properties, is used widely in medicine as a sedative and hypnotic. It is three to four times more potent than diazepam. Its onset of action is approximately 90 seconds when administered intravenously and 15 minutes when administered intramuscularly. Though midazolam has impressive amnestic properties, like the other benzodiazepines, it has no effect on pain.

Midazolam should not be administered to patients who are in shock, with depressed vital signs, or who are in alcoholic coma. Emergency resuscitative equipment must be available prior to the administration of midazolam. Vital signs must be continuously monitored during and after drug administration. Midazolam has more potential than the other benzodiazepines to cause respiratory depression and respiratory arrest. Flumazenil (Romazicon), a benzodiazepine antagonist, should be available to use as an antidote if required.

The sedative effects of midazolam may be enhanced by concomitant use of barbiturates, alcohol, or narcotics (and should, therefore, not be used in patients who have taken central nervous system [CNS] depressants).

When used for sedation, midazolam must be administered cautiously, as the amount of medication required to achieve sedation varies from individual to individual. Typically, 1–2.5 mg are administered by slow IV injection. Usually, it is best to dilute midazolam with normal saline or D_5W prior to IV administration. Midazolam can be administered intramuscularly at a dose of 0.07–0.08 mg/kg (average adult dose of 5 mg).

Midazolam is available in 2-, 5-, 10-mL vials (1 mg/mL) and 1-, 2-, 5-, 10-mL vials (5 mg/mL). Midazolam is administered in 2.5-mg increments.

Morphine Morphine sulphate is an opium alkaloid used to relieve pain (narcotic analgesic), to sedate, and to reduce anxiety. It is used with musculoskeletal injuries for its ability to reduce pain perception. Morphine may reduce vascular volume and cardiac preload by increasing venous capacitance and may thus decrease blood pressure in the hypovolemic patient. It should not be administered to a patient with hypovolemia or hypotension. Its major side effects are respiratory depression and possible nausea and vomiting.

Morphine is available in 10-mL single-use vials or Tubex® units of a 1-mg/mL solution or as 1 mL of a 10-mg/mL solution vial for dilution with 9 mL normal saline. Administer a 2-mg IV bolus slowly, repeating as necessary every few minutes to effect.

Naloxone hydrochloride (Narcan®) is a narcotic antagonist that can quickly reverse the effects of narcotics (morphine, meperidine, and fentanyl) and should be available any time you use morphine sulphate. Naloxone is administered as an IV bolus of 0.4 to 2 mg, repeated every two to three minutes until effective. Naloxone is a shorter-acting drug than morphine, and so repeat doses may be necessary.

Fentanyl Fentanyl (Sublimaze®) is a synthetic narcotic agonist analgesic with pharmacological action similar to those of morphine and meperidine, but its action is more prompt and less prolonged. On a weight basis, fentanyl is 50 to 100 times more potent than morphine. Its principal actions are analgesia and sedation. Its emetic effect is less than with either morphine or meperidine.

Vital signs should be monitored routinely. Fentanyl may produce bradycardia, which may be treated with atropine. However, fentanyl should be used with care in patients with cardiac bradydysrhythmias.

Fentanyl should be administered with caution to patients with liver and kidney dysfunction because of the importance of these organs in the metabolism and excretion of drugs.

As with other narcotic analgesics, the most common serious reactions reported to occur with fentanyl are respiratory depression, apnea, muscle rigidity, and bradycardia. If these side effects remain untreated, respiratory arrest, circulatory depression, or cardiac arrest may occur. Resuscitation equipment and a narcotic agonist, such as naloxone, should be readily available to manage apnea.

Fentanyl may be used in the management of severe pain, for maintenance of analgesia, and as a sedative agent in rapid sequence sedation/intubation.

Fentanyl is available in 100- and 250-µg vials.

Meperidine Meperidine hydrochloride (Demerol®) is a narcotic analgesic with properties similar to those of morphine, although it may produce less smooth muscle relaxation, constipation, and cough reflex suppression. As with morphine, it is used with musculoskeletal injuries for its ability to reduce the patient's perception of pain. It also may produce respiratory depression and hypotension, especially in the patient who is volume depleted.

Meperidine is supplied in single-dose vials and preloaded syringes and in concentrations of from 10 to 100 mg/mL. It may be administered in doses of 50 to 100 mg IM. For IV administration, use a concentration of 10 mg/mL diluted in normal saline or Ringer's Lactate solution, and inject slowly in doses of 50 to 100 mg. Narcan® will reverse its effects.

OTHER MUSCULOSKELETAL INJURY CONSIDERATIONS

Other areas for special consideration with musculoskeletal injuries include pediatric injuries, athletic injuries, patient refusals and referrals, and psychological support for the patient with musculoskeletal injury.

Pediatric Musculoskeletal Injury

Children are at higher risk than adults for musculoskeletal injuries due to their activity levels and incompletely developed coordination. Special injuries affecting them include greenstick fractures and epiphyseal fractures.

The incomplete nature of the greenstick fracture produces a stable but angulated limb in the young child. The injured limb is painful and will not bear weight. In these cases, do not attempt to realign the limb; understand that the orthopedic specialist will probably complete the fracture to permit proper healing.

Epiphyseal fractures disrupt the child's growth plate and endanger future bone growth. This injury is likely with fractures within a few centimetres of the joint because the epiphyseal plate is a point of skeletal weakness. Treat these fractures as you would in an adult, but recognize that they are potentially limb-threatening injuries.

Athletic Musculoskeletal Injuries

Athletes, especially those involved in contact sports, such as football, soccer, basketball, and wrestling, have a higher incidence of musculoskeletal injuries than the general public. Injuries to the joints, often serious knee and ankle sprains, are common reasons for calls to the EMS. Such injuries are especially important because they occur in individuals who are at least moderately well conditioned and result from the application of significant kinetic forces. When you are called to the side of an injured athlete, be especially sensitive to the potential for residual disability caused by these injuries, and be predisposed to transport instead of permitting the patient to remain at the scene.

Knowing the athletic trainers in your area may help your on-scene operations run more smoothly and efficiently.

Knowing the athletic trainers in your area may help your on-scene operations run more smoothly and efficiently. It is important for trainers to understand that once you are called to the scene, the injured athlete becomes a patient of the EMS system and will be treated under the system's medical direction and protocols. Also, as the representative of that system, you are likely to assume responsibility for decisions about care and transport of the patient. Ensuring that trainers understand these facts may eliminate confrontations over care of injured athletes.

Athletic trainers use the acronym RICE to identify the recommended treatment for sprains, strains, and other soft-tissue injuries. RICE stands for *R*est the extremity, *I*ce for the first 48 hours, *C*ompress with an elastic bandage, and *E*levate for venous drainage. This is consistent with standard emergency care for sprains and strains. (Note, however, that the application of the elastic bandage in this case is to strengthen the limb for further activity and is not recommended for prehospital care.)

Content Review

RICE PROCEDURE FOR STRAINS, SPRAINS, SOFT-TISSUE INJURIES
Rest the extremity.
Ice for the first 48 hours.
Compress with elastic bandage.
Elevate the extremity.

Patient Refusals and Referral

In some situations, you may encounter a patient suffering from an isolated sprain or strain with no significant mechanism of injury and no other signs, symptoms, or complaints. This patient may refuse your assistance or be a candidate for on-scene treatment and referral for follow-up medical care. Evaluate the need for immobilization and x-rays, and determine if the patient should seek immediate care in an emergency department or see a personal physician.

Follow local protocols with patient refusals and referrals, and document such cases thoroughly.

Psychological Support for the Musculoskeletal Injury Patient

Regardless of the specific type of injury sustained, patients need psychological as well as physiological support. Too often, we concentrate all efforts on the patient's injuries, forgetting the emotional impact that the incident and the emergency care measures employed have on the patient. Keep in mind that patients are not frequently exposed to injuries. They do not know what effects the injuries will have on their lives or what to expect from medical care in the prehospital, emergency department, or in-hospital setting. Remember that you can have a significant impact on a patient's emotional response to trauma. Displaying a concerned attitude and a professional demeanour and communicating frequently and compassionately with patients will go far to calm and reassure them. Simple attention paid to the patient may make the experience with prehospital emergency medical service one that is remembered positively.

Psychological support provided by the paramedic can have a significant impact on a patient's emotional response to trauma.

Summary

Injuries to the bones, ligaments, tendons, and muscles of the extremities rarely threaten your patient's life. Major exceptions are pelvic and serious or bilateral femur fractures, in which associated hemorrhage can contribute significantly to hypovolemia and shock. In addition, serious musculoskeletal trauma suggests the possibility of other, life-threatening trauma and, in fact, occurs in about 80 percent of cases of major multisystem trauma. The presence of serious musculoskeletal trauma should increase your index of suspicion for other serious internal injuries.

Care for isolated musculoskeletal trauma is usually delayed until the ABCs are stabilized and other patient life threats are dealt with. The goals of the care are to protect any open wounds, position affected limbs properly, immobilize the area of injury, and carefully monitor distal extremities to ensure neurovascular function.

Manage fractures by aligning the extremity with gentle traction and immobilizing it by splinting. In cases where you discover a loss of distal neurovascular function, move the extremity slightly to restore distal neurovascular function, and then splint.

Joint injuries carry a greater risk of damage to distal circulation, sensation, and motor function. Splint these injuries as you find them unless there is distal neurovascular compromise. If that is the case, employ gentle manipulation to restore circulation, motor function, or sensation. If gentle manipulation is unsuccessful and transport may be delayed, attempt reduction of any dislocation of the hip, knee, ankle, shoulder, or finger as permitted by local protocol.

Care for injuries to connective and muscular tissues by immobilizing the area of injury in the position of function. Evaluate distal extremities for pulse, capillary refill, colour, temperature, sensation, and motor function before, during, and after any immobilization or movement of a limb, and provide frequent monitoring thereafter.

CHAPTER 23

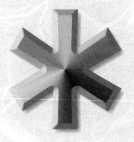

Head, Facial, and Neck Trauma

Objectives

After reading this chapter, you should be able to:

1. Describe the incidence, morbidity, and mortality of head, facial, and neck injuries. (p. 206)

2. Explain head and facial anatomy and physiology. (see Chapter 12)

3. Differentiate among the types of injuries to the following structures, highlighting the defining characteristics of each (see Chapter 12):
   a. Eye
   b. Ear
   c. Nose
   d. Throat
   e. Mouth

4. Predict head, facial, and other related injuries on the basis of mechanism of injury. (pp. 206–207)

5. Differentiate among facial injuries on the basis of the assessment and history. (pp. 219–223)

6. Explain the pathophysiology, assessment, and management for patients with eye, ear, nose, throat, and mouth injuries. (pp. 219–246)

7. Explain anatomy and relate physiology of the central nervous system (CNS) to head injuries. (pp. 211–219)

Continued

Objectives Continued

8. Distinguish among facial, head, and brain injury. (pp. 208–224)
9. Explain the pathophysiology of head/brain injuries. (pp. 206–219)
10. Explain the concept of increasing intracranial pressure (ICP). (pp. 210–216)
11. Explain the effect of increased and decreased carbon dioxide on ICP. (pp. 215–216)
12. Define and explain the process involved with each of the levels of increasing ICP. (pp. 215–216)
13. Relate assessment findings associated with head/brain injuries to the pathophysiological process. (pp. 206–219)
14. Classify head injuries (mild, moderate, severe) according to assessment findings. (pp. 213–214)
15. Identify the need for rapid intervention and transport of the patient with a head/brain injury. (pp. 225, 232)
16. Describe and explain the general management of the head/brain injury patient, including pharmacological and nonpharmacological treatment. (pp. 232–244)
17. Analyze the relationship between carbon dioxide concentration in the blood and management of the airway in the head/brain injured patient. (pp. 210–216)
18. Explain the pathophysiology, assessment, and management of a patient with the following:
    a. scalp injury (pp. 208–209, 227–228, 232–244)
    b. skull fracture (pp. 209–211, 227, 232–244)
    c. cerebral contusion (pp. 212, 232–244)
    d. intracranial hemorrhage (including epidural, subdural, subarachnoid, and intracerebral hemorrhage) (pp. 212–213, 232–244)
    e. axonal injury (including concussion and moderate and severe diffuse axonal injury) (pp. 213–214, 232–244)
    f. facial injury (pp. 219–223, 228–229, 232–244)
    g. neck injury (pp. 223–224, 229–230, 232–244)
19. Develop a management plan for the removal of a helmet for a head-injured patient. (p. 226)
20. Differentiate among the types of head/brain injuries on the basis of the assessment and history. (pp. 206–232)
21. Given several preprogrammed and moulaged head, face, and neck trauma patients, provide the appropriate scene assessment, primary assessment, rapid trauma or focused secondary assessment and history, detailed assessment, and ongoing assessment and provide appropriate patient care and transportation. (pp. 225–246)

INTRODUCTION TO HEAD, FACIAL, AND NECK INJURIES

Severe head injury is the most frequent cause of trauma death.

Head, facial, and neck injuries are common with major trauma. Each year in Canada, 34 000 people are admitted to hospital with brain injuries—that is almost 100 people injured per day. Although most of these hospitalizations are due to relatively minor injuries, severe head injury is the most frequent cause of trauma death. It is especially lethal in auto collisions and frequently produces significant long-term disability in patients who survive it. Gunshot wounds that penetrate the cranium result in a mortality of about 75 to 80 percent. Injuries to the face and neck threaten critical airway structures as well as the significant vasculature found in these regions.

The populations most at risk for serious head injury are males between the ages of 15 and 24, infants and young children, and the elderly. Education programs promoting safe practices in many different fields and the use of head protection, seat belts, and airbags have had major effects on reducing head injury mortality and morbidity. The use of helmets for bicycling, in-line skating, and motorcycling and in contact sports like football has also significantly reduced the incidence of serious head injury. In motorcycle collisions, for example, helmet use reduces serious head injury by more than 50 percent. Once a head injury occurs, however, time becomes a critical consideration. Intracranial hemorrhage and progressing edema can increase the intracranial pressure (ICP), hypoxia, and the internal and permanent damage done.

PATHOPHYSIOLOGY OF HEAD, FACIAL, AND NECK INJURY

Head, facial, and neck injuries are difficult to assess in the prehospital setting, and yet they commonly threaten life or may expose victims to lifelong disability. A clearer appreciation of the anatomy of these regions, of the various mechanisms of injury affecting them, and of the specific pathological processes related to head, facial, and neck injury can help you better anticipate, assess, and then manage these injuries and their effects on the human system.

MECHANISMS OF INJURY

Injuries to the head, neck, and face are divided by mechanisms of injury into blunt (closed) and penetrating (open).

Blunt Injury

The structures of the head, face, and neck protect very well against most blunt trauma. At times, however, the forces producing blunt trauma are of such magnitude as to compromise the body's well-designed protective mechanisms. For example, head injuries most frequently result from auto and motorcycle crashes and account for more than half of vehicle crash deaths. Sports-related impacts, falling objects, falls, and acts of violence, such as assault with a club, are other less common but still significant mechanisms of head injury (Figure 23-1).

The face is another area frequently subjected to blunt trauma. Significant facial injury occurs less frequently than head injury in auto impacts because, rather than the face, the head's frontal or parietal regions are more likely to hit the windshield. The same holds true for falls, as the arms, chest, or head absorb en-

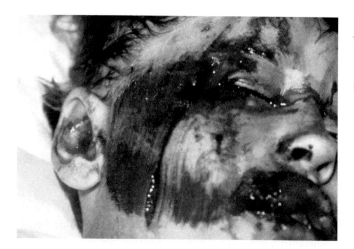

ergy as the conscious victim tries to protect the facial area from injury. Intentional violence is less likely to spare the facial region. The face is often the target of blows from a fist or from impact-enhancing objects, such as sticks or clubs. The middle and inner ear and the eyes are very well protected against most blunt trauma, though ear injury may be caused by compressional forces associated with diving or explosions. The eyes may occasionally be injured by impacts from smaller blunt objects, such as a racquetball, baseball, or tennis ball.

The neck is anatomically well protected from most blunt trauma because the head and chest protrude more anteriorly. Laterally, the neck is protected as the shoulders protrude a significant distance from the neck. The neck is, however, a point of impact in special situations. For example, during an auto collision the neck may strike the steering wheel or be injured by a shoulder strap that is worn without a lap belt. The region may also be struck by objects during fights or traumatically constricted or distracted during an attempted suicide by hanging.

Penetrating Injury

Penetrating injuries to the head, face, and neck are not as common as those resulting from blunt trauma, but they can be just as severe and potentially life threatening. In addition, a penetrating injury to the head suggests the meninges have been opened, producing a route for potentially serious infection.

Penetrating injuries to the head, face, and neck usually result from either gunshots or stabbings. Gunshot wounds are most common and especially hideous because bullets release tremendous energy as they slow during collision with skeletal and central nervous tissue. Similarly, explosions propel projectiles, either intrinsic to the explosive device or from debris produced by the blast, that may penetrate and damage this region. Knife wounds to the head and face tend to be superficial because of the region's extensive skeletal components. The anterior and lateral neck, however, are not as well protected, and wounds there may compromise both the airway and major blood vessels, quickly threatening the patient's life.

There are many other types of penetrating injuries that may involve the head, face, and neck. Some examples include the "clothesline" impact with a wire fence while a victim is riding an all-terrain vehicle or snowmobile; bites from humans, dogs, and other animals; or a tongue bitten when it is trapped between the teeth during an impact. Infrequently, a fall may impale a person on a fixed object, such as a concrete reinforcing bar, producing a penetrating injury.

Blunt and penetrating injury mechanisms have different impacts depending on the structures they involve. The following sections discuss the pathological processes of injuries as they affect the head, face, and neck.

HEAD INJURY

Head injury is defined as a traumatic insult to the cranial region that may result in injury to soft tissues, bony structures, and the brain. Let us look at head injury as it progresses from the exterior to the interior, examining scalp, cranial, and brain injuries.

Scalp Injury

The most superficial head injuries involve the scalp (Figure 23-2). A scalp injury may also be the only overt indication of deeper, more serious injury beneath. The scalp overlies the firm cranium and is very vascular. Its blood vessels lack the ability to constrict as effectively as those elsewhere in the body; hence, scalp wounds tend to bleed heavily. Some people believe that head injuries do not result in shock; this, however, assumes that the hemorrhage they cause is easy to control. In fact, any serious blood loss from scalp wounds can contribute to shock and, if left uncontrolled, may itself cause hypovolemia and shock. Scalp wounds further provide a route for infection because emissary veins drain from the dural sinuses, through the cranium, and into the superficial venous circulation. Because of rich circulation to the area, scalp wounds tend to heal well.

Scalp wounds may present in a manner that confounds assessment. Usually, blunt trauma creates a contusion that, because of the firm skull underneath, expands outwardly in a very rapid and noticeable way. However, blunt trauma may also tear underlying fascia and areolar tissue, causing it to separate. This can leave an elevated border surrounding a depression, mimicking the contour of a depressed skull fracture. However, the scalp's blood vessels may bleed into a depressed skull fracture, fill any depression, and conceal the injury's true nature.

The presentation of scalp wounds may make them difficult to assess.

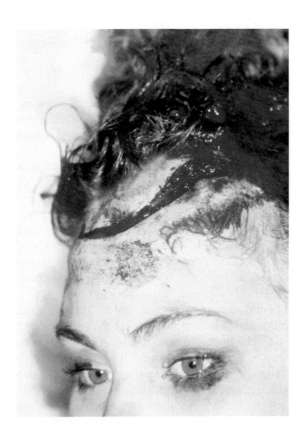

FIGURE 23-2 Scalp wounds can bleed heavily.

A common and special type of scalp wound is the avulsion. Areolar tissue is only loosely attached to the skull, and glancing blows can create a shearing force against the scalp's border. Such blows frequently tear a flap of scalp loose and fold it back against the uninjured scalp, exposing a portion of the cranium. The mechanism of injury may also seriously contaminate the wound and may cause moderate hemorrhage unless the avulsed tissue folds back sharply, compressing the blood vessels.

Cranial Injury

Because of its spherical shape and skeletal design, the skull does not fracture unless trauma is extreme. Such fractures may present as linear, depressed, comminuted, or basilar in nature (Figure 23-3). Linear fractures are small cracks in the cranium and represent about 80 percent of all skull fractures. The temporal bone is one of the thinnest and most frequently fractured cranial bones. If there are no associated intracranial injuries, a linear fracture poses very little danger to the patient. In contrast, a depressed fracture represents an inward displacement of the skull's surface and results in a greater likelihood of intracranial damage. Comminuted fractures involve multiple skull fragments that may penetrate the meninges and cause physical harm to the structures beneath.

A common type of skull fracture involves the base of the skull. This area is permeated with foramina (openings) for the spinal cord, cranial nerves, and various blood vessels. The basilar skull also has hollow or open structures, such as the sinuses, the orbits of the eye, the nasal cavities, the external auditory canals, and the middle and inner ears. These spaces weaken the skull and leave the basilar area prone to fracture.

The temporal bone is one of the thinnest and most frequently fractured cranial bones.

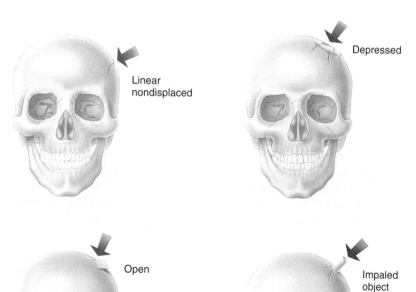

Linear nondisplaced

Depressed

Open

Impaled object

FIGURE 23-3 Various types of skull fractures.

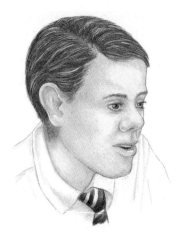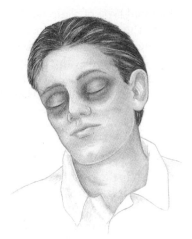

Retroauricular ecchymosis
(Battle's sign)

Bilateral periorbital ecchymosis
(raccoon eyes)

✳ retroauricular ecchymosis
black-and-blue discoloration
over the mastoid process (just
behind the ear) that is characteristic of a basilar skull fracture. (Also called Battle's sign.)

✳ bilateral periorbital ecchymosis
black-and-blue discoloration
of the area surrounding the
eyes. It is usually associated
with basilar skull fracture.
(Also called raccoon eyes.)

*The "halo sign" is most
reliable when associated with
fluid leaking from the ear.*

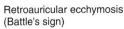

*The glucose level of CSF is
normally half that of the blood.
If you are unsure whether a
clear fluid is water or CSF,
check the glucose level of the
fluid and compare it with the
patient's blood glucose level.*

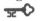

The signs of basilar skull fracture vary with the injury's location (Figure 23-4).
If the fracture involves the auditory canal and the lower lateral areas of the skull,
hemorrhage may migrate to the mastoid region (just posterior and slightly inferior to the ear). This causes a characteristic discoloration called **retroauricular
ecchymosis** or "Battle's sign." Another classic sign of basilar skull fracture is
bilateral periorbital ecchymosis, sometimes referred to as "raccoon eyes." This is
a dramatic discoloration around the eyes associated with orbital fractures and
hemorrhage into the surrounding tissue. Both retroauricular ecchymosis and
bilateral periorbital ecchymosis take time to develop; neither is likely to develop
during the period after an injury when the patient is under paramedic care.

Basilar skull fracture can tear the dura mater, opening a wound between the
brain and the body's exterior. Such a wound may permit cerebrospinal fluid
(CSF) to seep out through a nasal cavity or an external auditory canal and also
provide a possible route for infection to enter the meninges.

This type of wound may also provide an escape for CSF in the presence of
increasing intracranial pressure. Escaping CSF may mediate the rise in intracranial pressure (ICP) and somewhat limit damage to the brain. (While CSF is an
important medium, the body can regenerate it quite rapidly.) Blood mixed with
CSF and flowing from the nose, mouth, or ears will demonstrate the target or
"halo" sign (a dark red circle surrounded by a lighter yellowish one) when
dropped on a pillow or towel (Figure 23-5). Normal blood demonstrates a narrow concentric ring of yellowish coloration surrounding the red circle produced
by the less mobile erythrocytes. If CSF is mixed with the blood, this outer ring is
much larger. Be aware, however, that other fluids, like lacrimal or nasal fluids or
saliva, may cause a similar response. Hence, the halo sign is most reliable when
associated with fluid leaking from the ear.

Bullet impacts induce specific types of cranial fracture. The entrance wound
often produces a comminuted fracture and sends bone fragments into the brain.
Often, the bullet's kinetic energy is sufficient to permit the bullet to exit from the
cranium and cause a second fracture. This exit wound site is blown outward and
is often more severe in appearance than the entrance wound.

In many cases, the energy of the projectile's passage through the cranium
causes a cavitational wave of extreme pressure, which is contained and enhanced
by the rigid container of the skull. The result is extreme damage to the cranial
contents, and, if the transmitted kinetic energy is strong enough, the skull may
fracture and "explode" outward.

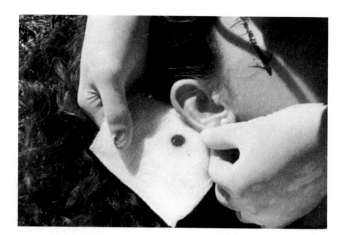

FIGURE 23-5 The "halo test" can detect the presence of cerebrospinal fluid (CSF). If CSF is present, it will diffuse faster across a paper towel or gauze because it is thinner than blood.

Another type of wound occurs when a bullet enters the cranium at an angle, is deflected within, and continues to move along the cranium's interior until its energy is completely exhausted. This process does devastating damage to the cerebral cortex and is rarely survivable.

A special type of cranial injury involves an impaled object. As is the case with objects impaled in most other regions of the body, any further motion of the object may cause additional hemorrhage and tissue damage. When the object is impaled in the cranium, the situation is especially serious. Brain tissue is much more delicate than other body tissue, does not immobilize the object as well, and is easily injured by the object's motion. As with objects impaled elsewhere, removal of the impaled object from the cranium may cause further injury and increase blood accumulation.

Note that a cranial fracture, by itself, is a skeletal injury that will heal with time; it does not, by itself, threaten the brain. Rather, it is the possibility of injury beneath and suggested by the skull fracture that is of greatest concern. The forces necessary to fracture the cranium are extreme and likely to cause injury within.

Brain Injury

Brain injury is defined by the National Head Injury Foundation as "a traumatic insult to the brain capable of producing physical, intellectual, emotional, social, and vocational changes." It is classified as a direct or an indirect injury to the tissue of the cerebrum, cerebellum, or brainstem.

Direct Injury Direct (or primary) injury is caused by the forces of trauma and can be associated with a variety of mechanisms. Rapid acceleration (or deceleration) or penetrating injury can cause mechanical injury to nervous system cells and impair their function. The forces causing direct injury can also disrupt blood vessels, both restricting blood flow through the injured area and causing irritation of nervous tissue as blood flows into it. Remember that the brain is specially protected from contact with some of the blood's content by the blood–brain barrier. Injury disrupts this barrier. Lastly, serious jarring may damage capillary walls, affect their permeability, and cause a fluid shift to the interstitial space, or tissue edema. Most frequently, there is a mixture of these mechanisms associated with direct brain injury.

Two specific types of direct brain injury are coup and contrecoup injury (Figure 23-6). **Coup injuries** are tissue disruptions that occur directly at the point of impact. These injuries are inflicted as the brain displaces toward the impact surface and collides with the interior of the cranium. They are most common in the frontal region because its interior surface is rough and irregular. In contrast, the occipital

A cranial fracture, by itself, is a skeletal injury that will heal with time. However, the forces necessary to fracture the skull are often sufficient to induce brain injury.

✱ coup injury an injury to the brain occurring on the same side as the site of impact.

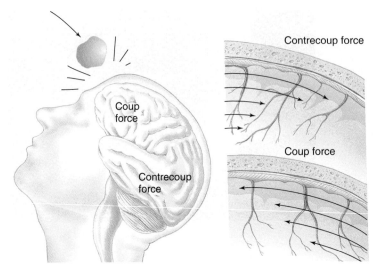

FIGURE 23-6   Coup and contrecoup movement of the brain.

* **contrecoup injury** occurring on the opposite side; an injury to the brain opposite the site of impact.

Content Review

TYPES OF DIRECT BRAIN INJURY

Focal
  Cerebral contusion
  Intracranial hemorrhage
    Epidural hematoma
    Subdural hematoma
    Intracerebral hemorrhage
Diffuse
  Concussion (mild to moderate diffuse axonal injury)
  Moderate diffuse axonal injury
  Severe diffuse axonal injury (formerly, brainstem injury)

* **epidural hematoma** accumulation of blood between the dura mater and the cranium.

areas are smooth and coup injuries occur there less frequently. Coup injury may also occur as the brain slides along the rough contours at the base of the skull.

Contrecoup injuries produce tissue damage away from the impact point as the brain, floating in CSF inside the cranium, "sloshes" toward the impact, then away from it, again striking the interior of the skull. For example, a blow to the forehead might result in injury to the occipital region (visual centre) and produce visual disturbances (seeing stars). Contrecoup injury to the frontal region of the brain is most common (from an impact to the occipital region) again because the frontal bones have an irregular inner surface.

Direct brain injuries can be further assigned to one of two specific categories—focal or diffuse.

Focal Injuries   Focal injuries occur at a specific location in the brain and include contusions and intracranial hemorrhages.

Cerebral Contusion   A cerebral contusion is caused by blunt trauma to local brain tissue that produces capillary bleeding into the substance of the brain. The contusion is relatively common with blunt head injuries and often produces prolonged confusion or other types of neurological deficit. This pathology may result from a coup or contrecoup mechanism and may occur at one or several sites in the brain. The localized form of the injury manifests with dysfunctions related to the site of the injury. For example, a patient who suffers a contusion of the frontal lobe after trauma to the forehead may experience personality changes. (Remember, the frontal lobe is the most commonly injured lobe.)

Intracranial Hemorrhage   Bleeding can occur at several locations within the brain, each presenting with a different pathological process. These injuries—proceeding from the most superficial to the deepest—are epidural, subdural, and intracerebral hemorrhages. In contrast to patients with concussions and contusions, expect the intracranial hemorrhage patient to deteriorate during your assessment and care because of associated indirect injury, such as increasing intracranial pressure.

Bleeding between the dura mater and the skull's interior surface is called **epidural hematoma** (Figure 23-7). It usually involves arterial vessels, often the middle meningeal artery in the temporal region. Because the bleeding is from a relatively high-pressure vessel, ICP builds rapidly, compressing the cerebrum and increasing the pressure within the skull. As pressure builds, the patient moves quickly toward unresponsiveness. The hemorrhage-induced increase in

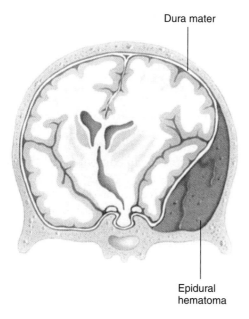

Dura mater

Epidural
hematoma

FIGURE 23-7   Epidural hematoma.

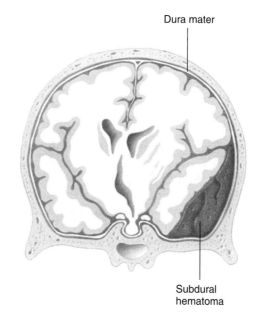

Dura mater

Subdural
hematoma

FIGURE 23-8   Subdural hematoma.

ICP reduces oxygenated circulation to the nerve cells (indirect injury). Bleeding may be so extensive that it displaces the brain away from the injury site, pushing it toward the foramen magnum. Although the progression is both rapid and life threatening, immediate surgery can frequently reverse it.

Bleeding within the meninges, specifically beneath the dura mater and within the subarachnoid space, is called **subdural hematoma** (Figure 23-8). This type of bleeding occurs very slowly and may have a subtle presentation because blood loss is usually due to rupture of a small venous vessel, often one of those bridging to the dural sinuses. The vessel most commonly involved is the superior sagittal sinus. Because the subdural hemorrhage occurs above the pia mater, it does not cause the cerebral irritation associated with intracerebral hemorrhage. The free blood in the cerebrospinal fluid may clog the structures responsible for the fluid's reabsorption, which can result in increasing ICP. The patient usually does not show overt signs and symptoms until hours or even days after the injury. Because of this delay, subdural hemorrhage is difficult to detect in the prehospital setting.

Suspect subdural hematoma in a medical (nontrauma) patient who demonstrates neurological signs and symptoms. Careful history taking may uncover a recent mechanism of injury, such as a fall, that could cause this presentation. You occasionally encounter such pathologies with the elderly or with chronic alcoholics. Because both the aging process and chronic alcoholism reduce the size of the brain, head impact causes greater and less controlled motion of the brain within the cranium. This increases the likelihood of injury and, specifically, subdural hematoma.

Intracerebral hemorrhage results from a ruptured blood vessel within the substance of the brain. Although blood loss is generally minimal, it is particularly damaging. Tissue edema results because free blood, outside the blood vessels, irritates the nervous tissue. Intracerebral hemorrhage often presents much like a stroke with the manifestations occurring very quickly. The particular presentation relates to the area of the brain involved. Normally, the signs and symptoms will progressively worsen with time.

Diffuse Injuries   Diffuse injuries involve a more general scenario of injury and include mild (concussions), moderate, and severe axonal disruptions. During

✳ **subdural hematoma** collection of blood directly beneath the dura mater.

Suspect subdural hematoma in a medical (nontrauma) patient who demonstrates neurological signs and symptoms.

✳ **intracerebral hemorrhage** bleeding directly into the tissue of the brain.

head impact, a shearing, tearing, or stretching force is applied to the nerve fibres and causes damage to the axons, the long communication pathways of the nerve cells. This pathology is frequently distributed throughout the brain and thus is called **diffuse axonal injury (DAI)**. Diffuse axonal injuries are common among occupants of vehicles involved in collisions and in pedestrians struck by vehicles because of the severe acceleration/deceleration mechanisms. DAIs can range from the mild (a concussion) to the severe and life threatening (a brainstem injury).

Concussion   A **concussion** is a mild to moderate form of DAI and is the most common outcome of blunt head trauma. It represents nerve dysfunction without substantial anatomical damage (i.e., a normal head computed tomography [CT] scan). Concussion results in a transient episode of neuronal dysfunction (confusion, disorientation, event amnesia), followed by a rapid return to normal neurological activity. Prehospital management of concussion consists of frequent neurological assessments with attention to the airway, respiratory effort, and subtle changes in the level of consciousness. Most patients survive with no neurological impairment.

Concussion, contusion, intracerebral hemorrhage, subdural hematoma, and epidural hematoma may occur alone or in combination with one another. For example, an injury may cause a patient to sustain a concussion and an epidural hematoma concurrently. The concussion results in immediate unconsciousness, which resolves after only a few minutes. The patient becomes conscious and alert but then later exhibits a deteriorating level of consciousness. This interim period of consciousness, called a lucid interval, occurs while the epidural hematoma expands.

Moderate Diffuse Axonal Injury   Here again, shearing, stretching, or tearing of the axons occurs, but now there is minute bruising of brain tissue. This type of injury is often referred to as the "classic concussion." If the cerebral cortex or reticular activating system of the brainstem is involved, the patient may be rendered unconscious. This type of injury is more severe than a mild concussion, occurs in 20 percent of all severe head injuries, and composes 45 percent of all DAI cases. Moderate DAI is commonly associated with basilar skull fracture. Although most patients survive this injury, some degree of residual neurological impairment is common.

Short- and long-term signs and symptoms associated with moderate DAI include immediate unconsciousness, followed by persistent confusion, inability to concentrate, disorientation, and retrograde and anterograde amnesia. The victim may also complain of headache, focal neurological deficits, light sensitivity (photophobia), and disturbances in smell and other senses. Anxiety may be present, and the patient may experience significant mood swings.

Severe Diffuse Axonal Injury   Severe DAI (previously known as brainstem injury) is a significant mechanical disruption of many axons in both cerebral hemispheres with extension into the brainstem. Approximately 16 percent of all severe head injuries and 36 percent of all cases of DAI are classified as severe. Many patients do not survive this type of injury; those who do have some degree of permanent neurological impairment. The patient experiencing severe DAI is unconscious for a prolonged period of time and displays the signs of increased ICP (Cushing's reflex) and decerebrate or decorticate posturing.

Indirect Injury   Indirect (or secondary) injuries are the result of factors that occur because of, though after, the initial (or primary) injury. These processes are progressive and cause the patient deterioration often associated with serious head injuries. The indirect injuries may be as damaging or more damaging than the initial injury because of the unique design of the skull and the especially delicate nature of central nervous system tissue.

Indirect injuries are caused by two distinct pathological processes. The first process is a diminishing circulation to brain tissue (intracranial perfusion) due to an increasing ICP and possibly exacerbated by hypoxia, hypercarbia, and systemic hypotension. The second process is progressive pressure against, or physical displacement of, brain tissue secondary to an expanding mass within the cranium. Both these pathologies continue, expand the nervous tissue injury, and cause some of the specific and progressive signs and symptoms associated with head injury.

Intracranial Perfusion The brain is one of the body's most perfusion-sensitive organs. Any injury that affects perfusion has a rapid and devastating effect on the brain and its control of body systems. Cerebral, cerebellar, and brainstem perfusion may be disrupted both by increasing ICP and by low systemic blood pressure (hypotension).

As mentioned earlier, the cranial volume is fixed and does not vary. The cerebrum, cerebellum, and brainstem account for 80 percent (1200 mL) of this volume. Venous, capillary, and arterial blood account for most of the remaining space, or about 12 percent (150 mL), while CSF accounts for roughly the remaining 8 percent (90 mL). Any increase in the size of one internal component must be matched by a similar reduction in another component. If it is not, the ICP will rise.

As a mass expands within the cranium, the first means of compensating for the expansion is compression of the venous blood vessels. If the mass continues to expand, the next intracranial volume affected is the CSF, which is pushed out of the cranium and into the spinal cord. These mechanisms respond very quickly and maintain an ICP very close to normal. However, once they reach their compensatory limits, the ICP rises quickly and begins to restrict arterial blood flow. The reduction in cerebral blood flow triggers a rise in the systemic blood pressure in an attempt to ensure adequate cerebral perfusion, a process known as autoregulation. The greater the pressure of arterial blood flow, the greater is the ICP. This increase in ICP further increases the resistance to cerebral blood flow, producing more hypoxia and hypercarbia. The resulting additional increase in systolic blood pressure and then ICP, leads to a worsening, eventually deadly, cycle (Figure 23-9). If the mass, injury (edema), or hemorrhage continues to expand, the ICP becomes so high that cerebral circulation all but stops.

Another factor affecting ICP and circulation through the brain is the level of carbon dioxide in the CSF. As the carbon dioxide level rises, the cerebral arteries dilate to encourage greater blood flow and reduce the hypercarbia. In the presence of an already high ICP, this process can have devastating results. The brain's response to high carbon dioxide concentrations and the increasing ICP causes the classic hyperventilation and hypertension associated with head injury. Low levels of carbon dioxide, conversely, can also have dire effects, triggering cerebral arterial constriction. In extreme cases, the resulting constriction can all but stop circulation through the brain.

Two systemic problems frequently associated with trauma and sometimes related to brain injury are low blood pressure and poor ventilation. These problems seriously compound any existing head injury through a tertiary injury mechanism.

Hypotension, especially in the brain-injured patient with increasing ICP, may contribute to poor cerebral perfusion pressure (CCP). In turn, diminished cerebral circulation causes increasing acidosis (retained carbon dioxide) and anaerobic metabolism. This induces further neural cell injury due to hypoxia and acidosis. At the same time, vasodilation (in response to increasing acidosis and carbon dioxide levels) elevates any existing ICP.

Hypoxia, secondary to shock or chest injury, increases the severity of any head injury. The reduced blood oxygen levels increase the cellular hypoxia at and around the injury site. Since central nervous tissue is extremely dependent on good cellular oxygenation, neural cell damage becomes more severe.

Pressure and Structural Displacement As hemorrhage accumulates or edema increases in a region of the brain, this expansion pushes uninjured tissue

Remember,
$CPP = MAP - ICP$

Low blood pressure and poor respiratory exchange seriously compound any existing head injury.

FIGURE 23-9 Pathway of deterioration following central nervous system insult.

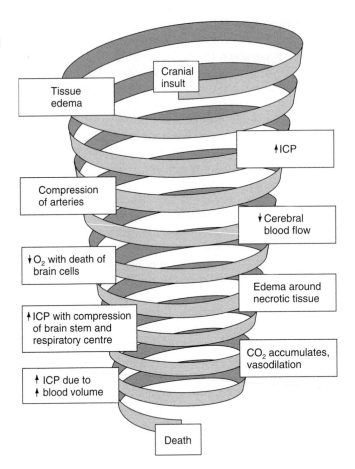

Cranial insult

Tissue edema

↑ICP

Compression of arteries

↓Cerebral blood flow

↓O₂ with death of brain cells

Edema around necrotic tissue

↑ICP with compression of brain stem and respiratory centre

CO₂ accumulates, vasodilation

↑ICP due to ↑ blood volume

Death

Content Review

SIGNS AND SYMPTOMS OF BRAIN INJURY

Altered level of consciousness
Altered level of orientation
Alterations in personality
Amnesia
 Retrograde
 Anterograde
Cushing's reflex
 Increasing blood pressure
 Slowing pulse rate
 Erratic respirations
Vomiting (often without nausea)
Body temperature changes
Changes in reactivity of pupils
Decorticate posturing

away from the injury site. Even in the absence of increased ICP, such expansion puts pressure on adjacent brain cells, most commonly along the brainstem. As the mass continues to increase in size, it may physically compress brainstem components. With further expansion, it may push the brain tissue against and around the falx cerebri and the tentorium cerebelli. Because these are basically immobile structures within the skull, the displacement results in a process called herniation. With herniation, a portion of a brain structure is pushed into and through an opening, physically disrupting the structure and compromising its blood supply. If the displacement affects the upper brainstem by pushing it through the tentorium incisura, it causes vomiting, changes in the level of consciousness, and pupillary dilation. If the displacement affects the medulla oblongata by pushing it into the foramen magnum, it results in disturbances in breathing, blood pressure, and heart rate.

Signs and Symptoms of Brain Injury

Direct injury, increasing ICP, and compression and displacement of brain tissue produce an altered level of orientation and of consciousness as well as specific signs and symptoms related to the CNS structure(s) affected. The actual process of brain injury can be mapped as the pressure increases and the injury moves from the cortical surface and down the brainstem.

As a portion of the cerebral cortex is disrupted by injury, the specific activity it controls is affected. For example, if the frontal lobe is injured, the patient will likely present with alterations in personality. If the occipital region is affected, visual disturbances can be expected. A large region of cortical disruption may reduce the patient's level of awareness. The patient may become unaware of the circumstances leading up to the incident (**retrograde amnesia**) or following it (**anterograde amnesia**) or disoriented (to time, place, and person), confused, or combative. Focal deficits, such as hemiplegia or weakness, or seizures may also result. When intracranial injury extends to components of the ascending reticular activating system in the brainstem, the patient may display an altered level of arousal, including lethargy, somnolence, or coma.

If the compression results from a building mass along the central region of the cerebrum, pressure is first directed to the midbrain, then to the pons, and finally to the medulla oblongata. The signs and symptoms of this progressive pressure and structural displacement are somewhat predictable and are known as the central syndrome.

In this syndrome, upper brainstem compression produces an increasing blood pressure to maintain CPP and a reflex decreasing heart rate in response to vagus nerve (parasympathetic) stimulation of the SA node and AV junction. The patient may also exhibit a characteristic cyclic breathing pattern called **Cheyne-Stokes respirations**. This consists of increasing, then decreasing respiratory volumes, followed by a period of apnea. The combination of an increasing blood pressure, slowing pulse, and erratic respirations is a classic sign of brainstem pressure or injury called **Cushing's reflex** (Figure 23-10). If the brain injury involves the hypothalamus, the patient may experience vomiting, frequently without nausea, and body temperature changes. The pupils remain small and reactive. Decorticate posturing (body extension with arm flexion) in response to painful stimuli may occur as the neural pathways through the upper brainstem are disrupted.

As the middle brainstem becomes involved, the pulse pressure widens and the heart rate becomes bradycardic. Respirations now may be deep and rapid (central neurological hyperventilation). Increasing ICP may also induce pupil sluggishness or nonreactivity (bilaterally, since the pathology involves compression from above) as the oculomotor nerve (CN-III) is compressed. The patient develops extension (decerebrate) posturing. Few patients ever function normally again once they have reached this ICP level.

Finally, as the pressure reaches the lower brainstem, the pupils become fully dilated and unreactive. Respirations become ataxic (erratic with no characteristic rhythm) or may even cease altogether. The pulse rate is often very irregular with great swings in rate. Electrocardiographic (ECG) conduction disturbances become

* **retrograde amnesia** inability to remember events that occurred before the trauma that caused the condition.

* **anterograde amnesia** inability to remember events that occurred after the trauma that caused the condition.

* **Cheyne-Stokes respirations** respiratory pattern of alternating periods of apnea and tachypnea.

* **Cushing's reflex** response due to cerebral ischemia that causes an increase in systemic blood pressure, which maintains cerebral perfusion during increased ICP.

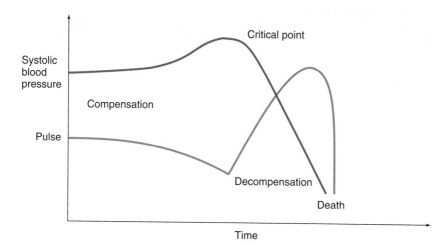

FIGURE 23-10 How systolic blood pressure and pulse rate respond to increasing intracranial pressure (ICP).

apparent, including QRS complex, S-T segment, and T-wave changes. As control over blood pressure is disrupted, the patient becomes hypotensive. The patient no longer responds to painful stimuli, and the skeletal muscles become flaccid. Patients rarely survive once the ICP rises to this level.

If the mass causing the compression is located more laterally than in the central syndrome described above, the signs and symptoms occur in a less predictable sequence. The pupillary responses, sluggishness, nonreactivity, and dilation, are usually ipsilateral (on the same side) as the expanding mass.

Pediatric Head Trauma

Pediatric head trauma has a very different pathology than that in the older patient. The skull is not fully formed at birth and is still rather cartilaginous. It will distort more easily with the force of an impact and transmit that force more directly to the delicate central nervous tissue. However, the incomplete formation of the skull with its "soft spots" (the anterior and posterior fontanelles) permits some intracranial expansion. The fontanelles bulge outward with increasing ICP. Generally, then, this softer skeletal structure increases the direct injury associated with head trauma in the very young pediatric patient but slows the progression of increasing ICP.

As noted earlier, the blood and CSF represent about 20 percent of the total volume of the adult cranium (about 240 mL). A blood loss into the cranium cannot account for a significant component of hypovolemia in the adult. A pediatric patient, however, has a proportionally larger head, the ability to accommodate increased fluids because of the fontanelles, and a much smaller total body fluid volume and fewer reserves. In the pediatric patient, therefore, intracranial hemorrhage may significantly contribute to hypovolemia.

When treating an infant with a head, face, or neck injury, pay particular attention to the airway. Infants are obligate nasal breathers and must have a patent nasal passage and pharynx to ensure a clear airway. Hyperextension of the head will obstruct the airway as the tongue pushes the soft pallet closed. Ensure proper head positioning, and ventilate using both the mouth and the nose.

In the pediatric patient, intracranial hemorrhage may significantly contribute to hypovolemia.

Glasgow Coma Scale

The **Glasgow Coma Scale** (GCS) is a standardized evaluation method used to measure a patient's level of consciousness. The scale assesses the best eye opening, verbal, and motor responses and awards points for the various responses. Responses must be determined for both sides of the patient and any side-to-side differences noted. (A fuller discussion of the scale is found later in this chapter.)

✱ **Glasgow Coma Scale** scoring system for monitoring the neurological status of patients with head injuries.

Eye Signs

Pay close attention to the eyes when evaluating a patient with possible head trauma. The eyes are a very specialized body tissue (such as CNS tissue) and a very visible special sense organ. The eyes can give indications of problems with cranial nerves CN-II, III, IV, and VI and with perfusion associated with cerebral blood flow. The surface of the eye is highly dependent on good perfusion and lacrimal fluid flow. If perfusion is diminished, the eyes lose their luster quickly. The eyes also give quick, highly visible signs of the patient's demeanour—anxiety, fear, anger, and so on.

Pupil size and reactivity also give clues to underlying conditions. Depressant drugs or cerebral hypoxia will reduce pupillary responsiveness, while extreme hypoxia causes them to dilate and fix. An expanding cranial lesion places progressive pressure on the oculomotor nerve (CN-III), causing the ipsilateral (same side) pupil to become sluggish, then dilated, and then fixed. This occurs because the

Evaluation of the eyes is very important in patients with suspected head injury.

outer oculomotor nerve contains parasympathetic fibres. As increasing pressure interferes with these nerve fibres, the pupil dilates and is unable to constrict. If one pupil is fixed and yet shows some response to consensual stimulation (light variations in the other eye), the problem most likely lies with the oculomotor nerve.

FACIAL INJURY

Facial injury is a serious trauma complication not only because of the cosmetic importance people place on facial appearance but also because of the region's vasculature and the location of the initial airway and alimentary canal structures and the organs of sight, smell, taste, and hearing present there. Remember, too, that serious facial injuries suggest associated head and spinal injuries.

Facial Soft-Tissue Injury

Facial soft-tissue injury is common and can threaten both the patient's airway and her physical appearance. Because of the ample supply of arterial and venous vessels, injuries in the region may bleed heavily, contributing to hypovolemia. Facial injuries are often the result of violence, as in the case of bullet or knife wounds. Superficial injuries and hemorrhage rarely affect the airway. With deep lacerations, however, blood may accumulate and endanger the airway or enter the digestive tract and induce vomiting. Serious blunt or penetrating injury to the soft tissues and skeletal structures supporting the pharynx may reduce the patient's ability to control the airway, increasing the likelihood of foreign body or fluid aspiration and airway compromise. Hypoxia due to aspiration is more likely caused by blood than by other fluids or physical obstruction.

Remember, the process of inspiration creates a less-than-atmospheric pressure in the lungs to draw air in. This reduction in pressure may collapse damaged structures along the airway that are normally held open by bony or cartilaginous formations. Soft-tissue swelling may also rapidly restrict the airway or close it completely. Swelling and deformity from trauma may distort the facial region so that landmarks are hard to recognize, making airway control even more difficult. In serious facial soft-tissue injury, always consider the likelihood of associated injury, especially basilar skull fracture and spine injury.

Patients with serious facial soft-tissue injuries are likely to have associated injury, especially basilar skull fractures and spine injuries.

Facial Dislocations and Fractures

Trauma may result in open or closed facial fractures with significant associated pain, swelling, deformity, crepitus, and hemorrhage. Common injuries include mandibular, maxillary, nasal, and orbital fractures and dislocations.

Mandibular dislocation occurs as the condylar process displaces from the temporomandibular joint, just anterior to the ear. This dislocation may result in the malocclusion of the mouth, misalignment of teeth, deformity of the facial region at or around the joint, immobility of the jaw, and pain. The patient's ability to control the airway may be decreased, but dislocation is not usually a significant threat to the airway or breathing.

Fractures of the mandible are painful, present with deformity along the jaw's surface, and may result in the loosening of a few teeth. An open mandibular fracture may produce blood-stained saliva. Mandibular fracture may represent a serious life threat if the patient is placed supine. With such a fracture, the tongue is no longer supported at its base and may displace posteriorly, blocking the airway even in a conscious patient. Always look for a second fracture site when you encounter a patient with a mandibular fracture.

Maxillary fractures are classified according to **Le Fort criteria** (Figure 23-11). A slight instability involving the maxilla alone usually presents with no associated

Content Review

LE FORT FACIAL FRACTURES

I—slight instability to maxilla; no displacement
II—fracture of both maxilla and nasal bones
III—fracture involving entire face below brow ridge (zygoma, nasal bone, maxilla)

 Le Fort criteria classification system for fractures involving the maxilla.

displacement and is classified as a Le Fort I fracture. A Le Fort II fracture results in fractures of both the maxilla and nasal bones. Le Fort III fractures characteristically involve the entire facial region below the brow ridge, including the zygoma, nasal bone, and maxilla. Le Fort II and III fractures usually result in CSF leakage and may endanger the patency of the nasal and oral portions of the airway.

Dental injury is commonly associated with serious blunt facial trauma. Teeth may chip, break, loosen, or dislodge from the mandible or maxilla. They may then become foreign objects drawn (aspirated) into the airway. Note that a dislodged tooth may be reimplanted if fully intact and handled properly during prehospital care. If possible, transport the tooth to hospital in a container of milk.

Orbital (blowout) fractures most commonly involve the zygoma or maxilla of the inferior shelf. Zygomatic arch fractures are painful and present with a unilateral depression over the prominence of one cheek. The fracture may entrap the extraocular muscles, reducing the eye's range of motion, and can cause blurred or double vision (**diplopia**). Zygomatic fractures may also entrap the masseter muscle and limit jaw movement. With a maxillary bone fracture, the patient often experiences significant swelling and pain in the maxillary sinus region. Although these injuries are not life threatening, they warrant evaluation by emergency department staff.

A special type of facial injury is that associated with a suicide attempt using a rifle or shotgun. The victim places the barrel under the chin but in an effort to push the trigger, stretches and tilts the head back. The gunshot blast is directed

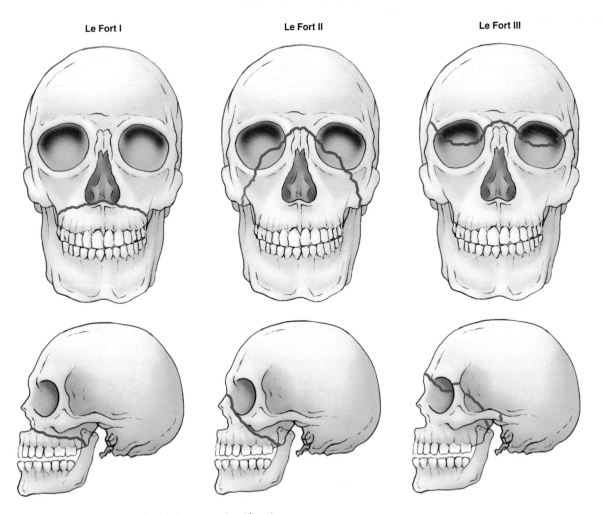

Le Fort I   **Le Fort II**   **Le Fort III**

FIGURE 23-11   Le Fort facial fracture classification.

under the chin and at the facial region but may be deflected from entering the cranium. The result is a very disrupted facial region with most of the structures of, and supporting, the airway destroyed. The patient may still be conscious; there is usually heavy bleeding, and the remains of the airway are hard to locate. With such a patient, the airway is in serious danger of obstruction and attempts to secure it are very challenging.

Nasal Injury

Nasal injuries are painful and often create a grossly deformed appearance, but they are not usually life threatening. While dislocation or fracture of the cartilage and nasal bone may interfere with nasal air movement, the swelling and associated hemorrhage are more likely threats to the airway. However, the conscious and alert patient is usually able to control the airway.

Epistaxis (nosebleed) is a common nasal problem. Bleeding can be spontaneous as well as traumatic and can be further classified as either anterior or posterior. Anterior hemorrhage comes from the septum and is usually due to bleeding from a network of vessels called Kisselbach's plexus. Such hemorrhage bleeds slowly and is usually self-limiting. Posterior hemorrhage may be severe and cause blood to drain down the back of the patient's throat. In epistaxis secondary to severe head trauma with likely basilar skull fracture, the integrity of the nasal cavity's posterior wall may be compromised. Attempts at nasal airway, nasogastric tube, or nasotracheal tube insertion may permit the tube to enter the cerebral cavity and directly damage the brain; therefore, it should be avoided with facial smash.

Ear Injury

The external ear, or pinna, which is exposed, is frequently subjected to trauma. It has a minimal blood supply and does not often bleed heavily when lacerated. In glancing blows, the pinna may be partially or completely avulsed. In a folding type of injury, the cartilage may separate. Due to the poor blood supply, external ear injuries do not heal as well as other facial wounds.

The internal portions of the ear—the external auditory canal and the middle and inner ear—are well protected from trauma by the structure of the skull. Injury only results from objects forced into the ear or from rapid changes in pressure as in diving accidents or explosions. With an explosion—even with repeated small arms fire—the pinna focuses the rapidly changing air pressure and directs it into the external auditory canal. This enhanced pressure irritates or ruptures the tympanum and, if strong enough, fractures the small bones of hearing (the ossicles). The result can be temporary or permanent hearing loss. In a diving injury, the changing pressure is not equalized by the eustachian tube (also called the pharyngotympanic passage) and eventually builds up until the eardrum ruptures. Water floods the middle ear and interferes with the functioning of the semicircular canals. The patient experiences vertigo, an extremely dangerous sensation when near-weightless under water.

Basilar skull fracture may also disrupt the external auditory canal and tear the tympanum. If the dura mater is torn, cerebrospinal fluid (CSF) may flood the middle ear and seep outward through the torn tympanum (Figure 23-12). As with the other mechanisms described earlier, hearing loss may result.

Tympanic injuries are not life threatening and, in many cases, repair themselves, even with a rupture that tears as much as half the tympanum. However, a victim with acute hearing loss can be quite apprehensive and anxious. The patient may be frustrated when unable to hear and understand questions or instructions. Such a patient may also be unable to hear sounds of approaching danger, such as traffic noise.

FIGURE 23-12 Blood or fluid draining from a patient's ear suggests basilar skull fracture.

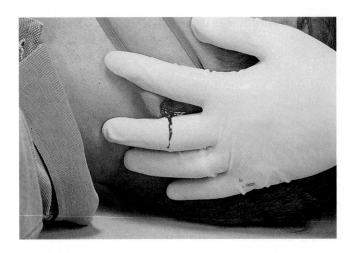

Eye Injury

Although the orbit is a very effective protective housing for the eye, penetrating trauma and some blunt trauma may cause serious injury. The anterior eye structures are extremely specialized and, like most specialized tissues, do not regenerate effectively. If significant penetrating injury occurs, especially if accompanied by loss of the eye's fluids—aqueous or vitreous humor—the patient's sight is threatened, possibly with permanent loss. A penetrating object is likely to disturb the integrity of the anterior and possibly the posterior chamber. In addition, removal of the object may allow fluids to leak from the chambers and further threaten the patient's vision. Penetrating injuries may be caused by foreign bodies so small that they are difficult to see with the naked eye. Suspect the presence of such bodies if the patient reports a history of sudden eye pain and the sensation of an impaled foreign body after using a power saw or grinder, especially when working with metal.

Similarly, small foreign particles that land on the eye's surface can also cause ocular injury. The object may embed in the surface of the eyelid and then drag across the cornea as the eye blinks. Corneal abrasions or lacerations result, often causing intense and continuing pain, even after the object is cleared from the eye. These lacerations are usually superficial but occasionally can be deep.

Blunt trauma may result in several ocular presentations. Hemorrhage into the anterior chamber pools, displaying a collection of blood in front of the iris and pupil. This condition, called **hyphema,** is a potential threat to the patient's vision and requires evaluation by an ophthalmologist and possibly hospital admission.

A less serious, but equally dramatic, eye injury is a subconjunctival hemorrhage. This may occur after a strong sneeze, vomiting episode, or direct eye trauma, such as orbital fracture. It occurs when a small blood vessel in the subconjunctival space bursts, leaving a portion of the eye's surface blood red (Figure 23-13). Subconjunctival hemorrhage often clears without intervention and rarely causes any residual scars or impairment.

Blunt trauma may fracture the orbital structures surrounding the eye and produce an injury called eye avulsion. In such a case, the eye is not really avulsed but appears to protrude from the wound as the structure of the orbit is crushed and depressed. If the eye as well as the nerves and vasculature remain intact, sight in the eye can usually be salvaged.

Two other, more serious ocular problems involve the retina. **Acute retinal artery occlusion** is not an injury but, rather, a vascular emergency caused when an

 hyphema blood in the anterior chamber of the eye, in front of the iris.

A hyphema is a sight-threatening injury.

Occasionally, blood will completely fill the anterior chamber resulting in what is called an "eight-ball" hyphema. This can be easily missed without close examination.

 acute retinal artery occlusion a nontraumatic occlusion of the retinal artery resulting in a sudden, painless loss of vision in one eye.

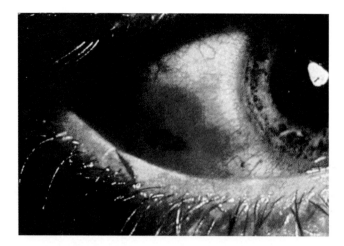

FIGURE 23-13   Subconjunctival hemorrhage.

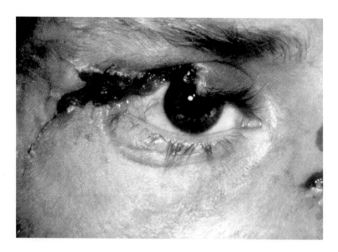

FIGURE 23-14   Laceration of the eyelid.

embolus blocks the blood supply to one eye. The patient complains of sudden and painless loss of vision in the eye. In **retinal detachment**, which may be traumatic in origin, the retina separates from the eye's posterior wall. The patient complains of a dark curtain obstructing part of the field of view. Both of these conditions are true emergencies in which the patient's eyesight is at risk.

Soft-tissue lacerations can occur around the eye and involve the eyelid (see Figure 23–14). If not properly identified and repaired, such an injury may disrupt the function of the lacrimal duct and interrupt lubrication and oxygenation of the cornea. Another soft-tissue problem may occur if a contact lens is left in the eye of an unconscious patient. The contact lens will then obstruct the normal lacrimal fluid flow across the eye. This loss of circulation may dry out the eye's surface and cause hypoxic injury. The result is usually severe eye pain and possible damage to the cornea.

✱ **retinal detachment** condition that may be of traumatic origin and present with patient complaint of a dark curtain obstructing a portion of the field of view.

NECK INJURY

The neck is protected from impact by the more anterior head and chest and by its own skeletal and muscular structures. The neck's major skeletal component is the cervical vertebral column, which is strengthened by interconnecting ligaments. The neck muscles provide additional protection to the vital structures in the neck. They include the muscles that support and move the head through a large range of motion as well as the shoulder muscles that help move the upper extremities and act as auxiliary breathing muscles. The skeletal structures and muscles of the neck protect the airway, carotid and jugular blood vessels, and the esophagus very well from all but anterior blunt trauma and deep penetrating trauma. Such trauma may result in serious injuries to the airway, cervical spine, blood vessels, and other structures in the region.

Most trauma surgeons feel that any neck injury that penetrates the most superficial muscle (platysma) should be surgically explored.

Blood Vessel Trauma

Blunt trauma to a blood vessel may produce a serious and rapidly expanding hematoma. This hematoma may be trapped within the fascia of the region and apply restrictive pressure to the jugular veins. Laceration of the external jugular vein, or deep laceration involving the internal jugular vein or the carotid arteries may result in severe hemorrhage due to the large size of the vessels and the volume of blood they carry (Figure 23-15). Their laceration and subsequent hemorrhage can rapidly lead to hypovolemia and shock. Arterial interruption may cause subsequent brain hypoxia and infarct, mimicking the signs and symptoms of a stroke. An open neck wound affecting the external jugular vein may permit formation of an air embolism as the venous pressure drops below atmospheric pressure with deep respirations.

Airway Trauma

Trauma may also injure the trachea. Severe blunt or penetrating trauma may separate the larynx from the trachea, fracture or crush either of these two structures, or open the trachea to the environment. These injuries may result in serious hemorrhage that threatens the airway, vocal cord contusion or swelling, destruction of the integrity of the airway and collapse on inspiration, disruption of normal airway landmarks, and restrictive soft-tissue swelling.

Cervical Spine Trauma

Severe blunt trauma and, in some cases, gunshot wounds to the neck may cause vertebral fracture and cervical spine instability. The wounds may cause pressure on the spinal cord, cord contusion, or severing of the cord. Such injuries will likely cause bilateral paresthesia, anaesthesia, weakness (paresis), or paralysis, generally at and below the dermatome controlled by the peripheral nerve branch leaving the vertebral column at the level of the injury. Neurogenic shock from these injuries may cause hypotension from vasodilation. (This is discussed in Chapter 24, "Spinal Trauma.") Blunt trauma may disrupt and injure the muscles and connective tissues of the region and result in serious pain and limited motion.

Other Neck Trauma

The neck may also demonstrate subcutaneous emphysema due to tension pneumothorax (air pushed into the skin from intrathoracic pressure that migrates to the neck) or from tracheal injury in the neck. Penetrating trauma may involve the esophagus, perforating it and permitting gastric contents or undigested material to enter the fascia. Since the fascia communicates with the mediastinum, this foreign material can physically harm mediastinal structures or provide the medium for infection, which may have devastating results. Deep penetrating trauma may disrupt the vagus nerve, causing tachycardia and gastrointestinal disturbances. More anterior and superficial injuries may damage the thyroid and parathyroid glands.

FIGURE 23-15   Laceration to the neck.

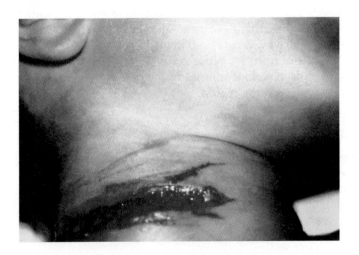

ASSESSMENT OF HEAD, FACIAL, AND NECK INJURIES

As with all trauma patients, assessment of head, facial, and neck injury patients follows the standard format, including the scene asssessment, primary assessment, rapid trauma assessment/secondary asseessment and history, and the detailed assessment as appropriate. Perform ongoing assessments frequently on these patients. With head, facial, and neck injuries, pay special attention to ensuring airway patency and monitoring breathing, level of consciousness and orientation, pupillary signs, and blood pressure. With these patients, be sure to consider the need for rapid transport to a trauma centre specializing in neurological care.

SCENE ASSESSMENT

Analysis of the mechanism of injury is a key part of the assessment of the patient with a possible head, face, or neck injury. During the scene assessment, consider the circumstances of injury, and identify the nature and extent of forces that caused the injury. In a vehicle collision, for example, look for evidence of head impact, such as the characteristic spider-web windshield. Look also for deformity of the upper steering wheel, which suggests head or neck trauma or the use of the shoulder belt without the lap belt. Identify the direction of the forces causing injury, and anticipate what body structures the forces may have damaged. In motorcycle collisions, remember that helmet use reduces head injury by about 50 percent but does not spare the neck from cervical spine injury. In shootings, try to determine the calibre and type of weapon, the distance from the gun to the victim, and the approximate angle of the bullet's entry into the patient's body.

With other types of impacts, try to determine what forces were involved and how they were directed to the head, face, and neck. Use this information to anticipate injuries to the brain, airway, and sense organs. Remember that many signs of head injury may be masked by the patient's use of alcohol or other drugs, by the nature of the injury, and/or by the slow development of the wound process. Consequently, a good analysis of the mechanism of injury (MOI) and the resulting indexes of suspicion are very important. Your thorough analysis must enable you to describe both the incident scene and the mechanism of injury to the attending physician at the emergency department. Remember that the mechanism of injury can often give a better indication of the seriousness of the injury than can the patient's signs and symptoms.

Rule out scene hazards, and request any additional resources needed at the scene as soon as you can. Use of gloves is the minimum level of body substance isolation (BSI) protection when approaching the potential head, face, and neck injury patient. Serious head injuries pose real risks of exposure to blood or other fluids propelled by air movement or by arterial or heavy venous bleeding. Anticipate such exposures, and don splash and eye protection when coming in contact with any patient with significant trauma to the head, face, or neck.

PRIMARY ASSESSMENT

As you approach, form an initial impression of the patient's condition. Is the patient alert? Does the patient show any signs of anxiety? If there is any reason to suspect that the head or neck sustained serious impact, provide immediate manual immobilization of the head and cervical spine (Figure 23-16). Quickly determine the patient's level of consciousness and then orientation to time, place, and persons early in the primary assessment. While determining the patient's level of orientation may add a few seconds to the primary assessment, assessing trends

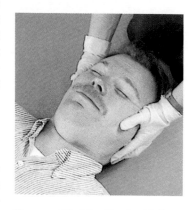

FIGURE 23-16 If spinal injury is suspected, immediately immobilize the head and neck manually.

in orientation can be critical to rapid identification of a brain injury patient. Be alert to the patient's facial skin colour, respiratory effort, pupil lustre, and level of responsiveness throughout the primary assessment, as these factors can help you recognize internal head injury. As you gather information about the patient, continue to build and modify your general patient impression and your index of suspicion for head injury.

Apply a cervical collar at the end of the primary assessment, and maintain manual head immobilization until the patient is fully immobilized in a Kendrick extrication device (KED), or on a long spine board with a cervical immobilization device. If there are any significant injuries to the neck, do not apply the collar until you complete the assessment and provide needed care. While the cervical collar provides some neck stabilization, it does not completely immobilize the region, and its placement may be delayed so long as manual immobilization is continued.

If the patient is wearing a helmet, consider whether or not to remove it as described in Chapter 24, "Spinal Trauma." A patient's use of a helmet reduces the likelihood of soft-tissue injury and skull and facial fractures. Helmet use can also significantly reduce the incidence of brain injury, but do not be lulled into a false sense of security by the absence of outward signs of trauma. Be watchful for the early signs of internal brain injury, and be sure to inform the emergency department staff that the patient was wearing a helmet. Also alert them to any signs of impact or helmet damage suggestive of the forces of trauma that the patient experienced.

Airway

Then, move quickly to evaluate the airway. Examine the face and neck for any deformity, swelling, hemorrhage, foreign bodies, or other signs of injury that may threaten the airway. Suction and insert an oral or nasal airway as necessary. Listen for unusual or changing voice patterns, as they may be indicative of airway injury and developing edema. Swelling can quickly occlude the airway, and any hemorrhage can complicate airway maintenance as the patient loses consciousness and the gag reflex. Anticipate vomiting, possibly without warning. Ensure that the airway is structurally sound and that the mandible supports the tongue well enough to keep it out of the airway. Have a large-bore suction catheter and strong suction ready to remove any fluids, and consider positioning the patient to enhance airway drainage (left lateral recumbent position) if doing so is not contraindicated by injuries. If the patient does not display a gag reflex or has an altered level of consciousness, consider early insertion of an endotracheal tube, if it is within your scope of practice.

If there is a serious neck injury, check the structural integrity of the trachea. If the trachea is open to the environment, keep the wound clear of blood to prevent aspiration, and seal the wound unless the patient's upper airway is blocked. If an impaled object obstructs the airway, remove it, anticipating that heavy bleeding may then threaten the airway. Blunt wounds may crush the cartilage of the trachea, causing it to close with the reduced pressure during inspiration. This type of crushing injury may require surgical opening of the trachea by needle cricothyrostomy or surgical cricothyrotomy to ensure air exchange.

Breathing

Closely monitor breathing to ensure that the patient is moving an adequate volume of air. Determine the rate of respirations and their rhythm. Estimate the amount of air moved with each breath, and from those numbers determine the minute volume:

$$\text{Minute volume} = \text{Tidal volume} \times \text{Respiratory rate}$$

If the patient is breathing less than 12 times per minute, moving less than 500 mL of air with each breath, or has a minute volume of less than 6 litres, consider overdrive ventilation. Remember that head injury is likely to produce erratic breathing patterns and that hypoxia and carbon dioxide (CO_2) retention both contribute to morbidity and mortality with brain injury. Ventilate at 12 to 14 full breaths per minute with a volume of between 800 and 1000 mL. Do not hyperventilate the patient if you suspect brain injury. Hyperventilation will blow off carbon dioxide and cause vasoconstriction, further decreasing cerebral perfusion. Remember to pause after ventilation to allow CO_2 to exit the lungs.

Apply oxygen via nonrebreather mask with a flow of 12 to 15 litres per minute, to ensure inspiration of high concentrations. It is advisable to apply pulse oximetry to monitor oxygenation. Attempt to keep oxygen saturation above 95 percent.

Head injury patients may need oxygen to overcome the effects of hypoxia and CO_2 retention associated with their injuries, but do not hyperventilate the patient if you suspect brain injury.

Circulation

Begin to monitor the patient's pulse rate and its rhythm early in your care, and continue to do so frequently thereafter. A slow and strong (bounding) pulse may be an early sign of building intracranial pressure (ICP). Apply an ECG monitor and watch for rhythm disturbances. Quickly look for any hemorrhage from the head, face, and neck, and control any moderate to severe bleeding with direct pressure and bandaging. Be cautious of open neck wounds because they may present a risk for air embolism. Cover any such wounds quickly with occlusive dressings and secure them in place.

A slow and strong (bounding) pulse may be an early sign of building ICP.

At the end of the primary assessment, you must determine whether to perform a rapid trauma assessment followed by gathering of vital signs and the patient history or to perform a focused history and secondary assessment followed by gathering of vital signs. With most head, face, and neck injury patients, you will perform a rapid trauma assessment because of the high likelihood of airway, vascular, special sense organ, or central nervous system injuries in these regions. If there is no significant mechanism of injury and injuries appear minor and superficial, perform an assessment focused on the specific area(s) of injury.

RAPID TRAUMA ASSESSMENT

The rapid trauma assessment calls for performance of a quick and directed head-to-toe examination of a patient with a significant MOI. When head, facial, or neck injury is suggested in such a patient, pay particular attention to the procedures described below as you carry out the assessment. Manage any life-threatening injuries and conditions as you find them during the rapid trauma assessment. If the patient shows any signs of pathology within the cranium, consider rapid transport. Brain injury patients can deteriorate quickly, but rapid neurosurgical intervention can frequently alleviate life-threatening problems.

Head

Look at, then sweep, each region of the skull, feeling for deformity and bleeding with the more sensitive tips of your fingers. Interlock your fingers to sweep the posterior head, and look at your gloves to check for any blood that indicates hemorrhage there. If you find any moderate or serious hemorrhage, apply direct pressure unless you suspect skull fracture. Control the hemorrhage with gentle pressure around the wound and place a loose dressing over it. Palpate gently for any deformities, being careful, however, not to palpate the interior of open wounds (Figure 23-17).

Shine a penlight into the external auditory canal and look for signs of escaping cerebrospinal fluid (CSF). This fluid loss may be difficult to notice early

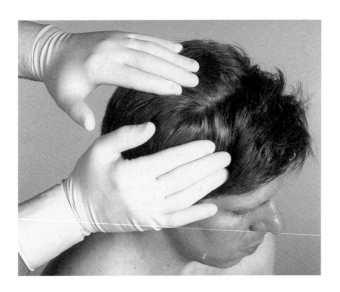

FIGURE 23-17 Carefully inspect and palpate the head for bleeding and other signs of injury.

during assessment, and so observe carefully. If blood or fluid drains from the auditory canal, cover the ear with a gauze dressing to permit fluid to move outward while providing a barrier to keep contaminants from entering. If the fluid drains on a gauze dressing or other fabric, look for the halo sign. However, you should presume (regardless of the presence or absence of halo sign) that any fluid draining from the ear contains CSF. Examine the pinnae for injury and, after you complete the rapid trauma assessment, bandage and dress as needed.

If you observe a skull deformity, palpate such a closed wound very gently. Try to determine the probability of skull fracture before swelling makes this determination more difficult. Cover any open wounds with dressings to restrict blood flow and prevent further contamination. The signs of basilar skull fracture—bilateral periorbital ecchymosis and retroauricular ecchymosis (raccoon eyes and Battle's sign)—are very late indications of this injury and are not likely to be recognizable during field assessment and care.

Bilateral periorbital ecchymosis and retroauricular ecchymosis are very late signs of basilar skull fracture and are not likely to be recognizable during field assessment and care.

Head injury may cause seizures. Seizures are serious complications because they may compromise the airway and respirations, increase ICP, and exacerbate any existing brain injury. If you observe a seizure or if the patient or bystanders describe one as you gather the history, find out as much about the episode as you can, and be prepared to describe the seizure in detail, including its origin and progression, to the attending physician. Protect the seizing patient from further injury, and be especially watchful of the airway. Consider the administration of diazepam, which reduces electrical impulse transmission across the cerebrum and may limit seizure activity.

Face

Study the patient's facial features carefully, looking for asymmetry, swelling, discoloration, or deformity. Palpate the facial region, including the brow ridge, nasal region, cheek, maxilla, and mandible, searching for any deformity, instability, or crepitus that suggest fracture and for any signs of soft-tissue swelling (Figure 23-18). Palpate the maxilla, and attempt, gently, to move it from left to right. It should be firmly attached to the facial bones and should display no crepitus. Do likewise with the mandible. It should be solid, yet very mobile from left to right and up and down. Note and investigate any patient report of pain during your palpation and movement. Open the patient's mouth, and

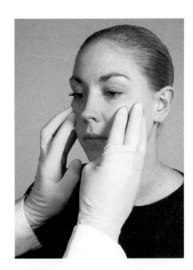

FIGURE 23-18 Carefully palpate the facial bones.

228 CHAPTER 23 *Head, Facial, and Neck Trauma*

examine for any signs of trauma, excessive secretions and bleeding, or swelling. All teeth should be firmly in place (loose teeth may suggest mandibular fracture). Find any displaced teeth and prepare them for transport with the patient, or suspect that missing teeth may have been aspirated. Ensure that the mandible is intact and supports the airway.

Carefully examine the eyes. In general, eye reactivity and lustre reflect the oxygenation status of the brain. Watch for bright and sparkling eyes and briskly reactive pupils. Shine a bright light into the eyes—or in bright sunlight, shade them—and watch for sluggishness, nonreactivity, and constriction (or dilation). Ensure that reactivity is bilateral. Note that both eyes should respond to changes in light intensity affecting only one eye (consensual reactivity). Both eyes should gaze together and, at rest, gaze directly forward. Watch for a down and out gaze. Usually, an affected pupil is on the same side (ipsilateral) as a head injury. If the patient is conscious and alert, have her follow your finger up and down and then left and right with each eye. Watch for and note any limited eye movement. Restricted eye movement suggests eye muscle entrapment and nerve compression or injury and paralysis.

Carefully examine the pupil, iris, and conjunctiva. The pupil and iris should be round, the anterior chamber clear, and the sclera free of accumulating blood. Check for contact lenses, especially in the unconscious patient. If they are found, remove them carefully.

Restricted eye movement suggests eye muscle entrapment or nerve compression or injury and paralysis.

Neck

Examine the anterior, lateral, and posterior aspects of the neck for signs of injury, including swelling, discoloration, wounds, blood loss, and frothy blood. Frothy blood is likely caused by bleeding in association with a tracheal injury and suggests serious airway compromise. Palpate the region, feeling for any changes in skin tension, deformities, or unusual masses underneath. Crepitus beneath the skin may be associated with subcutaneous emphysema from a tracheal or chest injury or a tracheal or laryngeal fracture. Identify the thyroid cartilage, beneath and posterior to the mandible. Palpate it, the cricoid cartilage, and then the trachea. Ensure that they are not deformed by trauma and remain midline in the neck. Visually examine the depth of neck wounds to anticipate those that may involve jugular or carotid blood vessels, and cover any open wounds with occlusive dressings.

Any penetration of the lateral neck muscles should heighten your index of suspicion for a serious neck injury.

While carrying out the rapid trauma assessment, question the responsive patient about headaches and increased light sensitivity (photophobia), which are common symptoms of head injury. Also, question the patient about her memory of the events preceding and following the injury to identify retrograde and anterograde amnesia. Note any repetitive questioning by the patient (inability to establish short-term memory) and any unusual behaviour or confusion. Ask if the patient has any unusual fullness in the throat and any difficulty swallowing. Ask about any visual disturbances, such as double vision (diplopia) and blurred vision, that may indicate eye muscle entrapment. Inquire about visual acuity (the ability to distinguish objects) both near and far, and note reports of any restriction to vision, which the patient might describe as a curtain drawn across the field of view. Patient complaints of eye pain are also important and may suggest conjunctival or corneal injury. You may also note patient complaints about focal deficits. Examine any area of paresthesia, anesthesia, weakness, or paralysis, noting the borders of the area and whether it is unilateral or bilateral. Question the patient frequently to identify any increase or decrease in awareness and any changes in injury symptoms.

Complete the rapid trauma assessment by examining the rest of the body, paying particular attention to any region where the MOI suggests serious injury

Question the head, face, or neck injury patient frequently to identify any increase or decrease in awareness and any changes in injury symptoms.

and in which the patient complains of serious symptoms. While examining the extremities, look for any signs of decreased muscle tone, flaccid muscles, and diminished sensation or muscle strength, and determine if any unusual findings are bilateral or unilateral and where the deficit begins. Then, gather the balance of the patient history, determine the patient's Glasgow Coma Scale score, and take a set of the patient's vital signs.

Glasgow Coma Scale Score

Determine the patient's best eye opening, motor, and verbal responses using the Glasgow Coma Scale (GCS). The Glasgow Coma Scale awards the patient points for different responses, with a total score that will range between 3 and 15 points (see Table 23-1). The scale is a moderately good predictor of head injury severity. A patient with a score of between 13 and 15 is considered to have a mild head injury. A score between 9 and 12 indicates moderate injury, while a score of 8 or less represents severe head injury. Most patients with GCS of 8 or less are in a coma.

When assessing eye-opening response, award 1 point for no response, 2 for eye opening in response to pain, 3 for response to verbal command, and 4 for spontaneous eye opening. With verbal response, award 1 point for no sound or response, 2 points for incomprehensible, garbled sounds, 3 points for inappropriate words and speech that makes no sense, 4 points for confused or disoriented speech, and 5 for clear and oriented speech. With motor response, award 1 point for no movement or response, 2 points for decerebrate posturing, 3 points for decorticate posturing, 4 points for purposeful motion (withdrawal of a body part from pain), 5 points for purposeful movement (of the hand) to localize pain, and 6 for following simple verbal commands. The lowest GCS value is 3, which represents a completely unresponsive patient. The maximum GCS value is 15, which represents the fully conscious and alert patient.

Patients with a Glasgow Coma Scale score of 8 or less should be immediately intubated.

Table 23-1   GLASGOW COMA SCALE

Eye Opening

Spontaneous	4
To verbal command	3
To pain	2
No response	1

Verbal Response

Oriented and converses	5
Disoriented and converses	4
Inappropriate words	3
Incomprehensible sounds	2
No response	1

Motor Response

Obeys verbal commands	6
Localizes pain	5
Withdraws from pain (flexion)	4
Abnormal flexion in response to pain (decorticate rigidity)	3
Extension in response to pain (decerebrate rigidity)	2
No response	1

Record the best response for each of the GCS criteria (for example, as E_3, V_4, M_5), and note any differences, either from side to side or in the upper versus lower extremities. Also, note the eye signs along with the GCS score results because they help identify the existence and nature of the patient's brain injury.

Vital Signs

Carefully monitor the vital signs for evidence of increasing ICP. Identify and record the pulse rate and strength. Note the blood pressure, especially the pulse pressure. Lastly, note the respiratory pattern. The vital signs change with increasing ICP or injury to the brainstem. Be watchful for a slowing pulse rate, increasing systolic blood pressure, and the development of erratic respirations (Cheyne-Stokes, central neurological hyperventilation, or ataxic respirations), which together are known as Cushing's reflex.

At the conclusion of the rapid trauma assessment, determine the need for rapid transport. A history of head trauma, coupled with any history of unconsciousness, a degradation in the level of orientation or consciousness, or any vital sign suggestive of brain injury, requires rapid transport to the closest appropriate facility. If such signs and symptoms of brain injury exist, begin rapid transport, and contact medical direction for approval to transport to the nearest neurocentre. Significant airway threats and uncontrolled hemorrhage are also indicators for rapid transport. Carefully monitor other head, face, and neck injury patients during further assessment, and care for any signs of increasing ICP or expanding lesions. Identify the wounds and other injuries you have found or suspect, and prioritize them for care.

At the conclusion of the rapid trauma assessment, determine the need for rapid transport.

FOCUSED HISTORY AND SECONDARY ASSESSMENT

If your head, face, or neck injury patient has no significant mechanism of injury and no other indications of serious injury, perform a focused history and secondary assessment, concentrating on the area of injury. During your assessment, however, carefully observe for any signs of a diminished level of consciousness or orientation or any evidence of previous unconsciousness or airway or vascular restriction or compromise. If you discover any of these things, complete a rapid trauma assessment, and consider the patient for rapid transport to the appropriate facility. Remember, the signs of significant brain injury may not develop for some time or may be masked by drug or alcohol use or by the patient's anxiety. It is always better to err on the side of more intensive patient care.

Direct the focused history and secondary assessment to the areas of specific patient complaint and to areas where the MOI suggests injury. Use the assessment techniques—inspection, palpation, and so on—suggested for the rapid trauma assessment.

When you have completed the focused assessment, obtain a set of baseline vital signs and gather a patient history. Then, provide emergency care for the injuries you have found, and prepare the patient for transport.

With superficial wounds to the head, face and neck, apply dressings and bandages as for minor soft-tissue injuries, but be alert for hemorrhage into the airway and the vomiting that may follow it and for any signs of progressive swelling that may restrict the airway. Watch also for open neck wounds that may permit air to enter the jugular vein. Cover such wounds with occlusive dressings held firmly in place.

Inspect any soft-tissue head, facial, or neck injury very carefully before bandaging it, and be prepared to describe the injury to the attending emergency department physician or nurse so that they do not have to remove and replace dressings and bandages unnecessarily.

DETAILED ASSESSMENT

You will normally perform a detailed assessment for the head, face, and neck injury patient during transport and only if and when you have cared for all other serious injuries. The detailed assessment is an in-depth, head-to-toe assessment searching for any other signs or symptoms suggestive of injury. Use your skills of questioning, inspection, palpation, and—as appropriate—auscultation to search out these additional injuries. Look for signs of neurological deficit in the extremities, including flaccidity, paresthesia, anesthesia, weakness, and paralysis. Remember that early in the course of trauma, serious injuries may be masked by other more painful ones, by patient anxiety, and by drug and alcohol use. Careful evaluation is required to identify injuries at this stage of patient care.

ONGOING ASSESSMENT

Perform ongoing assessments every five minutes for patients with potentially serious injuries. Be especially alert for slowing of the pulse, increasing systolic blood pressure (an increasing pulse pressure), and development of deeper, more rapid, or erratic respirations. Carefully observe the patient for changes in the level of consciousness and orientation as well. Finally, watch the eyes for signs of cerebral hypoxia—they become dull and lacklustre—or of increasing ICP—one pupil becomes sluggish, nonreactive, and then dilated. Note any changes in any element of patient presentation, and track any trends to identify whether the patient's condition is deteriorating, improving, or remaining the same.

Watch pulse oximetry and blood pressure readings to ensure that the patient becomes neither hypoxic nor hypovolemic. Both these conditions are associated with increased mortality and morbidity when associated with brain injury. If you notice any sign of deterioration, provide rapid transport.

HEAD, FACIAL, AND NECK INJURY MANAGEMENT

The management priorities for the patient sustaining head, face, or neck trauma include care directed at maintaining the patient's airway and breathing, ensuring circulation through hemorrhage control, addressing or taking steps to avoid hypoxia and/or hypovolemia, and providing appropriate medications. Once these priorities have been attended to, you may care for minor head, facial, and neck wounds.

AIRWAY

The airway is one of the most important care priorities with head, face, and neck injury patients. Head, face, and neck injuries can leave patients unable to control the airway due to either an altered mental status or damaged airway structures. In addition, soft-tissue trauma to the airway may cause edema that can quickly progress from restriction of the airway to its complete obstruction. Vigilant attention to the airway and aggressive airway care are the only means of ensuring that the airway remains protected and patent. Airway management techniques appropriate for such patients include suctioning, patient positioning, oral and nasal airway insertion, and endotracheal intubation. (You can review these techniques in Chapter 27, Part 2: "Airway Management and Ventilation.")

A slowing pulse rate, increasing systolic blood pressure, and the development of erratic respirations are signs of increasing ICP.

If the patient's eyes become dull and lacklustre, it is a sign of cerebral hypoxia; if one pupil becomes sluggish, nonreactive, and then dilated, that indicates intracranial injury.

Vigilant attention to the airway and aggressive airway care are vital with head, facial, and neck injury patients.

Suctioning

Airway tissues are extremely vascular, bleed profusely, and swell quickly. Soft-tissue injury may cause significant hemorrhage that can compromise the airway in two ways. First, the sheer volume of blood may block the airway. Note that aspiration of blood is more often responsible for hypoxia than physical obstruction of the airway; so be certain to suction as necessary in order to remove blood from the airway.

Secondly, blood is a gastric irritant that frequently induces emesis. If a large volume of blood is swallowed, the patient may vomit, thus endangering the airway. In addition, vomiting is common with head injury patients because emesis is a frequent result of brain injury or increasing ICP. Vomiting often occurs without warning (without nausea) and can be projectile in nature. Vomiting is especially dangerous with head injury patients because they commonly have a depressed or absent gag reflex. Gastric contents are very acidic and will quickly damage the tissues of the lower airway if aspirated. Aspiration of gastric contents is associated with a high mortality. Be ready to suction aggressively as needed in any patients with nasal, oral, or head trauma. Use a large-bore catheter or a suction hose without a tip to clear the airway of any blood or emesis.

Patient Positioning

Consider placing the patient in a position that protects the airway early in your care (during the primary assessment). The best position for the patient with suspected head injury is on the left side, with the head turned slightly and facing downward, the left lateral recumbent position. Remember, of course, that head injury patients require spinal precautions. Maintain manual immobilization until the patient is secured to a long spine board, and then be prepared to turn patient and board as a unit to facilitate airway drainage.

It is unlikely that suction alone will evacuate all emesis from the oral cavity before the unconscious or semiconscious patient attempts an inspiration. If the patient experiencing serious oral, nasal (epistaxis), or facial bleeding is conscious and alert and no serious spinal injury is suspected, have the patient sit leaning forward to promote drainage and keep fluids from flowing into the posterior airway. If the patient has sustained an open neck injury with the danger of air embolism, place the patient on a spine board in the Trendelenburg position, with the lower part of the patient's body elevated about 30 centimetres. Otherwise, position the patient with potential brain injury by elevating the head of the spine board to about 30 degrees to reduce both external hemorrhage and ICP.

Oropharyngeal and Nasopharyngeal Airways

Oro- and nasopharyngeal airways each have advantages and disadvantages when used with head, face, and neck injury patients. The nasal airway does not trigger the gag reflex as easily as the oral airway and is better tolerated by the semiconscious patient. Because there is less stimulation of the gag reflex, there is also a reduction in transient increases in ICP and in the chances of increasing the severity of head injury. One hazard of nasal airway use is the possible insertion of the tube directly into the cranium through a fracture of the posterior nasal border. Always insert the nasal airway straight back, through the largest of the nares (nostrils), and use only gentle force in its introduction. If you suspect basilar skull fracture, use an oral airway or endotracheal intubation to establish and maintain the airway.

While the oral and nasal airways help keep the respective pharynxes open, they can represent threats to the airway. The ends of the tubes sit just superior to the opening of the larynx. If a patient vomits, which frequently happens with brain injury, the vomitus is blocked from exiting the patient's mouth through the airway and remains just at the laryngeal opening. With the next breath, the patient can aspirate the gastric contents, which may have serious consequences. Whenever an oral or nasal airway is in place, monitor the patient's airway carefully, and be prepared to remove the airway and evacuate any emesis. Remember, an airway adjunct alone will not maintain a patent airway.

Endotracheal Intubation

Endotracheal intubation is the most definitive method of ensuring a clear and patent airway in the head injury patient. Intubate early in the care of the unresponsive patient, and consider intubation for any patient with a reduced level of consciousness. Techniques useful in caring for head injury patients include orotracheal, digital, nasotracheal, directed, and rapid sequence intubation.

Orotracheal Intubation Orotracheal, or oral, intubation is the most common and usually the most successful technique for placing an endotracheal tube. It does, however, pose some hazards for head, face, and neck injury patients. All patients who sustain serious injuries in these regions require spinal immobilization. Immobilization, however, limits the movement of the patient's head during intubation attempts, restricting you from manually bringing the oral opening, pharynx, and trachea in line. The result is often an inability to visualize the vocal folds and watch the endotracheal tube pass into the trachea, seriously reducing the chances of a successful oral intubation.

To improve visualization during oral intubation with spinal immobilization, employ a technique called Sellick's manoeuvre. Apply pressure directed posteriorly to the cricoid ring with the thumb and index finger, moving downward toward the vertebral column. This brings the trachea more in line with the oral cavity and pharynx and compresses the esophagus, thus reducing the likelihood of vomitus entering the upper airway during intubation. Exercise caution to prevent the pressure from flexing the cervical spine. Be aware that Sellick's manoeuvre may not align the airway enough to permit visualized oral intubation.

Attempts at endotracheal intubation can increase the parasympathetic (vagal) tone. This, in turn, may increase ICP and lower the heart rate or increase the severity of other cardiac dysrhythmias already induced by the brain injury. Therefore, carry out the intubation rapidly. If possible, have the most experienced care provider attempt the procedure to reduce both intubation time and vagal stimulation. Also consider use of a pharmacological agent, such as a topical anesthetic spray, to reduce both vagal stimulation and the retching associated with stimulation of the gag reflex.

Digital Intubation Another technique that may be effective when intubating a patient undergoing spinal precautions is digital intubation. In this procedure, the endotracheal tube is positioned without visualization; instead, the tube is directed into the trachea from the base of the tongue by the intubator's fingers. This is a procedure best attempted by a paramedic with long thin fingers.

A slightly smaller than usual endotracheal tube is shaped by a stylet into a "J" configuration. The patient's mouth is held open with a bite block while you insert the first two fingers of one hand and "walk" them back along the tongue to its base. Use these fingers to locate and lift the epiglottis. Advance the tube with your other hand along the back of the tongue, and direct it with your fingers past the epiglottis and toward the tracheal opening. Continue to advance the endotracheal tube with slight anterior pressure along the posterior surface of the epiglottis for

Intubate early in the care of the unresponsive patient, and consider intubation for any patient with a reduced level of consciousness.

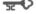

If possible, have the most experienced care provider attempt intubation to reduce both the length of the procedure and vagal stimulation.

about 3.5 to 6 cm. Remove the stylet and carefully confirm tube placement in the trachea, not the esophagus.

Nasotracheal Intubation A third procedure for intubation of the patient with possible spinal injury is nasotracheal, or nasal, intubation. Insert the endotracheal tube into the largest of the nares. Then, direct it posteriorly, curving it toward the floor of the nasal cavity. Advance the tube the length of an oral airway (the distance between the earlobe and the corner of the mouth). At this point, slowly continue insertion, while you, with your ear at the endotracheal tube opening, listen for the sounds of respirations. Gently manipulate the tube until the respiratory sounds are loudest, and then advance it during inspiration. The tube should pass directly into the trachea. The technique can be made somewhat easier using an endotracheal tube with a directable tip (such as an Endotrol). With this device, a small cord connected to the tube's end permits the user to increase or decrease the tube's curve.

The disadvantages to nasal intubation include the necessity of having a breathing patient and a quiet environment, and the danger of inserting the tube through a fractured cribiform plate and into the skull. The procedure has a lower rate of success than either oral or digital intubation. Nasal intubation also tends to raise ICP more than oral intubation because it generally takes longer and more aggressively stimulates the posterior nasal and oral pharynxes.

Directed Intubation In some cases of serious facial or upper neck trauma, as in a shotgun blast, the landmarks of the upper airway are disrupted or destroyed. In such cases, obtaining and maintaining an airway may be extremely difficult. Use strong suction over the area, and use the laryngoscope to attempt to visualize the elements of the oro- and laryngopharynx. If you cannot see airway landmarks themselves, look for bubbling air escaping from the trachea with expirations. If you believe you are close to the tracheal opening and can visualize the area, have an assistant compress the chest to induce bubbling. Attempt to pass the endotracheal tube along the route of bubbles and into the trachea. With this technique, it is critically important to confirm proper placement of the endotracheal tube.

Rapid Sequence Intubation Occasionally, a patient who is responsive or whose teeth are clenched (trismus) needs intubation. Such cases might involve brain injury patients or those with serious oral trauma with the risk of swelling and progressive airway obstruction. Rapid sequence intubation is a medication-facilitated procedure utilized by critical care paramedics that paralyzes the conscious or semiconscious patient to permit intubation. A sedative/amnestic is administered to sedate the patient and reduce anxiety. Then, a quick-acting paralytic agent is given to induce muscle relaxation, including the muscles of the oral and pharyngeal cavities. The patient must then be intubated and positive pressure ventilations provided quickly because the paralytic agent paralyzes all skeletal muscles, including those associated with breathing. The paralytic agent also eliminates the gag reflex and the patient's ability to maintain the airway.

The drugs most commonly used for this procedure are the paralytics succinylcholine, pancuronium, and vecuronium and the sedatives diazepam, midazolam, and morphine. Sedative antagonists are frequently used to reverse the effects of these drugs when given and include flumazenil (for diazepam or midazolam) and naloxone (for morphine). (See Chapter 27, Part 2: "Airway Management and Ventilation.")

The process for rapid sequence intubation begins with reconfirmation of the indications: a patient experiencing muscle spasm (trismus) or who has an intact gag reflex (semiconscious or conscious patient) and who needs a protected airway. Apply Sellick's manoeuvre and ventilate or be ready to ventilate the patient as needed. Premedicate the patient with the sedative, and then administer the

Confirmation of tube placement is especially important when the tube has been placed blindly.

If you hear good breath sounds bilaterally, detect no epigastric sounds, and see the chest wall move equally with each breath, the tube is most likely in the trachea.

Endotracheal intubation should be confirmed by the three different methods described in Chapter 27.

paralytic quickly. When the muscles relax and/or the gag reflex ceases, have the most experienced care provider attempt oral or digital intubation.

Confirmation of Tube Placement Once the endotracheal tube is inserted using one of the techniques described above, confirm its proper placement in the trachea. This is especially important when the tube has been placed blindly. Auscultate, at a minimum, the axillae and over the epigastrium. (Good breath sounds at the axillae reflect good ventilation to the distal alveoli.) Watch carefully for good, symmetrical chest wall excursion with each ventilation. If you hear good breath sounds bilaterally, detect no epigastric sounds, and see the chest wall move equally with each breath, the tube is most likely in the trachea. Inflate the cuff of the tube, and hyperventilate the patient for a short period of time. Use an end-tidal CO_2 monitor, pulse oximetry, and observation of the patient's skin colour to help confirm and monitor proper and continuing endotracheal tube placement. An esophageal detector device, although not as accurate as $ETCO_2$, can also be used for endotracheal tube placement. Remember that the endotracheal tube may dislodge from the trachea during any movement of the patient, as from the ground to the stretcher or as the stretcher is loaded into the ambulance. Reconfirm proper tube placement frequently.

Cricothyrotomy

In some cases of face and neck trauma, the region may be so distorted or blocked that oral and nasal intubations are impossible. Here, the only potential for providing a life-saving airway may be opening a surgical pathway for the air. There are two forms of this procedure: the needle cricothyrostomy and the surgical cricothyrotomy. Both needle cricothyrostomy and surgical cricothyrotomy are within the scope of practice of critical care paramedics but are practised very seldom in the treatment of patients in the field.

With needle cricothyrostomy, one or more large-bore catheters are inserted into the cricothyroid membrane to provide a temporary airway. This technique permits only limited air exchange and does not sustain the patient. Inspirations can be enhanced by oxygen-powered ventilation (termed transtracheal jet insufflation); however, exhalations are not adequate and the patient cannot be sustained by the technique for more than several minutes.

With surgical cricothyrotomy, an incision and opening is made in the cricothyroid membrane to provide an emergency airway. The soft tissue covering the membrane that separates the thyroid and cricoid cartilages is then held open by a small oral airway or a shortened #6 endotracheal tube. The chief dangers associated with surgical cricothyrotomy are serious bleeding from the soft tissue surrounding the site (and that bleeding's threat to the airway) and damage to the thyroid and parathyroid glands just below the incision site.

To begin either the needle cricothyrostomy or surgical cricothyrotomy, don gloves, goggles, and gown. Then, briskly cleanse the upper anterior neck with an alcohol swab in concentric circles outward from the base of the thyroid cartilage. Set out the needed equipment including a large-bore (14-gauge or larger) over-the-needle catheter and a syringe for the needle procedure or a sharp scalpel and a small oral airway or shortened endotracheal tube for the surgical cricothyrotomy. Palpate upward along the trachea, reaching the cricoid cartilage, then the thyroid cartilage, the membrane in between them, and the cricothyroid membrane. The first solid structure you feel as you palpate up the trachea is the cricoid ring. Just above it and before the next hard ring is the cricothyroid membrane (Figure 23-19).

For the needle cricothyrostomy, attach the catheter to the syringe and perforate the cricothyroid membrane by inserting the needle into the skin and membrane until you feel a "pop." Advance the catheter a few centimetres over the

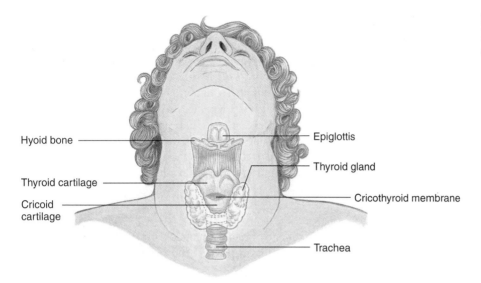

Hyoid bone

Epiglottis

Thyroid gland

Thyroid cartilage

Cricothyroid membrane

Cricoid cartilage

Trachea

needle, and then withdraw the needle. When using a single large-bore catheter, remove the tube from a 6.0 pediatric endotracheal tube, and connect it to the catheter hub. Attach the bag and valve, and ventilate or use a high-flow transtracheal jet insufflation device. Use of a demand valve is not acceptable, since the pressure of its oxygen flow is insufficient to adequately ventilate the patient through the needle. Give the patient a very long time to exhale, as the airway is now extremely restricted. Normally, expiration through the catheter takes about four times longer than inspiration. Watch carefully for the chest rising and good breath sounds.

For the surgical cricothyrotomy, insert the blade of a sterile scalpel into the skin and the cricothyroid membrane until you feel a "pop." Enlarge the opening, as needed, to accept the shortened endotracheal tube. Introduce an endotracheal tube, cut to about 10 cm in length and bent to a sharp curve, through the surgical opening. Ventilate the patient with a bag-valve-mask device using a child-sized mask; or connect the bag and valve to the endotracheal tube, and seal the area with sterile dressings. You may have to close the patient's mouth and nose, or seal the upper airway opening to ensure that the air reaches the lungs. If the airway obstruction is partial, open the mouth and nose during expiration to enhance the flow of air outward, especially when using needle cricothyrostomy.

Give the patient who has received a needle crichothyrostomy a very long time to exhale because the airway is now extremely restricted.

Placing a second needle adjacent to the first needle will help facilitate exhalation.

BREATHING

Ensuring of breathing is an important priority with any patient, but it becomes extremely critical with the head-injured patient. Not only is reduced air exchange a problem, but excessive air exchange and the excessive depletion of carbon dioxide can also endanger the patient. Providing supplemental oxygenation and appropriate ventilation are essential with such patients.

Oxygen

Any patient who has sustained a significant head injury or who displays any indication of lowered level of consciousness, orientation, or arousal is a candidate for high-flow, high-concentration oxygen. Administer oxygen at a rate of 12 to 15 L/min via a nonrebreather mask with a patient who is moving an adequate respiratory volume. If the patient is not breathing adequately, supplement any positive pressure ventilations with oxygen via reservoir, again flowing at 12 to 15 L/min.

Any patient who has sustained a significant head injury or who displays any indication of lowered level of consciousness, orientation, or arousal is a candidate for high-flow, high-concentration oxygen.

Ventilations

Provision of a good supply of oxygen is critical to the head injury patient, but so too is the removal of carbon dioxide. Assess the patient's respiratory status, and if the patient is not moving a normal volume of air, employ overdrive respiration. Ventilate 12 to 14 times per minute with full breaths (about 800 to 1000 mL). Be careful not to hyperventilate the patient because doing so reduces carbon dioxide levels in the blood and significantly reduces the cerebral blood flow. Endotracheal intubation makes ventilations easier and more efficient. Be careful not to accidentally hyperventilate the head injury patient once the tube is in place. Monitor the oxygen saturation with pulse oximetry to maintain a level of 95 percent or greater.

CIRCULATION

Your care of the patient with head, facial, and neck injuries includes both control of any serious hemorrhage and support of the body's attempts to maintain blood pressure and cerebral circulation.

Hemorrhage Control

Head and facial hemorrhage is usually easy to control because most of the injuries are to the tissues that lie over facial and cranial bones. Direct pressure is commonly an effective means of controlling such bleeding, though you should take care not to put pressure directly on suspected skull or facial fractures. Wrap bandaging circumferentially, but be careful to keep the airway clear. Allow the patient to vomit should emesis occur. Watch the airway, and be prepared to suction aggressively to limit danger from aspiration. Suctioning can also ensure that the patient does not swallow large volumes of blood, stimulating emesis. Permit the conscious and alert patient with no suspected spinal injury who is suffering epistaxis to sit leaning forward, allowing the blood to drain. This positioning keeps blood from flowing down the pharynx and entering the esophagus.

An open neck injury carries the risk of air entering the external jugular vein during strong inspiration, leading to cerebral embolism with stroke-like symptoms. Seal any open neck wound with an occlusive dressing held firmly in place by bandaging, and tilt the patient's body head down on a backboard or stretcher if possible. Carefully evaluate any other open wounds for frothy blood suggestive of tracheal involvement, seal those wounds with occlusive dressings, and monitor respirations.

Blunt trauma to the neck may produce the equivalent of compartment syndrome. Fasciae in the region compartmentalize muscle and anatomical structures and permit pressures to rise with rapid edema or blood accumulation. Any sign of neck edema or hematoma is an indication for rapid transport. Monitor the patient's skin tension and level of consciousness en route to the hospital.

Severe hemorrhage associated with open neck wounds can lead quickly to hypovolemia and shock. Control the blood loss by using a dressing and gloved fingers to apply direct pressure to the source of bleeding. You may have to maintain digital pressure throughout prehospital care because application of circumferential bandaging may restrict the airway and circulation.

Blood Pressure Maintenance

Another component of circulation care for the head, face, and neck injury patient is guarding against hypotension. The brain is highly dependent on receiving a continuous supply of oxygenated circulation. Any interruption of the supply, such as might be caused by hypotension in response to increasing intracranial pressure (ICP), will rapidly prove fatal. Care for the patient in whom you suspect increased

ICP with fluid resuscitation, even though the patient's other injuries might not suggest that step. For example, the patient with penetrating chest trauma might not receive aggressive fluid resuscitation until the systolic blood pressure drops to below 90 mmHg. If that patient also has a head injury with increasing ICP, waiting for the blood pressure to drop to a lower level would be life threatening. Hence, provide fluid (electrolyte) administration, and other shock care measures as with other trauma-induced hypovolemia hypotension.

HYPOXIA

It is very important to monitor the patient who has a head injury at all times in order to quickly identify and correct any hypoventilation. Hypoxia can further damage CNS tissue already affected by direct injury. If someone else is delivering ventilations, frequently monitor both that person's performance as well as the patient's oxygen saturation levels. Care providers often find it difficult to determine accurate ventilation rates while manually ventilating with a bag-valve mask during the emergency. Ensure that the patient is well oxygenated before any intubation attempt and hyperoxygenated for a short time after intubation. Also, be watchful for interruptions in ventilations that might occur during patient movement or when changing ventilation providers.

HYPOVOLEMIA

Like hypoxia, hypovolemia and the associated hypotension reduce oxygen transport to the brain. This condition also reduces circulation through the brain as well as the blood's ability to remove the by-products of metabolism. Since brain tissue is especially sensitive to oxygen deprivation, with head injury patients who have already suffered some damage to brain tissue, any further circulatory loss might prove devastating. The problems of hypovolemia and hypotension are compounded if there is any increase in ICP. Such an increase further restricts cerebral blood flow, and the body's autoregulatory mechanisms cannot compensate in a preexisting state of hypotension.

Provide aggressive fluid resuscitation for any patient with significant head injury in whom you suspect brain injury and who shows signs of shock compensation—rapid, thready pulse, slowed capillary refill, lowered level of consciousness, anxiety, or restlessness. Insert two large-bore catheters, and administer Ringer's Lactate solution or normal saline at a wide-open rate through nonrestrictive trauma IV tubing. Administer 20mL/kg of an isotonic solution to maintain a systolic blood pressure of 90 mmHg. Carefully monitor vital signs, and stop fluid boluses if pulmonary edema results.

Provide aggressive fluid resuscitation for any patient with significant head injury in whom you suspect brain injury and who shows signs of shock compensation.

MEDICATIONS

Several medications may be useful in the care of the head injury patient. These medications include oxygen, diuretics (mannitol, furosemide), paralytics (succinylcholine, pancuronium, vecuronium) sedatives (diazepam, midazolam, morphine, fentanyl), atropine dextrose, thiamine, and topical anesthetic sprays.

Oxygen

Oxygen administration is the primary first-line therapy used in the care of the patient with suspected head injury. Administration of high-flow oxygen provides a high inspired oxygen level and facilitates diffusion through the alveolar and capillary walls as well as the highest oxygen uptake by the hemoglobin of the red blood cells. Oxygen saturation is important for the head injury patient because

Oxygen administration is the primary first-line therapy used in the care of the patient with suspected head injury.

the brain is acutely dependent on a good supply of oxygen. There are no contraindications or side effects of concern for use of oxygen during prehospital emergency care. (Note, however, that hyperventilation is contraindicated in head injury patients because it reduces circulating CO_2 levels.)

Administer oxygen via a nonrebreather mask at a flow rate of between 12 and 15 L/min for the patient who is breathing adequately. If the patient is receiving positive pressure ventilations, supplement the ventilations with 12 to 15 L/min of oxygen flowing into the reservoir. Monitor oxygen administration using the pulse oximeter, and keep the saturation level above 95 percent. Also monitor skin colour, respiratory excursion, orientation, and anxiety to ensure that the patient is well oxygenated.

Diuretics

Mannitol should be used in the prehospital setting only on a consensus agreement with local neurosurgeons and the EMS system medical director and only by a certified critical care paramedic.

Mannitol Mannitol is a large glucose molecule that does not leave the bloodstream because of its size. It is an osmolar diuretic that draws water from body tissue into the bloodstream. Mannitol then is eliminated by the kidneys and, as it leaves the kidneys, takes both water and sodium with it, reducing the body's fluid load. Mannitol is especially effective in drawing fluid from the brain, thereby reducing cerebral edema and ICP. Although very effective in reducing cerebral edema, mannitol may reduce the ICP associated with intracranial hemorrhage. This may result in increased hemorrhage and, ultimately, more serious brain damage. Mannitol is contraindicated in patients with hypovolemia or hypotension because of its diuretic properties and in patients with a recent history of congestive heart failure because it transiently raises the cardiovascular fluid volume. Mannitol may be most useful in the patient who develops a dilated pupil during care or one who has pupillary dilation and a normal or elevated blood pressure.

Mannitol is usually supplied in a single-use vial with a concentration of 20 percent. It is given as a single slow bolus (over five minutes) of 1 g/kg of the patient's weight. It is highly hypertonic and forms crystals at low temperatures (below 7°C [45°F]). It can be reconstituted with rewarming and gentle agitation, although it should always be administered through an in-line filter to ensure that no particulate matter enters the bloodstream. Flush the IV line before and after the administration of mannitol to reduce the risk of precipitation.

Furosemide Furosemide (Lasix®) is a loop diuretic that inhibits the reabsorption of sodium in the kidneys. It results in the increased secretion of water and electrolytes, including sodium, chloride, magnesium, and calcium. Furosemide also causes venous dilation and a reduced cardiac preload. It is often given in combination with mannitol to increase the rate of diuresis. While it does not remove fluid from cerebral edema as effeciently as mannitol, it does cause more rapid fluid elimination by the kidneys. Furosemide is generally contraindicated in pregnant patients because it may cause fetal abnormalities. Since, like mannitol, furosemide causes diuresis, use it with caution, if at all, in patients with hypotension secondary to hypovolemia.

Furosemide often comes in a preloaded syringe or a single-use vial and is given as a slow IV bolus or intramuscular (IM) injection. It is administered at a dose of about 0.5 to 1.0 mg/kg, frequently in doses of either 40 or 80 mg. Administer the medication very slowly, over one to two minutes.

Paralytics

Paralytics are drugs that paralyze the skeletal muscles, permitting intubation in patients with whom the procedure would otherwise be impossible. Administration is a part of the rapid sequence intubation procedure, in which you must quickly sedate, paralyze, then intubate the patient while ensuring that the patient is well oxygenated and the airway remains clear. Rapid sequence intubation uses diazepam, midazolam, or morphine sulphate to sedate the patient; in some cases, atropine sulphate to limit muscle fasciculations; and succinylcholine chloride, pancuronium bromide, or vercuronium to paralyze the patient.

Succinylcholine Succinylcholine (Anectine®) is an ultra-short-acting depolarizing skeletal muscle relaxant. It acts on cholinergic receptors to cause the muscles to contract (depolarize). This action produces **fasciculations,** individual muscle contractions seen beneath the skin. Succinylcholine induces complete paralysis in 30 to 60 seconds and persists for about two to three minutes with IV administration. Onset of paralysis occurs in 75 seconds to three minutes with IM administration. Succinylchloline is frequently administered to achieve temporary paralysis for the intubation of patients with muscle tone, spasms, or seizures that may otherwise prevent the procedure. Succinylcholine paralyzes the muscles of respiration, and so care providers must be immediately ready to intubate and ventilate the patient when the drug takes effect. Succinylcholine does not affect the patient's level of consciousness, cerebration, anxiety, or pain perception, and so its use should follow the administration of a sedative/amnestic agent. Succinylcholine increases ICP and may induce vomiting and so should be used with caution, if at all, in cases of head injury. Because it slightly increases intraocular pressure, it is contraindicated patients with penetrating eye injuries and should be used with caution in patients who are taking digitalis.

 fasciculations involuntary contractions or twitchings of muscle fibres.

Succinylcholine is administered rapidly in an IV dosage of 1 to 1.5 mg/kg. It may be given IM if necessary. In that case, it is usually supplied in a single-use vial with 10 mL of a 20-mg/mL solution. Storage of succinylcholine requires refrigeration. If the patient is conscious, succinlycholine is given after administration of a sedative/amnestic to sedate the patient during the procedure. Frequently, 0.5 mg of atropine is administered prior to succinylcholine to halt the fasciculations.

Pancuronium and Vecuronium Pancuronium (Pavulon®) and vecuronium (Norcuron®) are nondepolarizing skeletal muscle relaxants. They induce paralysis without causing muscle contractions and fasciculations. Pancuronium is a longer-acting agent, taking from three to five minutes to become effective with effects lasting from 30 to 60 minutes. It is not used frequently in prehospital care and must be refrigerated for maximum shelf life. Vecuronium is a more effective agent with a more rapid onset (less than one minute) and shorter duration (25 to 40 minutes). It also has fewer cardiovascular side effects than either succinylcholine or pancuronium. Like succinylcholine, pancuronium and vecuronium are used to paralyze patients with muscle tone, spasms, or seizures in order to permit endotracheal intubation. They also do not have any effect on the level of consciousness, cerebration, anxiety, or pain perception, and so their use should follow administration of a sedative/amnestic agent.

It is important to remember that neuromuscular blockers do not affect the patient's level of consciousness. All conscious patients should be sedated before administration of one of these agents.

Pancuronium comes in single-use vials or preloaded syringes containing 1 mg/mL. It is administered by rapid IV bolus of 0.04 to 0.1 mg/kg. Vecuronium is administered rapidly in an IV bolus of 0.08 to 0.1 mg/kg. Vecuronium comes as 10-mg vials of powder that must be reconstituted with saline (either 5 or 10 mL) prior to administration.

Sedatives

Diazepam Diazepam (Valium®) is a benzodiazepine with both anti-anxiety and muscle relaxant qualities. In prehospital care, it is often used to premedicate patients to facilitate intubation. Diazepam is also a potent anticonvulsant. It is administered in a slow IV bolus of 5 to 10 mg, not to exceed 5 mg/min, into a large vein. Diazepam is rather fast acting, with IV effects occurring almost immediately and reaching peak effectiveness in 15 minutes. Its duration is from 15 to 60 minutes. Do not mix diazepam with any other drugs, and flush the IV line before and after administration. Administer it as close to the IV catheter as possible.

Do not inject it into a plastic IV bag because diazepam is readily absorbed by plastic, which quickly reduces its concentration.

Diazepam is usually supplied in single-use vials or preloaded syringes containing 2 mL of a 5-mg/mL solution (10 mg). Administer IV 5 to 10 mg every 10 to 15 minutes to a maximum of 30 mg. When an IV line is not immediately available, diazepam may be administered rectally for seizures with effects occurring as quickly as when given intravenously.

The effects of diazepam (and midazolam) may be reversed by the administration of flumazenil. Usually, 2 mL of a 0.1-mg/mL solution is given through IV (over 30 seconds) with a second dose repeated at 60 seconds. Be careful in its administration, as flumazenil may precipitate seizures in the head injury patient.

Midazolam Midazolam (Versed®) is a benzodiazepine similar to diazepam, though it is three to four times more potent. Onset of its effects occurs within three to five minutes. Administration of midazolam may cause cardiorespiratory arrest, and the drug does not protect against increasing ICP that follows succinylcholine and pancuronium administration. Midazolam is frequently paired with vecuronium to achieve rapid sedated paralysis. It may cause vomiting and nausea and many of the signs and symptoms of head injury.

Administer midazolam very slowly in small increments (at no more than 1 mg/min) titrated to the desired effect or the maximum administration of 2.5 mg. Midazolam is supplied in 2-, 5-, and 10-mL vials of a 1 mg/mL concentration and may be mixed in the same syringe with morphine, meperidine, or atropine or diluted with normal saline.

Morphine Morphine is an opium alkaloid used to relieve pain (narcotic analgesic), to sedate, and to reduce anxiety. It may mask the signs and symptoms of head injury and mildly increase ICP. It also reduces vascular volume and cardiac preload by increasing venous capacitance and thus may decrease blood pressure in the hypovolemic patient. Its major side effects are respiratory depression and possible nausea and vomiting.

Morphine is available in 10-mL single-use vials or Tubex® units of a 1 mg/mL solution or as 1-mL of a 10-mg/mL solution vial for dilution with 9 mL normal saline. Administer a 5- to 10-mg IV bolus, slowly, and repeat as necessary every few minutes until effective.

Naloxone (Narcan®) is a narcotic antagonist that can quickly reverse the effects of narcotics and should be at hand anytime you use morphine sulphate. Naloxone is administered as an IV bolus of 0.4 to 2 mg, repeated every two to three minutes until effective (up to 10 mg). Naloxone is a shorter-acting drug than morphine, and so repeat doses may be necessary.

Fentanyl Fentanyl (Sublimaze®) is a synthetic narcotic agonist analgesic with pharmacological action similar to those of morphine and meperidine, but its action is more prompt and less prolonged. On a weight basis, fentanyl is 50 to 100 times more potent than morphine. Its principal actions are analgesia and sedation. Its emetic effect is less than with either morphine or meperidine.

Vital signs should be monitored routinely. Fentanyl may produce bradycardia, which may be treated with atropine. However, fentanyl should be used with care in patients with cardiac bradydysrhythmias.

Fentanyl should be administered with caution to patients with liver and kidney dysfunction because of the importance of these organs in the metabolism and excretion of drugs.

As with other narcotic analgesics, the most common serious reactions reported to occur with fentanyl are respiratory depression, apnea, muscle rigidity, and bradycardia. If these side effects remain untreated, respiratory arrest, circulatory depression, or cardiac arrest may occur. Resuscitation equipment and a narcotic agonist, such as naloxone, should be readily available to manage apnea.

Fentanyl may be used in the management of severe pain, for maintenance of analgesia, and as a sedative agent in rapid sequence sedation/intubation.

Fentanyl is available in 100- and 250-µg vials.

Atropine

Atropine is an anticholinergic (parasympatholytic) agent sometimes administered as part of a rapid sequence intubation routine. It has the ability to reduce parasympathetic (vagal) stimulation associated with intubation attempts and the resultant decrease in heart rate. Atropine may reduce oral and airway secretions and limit the fasciculations associated with administration of succinylcholine. Atropine may cause pupillary dilation and other CNS signs frequently associated with head injury—headache, nausea, vomiting, and blurred vision.

Atropine is available in many concentrations from 0.05 and 0.1 mg/mL preloaded syringes to 10-mL vials of 1 mg/mL solution. For emergency administration, its usual form is 10-mL preloaded syringes of 0.1-mg/mL concentration. Atropine is usually administered as a 0.5 mg bolus for rapid sequence intubation.

Dextrose

In general, both hypoglycemia and hyperglycemia are detrimental to the patient with head injury. In the past, dextrose was given routinely to patients who were unresponsive with an undetermined cause. However, current practice calls for identifying the blood glucose level on all unresponsive patients, especially those with a possible history of chronic alcoholism or diabetes. If significant hypoglycemia is found, administer 25 gm of glucose and 100 mg of thiamine.

The empiric use of dextrose in the head-injured patient is contraindicated.

Dextrose is supplied in preloaded syringes containing 50 mL of a 500 mg/mL (50 percent) solution (D50W). It is to be administered slowly through a large vein because it is a very hypertonic solution. In severe cases of hypoglycemia, a second dose may be administered.

Thiamine

Thiamine, more commonly known as vitamin B_1, is a substance obtained from diet and needed for body metabolism. Thiamine is essential for the processing of glucose through the Kreb's cycle, from which the body gains its life-sustaining energy. In malnourished patients (like the chronic alcoholic), thiamine is depleted, and the body tissue cannot obtain energy from glucose. The brain is especially affected, since it does not store energy sources.

Thiamine is supplied in 1-mL single-use ampules, vials, and preloaded syringes containing a 100-mg/mL solution. It is administered as an IV bolus or IM. It should be administered before or with glucose.

Topical Anesthetic Spray

Topical sprays use an anesthetic agent, such as xylocaine or benzocaine, to anesthetize the oral and pharyngeal mucosa. This reduces the gag reflex, making endotracheal intubation easier and reducing the impact of retching on ICP. The agent is sprayed into the oral pharynx, where it is rapidly absorbed by mucosal tissue. It inhibits nerve sensation, thereby reducing the gag reflex. The effects of the agent are immediate (within 15 seconds), remain local, and last for about 15 minutes. These agents are usually supplied in two-ounce aerosol spray cannisters with long, hollow extension tubes to direct the spray down the throat. The agent is applied by directing a spray of the material into the posterior oral cavity and pharynx. While topical anesthetic sprays permit easier intubation and reduce the associated vagal effects, they also reduce the patient's ability to remove fluids from the airway and thus increase the danger of aspiration.

TRANSPORT CONSIDERATIONS

When transporting head injury patients, limit external stimulation, such as the use of red lights and sirens, and try to provide a smooth ride.

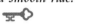

There are special considerations to observe when transporting the patient with serious head injury to the hospital. Limit any external stimulation, such as the use of red lights and sirens, and try to achieve a smooth ride. Stimulation may further agitate the patient, increase ICP, and induce seizures.

Be cautious in considering the head injury patient as a candidate for air medical service transport. While the time saved by helicopter transport may be very important, the head injury patient is prone to seizures, especially with the physical stimulation (noise and vibration) associated with this mode of transport. Seizures aboard any type of aircraft are very dangerous. If you elect to transport by air, ensure that the patient is firmly secured to a long spine board (including feet and hands) and that her airway is protected by endotracheal intubation.

EMOTIONAL SUPPORT

Identify someone to remain with the patient specifically for calming and reassuring her during care and transport. Have that person continuously reorient the patient to her environment. Remember, head injury patients may have trouble remembering events preceding and immediately following the incident as well as have difficulty retaining short-term memory. The person assigned the special role should describe what happened to the patient and help the patient remain oriented to the current location and what is happening. This simple step aids greatly in reducing the patient's anxiety and in helping a return to a normal level of orientation.

Head injury patients may be very confused, distressed, abusive, or even combative. Do not take their behaviour personally. Maintain a professional demeanour, and provide emotional support during assessment, care, and transport.

SPECIAL INJURY CARE

There are certain types of head, face, and neck trauma that deserve special care. They include scalp avulsion, injury to the pinna of the ear, eye injury, dislodged teeth, and impaled objects.

Scalp Avulsion

Avulsion occurs when a glancing blow tears the scalp's border and releases a flap of scalp. The flap may remain in anatomical position, fold back and expose the cranium, or be torn completely free. If the avulsion uncovers the cranium, cover both the open wound and the undersurface of the exposed scalp flap with a large bulky dressing. Also place padding under the fold of the scalp to prevent any sharp kinking along its border. If the region is seriously contaminated, remove gross contamination, and rinse the area with normal saline before applying the dressings. Scalp avulsions tend to heal very well unless grossly contaminated or the circulation to the flap is severely disrupted.

Pinnal Injury

Serious injury to the pinna, or exposed portion of the ear, often results from glancing blows and trauma, like a tearing or avulsion injury, that disrupts its structure. Such an injury is best treated by placing the pinna in as close to its anatomical position as possible. Then, place a dressing between the head and medial surface of the injured ear, and cover the exposed ear with a sterile dressing. Finally, bandage the dressed injury firmly to the head.

Eye Injury

Care for eye injuries involves careful assessment and protective care. Most eye wounds or injuries are best cared for by applying soft dressings to cover the closed, injured eye. The other eye, even if uninjured, is also dressed and the dressings on both eyes are held in place with gentle bandaging. This technique prevents sympathetic motion (one eye moving with the other), which may cause additional damage to the injured eye. If the eye injury is an open wound or torn eyelid, consider using a sterile dressing soaked in normal saline to reduce the pain and discomfort and prevent evaporative loss of lacrimal fluid. Place the patient in the supine position if other injuries do not prevent it.

If the patient complains of eye pain without apparent injury, suspect corneal abrasion or laceration, possibly caused by an object embedded in the conjunctiva or sclera. Gently invert the eyelid, and examine for any small embedded object (Figure 23-20a and b). If you observe one, you may attempt to remove it with a saline-moistened cotton swab. Even if you successfully remove the object, the patient is likely to continue reporting pain and the sensation of the impaled object. As with apparent wounds, cover both eyes with soft dressings and loose bandaging.

If the eye is avulsed or has an impaled object in it, cover the eye and the object with a cup or other protective material and again dress and bandage both eyes. If the patient is combative or has a significantly reduced level of consciousness,

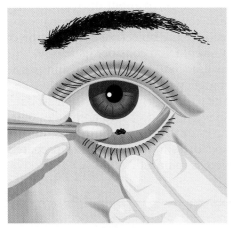

a.

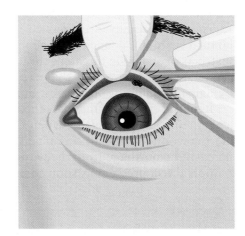

b.

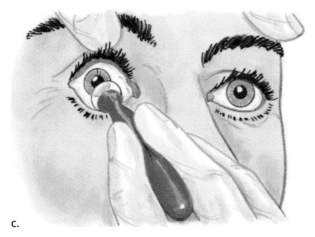

c.

FIGURE 23-20 To remove particles from the white of the eye, (a) pull down the lower lid while the patient looks up, or (b) pull up the upper lid while the patient looks down. (c) You can use a moistened suction cup to remove hard lenses.

secure her hands together and then to her waist or belt. This prevents accidental dislodging of the protective dressing and possible aggravation of the eye injury.

Eye injuries and the loss of eyesight in one or both eyes can create anxiety in most patients. Be sure to calm and reassure the patient, and explain in advance your actions as you move the patient from the scene to the ambulance and to the hospital.

If, during the assessment, you observe that the patient is wearing contact lenses and there is any possibility that she may become unresponsive, have the patient remove the lenses. If the patient is already unresponsive, try removing the lenses yourself with a contact removal suction cup (Figure 23-20c). This miniature suction cup seals against the contact lens and allows easy removal. Alternatively, lift the eyelid, which may cause the lens to dislodge, or, with the patient's eye closed, gently push the lens into the corner of the eye. Keep the lens in a contact lens case, where it should be soaked in a contact lens or sterile saline solution.

Dislodged Teeth

Locate any teeth that may have been dislodged by trauma and transport them to the hospital with the patient. Rinse the teeth in normal saline, and wrap them in saline-soaked gauze or a container of milk for transport to the emergency department. If a tooth is largely intact, it may be successfully reimplanted.

Impaled Objects

Any object impaled in the head, face, or neck should be left in place and dressed and bandaged to ensure that it does not move about during care and transport. Use bulky dressings to stabilize the object. Secure the patient's hands if there is a danger that she may dislodge the object. Only if the object obstructs or seriously threatens the airway should you consider its removal. In such cases, removal will likely increase the associated hemorrhage and possibly damage adjoining structures, but the patency of the airway is vital.

Removal of objects that pass through the patient's cheek pose the least danger for removal. With such a wound, you have ready access to both sides of it, and the wound involves no critical structures or organs. Nevertheless, expect increased hemorrhage from the wound, have dressings ready, and be prepared to apply direct pressure as soon as the object is removed.

Summary

The head, face, and neck contain very special and important structures—key elements of the central nervous system, the airway, the alimentary canal, and major organs of sensation. Serious trauma to the region endangers these structures and therefore demands special assessment and care. During the scene assessment, identify possible mechanisms of injury and the injuries they suggest. Confirm the injuries during the primary and rapid trauma assessments. Identify your patient's level of consciousness and orientation early, and watch the eyes carefully for signs of cerebral hypoxia and increasing intracranial pressure. Ensure that the spine is immobilized and the airway is clear and protected from aspiration and physical obstruction. Administer high-concentration oxygen, and ventilate as necessary, being careful not to under- or overventilate the patient. Secure rapid transport for the patient with possible intracranial hemorrhage or serious lesion. Once the central nervous system, the airway, and breathing are protected, address the skeletal structure fractures, minor bleeding, and open wounds. During all your care for the patient with injury to the head, face, or neck, provide emotional support.

CHAPTER 24

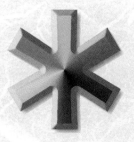

Spinal Trauma

Objectives

After reading this chapter, you should be able to:

1. Describe the incidence, morbidity, and mortality of spinal injuries in the trauma patient. (pp. 248–249)
2. Describe the anatomy and physiology of spinal structures and structures related to the spine, including the cervical spine, thoracic spine, lumbar spine, sacrum, coccyx, spinal cord, nerve tracts, and dermatomes. (see Chapter 12)
3. Predict spinal injuries on the basis of mechanism of injury. (pp. 249–252)
4. Describe the pathophysiology of spinal injuries. (pp. 249–255)

5. Identify the need for rapid intervention and transport of the patient with spinal injuries. (pp. 256–261)
6. Describe the pathophysiology of traumatic spinal injury related to the following:
   - Spinal shock (p. 254)
   - Neurogenic shock (p. 255)
   - Quadriplegia/paraplegia (pp. 253–254)
   - Incomplete and complete cord injury (pp. 253–254)
   - Cord syndromes:
     – Central cord syndrome (p. 254)

Continued

Objectives Continued

        – Anterior cord syndrome (p. 254)
        – Brown-Séquard's syndrome (p. 254)
7. Describe the assessment findings associated with and management for traumatic spinal injuries. (pp. 256–274)
8. Describe the various types of helmets and their purposes. (pp. 266–267)
9. Relate the priorities of care to factors determining the need for helmet removal in various field situations including sports-related incidents. (pp. 266–267)

10. Given several preprogrammed and moulaged spinal trauma patients, provide the appropriate scene assessment, primary assessment, rapid trauma or secondary assessment and history, detailed assessment, and ongoing assessment and provide appropriate patient care and transport. (pp. 256–274)

INTRODUCTION TO SPINAL INJURIES

A spinal cord injury can both threaten life and cause serious, lifelong disability. Statistics Canada reports that in 1998–1999 (the latest year for which statistics are available), young people between the ages of 15 and 34 accounted for 40 percent of the 1347 hospital injury admissions due to spinal cord injuries. Motor vehicle collisions (43 percent) and falls (36 percent) were the leading causes of hospitalizations for spinal cord injuries. These injuries are often severe enough to cause paraplegia or quadriplegia. Most spinal cord injuries are permanent.

During the years 1994–1999, there were 877 hospitalizations for injuries that resulted in paraplegia or quadriplegia, and the majority were seen in young men.

The Canadian Institute for Health Information (CIHI) reports that the number of spinal cord injury hospitalizations has dropped 15 percent, from 1580 in 1994–1995 to 1347 in 1998–1999. This trend was particularly evident in the number of hospitalizations for spinal cord injuries caused by motor vehicle collisions, which decreased from 709 to 547 (a 23-percent drop) over the five-year period.

In 1998–1999, motor vehicle collisions accounted for more than 53 percent of all admissions for spinal cord injuries in people between the ages of 15 and 34 years, compared with only 25 percent of admissions of people aged 65 years and older. In contrast, falls were the primary cause of admissions for spinal cord injuries in seniors (64 percent), while they accounted for only 25 percent of hospitalizations in the 15–34 age group.

Spinal cord injury is an especially devastating type of trauma. The spinal cord consists of highly specialized central nervous system tissue and does not repair itself when seriously injured. Permanent injury to it affects the body's major communications pathways and control over the lower extremities (paraplegia) or both upper and lower extremities (quadriplegia). Spinal cord injuries also af-

> *Of all patients who suffer neurological deficit from trauma, some 40 percent have experienced spinal cord injury.*
>

fect the body's control over internal organs and the body's internal environment (homeostasis). A patient with a serious spinal injury is left less able to care for himself, will have a significantly altered lifestyle, and will face increased expenses associated with care and support. In fact, lifelong care costs for the victim of a permanent spinal cord injury may well exceed $1 million dollars. This figure does not include the patient's lost earning power due to the disability.

As with most trauma, the best form of care is prevention. Recent advances in motor vehicle and highway designs have helped reduce the incidence of spinal injury in its most common category, motor-vehicle trauma. Proper use of lap and shoulder belts further reduces the incidence of spinal cord injury, as do programs to eliminate drunk driving. Educational programs aimed at teaching safe practices also reduce the potential for spinal cord injury. These programs can foster such behaviours as not diving into unknown waters, developing good physical conditioning, and wearing protective equipment in sports. Following good safety practices in the workplace and in the home can also reduce both temporary and permanent spinal column and cord injuries.

PATHOPHYSIOLOGY OF SPINAL INJURY

If you understand how the events of trauma affect the spinal cord and the body systems, you will be better prepared to anticipate and recognize spinal column and cord injuries. Traumatic events may cause immediate and devastating injury to the cord with no chance for the patient's recovery. Such events may also cause damage to bones or ligaments, resulting in spinal column instability and creating the potential for cord injury during patient care and transport. By understanding the mechanism of injury and the spinal problems it may produce (the pathophysiology), you can more quickly recognize and better protect the patient who has spinal cord trauma.

MECHANISMS OF SPINAL INJURY

The mechanisms of injury that affect the spinal column and cord include extremes of normal motion, such as flexion, extension, rotation, and lateral bending (Figure 24-1). Damaging mechanisms also include stresses along the axis of the spine: axial loading and distraction. Finally, spinal injury may occur as a direct result of either blunt or penetrating trauma or as an indirect effect of trauma—when an expanding mass (edema or hematoma) compresses the cord or when a disruption in the blood supply damages it.

Extremes of Motion

Hyperextension or hyperflexion bend the spine forcibly, most commonly in the cervical or lumbar regions. A classic example of an extension injury mechanism is a rear-impact auto collision. The patient's head remains stationary, while the upper torso moves rapidly and abruptly forward with the auto. The heavy head moves backward and hyperextends the neck. The hyperextension places compressing forces on the posterior vertebral structures (the spinous processes, laminae, and pedicles) and stretching forces on the anterior vertebral ligaments. Extremes of extension may cause disc disruption, compression of the interspinous ligaments, and fracture of the posterior vertebral elements. If the forces are great enough, ligaments may tear or the vertebra may fracture, resulting in instability and bone displacement.

In frontal-impact collisions, the shoulder strap may restrain the body, while the head continues its forward travel. The attachment of the neck restrains the head and

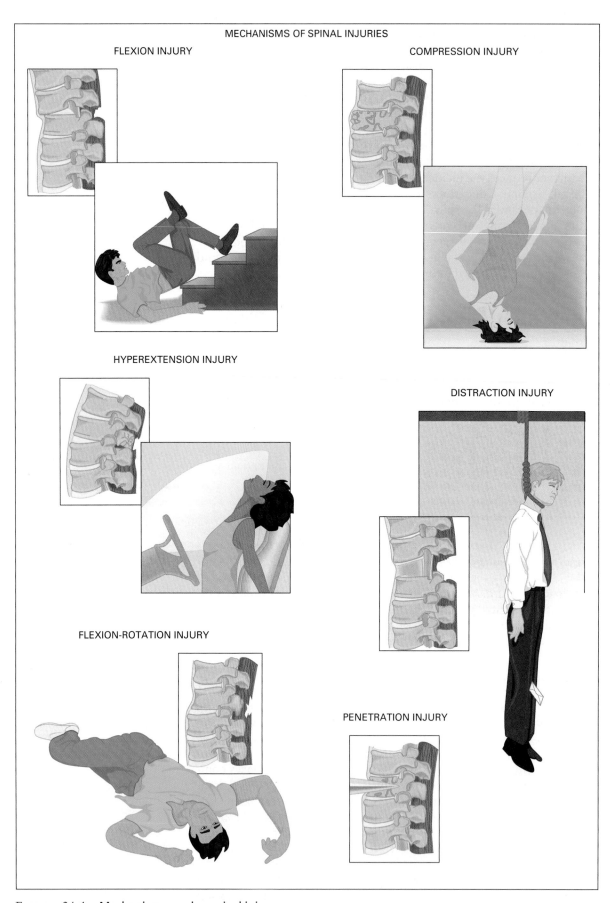

FIGURE 24-1   Mechanisms causing spinal injury.

flexes the spine with the movement. The process is frequently forceful enough to cause a patient to literally "kiss the chest" (sometimes demonstrated by a female patient's lipstick print on her shirt front). Extreme flexion may lead to wedge fractures of the anterior vertebral bodies, stretching or rupture of the posterior longitudinal and interspinous ligaments, compression injury to the cord, fracture of the pedicle(s), and disruption of the intervertebral discs with dislocation of the vertebrae.

Excessive rotation may occur in both the cervical and the lumbar regions of the spine. Anatomically, the head is attached to the vertebral column at the foramen magnum, located well posterior of the midline and the head's centre of mass. With lateral impact, the head turns toward the impacting force as the body moves out from under it. The cervical spine attachment restrains its motion and turns the head violently. Rotation injury normally affects the upper reaches of the cervical region but may also be transmitted to the lumbar spine, as, for example, when a tackled football player's thorax twists, while his feet are firmly planted. The result is a rotational injury that may include stretching or tearing of the ligaments, rotational subluxation or dislocation, and vertebral fracture.

Lateral bending may take place along the entire vertebral column, though it is most common and likely to cause injury in the cervical and lumbar regions. As one portion of the body moves sideways and the remaining portion stays fixed, the spine absorbs the energy. The movement may compress the vertebral structures inducing compression fracture on one side of the column (toward the impact), while it tears ligaments on the opposite side. The result may be compression of the vertebral pedicles with bone fragments driven into the spinal foramen, torn ligaments, and vertebral instability. An example of this mechanism is a lateral-impact auto collision, in which the forces of the crash move the thorax to the side and out from under the head, placing severe lateral stress on the cervical spine. Because of the structure of the spine, the forces necessary to induce injury from lateral bending are generally less than those needed to cause flexion/extension injury.

Axial Stress

Axial loading occurs as compressional stress is brought to bear along the axis of the spine. It may occur when a person lifts a weight too great for the strength of his lumbar spine or when a person falls and lands on his heels. The resulting force is transmitted up the lower extremities to the pelvis, the sacrum, and the lumbar spine. Another frequent mechanism of axial loading injury is the shallow water dive. In this case, the diver's head hits the pool bottom, while the weight of the lower portion of the body drives the thorax into the head, crushing the cervical spine. This mechanism also occurs in auto collisions, when an occupant is propelled into the windshield by the collision forces. With these mechanisms, impact is likely to compress, fracture, and crush the vertebrae and herniate (rupture) discs, releasing their semiliquid centres into the vertebral foramina and compressing the spinal cord. The most common sites of axial loading injuries are between T-12 and L-2 (in lifting injuries and heel-first falls) and the cervical region (in head impacts).

Distraction is the opposite of axial loading. A force, such as gravity applied during hanging or at the end of a bungee jumper's jump, stretches the spinal column and tears ligaments. The process may also stretch and damage the spinal cord without causing physical damage to the spinal column. The upper cervical region is most commonly affected by this mechanism of injury.

Often, the actual spinal injury process involves complicated combinations of the various injury mechanisms mentioned above. Hanging may suspend the victim from the side of the head, causing injury from distraction and severe lateral bending

> *Because of the structure of the spine, the forces necessary to induce injury from lateral bending are generally less than those needed to cause flexion/extension injury.*
>
>

> *Often, the spinal injury process involves a combination of mechanisms.*

directed at the C-1/C-2 region (causing a hangman's fracture). The lateral-impact auto collision may produce both lateral bending and rotational injury mechanisms affecting the cervical spine. The shallow water dive may result in both axial loading and hyperflexion as the body pushes against and bends the neck. Note that the cervical spine is posterior to the midline of both the head and the chest. In-line impacts frequently cause the head and neck to flex as the body pushes forward.

Be aware of the distinctions among connective tissue, skeletal, and spinal cord injuries. Connective tissue and skeletal injuries do not necessarily result in spinal cord injuries. They do, however, represent potential instability of the spinal column and the danger that any subsequent motion, even normal motion, may result in spinal cord injury. Spinal cord injury can also occur without noticeable injury to the ligaments, discs, and vertebra of the spinal column. This is why, whenever a patient shows any sign of spinal injury or has experienced a mechanism that suggests the possibility of spinal injury, you must provide manual immobilization immediately and full mechanical immobilization as soon as possible. Maintain immobilization during all of your assessment, care, and transport.

Connective tissue and skeletal injuries represent potential instability of the spinal column and the danger that any subsequent motion may result in spinal cord injury.

Other Mechanisms of Injury

Other mechanisms of spinal injury can involve both direct blunt and penetrating trauma. Kinetic forces may be directed at the spine when objects strike the spine posteriorly (or laterally in the neck) or when a person falls on or is thrown against an object (as in a blast). Penetrating injuries caused by such objects as knives and ice-picks or by missiles, such as blast fragments and bullets, may also apply the forces of trauma directly to the spinal column. The penetrating object may harm vertebral ligaments, fracture vertebral structures, drive bone fragments directly into the spinal cord, or directly damage the cord itself. However, unlike blunt trauma, penetrating injury rarely results in ligamentous instability of the vertebral column.

As a result of trauma, tissues adjacent to the spinal cord may swell or otherwise encroach on the vertebral foramen. With the close tolerance between the interior surfaces of the vertebral foramen and the cord, this swelling may place pressure on the cord, producing direct compression injury and halting blood flow through the compressed tissues. Such injury may also involve the spinal nerve roots that exit the vertebral column close to the injury.

Electrocution, on rare occasions, can cause spinal injury. The extreme and uncontrolled muscular contractions associated with electrocution can tear tendons and ligaments and fracture vertebrae, resulting in column instability and possible spinal cord injury.

A direct injury to the spinal or vertebral blood vessels or any soft-tissue or skeletal injury and the swelling associated with them may decrease the circulation to portions of the cord. This will likely result in tissue ischemia and compromise of cord function.

The coccygeal region of the spinal column can also be injured. Although it contains neither the spinal cord nor many peripheral nerve roots, injury to the region can be painful. Such injuries are usually related to direct blunt trauma, for example, that are caused by "falling on one's tailbone."

RESULTS OF TRAUMA TO THE SPINAL COLUMN

Spinal injuries may damage the musculoskeletal components of the spinal column, injure the spinal cord, or both. Spinal column injury alone may damage the ligaments and skeletal elements of the column, damaging its integrity and endangering the spinal cord. Injury to the cord may endanger or destroy the ability of the central nervous system to communicate with the body distal to the injury.

Column Injury

The spine is subject to numerous types of injury. The forces of trauma or the stresses of heavy lifting may tear tendons, muscles, and ligaments, resulting in pain and a reduction in the stability of the vertebral column. Those forces may cause movement of the vertebrae from their normal position, a subluxation (partial or incomplete dislocation), or dislocation. The injury process may fracture the spinous or transverse processes, the pedicles, the laminae, or the vertebral bodies. Trauma, especially axial loading, may damage the intervertebral discs. These injuries are to the connective or skeletal tissues of the vertebral column. They may or may not be associated with injury to the spinal cord itself.

Several sites along the spinal column are especially subject to injury. The cervical region accounts for more than half of all spinal injuries, with the atlas/axis (C-1/C-2) joint being most frequently involved. This is due to the very delicate nature of the two vertebrae, the mobility of the joint, and the great weight of the head it supports. C-7 is also injured frequently because it is located at the transition between the flexible cervical spine and the more rigid thoracic spine.

Similar injuries occur at the transition point between the thoracic and lumbar vertebrae (T-12/L-1), again due to the differences between the rigid thoracic spine and the flexible lumbar spine. The lumbosacral area (L-5/S-1) likewise is injured because the pelvis immobilizes the sacral spine. Spinal injuries not associated with the cervical spine are about equally divided between injuries to the thoracolumbar and lumbosacral regions.

Remember that the spinal cord ends at the L-1/L-2 region. Below this point, the spinal nerve roots extend until they exit the spinal column. These spinal nerve roots are more mobile than the cord and less likely to be injured within the spinal foramen during spinal column injury.

Cord Injury

The spinal cord can be injured through the mechanisms discussed earlier. Those injuries can be further described as either primary or secondary. A primary injury is one directly associated with the insult, and its effects occur immediately. For example, a primary injury may be caused by cord compression, stretching, or a direct injury. A secondary injury results when the initial injury causes swelling or ischemia, further injuring the cord tissue. It may also occur as an unstable spinal column is moved about and causes physical injury to the spinal cord. Primary and secondary injuries to the spinal cord can include concussion, contusion, compression, laceration, hemorrhage, and transection.

Concussion Concussion of the cord, like a cerebral concussion (see Chapter 23, "Head, Facial, and Neck Trauma"), causes a temporary and transient disruption of cord function. Without associated injuries, cord concussion generally does not produce any residual deficit.

Contusion Spinal cord contusion is simply a bruising of the cord. It is associated with some tissue damage, vascular leakage, and swelling. If blood crosses the blood–brain barrier, more significant edema may occur. But, in general, this injury is likely to repair itself with limited residual effects or none at all. The resolution of a cord contusion and its associated signs and symptoms is likely to take longer than is the case with a concussion.

Compression Spinal cord compression may occur secondary to the displacement of a vertebra, through herniation of an intervetebral disc, from displacement of a vertebral bone fragment, or from swelling of adjacent tissue. The pressure caused by these mechanisms results in restricted circulation, ischemic damage, and possibly physical damage to the cord.

Cervical spine injuries account for more than half of all spinal injuries.

Laceration Cord laceration can occur as bony fragments are driven into the vertebral foramen or the cord is stretched to the point of tearing. Laceration is likely to result in hemorrhage into the cord tissue, swelling due to the injury, and disruption of some portions of the cord and their associated communication pathways. In very minor lacerations, some recovery may be expected. Severe lacerations usually result in permanent neurological deficit.

Hemorrhage Spinal cord hemorrhage, often associated with a contusion, laceration, or stretching injury, produces injury by disruption of the blood flow, application of pressure from accumulating blood, and irritation by blood passing across the blood–brain barrier. Some of the arteries supplying the cord may affect circulation distant from the injury and result in ischemic injury above the level of physical injury.

Transection A cord **transection** is an injury that partially or completely severs the spinal cord. In a complete transection, the cord is totally cut and the potential to send and receive nerve impulses below the site of injury is lost. With transection injuries below the beginning of the thoracic spine, the results include incontinence and paraplegia, while injuries to the cervical spine cause quadriplegia, incontinence, and partial or complete respiratory paralysis.

Incomplete cord transection involves only a portion of the cord, and some spinal tracts remain intact. There is potential for some recovery of function. There are three particular types of incomplete spinal cord transection: anterior cord syndrome, central cord syndrome, and Brown-Séquard's syndrome.

Anterior cord syndrome is caused by bony fragments or pressure compressing the arteries that perfuse the anterior cord. The cord is damaged by vascular disruption and its potential for recovery is poor. The injury generally involves loss of motor function and of sensation to pain, light touch, and temperature below the injury site. The patient is likely to retain motion, positional, and vibration sensations.

Central cord syndrome is usually related to hyperextension of the cervical spine, as might occur with a forward fall and facial impact. It is often associated with a preexisting degenerative disease, such as arthritis, that has narrowed the vertebral canal. This syndrome results in motor weakness, more likely affecting the upper rather than the lower extremities, and possible bladder dysfunction. Of the three syndromes, central cord syndrome has the best prognosis for recovery.

Brown-Séquard's syndrome is usually caused by a penetrating injury that affects one side of the cord (hemitransection). The damage to one side results in sensory and motor loss to that side (ipsilateral) of the body. Pain and temperature perception are lost on the opposite (contralateral) side of the body because of the switching of the associated nerves that occurs as they enter the spinal cord. This injury is rare and is usually associated with some recovery, except in cases of direct penetrating trauma.

Spinal Shock

Spinal shock is a temporary insult to the cord that affects the body below the level of injury. The affected area becomes flaccid and loses feeling, and the patient is unable to move the extremities or other musculature (flaccid paralysis). There is frequently a loss of bowel and bladder control and, in the male, priapism (a prolonged, nonsexual penile erection). Body temperature control is affected, and hypotension is often present due to vasodilation. Spinal shock is often a transient problem if the cord is not seriously damaged.

Neurogenic Shock

Neurogenic (or spinal-vascular) shock results when injury to the spinal cord disrupts the brain's ability to exercise control over the body. The interruption of signals limits vasoconstriction, most noticeably in the skin below the level of injury. Lack of sympathetic tone causes the arteries and veins to dilate, expanding the vascular space, resulting in a relative hypovolemia. With the reduced cardiac preload, the atria fail to fill adequately, and their contraction does not stretch the walls of the ventricles. This reduces the strength of contraction (Frank-Starling reflex) and cardiac output. The problem is further compounded as the autonomic nervous system loses its sympathetic control over the adrenal medulla. It can then no longer control the release of epinephrine and norepinephrine. These hormones are responsible for increasing the heart rate against direct parasympathetic stimulation. Their absence restricts the increase in heart rate that normally follows reduced cardiac preload and falling blood pressure. The result of all these factors is relative hypovolemia. In addition, it is difficult for the patient to maintain blood pressure with a reduced cardiac output when the body is unable to increase peripheral vascular resistance through vasoconstriction. The patient in neurogenic shock is thus likely to present with a slow heart rate, low blood pressure, and shock-like symptoms (cool, moist, and pale skin) above the cord injury, and warm, dry, and flushed skin below the injury, as well as with priapism in the male.

Autonomic Hyperreflexia Syndrome

Autonomic hyperreflexia syndrome is associated with the body's resolution of the effects of neurogenic shock. It occurs in patients well after the initial spinal injury as the body begins to adapt to the problems associated with loss of neurologic control below the injury. After a time, the vascular system adjusts to the lack of sympathetic stimulation, and the blood pressure moves toward normal. However, the body now does not respond to increases in blood pressure with vasodilation below the cord injury so only bradycardia results. Autonomic hyperreflexia syndrome is most commonly associated with injuries at or above T-6. The syndrome presents with sudden hypertension, as high as 300 mmHg, bradycardia, pounding headache, blurred vision, and sweating and flushing of the skin above the point of injury. Nasal congestion, nausea, and bladder and rectum distention are also frequently present in autonomic hyperreflexia syndrome.

✱ **autonomic hyperreflexia syndrome** condition associated with the body's adjustment to the effects of neurogenic shock; presentations include sudden hypertension, bradycardia, pounding headache, blurred vision, and sweating and flushing of the skin above the point of injury.

Other Causes of Neurological Dysfunction

Not all injuries that result in neurological dysfunction affecting a dermatome or myotome are related to spinal cord injuries. An injury may occur anywhere along a nerve impulse's path of travel. For example, the C-7 nerve root travels from just below the seventh cervical vertebra through the shoulder, arm, and forearm before innervating the little finger. It may be injured by a vertebral fracture; soft-tissue injury and swelling; a shoulder, arm, or forearm fracture; penetrating trauma; or compartment syndrome.

Any of the injuries described above will interrupt sensory impulses to the brain from the little finger region and motor signals to the region from the brain (to initiate movement and maintain muscle tone). The most obvious difference between nerve root injury and spinal cord injury is the size of the region affected. Remember, however, that an injury that is currently affecting only a single dermatome may have created a vertebral column instability that threatens the entire cord.

There are also several nontraumatic processes that affect the spinal cord. Refer to Chapter 29 for further information on them.

The obvious difference between nerve root injury and spinal cord injury is that in the former a single dermatome is affected, while in the latter multiple dermatomes are affected.

ASSESSMENT OF THE SPINAL INJURY PATIENT

Put special emphasis on your analysis of the mechanism of injury in the case of a patient with a possible spinal injury.

Assessment and care for the patient with a potential spinal injury begins with special emphasis on the analysis of the mechanism of injury. During this analysis, make a conscious attempt to identify or rule out the likelihood of spinal injury. This is important because the patient who has suffered serious trauma may have other injuries that are much more painful and more obvious, which may distract you from the less obvious signs of spinal injury. Also, a seriously injured trauma patient may have a reduced level of consciousness due to intoxication or to other processes, such as shock or head injury, and thus be an unreliable reporter of the symptoms of spinal injury. For these reasons, you should consider the mechanism of injury to be the most critical indicator of spinal injury.

Scene Assessment

Analyze the mechanism of injury very carefully to identify what forces were transmitted to the patient and from which direction they came (Figure 24-2). Identify the likely movements of the spine during the crash or impact, and determine if severe flexion, extension, lateral bending, rotation, axial loading, or distraction was likely. Also, ensure that direct forces of blunt or penetrating trauma did not involve the spine. Be especially concerned about high-speed motor-vehicle collisions, falls from heights greater than three times the patient's height, any serious blunt injuries above the shoulders, and any penetrating wounds close to or directed toward the spine. Also, maintain a high level of suspicion in cases of athletic injuries, in which blunt and twisting forces are often transmitted to the spine. If there is any reason to suspect spinal injury, be prepared to employ immediate cervical immobilization as you begin the primary assessment.

Examine the scene to determine whether the patient used a helmet or other protective gear. Remember that helmets reduce the likelihood of head injury but neither increase nor decrease the likelihood of neck injury. Whenever a patient wearing a helmet sustains moderate or severe head impact, suspect spine injury, and employ spinal precautions. Also, bring the helmet to the emergency depart-

FIGURE 24-2 Often, the mechanism of injury will suggest the possibility of spinal column injury.

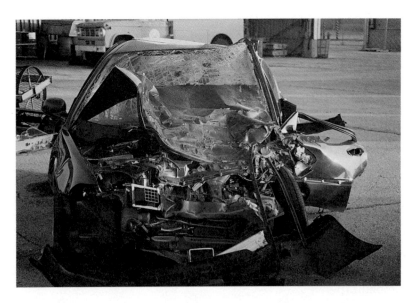

ment with the patient or relate the damages it displayed to the emergency department physician.

Even if the incident does not appear to involve a significant mechanism of injury or forces directed at the spine, ensure that there are no signs or symptoms of spinal injury during your early assessment. If you are unclear about the mechanism of injury or the potential for spinal involvement, always err on the side of protecting the patient. Full spinal precautions cause some patient discomfort and extend your time at the scene, but failure to provide needed immobilization may result in an unnecessary, devastating, and lifelong disability or even in death. Generally, a patient sustaining any serious injury receives immediate manual spinal immobilization, thereafter maintained by mechanical immobilization from your first moments at his side until arrival at the emergency department.

PRIMARY ASSESSMENT

As you approach the patient, begin to develop a general impression. Determine the patient's mental status; rule out the likelihood of spinal injury, or apply cervical spine precautions; and begin assessment of the ABCs (airway, breathing, circulation). The general impression and determination of mental status identify the patient's general condition and level of consciousness. Suspect and treat any trauma patient or possible trauma patient who is not conscious and alert and fully oriented to time, place, person, and self as though that patient has a spinal injury. Consider employing spinal precautions for any intoxicated or head-injured patients, any with significant injuries above the shoulders, any with painful injuries, or any one subject to the "fight-or-flight" response. Be aware that these circumstances can distract from or mask the symptoms of spinal injury.

Firmly apply manual immobilization to hold the patient's head in the neutral, in-line position before proceeding with the remaining assessment and care. Many sources in prehospital emergency care refer to the process of manually holding the head in the neutral, in-line position as "manual stabilization," while others refer to it as "manual immobilization." While both terms accurately describe the action, this volume will refer to the procedure as "manual immobilization." Manual immobilization should continue from the moment you arrive at the patient's side and suspect spinal injury until the patient receives full mechanical immobilization to a long spine board with a cervical immobilization device (or vest-type immobilization device).

Neutral, in-line positioning is very important in the care of a spinal injury patient as it maintains the best orientation of the spinal column and the greatest clearance between the cord and the interior of the spinal foramen. This positioning permits the best circulation and thus lessens the impact of local injury and edema. As your assessment progresses, gently and smoothly move any body segment that is out of alignment toward alignment as you examine it. If the patient feels any increase in pain or if you feel resistance to movement, immobilize the head and neck or other portion of the body in the position achieved. Do not continue movement as doing so may compromise the spinal cord. Maintain the patient's head and body using manual immobilization until you can secure the position with full mechanical immobilization using the spine board, firm padding, and a cervical immobilization device.

Once you assess the neck, consider applying a cervical collar. While the collar does not prevent flexion/extension, rotation, or lateral bending, it does limit cervical motion. However, manual immobilization of the head and neck is adequate until time and patient priorities permit you to apply the collar. Manual immobilization must continue even after a cervical collar has been applied until full mechanical immobilization is achieved.

As you move on to assess the airway, be sure that the patient's head remains in the neutral, in-line position. The airway is more difficult to control when you are required to observe spinal precautions. Be ready to carefully log roll the patient if he vomits or, if necessary, to drain the upper airway of fluids. Have adequate suction ready and anticipate the possible need to clear the airway during transport should vomiting occur. To prepare for this, secure the patient firmly to a spine board, and immobilize him well enough to permit 90-degree rotation of the board.

If handling by an advanced care paramedic (ACP) or the need for advanced airway procedures are indicated, consider orotracheal intubation with spinal precautions or digital intubation. Have the patient's head held firmly in the neutral, in-line position as you attempt to identify airway features, and insert the endotracheal tube. Anticipate that landmarks will be hard to visualize because the head cannot be brought into the sniffing position and the upper airway aligned. During the procedure, be careful not to displace the jaw anteriorly beyond the point at which it begins to lift the neck (extension) or to permit any rotation of the head. Digital intubation has the benefit of not requiring any displacement of the head and neck, although it requires a care provider who is skilled in the procedure and who has long fingers to direct the tube properly.

After using any modified or blind intubation technique like those just described, be very careful to ensure proper tube placement by assessing for the presence of good chest excursion and bilaterally equal breath sounds and the absence of epigastric sounds with ventilation. Check the depth of tube placement by noting the number on the side of the tube, and secure the tube firmly. Monitor both the tube's depth and the breath sounds frequently during your care and transport. Using the pulse oximeter or capnometer can help ensure that your patient remains effectively oxygenated.

Quickly evaluate your patient's respiratory effort. In the patient with a suspected spinal injury, watch the motion of the chest and abdomen carefully. They should rise and fall together. Exaggerated movement of the abdomen and limited chest excursion with motion opposite to that of the abdomen suggest diaphragmatic breathing. For such a patient, provide positive pressure ventilation coordinated with the patient's respiratory effort (overdrive ventilation), and employ spinal precautions immediately. Your assistance will make breathing more effective and less energy consuming. Use pulse oximetry to continuously evaluate the effectiveness of respirations.

Be extremely watchful of patients with bradycardia, especially when it is likely that they may be experiencing hypovolemia and shock.

During your check of the patient's circulation status, monitor the pulse carefully. Be extremely watchful of patients with bradycardia, especially when it is likely that they may be experiencing hypovolemia and shock. This bradycardia may be relative—for example, if a patient has a normal heart rate in the presence of low blood pressure and hypovolemia when a tachycardia might be expected. As you scan the body for other signs of vascular injury or shock, watch for warm and dry skin in the lower extremities and the upper portions of the body showing the cool, clammy skin associated with hypovolemic compensation. This is an indication of neurogenic injury and possible shock secondary to spinal cord damage. Spinal cord injury may also induce paralysis and anesthesia below the lesion, reducing the pain or other symptoms of blood loss from an abdominal or extremity injury.

RAPID TRAUMA ASSESSMENT

Once the primary assessment is complete, determine the need for the rapid trauma assessment or the secondary assessment and history. In patients with suspected or likely spinal column or cord injury, move directly to the rapid trauma assessment (Figure 24-3). Even if such patients are otherwise stable, consider rapid trauma assessment, expeditious employment of spinal precautions, and immediate transport to a trauma centre. These patients are likely to deteriorate and need neurological intervention.

SIGNS OF SYMPTOMS OF POSSIBLE SPINAL INJURY

- PAIN   Unprovoked pain in area of injury, along spine, in lower legs.

- TENDERNESS   Gentle touch of area may increase pain.

- DEFORMITY (rare)   There may be abnormal bend or bony prominence.

- SOFT-TISSUE INJURY   Injury to the head, neck, or face may indicate cervical spine injury. Injury to shoulders, back, and abdomen may indicate thoracic or lumbar spine injury. Injury to extremities may indicate lumbar or sacral spine injury.

- PARALYSIS   Inability to move or inability to feel sensation in some part of body may indicate spinal fracture with cord injury.

- PAINFUL MOVEMENT   Movement may cause or increase pain. Never try to move the injured area.

- ALSO   Loss of bowel or bladder control, priapism, impaired breathing.

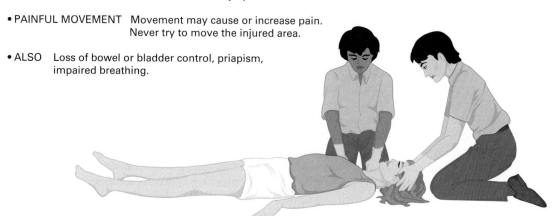

FIGURE 24-3   Provide immediate and continuing manual immobilization of the patient with possible spine injury while assessing for additional signs and symptoms.

During the rapid trauma assessment, palpate the entire posterior spine. Feel for any deformity, pain, crepitus, unusual warmth, or tenderness from C-1 through L-5. It may be beneficial to repeat palpation of the spine from L-5 to C-1, as pain or tenderness may be difficult to identify in the presence of other painful injuries when minor tenderness may be the only symptom of significant vertebral column instability.

Continue your assessment, inspecting each distal extremity and evaluating both motor and sensory functions. If there is any limb injury, perform what spinal assessment you can while working around the injuries and ensuring that you do not cause further harm to the limb.

For each upper extremity, test finger abduction/adduction (T-1) by having the patient spread the fingers of the hand, while you squeeze the second, third, and fourth fingers together. You should meet with bilaterally equal and moderate resistance to your effort. Test finger or hand extension (C-7) by having the patient hold the fingers and/or wrists fully extended. Place pressure against the back of the fingers, while you hold the forearm immobile. Again, you should meet bilaterally equal and moderate resistance. Finally, have the patient squeeze your first two fingers in his hand, and ensure that the grip is firm and bilaterally equal (Figure 24-4).

To assess for limb sensation, first ask the patient about any abnormal feelings in the limb—inability to move (paralysis), weakness, numbness (anesthesia),

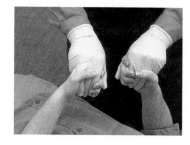

FIGURE 24-4   Compare grip strength bilaterally.

Assessment of the Spinal Injury Patient   **259**

tingling (paresthesia), or pain. Have the patient close both eyes, and check his ability to distinguish between sensations of pain and light touch. To check pain reception (the spinothalamic tract), induce slight point pain using the retracted tip of a ballpoint pen or another pointed object not likely to cause injury. To check for light touch (involving several tracts), use a cotton swab or a gentle touch with the pad of a finger. Responses to both pain and touch stimulation should be bilateral and equal.

Also, test the motor and sensory functions of the lower extremities (Figure 24-5). Place your hand against the ball of the patient's foot, and have him push firmly against it (plantar flexion, S-1 and S-2). Then, place your hand on top of the toes, and have the patient pull the toes and foot upward (dorsiflexion, L-5). To evaluate pain sensation, use the same techniques you used in testing the upper extremities. Lower limb strength and sensations should be present and bilaterally equal.

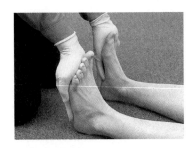

FIGURE 24-5   Compare lower limb strength bilaterally.

During the secondary assessment, look for any line of demarcation between normal sensation and paresthesia or anesthesia and any differences in muscle tone. Begin the assessment with the feet, and work up the body toward the head. Try not to alarm the patient because if he realizes that your touch is not felt, his anxiety may increase. Use a sharp object not likely to cause injury, such as a ballpoint pen with tip retracted, and feel upward. Note the level at which the patient first identifies sensation or pain, and relate it to the dermatomes. You might mark the level at which sensation is first noticed on the patient with a pen so that you can compare the results of later tests with your initial results.

Also, evaluate the myotomes to determine the level of muscular control. Suspect muscle flaccidity if a body area has muscle masses with a more relaxed tone than the rest of the body. These neurological signs give you a good indication of the level of spinal cord disruption. Examine both sides of the body, as there may be differences from side to side in both sensation and levels of voluntary and involuntary (muscle tone) motor activity.

You may also perform a test for Babinski's sign (Figure 24-6). Stroke the lateral aspect of the bottom of the foot, and watch for the movement of the toes and great toe. Fanning of the toes and dorsiflexion (lifting) of the great toe is a positive sign and suggests injury along the pyramidal (descending spinal) tracts.

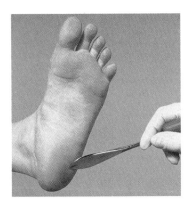

FIGURE 24-6   Test for Babinski's sign.

If discrete areas of nervous deficit exist, relate them to an injury along the nerve pathway or suspect injury to the spinal nerve root as it emerges from the spinal column. A nerve root injury suggests the possibility of a vertebral column injury and the need for spinal immobilization. Also, consider that the source of a deficit may be peripheral nerve damage related to soft-tissue or skeletal damage along its pathway to the affected area. Again, try to identify the associated dermatome and myotome and thus the likely location of the lesion along the spinal column, spinal root, or peripheral nerve.

Another sign of spinal injury is priapism. This prolonged, possibly painful erection of the penis is due to unopposed parasympathetic stimulation. Disruption of the sympathetic (thoracolumbar) pathways during a cervical spinal injury can produce this sign. In many cases, however, the pain sensation is lost due to disruption of the sensory pathways to the brain.

Occasionally, the patient with midcervical spinal injury presents with the "hold-up" position. The patient's arms spontaneously rise to a position above the shoulders and head. This occurs because the injury paralyzes the adductor and extensor muscles, while the patient maintains control over the abductors and flexors. Without the opposition of the adductors and extensors, normal muscle tone impulses or any attempt by the patient to move the limb cause it to move toward the flexed position. In such cases, simply tie the patient's wrists to his belt to hold the limbs down during transport.

If the patient does not show any signs or symptoms of spinal injury and the mechanism of injury does not suggest spinal injury, ask the patient to gently move his neck. If the patient experiences any pain or discomfort or shows any neurological deficit, employ spinal precautions, and consider transport to a neurocentre for further evaluation. Also, examine the extremities for signs of neurological impairment. If any are found, immediately employ spinal precautions.

Vital Signs

Evaluate the vital signs carefully in the patient with suspected spinal injury. Any signs of abnormally low blood pressure, slow heart rate, or absent, diaphragmatic, or shallow respirations indicate possible spinal cord injury.

Body temperature is an important consideration when evaluating the patient with suspected spinal injury. Spinal injury patients are subject to fluctuations in body temperature related to ambient temperature changes. This is because these patients lose the ability to control the skin's heat conservation/dissipation function below the lesion. While this does not result in an obvious sign in the patient, he is highly susceptible to body temperature fluctuations. Cover the patient with blankets in all but the warmest environments, and monitor the patient's temperature carefully.

At the conclusion of the rapid trauma assessment, consider the patient with any sign, symptom, or mechanism of injury suggestive of vertebral column or spinal cord injury for rapid transport to a nearby neurocentre or trauma centre. Employ full spinal precautions, monitor for neurogenic shock, and perform frequent ongoing patient assessments.

Any signs of abnormally low blood pressure, slow heart rate, or absent, diaphragmatic, or shallow respirations suggest possible spinal cord injury.

ONGOING ASSESSMENT

For the ongoing assessment, repeat the elements of the primary assessment, take vital signs, and reevaluate any signs or symptoms of spinal cord injury every five minutes (Figure 24-7). Monitor carefully for any changes in neurological signs, including levels of orientation, responsiveness, sensation, and motor function. Observe also for any changes in the dermatomes and myotomes affected by the injury. Look for any improvement or deterioration. Watch for a slowing pulse rate or a constant pulse rate in the presence of falling blood pressure. Watch for a dropping blood pressure without signs of shock compensation. Remember that spinal column injury may not produce any overt associated neurological signs or symptoms and yet may still threaten the spinal cord if the patient is moved without proper precautions.

MANAGEMENT OF THE SPINAL INJURY PATIENT

Spinal injury care steps (spinal precautions) performed during the primary assessment include moving the patient to the neutral, in-line position, maintaining that position with manual immobilization until the patient is fully immobilized by mechanical means, and applying the cervical collar once the neck assessment is complete. The remaining steps in management of the spinal injury patient are related to maintaining the neutral, in-line position while moving the patient to the long spine board and then firmly securing him to the board for transport to the hospital.

These skills have but one major objective: maintaining the neutral, in-line position. Although this might seem a simple objective, it is not. Remember that the spine is a chain of 33 small, rather delicate bones, which is attached to other

Spinal precautions have one major objective: maintaining the patient in the neutral, in-line position.

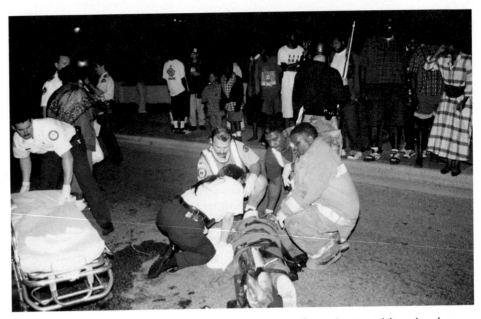

FIGURE 24-7   Repeat the ongoing assessment every five minutes with seriously injured patients.

skeletal members only at the head, thorax, and pelvis. These skeletal attachments may transmit forces that attempt to flex, extend, rotate, compress, distract, and laterally bend the spine during any patient movement. The procedures and devices discussed below are intended to ensure that the patient remains in the neutral, in-line position throughout care, movement, and transport.

Constantly calm and reassure the patient with suspected spinal injury. Spinal injury can produce extreme anxiety in patients because of the severity of its effects and their potentially lifelong implications. The application of spinal precautions can compound this anxiety. The patient must endure complete immobilization on a rigid and relatively uncomfortable device, the long spine board. He will be unable to move and protect himself during the processes of immobilization, assessment, care, and transport to the hospital. To alleviate some of the anxiety, be sure to communicate frequently with the patient. Tell the patient why you are employing spinal precautions and explain, in advance, what you will be doing in each step of the process. Do what you can to make the patient comfortable and to provide assurance that you and your team are caring for his needs.

SPINAL ALIGNMENT

The first step of the spinal precautions process is to bring the patient from the position in which he is found into a neutral, in-line position adequate for assessment, airway maintenance, and spinal immobilization. This process involves moving the patient to the supine position with the head facing directly forward and elevated 2 to 5 cm above the ground. Remember that the spine curves in an "S" shape through its length. This leaves the head displaced forward when the posterior thorax and buttocks (supporting the pelvis) rest on a firm, flat surface. Also, remember that the neutral position (also known as the position of function) is generally with the joints halfway between the extremes of their motion. In spinal positioning, this means that the hips and knees should be somewhat flexed for maximum comfort and minimum stress on the muscles, joints, and spine. For complete spinal immobilization, consider placement of a rolled blanket under the knees.

It is also important to ensure that there are no distracting or compressing forces on the spine. If the patient is seated or standing, support the head to leave only a portion of the head's weight on the spine. Be careful not to lift the entire head, as this places a distracting force on the spine. Lastly, bring the spine into line by aligning the nose, navel, and toes to ensure that there is no rotation along the spine's length. The head must face directly forward, and the shoulders and pelvis must be in a single plane with the body. This neutral, in-line positioning allows for the greatest spacing between the cord and inner lumen of the spinal foramen. Neutral, in-line positioning both reduces pressure on the cord and increases circulation to and through it, an especially important consideration in the presence of injury. There are many techniques for moving and immobilizing the patient with suspected spinal injury; whichever you employ, always focus on obtaining and then maintaining neutral, in-line positioning. Doing this ensures that you have the best opportunity to protect the vertebral column and the spinal cord of the patient during your time at his side.

The only contraindications to moving the patient with suspected spinal injury from the position in which he is found to the neutral, in-line position are as follows: when movement causes a noticeable increase in pain; when you meet with noticeable resistance during the procedure; when you identify an increase in neurological signs as you move the head; or when the patient's spine is grossly deformed. Pain and resistance both suggest that the alignment process may be moving the injury site and thus may be causing further injury. When you meet with resistance or increased pain during any positioning of the head or spine, immobilize the patient as found. The same rule applies when you note an increase in the signs of neurological injury in the patient with movement of the spine. Finally, in cases of severe deformity of the spine, do not move the patient because any movement will further compromise the column and the cord. Use whatever padding and immobilization devices are necessary to accommodate the patient's positioning, and ensure that no further movement occurs.

Ensure that any movement of the patient during assessment or care is toward alignment. If, for example, the patient is lying twisted on the ground when you find him, assess the exposed areas, then move the patient toward alignment. If the patient is found prone, assess the patient's posterior surfaces before you log roll him (to a long spine board) for further assessment and care. Never move a patient twice before you complete your mechanical immobilization if possible.

> *Move any body segment that is out of alignment toward alignment as you examine it, but if the patient feels any increase in pain or if you feel resistance to movement, immobilize the head and neck or other portion of the body in the position achieved.*
>
>

MANUAL CERVICAL IMMOBILIZATION

The typical trauma patient is found either seated (as in an auto) or lying on the ground. With the seated patient, initially approach from the front, and carefully instruct the patient not to move or turn the head. It is an almost reflexive act to turn to listen when we hear someone speak to us from behind. Such movement is dangerous in the patient with suspected spinal injury. Ask your patient to keep his head immobile, and explain to the patient that a caregiver is going to position himself behind the patient to immobilize the spine.

Then, the assigned caregiver should move behind the patient and bring his hands up along the patient's ears, using the little fingers to catch the mandible and the medial aspect of the heels of the hand to engage the mastoid region of the skull (Figure 24-8). Gentle pressure inward engages the head and prevents it from moving. A gentle lifting force of a few kilograms helps take some of the weight of the head off the cervical spine, but care should be taken not to lift the head or apply any traction to this critical region. The patient's head should then be moved slowly and easily to a position in which the eyes face directly forward and along a line central to and perpendicular to the shoulder plane.

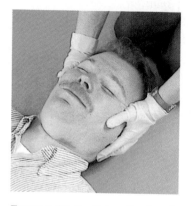

FIGURE 24-8 Bring the head to the neutral, in-line position, and maintain manual immobilization until the head, neck, and spine are mechanically immobilized.

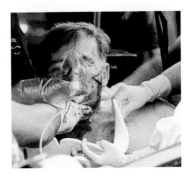

FIGURE 24-9 When you cannot access the patient from behind to apply manual immobilization, use alternative hand placement.

If there is no access to the seated patient from behind, employ the same techniques of movement and immobilization from the front with the little fingers engaging the mastoid region, while the heels of the hand support the mandible. When approaching from the patient's side, place one hand under the mandible while using the other to support the occiput (Figure 24-9).

If the patient is supine, support the head by placing your hands along the lateral and inferior surfaces of the head. Position the little fingers and heels of the hands just lateral to the occipital region of the skull to support the head. With gentle inward pressure, hold the patient's head immobile, and prevent flexion/extension, rotation, and lateral bending motions. Lift the head gently off the ground to approximate the neutral position, usually 2–5 cm for the adult. (If the surface on which the patient is found is not flat, adjust the height accordingly.) Position a small adult's or a large child's head at about ground level. Elevate the shoulders of infants or very small children because of their proportionally larger heads. Apply no axial pressure by either pushing or pulling the head toward or away from the body.

If a patient is found prone or on the side, position your hands according to the patient's position. If it will be some time until the patient can be moved to the supine position, place your hands such that they are comfortable during cervical immobilization. You should then reposition your hands just before the patient is moved to the final position. If the time until moving the patient to the supine position is expected to be short, place your hands such that they will be properly positioned at the conclusion of the move. This may involve initially twisting your hands into a relatively uncomfortable position.

Assessment, care, and patient movement may require the caregiver maintaining immobilization to reposition his hands. To accomplish this, another caregiver supports and immobilizes the patient's head and neck by bringing his hands in from an alternative position. This caregiver places one hand under the patient's occiput, while the other hand holds the jaw. Once the head is stable, have the original caregiver reposition his hands, reassume immobilization, and then have the second caregiver remove his hands.

CERVICAL COLLAR APPLICATION

A cervical collar by itself does not immobilize the cervical spine.

Always ensure that the cervical collar is correctly sized for the patient, or choose another one.

After a patient with suspected spinal injury has been manually immobilized, consider the application of the cervical collar. Apply the collar as soon as the neck is fully assessed, generally during the rapid trauma assessment. The cervical collar is only an adjunct to full cervical immobilization and should never be considered to provide immobilization by itself. The collar does limit cervical spine motion and reduce the forces of compression (axial loading), but it does not completely prevent flexion/extension, rotation, or lateral bending.

To apply the cervical collar, size it to the patient according to the manufacturer's recommendations. Position the device under the chin and against the chest. Contour it over the shoulders, and secure it firmly behind the neck. Be sure the Velcro® closures remain clear of sand, dirt, fabric, or the patient's hair and make a secure seal behind the neck (Figure 24-10). The collar should fit snugly around the neck but not place pressure against its anterior surface (carotid and jugular blood vessels and trachea). The collar should direct a limiting force against the jaw and occiput to restrict any flexion/extension of the head and neck. Ensure that the collar does not seriously limit the movement of the jaw, as this could prevent the patient from vomiting. Once the cervical collar is in place, do not release or relax manual cervical immobilization until the patient is fully immobilized either with a vest-type immobilization device or to a long spine board with a cervical immobilization device.

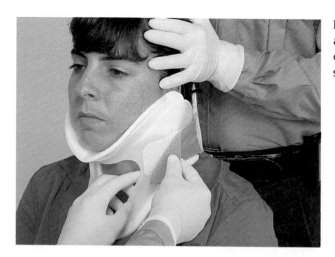

FIGURE 24-10 Properly place and secure the cervical collar on patients with suspected spinal injury.

STANDING TAKEDOWN

Often, at vehicle collision sites, you will find patients walking around when the mechanisms of injury suggest possible spinal injuries. These patients must receive spinal precautions, even though they are found standing. Your objective in such cases is to bring the patient to a fully supine position for further assessment, care, immobilization, and transport.

To accomplish this, employ a standing takedown procedure that maintains the spine in axial alignment. Have the patient remain immobile, while a caregiver approaches from the rear and assumes manual cervical immobilization. Quickly assess any areas that will be covered by the cervical collar or long spine board. Apply a cervical collar, and place a long spine board behind and against the patient, with the caregiver maintaining immobilization spreading his arms to accommodate the board. Position two other caregivers, one on each side of the spine board, and have each place a hand under the patient's axilla and with it grasp the closest (preferably next higher) handhold on the board. The team should then move the patient and spine board backward, tilting the patient on his heels until the patient and the board are supine (Figure 24-11).

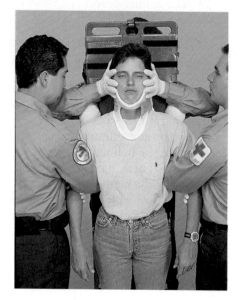

FIGURE 24-11 The standing takedown.

Management of the Spinal Injury Patient **265**

During the move, the hands in the handholds support the thorax, while the caregiver maintaining cervical immobilization rotates his hands against the patient's head without either flexing or extending the head and neck as the patient moves from standing to supine. During this manoeuvre, the hands holding the patient's head must move from grasping the mastoid and mandible (standing) to grasping the lateral occiput (supine). This is not easy, as the head must rotate while the caregiver's hands remain in the same relative position. As with all movement procedures, the caregiver at the patient's head should be in control and direct the process.

Once the patient and board are on the ground, continue to maintain manual immobilization while assessing and caring for the patient. Then, provide mechanical immobilization to the long spine board before moving the patient to the ambulance.

HELMET REMOVAL

Helmet removal may be a tricky endeavour. You should familiarize yourself with the types of helmets used by sporting teams in your area (e.g., high-school football).

Helmet use in contact sports, bicycling, skateboarding, in-line skating, and motorcycling has increased over the past decade. While these devices offer significant protection for the head during impact, they have not proven to reduce spinal injuries. Their use also complicates spinal injury care for the paramedics. Many helmets are of the partial variety (such as those worn for bicycling and skateboarding) and are easy to remove at the trauma scene. Some motorcycle and sports helmets, however, fully enclose the head and are very difficult to remove in the field. These helmets are also very difficult to secure to the spine board because of their spherical shapes. Further, most full helmets do not hold the head firmly within; so even fixing the helmet securely to the spine board does not result in effective cervical immobilization. Some newer contact sport helmets contain air bladders that expand and firmly hold the head in position within the helmet. These helmets immobilize the head well, but they are still difficult to firmly secure to a spine board. Consequently, most full-enclosure helmets must be removed to ensure adequate spinal immobilization.

The helmet must be removed if you find any of the following conditions:

- The helmet does not immobilize the patient's head within.
- You cannot securely immobilize the helmet to the long spine board.
- The helmet prevents airway care.
- The helmet prevents assessment of anticipated injuries.
- There are, or you anticipate, airway or breathing problems.
- Helmet removal will not cause further injury.

During helmet removal, have a caregiver initially stabilize the cervical spine by manually stabilizing the helmet. Remove the face mask, if present, either by unscrewing it or by cutting it off if possible. Remove or retract any eye protection or visor and unfasten or cut away any chin strap as well. Be careful not to manipulate the helmet or otherwise transmit movement to the patient through the helmet. Then, have another caregiver immobilize the head by sliding his hands under the helmet and placing them along the sides of the head, supporting the occiput, or by placing one hand on the jaw and the other on the occiput. This caregiver should choose the hand placement that works best for him and that can be accommodated by the helmet. The caregiver holding the helmet should then grasp the helmet and spread it slightly to clear the ears by pulling laterally just below and anterior to the ear enclosure. That caregiver then rotates the helmet to clear the chin, counter-rotates it to clear the occiput, and then rotates it to clear the nose and brow ridge (Figure 24-12). The clearance is usually very tight with a well-fitted helmet.

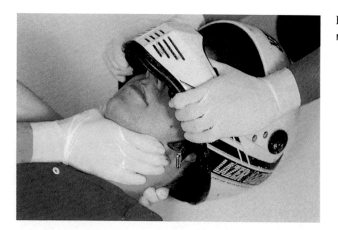

FIGURE 24-12 Helmet removal.

Execute the procedure slowly and carefully to prevent head and neck motion and to minimize patient discomfort. For helmets with air bladders, use the same procedure, but empty the bladder after someone stabilizes the head and before you begin the removal. Helmet removal is a complex skill that you must practise frequently before you can employ it successfully in the field.

MOVEMENT OF THE SPINAL INJURY PATIENT

Once you assess and provide the essential care for a patient with a suspected spinal injury, plan the movement to the long spine board carefully. If any step of assessment or patient care requires patient movement, consider moving the patient onto the long spine board. Movement techniques suitable for moving the spinal injury patient to the long spine board include the log roll, straddle slide, orthopedic stretcher lift, application of a vest-type device (or short spine board), and rapid extrication. Choose a technique that affords the least spinal movement depending on the conditions and equipment at hand. Also, select your movement technique and adjust its steps to accommodate the patient's particular injuries.

A key factor in all movement techniques for the patient with suspected spinal injury is the coordination of the move. It is essential that you move the patient as a unit with his head facing forward and in a plane with the shoulders and hips. This can best be accomplished if the caregiver at the head controls and directs the move. He is able to see the other rescuers and has a focused and limited function (holding the head), which permits that person to evaluate what the other caregivers are doing. The caregiver at the head directs the move by counting a cadence, such as, "Move on four—one, two, three, four." A four count is preferable as it gives the other caregivers a good opportunity to anticipate the actual start of movement. All moves must be executed slowly and be well coordinated among caregivers.

Consider what the final positioning of the patient will be when you choose a spinal movement technique. Most spinal injury patients are best served with supine positioning on a long spine board. However, a patient with a thoracic spine injury is frequently placed in a prone position on a soft stretcher. With this patient, any other positioning, such as supine on a firm spine board, puts pressure on the injury site from the body's weight, and any movement is more likely to cause movement of the injury site and compound any damage.

Choose a spinal movement technique that affords the least spinal movement.
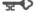

The caregiver at the head directs and controls the movement of the patient with a suspected spinal injury.

A four-count is a preferable cadence as it gives a good opportunity to anticipate the start of the move.

Log Roll

The log roll can be used to rotate the patient 90 degrees, insert the long spine board, and then roll the patient back. It can also be used to roll the patient 180 degrees from prone to supine or vice versa.

FIGURE 24-13 The four-person log roll.

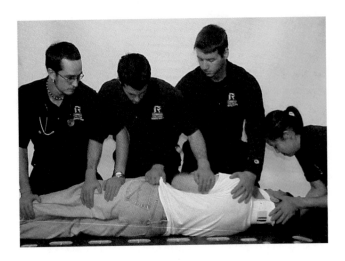

As you begin the 90-degree roll, ensure manual spinal immobilization, and apply a cervical collar. Note that anatomically the shoulders are wider than the hips and legs. To provide a uniform roll, extend the patient's arm above his head. Then, place a bulky blanket between the legs (with its bulkiest portion between the feet) and tie the legs together. This reduces pelvic movement and lateral bending of the lumbar spine.

It takes four caregivers to perform the log roll with a spinal injury patient (Figure 24-13). One caregiver holds the head, while one kneels at the patient's shoulder with the knees tight against the patient's chest. The third caregiver kneels at the patient's hip with the knees tight against the patient's hip. The last caregiver kneels at the patient's knees with his knees tight against the patient's knees.

The caregivers reach across the patient and around the opposite shoulder, hip, and knee, respectively, and grasp the patient firmly. On a count initiated by the caregiver at the head, the team, in unison, rolls the patient against their knees and past a 90-degree angle. With a free hand, the caregiver at the knees (or an additional caregiver) slides a long spine board under the patient from the patient's side or the foot end. The board should be positioned tightly against the patient so that the head, torso, and pelvis will eventually rest solidly on the board. Then, at the count of the caregiver at the head, the team rolls the patient back 90 degrees onto the board.

The 180-degree log roll begins with placement of the long spine board between the caregivers and the patient, with the board resting at an angle on the caregivers' thighs. The caregivers reach across the board and grasp the patient as for the 90-degree log roll. The caregiver at the head must be careful to anticipate the turning motion and position his hands so that they will be comfortably positioned at the end of the roll. On the count of the caregiver at the head, the team rolls the patient past 90 degrees until he is positioned against the tilted long spine board. Then, they reposition their hands against the other (lower) side of the patient and slowly back their thighs out from under the patient until the board rests on the ground.

Straddle Slide

Another technique effective for moving the patient with suspected spinal injury is the straddle slide. In this procedure, three caregivers are positioned at the patient's head, shoulders, and pelvis, while a fourth prepares to insert the long spine board from the side of the patient's head or feet. The caregiver at the head maintains cervical immobilization and guides the lift with a cadence. The second caregiver straddles the patient (facing the patient's head) and grasps the shoulders. The third caregiver straddles the patient (facing the head) and grasps the pelvis. All the caregivers keep their feet planted widely enough apart to permit the insertion of the long spine board. At the direction of the caregiver at the head, the three caregivers lift the patient just enough to permit the fourth caregiver to carefully position the long spine board underneath the patient. (Note: If the board is to be inserted from the side of the patient's feet, the caregiver inserting the board lifts the patient's feet with one hand and slides the board into place with the other.) On a signal from the caregiver at the head, the team gently lowers the patient to the long spine board.

Orthopedic Stretcher

The orthopedic stretcher, also known as the scoop stretcher, is a valuable device for positioning the patient on the spine board or helping secure the patient to the long spine board. To apply the device, lengthen it to accommodate the patient's height, and then separate it into its two halves. Maintain cervical immobilization while you gently negotiate each half of the stretcher under the patient from the sides and connect them at the top, and then the bottom. Be careful not to entrap the patient's skin or body parts while positioning the stretcher, especially on uneven ground. Once the device is connected, you may use the stretcher to lift the patient to the waiting spine board. Orthopedic stretchers are usually not rigid enough to be used by themselves as transport devices for spinal injury patients. Rather, they are most effective in moving patients to the long spine board, where they may remain as an adjunct to full immobilization, or you may disconnect the halves, remove them, and immobilize the patient to the long spine board in the usual way.

Vest–Type Immobilization Device (and Short Spine Board)

A specialized piece of EMS equipment that may be used with some spinal injury patients is the vest-type immobilization device (Figure 24-14). This device immobilizes the patient's head, shoulders, and pelvis to a rigid board so that you can move the patient from a seated position, as in an automobile, to a fully supine position. The vest-type device comes as a commercially made device that usually has the needed strapping already attached. The device is usually constructed of thin, rigid wood or plastic strips embedded in a vinyl or fabric vest. It is then wrapped and secured around the patient to provide immobilization.

To apply the vest-type device, manually immobilize the patient's cervical spine, and apply a cervical collar while the device is being readied for application.

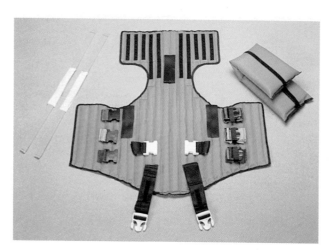

FIGURE 24-14   A vest-type immobilization device.

If the patient is positioned against a soft seat (as in an automobile), gently move the patient's shoulders and head a few inches forward to permit insertion of the vest. The caregiver holding cervical immobilization directs and coordinates the move, while a second caregiver guides and controls shoulder movement. Position the device behind the patient by either inserting the head portion under and through the arms of the caregiver providing cervical immobilization, or angling it, base first, and then moving it behind the patient's back. Position the device vertically so that the chest appendages fit just under the arms. This positioning permits you to fasten the straps and secure the shoulders without any upward or downward movement of the device. First, secure the device to the chest and pelvis with strapping, and ensure that the vest is immobile. Tighten the straps firmly, but be sure that they do not inhibit respiration. Secure the thigh straps as they hold the hips and thighs in the flexed position, limiting lumbar motion. Then, fill the space between the occiput and the device with noncompressible padding to ensure neutral positioning. Secure both the brow ridge and the chin to the device with straps, but be very careful to allow for vomiting by the patient and subsequent clearing of the airway, or be prepared to cut the chin strap immediately if vomiting occurs. Tie the patient's wrists together.

The vest-type immobilization device is not meant to lift the patient but rather to facilitate rotating him on the buttocks and then to tilt the patient to the supine position for further spinal immobilization (Figure 24-15). Once the patient is positioned on the long spine board, gently and carefully release the thigh straps and slowly and gently extend the hips and knees. If the patient's head remains firmly affixed to the vest-type device after transfer to the spine board, leave the vest on the patient, and secure the vest to the long spine board, since doing this effectively secures both head and torso. If the head becomes loose during the transfer, reapply manual cervical immobilization, secure the torso with strapping, and secure the head with a cervical immobilization device.

Rapid Extrication

Applying a vest-type immobilization device is a time-consuming process. Often, the circumstances of the emergency—either issues of scene safety or the need for rapid transport to the trauma centre—preclude spending the time required for standard spinal immobilization. In such cases, use a rapid extrication procedure.

With whatever personnel available, stabilize the patient's spine, shoulders, pelvis, and legs, with the patient's nose, navel, and toes in a straight line. Ensure that caregivers are coordinated and understand what move is to take place. One

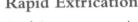

The vest-type device is not meant to lift the patient but rather to facilitate rotating and tilting the patient to the supine position.

FIGURE 24-15 The vest-type immobilization device is not intended for lifting the patient but for pivoting him.

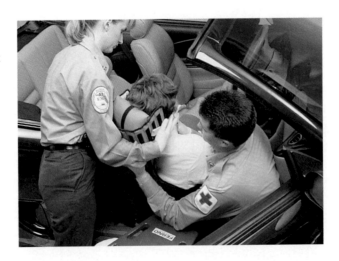

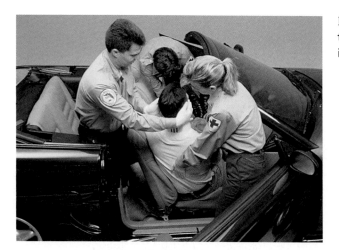

FIGURE 24-16 Rapid extrication of a patient with a spinal injury.

caregiver, usually at the patient's head, should direct the move, counting a cadence to enable the crew to work together (Figure 24-16). Ensure that personnel involved in the extrication move the patient but maintain the alignment of the patient's nose, naval, and toes. Then, on the leader's count, they should move the patient from a seated or other position to a waiting spine board.

Remember the objectives of movement and stabilization of the spine: keep the spine in the neutral, in-line position by keeping the patient's eyes facing directly forward and keeping the shoulders and pelvis in a plane perpendicular to that of the gaze. Be sure to prevent any flexion/extension, rotation, or lateral bending.

While the technique of rapid extrication does not provide maximum protection for the spine, it does permit rapid transport of the patient with a spinal injury when other considerations demand it. Use the procedure only when your patient cannot afford the time it would take for normal movement techniques. Rapid extrication from the confined space of a wrecked automobile is difficult at best. Plan your move carefully, and execute the rapid extrication by carefully explaining the process and individual responsibilities to your team members.

> *During all movement of a spinal injury patient, keep the spine in the neutral, in-line position by keeping the patient's eyes facing directly forward, and the shoulders, pelvis, and toes in the same plane.*
>
>

Final Patient Positioning

Centring the patient on the board is essential to ensuring that the patient's spine remains in line and he is effectively immobilized. Accomplish this by placing team members at the patient's head, shoulders, pelvis, and feet. The caregivers then place one hand on each side of the patient and prepare to move the patient toward the centre of the board. On a cadence signalled by the caregiver at the head, they slide the portion of the patient that is out of alignment to an in-line position, centred on the long spine board.

Long Spine Board

The long spine board is simply a reinforced flat, firm surface designed to facilitate immobilization of a patient in a supine or prone position (Figure 24-17). While the board may immobilize patients with multisystem trauma, pelvic and lower limb fractures, and many other types of trauma, it is primarily designed for patients with spinal injuries. The board has several hand and strap holes along its lateral borders. Using nylon web strapping, you can immobilize a patient with almost any combination of injuries to the board firmly enough to permit rotating the patient and the board 90 degrees to clear the airway in case vomiting occurs.

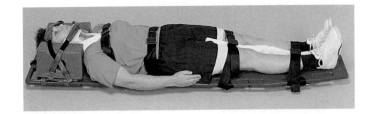

Secure the patient to the board with the strapping, immobilizing and holding the shoulders and pelvis firmly to the board. Such strapping may cross the body and capture the shoulder and pelvic girdles. Ensure that you firmly immobilize the patient to prevent lateral movement as well as cephalad (head-ward) and caudad (tail-ward) movement. Be sure that the pressure created by strapping does not come to bear on the central abdomen. That would cause forced extension of the lumbar spine. Immobilize the lower legs and feet with strapping or cravats. Tie the legs together, and place a rolled blanket under the patient's knees to immobilize them in a slightly flexed position.

Long spine board immobilization is made more effective by use of the cervical immobilization device (CID). This device is made up of two soft, padded lateral pieces that bracket the patient's head, maintaining its position, and a base plate that permits you to easily secure the device to the board. The base plate is affixed to the long spine board before the patient is moved to it. Once you position the patient on the board, fill the void between the occiput and the CID base plate with firm, noncompressible padding. Use no padding for the small adult or the older child, and pad the shoulders in the young child or infant to ensure proper spinal positioning. While a caregiver maintains manual immobilization of the head, bring the lateral components of the CID against the sides of the patient's head. Use medial pressure to hold the lateral CID components against the head and hold the head in position. Then, affix the lateral CID components to the Velcro® of the CID base plate. Secure the head in position and to the long spine board using forehead and chin straps or tape. Make sure the strapping catches the brow ridge and the mandible or the upper portion of the collar. The properly secured CID must hold the patient's head in the neutral position without movement while not placing undue pressure on the neck or restricting jaw movement (in case vomiting occurs). Be careful that the straps do not flex, extend, or rotate the head. Bulky blanket rolls, placed on each side of the head and secured both to the head and to the board will also effectively immobilize the head to the long spine board.

The long spine board does have drawbacks. Its firm surface places extreme pressure on the skin and tissues covering the ischial tuberosities and the shoulder blades. If a patient remains immobilized to the board for more than a couple of hours, ulceration injuries are likely to result.

The board also tends to encourage caregivers to immobilize the patient directly to it in a nonneutral position. In a proper neutral position, the head should be elevated about 2–5 cm above the board's surface and the knees should be bent at 15 to 30 degrees. This positioning relieves pressure on the cervical spine, lumbar spine, hips, and knees and increases patient comfort. You can obtain proper knee positioning by placing folded blankets under the patient's knees. Also, pad under the curves of the back. Do not overpad; just fill the gaps at the small of the back and neck with bulky soft dressing material.

Diving Injury Immobilization

Patients injured in shallow water dives are often paralyzed by the impact. They must rely on others to protect their airways and remove them from the water.

Immobilize the adult patient to the long spine board with the head elevated 2–5 cm, the knees slightly flexed, and with limited padding at the small of the back and the space behind the neck.

When carried out by untrained bystanders, however, these activities may compound any spinal injury. If you are present when such an accident occurs, be sure to carefully control any patient movement while he is still in the water. If necessary, turn him to a supine position, ensuring that the nose, navel, and toes remain in a single plane and that the eyes face directly forward. You may accomplish this by sandwiching the patient's chest between your forearms, while your arms and shoulders cradle the head. Once the patient is in the supine position, water provides an almost neutral buoyancy and, if the water is calm, helps immobilize the patient. Move the patient by pulling on the shoulders, while you cradle the head, in the neutral position, with your forearms. Float a long spine board under the patient to lift and carry him from the water.

MEDICATIONS

There are several conditions in which you may use medications to treat spinal injury patients, if permitted by your system's protocols. These conditions include neurogenic shock and the combative patient.

Medications and Neurogenic Shock

The loss of sympathetic control leads to both a relaxation of the blood vessels (vasodilation) below the level of the lesion and the inability of the body to increase the heart rate. This expanded vascular system leads to a relative hypovolemia and lower blood pressure. The problem is further compounded as the heart, without sympathetic stimulation and in the presence of this relative hypovolemia, displays a normal or bradycardic heart rate. Frequently, the hypovolemia is treated with a fluid challenge, followed by careful use of a vasopressor, such as dopamine. The slow heart rate is treated with atropine to reduce any parasympathetic stimulation.

The initial treatment for hypovolemia from suspected neurogenic shock is by fluid challenge. Establish an IV with a 1000-mL bag of Ringer's Lactate solution or normal saline, a nonrestrictive administration set, and a large-bore IV catheter. Administer 250 mL of solution quickly, monitor the blood pressure and heart rate, and auscultate the lungs for signs of developing pulmonary edema (crackles). If the patient responds with an increasing blood pressure, a slowing heart rate, and signs of improved perfusion, consider a second bolus. Monitor the patient, and administer a second bolus if the patient's signs and symptoms begin to deteriorate. If the patient does not improve with the fluid challenge, consider vasopressor therapy, as allowed by your protocols.

Dopamine (Intropin®) is a naturally occurring catecholamine that, in addition to its own actions, causes the release of norepinephrine. Dopamine increases cardiac contractility and hence cardiac output and, at higher doses, increases peripheral vascular resistance, venous constriction, cardiac preload, and blood pressure. While there are no contraindications for dopamine use in the emergency setting, its common side effects include tachydysrhythmias, hypertension, headache, nausea, and vomiting.

Dopamine is frequently packaged as either a premixed solution containing 800 or 1600 µg/mL or as a 5-mL vial containing 200 or 400 mg of drug. Vial contents are added to 250 mL of D5W to yield a concentration of either 800 or 1600 µg/mL. Dopamine is extremely light sensitive and once mixed should be discarded after 24 hours. If the solution is either pink or brown, discard it. Dopamine's onset of action is about five minutes, and its half-life is around two minutes; hence, it is administered via a continuous infusion. It should be run piggyback through an already well-established IV line, as infiltration can cause tissue necrosis. It is administered initially at 2.5 µg/kg/min, and then titrated to an increase in blood pressure or a maximum of 120 µg/kg/min. (Vasoconstriction usually begins at doses above 10 µg/kg/min)

Interruption of the sympathetic pathways by spinal cord injury causes unopposed parasympathetic stimulation and bradycardia (or at least prevents the compensatory tachycardia that occurs with decreased cardiac preload). The net result is a decrease in cardiac output. Atropine is administered to block the parasympathetic impulse that might contribute to slow down the heart rate.

Atropine is an anticholinergic agent most frequently used to treat symptomatic bradycardia and heart blocks in myocardial infarction. It is sometimes helpful in increasing the heart rate of patients with upper spinal cord injury due to unopposed vagal stimulation. It acts by inhibiting the actions of acetylcholine, the major parasympathetic neurotransmitter. Atropine has a quick onset of action and a half-life of just over two hours. It is available for emergency use in 5- and 10-mL preloaded syringes containing a concentration of 0.5 mg/mL. Atropine is administered rapidly in 0.5 mg (1 mL) intravenous doses every 3 to 5 minutes, up to a maximum of 2 mg. The only expected side effects in the emergency setting are dry mouth, blurred vision, and, possibly, tachycardia.

Medications and the Combative Patient

Frequently, the patient who has sustained potentially serious spinal injury has also sustained head injury, is intoxicated, or is otherwise very uncooperative or combative. In some of these cases, sedatives may be indicated to reduce anxiety and because the patient actively resists spinal precautions. Consider using meperidine (Demerol®) or diazepam (Valium®) to calm the patient. In extreme circumstances, consider use of the paralytics mentioned in Chapter 23, "Head, Facial, and Neck Trauma" in the discussion of facilitated intubation to paralyze the patient. Whenever you use these agents, you must carefully monitor the patient's level of consciousness and respirations. With use of paralytics, you must provide continuing ventilation for the patient during the action of the drug. Sedatives and paralytics should only be administered as permitted by your system's protocols and under the close and direct supervision of an online medical direction physician.

SUMMARY

Spinal injury is a frequent consequence of serious trauma and likely to cause serious disability or death. Injury to the spinal column may occur with only minimal signs and symptoms. So, prehospital care for any patient with a significant mechanism of injury or any trauma patient with a reduced level of consciousness must include spinal precautions. Throughout patient assessment, immobilization, and movement, provide emotional support and calming reassurance to lower patient anxiety, and carefully monitor the level of consciousness.

CHAPTER 25

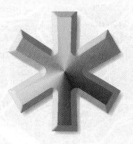

Thoracic Trauma

Objectives

After reading this chapter, you should be able to:

1. Describe the incidence, morbidity, and mortality of thoracic injuries in the trauma patient. (p. 277)
2. Discuss the anatomy and physiology of the thoracic organs and structures. (see Chapter 12)
3. Predict thoracic injuries on the basis of mechanism of injury. (pp. 278–280)
4. Discuss the pathophysiology of, assessment findings with, and the management and need for rapid intervention and transport of the patient with chest wall injuries, including the following:
   a. Rib fracture (pp. 281–282, 302–303)
   b. Flail segment (pp. 283–284, 303)
   c. Sternal fracture (pp. 282–283)

5. Discuss the pathophysiology of, assessment findings with, and management and need for rapid intervention and transport of the patient with injury to the lung, including the following:
   a. Simple pneumothorax (pp. 285–286)
   b. Open pneumothorax (pp. 286–287, 303)
   c. Tension pneumothorax (pp. 287–288, 304–305)
   d. Hemothorax (pp. 288–289, 305)
   e. Hemopneumothorax (p. 288)
   f. Pulmonary contusion (pp. 289–290)

Continued

Objectives Continued

6. Discuss the pathophysiology of, findings of assessment with, and management and need for rapid intervention and transport of the patient with myocardial injuries, including the following:
   a. Myocardial contusion (pp. 290–291, 306)
   b. Pericardial tamponade (pp. 291–293, 306)
   c. Myocardial rupture (pp. 293–294, 306)

7. Discuss the pathophysiology of, findings of assessment with, and management and need for rapid intervention and transport of the patient with vascular injuries, including injuries to the following:
   a. Aorta (pp. 294, 306)
   b. Vena cava (p. 294)
   c. Pulmonary arteries/veins (p. 294)

8. Discuss the pathophysiology of, findings of assessment with, and management and need for rapid intervention and transport of patients with diaphragmatic, esophageal, and tracheobronchial injuries. (pp. 295–296, 306)

9. Discuss the pathophysiology of, findings of assessment with, and management and need for rapid intervention and transport of the patient with traumatic asphyxia. (pp. 296, 306–307)

10. Differentiate among thoracic injuries on the basis of the assessment and history. (pp. 296–302)

11. Given several preprogrammed and moulaged thoracic trauma patients, provide the appropriate scene assessment, primary assessment, rapid trauma or secondary assessment and history, detailed assessment, and ongoing assessment and provide appropriate patient care and transport. (pp. 296–307)

INTRODUCTION TO THORACIC INJURY

The thoracic cavity contains many vital structures, including the heart, great vessels, esophagus, **tracheobronchial tree,** and lungs. Trauma to any one of these structures could lead to a life-threatening event. Twenty-five percent of all motor-vehicle deaths are due to thoracic trauma. The majority of these deaths are secondary to injury to the heart and great vessels. In addition, abdominal injuries are also common in patients with traumatic chest injury and can cause significant **co-morbidity.**

The incidence of blunt thoracic trauma has increased with the development of the modern automobile (Figure 25-1). Together with the development of a national highway system, more people are travelling greater distances, at greater speeds, and roadways are becoming more congested. This allows for an increased incidence of motor-vehicle collisions (MVCs) and thus an increase in the incidence of thoracic injuries and subsequent deaths, as most blunt thoracic trauma deaths are MVC related. An increase in penetrating trauma associated with violent crime has also been observed in urban areas. The weapons used in violent crime in years past were likely to be of the "Saturday night special" variety, cheap small-calibre revolvers, often producing just single wounds. The weapons of choice now are more likely to be large-calibre semi-automatic or automatic weapons that increase the likelihood of multiple missile injuries. With multiple wounds, there is a higher likelihood of injury to vital structures and therefore a higher mortality. Many advances in the treatment of penetrating thoracoabdominal trauma have been made in recent wars, and the incidence of mortality from these wounds has decreased from 8 to 40 percent in World War II to 3 to 18 percent today.

Prevention efforts include gun control legislation, firearm safety courses, seatbelt laws, and better design of automobiles, including passive restraint systems, such as airbags. Statistics indicate that these efforts have already decreased the incidence of these injuries and the related morbidity and mortality.

In this chapter, we will discuss thoracic trauma in relation to penetrating and blunt injuries. These mechanisms have more clinical significance than simple injury categories. Certain injuries are almost exclusively associated with one type of chest trauma but unlikely with the other. For example, pericardial tamponade is almost exclusively associated with penetrating thoracic trauma, while cardiac rupture is almost exclusively caused by blunt thoracic trauma. By considering the mechanism of injury, understanding the pathology of the various injuries, and by being aware of the patient's physical signs of injury and symptoms, you will be better able to predict, identify, and treat potential life threats.

Twenty-five percent of all motor-vehicle deaths are due to thoracic trauma.

✱ **tracheobronchial tree** the structures of the trachea and the bronchi.

✱ **co-morbidity** associated disease process.

Penetrating trauma is increasing in urban areas.

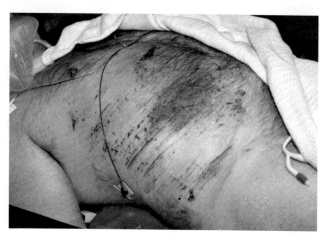

FIGURE 25-1 An example of blunt trauma to the chest.

PATHOPHYSIOLOGY OF THORACIC TRAUMA

Thoracic trauma is classified into two major categories by mechanism; blunt and penetrating. It is important to examine these injury mechanisms and their effects on the organs of the thorax.

BLUNT TRAUMA

Blunt thoracic trauma is injury resulting from kinetic energy forces transmitted through the tissues. These injuries may be further subdivided by mechanism into blast, crush (compression), and deceleration injuries.

Blast injuries result from an explosive chemical reaction that creates a pressure wave travelling outward from the epicentre. This pressure wave causes tissue disruption by dramatic compression and then decompression as the wave passes. In the thorax, this action may tear blood vessels and disrupt the alveolar tissue. These injuries may lead to hemorrhage, pneumothoraces, and air embolism (air entering the disrupted pulmonary vasculature and subsequently returning to the central circulation). Other injuries associated with a blast mechanism can include disruption of the tracheobronchial tree and traumatic rupture of the diaphragm. When the blast occurs in a confined space, the pressure wave may be contained and accentuated. The result is an increase in the incidence and severity of the associated injuries.

Crush injuries occur when the body is compressed between an object and a hard surface. This leads to direct injury or disruption of the chest wall, diaphragm, heart, or tracheobronchial tree. If the victim remains pinned between two objects, significant restriction in ventilation and venous return may occur, also known as traumatic asphyxia.

Deceleration injuries occur when the body is in motion and strikes a fixed object as, for example, the chest against the steering column in a front-end collision (Figure 25-2). This impact causes a direct blunt injury to the chest wall, while the internal organs of the thoracic cavity continue in motion. The organs and structures then collide with the internal surface of the thoracic cavity and may be compressed as more posterior structures collide with them. If the organ or structure has points of fixation, as with the aorta at the ligamentum arteriosum, the force of the organ moving against this point of fixation (shear force) can lead to a traumatic disruption. These sudden deceleration and shear forces can

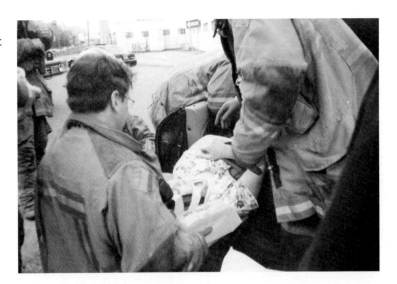

FIGURE 25-2 Frontal impact auto collisions frequently result in chest trauma.

cause disruption of the myocardium, great vessel, lung, trachea, and bronchi. The rapid compression of the chest, especially against a closed glottis, may also cause alveolar and tracheobronchial rupture and pneumothorax.

The age of the victim of blunt trauma may affect the trauma received and its seriousness. The cartilaginous nature of the pediatric thorax spares the infant or child from rib fractures but more easily transmits the energy of trauma to the vital organs below. The result is more minor signs of injury, few rib fractures, and a greater incidence of serious internal injury. The geriatric patient responds very differently to blunt chest trauma. That patient will suffer more frequent rib fracture than the younger adult due to calcification of the skeletal system. Though the greater incidence of rib fracture may somewhat protect the underlying organs, preexisting disease and the progressive reduction of respiratory and cardiac reserves result in a greater morbidity and mortality from serious chest trauma.

The age of the victim of blunt trauma may affect the seriousness of the trauma received.

PENETRATING TRAUMA

Penetrating thoracic trauma induces injury as an object enters the chest and causes either direct trauma or secondary injury from transmitted kinetic energy forces related to the cavitational wave of high velocity projectiles. Penetrating chest trauma can be subdivided into three categories: low-energy, high-energy, and shotgun wounds.

Low-energy wounds are those caused by arrows, knives, handguns, and other relatively slow moving objects (Figure 25-3). They cause injury by direct contact or very limited creation of temporary cavities. The injury that occurs from this type of wound is related to the direct path that the missile or object takes.

High-energy wounds are caused by military and hunting rifles (and some high-powered handguns at close range) that fire missiles at very high velocity. Their velocity gives the projectile very high kinetic energy. As the projectile passes through tissue, it creates a shock wave, tissue movement (including compression

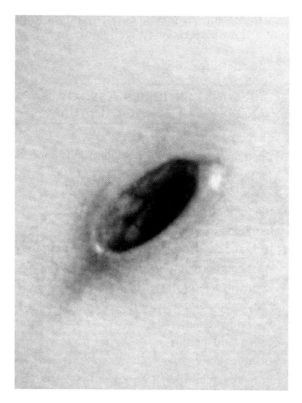

FIGURE 25-3   Penetrating (stab) wound to the chest.

and stretching), and a large temporary cavity. These wounds cause extensive tissue damage perpendicular to the track of the projectile.

Shotgun wounds are classified according to the distance between the victim and the shotgun. A smaller gauge (a larger calibre) of shotgun and a larger size of shot also increase the effective range and penetrating power of the weapon and its potential to cause tissue damage. Type I injuries are those where the target is greater than 7 m from the gun barrel at discharge. The pellets usually penetrate the skin and subcutaneous tissue but rarely penetrate the deep fascia to cause body cavity penetration. Type II injuries occur at a distance of 3–7 m and often permit the pellets to penetrate the deep fascia with internal organ injury possible. Type III injuries occur at a distance of less than 3 m and usually involve massive tissue destruction and life-threatening injury.

Penetrating thoracic trauma is often related to the structures involved. Lung tissue is very resilient when hit by high-energy projectiles. The "spongy" nature of the air-filled alveoli absorbs the energy of cavitation and reduces the size of the temporary cavity and injury associated with the compression and stretching. The great vessels and heart (if it is distended with blood) respond much differently. The fluid transmits the kinetic energy very well and may result in cardiac or vessel rupture. With slower moving projectiles or the heart in diastole, the result may be a simple penetration. While a projectile tends to move in a straight line, it is easily deflected by contact with a rib, clavicle, scapula, or the spinal column. Contact with skeletal structures may also fragment the projectile, increasing the rate of energy exchange and the seriousness of injury. Penetrating trauma frequently leads to pneumothorax, which may be bilateral, depending on the track of the missile or knife. Table 25-1 lists common injuries associated with penetrating thoracic trauma.

CHEST WALL INJURIES

Chest wall injuries are by far the most common injuries encountered in blunt chest trauma. As previously discussed, an intact and moving chest wall is necessary to develop the pressures essential for air movement into and out of the lungs (the bellows effect). Chest wall injury may disrupt this motion and result in res-

Shotgun wounds within 3 m of the discharging barrel cause serious tissue destruction and are frequently life threatening.

Chest wall injuries are by far the most common injuries encountered in blunt chest trauma.

Table 25-1	INJURIES ASSOCIATED WITH PENETRATING THORACIC TRAUMA

Closed pneumothorax

Open pneumothorax (including sucking chest wound)

Tension pneumothorax

Pneumomediastinum

Hemothorax

Hemopneumothorax

Laceration of vascular structures, including the great vessels

Tracheobronchial tree lacerations

Esophageal lacerations

Penetrating cardiac injuries

Pericardial tamponade

Spinal cord injuries

Diaphragmatic penetration/laceration/rupture

Intra-abdominal penetration with associated organ injury

piratory insufficiency. Closed injuries of the chest wall include contusions, rib fractures, sternal fractures/dislocations, and flail chest. Open injuries to the chest wall are almost entirely due to penetrating trauma and are often associated with deep structure injury in addition to disruption of the changing intrathoracic pressure necessary for respiration.

Chest Wall Contusion

Chest wall contusion is the most common result of blunt injury to the thorax. The injury damages the soft tissue covering the thoracic cage and causes pain with respiratory effort. Like contusions elsewhere, contusion of the chest wall may present with erythema initially, then ecchymosis. The discoloration may outline the object that caused the trauma, may outline the ribs as the soft tissue is trapped between the ribs and the offending agent, or may outline a combination of both. The most noticeable symptom of chest wall contusion is pain, made worse with deep breathing and possibly resulting in reduced chest expansion. The area will be tender at the contusion site, and you may observe decreased chest wall movement due to pain. You may auscultate limited breath sounds because of decreased air movement caused by limited chest expansion.

The pain of chest wall contusion and associated restriction of deep inspiration may lead to hypoventilation. Hypoventilation may not be apparent in a young, otherwise healthy, individual and may not pose a significant life threat due to the individual's significant pulmonary reserves. The aged patient, however, often has preexisting medical problems, has little pulmonary reserve, and does not tolerate this injury as well. Such a patient quickly becomes hypoxemic (low oxygen levels in the blood) without proper respiratory support. In a pediatric patient, the ribs are very flexible, resist fracture, and easily transmit the forces of trauma. The result may be chest wall contusion and internal injury without rib fracture.

Rib Fracture

Rib fractures are found in more than 50 percent of cases of significant chest trauma from blunt mechanisms. Rib fractures are likely to occur at the point of impact or along the border of the object that strikes the chest (Figure 25-4). Fractures may also occur at a location remote from the injury site. The thoracic cage is a hollow cylinder that has some flex to it. As the compressional force of blunt trauma deforms the thorax, the ribs flex and may fracture at their weakest point, the posterior angle (along the posterior axillary line).

Ribs 4 through 8 are the most commonly fractured, as they are least protected by other structures and are firmly fixed at both ends (to the spine and sternum). It takes great force to fracture the first three ribs because the shoulder, scapula, and the heavy musculature of the upper chest protect them. Their fracture is frequently associated with severe intrathoracic injuries (tracheobronchial tree injury, aortic rupture, and other vascular injuries), especially if multiple ribs are involved. Fracture of these ribs results in a mortality rate of up to 30 percent due to the associated injuries. Ribs 9 through 12 are less firmly attached to the sternum, are relatively mobile, and are thus less likely to fracture. However, they better transmit the energy of trauma to internal organs and may permit intra-abdominal injury without fracture. Fractures of ribs 9 through 12 are frequently associated with serious trauma and splenic or hepatic injury.

The incidence and significance of rib fracture varies with age. The pediatric patient has highly cartilaginous ribs that bend easily. The ribs resist fracture and transmit kinetic forces to the thoracic and abdominal structures underneath. The pediatric patient hence has a decreased incidence of rib fracture and an increased

Chest wall contusion is the most common result of blunt injury to the thorax.

Content Review

SIGNS AND SYMPTOMS OF CHEST WALL INJURIES

Blunt or penetrating trauma to chest
Erythema
Ecchymosis
Dyspnea
Pain on breathing
Limited breath sounds
Hypoventilation
Crepitus
Paradoxical motion of chest wall

Rib fractures are found in more than 50 percent of cases of significant chest trauma from blunt mechanisms.

Ribs 4 through 8 are the most commonly fractured.

In pediatric patients, more flexible ribs permit more serious internal injury before they fracture.

FIGURE 25-4   Rib fractures.

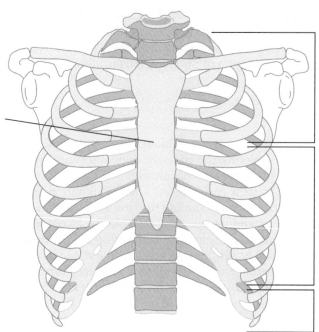

Great force is required for sternal fractures.

Ribs 1–3 are well protected by shoulder bones and muscles.

Ribs 4–8 are most frequently fractured.

Ribs 9–12 are relatively mobile and fracture less frequently.

incidence of underlying injury. The geriatric patient, conversely, has ribs that are calcified, less flexible, and more easily fractured. The geriatric patient is also more likely to have co-morbidity, such as chronic obstructive pulmonary disease (COPD), which reduces respiratory reserves and compounds the effects of rib injury. If multiple rib fractures are noted in a young adult, they are probably associated with severe trauma and may lead to significant pain, splinting, hypoventilation, and inadequate cough. They also are likely to be associated with significant internal injuries. The mortality associated with rib fractures increases with the number of fractures, extremes of age (the very young or very old), and associated chronic respiratory or cardiac problems, especially in the elderly trauma victim.

The rib fracture is likely to be associated with an overlying chest wall contusion and presents with those signs and symptoms. The fracture site may also demonstrate a grating sensation (crepitus) as the bone ends move against each other, either during chest wall movement or during direct palpation. The pain associated with rib fracture is greater than that with chest wall contusion and will more greatly limit respiratory excursion. This reduced chest wall excursion frequently leads to hypoxia, hypoventilation, and muscle spasms at the fracture site. Hypoventilation can result in a progressive collapse of alveoli called atelectasis. This collapse reduces the lung surface available for gas exchange and contributes to hypoxia. These atelectatic segments also may become filled with blood or tissue fluid due to the injury and set the stage for secondary infection, such as pneumonia. While pneumonia does not develop in the emergency setting, it is the cause of a significant mortality in blunt chest injury patients. Serious internal injuries may also result as the jagged rib ends move about and lacerate structures beneath them. Laceration of the intercostal arteries may result in hemothorax, while damage to the intercostal nerves may result in a neurological deficit. Fracture and displacement of the lower ribs may injure the liver (right) or spleen (left).

Rib fracture mortality increases with the number of fractures, extremes of age, and associated disease.

Sternal Fracture and Dislocation

Sternal fractures and dislocations are usually associated with blunt anterior chest trauma. Sternal fracture results only from severe impact, as this region of the chest is well supported by the ribs and clavicles. The most likely mech-

Sternal fracture is frequently associated with serious myocardial injury.

anism is a direct blow, a fall against a fixed object, or the blunt force of the sternum against the steering wheel or dashboard in a motor vehicle crash. The overall incidence of sternal fracture in thoracic trauma patients is between 5 and 8 percent. However, the mortality associated with it is between 25 and 45 percent because of underlying myocardial contusion, cardiac rupture, pericardial tamponade, and pulmonary contusion. If the surrounding ribs or costochondral joints are disrupted, the injury may result in a flail chest. The injury results in a noticeable deformity and possible crepitus with chest wall movement or palpation.

Dislocation at the sternoclavicular joint is uncommon and also requires significant force. It, too, may occur with blunt trauma to the anterior chest or with a lateral compression mechanism, as in side impact collisions or falls with the patient landing on the shoulder. The clavicle may dislocate from the sternum in one of two ways, anteriorly or posteriorly. The anterior dislocation creates a noticeable deformity anterior to the manubrium. The posterior dislocation displaces the head of the clavicle behind the sternum where it may compress or lacerate the underlying great vessels or compress or injure the trachea and esophagus. Tracheal compression may result in stridor and voice change, though any deformity is more difficult to identify, except that the shoulder may noticeably displace anteriorly and medially.

Flail Chest

Flail chest is a segment of the chest that becomes free to move with the pressure changes of respiration. The condition occurs when three or more adjacent ribs fracture in two or more places (Figure 25-5). It is one of the most serious chest wall injuries as it is often associated with severe underlying pulmonary injury (contusion) and reduces the volume of respiration and increases the effort associated with it. This underlying injury adds to mortality in serious thoracic trauma (between 20 and 40 percent), as does age, head injury, shock, and other associated injuries. The most common mechanisms of injury causing flail chest are blunt traumas from falls, motor vehicle crashes, industrial accidents, and assaults.

* **flail chest** defect in the chest wall that allows for free movement of a segment. Breathing will cause paradoxical chest wall motion.

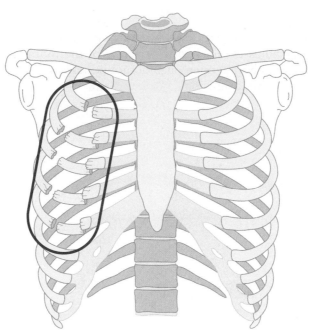

FIGURE 25-5　Flail chest occurs when three or more adjacent ribs fracture in two or more places.

The flail segment created by this injury is no longer a controlled component of the chest wall and bellows system. Increasing intrathoracic pressure associated with expiration moves the flail segment outward, while the rest of the chest moves inward, pushing air under the moving segment that would normally be exhaled. This reduces the change in chest volume caused by the breathing effort as well as the volume of air expired and draws the mediastinum toward the injury. During inspiration, the intrathoracic pressure falls as the respiratory muscles move the chest wall outward and the diaphragm drops caudally (tail-ward). The reduced pressure draws the flail segment inward. The lung beneath it moves away from the inward-moving segment, reducing the volume of air moving into the thorax and displacing the mediastinum away from the injury. In summary, the injury produces a segment of the chest wall that moves in opposition of the chest's normal respiratory effort (paradoxical movement), it reduces the volume of air moved with each breath, and it displaces the mediastinum toward and then away from the injury site with each breath (Figure 25-6). In flail chest, the patient takes more energy to move less air, and the respiratory volume is further reduced, as the rib fracture pain produces a natural splinting of the chest.

It takes tremendous energy to create these six fracture sites (three or more ribs fractured in two or more places) and, accordingly, flail chest is often associated with serious internal injury. In addition, the movement of the flail segment, which is opposite to the rest of the chest wall, is damaging to surrounding tissue. With each breath, the bone fracture sites move against one another causing further muscle damage, soft-tissue damage, and pain. Small flail segments may go undetected as the associated intercostal muscle spasm naturally splints the segment. With time, however, these muscles suffer further injury and fatigue, and the flail segment's paradoxical movement may become more and more apparent.

Positive pressure ventilation of the patient with flail chest reverses the mechanism that causes the paradoxical chest wall movement, restores the tidal volume, and reduces the pain of chest wall movement. It accomplishes this by pushing the chest wall and the flail segment outward with positive pressure. Passive expiration then may cause both the flail segment and the rest of the chest to move inward, again, together.

Over time, the muscles splinting the flail segment will fatigue, and paradoxical respiration will become more evident.

PULMONARY INJURIES

Pulmonary injuries are injuries to lung tissue or injuries that damage the system that holds the lung to the interior of the thoracic cavity. They include simple pneumothorax, open pneumothorax, tension pneumothorax, hemothorax, and pulmonary contusion.

FIGURE 25-6 Paradoxical movement of the chest wall seen in flail chest.

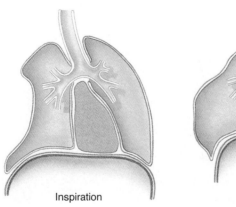
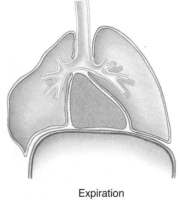

Inspiration

Expiration

Simple Pneumothorax

Simple **pneumothorax** (also known as closed pneumothorax) occurs when lung tissue is disrupted and air leaks into the pleural space (Figure 25-7). While there may be an external, and possibly penetrating, wound, there is no communication between the pleural space and the atmosphere. The pressure within the thorax does not exceed normal expiratory pressures, and there is no associated mediastinal shift. As more and more air accumulates in the pleural space, the lung collapses. With lung collapse, the alveoli collapse (atelectisis) and blood flowing past the collapsed alveoli does not exchange oxygen and carbon dioxide. As more and more of the alveoli collapse, this condition, called ventilation/perfusion mismatch becomes more pronounced and begins to lower the blood oxygen level (hypoxemia). This soon becomes life endangering, especially if there are other associated injuries or shock.

Simple pneumothorax can occur with penetrating and blunt mechanisms. Blunt trauma may cause a pneumothorax when a rib fracture directly punctures the lung. Another mechanism may cause alveolar rupture from a sudden increase in intrathoracic pressure as the chest strikes the steering column with fully expanded lungs and a closed glottis (much like a paper bag filled with air and compressed suddenly between two hands). The incidence of pneumothorax in serious thoracic trauma is between 10 and 30 percent, and its morbidity is related to the amount of atelectisis and the degree of perfusion mismatch. Penetrating trauma to the chest is frequently associated with simple pneumothorax or with an injury that allows air to enter the pleural space through an external wound (open pneumothorax).

A simple pneumothorax reduces the efficiency of respiration and quickly leads to hypoxia. The hypoxia and increase in blood levels of CO_2 cause the medulla to increase the respiratory rate (tachypnea) and volume. If only a very small portion of the lung is involved, there may be no apparent signs or symptoms. A larger pneumothorax may cause mild dyspnea, or complete lung collapse may result in severe dyspnea and hypoxia. The signs, symptoms, and significance of simple pneumothorax increase with preexisting disease. Pneumothorax may

* **pneumothorax** air in the pleural space.

Content Review

SIGNS AND SYMPTOMS OF PNEUMOTHORAX
Trauma to chest
Chest pain on inspiration
Hyperinflation of chest
Diminished breath sounds on affected side

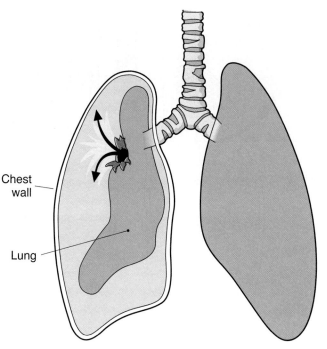

FIGURE 25-7 Simple (closed) pneumothorax.

Chest wall

Lung

produce local chest pain with respiration as the pleurae become irritated (pleuritic pain). The pathology may cause the chest to hyperinflate and breath sounds to diminish on the affected side (usually in the extremes of the upper and lower areas of the lung first). A small pneumothorax involving collapse of less than 15 percent of the affected lung may be difficult to detect clinically and requires only supportive measures. Often, the small pneumothorax will seal itself, and the air in the pleural cavity will be absorbed. A larger pneumothorax is often clinically apparent and requires more aggressive therapy, such as high-flow oxygen and chest tube placement (in the emergency department).

Open Pneumothorax

Open pneumothorax is most commonly noted in military conflicts when a high-velocity bullet creates a significant wound in the chest wall (usually the exit wound). Recently, use of high-velocity assault weapons has become more common in civilian settings, and thus the frequency of these injuries is on the increase. Another cause of open pneumothorax is a shotgun blast at close range resulting in an associated large wound to the chest wall. This chest wall disruption leads to the free passage of air between the atmosphere and the pleural space (Figure 25-8). Air is drawn into the wound as the chest moves outward and the diaphragm moves downward during inspiration. The internal thoracic pressure drops, and air rushes through the wound and into the chest cavity. This air replaces the lung tissue and causes its collapse, which results in a large functional dead space. The inspiratory effort of the intact side of the chest draws the mediastinum toward it and away from the injury. This prevents the uninjured lung from fully inflating. On exhalation, the contracting chest wall and rising diaphragm increase the internal pressure and force air outward through the wound. This movement of air into and out of the chest through the wound is the cause of the "sucking" sound that leads to the wound's common name, "sucking chest wound."

For air movement to occur through the opening in the chest wall, the opening must be at least two-thirds the diameter of the trachea. Remember, the size of the trachea is about the size of the patient's little finger. This must be the size of

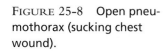

FIGURE 25-8 Open pneumothorax (sucking chest wound).

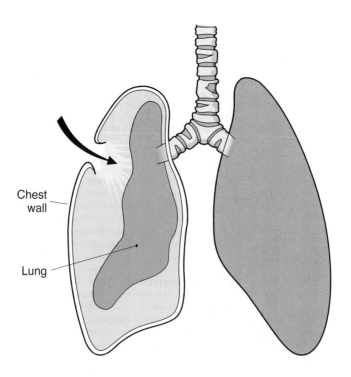

Chest wall

Lung

the opening into the chest, not the size of the wound. The thickness and resiliency of the chest wall often closes the wound to air movement unless the wound is quite large. The remaining defect may then permit the free movement of air and create an open pneumothorax.

The open pneumothorax can be recognized by the large open wound to the thorax and the characteristic air movement (or sound) it produces. Air passage through the wound and the wound's associated hemorrhage may produce frothy blood around the opening, another characteristic of the open pneumothorax. The patient is likely to experience severe dyspnea and possibly hypovolemia from associated injury and hemorrhage. The patient's condition is further compromised because the reduced intrathoracic pressures developed during inspiration do not complement venous return to the heart as they do with the intact thorax and respiratory effort.

Tension Pneumothorax

Tension pneumothorax is an open or simple pneumothorax that generates and maintains a pressure greater than atmospheric pressure within the thorax. It may be caused by a traumatic mechanism and injury or possibly by positive pressure ventilation of a patient with chest trauma or congenital defect affecting the respiratory tree. Tension pneumothorax may also occur as an open pneumothorax is sealed and an internal injury or defect permits the buildup of pressure.

Tension pneumothorax occurs because the mechanism of injury (either the external wound, or the internal injury) forms a one-way valve. Air flows into the pleural space through the defect during inspiration as the pressure within the pleural space is less than atmospheric. With expiration, the increasing pleural pressure closes the defect and does not permit air to escape. With each breath, the volume of air and the pressure within the pleural space increase. The increasing intrapleural pressure collapses the lung on the ipsilateral (same or injury) side, causes intercostal and suprasternal bulging, and begins to exert pressure against the mediastinum. As the pressure continues to build, it displaces the mediastinum, compressing the uninjured lung and crimping the vena cava as it enters the thorax through the diaphragm or where it attaches to the heart. This reduces venous return, results in an increase in venous pressure, causes jugular vein distention (JVD), and narrows the pulse pressure. Tracheal shift may occur as the mediastinal structures are pushed away from the increasing pressure. This is a very late and rare finding and more commonly seen in the young trauma victim, as the pediatric mediastinum is more mobile than the adult's. Atelectasis occurs in the ipsilateral side from the initial lung collapse and on the contralateral (uninjured or opposite) side from the mediastinal shift and compression of that lung. These mechanisms lead to ventilation/perfusion mismatch, further hypoxemia, and systemic hypoxia.

Tension pneumothorax begins with the presentation of a simple or open pneumothorax (Figure 25-9). As the pressure in the pleural space begins to increase, dyspnea, ventilation/perfusion mismatch, and hypoxemia develop. The ipsilateral side of the chest becomes hyperinflated, is hyperresonant to percussion, and respiratory sounds become very faint and then absent. The pressure may cause the intracostal tissues to bulge. The opposite or contralateral side of the chest becomes somewhat dull to percussion, with progressively fainter respiratory sounds as the tension pneumothorax becomes worse. Severe hypoxia results in cyanosis, diaphoresis, and an altered mental status, while the increased intrathoracic pressure reduces venous return and may cause JVD and hypotension. If the condition is not quickly recognized and promptly treated, it may lead to death.

Tension pneumothorax is a serious and immediate life threat. It can be corrected, by an ACP/CCP, by relieving the intrapleural pressure by inserting a needle through the chest wall to convert the tension pneumothorax to an open

* **tension pneumothorax** buildup of air under pressure within the thorax. The resulting compression of the lung severely reduces the effectiveness of respirations.

Content Review

SIGNS AND SYMPTOMS OF TENSION PNEUMOTHORAX
Chest trauma
Dyspnea
Ventilation/perfusion mismatch
Hypoxemia
Hyperinflation of affected side of chest
Hyperresonance of affected side of chest
Diminished, then absent breath sounds
Cyanosis
Diaphoresis
Altered mental status
Jugular venous distention
Hypotension
Hypovolemia

FIGURE 25-9 Physical findings of tension pneumothorax.

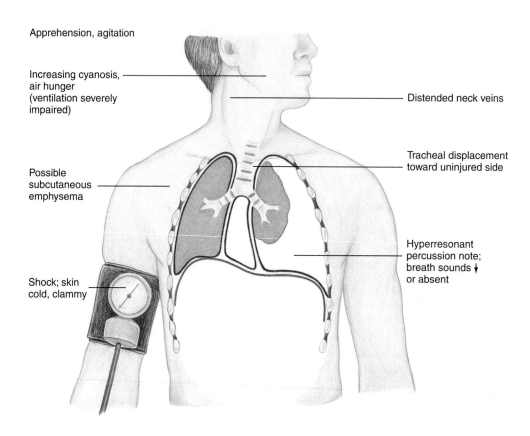

Apprehension, agitation

Increasing cyanosis, air hunger (ventilation severely impaired)

Distended neck veins

Tracheal displacement toward uninjured side

Possible subcutaneous emphysema

Hyperresonant percussion note; breath sounds ↓ or absent

Shock; skin cold, clammy

pneumothorax. If a valve is added to the decompression needle, it may permit only the escape of air during respiration. If there is no continuing internal defect, this may progressively reexpand the collapsed lung and return effective respiration.

Hemothorax

✱ **hemothorax** blood within the pleural space.

✱ **hemopneumothorax** condition where air and blood are in the pleural space.

Hemothorax is simply the accumulation of blood in the pleural space due to internal hemorrhage. It can be very minor and not detectable in the field or, when associated with serious or great vessel injury, may result in rapid patient deterioration. Serious hemorrhage may displace a complete lung, accumulate more than 1500 mL of blood quickly, and produce a mortality rate of 75 percent, with most (two-thirds) of the patients dying at the scene. Hemothorax is primarily a blood loss problem as both sides of the thorax may hold up to 3000 mL of blood (or half the total blood volume). However, the blood lost into the thorax reduces the tidal volume and efficiency of respiration in a patient who has already suffered trauma and is likely to move quickly into shock.

Hemothorax is frequently associated with rib fractures and can be associated with either blunt or penetrating mechanisms. It often accompanies pneumothorax (a **hemopneumothorax**) and occurs 25 percent of the time with penetrating trauma. Hemorrhage into the pleural space may occur from a lung laceration (most common) or laceration of the intercostal arteries, pulmonary arteries, great vessels, or internal mammary arteries. The intercostal arteries can bleed at a rate of 50 mL/min. The bleeding into the chest is more rapid than would occur elsewhere because the pressure within the chest is often less than atmospheric pressure (Laplace's law). The blood lost into the hemothorax contributes to hypovolemia and displaces lung tissue. If the accumulation is significant, it may cause significant hypovolemia and shock, hypoxemia, respiratory distress, and respiratory failure.

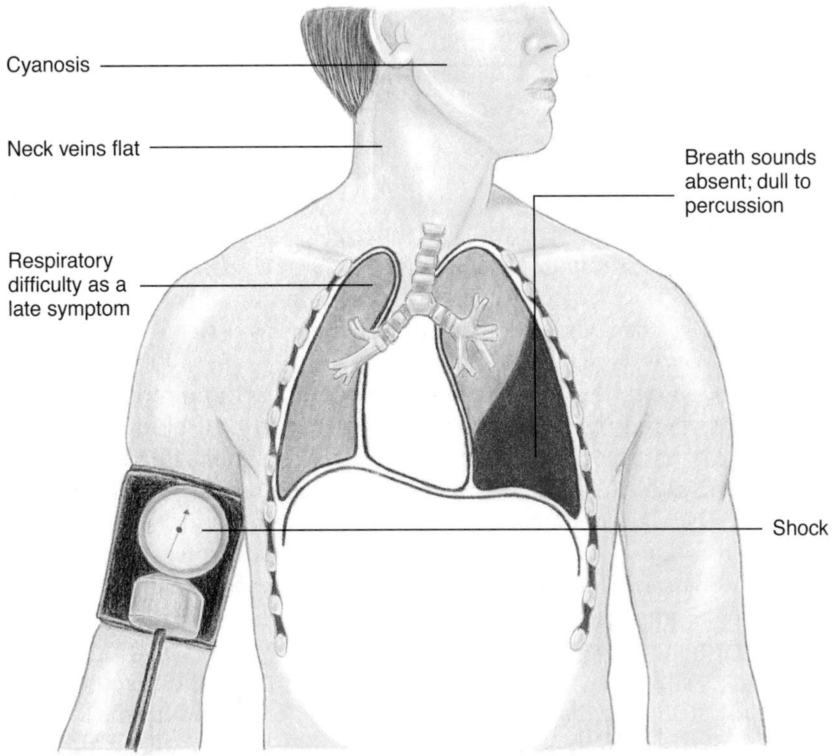

FIGURE 25-10 Physical findings of massive hemothorax.

Cyanosis

Neck veins flat

Respiratory difficulty as a late symptom

Breath sounds absent; dull to percussion

Shock

The patient with hemothorax will have either a blunt or penetrating injury, such as those associated with open or simple pneumothorax. The patient may also display the signs and symptoms of shock and some respiratory distress (Figure 25-10). The blood pools in the lower chest in the seated patient or posterior chest in the supine patient. The lungs present with normal breath sounds, except directly over the accumulating fluid. There the breath sounds are very distant, if they can be heard at all.

Pulmonary Contusion

Pulmonary contusions are simply soft-tissue contusions affecting the lung. They are present in 30 to 75 percent of patients with significant blunt chest trauma and are frequently associated with rib fracture. Pulmonary contusions range in severity from very limited, minor, and unrecognizable injuries to those that are extensive and quickly life threatening. They result in a mortality rate of between 14 and 20 percent in serious chest trauma patients.

There are two specific mechanisms of injury that allow the transfer of energy to the pulmonary tissue and result in pulmonary contusions. They are deceleration and the pressure wave associated with either passage of a high-velocity bullet or explosion. Deceleration injury occurs as the moving body strikes a fixed object. A common example of this mechanism is chest impact with the steering wheel during an auto crash. As the chest wall contacts the steering wheel and stops, the lungs continue forward, compressing and stretching the alveolar tissue or shearing it from the relatively fixed tracheobronchial tree. This causes disruption at the alveolar/capillary membrane, leading to microscopic hemorrhage and edema. The second mechanism, the pressure wave of an explosion or bullet's passage, dramatically compresses and stretches the lung tissue. Due to the nature of the lung tissue (air-filled sacs surrounded by delicate and vascular membranes), the passage of this

Content Review

SIGNS AND SYMPTOMS OF HEMOTHORAX
Blunt or penetrating chest trauma
Signs and symptoms of shock
Dyspnea
Dull percussive sounds over site of injury

Pathophysiology of Thoracic Trauma **289**

pressure is partially reflected at the gas/fluid (alveolar/capillary) interface. This leaves small, flame-shaped areas of disruption throughout the membrane leading to microhemorrhage and edema (called the Spalding effect). Pulmonary contusion is not generally associated with low-speed penetration of the chest and laceration of the lung tissues and structures.

The overall magnitude of pulmonary injury depends on the degree of deformity or stretch, and the velocity at which it occurs. Similar pulmonary contusions may result from different mechanisms. For example, an AK-47 round fired at 700 m/sec striking body armour and deforming the chest wall instantaneously by 1–2 cm (high velocity) may cause pulmonary contusions similar to chest impact during an MVC where the chest is deformed 50 percent as it strikes the steering wheel at 15 m/sec (low velocity).

Microhemorrhage into the alveolar tissue associated with pulmonary contusion may be extensive and result in up to 1000 to 1500 mL of blood loss. This hemorrhage into the tissue of the alveoli also causes irritation, initiates the inflammation process, and causes fluid to migrate into the region. The accumulation of fluid in the alveolar/capillary membrane (pulmonary edema) progressively increases its dimension and decreases the rate at which gases, and especially oxygen, can diffuse across it. The fluid accumulation also stiffens the membrane, makes the lung less compliant, and increases the work necessary to move air in to and out of the affected tissue.

The thickening wall reduces the efficiency of respiration and results in hypoxemia, while the stiffening makes respiration more energy consuming. The development of edema also increases the pressure necessary to move blood through the capillary beds. This increases the pressure within the pulmonary vascular system (pulmonary hypertension) and the workload of the right heart. In combination, these effects lead to atelectasis, hypovolemia, ventilation/perfusion mismatch, hypoxemia, hypotension and, possibly, respiratory failure and shock. Although isolated pulmonary contusions can occur, they are frequently associated with chest wall injury and injuries elsewhere (87 percent of the time).

The patient with pulmonary contusion presents with a mechanism of injury and evidence of blunt or penetrating chest impact. While the associated injuries may display immediate signs and symptoms (as in the pain of a rib fracture), the signs and symptoms of the pulmonary contusion take time to develop. The patient will likely complain of increasing dyspnea, demonstrate increasing respiratory effort, and show the signs of hypoxia. Oxygen saturation may gradually fall as the pathology develops. Careful auscultation of the chest may reveal increasing crackles and fainter breath sounds. Serious pulmonary contusion may cause **hemoptysis** (coughing up blood) and the signs and symptoms of shock.

✱ **hemoptysis** coughing of blood that has origin in the respiratory tract.

Cardiovascular injuries are the subset of thoracic trauma that leads to the most fatalities.

Cardiovascular Injuries

Cardiovascular injuries are the subset of thoracic trauma that leads to the most fatalities. They include myocardial contusion, pericardial tamponade, myocardial aneurysm or rupture, aortic aneurysm or rupture, and other vascular injuries.

Myocardial Contusion

Myocardial contusion is a frequent result of trauma and may occur in 76 percent of all serious chest trauma. It carries a high mortality rate and occurs most commonly with severe blunt anterior chest trauma. Here, the chest is struck by or strikes an object. The heart, which is relatively mobile within the chest, hits the inside of the anterior chest wall and then may be compressed between the sternum and the thoracic spine as the thorax flexes with impact. The resulting contusion will most likely affect the right atrium and right ventricle (Figure 25-11). This is related to the heart's position in the chest, rotated somewhat counterclockwise and presenting the right atrium and ventricle surfaces toward the sternum.

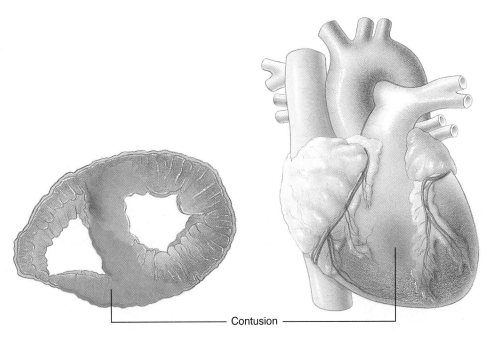

Contusion

FIGURE 25-11   Myocardial contusion most frequently affects the right atrium and ventricle as they collide with the sternum.

The cardiac contusion is similar to a contusion in any other muscle tissue. The injury disrupts the muscle cells and microcirculation, resulting in muscle fibre tearing and damage, hemorrhage, and edema. The injury may reduce the strength of cardiac contraction and reduce cardiac output. Because of the automaticity and conductivity of the cardiac muscle, contusion may also disturb the cardiac electrical system. If the injury is serious, it may lead to hematoma, hemopericardium (blood in the pericardial sac), and necrosis and may result in cardiac irritability, ectopic (irregularly occurring) beats, and conduction system defects, such as bundle branch blocks and dysrhythmias. If the injury is extensive, it may lead to tissue necrosis (death), decreased ventricular compliance, congestive heart failure, cardiogenic shock, myocardial aneurysm, and acute or delayed myocardial rupture. In contrast to a myocardial infarction from coronary artery disease, the cellular damage from myocardial contusions heals with less scarring, and there is no progression of the injury in the absence of associated coronary artery disease.

The patient experiencing myocardial contusion will have a history of significant blunt chest trauma, most likely affecting the anterior chest. The patient will likely complain of chest or retrosternal pain, very much like that of myocardial infarction and may have associated chest injuries, such as anterior rib or sternal fractures. Cardiac monitoring most frequently reveals sinus tachycardia (though it may be caused by pain, hypovolemia, or hypoxia from associated chest injury). Other dysrhythmias associated with myocardial contusions are atrial flutter or fibrillation, premature atrial or ventricular contractions, tachydysrhythmias, bradydysrhythmias, bundle branch patterns, T-wave inversions, and ST-segment elevations. A pericardial friction rub and murmur may be auscultated over the **precordium** but is more likely to occur weeks after the injury and is associated with the development of an inflammatory pericardial effusion.

Pericardial Tamponade

Pericardial tamponade is a restriction to cardiac filling caused by blood (or other fluid) within the pericardial sac. It occurs in less than 2 percent of all serious chest

Content Review

SIGNS AND SYMPTOMS OF CARDIAC CONTUSION

Blunt injury to chest
Bruising of chest wall
Rapid heart rate—may be irregular
Severe nagging pain not relieved with rest but may be relieved with oxygen.

✱ precordium area of the chest wall overlying the heart.

✱ pericardial tamponade a restriction to cardiac filling caused by blood (or other fluid) within the pericardial sac.

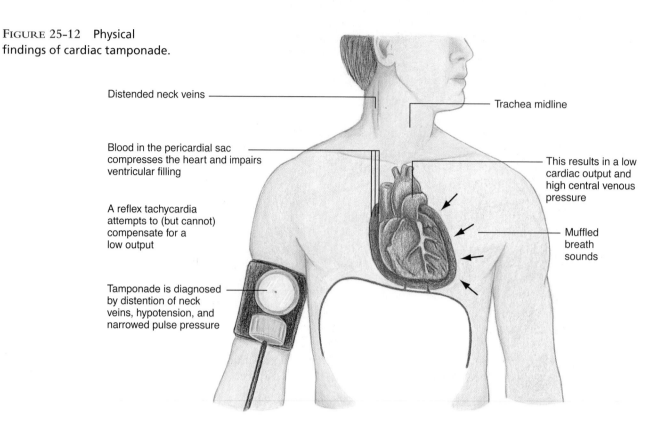

FIGURE 25-12 Physical findings of cardiac tamponade.

Distended neck veins

Blood in the pericardial sac compresses the heart and impairs ventricular filling

A reflex tachycardia attempts to (but cannot) compensate for a low output

Tamponade is diagnosed by distention of neck veins, hypotension, and narrowed pulse pressure

Trachea midline

This results in a low cardiac output and high central venous pressure

Muffled breath sounds

trauma patients and is almost always related to penetrating injury. Gunshot wounds are the most frequent mechanism and carry a high overall mortality, though they often result in rapid hemorrhage through the myocardial wall and then out through the defect in the pericardium. The frequency of gunshot wound mortality is probably related to the depth of injury, the degree of cardiac tissue damage caused by the cavitational wave, and a more rapid progression of the pathology.

The pathology of pericardial tamponade begins with a tear in a superficial coronary artery or penetration of the myocardium. Blood seeps into the pericardial space and accumulates (Figure 25-12). The fibrous pericardium does not stretch, and the accumulating blood exerts pressure on the heart. The pressure limits cardiac filling, first affecting the right ventricle, where the pressure of filling is the lowest. This restricts venous return to the heart, increases venous pressure, and causes jugular vein distention. The reduced right ventricular output limits outflow to the pulmonary arteries and then venous return to the left heart. The result is a decreasing cardiac output and systemic hypotension. The pressure exerted by the blood in the pericardium also restricts the flow of blood through the coronary arteries and to the myocardium. This may result in myocardial ischemia and infarct. It takes about 200 to 300 mL of blood to exert the pressure necessary to induce frank tamponade, while removing as little as 20 mL may provide significant relief. The progression of pericardial tamponade depends on the rate of blood flow into the pericardium. It may occur very rapidly and result in death before the arrival of emergency medical services or may gradually progress over hours.

The patient experiencing pericardial tamponade will likely have penetrating trauma to the anterior or posterior chest, though blunt trauma can also cause this problem. While the trajectories of missiles and knife blades are difficult to predict, consider pericardial tamponade with any thoracic or upper abdominal penetrating wound, especially if it is over the precordium (central lower chest). Pericardial tamponade will diminish the strength of pulses, decrease the pulse pressure, and distend the jugular veins (jugular vein distention, JVD). The patient will likely be agitated, tachycardic, diaphoretic, and ashen in appearance. Cyanosis may be noted in the head, neck, and upper extremities. Heart tones may be muffled or distant sounding. Beck's triad (JVD, distant heart tones, and hypotension) is indicative of pericardial tamponade but may not be recognized early in the injury's progression. Another sign of pericardial tamponade is Kussmaul's sign, the decrease or absence of JVD during inspiration. As the patient inspires, the reduced intrathoracic pressure increases venous return and decreases the pressure the accumulating pericardial fluid exerts on the heart. This then translates to a better venous return and cardiac output during inspiration and the effect is then seen in the jugular veins.

Other findings during pericardial tamponade may include pulsus paradoxus and electrical alternans. **Pulsus paradoxus** is a drop in systolic blood pressure of greater than 10 mmHg as the patient inspires during the normal respiratory cycle. (Normally the systolic blood pressure drops just slightly with each inspiration.) Pulsus paradoxus results because cardiac output increases with the minimal relief of the tamponade associated with the reduced intrathoracic pressure of inspiration. **Electrical alternans,** which is only rarely seen in acute pericardial tamponade, is noted on the cardiac rhythm strip as the P, QRS, and T amplitudes decreasing with every other cardiac cycle. In profound pericardial tamponade, the heart displays a rhythm without producing a pulse (PEA).

* **pulsus paradoxus** drop of greater than 10 mmHg in the systolic blood pressure during the inspiratory phase of respiration that occurs in patients with pericardial tamponade.

* **electrical alternans** alternating amplitude of the P, QRS, and T waves on the ECG rhythm strip as the heart swings in a pendulum-like fashion within the pericardial sac during tamponade.

* **aneurysm** a weakening or ballooning in the wall of a blood vessel.

Myocardial Aneurysm or Rupture

Myocardial **aneurysm** or rupture occurs almost exclusively in extreme blunt thoracic trauma as in automobile collisions. It also has been reported in cases where the blunt forces are not extreme, such as a result of cardiopulmonary resuscitation (CPR). The condition can affect any of the heart's chambers, the interatrial septum, the interventricular septum, or involve the valves and their supporting structures. Multiple heart chambers or structures are involved 30 percent of the time. Aneurysm and delayed myocardial rupture also occur secondary to necrosis from a myocardial infarction, repaired penetrating injury, or myocardial contusion. Necrosis usually develops around two weeks after the injury as inflammatory cells degrade the injured cells, weakening the tissue, and leading to aneurysm of the ventricular wall and/or subsequent rupture. Rupture can also occur with high-velocity projectile injury as the bullet impacts the distended heart chamber.

The patient who experiences myocardial rupture will likely have suffered serious blunt or penetrating trauma to the chest and may have severe rib or sternal fracture. Specific symptoms may depend on the actual pathology. The victim may have the signs and symptoms of pericardial tamponade if the rupture is contained within the pericardial sac. If the pathology only affects the valves, the patient may present with the signs and symptoms of right or left heart failure. If there is myocardial aneurysm, rupture may be delayed. When it happens, the patient will suddenly present with the absence of vital signs or the signs and symptoms of pericardial tamponade.

Traumatic Aneurysm or Rupture of the Aorta

Aortic aneurysm and rupture are extremely life-threatening injuries resulting from either blunt or penetrating trauma. The aorta is most commonly injured by blunt trauma, carries an overall mortality of 85 to 95 percent, and is responsible for 15 percent of all thoracic trauma deaths. Aneurysm and rupture are usually associated with high-speed automobile collisions (most commonly lateral impact) and, in some cases, with high falls. Unlike myocardial rupture, a significant number, possibly as high as 20 percent, of these victims will survive the initial insult and aneurysm. Some 30 percent of these initial survivors will die in six hours

Traumatic rupture of the thoracic aorta is almost always fatal.

if not treated, increasing to about 50 percent at 24 hours, and just under 70 percent by the end of the first week. This is the subset of patients that survive the initial impact and are alive at the scene that you can help the most by recognizing the injury and then by rapidly extricating, packaging, and transporting the patients to the trauma centre.

The aorta is a large high-pressure vessel that provides outflow from the left ventricle for distribution to the body. It is relatively fixed at three points as it passes through the thoracic cavity and, because of this, experiences shear forces secondary to severe deceleration of the chest. The areas of fixation are the aortic annulus (where the aorta joins the heart), the aortic isthmus (where it is joined by the ligamentum arteriosum), and the diaphragm (where it exits the chest) (see Table 25-2). Traumatic dissecting aneurysm occurs infrequently to the ascending aorta, and most commonly, to the descending aorta. With severe deceleration, shear forces separate the layers of the artery, specifically the interior surface (the tunica intima) from the muscle layer (the tunica media). This allows blood to enter and, because it is under great pressure, it begins to dissect the aortic lining like a bulging inner tube. It is likely to rupture if it is not surgically repaired.

The patient with aortic rupture will be severely hypotensive, quickly lose all vital signs, and die unless moved into surgery immediately. A dissecting aortic aneurysm progresses more slowly, though the aneurysm may rupture at any moment. The patient will probably have a history of a high fall or severe auto impact and deceleration. Lateral impact is an especially high-risk factor for aortic aneurysm. The patient may complain of severe tearing chest pain that may radiate to the back. The patient may have a pulse deficit between the left and right upper extremities and/or reduced pulse strength in the lower extremities. Blood pressure may be high (hypertension) due to the stretching of sympathetic nerve fibres present in the aorta near the ligamentum arteriosum, or the pressure may be low due to leakage and hypovolemia. Auscultation may reveal a harsh systolic murmur due to turbulence as the blood exits the heart and passes the disrupted blood vessel wall.

Serious lateral chest impact carries a high incidence of dissecting aortic aneurysm.

Other Vascular Injuries

The pulmonary arteries and vena cava are other thoracic vascular structures that can sustain injury during chest trauma. Their injury, and the resulting hemorrhage, may cause significant hemothorax, possibly leading to hypotension and respiratory insufficiency. The blood may also flow into the mediastinum and compress the great vessels, esophagus, and heart. Penetrating trauma is the primary cause of injury to the pulmonary arteries and vena cava.

The patient with pulmonary artery or vena cava injuries will likely have a penetrating wound to the central chest or elsewhere with a likelihood of central chest involvement. These injuries present with the signs and symptoms of hypovolemia and shock and result in hemothorax or hemomediastinum and then the signs and symptoms associated with those pathologies.

Table 25-2	INCIDENCE AND ANATOMIC LOCATION OF TRAUMATIC AORTIC RUPTURE	
Aortic annulus		9%
Aortic isthmus		85%
Diaphragm		3%
Other		3%

OTHER THORACIC INJURIES

Traumatic Rupture or Perforation of the Diaphragm

Traumatic rupture or perforation of the diaphragm can occur in both high-pressure blunt thoracoabdominal trauma as well as in penetrating trauma. Incidence is estimated from 1 to 6 percent of all patients with multiple trauma. It is more common in patients sustaining penetrating trauma to the lower chest, which has as much as a 30 to 40 percent incidence of abdominal organ and tissue involvement. Remember that during expiration, the diaphragm may move superiorly to the level of the fourth intercostal space (nipple level) anteriorly and the sixth intercostal space posteriorly. Any penetrating injuries at these levels or below may penetrate the diaphragm. Diaphragmatic perforation and herniation occur most frequently on the left side because assailants are most frequently right handed and the size and solid nature of the liver protect the diaphragm on the right. The liver is also unlikely to herniate through the torn diaphragm unless the injury is sizeable.

Suspect diaphragmatic perforation with any penetrating injury to the lower thorax.

If traumatic diaphragmatic rupture occurs, the abdominal organs may herniate through the defect into the thoracic cavity causing strangulation or necrosis of the bowel, restriction of the ipsilateral lung, and displacement of the mediastinum. Mediastinal displacement occurs when the displaced abdominal contents place pressure on the lung and mediastinal structures, moving them toward the contralateral side through much the same mechanism as is seen in tension pneumothorax.

Diaphragmatic rupture presents with signs and symptoms similar to tension pneumothorax, including dyspnea, hypoxia, hypotension, and JVD. The patient will have a history of blunt abdominal trauma or penetrating trauma to the lower thorax. The abdomen may appear hollow, and bowel sounds may be noted on one side of the thorax (most commonly the left). The patient may be hypotensive and hypoxic if the herniation is extensive. The patient may complain of upper abdominal pain, though this symptom is often overshadowed by other injuries. Diaphragmatic rupture may be recognized at the time of injury or may be missed if not extensive and present with delayed herniation months to years later.

Traumatic Esophageal Rupture

Traumatic esophageal rupture is a rare complication of blunt thoracic trauma. The incidence of it related to penetrating trauma of the thorax is somewhat higher but still only about 0.4 percent. Since the esophagus is rather centrally located within the chest, its injury usually coincides with other mediastinal injuries. (Esophageal rupture may also be the result of some medical problems, such as violent emesis, carcinoma, anatomical distortion, or gastric reflux.) Esophageal rupture carries a 30 percent mortality, even if quickly recognized, and mortality is much greater if this injury is not diagnosed promptly. The life threat from esophageal rupture is related to material entering the mediastinum as it passes down the esophagus or as emesis comes up. This results in serious infection or chemical irritation and serious damage to the mediastinal structures. Air may also enter the mediastinum through an esophageal rupture, especially during positive pressure ventilations.

The patient with espohageal rupture will probably have deep penetrating trauma to the central chest and may complain of difficult or painful swallowing, pleuritic chest pain, and pain radiating to the midback. The patient may also display subcutaneous emphysema around the lower neck.

Tracheobronchial Injury (Disruption)

Tracheobronchial injury is a relatively rare finding in thoracic trauma, with an incidence of less than 3 percent in patients with significant chest trauma. It may occur from either a blunt or a penetrating injury mechanism and carries a relatively high mortality similar to esophageal rupture of 30 percent. In contrast to patients with esophageal rupture who usually die days after injury, 50 percent of patients with tracheobronchial injury die within one hour of injury. Disruption can occur anywhere in the tracheobronchial tree but is most likely to occur within 2.5 cm of the carina.

The patient with disruption of the trachea or mainstem bronchi is generally in respiratory distress with cyanosis, hemoptysis, and, in some cases, massive subcutaneous emphysema. The patient may also experience pneumothorax and possibly, tension pneumothorax. Intermittent positive pressure ventilation drives air into the pleura or mediastinum and makes the condition worse.

Traumatic Asphyxia

Traumatic asphyxia occurs when severe compressive force is applied to the thorax and leads to backward flow of blood from the right heart into the superior vena cava and into the venous vessels of the upper extremities. (Traumatic asphyxia is not as much a respiratory problem as it is a vascular problem.) Traumatic asphyxia engorges the veins and capillaries of the head and neck with desaturated venous blood, turning the skin in this region a deep red, purple, or blue. The back flow of blood damages the microcirculation in the head and neck, producing petechiae (small hemorrhages under the skin) and stagnating blood above the point of compression. The back flow may damage cerebral circulation, resulting in numerous small strokes in the older patient whose venous vessels are not very elastic. If flow restriction continues, toxins and acids accumulate in the blood and may have a devastating effect when they return to the central circulation with the release of pressure. If the thoracic compression continues, it restricts venous return and may prevent the victim from ventilating. This results in hypotension, hypoxemia, and shock. Death may follow rapidly. Extrication of the patient may result in rapid hemorrhage from the injury site with release of the pressure. Release of the compression may likewise result in rapid patient deterioration and death.

> You must be ready to immediately handle the complications of traumatic asphyxia as soon as the patient is released from entrapment.

The traumatic asphyxia patient will have suffered a severe compression force to the chest that is likely to continue until extrication. The result of the compression—the back flow of blood and restricted blood flow—will be dramatic and cause the classic discoloration of the head and neck regions. The face appears swollen, the eyes bulge, and there are numerous conjunctival hemorrhages. The patient may have severe dyspnea related to the compression and injuries associated with severe chest impact. Once the pressure is released, the patient may show the signs of hypovolemia, hypotension, and shock as well as signs related to any coexisting respiratory problems.

ASSESSMENT OF THE THORACIC TRAUMA PATIENT

The proper assessment of the patient with a severe chest injury mechanism is critical to anticipating injury and providing the correct interventions. While the approach to this patient follows the standard format for assessment, special considerations regarding chest trauma occur during the scene assessment, primary assessment, and especially during the rapid trauma assessment. The ongoing assessment is also critical for monitoring the thoracic trauma patient for the progression of injuries sustained during serious chest trauma.

SCENE ASSESSMENT

Chest injury care, like that for any other serious trauma, requires body substance isolation procedures with gloves as a minimum. Consider a face shield if you will be attending to the airway and a gown for splash protection with serious penetrating thoracic trauma. Ensure that the scene is safe, including ensuring protection from the assailant, if penetrating trauma is suspected.

Examine the mechanism of injury carefully and try to determine if the central chest (heart, great vessels, trachea, and esophagus) might be in the pathway of penetrating trauma. In gunshot injuries, determine the type of weapon, calibre, distance between the gun barrel and the victim, and the probable pathway of the projectile. Determine the direction of blunt trauma impact as it may also have a bearing on which organs sustain injury. Anterior impact may rupture lung tissue and contuse the lung and heart. Lateral impact may tear the aorta as the heart displaces laterally and stresses the aorta's ligamentous attachments.

PRIMARY ASSESSMENT

During the primary assessment, determine the patient's mental status and the status of the airway, breathing, and circulation. Intervene as necessary to correct life-threatening conditions. It is during the primary assessment that you will first identify the signs and symptoms of serious chest trauma. Be especially watchful for any dyspnea; asymmetrical, paradoxical, or limited chest movement; hyperinflation of the chest; or an abdomen that appears hollow. Note any general patient colour reflective of hypoxia, such as cyanosis or an ashen discoloration. Look for distended jugular veins, costal or suprasternal retractions, and the use of accessory muscles of respiration.

Ensure that ventilation is adequate, and administer high-flow oxygen through nonrebreather mask. Administer any positive pressure ventilations with care, as thoracic injury may weaken the lung tissue and make the patient prone to pneumothorax or tension pneumothorax. Aggressive (or even cautious) ventilations may induce these problems. Be suspicious of internal hemorrhage and initiate at least one large-bore intravenous catheter and line in anticipation of hypovolemia, hypotension, and shock. With anterior blunt or penetrating trauma that may involve the heart, attach the ECG electrodes and monitor for dysrhythmias. Attach a pulse oximeter, and monitor oxygen saturation to evaluate the effectiveness of respiration. If there is any mechanism suggesting serious trauma to the chest or any physical signs of either hypoventilation or hypovolemia compensation, perform the rapid trauma assessment with a special focus on the chest, and prepare for rapid patient transport to a trauma centre.

Administer ventilations with care in the patient with chest trauma.

RAPID TRAUMA ASSESSMENT

During the rapid trauma assessment, you will examine the patient's chest in detail, carefully observing, questioning about, palpating, and auscultating the region.

Observe

Observe the chest for evidence of impact. Look for the erythema that develops early in the contusion process, especially as it outlines the ribs or forms a pattern reflecting the contours of the object that the chest hit. Look carefully for penetrating trauma, and try to determine the angle of entry and depth of penetration. Also, look for exit wounds. Lateral chest injury is likely to involve the lungs, while a pathway of energy through the central chest is likely to involve the heart, great vessels, trachea, or esophagus. Injury to the mediastinal structures is also likely to result in serious hemorrhage, hypovolemia, and shock. Look for intercostal and suprasternal retractions as well as external jugular vein distention (JVD). Remember, JVD is present in supine normotensive patients and may be exaggerated in them or may continue when the patient is moved to the seated position if venous pressure is elevated.

Watch chest movement carefully during respiration. The chest should rise and the abdomen should fall smoothly with inspiration and return to position during expiration. Any limited motion, either bilaterally or unilaterally, suggests a problem. Watch for the paradoxical motion of flail chest. That movement will be limited due to muscle spasm during early care, but continued motion will further damage the surrounding soft tissue, and the intracostal muscles will fatigue. This will lead to a more obvious paradoxical motion and greater respiratory embarrassment with time. Look, too, for any hyperinflation of one side of the chest and any deformity that may exist from rib fracture, sternal fracture or dislocation, or subcutaneous emphysema. Assess the volume of air effectively moved with each breath, and assure that the minute volume is greater than six litres. If not, consider overdrive ventilation with the bag-valve mask. Examine any open wound for air movement in or out, which is indicative of an open pneumothorax. Observe the patient's general colour. If a patient's skin is dusky, ashen, or cyanotic, suspect respiratory compromise. If the head and neck are red, dark red, or blue, suspect traumatic asphyxia.

Question

Question the patient about any pain, pain on motion, pain with breathing effort (pleuritic pain), or dyspnea. Note if the pain is crushing or tearing or is described otherwise by the patient. Have the patient describe the exact location of the pain, its severity, and any radiation of the pain. Question about other sensations, and carefully monitor the patient's level of consciousness and orientation.

Palpate

You may have to rely on your palpation skills to assess chest injuries when scene noise is excessive.

Palpate the thorax carefully, feeling for any signs of injury (Figure 25-13). Feel for any swelling, deformity, crepitus, or the crackling of subcutaneous emphysema. Compress the thorax between your hands with pressure directed inward. Then, apply downward pressure on the midsternum. Such pressure will flex the

FIGURE 25-13 Carefully palpate the thorax of a patient with a suspected injury to the region.

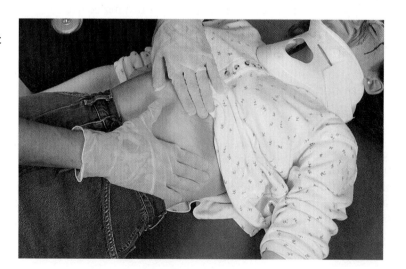

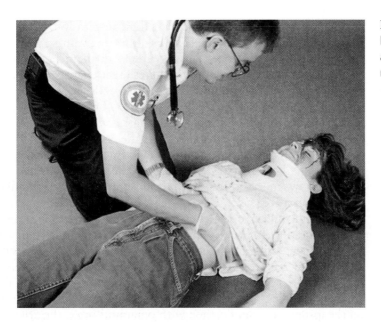

ribs and should elicit pain from any fracture site along the thorax. (Apply pressure only if you are unsure of chest injury. If you suspect rib or sternal fracture, provide appropriate care, but do not aggravate the injury.) Rest your hands on the lower thorax, and let the chest lift your hands with inspiration and let them fall with expiration (Figure 25-14). The motion should be smooth and equal. If not, determine the nature of any asymmetry.

Auscultate

Auscultate all lung lobes, both anteriorly and posteriorly (Figure 25-15). Listen for both inspiratory and expiratory air movement, and note any crackles, indicating edema from contusion or congestive heart failure, or any diminished breath sounds, suggesting hypoventilation. Compare one side with the other and one lobe with another. Be sensitive for distant or muffled respiratory or heart sounds.

Blunt Trauma Assessment

In blunt trauma, you commonly find slight discoloration of the surface of the chest indicative of contusions. The contusions also cause the patient pain, generally

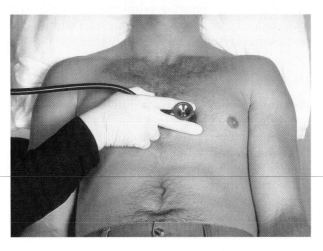

FIGURE 25-15 Auscultate all lung lobes, both anteriorly and posteriorly.

in an area or region, and somewhat limit respiration. As the impact energy increases, it may cause fractures of ribs 4 through 9 and a greater possibility of underlying injury. If the upper ribs, or ribs 10 through 12, fracture, suspect serious underlying injury. Sternal fracture takes great energy and is also associated with a higher incidence of internal injury. Rib fractures generate a point-specific pain (at the fracture site) and crepitus upon deep breathing or your flexing of the patient's chest during the rapid trauma assessment. That pain may further limit chest excursion during respiration. As the energy of trauma and the seriousness of chest trauma increase, more ribs may fracture, causing a flail chest. Remember that a flail chest's paradoxical motion is initially limited by muscular splinting and grows more noticeable and causes more respiratory distress as time since the collision increases.

In blunt injury to the chest, you must anticipate and assess for additional signs suggesting internal injury. Signs specific for lung injury include increasing dyspnea, signs of hypoxemia, accessory muscle use, and intracostal and suprasternal retractions. Auscultation will help you differentiate between pulmonary contusion and pneumothorax. Contusions demonstrate progressively increasing crackles, while pneumothorax presents with diminished breath sounds on the ipsilateral side. Further, with pneumothorax, the affected side may be hyperinflated and resonant to percussion. If the pneumothorax progresses to tension pneumothorax, you will likely note progressing dyspnea and hypoxia, use of accessory muscles, JVD, and tracheal shift toward the contralateral side (a late finding). Subcutaneous emphysema may develop, especially if the lung defect was caused by or is associated with a rib fracture that disturbs the integrity of the parietal pleura. Hemothorax is noticeable due to the vascular loss, more so than for the respiratory component of the pathology. Suspect it if you find the signs of hypovolemia associated with blunt chest trauma. Hemothorax, when sizeable, may cause dyspnea.

Blunt mediastinal injury will probably affect the heart, great vessels, and trachea. Heart injury may present with chest pain similar to that of myocardial infarction and, if serious enough, with the signs of heart failure or cardiogenic shock. The ECG may reveal tachycardia, bradycardia, cardiac irritability and, in cases of severe cardiac contusion, may demonstrate ST elevation. Cardiac rupture presents with the signs of imminent death, while pericardial tamponade is unlikely in blunt chest trauma. Injury to the great vessels (aneurysm) is most frequently associated with lateral impacts or feet-first high falls and may produce a tearing chest pain and pulse deficits in the extremities. If the aneurysm ruptures, rapidly progressing hypovolemia, hypotension, shock, and death ensue. Tracheobronchial injury results in rapidly developing pneumomediastinum or pneumothorax and possible subcutaneous emphysema, hemoptysis, dyspnea, and hypoxia. Positive pressure ventilations may increase the development and severity of signs. Traumatic asphyxia presents with JVD, discoloration of the head and neck, severe dyspnea, and possibly the signs of hypovolemia and shock.

Penetrating Trauma Assessment

Penetrating injury displays a different set of signs associated with different injuries. Inspect a chest wound for frothy blood or sounds of air exchange with respirations (open pneumothorax). Remember that a wound needs to be rather large (high-velocity bullet exit wound or close-range shotgun blast) for these signs to occur. A penetrating wound, however, commonly induces a simple pneumothorax with its associated signs and symptoms. A hyperinflated chest, JVD, tracheal shift away from the injury, distant or absent breath sounds, and severe dyspnea and hypotension suggest tension pneumothorax. The pressure of tension pneumothorax may push air outward through a penetrating wound or cause

Remember, the severity of internal injury associated with penetrating trauma may be great despite seemingly minor entrance and/or exit wounds.

subcutaneous emphysema around the wound. Some degree of hemothorax is likely to be associated with penetrating chest trauma and, if extensive, may reveal diminished or absent breath sounds. Hemothorax also causes or significantly contributes to hypovolemia and shock.

Penetrating trauma to the heart is likely to cause pericardial tamponade and present with JVD, distant heart sounds, and hypotension (Beck's triad). Pulsus paradoxus may be present, and jugular filling may occur with inspiration (Kussmaul's sign), both being indicative of pericardial tamponade. Heart sounds are distant, pulses are weak, and the patient experiences increasing hypotension and shock (Figure 25-16). Penetrating trauma to the heart may also cause myocardial rupture and associated pericardial tamponade or immediate death (Figure 25-17). The patient demonstrates vital signs that fall precipitously as the vascular volume is pumped into the mediastinum.

ONGOING ASSESSMENT

While the ongoing assessment simply repeats elements of the primary assessment, the taking of vital signs, and examination of any injury signs discovered during earlier assessment, it takes on great importance for the patient with chest trauma. With any serious chest impact or any penetrating injury to the chest, observe the respiratory depth, rate, and symmetry of effort. Auscultate the lung fields for equality and crackles and monitor the distal pulses, oxygen saturation, skin colour, and blood

Continuous reassessment of the patient with chest injury is essential as deterioration may occur in a matter of seconds.

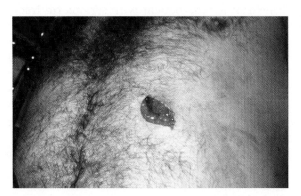

FIGURE 25-16 Penetrating stab wound to the chest involving the heart.

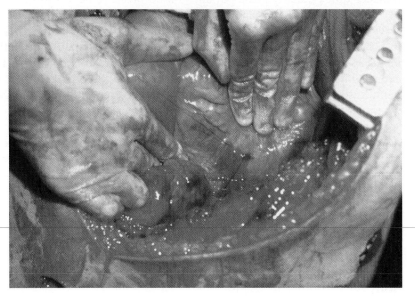

FIGURE 25-17 Stab wound that penetrated the pericardium.

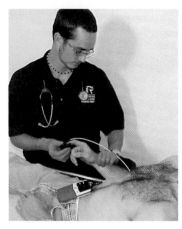

FIGURE 25-18 With pulse oximetry, you can continuously monitor the percentage of the patient's oxygen saturation.

General management of the patient with serious chest trauma requires ensuring good oxygenation and adequate respiratory volume and rate.

Remember, aggressive fluid resuscitation in the patient with chest trauma can result in hemodilution and loss of clotting factors.

pressure for signs of progressing hypovolemia (Figure 25-18). If any signs change between assessments, search out the cause, and rule out progressing chest injury. Be especially suspicious of developing tension pnuemothorax, pericardial tamponade, extensive and evolving pulmonary contusion, and hypovolemia associated with hemothorax. If any of these is found, institute the appropriate management steps.

MANAGEMENT OF THE CHEST INJURY PATIENT

The general management of the patient with significant chest injury focuses on ensuring good oxygenation and adequate respiratory volume and rate. Administer high-flow oxygen using the nonrebreather mask. Ensure that the airway is patent, and consider endotracheal intubation if there is any significant loss in the level of consciousness or orientation. Consider intubation early in your care, as patients with thoracic trauma are likely to get worse with time. Endotracheal intubation also makes ventilation of the patient with flail chest or pulmonary contusion easier.

Carefully evaluate the minute volume of the patient (breaths per minute times volume) and if it is less than 6000 mL consider overdrive ventilation. Bag-valve, mask the conscious patient with severe dyspnea at a rate of 12 to 16 full breaths per minute, trying to match the patient's respiratory rate. Closely monitor pulse oximetry, level of consciousness, and skin colour. Bag-valve-masking may also be beneficial for the patient with serious rib fractures and flail chest. The positive pressure displaces the chest outward, reducing the movement of the fracture site and moving the flail segment with the chest. It may also be beneficial to the patient who is exhausted from the increased breathing effort associated with pulmonary contusion. In this case, the ventilations help push any fluids back into the vascular system to relieve edema. Remember, however, that positive pressure ventilations change the dynamics of respiration from a less-than-atmospheric process to a greater-than-atmospheric process and may exacerbate respiratory problems, such as tracheobronchial injury, pneumothorax, and tension pneumothorax.

Anticipate heart and great vessel compromise with thoracic injury, and be ready to stabilize the patient's cardiovascular system. Initiate at least one large-bore IV site if the patient has a serious mechanism of chest trauma, and place two lines if there are any signs of hypovolemia or compensation. Be prepared to administer fluids quickly if the patient's blood pressure begins to fall.

Intravenous fluid infusion for the patient with chest trauma should be conservative. Rapid fluid administration may increase the rate of hemorrhage and dilute the clotting factors, further adding to the problem. Additional fluid also increases the edema associated with pulmonary contusion, increasing the rate and extent of its development. Any time you administer fluids to the chest trauma patient, auscultate all lung fields carefully, and reduce the fluid resuscitation rate whenever you hear respiratory crackles or the patient's dyspnea increases.

Care is specific for thoracic injuries, including rib fractures, sternoclavicular dislocation, flail chest, open pneumothorax, tension pneumothorax, hemothorax, cardiac contusion, pericardial tamponade, aortic aneurysm, tracheobronchial injury, and traumatic asphyxia.

RIB FRACTURES

Rib fractures, either isolated or associated with other respiratory injuries, may produce pain that significantly limits respiratory effort and leads to hypoventilation. In these patients, you may consider administering analgesics for greater patient comfort and improving chest excursion. Ensure that the patient is hemodynamically stable, that there is no associated abdominal or head injury, and that the patient is fully conscious and oriented. Note that use of nitrous oxide is contraindicated in chest trauma as the nitrogen may migrate into a pneumothorax or tension pneumothorax.

STERNOCLAVICULAR DISLOCATION

Supportive therapy with oxygen is usually all that is required for an isolated sternoclavicular dislocation. However, hemodynamic instability indicates associated injuries requiring rapid transport to a trauma centre, with aggressive resuscitation measures instituted en route.

FLAIL CHEST

Place the patient on the side of injury if spinal immobilization is not required, or secure a large and bulky dressing with bandaging against the flail segment to stabilize it (Figure 25-19). Employ high-flow oxygen therapy, monitor oxygen saturation with pulse oximetry, and monitor cardiac activity with the ECG. If there is significant dyspnea, evidence of underlying pulmonary injury, or signs of respiratory compromise, these measures will not suffice. Then, consider endotracheal intubation, positive pressure ventilations, and high-flow oxygen. Positive pressure ventilations internally splint the flail segment, expand atelectatic areas of the lung, and also treat underlying pulmonary contusion. Use of sandbags to support the flail segment is not indicated because it may diminish chest movement, adding to hypoventilation, atelectasis, and subsequent hypoxemia. Rapid transport to a trauma centre is indicated, as this injury, its complications, and associated injuries are life threatening.

Consider early intubation of the patient with flail chest, especially when oxygenation remains impaired despite the provision of high-flow oxygen.

OPEN PNEUMOTHORAX

Support the patient with open pneumothorax by administering high-flow oxygen and monitoring oxygen saturation and respiratory effort. If you find a penetrating injury, cover it with a sterile occlusive dressing (sterile plastic wrap) taped on three sides (Figure 25-20), or use an Asherman chest seal. This process converts the open pneumothorax into a closed pneumothorax, prevents further aspiration of air, and relieves any building pressure (tension pneumothorax) through the valve-like dressing. If the dyspnea diminishes somewhat but still continues, provide positive pressure ventilations and intubate as indicated. Carefully monitor the patient when you employ intermittent positive pressure ventilation because its use may lead to a tension pneumothorax. If after the dressing has been applied, the patient has progressive breathing difficulty, appears to be hypoventilating and hypoxemic, has decreasing breath sounds on the injured side and increasing JVD, remove the occlusive dressing. If you hear air rush out and the patient's respirations improve, reseal the wound, monitor respiration carefully, and again remove the dressing if any respiratory signs or symptoms redevelop. If removing the dressing does not relieve the increasing signs and symptoms, suspect and treat for tension pneumothorax.

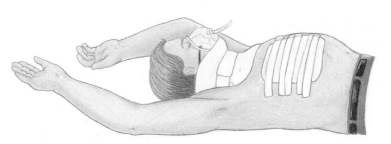

FIGURE 25-19 Flail chest should be treated with administration of oxygen and gentle splinting of the flail segment with a pillow or pad.

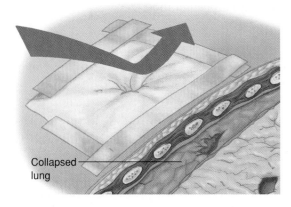

On inspiration, dressing seals
wound, preventing air entry

Collapsed
lung

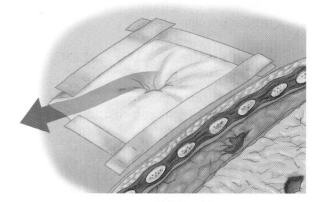

Expiration allows trapped air to escape
through untaped section of dressing

FIGURE 25-20   By taping the occlusive dressing on three sides, you create a flutter valve that helps prevent tension pneumothorax.

TENSION PNEUMOTHORAX

Confirm possible tension pneumothorax by auscultating the lung fields for diminished breath sounds and observing for severe dyspnea, hyperinflation of the chest, and JVD. Successful treatment depends on rapid recognition of this condition and then pleural decompression. This procedure is within the scope of practice of both advanced care paramedics (ACPs) and critical care paramedics (CCPs). As you prepare to decompress the affected (ipsilateral) side, apply high-flow oxygen if the airway is intact and the patient is able to demonstrate adequate ventilatory effort. Provide ventilations with the bag-valve mask and supplemental oxygen, and intubate if the patient is unable to maintain an airway or continues to show signs/symptoms of hypoxemia on high-flow oxygen. Perform needle thoracentesis by inserting a 14-gauge intravascular catheter into the second intercostal space, midclavicular line on the side of the thorax with decreased breath sounds and hyperinflation (Figure 25-21). Attach a syringe filled with sterile water or saline to the needle hub of the catheter. Then, advance the catheter through the chest wall while maintaining gentle traction on the syringe plunger. Ensure that you enter the thoracic cavity by passing the needle just over the rib. The intercostal artery, vein, and nerve pass just under each rib and may be injured if the needle's track is too high. As you enter the pleural space, you will feel a pop and note bubbling air through the fluid in the syringe. Advance the catheter into the chest and then withdraw the needle and syringe.

    If the patient remains symptomatic, place a second or third catheter to more rapidly facilitate decompression. Secure the catheter in place with tape, being careful not to block the port or kink the catheter. Leaving the catheter open to air converts the tension pneumothorax into a simple pneumothorax and stabilizes the patient. You may create a flutter valve by cutting the finger off a latex glove, making a small perforation in its tip, and securing it to the catheter hub, or by using as Asherman chest seal. Monitor the patient's respirations and breath sounds for a recurring tension pneumothorax. If signs and symptoms reappear, decompress the chest again. Frequently, the initial catheter will clog or kink and necessitate replacement by another.

    Rapidly transport the patient to a trauma centre for definitive treatment (usually with a chest tube). Be cautious in using IV crystalloid infusion if the patient is hemodynamically stable. An underlying pulmonary contusion may lead

Tension pneumothorax is an occasional complication of multiple trauma. Always assess for it, and decompress the chest when indicated.

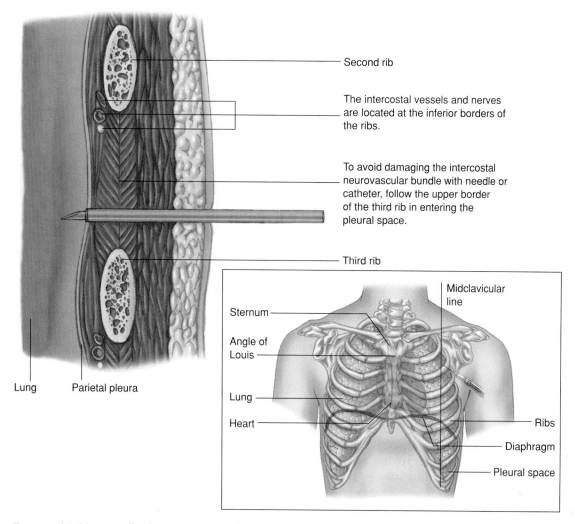

Second rib

The intercostal vessels and nerves are located at the inferior borders of the ribs.

To avoid damaging the intercostal neurovascular bundle with needle or catheter, follow the upper border of the third rib in entering the pleural space.

Third rib

Sternum

Angle of Louis

Lung

Heart

Midclavicular line

Ribs

Diaphragm

Pleural space

Lung   Parietal pleura

FIGURE 25-21   Needle decompression of a tension pneumothorax.

to edema, which is made worse by overaggressive fluid therapy. If your patient remains hypotensive after chest decompression and respirations do not become adequate, consider the possibility of internal hemorrhage and the need for (conservative) fluid resuscitation. If respirations do not dramatically improve, assess for a contralateral tension pneumothorax or pericardial tamponade as the cause.

HEMOTHORAX

Treat the patient with suspected hemothorax with oxygen administration and respiratory support as needed. Initiate two large-bore intravenous catheters, readied to infuse large volumes of fluid. Be conservative in fluid administration. Maintain systolic blood pressure (between 90 and 100 mmHg), but do not attempt to return it to preinjury levels. Carefully listen to breath sounds during any infusion because the increasing vascular volume may increase the edema and congestion of pulmonary contusion. It may also increase the pressure, rate, and volume of internal hemorrhage. If the pulmonary contusion is extensive and the patient cannot be adequately oxygenated with high-flow oxygen, positive pressure ventilations are indicated, which may limit further edema that contributes to the injury.

MYOCARDIAL CONTUSION

In serious frontal impact collisions, suspect myocardial contusion, and administer high-flow oxygen. Monitor cardiac electrical activity, and watch for tachycardia, bradycardia, ectopic beats, and conduction defects. Establish an IV line in the event that antidysrhythmics are needed, and monitor the patient for great vessel injury. Rapidly transport the patient to a trauma centre for further evaluation and continued monitoring.

PERICARDIAL TAMPONADE

If pericardial tamponade is suspected, consider diverting to the closest hospital with a physician-staffed emergency department where emergency pericardiocentesis can be performed.

Maintain a high index of suspicion for pericardial tamponade in the patient with central thoracic penetrating trauma. While there can be little prehospital care other than the administration of oxygen and some IV fluids to maximize venous return, definitive care is to remove some of the fluid accumulating in the pericardial sac. This action is not permitted in the field; hence the patient needs to be transported as rapidly as possible to the emergency department. Note that a relatively simple procedure can relieve this problem and can be adequately administered by an emergency physician. If a physician-staffed emergency department is closer to you than a trauma centre, it may be the best choice for the patient with pericardial tamponade. After the pericardiocentesis is performed, the patient may then be directed to the closest trauma centre.

AORTIC ANEURYSM

Care for the patient with dissecting aortic aneurysm is gentle but rapid transport to a trauma centre. Any jarring during extrication, assessment, care, packaging, or transport increases the risk of rupture and rapidly fatal exsanguination. Initiate IV therapy en route, but be very conservative in fluid administration. Mild hypotension may be protective of the injury site. If the aneurysm ruptures, as indicated by an immediate deterioration in vital signs, provide rapid administration of fluids. Anxiety and its effect on cardiac output and blood pressure may increase the likelihood of aneurysm rupture. Place a special emphasis on calming and reassuring the patient during very gentle care and transport.

TRACHEOBRONCHIAL INJURY

Support the patient with tracheobronchial injury with oxygen, and clear the airway of blood and secretions. If you are unable to maintain a patent airway or adequately oxygenate the patient, then intubate the trachea and provide positive pressure ventilations. Observe the patient carefully for the development of a tension pneumothorax, which may result as a complication of positive pressure ventilations, and treat as previously prescribed. Provide rapid transport as soon as the patient can be extricated and stabilized. This is important because these patients can rapidly destabilize and then require emergency surgical intervention.

TRAUMATIC ASPHYXIA

Administer oxygen, and support the airway and respiration of the traumatic asphyxia patient. This may require using positive pressure ventilations with the bag-valve mask to ensure adequate ventilation during the entrapment and possibly thereafter. Establish two large-bore IV lines for rapid infusion of crystalloid in anticipation of rapidly developing hypovolemia with chest decompression. Once the compressing force is removed, the direct effects of traumatic asphyxia spontaneously resolve; however, serious internal hemorrhage may begin. Prepare to transport the patient immediately after release from entrapment because the patient will likely have severe coexisting injuries.

Prolonged stagnant blood flow and a hypoxic cellular environment may cause accumulation of metabolic acids. As the compression is released, this blood returns to the central circulation, much as it does with entrapped limbs during crush injury.

SUMMARY

Thoracic trauma by either blunt or penetrating mechanisms has a great potential for posing a threat to a patient's life. In fact, 25 percent of all traumatic deaths are secondary to injuries in this region. In assessing these patients, the mechanism of injury, when considered along with the clinical findings, may help in differentiating among the many possible injuries. The assessment, in turn, helps guide your interventions and determines the need for rapid extrication and transport. Aggressive airway management, oxygenation, ventilation, and fluid resuscitation, when indicated, can make the difference between the patient's survival and death. Specific interventions, such as pleural decompression or stabilization of a flail segment, can also affect mortality and morbidity from chest trauma. Understanding the pathological processes affecting the chest during trauma and employing proper assessment and care measures will ensure the best possible outcome for your patients.

CHAPTER 26

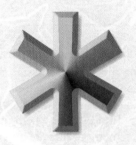

Abdominal Trauma

Objectives

After reading this chapter, you should be able to:

1. Describe the epidemiology, including morbidity/mortality, for patients with abdominal trauma as well as prevention strategies to avoid the injuries. (p. 310)

2. Apply the epidemiological principles to develop prevention strategies for abdominal injuries. (p. 310)

3. Describe the anatomy and physiology of the abdominal organs and structures. (see Chapter 12)

4. Predict abdominal injuries on the basis of blunt and penetrating mechanisms of injury. (pp. 310–318)

5. Describe open and closed abdominal injuries. (pp. 310–313)

6. Identify the need for rapid intervention and transport of the patient with abdominal injuries on the basis of assessment findings. (pp. 318–324)

7. Explain the pathophysiology of solid and hollow organ injuries, abdominal vascular injuries, pelvic fractures, and other abdominal injuries. (pp. 313–318)

8. Describe the assessment findings associated with and the management of solid and hollow organ injuries,

Continued

Objectives Continued

abdominal vascular injuries, pelvic fractures, and other abdominal injuries. (pp. 318–324)

9. Differentiate among abdominal injuries on the basis of the assessment and history. (pp. 318–323)

10. Given several preprogrammed and moulaged abdominal trauma patients, provide the appropriate scene assessment, primary assessment, rapid trauma or secondary assessment and history, detailed assessment, and ongoing assessment and provide appropriate patient care and transport. (pp. 318–326)

INTRODUCTION TO ABDOMINAL TRAUMA

Injury to the abdomen does not present as dramatically as it does elsewhere in the body and often occurs without overt signs.

The abdominal cavity is one of the body's largest cavities and contains many vital organs essential to life. Serious direct or secondary injury may damage these vital organs. In addition, large volumes of blood can be lost in the cavity before the loss becomes evident. In the abdomen, however, injury does not always present as dramatically as it does elsewhere in the body. Injury often occurs without overt signs because few skeletal structures protect the abdomen. The signs of transmitted injury—deformity, swelling, and the discoloration of contusions—take time to develop and are not often seen in the prehospital setting. These considerations make the anticipation of possible abdominal injuries and careful abdominal assessment critical for the patient with trauma to this region.

Over the past decade, the relative mortality and morbidity for the various abdominal injuries has declined due to improved surgical and critical care techniques. Reduced injury-to-surgery times have also contributed to this decline as emergency medical services (EMS) systems have recognized the necessity for rapid surgical intervention. The severity of injuries and the number of deaths associated with blunt trauma have also decreased, thanks to improvements in highway design and vehicle structure and to greater use of seat belts and other safety practices. However, the overall mortality and morbidity from penetrating trauma is on the rise due to the increasing violence in the society, most specifically, in the growing use and power of handguns.

Prevention of abdominal injuries, as with most other types of trauma, is the best way to reduce mortality and morbidity. As noted, highway and vehicle design improvements as well as safety practices at home and in the workplace play important roles in reducing both the incidence and the seriousness of abdominal injury.

There remains room for further improvements in safety practices, however. For example, many people still do not use seat belts. Failure to use the seat belt increases the incidence of abdominal injury secondary to impact with the steering wheel, dash, or other parts of the auto's interior and the incidence of impact after ejection. (Side-impact airbags have the potential to reduce the incidence of pelvic fracture and internal abdominal injuries frequently associated with this mechanism of injury.)

One area of special concern is the proper application of the lap belt. If the belt rides too high on the abdomen, with deceleration, the belt directs forces both to the contents of the abdominal cavity and to the lumbar spine. Severe compression may result in serious associated abdominal injury. Proper placement, in which the belt rests on the iliac crests, transmits the forces of severe deceleration to the pelvis and the body's skeletal structure, thus sparing the abdominal contents and the spine from injury. Proper positioning of seat belts is especially important with children.

Mortality and morbidity associated with penetrating trauma can also be reduced by reducing violence in society and by eliminating the availability of handguns on the streets.

PATHOPHYSIOLOGY OF ABDOMINAL INJURY

MECHANISM OF INJURY

Because the abdomen is bound by muscles, rather than skeletal structures, there is a freer transmission of the energy of trauma to the internal organs and structures.

Unlike the other major body containers (skull, spine, and thorax), the abdomen is bound by muscles, rather than skeletal structures. This results in a freer transmission of the energy of trauma to the internal organs and structures. Concurrently, the overt physical signs of this energy transmission are limited.

Penetrating trauma imparts its energy directly to the tissues touched by the offending object (Figure 26-1) or, as with high-velocity projectiles (from handguns, shotguns, and rifles), transmits energy and injury some distance from the projectile pathway. The bullet injury process causes damage as the projectile contacts tissue, sets that tissue and surrounding tissue in motion, then compresses and stretches surrounding tissue. The projectile adds to the damage as it draws debris and contaminants into the wound, causing wound infection and poor healing. The disruption of tissue from penetrating trauma may permit uncontrolled hemorrhage, organ damage, the spillage of hollow organ contents, and, eventually, irritation of the abdominal lining (peritoneum). Gunshot wounds to the abdomen, especially those from rifles, high-powered handguns, and shotguns at close range impart tremendous energy to the tissue and organs of the region and tend to cause mortality and morbidity about ten times greater than those associated with the lower velocity stab wounds. When penetrating trauma induces injury, it affects the liver 40 percent of the time, the small bowel about 25 percent of the time, and the large bowel about 10 percent of the time. Injuries to the spleen, kidneys, and pancreas follow in decreasing order of incidence.

Penetrating trauma most frequently involves the liver and small bowel.

A special type of penetrating trauma is induced by a blast from a shotgun. The shotgun delivers numerous round pellets (called shot) through the hollow gun barrel. The aerodynamics of the shot and the rapid expansion of their distribution (the pattern) cause the energy of impact to decrease rapidly when the projectiles move farther from the barrel. Generally, shotgun blasts at short range (under 3 metres) are extremely lethal. Between 3 and 7 metres, the penetration of the projectiles is great but often survivable. At distances greater than seven metres, the depth of penetration and subsequent injury fall off quickly. These parameters change somewhat with the decreasing gauge size (gun barrel diameter) and the size of the projectiles. (See Chapter 18, "Penetrating Trauma.")

Blunt trauma to the abdomen produces the least visible signs of injury and causes trauma through three mechanisms: deceleration, compression, and shear (Figure 26-2). As the exterior of the abdomen decelerates (or accelerates) during impact, its contents slam into one another in a chain reaction. They are first injured by the force changing their velocity and then by the forces of compression as they are trapped between the impacting energy and the more posterior organs. The entire contents of the cavity may be compressed between the force impacting the anterior abdominal cavity and the spinal column. Shear forces induce damage when one part of an organ is free to move while another part is restricted by the forces of trauma or by ligamentous or vascular attachments. Blunt trauma

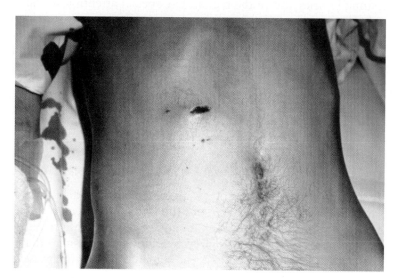

FIGURE 26-1 Stab wound to the right upper quadrant.

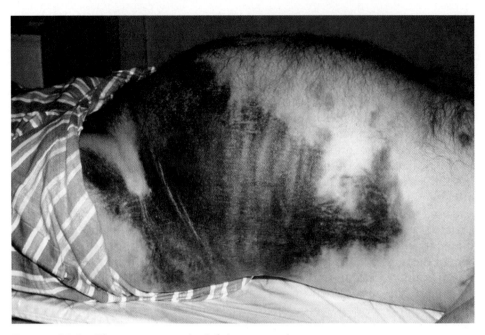

FIGURE 26-2   Blunt trauma to the left lower quadrant.

is responsible for about 40 percent of the incidences of splenic injury and a little more than 20 percent of hepatic (liver) injury. The bowel and kidneys are the next most frequently injured abdominal structures in blunt trauma.

Blast injuries to the abdomen involve both blunt and penetrating mechanisms. Shrapnel and debris propelled by the blast act as projectiles and create penetrating trauma. However, because of the irregular shapes of the objects and their poor aerodynamic properties, they tend to produce serious injury only in close proximity to the blast's centre. The pressure wave generated by the explosion causes blunt trauma as it dramatically compresses and relaxes air-filled organs and is likely to contuse organs or rupture them. Since the stomach and bowel are only occasionally distended with air, they are neither as frequently nor as seriously injured as the lungs by the blast pressure wave. Abdominal injury is a secondary concern with blast injury patients.

Careful evaluation of the mechanism of injury, including identification of the force and direction of impact as it relates to the abdomen, is important to anticipating injuries within the region. Pay special attention to the potential for seat belt injury or direct injury as the abdomen impacts the steering wheel in a vehicle crash, impacts with objects or the ground during a fall, or is struck during an assault. Remember that the early presentation of a contusion will likely be a simple reddening (erythema) of the affected area. Hence it is critically important to carefully analyze the mechanism of injury, maintain a high index of suspicion for intra-abdominal injury, and investigate the abdomen for signs and symptoms of injury. The abdominal wall, hollow organs, solid organs, vascular structures, mesentery, and peritoneum all respond differently to trauma.

INJURY TO THE ABDOMINAL WALL

Any injury to the contents of the abdomen must be disrupted or be transmitted through the abdominal wall. Since the skin and muscular lining of the abdomen are more resistant to injury than many of the internal organs, they are likely to be uninjured or minimally injured by blunt trauma forces that cause serious injury within. Even when injured, the skin and underlying muscle may only show erythema during the first hour or so. The more visible discoloration of ecchymosis and noticeable swelling require several hours to develop. Penetrating wounds may also be difficult to assess properly because the musculature and skin tension close the wound opening. Bullet and knife wounds look especially small and may appear much less lethal than they are.

Penetrating abdominal injury may cause the abdominal contents to protrude through the opening. This type of injury, called an **evisceration,** occurs most frequently through the anterior abdominal wall and is usually associated with a large and deep laceration. The omentum and/or small bowel are most likely to protrude. The evisceration endangers the protruding bowel because of compromised circulation and the drying of this delicate intra-abdominal tissue. However, replacing the protrusion risks introducing bacteria into the peritoneal space. If the bowel is torn, there is the additional danger of its contents leaking into the peritoneal space when the bowel is replaced.

Penetrating trauma to the thorax, buttocks, flanks, and back may also affect the abdomen and injure its contents. During deep expiration, the abdominal organs extend well into the thorax and move up to the nipple line anteriorly and to the tips of the scapulae posteriorly. Injury to the lower portion of the chest may lacerate the diaphragm and injure the stomach, liver, spleen, or gallbladder. The flank, back, and buttock muscles are thick and resist penetrating trauma very well. However, deep wounds in these locations can penetrate into the abdominal cavity and cause injury to adjacent organs. High-powered projectiles, especially those from hunting or military rifles, may have enough energy to deflect when striking bone and enter the abdomen from as far away as a proximal extremity wound.

Tears in the diaphragm may also disrupt the abdominal container. These tears may occur when the patient holds his breath just before an impact or with penetrating injury to the lower thorax or upper abdomen. Not only may such an injury compromise the important role of the diaphragm in respiration, but it may also permit or force abdominal contents (like those of the stomach, liver, or a portion of the small bowel) to enter the thoracic cavity. This reduces the volume of the thoracic cage available during respiration and compromises the blood supply to the herniated organs. Diaphragmatic injury occurs from stab injuries most frequently on the left side because this is where right-handed assailants strike. Gunshot wounds affect both sides equally. Small tears are unlikely to permit abdominal contents to enter the thorax and are unlikely to greatly affect respiration. Large tears are more likely to do both.

INJURY TO THE HOLLOW ORGANS

Hollow organs, such as the stomach, small bowel, large bowel, rectum, urinary bladder, gallbladder, and pregnant uterus, may rupture with compression from blunt forces, especially if the organ is full and distended. They may also tear as penetrating objects disrupt their structure. (The small bowel is the most frequently injured hollow abdominal organ during penetrating trauma because it rests anteriorly and just beneath the thin anterior abdominal muscles and omentum.) Damage to the hollow organs results in hemorrhage and in the spillage of their contents into the retroperitoneal, peritoneal, or pelvic spaces. The jejunum, ileum, colon, and rectum contain progressively higher bacterial concentrations, and their rupture and the subsequent leakage of material into the abdomen will likely induce severe but delayed infection (called sepsis). The other hollow organs are more likely to release contents that cause a chemical irritation of the abdominal lining. The urinary bladder will release urine; the gallbladder, bile; and the stomach and duodenum, chyme, which is acidic and rich in digestive enzymes. Injury to the hollow organs may result in frank blood in the stool (**hematochezia**), blood in emesis (**hematemesis**), and blood in the urine (**hematuria**).

* **evisceration** a protrusion of organs from a wound.

* **hematochezia** blood in the stool.

* **hematemesis** the vomiting of blood.

* **hematuria** blood in the urine.

INJURY TO THE SOLID ORGANS

Solid organs, such as the spleen, liver, pancreas, and kidneys, are also subject to blunt and penetrating trauma. These organs are especially dense and are not held together as strongly as the more muscular hollow organs of the body. They are prone to contuse, resulting in organ damage and minimal bleeding, or to rupture (also referred to as "fracture"). If the organ's capsule remains intact, it will limit the hemorrhage. However, if the capsule is disrupted by penetrating trauma or torn by the mechanism of blunt trauma, unrestricted hemorrhage may result.

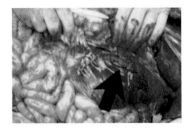

FIGURE 26-3   Penetrating trauma to the spleen.

The spleen is especially well protected by the lower ribs, the back and flank muscles, and the spinal column. It is not, however, protected by a strong peritoneal capsule and is very fragile in nature. It may be injured with severe abdominal compression, blunt left flank trauma, or penetrating injury to the region (Figure 26-3). The spleen then bleeds profusely, frequently resulting in shock and a life threat to the patient. The blood loss may accumulate against the diaphragm (especially in the supine patient) and result in referred pain to the left shoulder region.

The pancreas is central to the upper abdomen, somewhat less delicate than the spleen and well protected from blunt trauma by its location deep in the central abdominal cavity. Penetrating trauma may lacerate its structure and permit blood and digestive enzymes to flow into the abdominal cavity. These digestive juices may actually begin to digest pancreatic and surrounding tissues, leading to severe internal injury. Pancreatic injury does sometimes result from severe blunt trauma to the upper abdomen that compresses the pancreas between the trauma force and the vertebral column. This may occur when a patient strikes a steering wheel or the handlebars of a motorcycle during a crash. Such a patient frequently complains of upper abdominal pain that may radiate to the back.

The kidneys are equally well protected by their location deep in the abdominal cavity. They are somewhat more resistant to injury than the pancreas, have a more substantial serous capsule, and are attached by large renal arteries to the aorta. They are most frequently injured by trauma to the flanks. Renal injury may result in regional (back or flank) pain as well as hematuria.

The liver is the largest single organ within the abdomen. Being a peritoneal organ, it is surrounded by the strong visceral peritoneum, which resists injury and will hold the organ together if injured. The liver is firmer than the spleen and the pancreas and is somewhat protected by the inferior border of the thorax. When the forces of trauma are directed to this region, however, they are likely to damage the liver, especially if they induce lower rib fracture on the right side (Figure 26-4). The liver is restrained from forward motion by the ligamentum teres. During severe deceleration, the weight of the liver forces it into the liga-

FIGURE 26-4   Rupture of the liver.

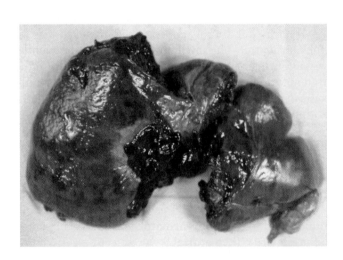

ment, causing shear forces, laceration, and hemorrhage. Liver injury often presents with tenderness along the right lower border of the thoracic cage and, as blood accumulates against the diaphragm, pain in the upper right shoulder.

INJURY TO THE VASCULAR STRUCTURES

Arteries and veins within the abdomen are prone to injury with serious consequences. The abdominal aorta and its major tributaries can be injured by direct blunt or penetrating trauma or may be injured as abdominal organs decelerate and pull on their vascular attachments during an auto crash or similar impact. Penetrating trauma does not frequently involve the very large vessels of the abdomen, but when the aorta or another major artery is damaged, internal hemorrhage can be severe. The vena cava and its tributaries can likewise be injured. Most vascular injuries (97 percent) are associated with penetrating trauma. As blood accumulates in the abdomen of a supine patient, it will come to rest against the diaphragm. There, it irritates the muscular structure and produces a referred pain in the shoulder region. However, other signs of significant hemorrhage may be limited.

Vascular injury in the peritoneal, retroperitoneal, and pelvic spaces can be serious for several reasons. These spaces are easily expandable, and hemorrhage may continue without the increase in pressure exerted by surrounding tissue that would occur if the vascular injury were within a mass of muscle elsewhere in the body. Without this pressure, both the rate and the volume of blood loss do not diminish. These spaces also contain organs that require significant circulation supplied by rather large arterial and venous vessels. The dynamic nature of the abdomen and its anatomical size mean that a greater volume of blood can be accommodated there before its presence becomes noticeable. Further, due to vagal stimulation caused by the presence of blood in the perotineal cavity, an increasing heart rate may not be present.

Most vascular trauma is associated with penetrating injury.

INJURY TO THE MESENTERY AND BOWEL

The mesentery provides the bowel with circulation, innervation, and attachment. Blunt injury occurs as the mesentery stretches during impact. This type of injury occurs most frequently at points of relative immobility as at the duodenal/jejunal juncture (where the small bowel is affixed by the ligament of Trietz) or where the small bowel joins the large bowel at the ileocecal junction. Injury involving the mesentery may disrupt blood vessels supplying the bowel and eventually cause ischemia, necrosis, and possible rupture. Mesenteric injuries do not usually bleed profusely because the peritoneal layers contain the hemorrhage. Deceleration or compression may tear or rupture the full bowel. With penetrating trauma, the omentum is frequently disrupted and the bowel may be torn anywhere along its length, though tears to the small bowel (jejunum and ileum) are the most likely because of its central–anterior location. Expect a tear to release bowel contents into the peritoneal space, but remember that signs and symptoms of such release are delayed. The duodenum is less frequently injured because of its location deep within the abdomen. Penetrating trauma to the lateral abdomen is likely to injure the large bowel (ascending colon on the right and descending colon on the left).

Expect a tear of the small bowel to release bowel contents into the peritoneal space, but remember that signs and symptoms of such release are delayed.

INJURY TO THE PERITONEUM

The peritoneum is the very delicate and sensitive lining of the anterior abdominal cavity. Its inflammation, called **peritonitis,** can be caused by two major mechanisms, bacterial irritation and chemical irritation. Bacterial peritonitis is an irritation due to infection, which is often released into the space by a torn bowel or open wound. It takes the bacteria between 12 and 24 hours to grow in sufficient

 peritonitis inflammation of the peritoneum caused by chemical or bacterial irritation.

When assessing the abdomen, be aware that local muscle injury caused by trauma may result in local or regional abdominal muscle tenderness and spasm that mimics peritonitis.

✳ rebound tenderness pain on release of the examiner's hands, allowing the patient's abdominal wall to return to its normal position; associated with peritoneal irritation.

✳ guarding protective tensing of the abdominal muscles by a patient suffering abdominal pain; may be a voluntary or involuntary response.

numbers to produce the inflammation, and hence the condition is usually not apparent during prehospital care. Chemical peritonitis occurs more rapidly than bacterial peritonitis because the caustic nature of the digestive enzymes and acids (from the stomach or duodenum) and, to a lesser degree, urine, quickly irritate the peritoneum and induce the inflammatory response. Blood does not induce peritoneal inflammation, and hence serious hemorrhage into the peritoneal cavity will not, by itself, cause this condition.

Peritonitis is a progressive process that presents with characteristic signs and symptoms. It usually begins with a slight tenderness at the location of injury. Over time, the area of inflammation expands, as does the area of tenderness. Any jarring of the abdomen, as occurs with percussion or when you quickly release the pressure of deep palpation, causes a twinge of pain (**rebound tenderness**). In response to pain induced by any movement of the irritated abdominal tissue, the anterior abdominal muscles contract, even in the unconscious patient. This is called **guarding.** If the pain becomes severe, the abdominal muscles assume an extreme contraction and leave the abdominal wall with a rigid, board-like feel. When assessing the abdomen, be aware that local muscle injury caused by trauma may result in local or regional abdominal muscle tenderness and spasm mimicking peritonitis. Tenderness or frank pain from the physical injury may coexist with the signs of peritonitis.

INJURY TO THE PELVIS

A pelvic fracture represents a serious skeletal injury, serious and often life threatening hemorrhage, and possible injury to the organs within the pelvic space. These organs—the ureters, bladder, urethra, female genitalia, prostate, rectum, and anus—can all be injured by the severe kinetic forces, the crushing nature of the injury, or by displaced bone fragments. Pelvic fracture can also cause serious injury to the pregnant uterus. Pelvic hemorrhage and fracture have been discussed in Chapter 22, "Musculoskeletal Trauma."

Sexual assault may also injure the reproductive structures located internally in the female and externally in the male. Direct trauma to the external female genitalia or injury caused by objects inserted into the vagina may tear the soft tissues of this region. Since these tissues are both very sensitive and vascular, the injury may bleed heavily and be very painful. The same is true for the male genitalia, though they are more prone to accidental injury because of their more external location.

INJURY DURING PREGNANCY

Trauma is the number one killer of pregnant females and penetrating abdominal trauma alone accounts for as much as 36 percent of overall maternal mortality.

Trauma is the number one killer of pregnant females. Penetrating abdominal trauma alone accounts for as much as 36 percent of overall maternal mortality. Gunshot wounds to the abdomen of the pregnant female also account for fetal mortality rates of between 40 and 70 percent. In blunt trauma, auto collisions are the leading cause of maternal and fetal mortality and morbidity. Proper seat belt placement can significantly reduce injury to the pregnant mother and to the fetus, while improper placement increases the incidence of both uterine rupture and separation of the placenta from the wall of the uterus. Mothers not wearing seat belts in serious auto collisions are four times more likely to lose their fetuses.

The physiological changes associated with pregnancy protect both the mother and her abdominal organs. With the increasing size of the uterus, most of the abdominal organs are displaced higher in the abdomen (Figure 26-5). This generally protects them unless blunt or penetrating trauma impacts the upper abdomen. If that happens, then the injury may involve numerous organs with increased morbidity and mortality. Direct penetrating injury to the central and

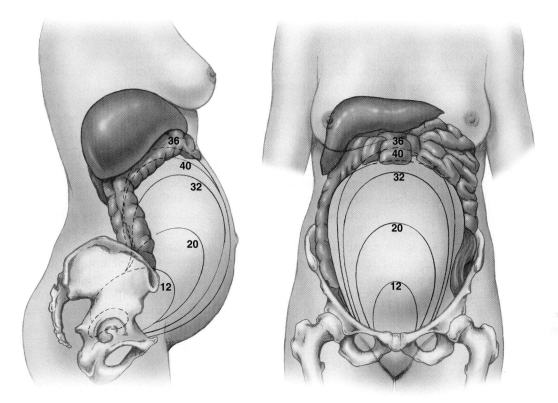

FIGURE 26-5 Changing dimensions of the pregnant uterus. Numbers represent weeks of gestation.

lower parts of the abdomen of the mother in late pregnancy often is not serious; the resulting injury, however, often damages the uterus and endangers the fetus.

The late-term pregnant female is at additional risk of vomiting and possible aspiration. Increasing uterine size increases intra-abdominal pressure, while the hormones of pregnancy relax the cardiac sphincter (the valve that prevents reflux of the stomach contents). The bladder is displaced superiorly early in pregnancy and then becomes more prone to injury and, when injured, bleeds more heavily.

The increasing size and weight of the uterus and its contents have several effects on the mother, especially when trauma occurs. The uterus of a supine patient in late pregnancy may compress the inferior vena cava and reduce the venous return to the heart. This may induce hypotension in the uninjured patient and have severe consequences in the hemorrhaging trauma patient. The increased intra-abdominal pressure along with the compression of the inferior vena cava by the uterus raise venous pressure in the pelvic region and lower extremities. This pressure engorges the vessels and increases the rate of venous hemorrhage from pelvic fracture or lower extremity wounds.

The increased maternal vascular volume (up by 45 percent) helps protect the mother from hypovolemia. However, this protection does not extend to the fetus because fetal blood flow is affected well before there are changes in the maternal blood pressure or pulse rate. In fact, it may take a maternal blood loss of between 30 and 35 percent before changes in maternal blood pressure or heart rate are evident. Therefore, it becomes very important to ensure early and aggressive resuscitation of the potentially hypotensive pregnant mother.

In the pregnant female, the thick and muscular uterus contains both the developing fetus and amniotic fluid. This container is strong, distributing the forces of trauma uniformly to the fetus and thereby reducing chances for injury.

While a pregnant mother is somewhat protected from hypovolemia, the fetus is not so protected.

Significant blunt trauma may cause the uterus to rupture or penetrating trauma may perforate or tear it. The dangers of severe maternal hemorrhage and disruption of the blood supply to the fetus present life threats to both. The potential release of amniotic fluid into the abdomen is also of great concern. The risk of uterine and fetal injury increases with the length of gestation and is greatest during the third trimester of pregnancy.

If an open wound to the uterus does occur, there may be added risk to the mother (in addition to hemorrhage) if she is Rh negative and the fetus is Rh positive. Penetrating or severe blunt trauma may cause some fetal/maternal blood mixing and lead to compatibility problems. Frank uterine rupture is a rare complication of trauma, but it does occur with severe blunt impact, pelvic fracture, and—very infrequently—with stab or shotgun wounds.

Blunt trauma to the uterus may cause the placenta to detach from the uterine wall because the placenta is rather inelastic, whereas the uterus is very flexible. This condition, called **abruptio placentae,** presents a life-threatening risk to both mother and fetus because the separation causes both maternal and fetal hemorrhage (Figure 26-6). More frequently than not, this hemorrhage is contained within the uterus and does not extend to the vaginal outlet. Blunt trauma may also cause the premature rupture of the amniotic sac (breaking of the "membranes" or "bag of waters") and may induce an early labour.

INJURY TO PEDIATRIC PATIENTS

Another special patient with regard to abdominal injuries is the child. Children have poorly developed abdominal musculature and a reduced anterior/posterior diameter. The rib cage is more cartilaginous and flexible and more likely to transmit injury to the organs beneath. These factors increase the incidence of pediatric abdominal injury, especially to the liver, spleen, and kidney. Children also compensate very well for blood loss and may not show any signs or symptoms until they have lost more than half of their blood volume. This is especially important with abdominal injuries because a great volume of blood may be lost into the abdomen with little pain or noticeable distention.

ASSESSMENT OF THE ABDOMINAL INJURY PATIENT

Assessment of the patient who has sustained abdominal trauma is somewhat abbreviated because definitive care for such injury is often surgical intervention. Hence, it is imperative that you quickly assess the patient and, if indications of serious abdominal injury exist, that you package and transport him expeditiously. Assessment of the abdominal injury patient is like that for any trauma patient, with pertinent and significant information gained during the scene assessment, primary assessment, rapid trauma assessment (or secondary assessment and history), and serial ongoing assessments.

SCENE ASSESSMENT

Ensure that the scene is safe for you, fellow rescuers, bystanders, and the patient. Be ready to use appropriate body substance isolation procedures before moving to the patient's side. Also, determine the number of expected patients and need for additional EMS, police, fire, and other service personnel.

For the patient who has sustained abdominal injury, the analysis of the mechanism of injury is the most important element of the scene assessment and

* **abruptio placentae** a condition in which the placenta separates from the uterine wall.

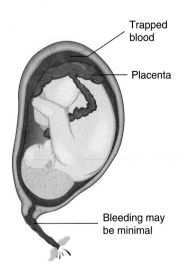

Trapped blood

Placenta

Bleeding may be minimal

FIGURE 26-6   Abruptio placenta.

possibly of the entire assessment. However, forming an index of suspicion for individual abdominal injuries is very difficult because the signs and symptoms are, for the most part, limited and nonspecific. In fact, more than 30 percent of patients with serious abdominal injury may present with no specific signs or symptoms of abdominal injury whatsoever. Additionally, other less life-threatening but more painful injuries may overshadow signs and symptoms of the patient's abdominal injury. Also, those signs and symptoms that are present may become less specific in nature with time and the progressive nature of peritonitis. Lastly, the patient's reporting of his condition may be unreliable due to the effects of alcohol or drug ingestion, head injury, or shock.

If the patient has suffered blunt trauma, identify the strength and direction of the forces and where on the body they were delivered. Focus your observation and palpation on that site during the primary and rapid trauma assessments, and place your highest suspicion of injury there. Begin to develop a list of possible organs injured (the index of suspicion) and the immediate and delayed effects they will have on the patient's condition. In serious blunt trauma or deep penetrating trauma, expect internal and uncontrolled hemorrhage.

If the patient was involved in an auto crash, find out if seat belts were used and if they were used properly (Figure 26-7). Remember that improper placement (above the iliac crests) may increase the likelihood of abdominal compression (and lumbar spine) injury. Lack of seat belt use increases the incidence and severity of all types of injuries, including abdominal injury. Examine the vehicle interior for signs of impact, such as the deformity of a bent steering wheel, a deflated airbag, or a structural intrusion into the passenger compartment. Frontal impact is most likely to compress the abdomen, injuring the liver and spleen and possibly rupturing distended hollow organs, such as the stomach and bladder. Right-side impact frequently causes liver, ascending colon, and pelvic injury, while left side impact causes splenic, descending colon, and pelvic injuries. Pedestrians, and especially children, are likely to sustain lower abdominal injury, especially if the vehicle hits the patient's midsection. It is important to determine the velocity of impact and the distance the patient was thrown. Motorcyclists and, to a lesser degree, bicyclists are likely to sustain abdominal injury as they are propelled forward, while the handlebars restrain the pelvis and lower abdomen. In assaults and other isolated impacts, be observant for left flank impact and splenic or renal damage and right-side impact causing renal or hepatic (liver) injury. If the impact involves the superior abdomen, suspect liver, stomach, spleen, and pancreatic injuries, while impact to the middle or lower abdomen will likely damage the small bowel, kidneys, and bladder.

With a patient who has experienced penetrating trauma, determine the nature of the offending agent. If it is a knife, arrow, or impaled object, determine

> *For the patient who has sustained abdominal injury, the analysis of the mechanism of injury is the most important element of the scene assessment and possibly of the entire assessment.*

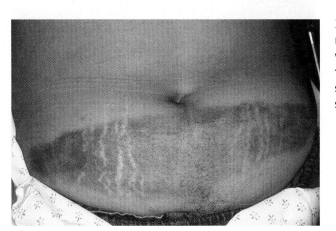

FIGURE 26-7 Use the mechanism of injury to identify where signs of injury might be found—for example, contusions resulting from compression by a seat belt.

the probable angle and depth of insertion (Figure 26-8). Do not move or remove the impaled object.

With gunshot wounds, determine whether the weapon was a handgun, shotgun, or rifle, the distance from the gun to the victim, and the gun's calibre. Also, determine the number of shots fired if possible and the angle from which the gun was fired. Be prepared to examine the flanks, the buttocks, and the back for any sign of additional or exit wounds. Attempt to estimate the amount of blood lost at the scene, and communicate this, with the other information listed above, to the emergency department physician.

Gunshot wounds provide a challenge to assessment. The damage done does not correlate well with the appearance of the entrance or exit wound. It is more related to the bullet's kinetic energy (velocity and mass) as it enters the body and to its energy exchange characteristics as it travels into and through tissue. Low-velocity bullets cause little damage beyond the bullet's actual path. However, these projectiles are easily deflected from their paths by contact with clothing, bone, or, in some cases, soft tissue. They also carry pieces of clothing and other debris into the body and tend not to pass through the body.

High-velocity weapons and the wounds they cause were once seen only in the military setting, but now more powerful handguns are causing similar wounds and internal injuries in civilian life. Their projectiles cause injury well beyond the bullet's path and injure tissue as the projectile creates a cavity and compresses and stretches neighbouring tissue (cavitation). The wounding process also draws debris into the wound, where the damaged and devitalized (without circulation) tissue forms a good medium for bacterial growth. The wounding process may create secondary projectiles as the bullet hits bone, breaks it apart, and then drives the fragments into adjacent tissue. The high-velocity bullet may also fragment and transmit its injuring potential to several pathways.

With either significant blunt or any penetrating trauma to the abdomen, suspect serious and continuing internal hemorrhage. Be especially watchful of the patient during your assessment, and initiate shock care at the first signs and symptoms of hypoperfusion. These signs and symptoms include diminishing level of consciousness or orientation, increasing anxiety or restlessness, thirst, increasing pulse rate, decreasing pulse pressure, and increasing capillary refill time.

The internal damage done by a bullet does not correlate well with the appearance of the entrance or exit wound.

With significant blunt or penetrating trauma, suspect serious and continuing internal hemorrhage.

FIGURE 26-8 Analyze the mechanism of a penetrating trauma in an attempt to determine the probable angle and depth of the wound.

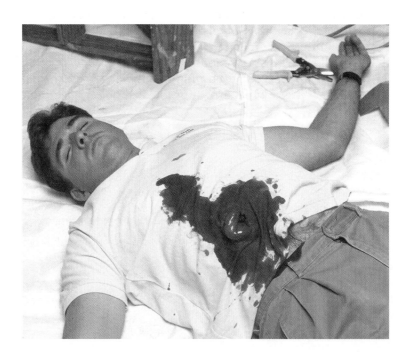

Information you gather at the scene is invaluable to the attending emergency department physician. That information, however, will be unavailable unless you document it carefully and report it upon your arrival at the hospital. Doing this is essential to ensuring that the patient receives the best care in both the prehospital and in-hospital settings.

PRIMARY ASSESSMENT

As you begin the primary assessment, carefully note your patient's level of consciousness and orientation as well as any indication that he may be affected by alcohol, drugs, head injury, or shock. These agents and conditions reduce the reliability of your patient's reporting of the signs and symptoms of abdominal injury. Any decrease in the level of orientation or consciousness should alert you to the need to maintain a higher index of suspicion for abdominal injury and to perform more careful initial and rapid trauma assessments. The patient may also complain of dizziness or lightheadedness when moving from a supine position to a seated or standing position. (Do not ask the patient to move: however, he may have moved on his own before your arrival.) Any of these signs and symptoms should lead you to suspect hypovolemia, possibly from an abdominal injury. Use your initial evaluation as a baseline against which to trend any changes in the patient's level of consciousness or orientation.

As you evaluate airway, breathing, and circulation, be observant for any associated signs and symptoms of hypovolemia, especially if they occur early in your care or are out of proportion with the obvious or expected injuries. Note any rapid shallow respirations, diminished pulse pressure, rapid pulse rate, slow capillary refill time, or thirst. Limited chest movement may be due to the pain of peritonitis or blood irritating the diaphragm. Shallow respirations may be due to spilling of abdominal contents in the thorax from a ruptured diaphragm. Be prepared to protect the airway because abdominal trauma patients are likely to vomit.

RAPID TRAUMA ASSESSMENT

Perform the usual full rapid trauma assessment, but if you have developed a high index of suspicion for abdominal injury, pay particular attention to that region. Carefully examine the abdomen for evidence of injury as suggested by the mechanism of injury or by signs or symptoms observed during the primary assessment. When you suspect that the patient has received blunt trauma, look carefully over the entire abdominal surface for the slight reddening of erythema or minor abrasions associated with superficial soft-tissue injury. Remember that any trauma must pass through the exterior of the abdomen before it can do damage within.

Quickly examine the anterior surface of the abdomen and then the flanks, then carefully and gently log-roll the patient to examine the back, looking for any signs of injury, erythema, ecchymosis, contusions, or open wounds, including eviscerations and impaled objects (Figure 26-9). Also look at the abdomen's general shape and any signs of distention. Visualize the inguinal area for signs of injury or hemorrhage. Jeans may contain hemorrhage without any indication of the accumulation and so should be cut away or removed to assess this region when injury is suspected. Remember that the abdominal cavity can contain a very large volume of blood (in the order of 1.5 litres) before it becomes noticeably distended. In obese patients the volume of blood loss may be even greater before distention is visible. Also, be aware that the signs and symptoms of hemoperitoneum or retroperitoneal hemorrhage are minimal.

The abdomen may contain up to 1.5 litres of blood before distention becomes noticeable.

FIGURE 26-9 Examine the abdomen for signs of injury.

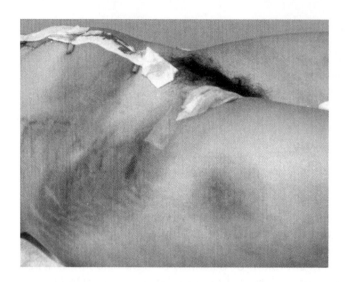

Visualize and palpate the pelvis for signs of injury or instability. Apply gentle pressure directed posteriorly, then medially, on the iliac crests, then place pressure downward on the symphysis pubis. If you note any crepitus or instability, suspect pelvic fracture and both injury to the organs of the lower abdomen and severe internal hemorrhage. If you already suspect pelvic injury, do not test or apply any pressure, and be very careful during movement to the ambulance and transport to the hospital. Any manipulation of the fracture site may restart or increase hemorrhage.

Question the patient about pain or discomfort in each quadrant, and then palpate the quadrants individually, leaving any quadrant with anticipated injury or patient complaint of pain to last. If you palpate an injured quadrant first, the pain may lead the patient to guard during any remaining palpation. Feel for any spasm or guarding as you palpate, then note any patient report of pain when you quickly release the pressure of your palpation (rebound tenderness). If you palpate an abdomen that is board hard, expect injury to the pancreas, duodenum, or stomach, especially if the time since the injury has been short.

Also, note any unusual pulsations in the abdomen. You may visualize some pulsing in the slim, young, healthy, athletic patient, but most patients will not have any visible or palpable pulses in the abdomen. Abnormal pulsation suggests arterial injury. Injuries to the thorax or pelvis also suggest abdominal injury, especially if there are lower rib fractures or the pelvic ring is unstable. Auscultation is not recommended during assessment of the abdominal trauma patient. It takes a great deal of time to adequately listen for bowel sounds, and their presence or absence neither confirms nor rules out possible injury.

When evaluating the patient with penetrating trauma to the abdomen, look carefully at the entrance wound, and note its appearance, size, and depth. Point-blank discharge of a gun against tissue will introduce the barrel exhaust into the wound created by the bullet. You may notice powder debris and the crackling of subcutaneous emphysema. Look for contamination and any signs of serious blood loss. Then, examine the patient for an exit wound. Exit wounds may look more "blown out" in nature and are generally larger and more serious in appearance than entrance wounds. Count the number of entry and exit wounds and note whether they are paired or if an inequality suggests that some projectiles did not exit. The wounds from a projectile may be very small and difficult to see, while still carrying the potential to cause lethal injury. Anticipate the injuries that occurred as the object or bullet sped into and through the body, but remember that it is not uncommon for a bullet to alter its path. Be suspicious of any pro-

Abnormal pulsations in the abdomen suggest arterial injury.

Auscultation is not recommended during assessment of the abdominal trauma patient.

jectile wound in the proximal extremities because the projectile may travel along the limb and into the body's interior. Also, keep in mind that a bullet wound to the thorax may then deflect and penetrate the abdomen, and vice versa.

While performing the rapid trauma assessment, carefully question the patient about the characteristics of any pain he feels, and ask specifically about any abdominal sensations or other symptoms. Serious injury may result while the patient feels limited pain or injury sensation, especially when other more painful injuries elsewhere might be distracting him. The evaluation of abdominal pain from the patient's complaint may, however, be subjective, as patients often vary in their responses to pain. In the male, retroperitoneal pain may be referred to the testicular region. Thirst may be one of the few symptoms of abdominal injury, as significant hemorrhage draws down the body's blood volume. Be sure to record any symptoms in the patient's own words, and ensure that these comments and your findings are documented on the prehospital care report and reported to the attending physician.

When investigating the rest of the patient history, give special consideration to the last oral intake. The bladder, bowel, and stomach are much more likely to rupture if full and distended. Ask about when the patient last ate or drank and how much he consumed. Relate the intake to the type of impact received, especially blunt trauma to the trunk.

Conclude the rapid trauma assessment by gathering a set of baseline vital signs.

At the end of the rapid trauma assessment, reevaluate the patient's priority for transport. The potential for an abdominal injury must factor into this determination. Remember that serious internal hemorrhage from blunt or penetrating trauma frequently occurs with few overt signs and symptoms. Any patient with a history of significant blunt or any penetrating trauma to the torso is a candidate for rapid transport to the trauma centre. Always err on the side of providing more patient care and early transport, rather than underestimating the seriousness of trauma to the abdomen.

Any patient with a history of significant blunt or any penetrating trauma to the torso is a candidate for rapid transport to the trauma centre.

Special Assessment Considerations with Pregnant Patients

If the patient you are treating is pregnant, pay special attention to the abdomen and the possibility of injury. Remember that the maternal blood volume is increased by up to 45 percent in the third trimester and blood loss can exceed 30 percent before the normal signs and symptoms of hypovolemia reveal themselves. Watch for the earliest signs of shock. To ensure that the uterus does not compress the vena cava, place the noticeably pregnant mother in the left lateral recumbent position. If spinal injury is also suspected, immobilize her firmly to the spine board, and when she is placed on the stretcher, rotate her onto her left side. Carefully evaluate the maternal vital signs, and remember that the fetus is likely to experience distress before the mother shows any signs of hypotension or hypoperfusion.

Place the late pregnancy patient on her left side to prevent compression of the inferior vena cava.

Trauma to the abdomen in late pregnancy may cause several specific uterine injuries and requires careful assessment. The normal uterus will be firm and round to palpation. It will be palpable above the iliac crests after the first 12 weeks of pregnancy and progress upward in the abdominal cavity until it reaches the costal border at about 32 weeks. Your palpation may result in tenderness and muscular contractions of the uterus, which are normal secondary to uterine contusions. These contractions will often be self-limiting; however, any tenderness, pain, or contractions should raise your suspicions of abruptio placentae. The mother may complain of cramping, generally related to palpable uterine contractions and, in some cases, experience vaginal hemorrhage. Abruptio placentae represents a serious risk to the fetus and mother and is a true emergency requiring rapid transport.

Palpation of the uterus that reveals an asymmetrical uterus or permits you to recognize the irregular features of the fetus suggests uterine rupture. This condition may also present with uterine contractions, but the fundus of the uterus is not palpable, and the mass does not harden with the contractions.

If uterine rupture or abruptio placentae are suspected or if you suspect any serious injury to the abdomen of the pregnant patient, report it to the emergency department. Alert the emergency department well before your arrival if you are transporting an injured pregnant mother. This allows department personnel to prepare for the special monitoring necessary for both the mother and the fetus.

ONGOING ASSESSMENT

The ongoing assessment is an essential part of the continuing care process for the patient with possible abdominal injury. During it, you will look for the signs of progressing abdominal injury or continuing hemorrhage. Perform it every five minutes in patients with any significant suggestion of abdominal injury. Often, the progressive nature of peritonitis leads to greater and greater patient complaints or may make abdominal signs and symptoms more evident as you care for and reduce the pain of other injuries. The signs of ongoing hemorrhage are equally progressive and may not clearly present until well into your patient care.

Pay close attention to the signs of hidden hemorrhage during ongoing assessments of the patient with suspected abdominal injury. Watch the blood pressure, pulse rate, capillary refill time, and the patient's appearance and level of consciousness and orientation. A decrease in the difference between the systolic and the diastolic blood pressures (the pulse pressure) suggests the body is compensating for shock. An increasing pulse rate (especially if the strength of the pulse is diminishing) and an increasing capillary refill time both suggest hypovolemic compensation. Also, observe for the skin becoming cool, clammy, cyanotic, or ashen, and watch for pulse oximetry readings that become more erratic. A change in either the level of consciousness or, more subtly, a lowering of the patient's orientation suggests that the brain is being hypoperfused. These findings all indicate that the body is employing increasing levels of shock compensation. If you cannot account for a continuing blood loss elsewhere, suspect internal and continuing abdominal hemorrhage. Subtle changes may be the only apparent signs of gradually worsening shock.

Another sign of continuing blood loss from an abdominal hemorrhage is aggressive fluid resuscitation that appears ineffective.

Another sign of continuing blood loss from an abdominal hemorrhage is aggressive fluid resuscitation that appears ineffective. Note your patient's response to fluid resuscitation. If his vital signs do not improve and all external hemorrhage is controlled, suspect continuing internal hemorrhage.

MANAGEMENT OF THE ABDOMINAL INJURY PATIENT

Management of the patient with abdominal injuries is supportive, with the major emphasis placed on bringing the patient to surgery as quickly as possible. Prehospital care centres on rapid packaging and transport and aggressive fluid resuscitation as needed. Specific care steps for the abdominal injury patient include proper positioning, general shock care, fluid resuscitation, and care for specific injuries (open wounds and eviscerations).

The patient with minor or severe abdominal pain should be positioned for comfort (unless the positioning is contraindicated by suspicion of spinal injury).

Flex the patient's knees to relax the abdominal muscles, and if the injuries permit, place the patient in the left lateral recumbent position to maintain knee flexure and the relaxed state of the abdominal muscles, and facilitate the clearing of vomitus from the airway.

Ensure good ventilation, and consider early administration of high-flow oxygen for the abdominal injury patient. The pain associated with peritonitis or diaphragmatic irritation may reduce respiratory excursion, adding to the potential for early shock development in these patients.

Control any moderate or serious external hemorrhage with direct pressure and bandaging. Minor bleeding may be controlled during transport, if at all.

When a serious mechanism of injury is found and the patient does not present with the signs and symptoms of shock, act in anticipation of it. Start a large-bore IV line with Ringer's Lactate solution or normal saline. Be prepared to run it wide open to deliver a bolus of 20 cc/kg of fluid if any signs of shock develop. Monitor the pulse rate and blood pressure. Institute a second line with a non-flow-restrictive saline lock using a large-bore catheter. Use this access if the patient's blood pressure begins to drop. Do not delay transport just to initiate any IV access. Start the IV access en route to the hospital if necessary. Prehospital infusion is usually limited to 2000 mL of fluid. Titrate your administration rate to maintain a systolic blood pressure of 90 mmHg, and ensure that you do not run out of fluid during field care and transport.

As you should with all serious trauma patients, communicate frequently with the abdominal injury patient to reduce anxiety and provide emotional support. Also, watch for any changes in the patient's description of the pain or injury's character or intensity. Be wary of patient hypothermia, especially when providing aggressive fluid resuscitation. Provide ample blankets, keep the patient compartment of the vehicle warm, take patient complaints of being cold seriously, and warm infusion fluids when possible. Hypothermia is a special consideration with pediatric patients because they have a disproportionately large body surface area to body volume and will rapidly lose heat to the environment.

Cover any exposed abdominal organs with a dressing moistened with sterile saline. Be careful to keep the region clean, and do not reposition any exposed organs. Cover the wet dressing with a sterile occlusive dressing, such as clear plastic wrap, to keep the site as clean as possible and yet retain the moisture. If the transport takes time, check the dressing periodically, and remoisten as necessary.

Another wound that deserves special attention is that caused by an impaled object. Do all that you can to keep the object from moving, and do not remove it from the victim. Any motion causes further injury, disrupts the clotting mechanisms, and continues the hemorrhage. Removal may withdraw the object from a blood vessel, thereby permitting increased internal and uncontrollable hemorrhage. Pad around the object with bulky trauma dressings, and wrap around the trunk with soft, self-adherent roller bandaging to secure it firmly. Apply direct pressure around the object if hemorrhage is anything but minor. If the object is too long to accommodate during transport or is affixed to an immovable object, attempt to cut it. Use a saw, cutter, or torch, but be very careful to ensure that vibration, jarring, and heat are not transmitted to the patient.

Carefully observe and care for penetrating wounds that may traverse both the abdominal and thoracic cavities. If the wound is large and may have penetrated the diaphragm or otherwise entered the thoracic cavity, seal the wound with an occlusive dressing taped on three sides or use an Asherman chest seal to permit the release of the buildup of air pressure that occurs in a tension pneumothorax. Be especially watchful of respiratory excursion and effort.

Content Review

MANAGEMENT OF THE ABDOMINAL INJURY PATIENT

Position the patient properly.
Ensure oxygenation and ventilation.
Control external bleeding.
Be prepared for aggressive fluid resuscitation.

When a serious mechanism of injury is found and the patient does not present with the signs and symptoms of shock, act in anticipation of it.

Stabilize impaled objects to prevent further injury and reduce associated hemorrhage.

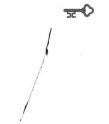

MANAGEMENT OF THE PREGNANT PATIENT

Special care is offered to the pregnant patient because of the anatomical and physiological changes induced by pregnancy. Place the late-term mother, when possible, in the left lateral recumbent position. This ensures that the weight of the uterus does not compress the vena cava, reduce blood return to the heart, and cause hypotension. It also facilitates airway care. Administer high-flow oxygen early in your care because the mother's respiratory reserve volume is diminished, as the work necessary for her to move air is greater due to the increased intra-abdominal pressure and because the fetus is especially susceptible to hypoxia. If necessary, employ intermittent positive pressure ventilation early in your care. Also, consider aggressive airway care. The pregnant mother is prone to vomiting and aspiration.

Maintain a high index of suspicion for internal hemorrhage, since the increased blood volume in the third-term of pregnancy may permit an increased blood loss before the signs and symptoms of hypovolemia become evident. The fetus may be at risk early in the blood loss, well before the mother displays any signs. Initiate IV therapy early, but remember that pregnancy induces a relative anemia and that aggressive fluid resuscitation may further dilute the erythrocyte concentrations and lead to ineffective circulation.

SUMMARY

Blunt or penetrating abdominal trauma can result in serious organ damage and life-threatening hemorrhage. Concurrently, the signs of injury are limited, non-specific, and do not reflect the seriousness of abdominal pathology. It is thus very important that your assessment carefully determine the mechanism of injury and the region of the abdomen it affects. This information must be communicated to the emergency department to ensure that its personnel acknowledge the significance of your first-hand knowledge of the mechanism of injury.

Care for significant abdominal injury is rapid transport to the trauma centre. Most significant abdominal injury results in serious internal bleeding or organ injury that can be neither cared for nor stabilized in the prehospital setting. Further, the definitive care for the patient with serious abdominal injury is provided through surgery. The patient must be transported to a facility capable of providing immediate surgical intervention when needed. This is a trauma centre. Prehospital care is supportive of the airway and breathing and preventive for shock.

The pregnant patient with abdominal injury deserves special attention because her vascular volume is increased and she will likely not show the signs of shock until the fetus is at risk. Careful observation while preparation for rapid transport to the trauma centre is in order. If any of the slightest signs of hypoperfusion is noted, initiate aggressive fluid resuscitation.

DIVISION 4

MEDICAL EMERGENCIES

Chapter 27   Pulmonology   328

Chapter 28   Cardiology   442

Chapter 29   Neurology   568

Chapter 30   Endocrinology   606

Chapter 31   Allergies and Anaphylaxis   622

Chapter 32   Gastroenterology   633

Chapter 33   Urology and Nephrology   657

Chapter 34   Toxicology and Substance Abuse   680

Chapter 35   Hematology   723

Chapter 36   Environmental Emergencies   741

Chapter 37   Infectious Disease   780

Chapter 38   Psychiatric and Behavioural Disorders   833

Chapter 39   Gynecology   857

Chapter 40   Obstetrics   867

CHAPTER 27

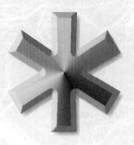

Pulmonology

Objectives

**Part 1: Pathophysiology and Respiratory Disorders
(begins on p. 331)**

After reading this chapter, you should be able to:

1. Discuss the epidemiology of pulmonary diseases and pulmonary conditions. (p. 331)
2. Identify and describe the function of the structures located in the upper and lower airway. (see Chapter 12)
3. Discuss the physiology of ventilation and respiration. (see Chapter 12)
4. Identify common pathological events that affect the pulmonary system. (pp. 334–337)

5. Compare various airway and ventilation techniques used in the management of pulmonary diseases. (pp. 347–369)
6. Review the use of equipment utilized during the physical assessment of patients with complaints associated with respiratory diseases and conditions. (pp. 345–347)
7. Identify the epidemiology, anatomy, physiology, pathophysiology, assess-

Continued

ment findings, and management (including prehospital medications) for the following respiratory diseases and conditions:

a. Adult respiratory distress syndrome (pp. 349–351)
b. Bronchial asthma (pp. 356–358)
c. Chronic bronchitis (pp. 354–355)
d. Emphysema (pp. 352–353)
e. Pneumonia (pp. 360–361)
f. Pulmonary edema (pp. 349–351)
g. Pulmonary thromboembolism (pp. 364–366)
h. Neoplasms of the lung (pp. 361–362)
i. Upper respiratory infections (pp. 358–360)
j. Spontaneous pneumothorax (pp. 366–367)
k. Hyperventilation syndrome (pp. 367–368)

8. Given several preprogrammed patients with nontraumatic pulmonary problems, provide the appropriate assessment, prehospital care, and transport. (pp. 348–369)

Part 2: Airway Management and Ventilation (begins on p. 370)

After reading this chapter, you should be able to:

9. Describe the anatomy of the airway and the physiology of respiration. (see Chapter 12)
10. Explain the primary objective of airway maintenance. (p. 370)
11. Identify commonly neglected prehospital skills related to the airway. (p. 380)
12. Describe assessment of the airway and the respiratory system. (pp. 372–380)
13. Describe the modified forms of respiration and list the factors that affect respiratory rate and depth. (pp. 374–377)
14. Discuss the methods for measuring oxygen and carbon dioxide in the blood and the prehospital use of these methods. (pp. 377–380)
15. Define and explain the implications of partial airway obstruction with good and poor air exchange and complete airway obstruction. (p. 370)

16. Describe the common causes of upper airway obstruction, including the following:
    • the tongue (p. 371)
    • foreign body aspiration (p. 371)
    • laryngeal spasm (p. 371)
    • laryngeal edema (p. 371)
    • trauma (p. 371)
17. Describe complete airway obstruction manoeuvres, including the following:
    • Heimlich manoeuvre (p. 422)
    • removal with Magill forceps (p. 422)
18. Describe causes of respiratory distress, including the following:
    • upper and lower airway obstruction (pp. 370–372)
    • inadequate ventilation (p. 372)
    • impairment of respiratory muscles (p. 372)
    • impairment of nervous system (p. 372)

Continued

19. Explain the risk of infection to EMS providers associated with airway management and ventilation. (pp. 380, 437)

20. Describe manual airway manoeuvres, including the following:
    - head-tilt/chin-lift manoeuvre (pp. 380–382)
    - jaw-thrust manoeuvre (p. 382)
    - Sellick's manoeuvre (p. 382)

21. Discuss the indications, contra-indications, advantages, disadvantages, complications, special considerations, equipment, and techniques of the following:
    - upper airway and tracheobronchial suctioning (pp. 432–433)
    - nasogastric and orogastric tube insertion (p. 434)
    - oropharyngeal and nasopharyngeal airway (pp. 384–386)
    - ventilating a patient by mouth-to-mouth, mouth-to-nose, mouth-to-mask, one/two/three person bag-valve mask, flow-restricted oxygen-powered ventilation device, automatic transport ventilator (pp. 437–441)

22. Compare the ventilation techniques used for an adult patient with those used for pediatric patients and describe special considerations in airway management and ventilation for the pediatric patient. (pp. 410–414, 439–440)

23. Identify types of oxygen cylinders and pressure regulators and explain safety considerations of oxygen storage and delivery, including steps for delivering oxygen from a cylinder and regulator. (p. 435)

24. Describe the indications, contra-indications, advantages, disadvantages, complications, litre flow range, and concentration of delivered oxygen for the following supplemental oxygen delivery devices (p. 436):
    - nasal cannula
    - simple face mask
    - partial rebreather mask
    - nonrebreather mask
    - Venturi mask

25. Describe the use, advantages, and disadvantages of an oxygen humidifier. (p. 436)

26. Describe the indications, contra-indications, advantages, disadvantages, complications, equipment, and technique for the following:
    - endotracheal intubation by direct laryngoscopy (pp. 396–399)
    - digital endotracheal intubation (pp. 402–404)
    - dual lumen airway (pp. 417–419)
    - nasotracheal intubation (pp. 414–416)
    - rapid sequence intubation (pp. 405–410)
    - endotracheal intubation using sedation (pp. 407–410)
    - open cricothyrotomy (pp. 427–430)
    - needle cricothyrostomy (translaryngeal catheter ventilation) (pp. 423–427)
    - extubation (pp. 416–417)

27. Describe the use of cricoid pressure during intubation. (pp. 382–383, 396, 409)

28. Discuss the precautions that should be taken when intubating the trauma patient. (pp. 405)

29. Discuss agents used for sedation and rapid sequence intubation. (pp. 405–410)

30. Discuss methods to confirm correct placement of the endotracheal tube. (pp. 399–400)

Part 1: Pathophysiology and Respiratory Disorders

INTRODUCTION

According to one study, respiratory complaints accounted for more than 28 percent of all emergency medical services (EMS) calls. More than 20 000 people die each year as a result of respiratory emergencies. Several factors increase the risk of developing respiratory disease. Intrinsic risk factors are those within or influenced by the patient. The most important of these is genetic predisposition. For example, bronchial asthma, **chronic obstructive pulmonary disease (COPD)**, and lung cancer are more common in those who have family members with these diseases.

Certain respiratory conditions are increased in patients with underlying cardiac or circulatory problems. Cardiac conditions that result in ineffective pumping of blood tend to cause pulmonary edema. Cardiac and circulatory diseases may allow blood to pool in the large veins of the pelvis and lower extremities, causing pulmonary emboli. Stress may increase the severity of any respiratory complaint and can precipitate acute episodes of asthma or COPD.

Extrinsic risk factors are those that are external to the patient. The most important of these is cigarette smoking. There is a strong link between cigarette smoking and the development of pulmonary diseases, such as lung carcinoma and COPD. Also, such diseases as pneumonia and pulmonary emboli are more likely in patients who smoke. Finally, cigarette smoking has been implicated as a risk factor in the development of cardiac disease. In any case, underlying lung damage caused by cigarette smoking worsens virtually all lung disorders.

Another key extrinsic risk factor is environmental pollutants. The prevalence of COPD is markedly increased in areas with high environmental pollutants, as are the number and severity of acute attacks of asthma and COPD.

This chapter explores the pathophysiology of respiratory disease and how to integrate this knowledge with your assessment findings to develop a field impression and manage the patient with respiratory problems.

PHYSIOLOGICAL PROCESSES

The major function of the respiratory system is to exchange gases with the environment. Oxygen is taken in and carbon dioxide eliminated, a process known as gas exchange.

Oxygen is vital to our bodies, allowing us to generate the energy that drives our many body functions. Oxygen from the atmosphere diffuses into the bloodstream through the lungs. Oxygen is then available for use in cellular metabolism by the body's 100 trillion cells. Waste products, including carbon dioxide, produced by cellular metabolism, must be eliminated from the body. In the lungs, carbon dioxide is exchanged for oxygen, and the carbon dioxide is excreted from the lungs.

Three important processes allow gas exchange to occur:

- Ventilation
- Diffusion
- Perfusion

The most important intrinsic factor in the development of respiratory disorders is genetic predisposition. The most important extrinsic factor is smoking.

* **chronic obstructive pulmonary disease (COPD)** a disease characterized by a decreased ability of the lungs to perform the function of ventilation.

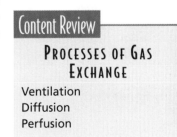

Content Review

PROCESSES OF GAS EXCHANGE
Ventilation
Diffusion
Perfusion

Ventilation

Ventilation is the mechanical process of moving air in and out of the lungs. In order for ventilation to occur, several body structures must be intact, including the chest wall, the nerve pathways, the diaphragm, the pleural cavity, and the brainstem.

Ventilation is divided into two phases: inspiration and expiration. During inspiration, air is drawn into the lungs. During expiration, air leaves the lungs. These phases of ventilation depend on changes in the volume of the thoracic cavity, as discussed in Chapter 12.

Diffusion

Diffusion is the process by which gases move between the alveoli and the pulmonary capillaries. Remember that gases tend to flow from areas in which there is a high concentration of gas into an area of low concentration. The normal concentration of oxygen in the alveoli is 104 mmHg as opposed to a concentration of 40 mmHg in the pulmonary arterial circulation. Therefore, oxygen will move from the oxygen-rich alveoli into the oxygen-poor capillaries in response to the gradient that exists in the concentration of gases. As the red blood cells move through the pulmonary capillaries, they become enriched with oxygen. Less oxygen will pass into the bloodstream as the gradient between alveolar and capillary oxygen concentration decreases.

Similarly, carbon dioxide passes out of the blood in response to a gradient that exists between the concentration of carbon dioxide in the blood in the pulmonary capillaries (45 mmHg) and in the alveoli (40 mmHg). By the time blood leaves the pulmonary capillaries, it has a dissolved concentration of oxygen of 104 mmHg and a carbon dioxide concentration of 40 mmHg.

The respiratory membrane, which normally measures 0.5 to 1.0 micrometre in thickness, must remain intact for gas exchange to occur. Any disorder that damages the alveoli or allows them to collapse will impede oxygen from entering the body and reduce carbon dioxide elimination. Changes in the respiratory membrane or any increase in the interstitial space will also impede the process of diffusion. For example, fluid accumulation in the interstitial space as the result of pulmonary edema or pneumonia will prevent proper diffusion of gases. Finally, the endothelial lining of the capillaries must be intact for exchange of oxygen and carbon dioxide to occur. Diseases that cause thickening of the endothelial lining will also interfere with the process of diffusion.

Provide oxygen to a patient with a lung diffusion problem to increase the concentration gradient that drives oxygen into the capillaries.

There are certain measures that you can take to address problems with lung diffusion. Providing the patient with high concentrations of oxygen is one simple step that can be utilized. Remember that the concentration gradient provides the driving force in moving oxygen into the capillaries. Therefore, the larger the difference between the concentration of oxygen in the alveoli and in the capillaries, the greater is the diffusion of oxygen into the bloodstream. Similarly, when fluid accumulation or inflammation is the underlying cause of the thickening of the interstitial space within the alveoli, such medications as diuretic agents or anti-inflammatory drugs (corticosteroids, antibiotics) are given to reduce fluid and inflammation.

Perfusion

One additional process that occurs in the lungs is **perfusion.** Lung perfusion is the circulation of blood through the lungs or, more specifically, the pulmonary capillaries. Lung perfusion is dependent on three conditions:

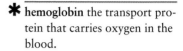

✱ **perfusion** the circulation of blood through the capillaries.

- Adequate blood volume
- Intact pulmonary capillaries
- Efficient pumping of blood by the heart

For perfusion to proceed effectively, there must be an adequate volume of blood in the bloodstream. Equally important is the concentration of **hemoglobin,** which is the transport protein that carries oxygen in the blood. Remember that oxygen is transported in the bloodstream in one of two ways: bound to hemoglobin or dissolved in the plasma. Under normal conditions, less than 2 percent of all oxygen is transported dissolved in plasma (this is what is measured by the oxygen partial pressure, PO_2), whereas more than 98 percent is carried by hemoglobin.

✱ **hemoglobin** the transport protein that carries oxygen in the blood.

Hemoglobin (Hb) has some unique properties. It is made up of four iron-containing heme molecules and a protein-containing globin portion. Oxygen molecules bind to the heme portion of the hemoglobin molecule. As oxygen binds to hemoglobin, its structure changes so that it more readily binds additional oxygen molecules. Similarly, as the fully oxygen-bound hemoglobin begins to release oxygen, it more readily sheds additional oxygen. The relationship is described by the *oxygen dissociation curve* (Figure 27-1). You can see that between 10 and 50 mmHg, there is a marked increase in the saturation of hemoglobin. However, as the PO_2 increases above 70 mmHg, there is only a small change in the saturation of hemoglobin, which is already near 100 percent.

Changes in the body temperature, the blood pH, and the carbon dioxide partial pressure (PCO_2) can all alter the oxygen dissociation curve. Within the tissues, as hemoglobin becomes bound with carbon dioxide, it loses its affinity for oxygen. As a result, more oxygen is released and is thus available to cells for metabolism (called the Bohr effect).

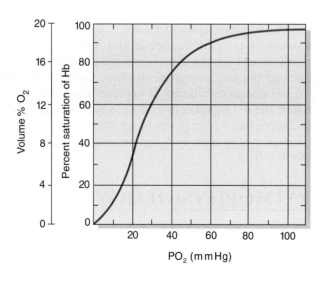

FIGURE 27-1 Oxygen dissociation curve.

Carbon dioxide is transported from the cells to the lungs in one of three ways:

- As bicarbonate ions
- Bound to the globin portion of the hemoglobin molecule
- Dissolved in plasma (measured as PCO_2)

The greatest portion of CO_2 produced during metabolism in cells is converted into bicarbonate ions. As the CO_2 is released into the capillaries, it enters the red blood cell, where an enzyme (carbonic anhydrase) combines carbon dioxide with water to form two ions, hydrogen (H^+) and bicarbonate (HCO_3^-). Bicarbonate is then released from the red blood cell and transported in plasma. In the lungs, the reverse process takes place, producing water and carbon dioxide. The carbon dioxide then diffuses into the alveoli, where it is eliminated during exhalation.

The carbon dioxide that is bound to hemoglobin is released in the lung because of the lower concentration of this gas in the alveoli. Additionally, as the heme portion of the hemoglobin molecule becomes saturated with oxygen, more carbon dioxide is released (called the Haldane effect). Finally, the approximately 10 percent of carbon dioxide that is dissolved in the plasma flows into the alveoli due to the gradient that exists between the concentration of gases (PCO_2 of 45 mmHg in the pulmonary artery versus 40 mmHg in the alveoli).

For perfusion to take place, in addition to having adequate blood volume, the pulmonary capillaries must be able to transport blood through all portions of the lung tissue. These vessels must be open and not occluded, or blocked. For example, a pulmonary embolism will occlude the pulmonary artery in which it lodges, making that artery unavailable for perfusion of the portion of the lung it usually supplies with blood. Finally, the heart must pump efficiently in order to push blood effectively through the pulmonary capillaries to perfuse the lung tissues.

In order to maintain perfusion, you must ensure that the patient has an adequate circulating blood volume. In addition, take all the necessary steps to improve the pumping action of the heart. For example, in patients with acute pulmonary edema, the use of diuretic agents reduces the blood return (preload) to an ineffectively pumping heart and improves cardiac efficiency.

The entire system we have just discussed provides for **respiration,** which is the exchange of gases between a living organism and its environment. Pulmonary respiration occurs in the lungs when the respiratory gases are exchanged between the alveoli and the red blood cells in the pulmonary capillaries through the respiratory membranes. Cellular respiration, conversely, occurs in the peripheral capillaries. It involves the exchange of the respiratory gases between the red blood cells and the various tissues. Many of the principles of gas exchange that occur in the lungs are reversed in the tissues, with oxygen being released to the cells and carbon dioxide accumulating in the plasma and red blood cells.

In order to maintain perfusion, ensure that the patient has an adequate circulating blood volume. Also, take all necessary steps to improve the pumping action of the heart.

✱ **respiration** the exchange of gases between a living organism and its environment.

PATHOPHYSIOLOGY

Remember that many disease states affect the pulmonary system and interfere with its ability to acquire the oxygen required for normal cellular metabolism. Additionally, respiratory diseases limit the body's ability to get rid of waste products, such as carbon dioxide. Your understanding of normal anatomy and physiology—ventilation, diffusion, and perfusion—will aid in understanding the mechanism of each disease process and will direct you toward the appropriate corrective actions. Ultimately, any disease process that impairs the pulmonary system will result in a derangement in ventilation, diffusion, perfusion, or a combination of these processes.

DISRUPTION IN VENTILATION

Diseases that affect ventilation will result in obstruction of the normal conducting pathways of the upper or lower respiratory tract, impairment of the normal function of the chest wall, or abnormalities involving the nervous system's control of ventilation.

Upper and Lower Respiratory Tracts

Disease states that affect the upper respiratory tract will result in obstruction of air flow to the lower structures. Upper airway trauma, for example, produces both significant hemorrhage and swelling. Infections of the upper airway structures, including epiglottitis, soft-tissue infections of the neck, tonsillitis, and abscess formation within the pharynx (peritonsillar abscess and retropharyngeal abscess), can all obstruct airflow. Similarly, lower airway obstruction may be produced by trauma, foreign body aspiration, mucus accumulation (as in asthmatics), smooth muscle constriction (in asthma and COPD), and airway edema produced by infection or burns.

Chest Wall and Diaphragm

As you read earlier, the chest wall and diaphragm are mechanical components that are essential for normal ventilation. Traumatic injuries to these areas will disrupt the normal mechanics, causing loss of negative pressure within the pleural space. This occurs in patients with **pneumothorax,** including open pneumothorax, tension pneumothorax, or **hemothorax.** Infectious processes, such as empyema (pus accumulation in the pleural space), or inflammatory conditions produce similar effects. Chest wall injuries, including rib fractures or **flail chest** and diaphragmatic rupture, limit the patient's ability to expand the thoracic cavity. Certain neuromuscular diseases, such as muscular dystrophy, multiple sclerosis, or amyotrophic lateral sclerosis (ALS, or Lou Gehrig's disease), impair muscular function so as to limit the ability to generate a negative pressure within the chest cavity.

Nervous System

Finally, any disease process that impairs the nervous system's regulation of breathing may also alter ventilation. Central nervous system depressants, such as alcohol, benzodiazepines, or barbiturates, alone or in combination, can alter the brain's response to important signals, such as rising PCO_2. Similarly, stroke, diseases, or injuries that involve the respiratory centres within the central nervous system can change the normal ventilatory pattern. In fact, certain abnormal respiratory patterns are produced by specific brain injury (Figure 27-2).

- *Cheyne-Stokes respirations* describes a ventilatory pattern with progressively increasing tidal volume, followed by a declining volume,

✱ **pneumothorax** a collection of air in the pleural space, causing a loss of the negative pressure that binds the lung to the chest wall. In an *open pneumothorax,* air enters the pleural space through an injury to the chest wall. In a *closed pneumothorax,* air enters the pleural space through an opening in the pleura that covers the lung. A *tension pneumothorax* develops when air in the pleural space cannot escape, causing a buildup of pressure and collapse of the lung.

✱ **hemothorax** a collection of blood in the pleural space.

✱ **flail chest** one or more ribs fractured in two or more places, creating an unattached rib segment.

FIGURE 27-2 Abnormal
respiratory patterns.

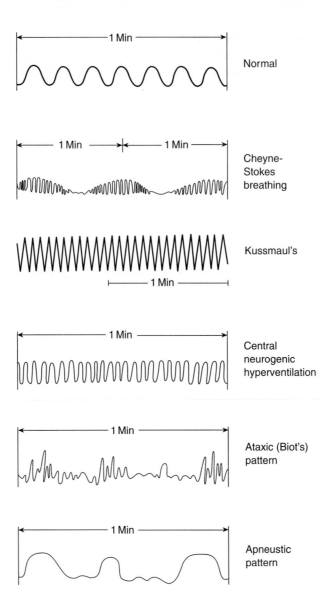

★ apnea absence of breathing.

separated by periods of **apnea** at the end of expiration. This pattern is typically seen in older patients with terminal illness or brain injury.

- *Kussmaul's respirations* are deep, rapid breaths that result as a corrective measure against such conditions as diabetic ketoacidosis that produce metabolic acidosis.

- *Central neurogenic hyperventilation* also produces deep, rapid respirations that are caused by stroke or an injury to the brainstem. In this case, there is loss of normal regulation of ventilatory controls and respiratory alkalosis is often seen.

- *Ataxic (Biot's) respirations* are characterized by repeated episodes of gasping ventilations separated by periods of apnea. This pattern is seen in patients with increased intracranial pressure.

- *Apneustic respiration* is characterized by long, deep breaths that are stopped during the inspiratory phase and separated by periods of apnea. This pattern is a result of stroke or severe central nervous system disease.

Also, remember that damage to the major peripheral nerves that supply the diaphragm and intercostal muscles, the phrenic nerve, and the intercostal nerves will also affect normal ventilatory mechanics. Traumatic disruption of the phrenic nerve during chest surgery, with penetrating trauma, or by neoplastic (cancerous, tumourous) invasion of the nerve can paralyze the diaphragm on the side of involvement.

DISRUPTION IN DIFFUSION

Other disease states can disrupt the diffusion of gases. Any change in the concentration of oxygen in the alveoli, such as occurs when a person ascends to high altitudes, can limit the diffusion of oxygen and produce **hypoxia.** Similarly, any disease that alters the structure or patency of the alveoli will limit diffusion. Destruction of alveoli by certain environmental pathogens, such as asbestos or coal (black lung disease), by COPD, or by inhalation injury reduces the capacity of the lungs to diffuse gases.

✱ hypoxia state in which insufficient oxygen is available to meet the oxygen requirements of the cells.

Finally, disease states that alter the thickness of the respiratory membrane will limit the diffusion of gases. The most common cause of this alteration is accumulation of fluid and inflammatory cells in the interstitial space. Fluid can accumulate in the interstitial space if high pressure within the pulmonary capillaries forces fluid out of the circulatory system. This is seen in patients with left-sided heart failure (cardiogenic causes) and is due to increased venous pressure as a result of poor functioning of the left ventricle. Patients with pulmonary hypertension have high resting pressures in the pulmonary circulation that ultimately lead to fluid accumulation in the interstitial space, causing right heart failure.

Similar effects can be produced by changes in the permeability (or leakiness) of the pulmonary capillaries (noncardiogenic causes). Permeability can be affected by adult respiratory distress syndrome, asbestos and other environmental pathogens, near-drowning, prolonged hypoxia, and inhalation injury. Also, remember that disease states that alter the pulmonary capillary endothelial lining, such as advanced atherosclerosis or vascular inflammatory states, can affect diffusion.

DISRUPTION IN PERFUSION

As detailed earlier, any alteration in appropriate blood flow through the pulmonary capillaries will limit normal gas exchange in the lungs. Any problem that reduces the normal circulating blood volume, such as trauma, hemorrhage, dehydration, or shock or other causes of hypovolemia, will limit normal perfusion of the lungs. Remember that hemoglobin is the major transport protein for oxygen and plays a significant role in the elimination of carbon dioxide. Therefore, any reduction in the normal circulating hemoglobin will also affect perfusion. All causes of anemia, a condition in which the number of red blood cells or amount of hemoglobin in them is below normal, must be considered. Such causes include acute blood loss, iron or vitamin deficiency, malnutrition, and chronic disease states.

Remember that blood must be available to all of the lung segments for maximum gas exchange to occur. When an area of lung tissue is appropriately ventilated but no capillary perfusion occurs, available oxygen is not moved into the circulatory system. This is referred to as *pulmonary shunting*. In patients with pulmonary embolism, a blockage of a division of the pulmonary artery by a clot prevents perfusion of the lung segments supplied by that branch of the artery. As a result, there may be significant shunt with return of unoxygenated blood to the pulmonary venous circulation.

ASSESSMENT OF THE RESPIRATORY SYSTEM

Assessment of the respiratory system is a vital aspect of prehospital care. You must quickly assess the airway and ventilation status during the primary assessment. If the patient's complaints suggest that the respiratory system is involved in the patient's problem, the focused history and secondary assessment should be directed to this aspect of the assessment.

If the patient's complaints suggest respiratory system involvement, direct the focused history and secondary assessment to this aspect.

SCENE ASSESSMENT

When you approach the scene, you should consider two major questions: (1) Is the scene safe for you to approach the patient? (2) Are there visual clues that might provide information regarding the patient's medical complaint?

When you approach the scene, consider these questions: (1) Is the scene safe? (2) Are there visual cues to the patient's medical complaint?

Remember that several hazards that may result in respiratory complaints indicated by the patient are also potentially dangerous for emergency care providers. Certain gases and toxic products that are causing respiratory complaints from your patient may also present a significant risk to you. Carbon monoxide, for example, is a colourless and odourless gas that may be present in quantities enough to overcome unsuspecting emergency care personnel. Other toxins from incomplete combustion produced in fires or industrial processes pose a similar risk. Recent incidents involving chemical agents, such as saran gas, or biologic agents, such as anthrax, highlight the need for emergency care providers to be aware of hazards to themselves as well as to their patients.

You should also be aware that there are certain rescue environments in which the concentration of available oxygen is significantly reduced. These would include such areas as grain silos, enclosed storage containers, or any enclosed space in which there is an active fire. You must take the appropriate precautions before entering such environments, including using your own supplemental oxygen supply.

In any situation where you believe there is a hazard to you as a care provider, make sure that the scene is appropriately secured before you enter. If specific protective items, such as hazardous materials suits, self-contained breathing apparatus, or supplemental oxygen, are needed, make sure they are available before you attempt to care for your patient. Similarly, if other personnel, such as fire suppression units or hazmat (hazardous materials) teams, are required, contact dispatch, and have them available on scene before putting yourself at risk.

Once it is safe to enter the scene, look for clues that will provide information to explain the patient's complaints. Do you see such evidence as cigarette packs or ashtrays that suggests that the patient or family members are smokers? Look for any home nebulizer machines or supplemental oxygen tanks that may suggest a patient with underlying COPD or asthma. If the patient is a small child, look for small items lying around the house that could suggest ingested foreign bodies. Your eyes, ears, and nose can lead you to several important clues that are useful as you begin your assessment of the patient.

PRIMARY ASSESSMENT

General Impression

Take the following considerations and steps to help form your initial impression of the patient's respiratory status:

- *Position.* Consider the patient's position. Patients with respiratory diseases tend to tolerate an upright posture better than lying flat. Indications of severe respiratory distress include a patient who is sit-

Content Review

GENERAL IMPRESSION OF RESPIRATORY STATUS
Position
Colour
Mental status
Ability to speak
Respiratory effort

ting upright with feet dangling over the side of the bed. In the most severe cases, the patient will assume the "tripod" position in which the patient leans forward and supports her weight with the arms extended (Figure 27-3).

- *Colour.* Patients with severe respiratory distress display **pallor** and **diaphoresis. Cyanosis** is a late finding and may be absent even with significant hypoxia. Peripheral cyanosis (bluish discoloration involving only the distal extremities) is not a specific finding and is also found in patients with poor circulation. Peripheral cyanosis reflects the slowing of blood flow and increased extraction of oxygen from red blood cells. Central cyanosis (involving the lips, tongue, and truncal skin) is a more ominous finding seen in hypoxia.

- *Mental Status.* Briefly assess the patient's mental status. The hypoxic patient is restless and agitated. Confusion is seen with both hypoxia (deficiency of oxygen) and hypercarbia (excess of carbon dioxide). When respiratory failure is imminent, the patient will appear extremely lethargic and somnolent. The eyelids will begin to droop, and the head will bob with each respiratory effort.

- *Ability to Speak.* Assess the patient's ability to speak in full, coherent sentences. Determine the ease with which the patient can discuss symptoms. Patients with respiratory distress will be able to speak only one to two words before they need to pause to catch their breath. Rambling, incoherent speech indicates fear, anxiety, or hypoxia.

- *Respiratory Effort.* As we have already described, normal ventilation is an active process. However, the use of accessory muscles in the neck (scalenes and sternocleidomastoids) and visible contractions of the intercostal muscles indicate significant breathing effort.

As you form your general impression, also make specific note of any of the following signs of respiratory distress:

- **Nasal flaring**
- Intercostal muscle retraction
- Use of the accessory respiratory muscles
- Cyanosis
- Pursed lips
- **Tracheal tugging**

Your initial assessment of the patient is directed at identification of any life-threatening conditions resulting from the compromise of airway, breathing, and circulation (the ABCs). Because this chapter concerns the respiratory system, we will focus here on assessment of airway and breathing.

Airway

Remember that oxygen is one of the most basic necessities for life and that the respiratory system is responsible for supplying it to the body tissues. As a result, any significant abnormality in the respiratory tract must be viewed as potentially life threatening.

After quickly forming your general impression, immediately focus on the patient's airway. When assessing the airway, keep these principles in mind:

- Noisy breathing nearly always means partial airway obstruction.

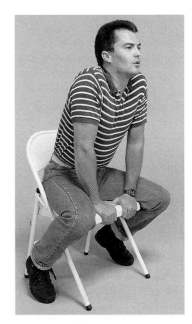

FIGURE 27-3   Tripod position.

✳ **pallor** paleness.

✳ **diaphoresis** sweatiness.

✳ **cyanosis** bluish discoloration of the skin due to significantly reduced hemoglobin in the blood. The condition is directly related to poor ventilation.

✳ **nasal flaring** excessive widening of the nares with respiration.

✳ **tracheal tugging** retraction of the tissues of the neck due to airway obstruction or dyspnea.

Any significant abnormality in the respiratory tract must be viewed as potentially life threatening.

* **asphyxia** a decrease in the amount of oxygen and an increase in the amount of carbon dioxide as a result of some interference with respiration.

If the airway is compromised, quickly institute basic airway management techniques. Once you have secured a patent airway, ensure that the patient has adequate ventilation.

* **dyspnea** difficult or laboured breathing; a sensation of "shortness of breath."

* **tachycardia** rapid heart rate.

If a patient complains of dyspnea, obtain a SAMPLE history. If the chief complaint suggests respiratory disease, ask the OPQRST questions about current symptoms.

* **orthopnea** dyspnea while lying supine.

* **paroxysmal nocturnal dyspnea** short attacks of dyspnea that occur at night and interrupt sleep.

* **hemoptysis** expectoration of blood from the respiratory tree.

- Obstructed breathing is not always noisy.
- The brain can survive only a few minutes in **asphyxia.**
- Artificial respiration is useless if the airway is blocked.
- A patent airway is useless if the patient is apneic.
- If you note airway obstruction, do not waste time looking for help or equipment. Act immediately.

If the airway is compromised, quickly institute basic airway management techniques. Once you have secured a patent airway, ensure that the patient has adequate ventilation. Your primary assessment of the respiratory system should be brief and directed. A more detailed assessment should be conducted once you have been able to establish that there is no immediate threat to life.

Breathing

The following signs should suggest a possible life-threatening respiratory problem in adults. They are listed in order from the most ominous to the least severe.

- Alterations in mental status
- Severe central cyanosis
- Absent breath sounds
- Audible stridor
- One-to-two-word **dyspnea** (need to breathe after every word or two)
- **Tachycardia** ≥ 130 beats per minute
- Pallor and diaphoresis
- The presence of intercostal and sternocleidomastoid retractions
- Use of accessory muscles

If any of these signs are present, you should direct your efforts toward immediate resuscitation and transport of the patient to a medical facility.

FOCUSED HISTORY AND SECONDARY ASSESSMENT

History

The history and secondary assessment should be directed at problem areas as determined by the patient's chief complaint or primary problem. Patients with respiratory diseases will often present with a complaint of "shortness of breath" (dyspnea). Obtain a SAMPLE history. If the chief complaint suggests respiratory disease, ask the OPQRST questions, including the following about the current symptoms. The answers to these or similar questions will provide you with a pertinent patient history.

- How long has the dyspnea been present?
- Was the onset gradual or abrupt?
- Is the dyspnea better or worse by position? Is there associated **orthopnea** or **paroxysmal nocturnal dyspnea**?
- Has the patient been coughing?
  - If so, is the cough productive?
  - What is the character and colour of the sputum?
  - Is there any **hemoptysis** (coughing up of blood)?

- Is there any chest pain associated with the dyspnea?
  - If so, what is the location of the pain?
  - Was the onset of pain sudden or slow?
  - What was the duration of the pain?
  - Does the pain radiate to any area?
  - Does the pain increase with respiration?
- Are there associated symptoms of fever or chills?
- What is the patient's past medical history?
- Has the patient experienced wheezing?
- Is the patient or close family member a smoker?

It is also important to ask the patient if she has ever experienced similar symptoms in the past. Patients with chronic medical conditions, such as COPD or asthma, can usually relate the severity of their current presenting complaints to episodes that they have experienced in the past. Question the patient or family about prior hospitalizations for respiratory disease. In particular, you should try to determine whether the patient required care in the intensive care unit (ICU) for breathing problems. Ask if the patient has ever required endotracheal intubation and ventilatory support. Consider patients who have been previously intubated to be potentially seriously ill, and approach their care with great caution.

Similarly, it is important to ask the patient if she already has a history of respiratory disease. The most common reason for a call to emergency care personnel is a worsening of an already present respiratory disease. This is typical in the case of patients with COPD, asthma, or lung cancer. If you are not familiar with the patient's diagnosis (for example, alpha-2 anti-trypsin deficiency), try to determine if the disease is affecting the process of ventilation, diffusion, or perfusion.

Continue history taking by determining the following:

- What current medications is the patient taking? (Pay particular attention to oxygen therapy, oral bronchodilators, corticosteroids, and antibiotics.)
- Does the patient have any allergies?

A good history of medication use is essential and may provide useful clues to the diagnosis. If time permits, gather the patient's current medications and transport them with the patient. This is a great benefit to the Emergency Department personnel who will be evaluating the patient. Pay particular attention to any medications that suggest pulmonary disease. These would include inhaled or oral sympathomimetics such as salbutamol and related agents that are used to treat diseases such as COPD or asthma. Ask about steroid preparations, which are also used in these conditions. Other common medications used by patients with COPD or asthma include Atrovent® (ipratropium bromide), Flovent® (fluticasone), Beclovent® (beclomethasone), Combivent® (ipratropium and salbutamol), Advair® (fluticasone and salmeterol), and antibiotic agents.

Also ask about drugs used for cardiac conditions, since cardiac patients often present with dyspnea. Nitrates, calcium channel blockers, diuretic agents, digoxin, and anti-dysrhythmic agents are all commonly used by patients with cardiac disease.

Finally, inquire about medication allergies. This is important information, since it helps to avoid administering agents to which the patient is allergic. Also, it's possible that a specific medication may be the cause of an allergic reaction that has resulted in upper airway edema and respiratory complaints.

PHYSICAL EXAM OF RESPIRATORY SYSTEM

Head
Neck
Chest
    Inspection
    Palpation
    Percussion
    Auscultation
Extremities

✳ **crepitus** crackling sounds.

✳ **subcutaneous emphysema** presence of air in the subcutaneous tissue.

FIGURE 27-4   Jugular vein distention.

Secondary Assessment

First, examine the patient's head and neck. Look at the lips. Pursed lips indicate significant respiratory distress. This is the patient's way of maintaining positive pressure during expiration and preventing alveolar collapse. Also, examine the nose, mouth, and throat for any signs of swelling or infection that might be causing upper airway obstruction.

Occasionally, the patient may also produce sputum, which can suggest an underlying cause of the patient's complaints. An increase in the amount of sputum produced suggests infection of the lungs or bronchial passages (bronchitis). Thick, green or brown sputum is characteristic of these infections. Thin, yellow or pale-grey sputum is more typical of inflammation or an allergic cause. Pink, frothy sputum is a sign of severe pulmonary edema. Truly bloody sputum (hemoptysis) may be seen with cancer, tuberculosis, and bronchial infection.

Assess the neck for signs of swelling or infection. Remember to look at the jugular veins for evidence of distention (Figure 27-4). This occurs when the right side of the heart is not pumping blood effectively, causing a "backup" in the venous circulation. Such findings are often accompanied by those of left-sided heart failure and pulmonary edema.

Physical examination of the respiratory system should follow the standard steps of patient assessment: *inspection, palpation, percussion,* and *auscultation.*

- *Inspection.* Inspection should include an examination of the anteroposterior dimensions and general shape of the chest. An increased anteroposterior diameter is suggestive of chronic obstructive pulmonary disease (COPD). Inspect the chest for symmetrical movement. Any asymmetry may be suggestive of trauma. A paradoxical movement (moving in a fashion opposite to that expected) is suggestive of flail chest. Note any chest scars, lesions, wounds, or deformities.

- *Palpation.* Palpate the chest, both front and back, for any abnormalities. Note any tenderness, **crepitus,** or **subcutaneous emphysema.** Palpate the anterior chest first and then the posterior.

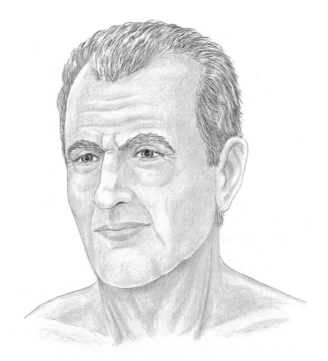

Inspect your gloved hands for blood each time they are removed from behind the patient's chest. In some instances, it may be appropriate to evaluate **tactile fremitus,** the vibration felt in the chest during speaking. When evaluating tactile fremitus, compare one side of the chest with the other. Simultaneously, palpate the trachea for **tracheal deviation,** which is suggestive of a tension pneumothorax.

* *Percussion.* If indicated, quickly percuss the chest. Limit percussion to suspected cases of pneumothorax and pulmonary edema. A hollow sound on percussion is often indicative of pneumothorax or emphysema. In contrast, a dull sound is indicative of pulmonary edema, hemothorax, or pneumonia. Remember, however, that percussion may be of little value in the noisy environment typical of most emergency scenes and is not usually performed in the prehospital setting.
* *Auscultation.* Auscultate the chest. Begin by listening without a stethoscope and from a distance. Note any loud stridor, wheezing, or cough. If possible, the patient should be in the sitting position and the chest auscultated in a symmetrical pattern. If the patient cannot sit up, auscultate the anterior and lateral parts of the chest. Each area should be auscultated for one respiratory cycle.

✱ **tactile fremitus** vibratory tremours felt through the chest by palpation.

✱ **tracheal deviation** any position of the trachea other than midline.

Normal breath sounds heard during auscultation can be characterized according to the following descriptions:

Normal Breath Sounds

* Bronchial (or tubular)
  – Loud, high-pitched breath sounds heard over the trachea
  – Expiratory phase lasts longer than inspiratory phase
* Bronchovesicular
  – Softer, medium-pitched breath sounds heard over the mainstem bronchi (below clavicles or between scapulae)
  – Expiratory phase and inspiratory phase equal
* Vesicular
  – Soft, low-pitched breath sounds heard in the lung periphery

While the patient breathes in and out deeply with the mouth open, note any abnormal breath sounds and their location. Many terms are used to describe abnormal breath sounds. The following list includes some of the more common terms:

Abnormal Breath Sounds

* *Snoring.* Occurs when the upper airway is partially obstructed, usually by the tongue.
* *Stridor.* Harsh, high-pitched sound heard on inspiration and characteristic of an upper airway obstruction, such as in croup.
* *Wheezing.* Whistling sound due to narrowing of the airways by edema, bronchoconstriction, or foreign materials.
* *Rhonchi.* Rattling sounds in the larger airways associated with excessive mucus or other material.
* *Crackles* (also called *rales*). Fine, moist crackling sounds associated with fluid in the smaller airways.
* *Pleural Friction Rub.* Sounds like dried pieces of leather rubbing together; occurs when the pleurae become inflamed, as in pleurisy.

Also, examine the extremities. Look for peripheral cyanosis, which may indicate hypoxia. Examine the extremities for swelling, redness, and a hard, firm cord indicating a venous clot. This may suggest a possible cause for pulmonary embolism. Look for clubbing of the fingers (Figures 27-5a and b), suggesting longstanding hypoxemia. This is typical of patients with COPD or cyanotic heart disease. Finally, the patient may demonstrate *carpopedal spasm*, in which the fingers and toes are contracted in flexion. This is found in patients with hyperventilation and is caused by transient shifts in the blood calcium concentration caused by changes in the serum CO_2 and pH (alkalinity or acidity) levels.

Vital Signs

The patient's vital signs may also provide information regarding the severity of the respiratory complaints. In general, tachycardia (rapid heart rate) is a highly nonspecific finding, caused by fear, anxiety, and fever. In patients with respiratory complaints, however, tachycardia may also indicate hypoxia. Remember that the patient may have recently used sympathomimetic drugs, such as salbutamol, which will accelerate the patient's heart rate. These same drugs will elevate the patient's blood pressure as well. During your assessment of the blood pressure, a patient will occasionally exhibit *pulsus paradoxus,* a drop in the systolic blood pressure of 10 mmHg or more with each respiratory cycle. Pulsus paradoxus is associated with chronic obstructive pulmonary disease (COPD) and cardiac tamponade. As a rule, however, you should not spend any time looking for pulsus paradoxus.

A change in a patient's respiratory rate may be one of the earliest indicators of respiratory disease. The patient's respiratory rate can be influenced by several factors, including respiratory difficulty, fear, anxiety, fever, and underlying metabolic disease. Assume that an elevated respiratory rate in a patient with dyspnea is caused by hypoxia. Although fluctuations in the respiratory rate are common, a persistently *slow* rate indicates impending respiratory arrest.

Continually reassess the patient's respiratory rate during the time that you are caring for the patient. Trends in the respiratory rate (for example, an increasing rate) can give you an overall assessment of the effectiveness of any intervention you

Assume that an elevated respiratory rate in a patient with dyspnea is caused by hypoxia. A persistently slow rate indicates impending respiratory arrest.

Constantly reassess the patient's respiratory rate and pattern.

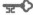

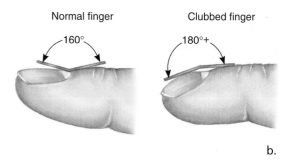

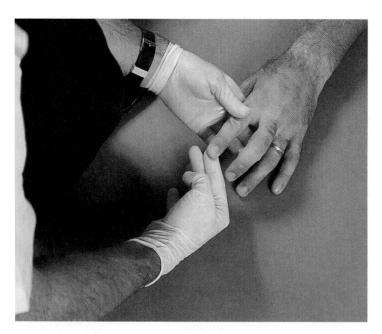

FIGURE 27-5 (a) Inspect for finger clubbing. Any clubbing may indicate chronic respiratory or cardiac disease. (b) Characteristics of finger clubbing include large fingertips and a loss of the normal angle at the nail bed.

a.

have made. Also, assess the patient's respiratory pattern. The normal respiratory pattern (eupnea) is steady, even breaths occurring 12 to 20 times per minute with an expiratory phase that lasts three to four times the inspiratory phase. **Tachypnea** describes a respiratory pattern with a rate that exceeds 20 breaths per minute. **Bradypnea** describes a respiratory pattern with a rate slower than 12 breaths per minute. Also, look for any abnormal respiratory patterns (e.g., Cheyne-Stokes, Kussmaul, or other) that were discussed earlier in the chapter.

✱ **tachypnea** rapid respiration.

✱ **bradypnea** slow respiration.

Diagnostic Testing

Three diagnostic measurements are of value in assessing the patient's respiratory status: *pulse oximetry, peak flow,* and *capnometry.*

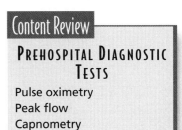

- *Pulse Oximetry.* Pulse oximetry offers a rapid and accurate means for assessing oxygen saturation. The pulse oximeter can be quickly applied to a finger or an earlobe. The pulse rate and oxygen saturation can be continuously recorded. Use of the pulse oximeter, if available, is encouraged in the care for any patient complaining of dyspnea or respiratory problems (Figure 27-6). Remember that the pulse oximetry reading may be difficult to obtain in a patient with peripheral vasoconstriction (as in sepsis or hypothermia). It may also be inaccurate under conditions in which an abnormal substance, such as carbon monoxide, binds to hemoglobin, since the instrument measures the saturation of hemoglobin without indicating what substance has saturated it.

  The oxygen saturation measurement obtained through pulse oximetry is abbreviated as SaO_2 (oxygen saturation). When pulse oximetry first came into use, some authors abbreviated the oxygen saturation measurement as SpO_2. However, this was sometimes confused with the PaO_2 obtained during blood gas measurement. SaO_2 is recognized throughout the paramedic profession.

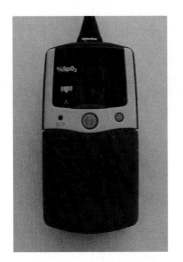
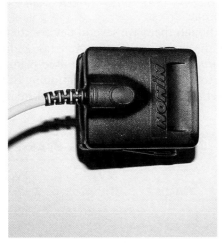
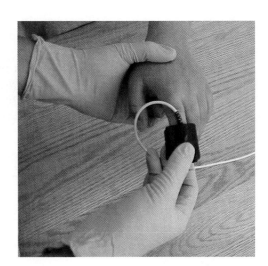

FIGURE 27-6   Sensing unit for pulse oximetry. This device transmits light through a vascular bed, such as in the finger, and can determine the oxygen saturation of red blood cells. To use the pulse oximeter, it is only necessary to turn the device on and attach the sensor to a finger. The desired graphic mode on the oximeter should be selected. The oxygen saturation and pulse rate can be continuously monitored.

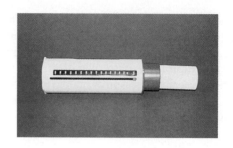

FIGURE 27-7　Wright Spirometer for determining peak expiratory flow rate (PEFR).

- *Peak Flow.* Small portable handheld devices are available for use in determining the patient's peak expiratory flow rate (PEFR). The normal expected peak flow rate is based on the patient's sex, age, and height. Remember that the measurement of the peak expiratory flow rate is somewhat effort dependent; you must have a cooperative patient who understands the use of the device in order to get an accurate reading.

  The PEFR is obtained using a Wright Spirometer (Figure 27-7), which is inexpensive and easy to use. Place the disposable mouth piece into the meter. First, have the patient take the deepest possible inspiration. Then, encourage the patient to seal her lips around the device and forcibly exhale. The peak rate of exhaled gas is recorded in litres per minute. This should be repeated twice, with the highest reading recorded as the patient's PEFR (Table 27-1).

- *Capnometry.* Devices that detect carbon dioxide at the end of the expiratory phase are now available. If gases are sampled at the end of an endotracheal tube, the level of measured carbon dioxide is highest at the end of expiration. This is referred to as end-tidal CO_2 measurement. The fact that carbon dioxide is detected implies that the metabolic processes of the body are active in producing CO_2 and that this gas is adequately exchanged in the lungs. Remember that almost no carbon dioxide is present in the esophagus and stomach. As a result, none would be detected by capnometry if the endotracheal tube is improperly placed into the esophagus. However, even a properly placed capnometry device will not detect CO_2 if the patient is in cardiac arrest.

  Although there are several devices that measure the level of CO_2 during the entire ventilatory cycle (as a continuous waveform called *capnography*), most devices are used primarily in the prehospital setting to ensure the proper positioning of the endotracheal tube in the trachea. These devices, called end-tidal CO_2 detectors, focus

Table 27-1	SPIROMETRY AND PEAK FLOW VALUES FOR ADULTS		
FEV$_1$* Severity	FEV$_1$ (Litres)	FVC† (%)	Peak Flow (Litres/Min)
Normal	4.0–6.0 L	80–90%	550–650 (Male)
			400–500 (Female)
Mild	3.0 L	70%	300–400
Moderate	1.6 L	50%	200–300
Severe	0.6 L	40%	100

*forced expiratory volume
†forced vital capacity

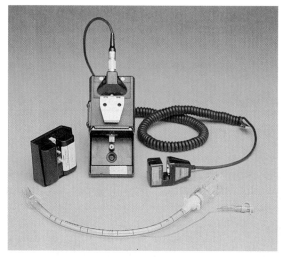

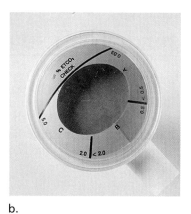

FIGURE 27-8　End-tidal CO_2 devices: (a) electronic (b) colorimetric.

a.

b.

only on the presence or absence of carbon dioxide in the sampled gas (*capnometry*). If the endotracheal tube becomes dislodged from its proper position, there is an almost immediate change in the readings from the end-tidal CO_2 device. This is in contrast to measurement of pulse oximetry, which may take several minutes to reflect the hypoxia produced by tube dislodgement.

Two types of devices are commonly used for capnometry. The first device gives a numerical readout of the level of carbon dioxide detected by the device (Figure 27-8a). The other device relies on a colour change produced by CO_2 to demonstrate the presence of the gas during exhalation (Figure 27-8b).

MANAGEMENT OF RESPIRATORY DISORDERS

The following sections will address the pathophysiology, assessment, and management of the more common respiratory disorders encountered in prehospital care. The discussion begins with a look at some general principles that can and should be applied to all respiratory emergencies.

MANAGEMENT PRINCIPLES

In cases of acute respiratory insufficiency, several principles should guide your actions in the prehospital setting.

- The airway always has first priority. In trauma victims who may have associated cervical spine injuries, protect and maintain the airway without extending the patient's neck.
- Any patient with respiratory distress should receive oxygen.
- Any patient whose illness or injury suggests the possibility of hypoxia should receive oxygen.
- If there is a question whether oxygen should be given, as in chronic obstructive pulmonary disease (COPD), administer it anyway. *Oxygen should never be withheld from a patient suspected of suffering hypoxia.*

Principles of management for respiratory disorders include the following: (1) Give first priority to the airway, and (2) always provide oxygen to patients with respiratory distress or the possibility of hypoxia, including patients with COPD.

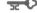

Keep these precautions in mind as you read through the descriptions of the pathophysiology, assessment, and management of respiratory disorders frequently encountered in the field.

SPECIFIC RESPIRATORY DISEASES

UPPER AIRWAY OBSTRUCTION

The most common cause of upper-airway obstruction is the relaxed tongue. In an unconscious patient in the supine position, the tongue can fall into the back of the throat and obstruct the upper air way. Additionally, the upper airway can become obstructed by such common materials as food, dentures, or other foreign bodies. A typical example of upper airway obstruction is the "café coronary," which tends to occur in middle-aged or elderly patients who wear dentures. These people often are unable to sense how well they have chewed their food. Therefore, they may accidentally inhale a large piece of food (often meat) that obstructs their airway. Concurrent alcohol consumption is often implicated in the "café coronary." Also, obstruction of the upper airway can be the result of facial or neck trauma, upper-airway burns, and allergic reactions. In addition, the upper airway can become blocked by an infection that causes swelling of the epiglottis (epiglottitis) or subglottic area (croup).

Assessment

Assessment of the patient with an upper airway obstruction varies, depending on the cause of the obstruction and the history of the event. The unresponsive patient should be evaluated for snoring respirations, possibly indicating tongue or denture obstruction. If confronted by a patient suffering a "café coronary," determine whether the victim is able to speak. Speech indicates that, at present, the obstruction is incomplete. If the victim who is unresponsive had been eating, strongly suspect a food bolus lodged in the trachea. If a burn is present or suspected, assume laryngeal edema until proven otherwise.

Patients who may be having an allergic reaction to food or medications will often report an itching sensation in the palate followed by a "lump" in the throat. The situation may progress to hoarseness, inspiratory stridor, and complete obstruction. Pay particular attention to the presence of urticaria (hives). Intercostal muscle retraction and use of the strap muscles of the neck for breathing suggest attempts to ventilate against a partially closed airway.

Management

Management of the obstructed airway is based on the nature of the obstruction. Blockage by the tongue can be corrected by opening the airway, using either the head-tilt, chin-lift, the jaw-thrust, or the modified jaw-thrust manoeuvre. The airway can be maintained by employing either a nasopharyngeal or oropharyngeal airway. If possible, remove obstructing foreign bodies using the following basic airway manoeuvres:

Conscious Adult In an adult patient who is conscious:

1. Determine whether there is a complete obstruction or poor air exchange. Ask the patient: "Are you choking?" "Can you speak?" If the patient is able to speak, she should be asked to produce a forceful cough to expel the foreign body.

Content Review

COMMON CAUSES OF AIRWAY OBSTRUCTION

Tongue
Foreign matter
Trauma
Burns
Allergic reaction
Infection

2. If the patient has complete obstruction or poor air exchange, perform the Heimlich manoeuvre until the obstruction is removed. In very obese or pregnant patients, use chest thrusts in lieu of the Heimlich manoeuvre or abdominal thrusts.

Unconscious Adult If the patient is unconscious or is losing consciousness:

1. Use the head-tilt, chin lift, the jaw-thrust, or the modified jaw-thrust in an attempt to open the airway.
2. Insert an NPA (nasopharyngeal airway) and attempt to give two ventilations via a bag-valve mask. If the attempts to ventilate fail, reposition the head, and repeat the attempt.
3. If steps 1 and 2 fail, perform chest compressions, similar to cardiopulmonary resuscitation (CPR), to be completed at the end of three sets of five.
4. If step 3 fails, try the tongue-jaw lift. If the foreign body can be visualized, attempt finger sweeps. If successful, resume ventilation. If unsuccessful, contact dispatch, and request an ACP or CCP while initiating transport of the patient to the hospital.
5. If you are an ACP or CCP, continue the chest compressions and finger sweeps while setting out the laryngoscope and the Magill forceps. Visualize the airway with the laryngoscope. If the foreign body can be seen, grasp it with the Magill forceps and remove it. Once the obstruction is removed, begin ventilating the patient and administer supplemental oxygen following airway adjunct insertion.

In cases of airway obstruction caused by laryngeal edema (e.g., anaphylactic reactions, angioedema), establish the airway by the head-tilt, chin-lift, jaw-thrust, or triple-airway manoeuvre. Then, administer supplemental oxygen. Attempt bag-valve-mask ventilation. Often, air can be forced past the obstruction and the patient adequately ventilated using this technique. Next, start an IV with a crystalloid solution, and administer subcutaneous epinephrine. See Chapter 42 for pediatric techniques.

NONCARDIOGENIC PULMONARY ADULT/EDEMA RESPIRATORY DISTRESS SYNDROME

Adult respiratory distress syndrome (ARDS) is a form of pulmonary edema that is caused by fluid accumulation in the interstitial space within the lungs. Patients with *cardiogenic* pulmonary edema have a poorly functioning left ventricle. This leads to increases in hydrostatic pressure and fluid accumulation in the interstitial space. In patients with ARDS, however, fluid accumulation occurs as the result of increased vascular permeability and decreased fluid removal from the lung tissue. This occurs in response to a wide variety of lung insults, including the following:

✱ **adult respiratory distress syndrome (ARDS)** form of pulmonary edema that is caused by fluid accumulation in the interstitial space within the lungs.

- Sepsis, particularly with gram-negative organisms
- Aspiration
- Pneumonia or other respiratory infections
- Pulmonary injury
- Burns
- Inhalation injury

- Oxygen toxicity
- Drugs, such as aspirin or opiates
- High altitude
- Hypothermia
- Near-drowning
- Head injury
- Emboli from blood clot, fat, or amniotic fluid
- Tumour destruction
- Pancreatitis
- Procedures, such as cardiopulmonary bypass or hemodialysis
- Other insults, such as hypoxia, hypotension, or cardiac arrest

The mortality in patients who develop ARDS is quite high, approaching 70 percent. While many patients die as the result of respiratory failure, many succumb to failure of several organ systems, including the liver and kidneys.

Pathophysiology

ARDS is a disorder of lung diffusion that results from increased fluid in the interstitial space. Each of the underlying conditions cited above results in the inability to maintain a proper fluid balance in the interstitial space. Severe hypotension, significant hypoxemia as the result of cardiac arrest, drowning, seizure activity or hypoventilation, high altitude exposure, and environmental toxins and endotoxins released in septic shock—all can cause disruption of the alveolar–capillary membrane. Increases in pulmonary capillary permeability, destruction of the capillary lining, and increases in osmotic forces all act to draw fluid into the interstitial space and contribute to interstitial edema. This increases the thickness of the respiratory membrane and limits diffusion of oxygen. In advanced cases, fluid also accumulates in the alveoli, causing loss of surfactant, collapse of the alveolar sacs, and impaired gas exchange. This results in a significant amount of pulmonary shunting with unoxygenated blood returning to the circulation. The result is significant hypoxia.

Assessment

With ARDS, symptoms are related to the underlying cause.

Specific clinical symptoms are related to the underlying cause of ARDS. For example, patients who develop ARDS as the result of sepsis will have symptoms related to their underlying infection. Determine if there is a history of prolonged hypoxia, head or chest trauma, inhalation of gases, or ascent to a high altitude without prior acclimation, all of which can suggest an underlying cause for the respiratory complaints.

Patients with ARDS experience a gradual decline in their respiratory status. In rare cases, a seemingly healthy patient has a sudden onset of respiratory failure and hypoxia. Such a presentation is characteristic of patients with high altitude pulmonary edema (HAPE).

Dyspnea, confusion, and agitation are often found in patients with noncardiogenic pulmonary edema. Patients may also report fatigue and reduced exercise ability. Symptoms, such as orthopnea, paroxysmal nocturnal dyspnea, or sputum production, are not commonly reported but may be seen.

The prominent physical findings are generally those associated with the underlying lung insult. Tachypnea and tachycardia are often found in association with ARDS. Crackles (rales) are audible in both lungs. Wheezing may also be heard if there is any degree of bronchospasm. Severe tachypnea, central cyanosis, and signs of imminent respiratory failure are seen in severe cases. Pulse oximetry will demonstrate low oxygen saturations in those patients with advanced disease. In those patients requiring ventilatory support, a decreased lung compliance will be noted. (It will require more operator force to deliver an adequate lung volume.)

Management

Specific management of the patient's underlying medical condition is the hallmark of treatment for this disorder. Treatment of gram-negative sepsis with appropriate antibiotics, removal of the patient from any offending toxin, or rapid descent to a lower altitude in patients with HAPE are the most important therapies for this condition. The patient will usually tolerate an upright position with the legs dangling off the stretcher.

Since the hypoxia seen in ARDS is the result of diffusion defects, oxygen supplementation is essential for all patients with this condition. Establish intravenous access, but provide fluids only if hypovolemia exists. Establish cardiac monitoring. Suctioning of lung secretions is often required to maintain airway patency.

Use positive pressure ventilation to support any ARDS patient who demonstrates signs of respiratory failure. Use bag-valve-mask ventilation for initial respiratory support, but note that these patients generally require endotracheal intubation and support using a mechanical ventilator for early management. **Positive end expiratory pressure (PEEP)** is often required to maintain patency of the alveoli and adequate oxygenation. Diuretics and nitrates, which are used in patients with cardiogenic pulmonary edema, are usually not helpful in patients with ARDS. Treatment occasionally includes corticosteroids for patients with ARDS/noncardiogenic pulmonary edema. Corticosteroids are thought to stabilize the alveolar–capillary membrane, although clinical studies have not demonstrated any benefit to their use.

Maintain cardiac monitoring and pulse oximetry throughout transport of the patient. Transport patients to a facility capable of advanced hemodynamic monitoring (including Swan-Ganz catheter) and mechanical ventilation support.

OBSTRUCTIVE LUNG DISEASE

Obstructive lung disease is widespread in our society. The most common obstructive lung diseases encountered in prehospital care are asthma, emphysema, and chronic bronchitis (the last two are often discussed together as chronic obstructive pulmonary disease, or COPD). COPD is found in 25 percent of all adults. Chronic bronchitis alone affects one in five adult males. Patients with COPD have a 50-percent mortality within 10 years of the diagnosis. Asthma afflicts 7.1 percent of Canadian men, 5.5 percent of Canadian women, and 10 to 15 percent of Canadian children. Experts believe that the figure may be as high as 20 percent. Asthma is the leading cause of hospital admission for children.

Although asthma may have a genetic predisposition, COPD is known to be directly caused by cigarette smoking and environmental toxins. Other factors have been shown to precipitate symptoms in patients who already have obstructive airway disease. Intrinsic factors include stress, upper respiratory infections, and exercise. Extrinsic factors include tobacco smoke, drugs, occupational hazards (chemical fumes, dust, and so on), and allergens, such as food, animal dander, dust, and mould.

Obstructive lung diseases have abnormal ventilation as a common feature. This abnormal ventilation is a result of obstruction that occurs primarily in the bronchioles. Several changes occur within these air conduits. Bronchospasm (sustained smooth muscle contraction) occurs, which may be reversed by beta-adrenergic receptor stimulation. Such agents as salbutamol and epinephrine are used to accom-

Management of the patient's underlying medical condition is the hallmark of treatment for ARDS.

Oxygen supplementation is essential for all ARDS patients.

* positive end expiratory pressure (PEEP) a method of holding the alveoli open by increasing expiratory pressure. Some bag-valve units used in EMS have PEEP attachments. Also, EMS personnel sometimes transport patients who are on ventilators with PEEP attachments.

plish this stimulation. Increased mucus production by goblet cells that line the respiratory tree also contribute to obstruction. This effect may be worsened by the fact that in many patients the cilia are destroyed, resulting in poor clearance of excess mucus. Finally, inflammation of the bronchial passages results in the accumulation of fluid and inflammatory cells. Depending on the underlying cause, some elements of bronchial obstruction are reversible, whereas others are not.

During inspiration, the bronchioles will naturally dilate, allowing air to be drawn into the alveoli. As the patient begins to exhale, the bronchioles constrict. When this natural constriction occurs—in addition to the underlying bronchospasm, increased mucus production, and inflammation that exist in patients with obstructive airway disease—the result is significant air trapping distal to the obstruction. This is one of the hallmarks of obstructive lung disease. This section will discuss each of these disease processes—emphysema, chronic bronchitis, and asthma—detailing the pathophysiology, assessment, and treatment.

EMPHYSEMA

Emphysema results from destruction of the alveolar walls distal to the terminal bronchioles. It is more common in men than in women. The major factor contributing to emphysema is cigarette smoking. Significant exposure to environmental toxins is another contributing factor.

Pathophysiology

Continued exposure to noxious substances, such as cigarette smoke, results in the gradual destruction of the walls of the alveoli. This process decreases the alveolar membrane surface area, thus lessening the area available for gas exchange. The progressive loss of the respiratory membrane results in an increased ratio of air to lung tissue. The result is diffusion defects. Additionally, the number of pulmonary capillaries in the lung is decreased, thus increasing resistance to pulmonary blood flow. This condition ultimately causes pulmonary hypertension, which, in turn, may lead to right-heart failure, **cor pulmonale,** and death (Figure 27-9).

Emphysema also causes weakening of the walls of the small bronchioles. When the walls of the alveoli and small bronchioles are destroyed, the lungs lose their capacity to recoil and air becomes trapped in the lungs. Thus, residual volume increases, while vital capacity remains relatively normal. The destroyed lung tissue (called *blebs*) results in alveolar collapse. To counteract this effect, patients tend to breathe through pursed lips. This creates continued positive pressure similar to PEEP (positive end expiratory pressure) and prevents alveolar collapse.

As the disease progresses, the PaO_2 further decreases, which may lead to increased red blood cell production and **polycythemia** (an excess of red blood cells resulting in an abnormally high hematocrit). The $PaCO_2$ also increases and becomes chronically elevated, forcing the body to depend on hypoxic drive to control respirations. Finally, remember that emphysema is characterized by irreversible airway obstruction.

Patients with emphysema are more susceptible to acute respiratory infections, such as pneumonia, and to cardiac dysrhythmias. Chronic emphysema patients ultimately become dependent on bronchodilators, corticosteroids, and, in the final stages, supplemental oxygen.

Assessment

The patient with emphysema may report a history of recent weight loss, increased dyspnea on exertion, and progressive limitation of physical activity. Unlike chronic bronchitis, discussed in subsequent sections, emphysema is rarely associated with a cough, except in the morning. Question the patient

* **cor pulmonale** hypertrophy of the right ventricle resulting from disorders of the lung.

* **polycythemia** an excess of red blood cells.

Emphysema is rarely associated with a cough except in the morning.

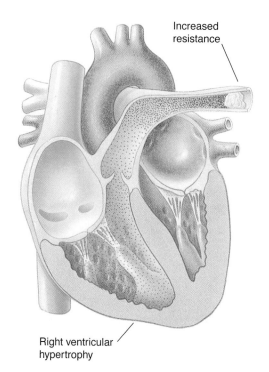

Increased resistance

Right ventricular hypertrophy

FIGURE 27-9 Longstanding chronic obstructive pulmonary disease can cause pulmonary hypertension, which, in turn, may lead to cor pulmonale.

about smoking or other tobacco use. This is generally reported in pack/years. Ask the number of cigarette packs (25 cigarettes/pack) smoked per day and the number of years the patient has smoked. Multiply the number of packs smoked per day by the number of years. For example, a man who has smoked two packs per day for 15 years would have a 30-pack/year smoking history. Medical problems related to smoking, such as emphysema, chronic bronchitis, and lung cancer, usually begin after a patient surpasses a 20-pack/year history, although this can vary significantly.

Secondary assessment of the emphysema patient usually reveals a barrel chest evidenced by an increase in the anterior/posterior chest diameter. You may also note decreased chest excursion with a prolonged expiratory phase and a rapid resting respiratory rate. Patients with emphysema are often thin, since they must use a significant amount of their caloric intake for respiration. They tend to have pink skin colour due to polycythemia (excess of red blood cells) and are referred to as "pink puffers." Emphysema patients often have hypertrophy of the accessory respiratory muscles (Figure 27-10).

The patient will often involuntarily purse her lips to create continuous positive airway pressure. Clubbing of the fingers is common. Breath sounds are usually diminished. Wheezes and rhonchi may or may not be present, depending on the amount of obstruction to air flow. The patient may exhibit signs of right-heart failure as evidenced by jugular vein distention, peripheral edema, and hepatic congestion. Signs of severe respiratory impairment in all patients with obstructive lung disease include confusion, agitation, somnolence, one-to-two-word dyspnea, and use of accessory muscles to assist ventilation.

Emphysema patients usually have a barrel chest, are often thin, and have a pink skin colour ("pink puffers").

Management

Although emphysema differs in the disease process from chronic bronchitis, the two respiratory disorders share several of the same symptoms and pathophysiology. As a result, you will treat the two disorders in a similar manner. The discussion of management of emphysema will be taken up with that of chronic bronchitis. (See next section.)

FIGURE 27-10 Typical appearance of patient with emphysema. There are well-developed accessory muscles and suprasternal retraction.

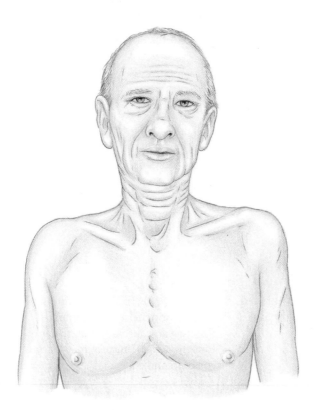

CHRONIC BRONCHITIS

Chronic bronchitis results from an increase in the number of the goblet (mucus-secreting) cells in the respiratory tree (Figure 27-11). It is characterized by the production of a large quantity of sputum. This often occurs after prolonged exposure to cigarette smoke.

FIGURE 27-11 Chronic mucus production and plugging of the airways occur in chronic bronchitis.

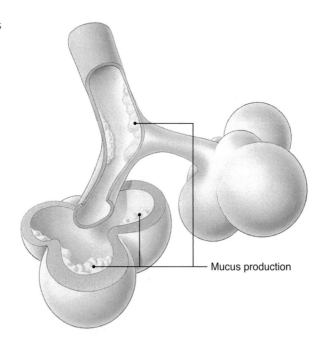

Mucus production

Pathophysiology

Unlike in emphysema, in chronic bronchitis, the alveoli are not severely affected, and diffusion remains normal. Gas exchange is decreased because there is lowered alveolar ventilation, which ultimately results in hypoxia and hypercarbia. Hypoxia may increase red blood cell production, which, in turn, leads to polycythemia (as occurs in emphysema). Increased $PaCO_2$ levels may lead to irritability, somnolence, decreased intellectual abilities, headaches, and personality changes. Physiologically, an increased $PaCO_2$ causes pulmonary vasoconstriction, resulting in pulmonary hypertension and, eventually, cor pulmonale. Unlike emphysema, the vital capacity is decreased, while the residual volume is normal or decreased.

Assessment

The patient with chronic bronchitis often will have a history of heavy cigarette smoking, but the disease may also occur in nonsmokers. There may also be a history of frequent respiratory infections. In addition, these patients usually produce considerable quantities of sputum daily. Clinically, the patient is described as having a productive cough for at least three months per year for two or more consecutive years.

Patients with chronic bronchitis tend to be overweight and can be cyanotic. Because of this, they are often referred to as "blue bloaters." This can be contrasted with the "pink puffer" image of emphysema patients described above. Auscultation of the thorax often will reveal rhonchi due to occlusion of the larger airways with mucus plugs. The patient may also exhibit signs and symptoms of right heart failure, such as jugular vein distention, ankle edema, and hepatic congestion.

Chronic bronchitis is usually associated with a productive cough and copious sputum production.

Chronic bronchitis patients tend to be overweight and are often cyanotic ("blue bloaters").

Content Review

EMPHYSEMA AND CHRONIC BRONCHITIS: MANAGEMENT GOALS

Relieve hypoxia
Reverse bronchoconstriction

Management

The primary goals in the emergency management of the patient with either emphysema or chronic bronchitis are to relieve hypoxia and reverse any bronchoconstriction that may be present. However, many of these patients are dependent on hypoxic respiratory drive. As a result, the supplemental administration of oxygen may decrease respiratory drive and inhibit ventilation. You must continually monitor the patient and be prepared to assist ventilations if signs of respiratory depression develop.

The first step in treating a patient suffering an exacerbation of emphysema or chronic bronchitis is to establish an airway. Then, place the patient in a seated or semi-seated position to assist the accessory respiratory muscles. Apply a pulse oximeter, and determine the blood oxygen saturation (SaO_2). Administer supplemental oxygen at a low-flow rate while maintaining an oxygen saturation above 90 percent. A nasal cannula can often be used, but you must constantly monitor the respiratory rate and depth as well as oxygen saturation. If hypoxia or respiratory failure is evident, increase the concentration of delivered oxygen. Be prepared to support the ventilation with bag-valve-mask assistance. Intubation may be required if respiratory failure is imminent.

Establish an intravenous line with Ringer's Lactate or normal saline at a "to-keep-open" rate. More aggressive fluid administration is suggested if signs of dehydration are present. This may also aid in loosening thick mucus secretions. Then, if warranted under local protocol, administer a bronchodilator medication, such as salbutamol, through a small-volume nebulizer.

Administer oxygen to the COPD patient who needs it to relieve hypoxia. Since this may decrease the respiratory drive, monitor the patient, and be prepared to assist ventilations if necessary.

ASTHMA

Asthma is a common respiratory illness that affects many persons, including approximately two million Canadians, or 6.4 percent of the adult population. In Canada, approximately 20 children and 500 adults die each year from asthma. It is estmated that more than 80 percent of asthma deaths could be prevented with proper asthma education. While the death rate from asthma in Canada has slowly decreased since 1990, there are still approximately 10 asthma deaths per week. In addition, the mortality rate for asthma among Blacks has been twice as high as among Caucasians. Approximately 50 percent of patients who die from asthma do so before reaching the hospital. Thus, EMS personnel are frequently called on to treat patients suffering an asthma attack. Prompt recognition followed by appropriate treatment can significantly improve the patient's condition and enhance her chance of survival.

Pathophysiology

Asthma is a chronic inflammatory disorder of the airways. In susceptible individuals, this inflammation causes symptoms usually associated with widespread but variable airflow obstruction. In addition to airflow obstruction, the airway becomes hyperresponsive. The airflow obstruction and hyperresponsiveness are often reversible with treatment. These conditions may also reverse spontaneously.

Asthma may be induced by any of several different factors. These factors, commonly referred to as "triggers" or "inducers," vary from one individual to the next. In allergic individuals, environmental allergens are a major cause of inflammation. These allergens may occur both indoors and outdoors. In addition to allergens, asthma may be triggered by cold air, exercise, foods, irritants, stress, and certain medications. Often, a specific trigger cannot be identified. Extrinsic triggers predominantly tend to affect children, whereas intrinsic factors trigger asthma in adults.

Within minutes of exposure to the offending trigger, a two-phase reaction occurs. The first phase of the reaction is characterized by the release of chemical mediators, such as histamine. These mediators cause contraction of the bronchial smooth muscle and leakage of fluid from peribronchial capillaries. This results in both bronchoconstriction and bronchial edema. These two factors can significantly decrease expiratory airflow, which results in the typical "asthma attack."

Often, the asthma attack will resolve spontaneously in 1–2 hours or may be aborted by the use of inhaled bronchodilator medications, such as salbutamol. However, within 6–8 hours after exposure to the trigger, a second reaction occurs. This late phase is characterized by inflammation of the bronchioles as cells of the immune system (eosinophils, neutrophils, and lymphocytes) invade the mucosa of the respiratory tract. This leads to additional edema and swelling of the bronchioles and a further decrease in expiratory airflow.

The second phase reaction will not typically respond to inhaled beta-agonist drugs. Instead, anti-inflammatory agents, such as corticosteroids, are often required. It is important to point out that the severe inflammatory changes seen in an acute asthma attack do not develop over a few hours or even a few days. The inflammation will often begin several days or several weeks before the onset of the actual asthma attack.

Assessment

Begin the primary prehospital assessment of the asthmatic by considering immediate threats to the airway, breathing, and circulation. Then, turn your attention to the focused history and secondary assessment.

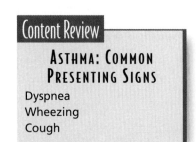

Content Review

ASTHMA: COMMON PRESENTING SIGNS
Dyspnea
Wheezing
Cough

The most common presenting symptoms of asthma are dyspnea, wheezing, and cough. Wheezing results from turbulent airflow through the inflamed and narrowed bronchioles. Many asthmatics will have a persistent cough. This is primarily due to the hyperresponsiveness of the airway. It is important to point out that some asthmatics do not wheeze. Instead, their initial presentation may be a frequent and persistent cough. As asthma severity increases, the patient may exhibit hyperinflation of the chest due to trapping of air in the alveoli. In addition, tachypnea (rapid respiration) will occur. The patient may start to use accessory muscles to aid respiration.

Note that some asthmatics do not wheeze, instead presenting with a frequent, persistent cough.

Symptoms of a severe asthma attack include one-to-two-word dyspnea (the inability to complete a phrase or sentence without having to stop to breathe), pulsus paradoxus (a drop of systolic blood pressure of 10 mmHg or more with inspiration), tachycardia, and decreased oxygen saturation on pulse oximetry. As hypoxia develops, the patient may become agitated and anxious.

When conducting the focused history and secondary assessment, start by obtaining a brief patient history. Most asthmatics will report that they suffer from asthma. In addition, the patient's home medications may help confirm a history of asthma. Common asthma medications include inhaled beta-agonists (salbutamol), inhaled corticosteroids (betamethasone, beclomethasone), inhaled cromolyn sodium, and inhaled anticholinergics (ipratropium bromide). Often, the patient will be taking oral bronchodilators, such as theophylline, or may be taking oral corticosteroids (prednisone).

Determine when the symptoms started and what the patient has taken in an attempt to abort the attack. Also, find out whether the patient is allergic to any medications. Question the patient about hospitalizations for asthma. If the patient has been hospitalized, ask whether the patient has ever required intubation and mechanical ventilation. A prior history of intubation and mechanical ventilation should heighten your index of suspicion. Similarly, an asthmatic who is on continuous corticosteroid therapy is also a high-risk patient.

After you obtain the pertinent history, perform a brief secondary assessment. Place particular emphasis on the chest and neck. Examination of the chest should begin with inspection. Note any increase in the diameter of the chest that may indicate air trapping. Also, note the use of accessory muscles, including retraction of the intercostal muscles or use of the strap muscles of the neck. Following inspection, palpate the chest, noting any deformity, crepitus, or asymmetry. Next, auscultate the posterior chest. Note any abnormal breath sounds, such as wheezing or rhonchi. Listen to the symmetry of breath sounds. Unilateral wheezing may indicate an aspirated foreign body or a pneumothorax.

Obtain accurate vital signs. One of the most important vital signs is the respiratory rate. An increase in the respiratory rate is one of the earliest symptoms of a respiratory problem. Many EMS personnel inaccurately measure the respiratory rate. The easiest method is to simply place your fingers on the patient's radial artery as if you were measuring the pulse rate. This will make the patient think you are obtaining the pulse rate, and she will not alter her breathing pattern. Measure the respiratory rate for at least 30 seconds. At the same time, note any alterations in the respiratory pattern. Pulse oximetry is an excellent adjunct to respiratory assessment. It will provide you with data regarding the oxygen saturation status (SaO_2) as well as an audible measure of the pulse rate.

EMS systems should be able to measure the peak expiratory flow rate (PEFR). (Review Figure 27-7 and Table 27-1.) The PEFR is a reliable indicator of airflow. If possible, measure peak flow rates to determine the severity of an asthma attack and the degree of response to treatment. The more severe the asthma attack, the lower will be the PEFR.

Management

Treatment of asthma is designed to correct hypoxia, reverse any bronchospasm, and treat the inflammatory changes associated with the disease. Administer oxygen at a high concentration (100 percent). Establish intravenous access, and place the patient on an ECG monitor. Direct initial treatment at reversing any bronchospasm present. The most commonly used drugs are the inhaled beta-agonist preparations, such as salbutamol (Ventolin). This can be easily administered with a small-volume, oxygen-powered nebulizer. Monitor the patient's response to the medication by noting improvement in PEFR and pulse oximetry readings.

Many asthma patients will wait before summoning EMS. The longer the time interval from the onset of the asthma attack until treatment, the less likely it will be that bronchodilator medications will work. Often, after a prolonged asthma attack, the patient may become fatigued. A fatigued patient can quickly develop respiratory failure and subsequently require intubation and mechanical ventilation. Always be prepared to provide airway and respiratory support to the asthmatic.

Special Cases

While most cases of asthma conform to the preceding descriptions, you may run into several special cases in the field. Asthma conditions that require special concern include status asthmaticus and asthmatic attacks in children.

Status Asthmaticus *Status asthmaticus* is a severe, prolonged asthma attack that cannot be broken even by repeated doses of bronchodilators. It is a serious medical emergency that requires prompt recognition, treatment, and transport. The patient suffering status asthmaticus frequently will have a greatly distended chest from continued air trapping. Breath sounds, and often wheezing, may be absent. The patient is usually exhausted, severely acidotic, and dehydrated. The management of status asthmaticus is basically the same as for asthma. *Recognize that respiratory arrest is imminent, and be prepared for endotracheal intubation.* Transport the patient immediately, and continue aggressive treatment en route.

Asthma in Children Asthma in children is common. The pathophysiology and treatment are essentially the same as in adults, with altered medication dosages. Several additional medications are used in the treatment of childhood asthma. (Asthma in children is discussed in greater detail in Chapter 42.)

UPPER RESPIRATORY INFECTION (URI)

Infections involving the upper airway and respiratory tract are among the most common infections for which patients seek medical attention. Although these conditions are rarely life threatening, upper respiratory infections (URIs) can make many existing pulmonary diseases worse or lead to direct pulmonary infection. The best defence against the spread of URI is such common practices as good handwashing and covering the mouth during coughing and sneezing. Attention to such details is important when caring for patients with underlying pulmonary disease or those who are immunosuppressed (human immunodeficiency virus [HIV] infection, cancer) because URIs are more severe in these populations. Because of the prevalence of such infections, complete protection is impossible.

Pathophysiology

Remember that the upper airway begins at the nose and mouth, passes through the pharynx and ends at the larynx. Other related structures are the paranasal sinuses and the eustachian tubes that connect the pharynx and the middle ear. In addition, several collections of lymphoid tissue found in the pharynx (palatine, pharyngeal, and lingual tonsils) produce antibodies and provide immune protection.

The vast majority of URIs are caused by viruses. A variety of bacteria may also produce infection of the upper respiratory tract. The most significant is Group A *Streptococcus*, which is the causative organism in "strep throat" and accounts for up to 30 percent of URIs. This bacterium is also implicated in sinusitis and middle ear infections. Up to 50 percent of patients who have pharyngitis (inflammation of the pharynx) are not found to have a viral or bacterial cause. Fortunately, most URIs are self-limiting illnesses that resolve after several days of symptoms.

Assessment

The major symptoms of URI are dependent on the portion of the upper respiratory tract that is predominantly affected (Table 27-2). Patients with URIs will often have accompanying symptoms, such as fever, chills, myalgias (muscle pains), and fatigue.

Remember that any child with suspected epiglottitis (see Chapter 42) should be supported in a position of comfort. Do not attempt examination of the throat as this may produce severe laryngospasm. Although most paramedic courses focus on children with epiglottitis, more cases each year are arising involving adults. This is a true emergency, regardless of the age of the patient.

Support the child with suspected epiglottitis in a position of comfort. Do not attempt examination of the throat, which may produce severe laryngospasm.

Management

In most cases, the diagnosis and treatment of upper respiratory conditions are based on the history and physical findings. Patients with pharyngitis are often diagnosed by obtaining a throat culture that confirms a bacterial cause of symptoms. A rapid test is also available. In patients with sinusitis and otitis media, treatment is based on a presumed bacterial cause.

As with other medical conditions, focus your attention on the patient's airway and ventilation. Generally, no intervention is required, except in children with epiglottitis and in some complicated URIs where a collection of pus may occlude the airway. Give supplemental oxygen to any patient who has underlying pulmonary disease.

In URI, as with other medical conditions, focus attention on the patient's airway and ventilation. Give supplemental oxygen to any patient with underlying pulmonary disease.

Table 27-2 LOCATIONS, SYMPTOMS, AND SIGNS OF UPPER RESPIRATORY INFECTIONS

Structure	Infection	Symptoms	Signs
Nose	Rhinitis	Runny nose, congestion, sneezing	Rhinorrhea
Pharynx	Pharyngitis	Sore throat, pain on swallowing	Erythematous pharynx, tonsil enlargement, pus on tonsils, cervical lymph node enlargement
Middle ear	Otitis media	Ear pain, decreased hearing	Red, bulging eardrum, pus behind ear drum, lymph node enlargement in front of or behind ear
Larynx	Laryngitis	Sore throat, hoarseness, pain on speaking	Red pharynx, hoarse quality to voice, cervical lymph node enlargement
Epiglottis	Epiglottitis	Sore throat, drooling, ill appearance	Upright position, drooling, ill appearance
Sinuses	Sinusitis	Headache, congestion	Tenderness over the sinuses, worsening of pain with leaning forward, yellow nasal discharge

Most URIs are treated symptomatically. Acetaminophen or ibuprofen is prescribed for fever, headache, and myalgias. Encourage patients to drink plenty of fluids. Salt water gargles may be beneficial in throat discomfort. Decongestants and antihistamines may be used to reduce mucus secretion. Encourage patients being treated with antibiotics to continue these agents.

In some patients with asthma or COPD, a URI may produce a worsening of their underlying medical condition. Use inhaled bronchodilators according to local protocol or on advice of medical direction. Transport patients with underlying medical conditions to a health-care facility capable of continued evaluation and management of the underlying condition. Continue appropriate monitoring with pulse oximetry and ECG during transport.

PNEUMONIA

Pneumonia is an infection of the lungs and a common medical problem, especially in the aged and those infected with HIV. In fact, pneumonia is one of the leading causes of death in both groups of patients, with a mortality rate of 24 per 100 000 in Canada. Total respiratory deaths account for 661 per 100 000.

Patients with HIV infection and those on immunosuppressive therapy (cancer patients) are at high risk of developing pneumonia. In addition, the very young and very old are at higher risk of acquiring pneumonia because of ineffective protective mechanisms. Other risk factors include a history of alcoholism, cigarette smoking, and exposure to cold temperatures.

Pathophysiology

Pneumonia is a collection of related respiratory diseases caused by a variety of infectious agents invading the lungs. Mucus production and the action of respiratory tract cilia play a role in protecting the body against bacterial invasion. When considering which patients are at risk, the unifying concept is that there is a defect in mucus production, ciliary action, or both.

Bacterial and viral pneumonias are the most frequent, although fungal and other forms of pneumonia do exist. More unusual forms of pneumonia are seen in those patients who are currently or recently have been hospitalized where they are exposed to a more unusual variety of microorganisms. This is referred to as hospital-acquired pneumonia. (The form that develops in the out-of-hospital setting is described as community-acquired pneumonia.)

The infection begins in one part of the lung and often spreads to nearby alveoli. The infection may ultimately involve the entire lung. As the disease progresses, fluid and inflammatory cells collect in the alveoli, and alveolar collapse may occur. Pneumonia is primarily a ventilation disorder. Occasionally, the infection will extend beyond the lungs into the bloodstream and to more distant sites in the body. This systemic spread may lead to septic shock.

Assessment

A patient with pneumonia will generally appear ill. She may report a recent history of fever and chills. These chills are commonly described as "bed shaking." There is usually a generalized weakness and malaise. The patient will tend to complain of a deep, productive cough and may expel yellow to brown sputum, often streaked with blood. Many cases involve associated **pleuritic** chest pain. Therefore, pneumonia should be considered in any patient who presents complaining of chest pain, especially if accompanied by fever and/or chills. In pneumonia involving the lower lobes of the lungs, a patient may complain of nothing more than upper abdominal pain.

✱ pleuritic sharp or tearing, as a description of pain.

Secondary assessment will commonly reveal fever, tachypnea, tachycardia, and a cough. Respiratory distress may be present. Auscultation of the chest usually demonstrates crackles (rales) in the involved lung segment, although wheezes or rhonchi may be heard. There usually is decreased air movement in the areas filled with infection. *Egophony* (a change in the spoken "E" sound to an "A" sound on auscultation) may also be noted.

In the forms of pneumonia involving viral, fungal, and rare bacterial causes, the typical symptoms described above are not seen. Instead, these patients may report a nonproductive cough with less prominent lung findings. Systemic symptoms, such as headache, malaise, fatigue, muscle aches, sore throat, and abdominal complaints, including nausea, vomiting, and diarrhea, are more prominent. Fever and chills are not as significant as in bacterial pneumonia.

Management

Pneumonia is generally diagnosed on the basis of physical assessment, x-ray findings, and laboratory cultures. Therefore, diagnosis in the field is unlikely. The primary treatment is antibiotics to which the causative organism is susceptible. In the field, however, antibiotics are not indicated, and treatment is purely supportive.

Place the patient in a comfortable position, and administer high-flow oxygen. Use pulse oximetry to assess the patient's oxygen requirements. In severe cases, ventilatory assistance is needed, and endotracheal intubation may be required. Establish intravenous access, and base fluid resuscitation on the patient's hydration status. Administering fluids for dehydration is appropriate, but overhydration can also worsen the respiratory condition. Breathing treatment with a beta agonist, particularly if wheezing is present, may be beneficial. Because patients with pneumonia often have some bronchospasm, these drugs will afford the patient some symptomatic relief. A cool, moistened wash cloth may soothe the patient.

Remember to be extremely careful when caring for the patient over age 65 with suspected pneumonia. In these patients, mortality and complication rates are high. Transport them to a facility capable of handling the significant complications associated with the disease in this population.

LUNG CANCER

Lung cancer (neoplasm) is the leading cause of cancer-related death in both men and women. Most patients with lung cancer are between the ages of 55 and 65 years. There is a high mortality rate for patients with lung cancer after only one year with the disease.

There are currently four major types of lung cancer based on the predominant cell type. Twenty percent of cases involve only the lung tissue. Another 35 percent involve spread to the lymphatic system, and 45 percent have distant metastases (cancer cells spreading to other tissues). In those cases where there is lung tissue invasion, the primary problem is disruption of diffusion. In some larger cancers, there may also be alterations in ventilation due to obstruction of the conducting bronchioles.

Cigarette smoking has long been known to be a risk factor for development of lung cancer. Environmental exposure to asbestos, hydrocarbons, radiation, and fumes from metal production have also been identified as risk factors. Finally, home exposure to radon has been implicated in the development of lung cancer. Preventive strategies include educating teenagers about the dangers of cigarette smoking and encouraging current smokers to quit. Implementing environmental safety standards that reduce the risk of exposure to such substances as asbestos will also reduce the risk of lung cancer. Finally, cancer screening of populations at risk will be an effective preventive measure.

Pathophysiology

Although cancers that start elsewhere in the body can spread to the lungs, the vast majority of lung cancers are caused by carcinogens (cancer-producing substances) from cigarette smoking. A small portion of lung cancers are caused by inhalation of occupational agents, such as asbestos and arsenic. These substances irritate and adversely affect the various tissues of the lung, ultimately leading to the development of abnormal (cancerous) cells.

There are four major types of lung cancers, depending on the type of lung tissue involved. The most common type of lung cancer is referred to as *adenocarcinoma*. This cancer arises from glandular-type (i.e., mucus-producing) cells found in the lungs and bronchioles. The next most frequently encountered type of lung cancer is *small cell carcinoma* (also called "oat cell" carcinoma). Small cell carcinoma arises from bronchial tissues. The third type of lung cancer is referred to as *epidermoid carcinoma*. Finally, *large cell carcinoma* is the fourth major type of lung cancer. Like small cell carcinoma, epidermoid and large cell carcinomas typically arise from the bronchial tissues. Lung cancers generally have a bad prognosis, with most patients dying within a year of the diagnosis.

Assessment

In lung cancer, as with other respiratory diseases, your first priority is to address signs of respiratory distress.

Many patients with lung cancer will have coexisting COPD from years of tobacco smoking.

As with other respiratory diseases, your first priority is to address signs of severe respiratory distress. Look for altered mental status, one-to-two-word dyspnea, cyanosis, hemoptysis, and hypoxia as indicated by pulse oximeter. Severe uncontrolled hemoptysis can be a particularly life-threatening presentation.

Patients with lung cancer will present with a variety of complaints, depending on whether they are related to direct lung involvement, invasion of local structures, or metastatic spread. Patients with localized disease will present with cough, dyspnea, hoarseness, vague chest pain, and hemoptysis. Fever, chills, and pleuritic chest pain are seen in patients who develop pneumonia. Symptoms related to local invasion include pain on swallowing (dysphagia), weakness or numbness in the arm, and shoulder pain. Metastatic symptoms are related to the area of spread and include headache, seizures, bone pain, abdominal pain, nausea, and malaise.

Physical findings are nonspecific. Patients with advanced disease have profound weight loss and cachexia (general physical wasting and malnutrition). Crackles (rales), rhonchi, wheezes, and diminished breath sounds may be heard in the affected lung. Venous distention in the arms and neck may be present if there is occlusion of the superior vena cava (called *superior vena cava syndrome*).

Management

Content Review

LUNG CANCER: MANAGEMENT GOALS

Administer oxygen.
Support ventilation.
Be aware of any DNR order.
Provide emotional support.

Administer supplemental oxygen as needed, depending on the clinical status and pulse oximetry measurement. Support the patient's ventilation as needed, and intubate as necessary. Be attentive, however, for any do not resuscitate (DNR) order or other advance directive, such as a living will, and follow your local protocol regarding these legal instruments. Consult medical direction if questions arise.

Initiate an IV of 0.9 percent normal saline and provide fluids if signs of dehydration are present.

Out-of-hospital drug therapy consists of bronchodilator agents when signs of obstructive lung disease are present. Transport the patient and en route monitor mental status, vital signs, and oxygen status as appropriate. Be prepared to provide emotional support to both the patient and the family during transport.

Toxic Inhalation

Inhalation of toxic substances into the respiratory tract can cause pain, inflammation, or destruction of pulmonary tissues. Significant inhalations can affect the ability of the alveoli to exchange oxygen, which leads to hypoxemia.

Pathophysiology

The possibility of inhalation of products toxic to the respiratory system should be considered in any dyspneic patient. Causes of toxic inhalation include superheated air, toxic products of combustion, chemical irritants, and inhalation of steam. Each of these agents can result in upper airway obstruction due to edema and laryngospasm. In such cases, bronchospasm and lower airway edema may additionally appear. In severe inhalations, disruption of the alveolar–capillary membranes may result in life-threatening pulmonary edema.

Assessment

When assessing the patient with possible toxic inhalation exposure, determine the nature of the inhalant or the combusted material. Several products can result in the formation of corrosive acids or alkalis that irritate and damage the airway. These include the following:

- Ammonia (ammonium hydroxide)
- Nitrogen oxide (nitric acid)
- Sulphur dioxide (sulphurous acid)
- Sulphur trioxide (sulphuric acid)
- Chlorine (hydrochloric acid)

> *When assessing the patient with possible toxic inhalation, determine the nature of the inhalant or combusted material.*
>

It is also crucial to determine the duration of the exposure, whether the patient was in an enclosed area at the time of the exposure, or if she experienced a loss of consciousness. Loss of consciousness may cause the airway to became vulnerable as a result of the loss of airway protective mechanisms.

During secondary assessment, pay particular attention to the face, mouth, and throat. Note any burns or particulate matter. Next, auscultate the chest for the presence of any wheezes or crackles (rales). Wheezing may indicate bronchospasm, while crackles may suggest pulmonary edema.

Management

After ensuring the safety of rescue personnel, remove the patient from the hazardous environment. Next, establish and maintain an open airway. Remember that the airway is often irritable, and attempts at endotracheal intubation may result in laryngospasm, completely obstructing the airway. Laryngeal edema, as evidenced by hoarseness, brassy cough, and stridor, is ominous and may require prompt endotracheal intubation. Administer humidified oxygen at high concentration. As a precaution, start an IV of a crystalloid solution to provide rapid venous access. Transport the patient promptly.

Carbon Monoxide Inhalation

Carbon monoxide is an odourless, tasteless, colourless gas produced from the incomplete burning of fossil fuels and other carbon-containing compounds.

Content Review

TOXIC INHALATION: MANAGEMENT SEQUENCE
Ensure safety of rescue personnel.
Remove patient from toxic environment.
Maintain an open airway.
Provide humidified, high-concentration oxygen.

Carbon monoxide can be encountered in industrial sites, such as mines and factories. It is present in the environment in various concentrations primarily because of automotive exhaust emissions. Most poisonings occur from automobile emissions and home-heating devices used in poorly ventilated areas. Carbon monoxide is often used in suicide attempts. In addition, it is a particular hazard for firefighters and rescue personnel.

Pathophysiology

Carbon monoxide exposure is potentially life threatening because it easily binds to the hemoglobin molecule. It has an affinity for hemoglobin 200 times that of oxygen. Once bound, receptor sites on the hemoglobin can no longer transport oxygen to the peripheral tissues. The result is hypoxia at the cellular level and, ultimately, metabolic acidosis. Additionally, carbon monoxide binds to iron-containing enzymes within the cells, leading to worsening cellular acidosis.

Assessment

With carbon monoxide poisoning, determine the source of exposure, its length, and the location.

When confronted by a patient suffering possible carbon monoxide poisoning, determine the source of exposure, its length, and the location. Less time is required to develop a significant exposure in a closed space compared with one in an area that is fairly well ventilated.

Signs and symptoms of carbon monoxide poisoning include headache, nausea and vomiting, confusion, agitation, loss of coordination, chest pain, loss of consciousness, and even seizures. On secondary assessment, the skin may be cyanotic, or it may be bright cherry red (a very late finding). There may be other signs of hypoxia, such as peripheral cyanosis or confusion.

Management

On detection of carbon monoxide poisoning, first ensure the safety of rescue personnel, and then remove the patient from the site of exposure. Ensure and maintain the airway. Administer supplemental oxygen at the highest possible concentration. If the patient is breathing spontaneously, apply a nonrebreather mask. If respiratory depression is noted, assist respirations. If shock is present, treat it. Prompt transport is essential.

Hyperbaric oxygen therapy may be used in the treatment of severe carbon monoxide poisoning. Hyperbaric oxygen increases the PaO_2, thus promoting increased oxygen uptake and displacement of the carbon monoxide from the hemoglobin.

PULMONARY EMBOLISM

A pulmonary embolism is a blood clot (thrombus) or some other particle that lodges in a pulmonary artery, effectively blocking blood flow through that vessel. This condition is potentially life threatening because it can significantly decrease pulmonary blood flow, which leads to hypoxemia (inadequate levels of oxygen in the blood). Pulmonary thromboembolism accounts for 5000 deaths annually in Canada. In fact, one in five cases of sudden death are caused by pulmonary emboli. The great majority of patients with pulmonary emboli survive; only 1 in 10 cases of documented pulmonary emboli are fatal.

The incidence of pulmonary emboli is high in certain populations. Any condition that results in immobility of the extremities can increase the risk of thromboembolism. Such conditions include recent surgery, long-bone fractures (with

Content Review

CARBON MONOXIDE INHALATION: MANAGEMENT SEQUENCE

Ensure the safety of rescue personnel.
Remove the patient from the exposure site.
Maintain an open airway.
Provide high-concentration oxygen.

immobilization in casts or splints), bedridden condition, or prolonged immobilization, as with long-distance travel. Venous pooling that occurs during pregnancy can also lead to pulmonary emboli. Certain disease states increase the likelihood of blood clot formation. These include cancer, infections, thrombophlebitis, atrial fibrillation, and sickle cell anemia. Also, the incidence of thromboembolic disease is high in patients taking oral birth control pills, particularly those who are smokers.

Pathophysiology

Sources of pulmonary emboli include air embolism, such as can occur during the placement of a central line; fat embolism, which can occur following a fracture; amniotic fluid embolism; and blood clots. It is also possible for a foreign body (such as part of a venous catheter) to become dislodged in the venous circulation. The vast majority of cases, however, are caused by blood clots that develop in the deep venous system of the lower extremities.

As a rule, a significant amount of blood passes through the veins of the lower extremity. During normal use of our legs, muscular contractions propel the blood through the venous system with the aid of valves that are present in the lower extremity veins. This action prevents blood from flowing backward through the venous system. When there is infection, venous injury, or any other condition that leads to pooling of blood in the deep veins of the lower extremity, clot formation occurs. If a portion of the clot becomes dislodged, it will pass through the right side of the heart and become lodged in the pulmonary vasculature.

When a pulmonary embolism occurs, the blockage of blood flow through the affected artery causes the right heart to pump against increased resistance. This results in an increase in pulmonary capillary pressure. The area of the lung supplied by the occluded pulmonary vessel can no longer effectively function in gas exchange, since it receives no effective blood supply. The major derangement in patients with pulmonary emboli is a perfusion disorder. The involved lung segment is still ventilated, producing a ventilation–perfusion mismatch.

Assessment

Signs and symptoms of a patient suffering a pulmonary embolism will vary, depending on the size and location of the obstruction. The patient suffering acute pulmonary embolism may report a sudden onset of severe unexplained dyspnea, which may or may not be associated with pleuritic chest pain. The patient may also report a cough, which is usually not productive but may occasionally produce blood (hemoptysis). There may be a recent history of immobilization, such as hip fracture, surgery, or debilitating illness.

The secondary assessment may reveal laboured breathing, tachypnea, and tachycardia. In massive pulmonary emboli, there may be signs of right heart failure, such as jugular vein distention and, in some cases, falling blood pressure. In many cases, auscultation of the chest may reveal no significant lung findings, although rare crackles (rales) and wheezing may be noted. Occasionally, a pleural friction rub (leathery sound heard with inspiration) may be heard.

Always examine the extremities. In up to 50 percent of cases, findings suggestive of deep venous thrombosis will be evident. These include a warm, swollen extremity with a thick cord palpated along the medial thigh and pain on palpation or when extending the calf.

In extreme cases, the patient may present with extreme confusion as the result of hypoxia, severe cyanosis, profound hypotension, and even cardiac arrest. Physical examination may reveal petechiae (small hemorrhagic spots) on the arms and chest wall in these cases.

The patient with acute pulmonary embolism may have a sudden onset of severe unexplained dyspnea, with or without pleuritic chest pain.

With suspected pulmonary embolism, always examine the extremities. In up to 50 percent of cases, findings suggestive of deep venous thrombosis will be evident.

Management

With pulmonary embolism, as with all respiratory conditions, your first priorities are maintaining airway, breathing, and circulation. Remember that a large pulmonary embolism may lead to cardiac arrest. Be prepared to perform CPR if needed.

As with all respiratory conditions, your first priorities are the airway, breathing, and circulation. Remember that a large pulmonary embolism may lead to cardiac arrest. Perform cardiopulmonary resusitation (CPR) if needed.

If you suspect a patient is suffering a pulmonary embolism, establish and maintain an airway. Assist ventilations as required. Administer supplemental oxygen at the highest possible concentration. Endotracheal intubation by an ACP or a CCP may be required.

Establish an IV of Ringer's Lactate or normal saline at a "to-keep-open" rate. The diagnosis of pulmonary embolism is often difficult and requires a high index of suspicion. Remember that patients with suspected pulmonary embolism may require a significant amount of care. This disorder has a high complication rate and a significant mortality rate. Carefully monitor the patient's vital signs and cardiac rhythm. Quickly transport the patient to a facility with the capabilities to care for the critical needs of the patient. Treatment in the hospital setting may include the use of various medications, such as thrombolytic agents and blood thinners (e.g., heparin).

Pulmonary embolism has a high complication rate and significant mortality rate. Carefully monitor vital signs and cardiac rhythm. Transport to a facility with the capability of caring for the critical needs of the patient.

Spontaneous Pneumothorax

A **spontaneous pneumothorax** is defined as a pneumothorax that occurs in the absence of blunt or penetrating trauma. Spontaneous pneumothorax is a common clinical condition, with 18 cases occurring for every 100 000 population. There is also a high recurrence rate. Fifty percent of patients will have a recurrent episode within two years.

There is a 5:1 ratio of male to female patients with spontaneous pneumothorax. Other risk factors include tall, thin stature and a history of cigarette smoking. This disorder tends to develop in patients between the ages of 20 and 40 years. Patients with COPD have a higher incidence of spontaneous pneumothorax, presumably because of the presence of thinned lung tissue (blebs) that may rupture.

* **spontaneous pneumothorax** a pneumothorax (collection of air in the pleural space) that occurs spontaneously, in the absence of blunt or penetrating trauma.

Pathophysiology

The primary derangement is one of ventilation as the negative pressure that normally exists in the pleural space is lost. This prevents proper expansion of the lung in concert with the chest wall. A pneumothorax occupying 15–20 percent of the chest cavity is generally well tolerated by the patient unless there is significant underlying lung disease.

Assessment

The patient with a spontaneous pneumothorax will have a sudden onset of pleuritic chest or shoulder pain, often precipitated by coughing or lifting.

The patient with a spontaneous pneumothorax presents with a sudden onset of sharp, pleuritic chest or shoulder pain. Often, the symptoms are precipitated by coughing or lifting. Dyspnea is commonly reported. The degree of symptoms is not strictly related to the size of the pneumothorax.

The secondary assessment is usually not significant. Decreased breath sounds on the involved side may be difficult to note. They may be best heard at the lung apex. Occasionally, the patient may have subcutaneous emphysema, which may be palpated as a crackling under the skin overlying the chest. Tachypnea, diaphoresis, and pallor are also seen. Cyanosis is rarely found.

Management

Use the patient's symptoms and pulse oximetry readings as guides to therapy. For most cases of spontaneous pneumothorax, supplemental oxygen is all that is required. Ventilatory support and endotracheal intubation are rarely required.

Be very careful when managing patients with a spontaneous pneumothorax who require positive pressure ventilation by mask or endotracheal tube. They are at risk for the development of a *tension pneumothorax*. You may note that the patient will become physically difficult to ventilate. Hypoxia, cyanosis, and hypotension may also develop. In addition to the usual signs of a pneumothorax, the patient will develop jugular vein distention and deviation of the trachea away from the pneumothorax. Needle decompression of a tension pneumothorax may be required.

Other management measures should include placing the patient in a position of comfort. Reserve intravenous access and electrocardiographic (ECG) monitoring for patients with significant symptoms or severe underlying respiratory disease. Carefully monitor such patients during transport.

Most cases of spontaneous pneumothorax require only supplemental oxygen.

Be careful when ventilating a patient with suspected spontaneous pneumothorax. Too much pressure may result in a tension pneumothorax.

HYPERVENTILATION SYNDROME

Hyperventilation syndrome is characterized by rapid breathing, chest pains, numbness, and other symptoms usually associated with anxiety or a situational reaction. However, as shown in Table 27-3, many serious medical problems can cause hyperventilation. To avoid improper treatment, consider hyperventilation to be indicative of a serious medical problem until proven otherwise.

Consider hyperventilation indicative of a serious medical problem until proven otherwise.

Pathophysiology

Hyperventilation syndrome frequently occurs in anxious patients. The patient often senses that she cannot "catch her breath." The patient will then begin to breathe rapidly. Hyperventilation in a purely anxious patient results in the excess elimination of CO_2, causing a respiratory alkalosis. This increases the amount of bound calcium, producing a relative hypocalcemia. This results in cramping of the muscles of the feet and hands, which is called *carpopedal spasm*.

Table 27-3	CAUSES OF HYPERVENTILATION SYNDROME
Acidosis	Interstitial pneumonitis, fibrosis, edema
Beta-adrenergic agonists	Metabolic disorders
Bronchial asthma	Methyxanthine derivatives
Cardiovascular disorders	Neurological disorders
Central nervous system infection or tumours	Pain
Congestive heart failure	Pregnancy
Drugs	Pneumonia
Fever, sepsis	Progesterone
Hepatic failure	Psychogenic or anxiety hypertension
High altitude	Pulmonary disease
Hypotension	Pulmonary emboli, vascular disease
Hypoxia	Salicylate

Assessment

With a hyperventilating patient, you may elicit a history of fatigue, nervousness, dizziness, dyspnea, chest pain, and numbness and tingling around the mouth, hands, and feet. The secondary assessment will reveal an anxious patient with tachypnea and tachycardia. As noted above, spasm of the fingers and feet may also be present. If the patient has a history of seizure disorder, the hyperventilation episode may precipitate a seizure. Other symptoms are related to the underlying cause of the hyperventilation syndrome.

Management

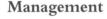

The primary treatment for hyperventilation is reassurance. Instruct the patient to reduce her respiratory rate and depth.

The primary treatment for hyperventilation syndrome is reassurance. Instruct the patient to voluntarily reduce her respiratory rate and depth of breathing. Mechanisms that will assist in increasing the PCO_2, such as breath holding or breathing into a paper bag, are discouraged in prehospital care. Hyperventilating patients require oxygen. Allowing them to rebreathe into a paper bag can be deadly. Many EMS systems permit paramedics to use rebreathing techniques only on physician orders. It is important to exclude other medical causes before determining that a patient is hyperventilating. Check the oxygen saturation by applying a pulse oximeter. Do not withhold oxygen.

The hyperventilating patient can often present a dilemma for prehospital care personnel. Although anxiety is the most common cause of hyperventilation, other more serious diseases can present in exactly the same manner. For example, pulmonary embolism or acute myocardial infarction can exhibit symptoms similar to hyperventilation syndrome.

CENTRAL NERVOUS SYSTEM DYSFUNCTION

Except in the case of drug overdose or massive stroke, central nervous system dysfunction is rarely the cause of respiratory emergencies.

Central nervous system (CNS) dysfunction, with the exception of drug overdose and massive stroke, is a relatively rare cause of respiratory emergencies. However, always consider the possibility of CNS dysfunction in any dyspneic patient.

Pathophysiology

CNS dysfunction can be a causative factor in respiratory depression and arrest. Causes include head trauma, stroke, brain tumours, and various drugs. Several medications, such as narcotics and barbiturates, make the respiratory centres in the brain less responsive to increases in $PaCO_2$. These agents also depress areas of the brain responsible for initiating respirations.

Assessment

With suspected central nervous system dysfunction, establish and maintain an open airway. If respiratory depression is noted or respirations are absent, initiate mechanical ventilation with supplemental oxygen and establish an IV of normal saline at a "to-keep-open" rate.

The assessment of patients with CNS dysfunction should follow the same approach as for any respiratory emergency. However, you should be alert for non-respiratory system problems, such as CNS trauma or drug ingestion. Be careful to note any variation in the respiratory pattern, which can be an indication of CNS dysfunction.

Management

If CNS dysfunction is suspected, establish and maintain an open airway. If respiratory depression is noted or if respirations are absent, initiate mechanical ventilation. Administer supplemental oxygen, and establish an IV of normal saline at a "to keep open" rate. Direct the specific therapy at the underlying problem if it is known.

DYSFUNCTION OF THE SPINAL CORD, NERVES, OR RESPIRATORY MUSCLES

Several disease processes can affect the spinal cord, nerves, and/or respiratory muscles. Dysfunction of these structures can lead to hypoventilation and progressive hypoxemia.

Pathophysiology

Numerous disorders can interfere with respiratory function. These include spinal cord trauma, poliomyelitis, amyotrophic lateral sclerosis (ALS or Lou Gehrig's disease), and myasthenia gravis. Viral infections, in certain cases, can cause dysfunction of the nervous system. An example of this is *Guillian-Barré Syndrome (GBS)*. In GBS, the myelin-covering of the nerve is damaged, resulting in relative loss of nerve impulse conduction. This affects virtually every peripheral nerve. Approximately 30 percent of patients with GBS will require ventilatory assistance, as the nerves that stimulate respiration are impaired.

Certain tumours can impinge on the spinal cord, depressing respiratory function. These disorders result in an inability of the respiratory muscles to contract normally, thus causing hypoventilation. Tidal volume and minute volume are decreased. You should also be aware that patients with these disorders do not have the ability to generate an adequate cough reflex and, as a result, are at risk of developing pneumonia.

Disorders that affect the spinal cord, nerves, or respiratory muscles and can interfere with respiratory function include spinal cord trauma, polio, ALS, myasthenia gravis, and tumours that impinge on the spinal cord.

Assessment

Patients with possible dysfunction of the spinal cord, nerves, or respiratory muscles may have a history of trauma that is not readily apparent. Always question the patient about injuries or falls. If there is any doubt about a possible injury, act accordingly, and immobilize the cervical spine. Also, inquire about signs or symptoms that may suggest a problem with the peripheral nerves. These include such findings as numbness, pain, or sensory dysfunction. The assessment of patients with possible dysfunction of the spinal cord, nerves, or respiratory muscles should follow the same approach as for any respiratory emergency. However, be alert for subtle findings that may indicate a problem with the peripheral nervous system. Always be ready to protect the airway and support ventilation if the patient has symptoms of possible airway obstruction or respiratory failure.

Management

Management of spinal cord and respiratory muscle dysfunction is purely supportive. Establish an airway, and provide ventilatory support. If myasthenia gravis is present and if transport time is long, the physician may request the administration of one of several agents effective in treating such patients.

Management of spinal cord and respiratory muscle dysfunction is purely supportive.

Part 2: Airway Management and Ventilation

Airway management and ventilation are the first and most critical steps in the primary assessment of every patient you will encounter. You must immediately establish and maintain an open airway while providing adequate oxygen delivery and carbon dioxide elimination for all patients. Without adequate airway maintenance and ventilation, the patient will succumb to brain injury or even death in as little as six to ten minutes. Early detection and intervention of airway and breathing problems, including bystander action, are vital to patient survival.

Your deliberate and precise use of simple, basic airway skills is the key to successful airway management and good patient outcome. Once you have applied the basic airway techniques to properly provide oxygenation and ventilation for your patient, you can use more sophisticated airway manoeuvres and skills to further stabilize her airway. You must continually monitor and reassess the airway, being careful to watch for displacement of the endotracheal tube, mucus plugging, equipment failure, or the development of a pneumothorax.

This part will provide the information and skills you will need to manage even the most difficult airway. It begins with a review of respiratory problems and then explores the primary assessment and management of the airway and ventilation in more detail. Finally, it details enhanced airway management options for the more experienced paramedic.

RESPIRATORY PROBLEMS

Respiratory emergencies can pose an immediate life threat to the patient. You must calmly and quickly assess the severity of the patient's illness or injury while considering the potential causes of and treatment for her respiratory distress. Often, the patient will give you little help, either because of anxiety or difficulty speaking. Her respiratory difficulty may be due to airway obstruction, injury to upper or lower airway structures, inadequate ventilation caused by worsening of an underlying lung disease and fatigue, or central nervous system (CNS) problems that threaten the airway or respiratory effort.

AIRWAY OBSTRUCTION

✱ **upper airway obstruction** an interference with air movement through the upper airway.

> **Content Review**
>
> ### CAUSES OF AIRWAY OBSTRUCTION
> - Tongue
> - Foreign bodies
> - Trauma
> - Laryngeal spasm and edema
> - Aspiration

Blockage of the airway is an immediate threat to the patient's life and a true emergency. **Upper airway obstruction** may be defined as an interference with air movement through the upper airway. The tongue, foreign bodies, vomitus, blood, or teeth can all obstruct the upper airway.

Airway obstruction may be either partial or complete. Partial obstruction allows either adequate or poor air exchange. Patients with adequate air exchange can cough effectively; those with poor air exchange cannot. They often emit a high-pitched noise while inhaling (stridor), and their skin may have a bluish appearance (cyanosis). They also may have increased breathing difficulty, which can manifest as choking, gagging dyspnea, or difficulty speaking (dysphonia). When you cannot feel or hear airflow from the nose and mouth, or when the patient cannot speak (aphonia), breathe, or cough, the airway is completely obstructed. The patient will quickly become unconscious and die if you do not relieve the obstruction. In the absence of breathing, difficulty ventilating the patient will indicate complete airway obstruction.

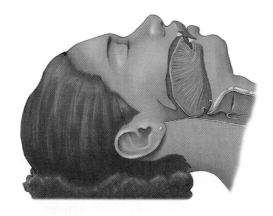

FIGURE 27-12　The tongue as airway obstruction.

The Tongue The tongue is the most common cause of airway obstruction (Figure 27-12). Normally, the submandibular muscles directly support the tongue and indirectly support the epiglottis. Without sufficient muscle tone, though, the relaxed tongue falls back against the posterior pharynx, thus occluding the airway. This may produce snoring respiratory noises. At the same time, the epiglottis also may block the airway at the larynx. This at least diminishes airflow into the respiratory system, and the patient's breathing efforts may inadvertently suck the base of her tongue into an obstructing position. The patient's tongue can block the airway whether she is in the lateral, supine, or prone position; however, the blockage depends on the position of the patient's head and jaw, and so simple airway manoeuvres, such as the jaw-thrust, can usually open her airway.

Foreign Bodies Large, poorly chewed pieces of food can obstruct the upper airway by getting lodged in the hypopharynx. These cases often involve alcohol consumption and denture dislodgement. Because they frequently occur in restaurants and are mistaken for heart attacks, they are commonly called "café coronaries." The patient may clutch her neck between the thumb and fingers, a universal distress signal. Children, especially toddlers, often aspirate foreign objects, as they have the tendency to put objects into their mouths.

Trauma In trauma, particularly when the patient is unresponsive, loose teeth, facial bone fractures, and avulsed or swollen tissue may obstruct the airway. Secretions, such as blood, saliva, and vomitus, may compromise the airway and risk aspiration. Additionally, penetrating or blunt trauma may obstruct the airway by fracturing or displacing the larynx, allowing the vocal cords to collapse into the tracheal lumen.

Laryngeal Spasm and Edema Since the glottis is the narrowest part of an adult's airway, edema (swelling) or spasm (spasmotic closure) of the vocal cords is potentially lethal. Even moderate edema can severely obstruct airflow and cause asphyxia (the inability to move air into and out of the respiratory system). Just beneath the mucous membrane that covers the vocal cords is a layer of loose tissue where blood or other fluids can accumulate. This tissue may swell following injury, and the swelling will be slow to subside. Causes of laryngeal spasm and edema include trauma, anaphylaxis, epiglottitis, and inhalation of superheated air, smoke, or toxic substances. The most common cause of spasm is overly aggressive intubation. Spasm often occurs, too, immediately on **extubation,** especially when the patient is semiconscious. Some authors propose that laryngeal spasm can sometimes be partially overcome by strengthening ventilatory effort, forceful upward pull of the jaw, or the use of muscle relaxants, although the success of these manoeuvres is quite variable.

The tongue is the most common airway obstruction.

Since the glottis is the narrowest part of an adult's airway, edema or spasm of the vocal cords is potentially lethal.

✱ extubation removing a tube from a body opening.

Aspiration Vomitus is the most commonly aspirated material. Patients most at risk for this are those who are so obtunded (drowsy) that they cannot adequately protect their airways. This can occur with hypoxia, CNS toxins, or brain injury, among other causes. In addition to obstructing the airway, aspiration's other effects also significantly increase patient mortality. Vomitus consists of food particles, protein-dissolving enzymes, hydrochloric acid, and gastrointestinal bacteria that have been regurgitated from the stomach into the hypopharynx and oropharynx. If this mixture enters the lungs, it can result in increased interstitial fluid and pulmonary edema. The consequent marked increase in alveolar–capillary distance seriously impairs gas exchange, thus causing hypoxemia and hypercarbia. Aspirated materials can also severely damage the delicate bronchiolar tissue and alveoli. Gastrointestinal bacteria can produce overwhelming infections. These complications occur in 50–80 percent of patients who aspirate foreign matter.

INADEQUATE VENTILATION

Insufficient minute volume respirations can compromise adequate oxygen intake and carbon dioxide removal. Additionally, oxygenation may be insufficient when conditions increase metabolic oxygen demand or decrease available oxygen. A reduction of either the rate or the volume of inhalation leads to a reduction in minute volume. In some cases, the respiratory rate may be rapid but so shallow that little air exchange takes place. Among the causes of such decreased ventilation are depressed respiratory function (as from impairment of respiratory muscles or nervous systems), bronchospasm from intrinsic disease, fractured ribs, pneumothorax, hemothorax, drug overdose, renal failure, spinal or brainstem injury, or head injury. In some conditions, such as sepsis, the body's metabolic demand for oxygen can exceed the patient's ability to supply it. Additionally, the environment may contain a decreased amount of oxygen, as in high-altitude conditions or a house fire, which also produces toxic gases, such as cyanide and carbon monoxide. These situations of inadequate ventilation can lead to hypercarbia and hypoxia.

RESPIRATORY SYSTEM ASSESSMENT

Vigilance is the key to airway management in every patient.

Vigilance is the key to airway management in every patient. The trauma patient whose airway and breathing initially looked fine on assessment may become symptomatic with the pneumothorax that was not initially evident. The asthma patient who initially responded to nebulizer treatment may have a sudden bronchospasm and worsen acutely. Minute-by-minute reassessment of the adequacy of every patient's airway and breathing is essential. The changes may be subtle increases in rate, worsening or onset of irregularity, or increased difficulty speaking.

PRIMARY ASSESSMENT

✳ **ABCs** airway, breathing, and circulation.

The primary assessment's purpose is to identify any immediate threats to the patient's life, specifically **a**irway, **b**reathing, and **c**irculation problems (**ABCs**). First, assess the airway to ensure that it is patent. Snoring or gurgling may indicate potential airway problems. Next, determine the adequacy of breathing. If the patient is comfortable, with a normal respiratory rate, alert, and speaking without difficulty, you may generally assume that breathing is adequate.

Patients with altered mental status warrant further evaluation. Feel for air movement with your hand or cheek. Look for the chest to rise and fall normally with each respiratory cycle. Listen for air movement and equal bilateral breath sounds. The absence of breath sounds on one side may indicate a pneumothorax or hemothorax in the trauma patient. In an adult patient, the respiratory rate generally ranges between 12 and 20 breaths per minute. Breathing should be spontaneous, effortless, and regular. Irregular breathing suggests a significant problem and usually requires ventilatory support. Observe the chest wall for any asymmetrical movement. This condition, known as **paradoxical breathing,** may suggest a flail chest. Patients who show increased respiratory effort, insisting on upright, sniffing, or semi-Fowler's positioning, or those refusing to lie supine, should be considered to be in significant respiratory distress.

If the patient is not breathing, or if you suspect airway problems, open the airway using the head-tilt/chin-lift or jaw-thrust manoeuvre, as described later in this chapter. If trauma is possible, use the jaw-thrust manoeuvre while stabilizing the cervical spine in neutral position. Once the airway is open, reevaluate the breathing status. If breathing is adequate, provide supplemental oxygen, and assess circulation. Consider the use of airway adjuncts, as discussed later. If breathing is inadequate or absent, begin artificial ventilation (Figure 27-13). When assisting a patient's breathing with a ventilatory device (bag-valve mask or other positive-pressure device), or after placing an airway adjunct, (nasopharyngeal airway or oropharyngeal airway), or endotracheally intubating, monitor the chest's rise and fall to determine correct usage and placement. (We will discuss these ventilatory devices and mechanical airways in detail later in this part.)

✱ paradoxical breathing assymetrical chest wall movement that lessens respiratory efficiency.

FOCUSED HISTORY AND SECONDARY ASSESSMENT

As discussed in Part 1, after you complete the primary assessment and correct any immediate life threats, conduct a focused history and secondary assessment while continuously monitoring the patient's ABCs.

Focused History

The time when the patient and her family noted the onset of symptoms is important information, as is whether the acute event occurred suddenly or gradually. Identifying possible triggers, such as allergens or heat, also can help the patient avoid them in the future. Additionally, the symptoms' course of development since onset will help direct diagnosis and treatment. Have the symptoms been progressively worsening, recurrent, or continuous? Associated symptoms will further help assess the cause of the patient's problem. Has she had fever or chills, productive cough, chest pain, nausea or vomiting, or diaphoresis? Does the patient think her voice sounds normal?

The patient's past medical history will put her present complaints into perspective and help identify the risk factors for a variety of likely diagnoses.

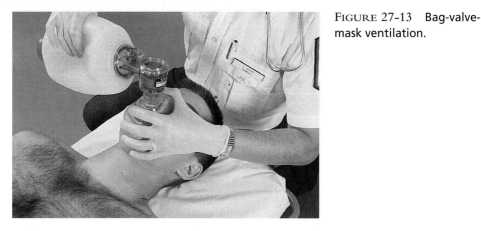

FIGURE 27-13   Bag-valve-mask ventilation.

Determine whether the present episode is similar to any past episodes of shortness of breath, what medical evaluations have been done, and what they have revealed. Has the patient ever been admitted to the hospital for her complaints? Has she ever been intubated?

The recent history leading to the onset of symptoms is also important. Did the patient run out of medication? Has she been noncompliant with (not taken) medications? Did she drink too much fluid or alcohol? Seize or vomit? Eat something that might induce an allergy? Receive any trauma? If an injury is involved, evaluate the mechanism of injury. Keep in mind that blunt trauma to the neck may have injured the larynx. Anything that makes the patient's condition better (ameliorates) or worse (exacerbates, aggravates) is also significant.

Secondary Assessment

Your secondary assessment of a patient with respiratory problems should continue the evaluation of her ABCs begun during your primary assessment. Now you will use the secondary assessment techniques of inspection, auscultation, and palpation to evaluate the patient's injury or illness in more detail and determine your plan of action. (Chapter 6 explains these techniques in detail.)

Inspection Begin the secondary assessment by inspecting the patient. Evaluate the adequacy of her breathing. Note any obvious signs of trauma. Always remember to assess the skin colour as an indicator of oxygenation status. Early in respiratory compromise, the sympathetic nervous system will be stimulated to help offset the lack of oxygen. When this happens, the skin will often appear pale and diaphoretic. Cyanosis (bluish discoloration) is another sign of respiratory distress. When oxygen binds with the hemoglobin, the blood appears bright red. Deoxygenated hemoglobin, conversely, is blue and gives the skin a bluish tint. This is not a reliable indicator, however, since severe tissue hypoxia is possible without cyanosis. In fact, cyanosis is considered a late sign of respiratory compromise. When it does appear, it usually affects the lips, fingernails, and skin. A red skin rash, especially if accompanied by hives, may indicate an allergic reaction. A cherry-red skin discoloration may, on rare occasions, be associated with carbon monoxide poisoning, as can bullae (large blisters).

Observe the patient's position. Tripod positioning (seated, leaning forward, with one arm forward to stabilize the body) may indicate COPD or asthma exacerbation; orthopnea (increased difficulty breathing while lying down) may indicate congestive heart failure or asthma.

Next, inspecting for dyspnea—an abnormality of breathing rate, pattern, or effort—is essential. Dyspnea may cause or be caused by hypoxia. Prolonged dyspnea without successful intervention can lead to **anoxia** (the absence or near-absence of oxygen), which, without intervention, is a premorbid (occurring just before death) event, as the brain can survive only four to six minutes in this state. Remember that all interventions are useless if you do not establish a patent airway.

Also, observe for the following modified forms of respiration:

* *Coughing*—forceful exhalation of a large volume of air from the lungs. This performs a protective function in expelling foreign material from the lungs.
* *Sneezing*—sudden, forceful exhalation from the nose. It is usually caused by nasal irritation.
* *Hiccoughing* (hiccups)—sudden inspiration caused by spasmodic contraction of the diaphragm with spastic closure of the glottis. It

✱ **anoxia** the absence or near-absence of oxygen.

serves no known physiological purpose. It has, occasionally, been associated with acute myocardial infarctions on the inferior (diaphragmatic) surface of the heart.

- *Sighing*—slow, deep, involuntary inspiration followed by a prolonged expiration. It hyperinflates the lungs and reexpands atelectatic alveoli. This normally occurs about once a minute.
- *Grunting*—a forceful expiration that occurs against a partially closed epiglottis. It is usually an indication of respiratory distress.

Note any decrease or increase in the respiratory rate, one of the earliest indicators of respiratory distress. Also, look for use of the accessory respiratory muscles—intercostal, suprasternal, supraclavicular, and subcostal retractions—and the abdominal muscles to assist breathing. This indicates increased respiratory effort secondary to respiratory distress. In infants and children, nasal flaring and grunting indicate respiratory distress. COPD patients having difficulty breathing will purse their lips during exhalation. Monitor the patient's blood pressure, including any differences noted during expiration and inspiration. Patients with severe chronic obstructive pulmonary disease may sustain a drop in blood pressure during inspiration. This drop is due to increased pressure within the thoracic cavity that impairs the ability of the ventricles to fill. Thus, decreased ventricular filling leads to decreased blood pressure. A drop in blood pressure of greater than 10 mmHg is termed **pulsus paradoxus** and may be indicative of severe obstructive lung disease.

✱ **pulsus paradoxus** drop in blood pressure of greater than 10 mmHg during inspiration.

Determine if the pattern of respirations is abnormal—deep or shallow in combination with a fast or slow rate. Keep in mind some of the common abnormal respiratory patterns discussed in Part 1:

- *Kussmaul's respirations*—deep, slow or rapid, gasping breathing, commonly found in diabetic ketoacidosis
- *Cheyne-Stokes respirations*—progressively deeper, faster breathing alternating gradually with shallow, slower breathing, indicating brainstem injury
- *Biot's respirations*—irregular pattern of rate and depth with sudden, periodic episodes of apnea, indicating increased intracranial pressure
- *Central neurogenic hyperventilation*—deep, rapid respirations, indicating increased intracranial pressure
- *Agonal respirations*—shallow, slow, or infrequent breathing, indicating brain anoxia

Finally, observing altered mentation may be key in determining if breathing is adequate or if significant hypoxia may be present. If the patient's mental status is not normal, you must determine her usual baseline mental status before you can make this assessment.

Auscultation Following inspection, listen at the mouth and nose for adequate air movement. Then, listen to the chest with a stethoscope (auscultate) (Figure 27-14). In a prehospital setting, you should auscultate the right and left apices (just beneath the clavicle), the right and left bases (eighth or ninth intercostal space, midclavicular line), and the right and left areas of the lower thoracic back or right and left midaxillary line (fourth or fifth intercostal space, on the lateral aspect of the chest). If the patient's condition permits, you can monitor six locations on the posterior chest—three right and three left. The posterior surface is preferable because heart sounds do not interfere with auscultation at this location.

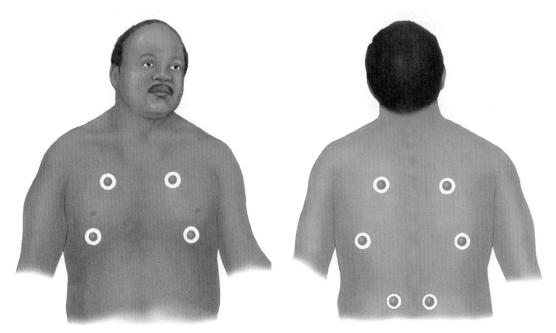

FIGURE 27-14   Positions for auscultating breath sounds.

However, since patients are usually supine during airway management, the anterior and lateral positions usually prove more accessible. Breath sounds should be equal bilaterally. Sounds that point to airflow compromise include the following:

- *Snoring*—results from partial obstruction of the upper airway by the tongue
- *Gurgling*—results from the accumulation of blood, vomitus, or other secretions in the upper airway
- *Stridor*—a harsh, high-pitched sound heard on inhalation, associated with laryngeal edema or constriction
- *Wheezing*—a musical, squeaking, or whistling sound heard on inspiration and/or expiration, associated with bronchiolar constriction
- *Quiet*—diminished or absent breath sounds are an ominous finding and indicate a serious problem with the airway, breathing, or both

Beware of the quiet chest!

Sounds that may indicate compromise of gas exchange include the following:

- *Crackles* (rales)—a fine, bubbling sound heard on inspiration, associated with fluid in the smaller bronchioles
- *Rhonchi*—a coarse, rattling noise heard on inspiration, associated with inflammation, mucus, or fluid in the bronchioles

When you assess the effectiveness of ventilatory support or the correct placement of an airway adjunct, remember that air movement into the epigastrium may sometimes mimic breath sounds. Thus, listening to the chest should be only one of several means that you use to assess air movement. Another method of checking correct placement of an airway adjunct is to auscultate over the epigastrium; it should be silent during ventilation. When you provide ventilatory support, watch for signs of gastric distention. They suggest inadequate hyperextension of the neck, undue pressure generated by the ventilatory device, or improper placement of airway adjuncts.

Palpation Finally, palpate. First, using the back of your hand or your cheek, feel for air movement at the mouth and nose. (If an endotracheal tube is in place, you can check for air movement at the tube's adapter.) Next, palpate the chest for rise and fall. In addition, palpate the chest wall for tenderness, symmetry, abnormal motion, crepitus, and subcutaneous emphysema.

When ventilating with a bag-valve device, gauge airflow into the lungs by noting compliance. **Compliance** refers to the stiffness or flexibility of the lung tissue, and it is indicated by how easily air flows into the lungs. When compliance is good, airflow meets minimal resistance. When compliance is poor, ventilation is harder to achieve. Compliance is often poor in diseased lungs and in patients suffering from chest wall injuries or tension pneumothorax. If a patient shows poor compliance during ventilatory support, look for potential causes. Upper airway obstructions, which cause difficulty with mechanical ventilation, can mimic poor compliance. If ventilating the patient is initially easy but then becomes progressively more difficult, repeat the initial assessment and look for the development of a new problem, possibly related to the mechanical airway manoeuvres. The following questions will aid this assessment:

* * **compliance** the stiffness or flexibility of the lung tissue.

* Is the airway open?
* Is the head properly positioned in extension (nontrauma patients)?
* Is the patient developing tension pneumothorax?
* Is the endotracheal tube occluded (a mucous plug or aspirated material)?
* Has the endotracheal tube been inadvertently pushed into the right or left mainstem bronchus?
* Has the endotracheal tube been displaced into the esophagus?
* Is the mechanical ventilatory equipment functioning properly?

Pulse rate abnormalities may also suggest respiratory compromise. Tachycardia (an abnormally fast pulse) usually accompanies hypoxemia in an adult, while bradycardia (an abnormally slow pulse) hints at anoxia with imminent cardiac arrest.

A fall in the pulse rate in a patient with airway compromise is an ominous finding.

Noninvasive Respiratory Monitoring

Several available devices will help you measure the effectiveness of oxygenation and ventilation. Those measurements used most commonly in prehospital care are pulse oximetry, capnography (both discussed briefly in Part 1 and in greater detail here), and esophageal detection devices. As already described, peak expiratory flow testing can also be useful in the prehospital setting for some respiratory diseases.

Pulse Oximetry Pulse oximetry is widely used in prehospital emergency care. A pulse oximeter measures hemoglobin oxygen saturation in peripheral tissues (Figure 27-15). It is noninvasive (does not require entering the body), rapidly applied, and easy to operate. Pulse oximetry readings are accurate and continually reflect any changes in peripheral oxygen delivery. In fact, oximetry often detects problems with oxygenation faster than do assessments of blood pressure, pulse, and respirations.

To determine peripheral oxygen saturation, you place a sensor probe over a peripheral capillary bed, such as a fingertip, toe, or earlobe. In infants, you can wrap the sensor around the heel and secure it with tape. The sensor contains two light-emitting diodes and two sensors. One diode emits near-red light, a wavelength specific for oxygenated hemoglobin; the other emits infrared light,

* **pulse oximetry** a measurement of hemoglobin oxygen saturation in the peripheral tissues.

FIGURE 27-15 Pulse oximeter.

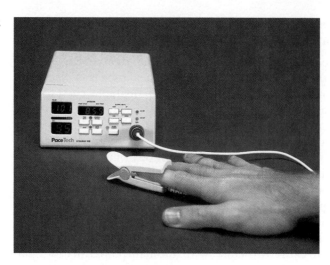

a wavelength specific for deoxygenated hemoglobin. Each hemoglobin state absorbs a certain amount of the emitted light, preventing it from reaching the corresponding sensor. Less light reaching the sensor means more of its type of hemoglobin is in the blood. The oximeter then calculates the ratio of the near-red and infrared light it has received to determine the *oxygen saturation percentage* (SaO_2).

Pulse oximeters display the SaO_2 and the pulse rate as detected by the sensors. They show the SaO_2 either as a number or as a visual display that also shows the pulse's waveform. The relationship between SaO_2 and the partial pressure of oxygen in the blood (PaO_2) is very complex. However, the SaO_2 does correlate with the PaO_2. The greater the PaO_2, the greater will be the oxygen saturation. Since hemoglobin carries 98 percent of oxygen in the blood while plasma carries only 2 percent, pulse oximetry accurately analyzes peripheral oxygen delivery.

Pulse oximetry is often called the "fifth vital sign." When available, you should use it in virtually any situation to determine the patient's baseline value, to guide patient care, and to monitor the patient's responses to your interventions. As a guide, normal SaO_2 varies between 95 and 99 percent. Readings between 91 and 94 percent indicate mild hypoxia and warrant further evaluation and supplemental oxygen administration. Readings between 86 and 91 percent indicate moderate hypoxia. You should generally give these patients 100-percent supplemental oxygen, exercising caution in those with COPD. Readings of 85 percent or lower indicate severe hypoxia and warrant immediate intervention, including the administration of 100-percent oxygen, ventilatory assistance, or both. Your goal is to maintain the SaO_2 in the normal (95–99 percent) range.

False readings with pulse oximetry are infrequent. When they do occur, the oximeter often generates an error signal or a blank screen. Causes of false readings include carbon monoxide poisoning, high-intensity lighting, and certain hemoglobin abnormalities. The absence of a pulse in an extremity also will cause a false reading. In hypovolemia and in severely anemic patients, the pulse oximetry reading may be misleading. While the SaO_2 reading may be normal, the total amount of hemoglobin available to carry oxygen may be so markedly decreased that the patient will remain hypoxic at the cellular level.

Pulse oximetry provides key information about the patient and is an important part of emergency care, including prehospital care. However, it is only one more assessment tool and does not replace other physical assessment or monitoring skills. Do not depend solely on pulse oximetry readings to guide care. Always consider and treat the whole patient.

Capnography Capnography is the measurement of exhaled carbon dioxide concentrations. The devices that make such measurements are called end-tidal carbon dioxide ($ETCO_2$) detectors. Their use in prehospital care is increasing, most commonly to assess proper placement of an endotracheal tube. The absence of CO_2 from the exhaled air strongly indicates that the tube is in the esophagus; its presence indicates proper tracheal placement.

End-tidal CO_2 detectors are available either as disposable colorimetric devices or as electronic monitors (Figures 27-16 and 27-17). They are attached either in-line or alongside the endotracheal tube and the ventilation device. A colour change in the colorimetric device or a light on the electronic monitor confirms proper tube placement. On the colorimetric device, the low CO_2 content of inspired air makes the device purple, while the higher CO_2 content of expired air makes it yellow. Some electronic devices now combine pulse oximetry, $ETCO_2$ detection, blood pressure, pulse rate, respiratory rate, and temperature monitors in one unit (Figure 27-18).

Although the $ETCO_2$ detector is accurate, the $ETCO_2$ level falls precipitously during cardiac arrest. Therefore, these patients may not cause a colour change on the $ETCO_2$ detector despite proper placement of the endotracheal tube.

✱ **capnography** the measurement of exhaled carbon dioxide concentrations.

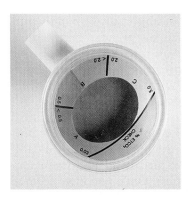

FIGURE 27-16 Colorimetric end-tidal CO_2 detector.

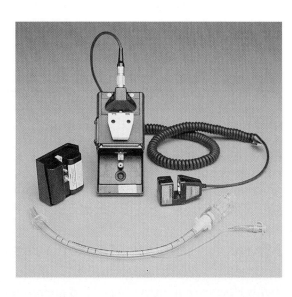

FIGURE 27-17 Electronic end-tidal CO_2 detector.

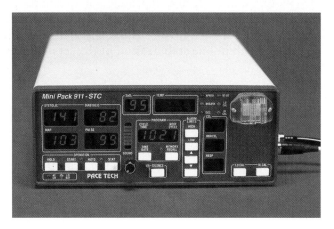

FIGURE 27-18 Combined devices check pulse oximetry, $ETCO_2$, blood pressure, pulse, respiratory rate, and temperature.

As with pulse oximetry, you should use an $ETCO_2$ detector only in conjunction with other methods of assessing endotracheal placement. It does not replace actually visualizing the endotracheal tube's passage through the vocal cords.

Esophageal Detector Device The esophageal detector device (EDD) is a simple and inexpensive tool to help determine whether an endotracheal tube is in the trachea or the esophagus. It uses the anatomical principle that the trachea is a rigid tube and will not collapse with negative pressure, while the esophagus is a collapsible tube that flattens with negative pressure and does not allow air to enter the syringe. The EDD may be either a rigid syringe or a bulb syringe (Figure 27-19). Once you have intubated the patient, you should attach the EDD to the proximal end of the endotracheal tube (ETT). Then, you should quickly pull back the syringe, aspirating air from the endotracheal tube. Easily withdrawn air confirms ETT placement in the trachea. If air is difficult or impossible to withdraw, the ETT is in the esophagus.

Peak Expiratory Flow Testing Peak expiratory flow testing (described more fully in Part 1) utilizes a disposable plastic chamber into which the patient exhales forcefully after maximal inhalation. It can be used as a crude measure of respiratory efficacy. Improving measurements can indicate good response to treatment.

BASIC AIRWAY MANAGEMENT

Deciding if a patient has a patent airway is the most important step in the primary assessment. Airway management is one of the few prehospital interventions that is known to improve patient survival rates. Once you have determined that intervention is needed, you must use simple manual airway manoeuvres and equipment before proceeding with more advanced techniques, such as endotracheal intubation or placement of a CombiTube. Always provide supplemental oxygen to all patients for whom it is indicated; never withhold it, even from the COPD patient. Be sure to always wear protective eyewear and gloves to avoid contact with the patient's body fluids. If you suspect cervical spine injury, perform modified airway techniques in conjunction with appropriate cervical spine stabilization. Once you have secured the airway, frequently reassess for an adequate airway and ventilation.

MANUAL AIRWAY MANOEUVRES

Manual manoeuvres are the simplest airway management techniques and are highly effective but often neglected in prehospital care. The head-tilt/chin-lift and the jaw-thrust are safe and dependable manoeuvres for relieving obstruction by the tongue. Perform one of these techniques on all unconscious patients but not on responsive patients. If you suspect cervical spine injury, perform the modified jaw-thrust with in-line stabilization of the cervical spine.

Head-Tilt/Chin-Lift

In the absence of cervical spinal trauma, the head-tilt/chin-lift is the best technique for opening the airway in an unresponsive patient who is not protecting her own airway.

In the absence of cervical spine trauma, the head-tilt/chin-lift is the best technique for opening the airway in an unresponsive patient who is not protecting her own airway. The head-tilt is hazardous to patients with cervical spine injuries; do not use it for those patients. To perform the head-tilt/chin-lift follow these steps:

1. Place the patient supine, and position yourself at the side of the patient's head.

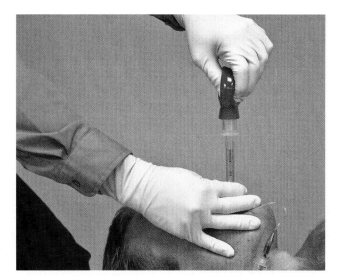

a.

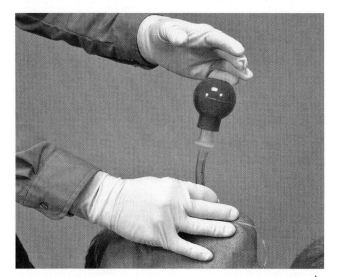

b.

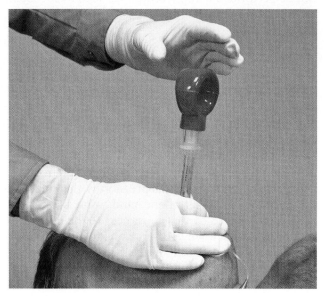

c.

FIGURE 27-19 An esophageal intubation detector—bulb style. **a.** Squeeze the device, and then attach it to the endotracheal tube. **b.** If the bulb refills easily on release, it indicates correct placement. **c.** If the bulb does not refill, the tube is improperly placed.

2. Place one hand on the patient's forehead, and using firm downward pressure with your palm, tilt the head back.
3. Put two fingers of the other hand under the bony part of the chin, and lift the jaw anteriorly to open the airway.

Caution: Avoid compressing the soft tissues of the neck and chin.

Jaw–Thrust Manoeuvre

A jaw-thrust is also acceptable for an unresponsive patient who isn't at risk of cervical spine injury and who cannot protect her airway.

1. Place the patient supine, and kneel behind her head.
2. Apply fingers on each side of the jaw at the mandibular angles.
3. Lift the jaw forward (anterior) with a gentle tilting of the patient's head to open the airway.

For trauma patients, maintain the cervical spine in neutral position, and use either the jaw-thrust without head-tilt or the modified jaw-thrust. You can perform both of these manoeuvres with a cervical collar in place:

1. Jaw-thrust without head-tilt: lift the jaw by grasping under the chin and behind the teeth, without tilting the head. Use extreme caution with this technique, as even unresponsive patients can clench their teeth shut; do not use this method if the patient's mouth resists opening.
2. Modified jaw-thrust: lift the jaw using fingers behind the mandibular angles; do not tilt the head. Use this method if the patient's mouth resists opening.

Although they are simple and effective, none of these manual airway manoeuvres protects the airway from aspiration. Additionally, the jaw-thrust and modified jaw-thrust are difficult to maintain for an extended time. The jaw-thrust is impossible to maintain if the patient becomes responsive or combative. Using them in conjunction with a bag-valve mask is often difficult and typically requires a second rescuer. Ventilation while maintaining a modified jaw thrust can be performed using a ventilator, such as the Genesis II in automatic mode.

Sellick's Manoeuvre

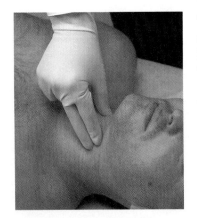

FIGURE 27-20 Sellick's manoeuvre (cricoid pressure).

To help prevent regurgitation and reduce gastric distention, Sellick's manoeuvre applies gentle pressure posteriorly on the anterior cricoid cartilage (Figures 27-20, 27-21a, and 27-21b). Since the esophagus lies just behind the cricoid cartilage, this manoeuvre will effectively close the esophagus to pressures as high as 100 cm/H_2O. It also facilitates intubation by moving the larynx to a posterior position, bringing it into view.

To locate the cricoid cartilage, palpate the thyroid cartilage (Adam's apple), position and feel the depression just below it (cricothyroid membrane). The prominence just inferior to this depression is the ring of cricoid cartilage. Using the thumb and index finger of one hand, apply pressure to the anterior and lateral aspects of the cricoid cartilage just next to the midline. In infants, use one fingertip, and apply gentle downward pressure, taking care to avoid excessive pressure.

When you use this technique during bag-valve-mask ventilation and endotracheal intubation, a second rescuer is required, and you must remember that the patient will likely regurgitate when you release cricoid pressure. Ideally, therefore,

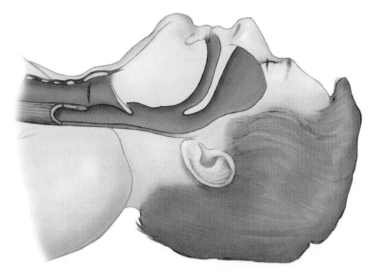

Figure 27-21a   Airway before applying Sellick's.

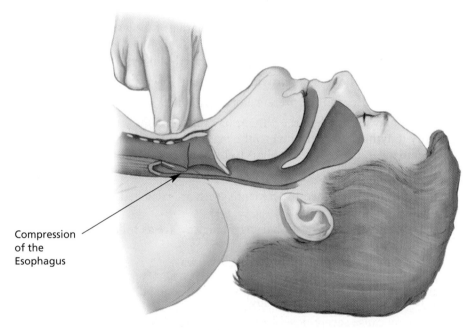

Figure 27-21b   Airway with Sellick's applied (note compression of the esophagus).

Compression of the Esophagus

once you have applied Sellick's manoeuvre, you must maintain it until endotracheal intubation is confirmed and personnel are ready to suction the oropharynx or place a nasogastric tube to decompress the stomach. Additionally, use caution in any patient with a suspected cervical spine injury, as movement of the neck in these patients could cause further spinal cord injury. Complications of Sellick's manoeuvre include esophageal rupture from unrelieved gastric pressure and obstruction of the trachea or laryngeal trauma from excessive manual pressure.

BASIC MECHANICAL AIRWAYS

In the absence of trauma, secretions, foreign bodies, and edema, basic manual airway manoeuvres should clear the tongue from the air passages. However, the tongue often falls back to block the airway again. Two available airway adjuncts—the nasopharyngeal airway and the oropharyngeal airway—correct this. These adjuncts cannot replace good head positioning, but they do help lift the base of the tongue forward and away from the posterior oropharynx, establishing a patent airway. Always attempt any appropriate manual manoeuvres before placing a mechanical airway.

Nasopharyngeal Airway

The **nasopharyngeal airway** is an uncuffed tube made of soft rubber or plastic. The nasopharyngeal airway follows the natural curvature of the nasopharynx, passing through the nose and extending from the nostril to the posterior pharynx just below the base of the tongue. It varies from 17 to 20 cm long, and its diameter ranges from 20 F to 36 F (**French**). A funnel-shaped projection at its proximal end helps prevent the tube from slipping inside a patient's nose and becoming lost or aspirated. The distal end is bevelled to facilitate passage. You will use the nasopharyngeal airway to relieve soft-tissue upper airway obstruction in cases where an oropharyngeal airway is not advised. Specific indications for the use of the nasopharyngeal airway include obtunded patients (with or without a suppressed gag reflex) and unconscious patients. If the patient does not tolerate the nasopharyngeal airway, you should remove it.

The nasopharyngeal airway's advantages are as follows:

- It can be rapidly inserted and safely placed blindly.
- It bypasses the tongue, providing a patent airway.
- You may use it in the presence of a gag reflex.
- You may use it when the patient has suffered injury to her oral cavity (anything from trauma to the mandible to significant soft-tissue damage to the tongue or pharynx).
- You may suction through it.
- You may use it when the patient's teeth are clenched.

Disadvantages of the nasopharyngeal airway are as follows:

- It is smaller than the oropharyngeal airway.
- It does not isolate the trachea.
- It is difficult to suction through.
- It may cause severe nosebleeds if inserted too forcefully.
- It may cause pressure necrosis of the nasal mucosa.
- It may kink and clog, obstructing the airway.
- Inserting it is difficult if nasal damage (old or new) is present.
- You may not use it if the patient has or is suspected to have a basilar skull fracture.

Do not use the nasopharyngeal airway in patients who are predisposed to nosebleeds or who have a nasal obstruction. Also, never use it when you suspect a basilar skull fracture, as the tube can inadvertently pass into the cranium.

The properly sized nasopharyngeal tube is slightly smaller in diameter than the patient's nostril, and in adults it is equal to or slightly longer than the distance from the patient's nose to her earlobe. Selecting the appropriate size is important. Too small a tube will not extend past the tongue; too long a tube may pass into the esophagus and result in hypoventilation and gastric distention with artificial ventilation (Figures 27-22 and 27-23). To insert the nasopharyngeal airway, follow these guidelines:

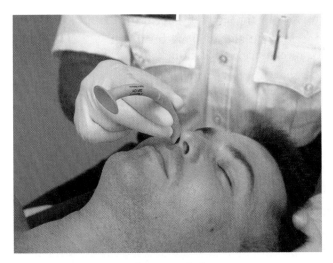

FIGURE 27-22   Nasopharyngeal airway.

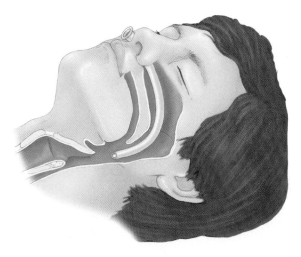

FIGURE 27-23   Nasopharyngeal airway, inserted.

1. If the patient has no history of trauma, hyperextend her head and neck.

2. Ensure or maintain effective ventilation. If indicated, hyperoxygenate the patient with 100-percent oxygen.

3. Lubricate the exterior of the tube with a water-soluble gel to prevent trauma during insertion.

4. Push the tube gently up on the tip of the nose and pass the tube into the right nostril. If the septum is deviated and you cannot easily insert the tube into the right nostril, use the left nostril. With the bevel oriented toward the septum, insert the tube gently along the nasal floor, parallel to the mouth. Avoid pushing against any resistance, as this may cause tissue trauma and airway kinking.

5. Verify appropriate position of the airway. Clear breath sounds and chest rise indicate correct placement. Also, feel at the airway's proximal end for airflow on expiration.

6. Hyperoxygenate the patient with 100-percent oxygen, if indicated.

While semiconscious patients tolerate a nasopharyngeal airway better than an oropharyngeal airway, it too may cause vomiting and laryngospasm. Insertion of the nasopharyngeal airway may injure the nasal mucosa, leading to bleeding, aspiration of clots, and the need for suctioning. Forceful insertion of the airway may lacerate the adenoids, causing considerable bleeding.

Oropharyngeal Airway

The **oropharyngeal airway** is a noninvasive semicircular plastic or rubber device designed to follow the palate's curvature. It holds the base of the tongue away from the posterior oropharynx, thus preventing it from obstructing the glottis. Its use is indicated in patients with no gag reflex.

When properly positioned, this device has several advantages:

* It is easy to place using proper technique.
* Air can pass around and through the device.

✴ **oropharyngeal airway** semicircular device that follows the palate's curvature.

- It helps prevent obstruction by the teeth and lips.
- It helps manage unconscious patients who are breathing spontaneously or need mechanical ventilation.
- It makes suction of the pharynx easier, as a large suction catheter can pass on either side of the device.
- It serves as an effective bite block in case of seizures or to protect the endotracheal tube.

Disadvantages of the oropharyngeal airway are as follows:

- It does not isolate the trachea or prevent aspiration.
- It cannot be inserted when the teeth are clenched.
- It may obstruct the airway if not inserted properly.
- It is easily dislodged.
- Return of the gag reflex may produce vomiting.

Do not use an oropharyngeal airway in conscious or in semiconscious patients who have a gag reflex, as it may cause vomiting or laryngospasm.

Do not use an oropharyngeal airway in conscious or in semiconscious patients who have a gag reflex, as it may cause vomiting (by stimulating the posterior tongue gag reflexes) or laryngospasm.

Oropharyngeal airways are available in sizes ranging from 40 mm (for infants) to 110 mm (for adults). Selecting the proper size is important. If the airway is too long, it can press the epiglottis against the entrance of the larynx, resulting in airway obstruction. If it is too small, it will not adequately hold the tongue forward. To measure for the appropriate oropharyngeal airway, place the flange beside the patient's cheek, parallel to the front of the teeth. A properly sized airway will extend from the patient's mouth to the angle of her jaw (Figure 27-24). To place the oropharyngeal airway, follow these guidelines:

1. If the patient has no history of trauma, hyperextend her head and neck. Open the mouth and remove any visible obstructions.
2. Ensure or maintain effective ventilation; if indicated, hyperoxygenate the patient with 100-percent oxygen.
3. Grasp the patient's jaw, and lift anteriorly.
4. With your other hand, hold the airway device at its proximal end, and insert it into the patient's mouth. Make sure the curve is reversed, with the tip pointing toward the roof of the mouth.
5. Once the tip reaches the level of the soft palate, gently rotate the airway 180 degrees until it comes to rest over the tongue.
6. Verify appropriate position of the airway. Clear breath sounds and chest rise indicate correct placement.
7. Hyperoxygenate the patient with 100-percent oxygen if indicated.

Make sure the airway is correctly positioned. Improper placement can obstruct the airway by pushing the tongue back against the posterior oropharynx (Figure 27-25). The device's advancing out of the mouth during ventilatory efforts indicates improper placement. Improper technique can also cause dental or pharyngeal trauma. An alternative insertion method useful in both pediatric and adult patients is to press the tongue upward and forward with a tongue blade. Then, the airway can be advanced until the flange is seated at the teeth. This is the preferred method of airway insertion in infants and children.

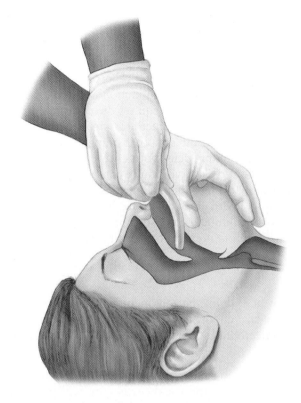

FIGURE 27-24a Insert the oropharyngeal airway with the tip facing the palate.

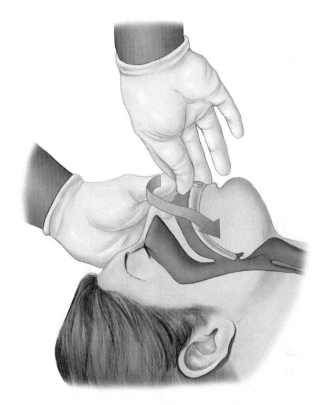

FIGURE 27-24b Rotate the airway 180° into position.

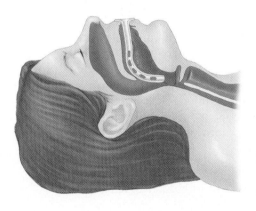

FIGURE 27-25 Improper placement of oropharyngeal airway.

ADVANCED AIRWAY MANAGEMENT

Inserting advanced mechanical airways requires special training. The preferred method of airway management is endotracheal intubation, as it is the only procedure that effectively isolates the trachea. Intubation is performed in emergency medical services that employ advanced care paramedics (ACPs) or critical care paramedics (CCPs). In services that employ primary care paramedics (PCPs), endotracheal intubation is not available. These services or systems use other airway devices, such as the esophageal tracheal CombiTube (ETC), laryngeal mask airway (LMA), or the pharyngo-tracheal lumen (PtL).

ENDOTRACHEAL INTUBATION

Endotracheal intubation involves inserting an endotracheal tube into the trachea in order to provide the patient with a definitive, protected airway. It is clearly the preferred method of advanced airway management in prehospital emergency care, as it allows the greatest control of the airway in conjunction with a bag-valve mask unit or ventilator. Under most circumstances, it requires direct visualization of the larynx with a laryngoscope, though alternative methods are available. Successfully instituting endotracheal intubation requires more training than do other techniques, and you must maintain ongoing proficiency to ensure patient safety. To ensure the quality of your judgment and skill, you must continuously review field intubations and the criteria for performing them. You must also remember that although endotracheal intubation affords the most effective airway control, you are bypassing important physiological functions of the upper airway—warming, filtering, and humidifying the air before it enters the lower airway.

Equipment

The equipment needed for endotracheal intubation includes a laryngoscope (handle and blade), an appropriate-size endotracheal tube, a 10-mL syringe, a stylet, a bag-valve mask, a suction device, a bite block, Magill forceps, and tape or a commercial tube-holding device.

Laryngoscope The **laryngoscope** is an instrument for lifting the tongue and epiglottis out of the way so that you can see the vocal cords. You will typically use it to place an endotracheal tube, but you may also use it in conjunction with Magill forceps to retrieve a foreign body obstructing the upper airway.

A laryngoscope consists of a handle and a blade. The handle may be either reusable or disposable. It houses batteries that power a light in the blade's distal tip. This light illuminates the airway, making it easier to see upper airway structures. The point attaching the handle and the blade is called the fitting. It locks the blade in place and provides electrical contact between the batteries and the bulb (Figure 27-26).

To prepare for intubation, attach the indentation on the proximal end of the laryngoscope's blade to the bar of the handle. It will click into place when properly seated. To determine if the laryngoscope is functional, raise the blade to a right angle with the handle until it clicks into place (Figure 27-27). The light

Endotracheal intubation is clearly the preferred method of advanced airway management in prehospital emergency care, as it allows the greatest control of the airway.

Content Review

ENDOTRACHEAL INTUBATION EQUIPMENT

- Laryngoscope (handle and blade)
- Endotracheal tube
- 10-mL syringe
- Stylet
- Bag-valve mask
- Suction device
- Bite block or oropharyngeal airway
- Magill forceps
- Tape or tube-holding device

✳ **laryngoscope** instrument for lifting the tongue and epiglottis in order to see the vocal cords.

FIGURE 27-26 Engaging the laryngoscope blade and handle.

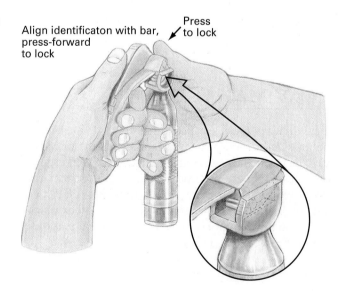

Align identification with bar, press-forward to lock

Press to lock

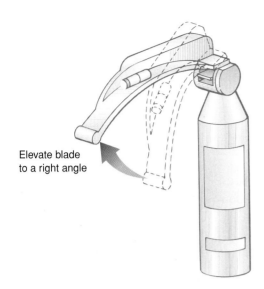

Elevate blade
to a right angle

FIGURE 27-27 Activating the
laryngoscope light source.

should turn on and be bright and steady. A yellow, flickering light will not sufficiently illuminate the anatomical structures. If the light fails to go on, the problem may be either dead batteries or a loose bulb. Every airway kit should include
spare parts. Infrequently, the contact points or the wire that runs through the
blade to the bulb will fail.

Like the handle, the blade may be reusable or disposable. Two common types
of blades are the curved blade (Macintosh blade) and the straight blade (often referred to as the Miller, Miller-Abbott, Wisconsin, or Flagg blade). Laryngoscope
blades range in size from 0 for infants to 4 for large adults (Figure 27-28).

The curved blade is designed to fit into the vallecula (Figure 27-29). When
you lift its handle anteriorly, the blade elevates the tongue and, indirectly, the
epiglottis, allowing you to see the glottic opening. Because the curved blade does
not touch the larynx itself, it should not traumatize or stimulate the very sensitive gag receptors on the posterior surface of the epiglottis. The curved blade also
permits more room for viewing and endotracheal tube (ETT) insertion. The
straight blade is designed to fit under the epiglottis (Figure 27-30). When you lift
its handle anteriorly, the blade directly lifts the epiglottis out of the way.

Which blade you use is largely a matter of individual preference, but you
should be skilled with both in order to accommodate patients' anatomical differences. A straight blade is better for endotracheal intubation in infants because
it stabilizes their floppier epiglottises and provides greater displacement of their
relatively larger tongues. It also is better for the occasional adult patient with a
floppy epiglottis or large tongue.

Endotracheal Tubes The endotracheal tube (**ETT**) is a flexible, translucent tube
open at both ends and available in lengths ranging from 12 cm to 32 cm, with
centimetre markings along its length (Figure 27-31). The proximal end has a
standard 15-mm inside diameter/22-mm outside diameter connector that
attaches to the ventilatory device, usually a bag-valve mask. The ETT is available
with internal tube diameters ranging from 2.5 mm to 4.5 mm (uncuffed) and
from 5.0 mm to 9.0 mm (cuffed). The distal end has a bevelled tip to facilitate
smooth movement through airway passages. When present, an inflatable
5–10 mL cuff at the distal end of ETT sizes from 5.0 mm to 9.0 mm provides a
seal between the ETT and the trachea. A thin inflation tube runs the length of the
main tube from the distal cuff to a syringe. A one-way valve at the proximal end
of the inflation tube permits the syringe to push air into the distal cuff or pull it

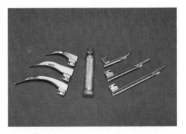

FIGURE 27-28 Laryngoscope
blades.

✱ ETT endotracheal tube.

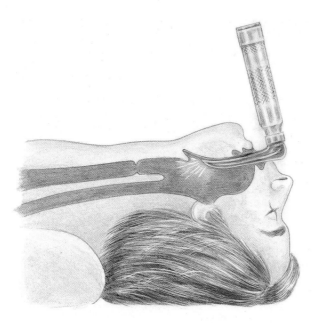

FIGURE 27-29 Placement of Mcintosh blade into vallecula.

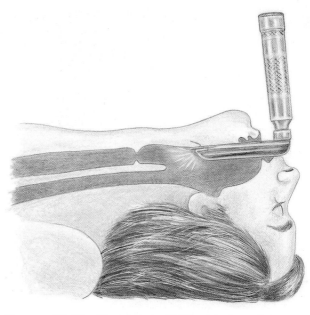

FIGURE 27-30 Placement of Miller blade under epiglottis.

out but prevents air from escaping the cuff when the syringe is removed. A pilot balloon at the inflation tube's proximal end indicates whether the distal cuff is properly inflated. The pilot balloon should be partially inflated but soft, to avoid overinflating the distal cuff and inadvertently pressuring the tracheal mucosa. This could cause ischemia of the tracheal wall. Always check the distal cuff for leaks before insertion.

Suppliers typically wrap an ETT in a curved shape. This is because the trachea lies anteriorly in the neck, and the tube must be directed upward to en-

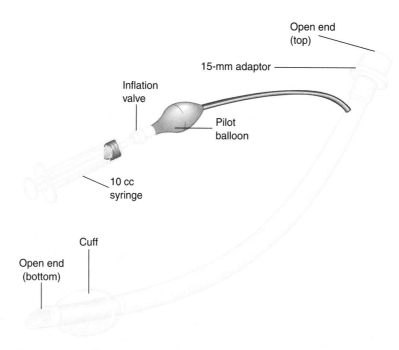

FIGURE 27-31 ETT and syringe.

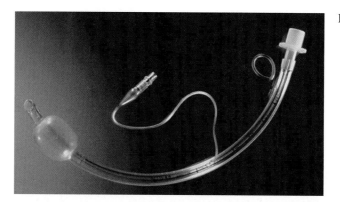

FIGURE 27-32 Endotrol ETT.

ter the glottic opening. On the Endotrol ETT, an O-shaped ring attaches to a plastic wire that runs the length of the tube and terminates distally (Figure 27-32). Pulling the ring bends the distal end of the tube upward and directs it into the glottic opening. This can facilitate placement of the tube without the need for a stylet.

Endotracheal tubes come in a variety of sizes. Markings on the tubes indicate their internal diameter in millimetres. The typical tube sizes for average-sized adult patients are 7.0–9.0 mm (females, 7.0–8.0 mm; males, 7.5–8.5 mm). A generally acceptable size for both male and female adults is 7.5 mm. (We discuss endotracheal intubation of children in detail later in this chapter.)

Stylet The malleable **stylet** is a plastic-covered metal wire used to direct the ETT anteriorly by bending its distal end into a J or hockey-stick shape (Figures 27-33 and 27-34). It is particularly useful in patients with extremely anterior laryngeal anatomy or those with short, thick necks with which head positioning can be difficult. Although using stylets is not mandatory, many paramedics prefer to use them in the prehospital setting because they afford greater control of the ETT. The wire stylet may damage tissues during intubation if it extends past the distal end of the ETT; therefore, you should keep it recessed at least 1 cm from the tip of the tube.

✱ Stylet plastic-covered metal wire used to bend the ETT into a J or hockey-stick shape.

10-mL Syringe The syringe allows you to inflate the distal cuff just enough to avoid air leaks around the ETT without causing tracheal ischemia.

Tube-Holding Devices Tie down or tape secure the endotracheal tube once it is in the trachea. The reasons for securing the ETT are twofold. First, moving the patient during resuscitation or transportation can easily dislodge the tube. Even if the ETT is not actually dislodged, its movement can still cause cardiovascular stimulation, an elevation in intracranial pressure, or injury to the tracheal mucosa.

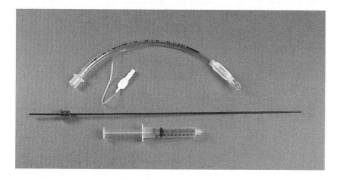

FIGURE 27-33 ETT, stylet, and syringe, unassembled.

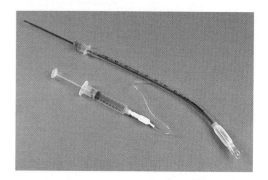

FIGURE 27-34 ETT, stylet, and syringe, assembled for intubation.

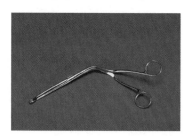

FIGURE 27-35   Magill forceps.

Second, the person providing ventilatory support may inadvertently push down on the ETT, forcing it into the right or left mainstem bronchus. Using tape requires extra care, as it can loosen when either the patient's face or the tube is moist. A number of commercial tube-holding devices are available.

Magill Forceps The **Magill forceps** are scissor-style clamps with circular tips. You will use them to remove foreign bodies or to redirect the endotracheal tube during nasotracheal intubation (Figure 27-35).

Lubricant Water-soluble lubricants facilitate inserting the ETT. Do not use petroleum-based lubricants; they may damage the ETT and cause tracheal inflammation.

Suction Unit A suction unit helps to remove secretions and foreign materials from the oropharynx during intubation attempts. It is a vital element that you must never forget. (We discuss suction units in more detail later in this chapter.)

End–Tidal CO$_2$ Detector or Other Confirmation Device These adjuncts to intubation are becoming the standard of care in most areas. You must be familiar with the devices, their role in intubation, and your local protocols' requirements for their use.

Additional Airways You should also have an oropharyngeal airway available during endotracheal intubation. You will occasionally use it as a block to prevent the patient from biting down on and collapsing the ETT.

Protective Equipment Endotracheal intubation, like many airway procedures, carries the risk of exposure to body substances. Because of this, it is essential to employ body substance isolation procedures. These include, but are not limited to, gloves, mask, protective eyewear, and possibly a gown. Remember, personal safety comes first!

Endotracheal Intubation Indications

Monitoring success rates for particular skills is not hard with an appropriate quality assurance program. Evaluating your ability to judge which patients you should intubate is considerably more difficult. Often, the patient's condition may warrant trying nebulizer treatments or supplemental oxygen before deciding to intubate. A patient's continued distress and failure to respond to treatment clearly indicate intubation. In conjunction with the medical director, you are responsible for continually improving your judgment regarding the use of advanced airway management techniques. This includes recognizing subtle indicators that the patient's condition is worsening, before the onset of respiratory arrest.

Endotracheal intubation provides a definitive, secure, open airway for patients who are experiencing, or are likely to experience, upper airway compromise. Some of the indications for endotracheal intubation in these patients include respiratory or cardiac arrest; unresponsiveness without a gag reflex; inability to protect the airway, resulting in an increased risk of aspiration; and obstruction due to foreign bodies, trauma, burns, or anaphylaxis. Endotracheal intubation also improves oxygenation and ventilation in patients with extreme lower airway difficulty. Some lower airway indications include severe respiratory distress due to such diseases as asthma, COPD, congestive heart failure (CHF), or pneumonia, as well as pneumothorax, hemothorax, or hemopneumothorax with respiratory difficulty. Clearly, then, endotracheal intubation may be indicated in breathing and apneic patients, though caution must be used in any patient with an intact gag reflex.

You are responsible for continually improving your judgment regarding airway management.

Content Review

ENDOTRACHEAL INTUBATION INDICATORS
- Respiratory or cardiac arrest
- Unconsciousness or obtusion without gag reflex
- Risk of aspiration
- Obstruction due to foreign bodies, trauma, burns, or anaphylaxis
- Respiratory extremis due to disease
- Pneumothorax, hemothorax, or hemopneumothorax with respiratory difficulty

Do not attempt endotracheal intubation in the prehospital setting if epiglottitis is present, unless airway failure is imminent. Attempts to manipulate the airway in epiglottitis are very likely to result in vigorous laryngospasm. The most prudent management of epiglottitis is oxygenation of the patient without agitation. The preferred treatment for epiglottitis is rapid transport to the operating room for endotracheal intubation under more controlled conditions. This is carried out with the necessary equipment for emergency tracheostomy opened and ready for immediate use. Sometimes, these patients steadily worsen, and loss of their airway is imminent and inevitable. In this case, the benefits from endotracheal intubation outweigh the risks. Regardless, the most experienced member of the crew should perform the procedure. Also, it is important to remember that there may be significant laryngeal edema and it may be necessary to insert a smaller than normal endotracheal tube. This should be kept in mind before undertaking this procedure. Always follow local protocols and contact medical direction regarding endotracheal intubation in cases where epiglottitis is present or suspected.

Advantages of Endotracheal Intubation

- It isolates the trachea and permits complete control of the airway.
- It impedes gastric distention by channelling air directly into the trachea.
- It eliminates the need to maintain a mask seal.
- It offers a direct route for suctioning of the respiratory passages.
- It permits administration of the medications naloxone (Narcan), atropine, Ventolin (salbutamol), epinephrine, and lidocaine via the endotracheal tube (use the mnemonic NAVEL to remember these medications)

Disadvantages of Endotracheal Intubation

- The technique requires considerable training and experience.
- It requires specialized equipment.
- It requires direct visualization of the vocal cords.
- It bypasses the upper airway's function of warming, filtering, and humidifying the inhaled air.

Complications of Endotracheal Intubation

Intubation presents a number of potential complications. Properly attending to detail and taking appropriate precautions will help you avoid these problems.

Equipment Malfunction Equipment malfunctions consume valuable time when you are establishing a definitive airway and effective oxygenation and ventilation. Having a preassembled airway kit that is checked regularly will lessen the chances of this occurring. Ideally, someone should check the airway kit daily to be sure that all needed supplies are present and that the bulb, batteries, and blade are in good working condition.

Teeth Breakage and Soft-Tissue Lacerations Endotracheal intubation can injure the lips and teeth, but you can eliminate this hazard by carefully using the laryngoscope as an instrument, not a tool. When inserting the blade into the mouth and pharynx, guide it gently into place, avoiding pressure on the teeth. When manipulating the jaw anteriorly, use gentle traction upward and toward the feet, rather than rotating and flexing your wrist, which will make the laryngoscope function as a lever. All levers require a fulcrum—and the only fulcrums available in your patient's mouth will be her upper incisors. A rotating/flexing action may thus break teeth. To avoid this hazard, lift the laryngoscope's handle (exposing the epiglottis) after you have applied the blade to the base of the tongue. After this, keep your wrist straight, and do any lifting with your shoulder and arm.

If you use the laryngoscope too roughly, you can lacerate the patient's lips, tongue, or pharyngeal structures, producing profuse bleeding that is hard to control. This can also happen if you direct the tube away from midline into the pyriform sinuses or allow the stylet to protrude from the distal end of the ETT. In the larynx and lower airway, you might damage the vocal cords, cause laryngeal edema, or tear the trachea if you are not careful. A gentle technique and attention to detail are the keys to avoiding these complications.

Hypoxia Delays in oxygenation, either from interruption of basic airway techniques and BVM ventilation with 100-percent oxygen or from prolonged intubation attempts, can produce profound, life-threatening hypoxia. Each patient's unique anatomy and unusual clinical situations can challenge even the most experienced paramedic. One basic rule that helps avoid hypoxia during intubation is to limit each intubation attempt to no more than 30 seconds before reoxygenating the patient. To gauge this interval, some paramedics hold their breath from the time they stop ventilating the patient until they start again.

If you cannot pass the tube through the vocal cords on the first attempt, at least identify your landmarks and note any unique or difficult features that you may need to address. For example, too much edema might indicate a smaller ETT. Or the patient's larynx might be more anterior than you realized from her external anatomy, and you will need to use a different blade or change the ETT angle. You can then pass the tube on a subsequent attempt, after hyperoxygenating the patient with basic airway techniques and 100-percent oxygen using a bag-valve-mask device.

Esophageal Intubation Misplacement of the ETT into the esophagus deprives the patient of oxygenation and ventilation. It is potentially lethal, resulting in severe hypoxia and brain death if you do not recognize it immediately. It also directs air into the stomach, encouraging regurgitation, which can lead to aspiration. Indicators of esophageal intubation include the following:

- An absence of chest rise and absence of breath sounds with mechanical ventilation
- Gurgling sounds over the epigastrium with each breath delivered
- Distention of the abdomen
- An absence of breath condensation in the endotracheal tube
- A persistent air leak, despite inflation of the tube's distal cuff
- Cyanosis and progressive worsening of the patient's condition
- Phonation (noise made by the vocal cords)
- No colour change with colorimetric $ETCO_2$ detector
- A falling pulse oximetry reading
- An esophageal intubation detector (bulb) that does not refill or that refills slowly

If you have any suspicion that the tube is in the esophagus, remove it immediately. Hyperoxygenate the patient with 100-percent oxygen, and attempt endotracheal intubation with another tube.

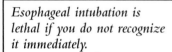

To avoid hypoxia during intubation, limit each intubation attempt to no more than 30 seconds before reoxygenating the patient.

Esophageal intubation is lethal if you do not recognize it immediately.

Endobronchial Intubation If you pass the endotracheal tube successfully through the vocal cords and advance it too far, it likely will enter either the right or left mainstem bronchus. As discussed earlier, the ETT may be misplaced to either side, but it is more likely to pass into the right mainstem, which angles away from the trachea less acutely than does the left. In either case, the ETT ventilates only one lung and the result is hypoventilation and hypoxia from inadequate gas exchange. Also, when the bag-valve device **insufflates** enough air for two lungs into the smaller area of only one lung, it can create enough pressure to cause barotrauma, such as a pneumothorax, worsening the patient's condition.

✱ **insufflate** to blow into.

You can avoid inserting the ETT too far by following these guidelines:

1. Advance the distal cuff no more than 1–2 cm past the vocal cords.
2. Once the tube is positioned, hold it in place with one hand to prevent it from being pushed any farther.
3. Inflate the cuff, and firmly secure the tube in place with tape or a commercial tube-holding device.
4. Note the number marking on the side of the ETT where it emerges from the patient's mouth at the teeth, gums, or lips. This will allow you to quickly recognize any changes in tube placement. Approximate ETT depth for the average adult is 21 cm at the teeth for women and 23 cm at the teeth for men, though this will vary.

Findings in endobronchial intubation include the following:

• Breath sounds present on one side of the chest but diminished or absent on the other
• Poor compliance (resistance to ventilations with the bag-valve device)
• Cyanosis, cardiac dysrhythmias, or other evidence of hypoxia

To resolve the problem, loosen or remove any securing devices and withdraw the ETT until breath sounds are present and equal bilaterally. Be certain to deflate the cuff when pulling back on the ETT.

Tension Pneumothorax Any tear in the lung parenchyma can cause a pneumothorax. If this is allowed to progress untreated, a tension pneumothorax, an accumulation of air or gas in the pleural cavity, may develop. A tension pneumothorax is a large pneumothorax that affects other structures in the chest. The expanding tension pneumothorax will adversely affect the other lung, the heart, and the structures of the mediastinum. It will eventually displace these structures away from the side of the chest with the tension pneumothorax. In addition to mainstem bronchus intubation, tension pneumothorax can result if you use too much of the bag-valve device's volume on a small adult or child or use the full bag-valve-device volume against diseased lungs with poor compliance. Tension pneumothorax is marked by progressively worsening compliance (more difficulty in ventilating), diminished unilateral breath sounds, hypoxia with hypotension, and distended neck veins. Often, the trachea will deviate away from the side of the chest with the pneumothorax. Also, the marked increase in intrathoracic pressure resulting from the tension pneumothorax can prevent the ventricles from filling adequately. This can cause a decrease in cardiac output and will worsen the patient's overall condition. If you suspect tension pneumothorax, needle decompression of the chest is indicated, as described in Chapter 25 on thoracic trauma.

Orotracheal Intubation

The most widely preferred and, therefore, the most commonly used path for endotracheal intubation is the orotracheal route. Many medical personnel favour this route because it involves direct visualization of the vocal cords and a clear view of the ETT's passage through them. It is thus the most accurate method of intubation and the least likely to induce trauma to the airway. To perform orotracheal intubation in the absence of suspected trauma, follow these steps (Procedure 27-1):

1. Place the patient supine.

2. After using basic manual and adjunctive airway manoeuvres to open the airway and ventilate, hyperoxygenate the patient with 100-percent oxygen.

3. While your partner ventilates the patient, prepare your intubation equipment, including suction, and be certain that all needed equipment is present and in good working order. Assemble and check the laryngoscope blade and handle to be certain you have a steady, bright light, and then close the handle. Insert the stylet into the ETT, making sure to keep the distal end of the stylet at least 2 cm proximal to the distal tip of the ETT. You may choose to bend the distal end of the ETT into a "hockey stick" shape just proximal to the distal cuff to help direct the ETT anteriorly. Apply water-soluble lubricant to the distal end of the ETT and reinsert. Leaving the ETT partially in its packaging until you are ready to insert it helps keep it as clean as possible. Fill the 10 cc syringe with 5 to 10 mL of air and attach it to the valve at the proximal end of the ETT, using a twisting motion to lock it in place. Check the cuff for air leaks.

4. Turn on the suction, and attach an appropriate tip.

5. Position the patient's head and neck. Remove any dentures or partial dental plates. To visualize the larynx, you must align the three axes of the mouth, the pharynx, and the trachea. To do this, place the patient's head in a "sniffing position" by flexing the neck forward and the head backward. Inserting a rolled towel or sheet under the patient's shoulders or the back of the head may help. Establishing this position is extremely difficult in patients with short, thick necks or whose motion is limited by such conditions as arthritis.

6. Hold the laryngoscope in your left hand whether you are right- or left-handed. Most laryngoscopes are designed for right-handed people; that is, the right-handed person must hold the laryngoscope in her left hand in order to manipulate the endotracheal tube with her right.

7. If you have not already done so, have your partner apply Sellick's manoeuvre (cricoid pressure) and maintain it until you confirm ETT placement in the trachea.

8. Insert the laryngoscope blade gently into the right side of the patient's mouth. With a gentle sweeping action, displace the tongue to the left. This pushes the tongue out of your line of vision and allows more room to manipulate the ETT.

9. Move the blade slightly toward the midline. Advance the Macintosh (curved) blade until the distal end is at the base of the tongue in the vallecula; advance the Miller (straight) blade until the distal end is under the epiglottis. As you advance the blade, move the patient's lower lip away from the blade using the index finger of your right hand.

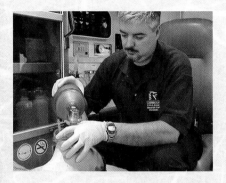

27-1a   Hyperoxygenate the patient.

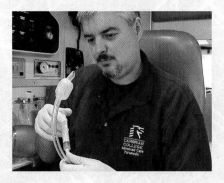

27-1b   Prepare the equipment.

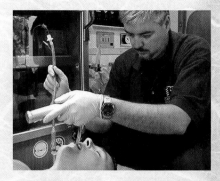

27-1c   Apply Sellick's manoeuvre (if required) and insert laryngoscope.

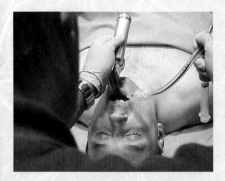

27-1d   Visualize the larynx and insert the ETT.

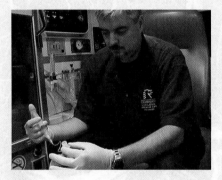

27-1e   Inflate the cuff, ventilate, and auscultate.

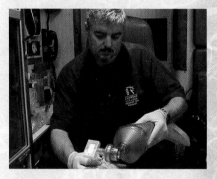

27-1f   Confirm placement with an $ETCO_2$ detector or an EDD.

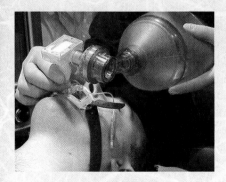

27-1g   Secure the tube.

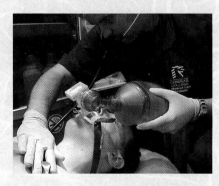

27-1h   Reconfirm ETT placement.

10. Lift the laryngoscope handle slightly upward and toward the feet to displace the jaw. Be careful not to put pressure on the teeth. At this point, you can see any vomitus, blood, or secretions in the posterior pharynx. You likely will have to suction the airway clear. If the secretions are thick or copious, you may need to remove the suction tip and use the suction hose.

11. On lifting the jaw, determine whether the laryngoscope blade is in proper position. You may need to adjust it before you can visualize the vocal cords. If you cannot see landmarks clearly, gently withdraw the blade, slowly and slightly. This may bring the vocal cords into view. If it does not, you might need to gently advance the blade farther into the hypopharynx.

12. Keeping your left wrist straight, use your left shoulder and arm to continue lifting the mandible and tongue to a 45-degree angle to the ground (up and toward the feet) until the glottis is exposed (Figure 27-36). Often, you may not see the entire glottis, but you should see at least its posterior third or half. If the larynx lies anteriorly, a slight increase in your partner's pressure on the Sellick's manoeuvre should improve your view of the vocal cords. Occasionally, your partner will need to lessen the cricoid pressure slightly to allow you to visualize the vocal cords. Be ready to instruct her to apply more or less cricoid pressure.

13. Hold the ETT in your right hand with your fingertips as you would a dart or a pencil; this gives you control to gently manoeuvre the ETT. Advance the tube through the right corner of the patient's mouth, and direct it toward the midline.

14. Directly visualizing the vocal cords, pass the ETT gently through the glottic opening until its distal cuff disappears beyond the vocal cords; then, advance it another 1–2 cm.

15. Hold the tube in place with your hand to prevent its displacement; do not let go under any circumstance until it is taped or tied securely in place. Attach a bag-valve device to the 15/22-mm connector on the tube; attach the ETCO$_2$ detector to the bag-valve device as your local protocols require.

16. Inflate the distal cuff with 5–10 mL of air. To avoid tracheal trauma or ischemia from excessive cuff pressure, apply only enough pressure to prevent air leakage around the ETT during ventilation. Listen for any air leak and adjust the cuff's pressure as needed. When cuff pressure is correct, remove the syringe, using a twisting motion to prevent any air leak.

17. Check for proper tube placement. While listening for equal bilateral breath sounds over the chest, watch to see that the chest rises and falls symmetrically. Listen over the epigastrium to be certain you hear no gastric sounds. Look for moisture condensation in the exhaled breath; it should appear in the ETT during each exhalation.

18. Hyperoxygenate the patient with 100-percent oxygen. Gently insert an oropharyngeal airway to serve as a bite block.

19. Secure the ETT with an ETT tie while maintaining ventilatory support. Loop the tape around the tube at the level of the patient's teeth, attaching it tightly to the tube without kinking or pinching it. Then, wrap the tape around the patient's head, and tie it at the side of her neck. Alternatively, use a commercial tube-holding device.

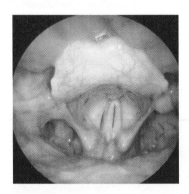

FIGURE 27-36   Glottis visualized through laryngoscopy.

20. Repeat step 17 periodically to confirm proper ETT placement. Also, repeat step 17 after any major movement of the patient or movement of her head or neck. (Neck manipulation can displace the tube by up to 5 cm.) Continue to support the tube manually while maintaining ventilatory support.

Verification of Proper Endotracheal Tube Placement Continuously checking and rechecking tube placement is an important responsibility during endotracheal intubation. The hypervigilance with which you must monitor the patient's clinical condition cannot be overemphasized. You can employ a number of methods in the field to confirm correct ETT placement. You should put them to maximum use, but do not become overly reliant on technology. The patient's clinical condition should be the deciding factor in your patient management decisions.

The most reliable method of confirming proper ETT placement is direct visualization of its passage through the vocal cords. This requires the proper use of a laryngoscope and continued visualization of the vocal cords throughout intubation. If you do this, you have little chance of inadvertently intubating the esophagus.

Following ETT placement, watch to be sure that the patient's chest rises with ventilations. If the ETT is misplaced in the esophagus, the chest will not rise. You also should auscultate for breath sounds. Their equal presence on both sides (apices and bases) of the chest and their absence over the epigastrium helps to confirm proper ETT placement. Conversely, their absence over the chest and their presence over the epigastrium indicates an esophageal intubation. Breath sounds present on one side but absent or diminished on the other indicate that the ETT may be advanced too deeply into one of the mainstem bronchi, that bronchial obstruction may be present, or that a pneumothorax is present. Absent breath sounds bilaterally may indicate esophageal intubation.

End-tidal CO_2 detectors and esophageal detector devices can be helpful. Adequate levels of exhaled carbon dioxide, as detected by an end-tidal CO_2 detector, confirm proper endotracheal tube placement. The ability to withdraw air readily from an esophageal detector device's syringe further confirms placement of the ETT in the trachea. Resistance to air withdrawal, or the creation of a vacuum, denotes esophageal intubation.

Also, observe the endotracheal tube's contents. Exhaled air approaches 100-percent humidity. Usually, the ambient relative humidity is less than 100 percent. Thus, condensation inside the ETT suggests its proper placement. Because the gastric sphincter relaxes in critically ill patients and the high pressures of a bag-valve mask create gastric distention, patients frequently vomit and aspirate during resuscitation. If you misplace the ETT into the esophagus, you may observe an efflux of gastric contents through the ETT, particularly with subsequent ventilation attempts. Because aspiration into the trachea also may have occurred, you might see vomitus in the ETT even with proper endotracheal intubation; nonetheless, this finding always should raise suspicion of esophageal intubation and prompt further investigation.

It is important to verify *and document* proper ETT placement. In fact, it is ideal to verify and document at least three different indicators of proper placement. These may include the following:

- Visualization of the tube passing between the cords
- Presence of bilateral breath sounds
- Absence of breath sounds over the epigastrium
- Positive end-tidal CO_2 change on an $ETCO_2$ device
- Verification of endotracheal placement by an esophageal detector device
- Presence of condensation inside the ETT

The hypervigilance with which you must monitor the patient's clinical condition cannot be overemphasized.

- Absence of vomitus inside the ETT
- Absence of phonation, or vocal sounds, once the tube is placed

In addition, an increase in the oxygen saturation will help support proper placement of the endotracheal tube. Likewise, a rise and fall of the chest indicates endotracheal intubation. Worsening gastric distention may indicate possible esophageal placement. Any gastric distention should be investigated. Remember, though, it is not uncommon for gastric distention to develop prior to endotracheal intubation due to mechanical ventilation. Even in experienced hands, it is extremely difficult to avoid gastric distention with mechanical ventilation until an endotracheal tube is placed.

Transillumination Intubation Since a bright light in the trachea is visible (transilluminates) through the soft tissue of the anterior neck, an ETT with a lighted stylet can facilitate correct intubation (Figure 27-37). The stylet is a plastic cable with a malleable, retractable wire running through its centre and a small, high-intensity bulb at its distal end. An on-off switch and power supply at the stylet's proximal end control the bulb, which begins to blink about 30 seconds after it is turned on. This blinking makes detecting the light's transilluminations easier.

You can confirm correct ETT placement by observing the stylet's light through the anterior neck's soft tissue; esophageal intubation results in little or no light being visible. Because you can place the ETT safely and correctly without directly visualizing the glottic opening, you can perform endotracheal intubation without manipulating a trauma patient's head and neck. Several studies have shown the transillumination technique to be fast, dependable, and atraumatic.

This technique's biggest limitation is that bright ambient light can make the transillumination difficult to see. Therefore, it works best in a darkened room and with thin patients. When attempting this procedure, reduce ambient light; in direct or bright daylight, shade the patient's neck.

To perform transillumination intubation, do the following:

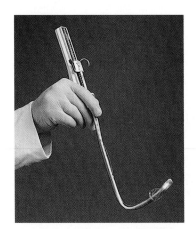

FIGURE 27-37   Lighted stylet for endotracheal intubation.

1. While maintaining ventilatory support, hyperoxygenate the patient with 100-percent oxygen.
2. Prepare and check your equipment. The ETT diameter should be 7.5–8.5 mm. You will need to cut the ETT to a length of 25–27 cm to accommodate the stylet. Place the stylet in the ETT, and lock the ETT in place at its proximal end. Using the sliding mechanism on the handle, adjust the stylet, and bend it into a hockey-stick shape just proximal to the distal cuff.
3. With the patient supine and her head in neutral position, kneel along either her right or left side, facing her head.
4. Turn on the stylet light.
5. With your index and middle fingers inserted deeply into the patient's mouth and your thumb under her chin, lift her tongue and jaw forward (Figure 27-38).
6. With the proximal end of the ETT directed toward the patient's feet, insert the tube/stylet into the mouth, and advance it gently through the oropharynx into the hypopharynx.
7. Use a "hooking" action with the tube/stylet to lift the epiglottis out of the way (Figure 27-39).
8. When you see a circle of light at the patient's Adam's apple, the stylet is placed correctly (Figure 27-40). A diffuse, dim, hard-to-see, or absent light indicates that the ETT/stylet combination is in

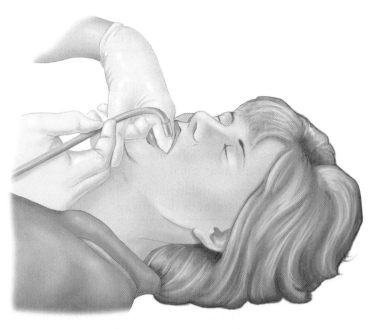

FIGURE 27-38 Insertion of lighted stylet/ETT.

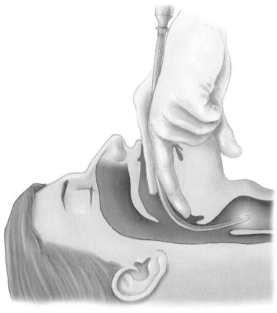

FIGURE 27-39 Lighted stylet/ETT in position.

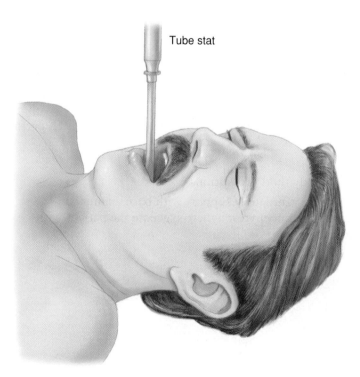

FIGURE 27-40 Transillumination of a lighted stylet.

the esophagus. A bright light lateral and superior to the Adam's apple indicates that it has moved into the right or left pyriform fossa. To correct either of these placements, withdraw the tube and, after ventilating the patient with 100-percent oxygen for several minutes, reattempt intubation using proper basic manual and adjunct airway manoeuvres.

9. After the ETT is properly placed, hold the stylet stationary. Advance the tube off the stylet into the larynx approximately 1–2 cm, simultaneously retracting the internal wire from the stylet using the O-ring at its proximal end.

10. Once the light is in the correct position and you have partially advanced the ETT while partially retracting the stylet wire, hold the tube firmly in place with one hand, and remove the stylet.

11. Attach the bag-valve device to the endotracheal tube's 15/22-mm connector, and deliver several breaths, inflating the distal ETT cuff and checking for proper placement as usual.

12. Secure the ETT, recheck placement, and maintain ventilatory support. Continue periodic assessment of the airway.

Digital Intubation Some situations may require you to perform digital intubation. This technique dates to the eighteenth century, when people performed intubations without the benefit of a laryngoscope. Instead, they used digital (finger), or tactile (touch), intubation (Figure 27-41).

Digital intubation is still useful for a number of situations in the prehospital setting. It is suggested when a patient is deeply comatose or in cardiac arrest and when proper positioning is difficult. The classic example is an unresponsive trauma patient with a suspected cervical spine injury. Since the digital technique does not require manipulation of the head and neck, it is of great value here. It may also be useful in extrication situations where the confined space prevents properly positioning the patient. Also, because digital intubation does not require visualization, it may be helpful when facial injuries distort the patient's anatomy or when you cannot suction copious amounts of blood, vomitus, or other secretions for a proper view of the airway.

Digital intubation is risky for the paramedic; it may stimulate even a deeply comatose patient to clamp down and bite your finger. Do not use it with conscious patients or with unconscious patients who have a gag reflex. To perform digital intubation:

1. Use blood and body fluid precautions.

2. While maintaining ventilatory support with basic manual and adjunctive airway manoeuvres, hyperoxygenate the patient with 100-percent oxygen.

FIGURE 27-41 Blind oro-tracheal intubation by digital method.

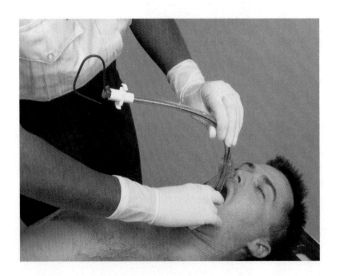

3. Prepare and check your equipment. You will need the following items: an appropriately sized ETT, a malleable stylet, water-soluble lubricant, a 5–10-mL syringe, a bite block, and an ETT tie or a commercial anchoring device. Insert the stylet into the endotracheal tube, and bend the ETT/stylet into a J shape.

4. While another team member stabilizes the patient's head and neck in an in-line (neutral) position, kneel at the patient's left shoulder, facing her head. Place a bite block device between the patient's molars to help protect your fingers.

5. Insert your left middle and index fingers into the patient's mouth (Figure 27-42). By alternating fingers, "walk" your hand down the midline while simultaneously tugging gently forward on the tongue. You may also use gauze to hold and extend the tongue more effectively, which may facilitate palpation of the glottis. This lifts the epiglottis up and away from the glottic opening, within reach of your probing fingers.

6. Palpate the arytenoid cartilage posterior to the glottis and the epiglottis anteriorly with your middle finger (Figure 27-43). Press the epiglottis forward, and insert the endotracheal tube into the mouth, anterior to your fingers (Figure 27-44).

7. Advance the tube, pushing it gently with your right hand. Use your left index finger to keep the tip of the ETT against your middle finger. This will direct the tip to the epiglottis.

8. Use your middle and index fingers to direct the tip of the ETT between the epiglottis (in front) and your fingers (behind). Then, with your right hand, advance the ETT through the cords, simultaneously manoeuvring it forward with your left index and middle fingers. This will prevent it from slipping posteriorly into the esophagus.

9. Hold the tube in place with your hand to prevent its displacement. Attach a bag-valve device with an $ETCO_2$ detector to the 15/22-mm connector on the ETT; inflate the distal cuff with 5–10 mL of air; check for proper tube placement.

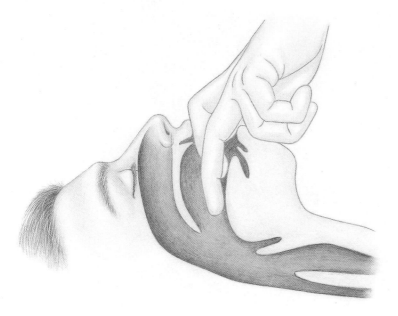

FIGURE 27-42 Digital intubation. Insert your middle and index fingers into the patient's mouth.

10. Hyperoxygenate the patient with 100-percent oxygen. Gently insert an oropharyngeal airway to serve as a bite block. Secure the ETT with umbilical tape. Repeat the steps to confirm proper ETT placement, and maintain ventilatory support. Continue your airway assessment periodically.

FIGURE 27-43 Digital intubation. Walk your fingers and palpate the patient's epiglottis.

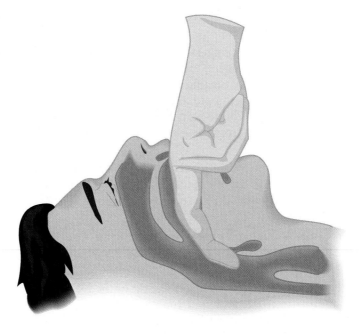

FIGURE 27-44 Digital intubation—insertion of the ETT.

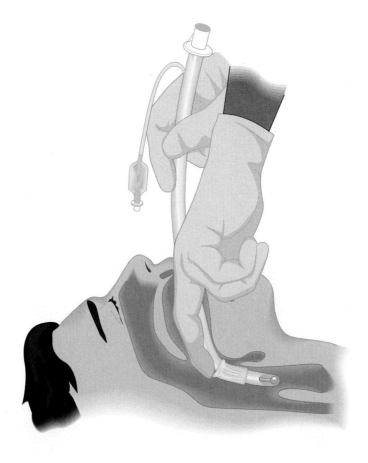

Trauma Patient Intubation Airway management and ventilatory support in the trauma patient are essential for a successful outcome. Appropriate treatment of all other injuries is meaningless if you do not ensure a patent airway and adequate oxygenation and ventilation.

The trauma patient presents a number of obstacles to effective airway management and ventilation. Some of them may be the need for extrication, blood in the oropharynx, distorted anatomy due to injury, and the need to protect the cervical spine. Getting an adequate seal on a mask is very difficult when the patient is being extricated or has significant facial trauma. You must keep the cervical spine in a neutral, in-line position throughout your management of all patients with known or suspected cervical spine trauma. Digital intubation, transillumination intubation, and nasotracheal intubation (described later in this chapter) provide potential solutions for some patients when trauma complicates airway management, but visualizing the vocal cords is still preferable. You can do this effectively using direct laryngoscopy-assisted orotracheal intubation with manual in-line stabilization of the cervical spine (Procedure 27-2).

To perform orotracheal intubation with in-line stabilization, follow these steps:

1. After basic manual and adjunctive airway manoeuvres, have your partner maintain in-line stabilization while kneeling at the patient's side, facing her head. This is done by placing both hands over the patient's ears with the little, ring, and middle fingers under the occiput, the index fingers anterior to the ears, and the thumbs on the face over the maxillary sinuses.

2. Apply slight pressure in a caudal direction (toward the feet) to support and immobilize the head.

3. Proceed gently with orotracheal intubation, keeping in mind the need to minimize movement of the cervical spine.

Rapid Sequence Intubation Your most immediate concern with every patient you treat is to maintain a patent airway and adequate oxygenation and ventilation. Clearly, if a patient is in cardiac or respiratory arrest or is unconscious or obtunded and not protecting her airway, endotracheal intubation is indicated. Quite commonly, however, you may have an awake patient, perhaps with significantly altered mental status, who is hypoxic even on 100-percent oxygen because of respiratory distress or a worsening airway disorder. This patient is working her hardest to breathe but does not have adequate gas exchange to support life. Her altered mental status indicates that some level of significant hypoxia is putting essential brain functions at risk.

You cannot perform orotracheal intubation on this patient until she fatigues enough to have respiratory failure, with resultant unconsciousness and decreased muscle tone. By then, however, she will have suffered prolonged hypoxia, possibly accompanied by myocardial infarction, brain damage, or vomiting with aspiration. If a patient clearly is precipitously failing in spite of maximal aggressive medical management, or if the history of her problem clearly indicates that she will not be able to or already cannot protect her airway, then active intervention is appropriate to control the airway and provide adequate ventilation. The safest way to do this is an advanced airway procedure called rapid sequence induction or **rapid sequence intubation** (RSI). Classic RSI is an anesthetic procedure whereby patients rapidly receive induction of general anesthesia followed by endotracheal intubation. In emergency medicine, we do not administer general anesthesia, but we have borrowed other elements of this technique in order to rapidly obtain an airway in a patient who has altered mental status. Although the term *rapid sequence induction* describes the classic procedure, it has been modified

Appropriate treatment of a trauma patient's other injuries is meaningless if you do not ensure a patent airway and adequate oxygenation and ventilation.

✱ **rapid sequence intubation** giving medications to sedate (induce) and temporarily paralyze a patient and then performing orotracheal intubation.

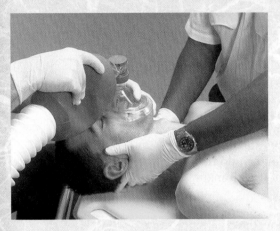

27-2a Hyperoxygenate the patient, and apply manual C-spine stabilization.

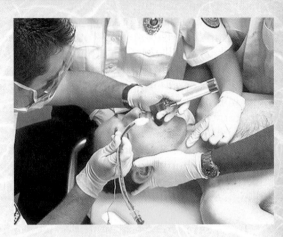

27-2b Apply Sellick's manoeuvre, and intubate.

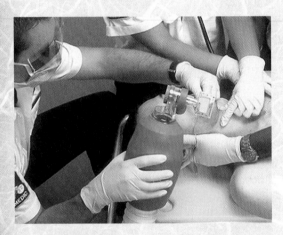

27-2c Ventilate the patient, and confirm placement.

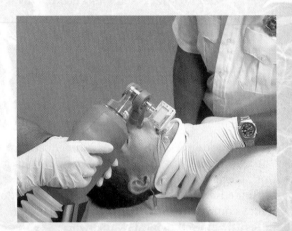

27-2d Secure the ETT, and place a cervical collar.

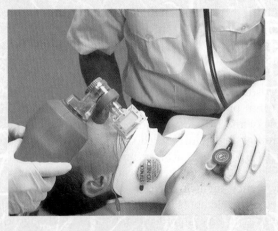

27-2e Reconfirm placement.

in the emergency medicine setting to *rapid sequence intubation*. Again, the difference is that the latter does not utilize a general anesthetic agent.

Rapid sequence intubation involves oxygenating the patient to the best level possible given her condition, monitoring carefully, and giving medications to induce (sedate) and temporarily paralyze the patient. You then proceed with orotracheal intubation in a controlled manner. Patients who are candidates for RSI are either awake, responsive, agitated, or combative or have a significant gag reflex, clenched teeth, or too much airway muscle tone to allow intubation. Indications for RSI include the following:

- Impending respiratory failure due to intrinsic pulmonary disease, such as COPD, CHF, asthma, or pneumonia

- Acute airway disorder that threatens airway patency, such as facial burns, laryngeal or upper airway trauma, and epiglottitis

- Altered mental status with significant risk of vomiting and aspiration, as in head trauma (a Glasgow Coma Scale score of 8 or less), drug or alcohol intoxication, status epilepticus

The basic physiology involved in RSI centres on the neuromuscular junction—the connection between peripheral nerves and skeletal muscle. Nerve impulses travel down the nerve and release a chemical (neurotransmitter) which stimulates (depolarizes) skeletal muscle, resulting in contraction. Acetylcholine is the primary neurotransmitter, and blocking its action results in relaxation of skeletal (voluntary) muscle. There are two ways to block the neuromuscular junction. Depolarizing agents substitute themselves into the neuromuscular junction in place of acetylcholine. They have a stimulating effect as they work, which produces fasciculations (generalized involuntary muscle twitching). Succinylcholine is a depolarizing agent and is the most commonly used paralytic agent for RSI. Nondepolarizing agents block the uptake of acetylcholine and do not allow stimulation of the muscle. Thus, they do not cause fasciculations. Vecuronium, atracurium, and pancuronium are typical examples of nondepolarizing neuromuscular blocking agents.

Paralyzing the patient causes complete muscular relaxation and allows you to take control of her precarious clinical condition. In addition to paralyzing the airway muscles, these agents also immobilize the respiratory muscles, and so the patient becomes apneic and requires mechanical ventilation. Esophageal and stomach muscles, and therefore sphincter tone, also relax, posing the risk of vomiting and aspiration. Succinylcholine (Anectine®), the agent preferred for neuromuscular blockade in emergency medical care, is a depolarizing drug. As mentioned, it causes fasciculations just before initiating paralysis. These fasciculations may increase the tendency to vomit and may increase intracranial pressure. Conditions that elevate serum potassium preclude the use of succinylcholine, which transiently increases serum potassium and thus can lead to life-threatening hyperkalemia. Side effects, which are dose related, include bradycardia and other dysrhythmias, as well as hypertension. The guidelines for using succinylcholine include the following:

- Dose: 1.5 mg/kg, IV bolus in adults; 2.0 mg/kg, IV bolus in children less than 10 years old

- Onset of action: 60–90 seconds

- Duration: 3–5 minutes

- Contraindications: penetrating eye injuries, patients with burns greater than eight hours' duration, massive crush injuries, and neurological injuries greater than one week out

Vecuronium (Norcuron) is a nondepolarizing agent; thus, it does not cause fasciculations. It is generally the second-line paralytic when succinylcholine is

Succinylcholine is the preferred neuromuscular blocking agent for emergency RSI.

Content Review

COMMON PARALYTIC AGENTS
- Succinylcholine
- Vecuronium
- Atracurium
- Pancuronium

contraindicated because vecuronium has fewer cardiac and hypotensive side effects than other nondepolarizing agents. In much smaller doses as a premedication, or priming dose, to succinylcholine or to a paralyzing dose of vecuronium, it effectively lessens or prevents fasciculations. It also blunts succinylcholine's bradycardic effect. This priming (or premedication) dose is given two minutes before the paralytic agent. Guidelines for using vecuronium include the following:

- Dose: 0.15 mg/kg IV bolus (paralyzing)
    0.01 mg/kg IV bolus (priming)
- Onset: 2–3 minutes
- Duration: 45 minutes

Atracurium (Tracrium) is a nondepolarizing paralytic useful for patients with kidney or liver disease because these conditions do not prolong its duration. Some patients experience hypotension from the histamine release that this drug causes. The usual dosage of 0.5 mg/kg IV has a duration of 20–30 minutes.

Pancuronium (Pavulon) is a nondepolarizing paralytic that has been used frequently in the past. The advantage of its relatively rapid onset (3–5 minutes), is offset by its major disadvantage, a long (60-minute) duration. It also produces tachycardia due to its effects on the heart. Better agents are currently available.

If you cannot intubate a paralyzed patient, she has no definitive airway. You must ventilate her mechanically for the duration of the paralysis (assuming you can mechanically maintain a patent airway). If the airway is lost during the procedure, you must be prepared to initiate a surgical airway (cricothyrotomy). Nothing works as fast as succinylcholine or is of as short a duration; therefore, it is the preferred neuromuscular blocking agent for emergency RSI.

Neuromuscular blocking agents do not affect mental status or pain sensation; therefore, you must use sedating and amnestic drugs to ease the awake, aware patient's anxiety and discomfort and to decrease her gag reflex, thereby increasing patient compliance and enhancing the ease of intubation. If the patient is already obtunded (from a drug overdose or head injury, for example), sedating her is pointless; omit that step. If the patient's injuries are causing significant pain and her clinical condition does not contraindicate their use, give small doses of pain medications as indicated.

When hypovolemia is present or when significant trauma is present with hypotension or a strong likelihood for hypotension, avoid induction agents that cause hypotension. Agents that blunt ICP response are good choices for the patient with head injury. Table 27-4 details general guidelines for common sedative (induction) agents. If you are able to identify that the patient has an allergy or sensitivity to a particular agent, you should not administer that agent.

Two other agents, atropine and lidocaine, are appropriate for use as premedication agents in RSI if indicated. Table 27-5 outlines their use.

Most patients with emergent airway conditions have eaten or drunk something within a few hours before the onset of their emergency conditions. Thus, you should consider every emergency patient to have a full stomach and be at risk of vomiting and aspiration. This is another reason that you should expediently intubate the patient after the onset of paralytic effect and apnea. Remember to always have a working suction device at the patient's side during airway manoeuvres. Likewise, application of Sellick's manoeuvre will help prevent aspiration.

To perform rapid sequence intubation, follow these steps:

1. Preoxygenate the patient with 100-percent oxygen using basic manual and adjunctive manoeuvres, and using a bag-valve mask if indicated.

Table 27-4 GUIDELINES FOR SEDATIVE (INDUCTION) AGENTS

Induction Agent	Dose	Onset	Duration (min)	Advantages	Disadvantages
Midazolam (Versed)	0.1–0.3 mg/kg	1–3 min	20–30 min	Amnesia effects, good sedative	Hypotension
Diazepam (Valium)	0.2–0.5 mg/kg	2–3 min	30–40 min	Amnesia effects	Hypotension, respiratory depression
Etomidate (Amidate)	0.3 mg/kg	1–2 min	5 min	Little effect on blood pressure, decreases intracranial pressure (ICP)	Suppresses cortisol → not good for head injured patients
Ketamine (Ketalar)	1–2 mg/kg	≤ 1 min	10–20 min	Decreases bronchospasm, little hypotension, amnesia	Increases ICP
Sodium Thiopental	3–5 mg/kg	≤ 1 min	5 min	Blunts ICP changes	Significant hypotension, bronchospasm
Propofol (Diprivan)	1–1.5 mg/kg	≤ 1 min	3–5 min	Rapid onset, good sedative effects	Significant hypotension
Fentanyl	3–5 µg/kg	1–2 min	30–40 min	Little effect on blood pressure; blunts ICP changes	Can cause muscle rigidity in chest wall

Table 27-5 ALTERNATIVE SEDATIVE (INDUCTION) AGENTS

Agent	Dose	Indication	Contraindication Precaution
Atropine	0.01-0.02 mg/kg (min.–max./0.1–0.4)	Pediatric patients, bradycardia	Cannot give less than 0.1 mg
Lidocaine	1 mg/kg	Head injury	Allergy

2. Prepare your equipment, supplies, and patient. In addition to the usual intubation equipment, be certain you have at least one, and preferably two, secure and working IV lines. Place the patient on a cardiac monitor and pulse oximeter. Draw the appropriate doses of medications into syringes and label them.

3. If the patient is alert, administer a sedative (induction) agent, such as midazolam (Versed) prior to administering any neuromuscular blocking agents.

4. Apply Sellick's manoeuvre (cricoid pressure), and maintain it until you confirm proper ETT placement.

5. According to local protocols, consider premedicating the patient with a priming dose of vecuronium. This is especially important in children, in whom fasciculations from succinylcholine can cause musculoskeletal trauma. Also, if indicated in local protocols, consider premedicating with lidocaine and atropine.

6. Paralyze the patient, administering succinylcholine 1.5 mg/kg IV bolus, and continue oxygenation. Alternatively, vecuronium (Norcuron) can be used as a blocking agent. It has a slower onset of action.

7. Once adequate relaxation is obtained, insert the ETT through the patient's vocal cords at the onset of apnea and jaw relaxation, using the orotracheal intubation procedure previously explained. Because you have preoxygenated the patient, bag-valve-mask ventilation is generally not indicated before the first intubation attempt, unless prolonged. Not ventilating the patient at this juncture will help prevent gastric distention and regurgitation. If you are unable to pass the tube after 20–30 seconds, stop, hyperoxygenate the patient with 100-percent oxygen for two minutes, and then try again. Remember that the patient's lower esophageal sphincter tone is decreased, and so ventilating during paralysis makes gastric distention and vomiting more likely, even with cricoid pressure. Your goal is to rapidly place the ETT properly in the trachea to minimize these complications, but do not avoid bag-valve-mask hyperoxygenation with 100-percent oxygen in the hypoxic patient.

8. Confirm proper placement of the ETT into the trachea. Inflate the distal cuff, ventilate with a bag-valve device with a CO_2 detector attached, and look for the appropriate colour change. Watch for the chest to rise and fall with ventilations. Auscultate with each ventilation for bilateral breath sounds over the chest and no gastric sounds over the stomach.

9. Release Sellick's manoeuvre.

10. Insert a bite block device, secure the ETT in place, reconfirm placement, and continue ventilating the patient. Continually assess the patient's condition, and recheck ETT placement.

11. Check with medical direction or follow your local protocol for indications for continuing paralysis with vecuronium during transport. This will depend largely on your patient's medical condition, her combativeness after the paralytic and induction agents wear off, and your anticipated transport time to the hospital.

Retrograde Intubation

Walters first described retrograde intubation in 1963 for use in patients with a drastically altered airway. This is also referred to in some literature as the Seldinger technique, so called because the Seldinger guide wires may be used. Indications for use include the patient with facial trauma and a suspected neck injury or patients in whom vomitus or bloody drainage obstructs the view or obscures the light in standard intubation. In these patients, blind nasotracheal intubation is not recommended, and there is concern with orotracheal intubation with movement of the head and cervical spine.

Retrograde intubation is accomplished by passing a needle and threaded long wire stylet through the cricoid membrane cephalad (toward the head) the vocal cords. When the guide wire reaches the oropharynx, it is retrieved, and the endotracheal tube is placed over the guide wire and then passed into the trachea past the vocal cords. The technique is no different in the child from that in the adult.

This techniques does take time to perform and is not considered a first- or even second-line airway management tool. Complications of this procedure are related to the needle stick, and bleeding may occur due to trauma caused by the guide wire. This procedure is not used routinely in EMS or in the emergency department.

Pediatric Intubation

Pediatric airway emergencies generally produce more anxiety than adult emergencies among both medical care providers and family. It is important to take appropriate steps to separate the parent from the pediatric patient with significant respiratory distress or apnea in order to effectively manage the airway. While the indications, procedures, and precautions for airway management in children are fundamentally the same as in adults, you must take additional precautions and remember several significant differences. These concerns revolve around variances in anatomy, as discussed in Chapter 12. A review of the anatomical features of the pediatric airway is given below:

- The structures are proportionally smaller and more flexible than an adult's.
- The tongue is larger in relation to the oropharynx.
- The epiglottis is floppy and round ("omega" shaped).
- The glottic opening is higher and more anterior in the neck.
- The vocal cords slant upward, toward the back of the head, and are closer to the base of the tongue.
- The narrowest part of the airway is the cricoid cartilage, not the glottic opening as in adults.

A straight laryngoscope blade is preferred for most pediatric patients, although straight or curved may be useful for adolescents. Also, selecting the appropriate tube diameter for children is critical. Too large a tube can cause tracheal edema and/or damage to the vocal cords, while too small a tube may not allow exchange of adequate ventilatory volumes. Table 27-6 lists general guidelines for selecting ETT size according to the child's age. Another guide for children's sizes is:

$$\text{ETT size (mm)} = (\text{Age in years} + 16) \div 4$$

or

$$\text{ETT size (mm)} = (\text{Age in years} \div 4) + 4$$

Correct tube size for an eight-year-old, for instance, would be $(8 + 16) \div 4$, or 6 mm. You can also measure tube size by matching it to the diameter of the child's smallest finger. Usually, you will use noncuffed endotracheal tubes with infants and children under the age of eight years because the round narrowing of these patients' cricoid cartilage forms a suitable cuff.

The depth of insertion of the distal tip for pediatric endotracheal tubes should be 2–3 cm below the vocal cords, as deeper insertion may result in mainstem intubation or injury to the carina. The uncuffed ETT has a black glottic marker at its distal end that should be placed at the level of the vocal cords. The cuffed ETT should be placed so that the cuff is just below the vocal cords. For detailed guidelines regarding depth of insertion for different age groups, refer to Table 27-6. Alternatively, you can use the formula $(3 \times \text{ETT inside diameter}) - 1$.

Table 27-6 APPROXIMATE SIZE OF ETT FOR PEDIATRIC PATIENTS

Patient's Age	ETT Size	Type	Depth of ETT Insertion	Laryngoscope Blade Size
Premature infant	2.5–3.0	Uncuffed	8 cm	0 straight
Full-term infant	3.0–3.5	Uncuffed	8–9.5 cm	1 straight
Infant to one year	3.5–4.0	Uncuffed	9.5–11 cm	1 straight
Toddler	4.0–5.0	Uncuffed	11–12.5 cm	1–2 straight
Preschool	5.0–5.5	Uncuffed	12.5–14 cm	2 straight
School aged	5.5–6.5	Uncuffed	14–20 cm	2 straight
Adolescent	7.0–8.0	Cuffed	20–23 cm	3 straight or curved

Also, remember that infants and small children have greater vagal tone than adults. Therefore, laryngoscopy and passage of an endotracheal tube are more likely to precipitate a vagal response, dramatically slowing the child's heart rate and decreasing cardiac output and blood pressure. If heart rate falls below 60 beats per minute (or below 80 beats per minute in an infant), stop the procedure, and reinitiate ventilations with 100-percent oxygen.

The indications for endotracheal intubation in a pediatric patient are the same as those for adults:

- When ventilatory support with a bag-valve mask is inadequate
- Cardiac or respiratory arrest
- When it is necessary to provide a route for drug administration (NAVEL) or ready access to the airway for suctioning
- When prolonged artificial ventilation is needed

Additionally, if local protocols allow, you may use endotracheal intubation in a child with epiglottitis if her condition is rapidly deteriorating.

To perform endotracheal intubation on a pediatric patient, follow these guidelines (Procedure 27-3):

1. After initiating basic manual and adjunctive manoeuvres, hyperoxygenate the patient with 100-percent oxygen, using the appropriately sized bag-valve mask.

2. Prepare and check your equipment. As stated earlier, a straight blade laryngoscope is usually preferred in infants and small children, since it provides greater displacement of the tongue and better visualization of the relatively cephalad and anterior epiglottis. Also, with children younger than eight years old, use an uncuffed endotracheal tube. Due to the short distance between the mouth and the trachea, you rarely need a stylet to position the tube properly. Remember to lubricate the ETT with water-soluble gel.

3. Place the patient's head and neck in an appropriate position. You should maintain a pediatric patient's head in a sniffing position (perhaps by placing a towel under her head) unless you know of or suspect trauma. In case of trauma, proceed with manual in-line stabilization of the cervical spine.

4. Have your partner apply gentle cricoid pressure (Sellick's manoeuvre).

5. Hold the laryngoscope in your left hand, and insert it gently into the right side of the patient's mouth. With a sweeping action, displace the tongue to the left.

6. Move the blade slightly toward the midline, and then advance it until the distal end reaches the base of the tongue.

7. Look for the tip of the epiglottis, and position the laryngoscope properly. Keep in mind that a child—particularly an infant—has a shorter airway and a higher glottis than an adult. Because of this, you may see the cords much sooner than you expect.

8. If you cannot see the glottis, bring the blade gently and slowly out until the vocal cords come into view. Lift the epiglottis gently with the tip of the laryngoscope. Be certain not to use the teeth or gums as a fulcrum.

9. Grasp the endotracheal tube in your right hand, and under direct visualization of the vocal cords, insert it through the right corner

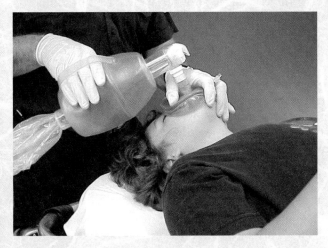

27-3a Hyperoxygenate the child.

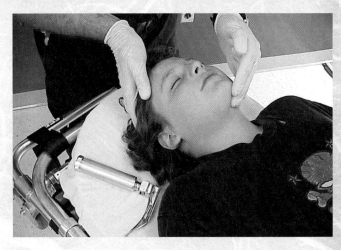

27-3b Position the head.

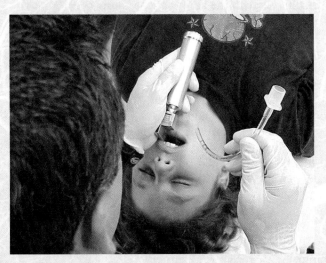

27-3c Insert the laryngoscope.

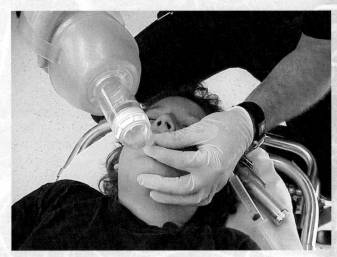

27-3d Insert the ETT and ventilate the child.

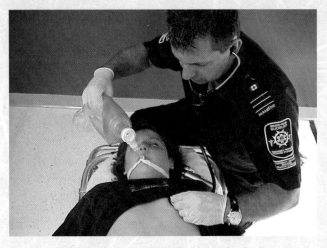

27-3e Confirm placement and secure the ETT.

of the patient's mouth into the glottic opening. Pass it through until the distal 10 mm or distal cuff of the ETT disappears 2–3 cm beyond the vocal cords. In some cases, advancing an ETT will be difficult at the level of the cricoid. Do not force the ETT through this region, as it may cause laryngeal edema and bleeding.

10. Hold the tube in place with your left hand, attach an infant- or child-sized bag-valve device to the 15/22-mm connector, and deliver several breaths, checking for proper tube placement. Watch for the chest to rise and fall symmetrically with each ventilation. Auscultate for equal, bilateral breath sounds at the lateral chest wall, high in the axilla. Breath sounds over the epigastrium should be absent with ventilations. The patient should improve clinically, with pinker colour and increased heart rate. Additionally, use the end-tidal CO_2 detector as previously discussed.

11. If the tube has a distal cuff, inflate it with just enough air to prevent any air leaks.

12. Secure the ETT with tape or a commercial device as with an adult patient, note placement of distance marker at teeth/gums, recheck for proper placement, and continue ventilatory support. Periodically reassess ETT placement, and watch the patient carefully for any clinical signs of difficulty. As with the adult patient, allow no more than 30 seconds to pass without ventilating your patient.

NASOTRACHEAL INTUBATION

✱ **nasotracheal route** through the nose and into the trachea.

The orotracheal route is usually preferred for intubation as it affords more control over the airway. In a few circumstances, however, the **nasotracheal route** (through the nose and into the trachea) may be useful. As a rule this is a "blind" procedure without direct visualization of the vocal cords. To perform nasotracheal intubations, you can often visualize the vocal cords with a laryngoscope and guide the ETT with Magill forceps. But if this is possible, orotracheal intubation is generally feasible and preferred. Potential indications for blind nasotracheal intubation include the following:

* Possible spinal injury
* Clenched teeth, preventing opening the patient's mouth
* Fractured jaw, oral injuries, or recent oral surgery
* Significant angioedema (facial and airway swelling)
* Obesity
* Arthritis, preventing placement in the sniffing position

Nasotracheal intubation is not recommended in the following situations:

* Suspected nasal fractures
* Suspected basilar skull fractures
* Significantly deviated nasal septum or other nasal obstruction
* Cardiac or respiratory arrest
* Unresponsive patient

Advantages of Nasotracheal Intubation When the patient's condition indicates its use, nasotracheal intubation offers the following advantages:

* The head and neck can remain in neutral position.

- It does not produce as much gag response and is better tolerated by the awake patient.
- It can be secured more easily than an orotracheal tube.
- The patient cannot bite the ETT.

Disadvantages of Nasotracheal Intubation The following disadvantages of nasotracheal intubation discourage its use unless clearly indicated by the patient's condition:

- It is more difficult and time consuming to perform than orotracheal intubation.
- It is potentially more traumatic for patients. Passage of the tube may lacerate the pharyngeal mucosa or larynx during insertion.
- The tube may kink or clog more easily than an orally placed endotracheal tube.
- It poses a greater risk of infection because the ETT introduces nasal bacteria into the trachea.
- Improper placement is more likely when performing blind nasotracheal intubation, as the tube's passage through the glottic opening cannot be visualized.
- Blind nasotracheal intubation requires that the patient be breathing.

Nasotracheal Intubation Technique To perform blind nasotracheal intubation, follow these steps (Figure 27-45):

1. Using basic manual and adjunctive manoeuvres, open the airway and ventilate the patient with 100-percent oxygen.
2. Prepare your equipment, and place the patient supine. If you suspect cervical spine injury, maintain the head and neck in neutral position with manual in-line stabilization.
3. Inspect the nose, and select the larger nostril as your passageway.

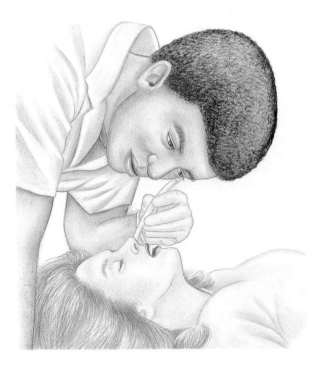

FIGURE 27-45 Blind naso-tracheal intubation.

4. Apply topical anesthesia or topical lidocaine in each nostril.

5. Insert the ETT into the nostril, with the bevel along the floor of the nostril or facing the nasal septum. This will help avoid damage to the turbinates. Next, gently guide the ETT from anterior to posterior.

6. As you feel the tube drop into the posterior pharynx, listen closely at its proximal end for the patient's respiratory sounds. These sounds are loudest when the ETT is proximal to the epiglottis. When the ETT's tip reaches the posterior pharyngeal wall, you must take care to direct it toward the glottic opening. At this point, the tip of the ETT may catch in the pyriform sinus. If it does, you will feel resistance, and the skin on either side of the Adam's apple will tent. To resolve pyriform sinus placement, slightly withdraw the ETT, and rotate it to the midline.

7. With the patient's next inhaled breath, advance the ETT gently but quickly into the glottic opening. Continue passing the ETT until the distal cuff is just past the vocal cords. At this point, the patient may cough, buck, or strain. Gagging or vocal sounds are signs of esophageal placement, while slight bulging and anterior displacement of the larynx usually indicate correct tracheal placement. When you place the ETT correctly in the trachea, you will see the patient's exhaled air as condensation in the ETT and feel it coming from the proximal end of the ETT.

8. Holding the ETT with one hand to prevent displacement, inflate the distal cuff with 5–10 mL of air, connect a bag-valve device with an ETCO$_2$ detector attached, hyperoxygenate the patient with 100-percent oxygen, and confirm proper placement of the ETT. Observe the chest rise and fall with ventilations, auscultate breath sounds over the chest bilaterally, and verify no gastric sounds with each ventilation.

9. Secure the ETT, and reconfirm proper placement. Continue to observe the patient's condition, maintain ventilatory support, and frequently recheck ETT placement.

Field Extubation

Infrequently, an intubated patient will awaken and be intolerant of the ETT. This happens most often with respiratory distress patients who undergo rapid sequence intubation (RSI). When the paralytic medications wear off and they awaken from the induction medications, they may struggle against the intubation and ventilation. This usually indicates sedation and, perhaps, repeat paralysis, as extubation will cause continued respiratory distress with loss of a definitive airway. If the patient is clearly able to maintain and protect her airway and accomplish adequate spontaneous respirations and is not under the influence of any sedating agents, and if reassessment indicates the problem that led to endotracheal intubation is resolved, extubation may be indicated. However, you must consider the high risk of laryngospasm, involuntary closure of the glottis on extubation, especially in the awake patient. Laryngospasm may prohibit successful reintubation attempts. Additionally, in repeat attempts at rapid sequence intubation, the medications will produce variable responses and will not ensure relaxation of the laryngospasm. The need for field extubation is extremely rare.

To perform field extubation, follow these steps:

1. Continue blood and body fluid precautions. Ensure patient's oxygenation. A crude method for accomplishing this in the field

is to be certain that the patient's mental status, skin colour, and pulse oximetry are optimal on room air with the ETT in place.

2. Prepare intubation equipment and suction.
3. Confirm patient responsiveness.
4. Suction the patient's oropharynx.
5. Deflate the ETT cuff.
6. Remove the ETT on cough or expiration.
7. Provide supplemental oxygen as indicated.
8. Reassess the adequacy of the patient's ventilation and oxygenation.

ESOPHAGEAL TRACHEAL COMBITUBE

The **Esophageal Tracheal CombiTube** (ETC) is a dual-lumen airway with a ventilation port for each **lumen.** The longer, blue port is the distal port; the shorter, clear port is the proximal port, which terminates in the hypopharynx. The ETC has two inflatable cuffs—a 15-mL cuff just proximal to the distal port and a 100-mL cuff just distal to the proximal port.

The ETC is inserted blindly through the mouth into the posterior oropharynx and then gently advanced. Upon insertion, the tube may enter the trachea or the esophagus, and should be inserted so that the black marks on the ETC are aligned with the patient's teeth. This will position the large cuff in the posterior pharynx (Figures 27-46 and 27-47). To determine which port has entered the trachea and is to be ventilated, first ventilate the longer external port, since esophageal insertion is highly likely. Now auscultate the chest. If you hear breath sounds over the chest and none over the stomach, continue ventilating through the longer external port. If you hear ventilation sounds over the stomach without breath sounds over the chest, stop ventilating through the longer port and at-

✱ **Esophageal Tracheal CombiTube** dual-lumen airway with a ventilation port for each lumen.

✱ **lumen** the tunnel through a tube.

Content Review

INTUBATION DEVICES

- Endotracheal tube (ETT)
- Esophageal Tracheal CombiTube (ETC)
- Laryngeal mask airway (LMA)
- Pharyngo-tracheal lumen airway (PtL)

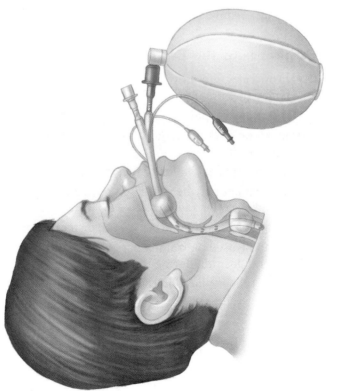

FIGURE 27-46 ETC airway—tracheal placement.

FIGURE 27-47   ETC airway—
esophageal placement.

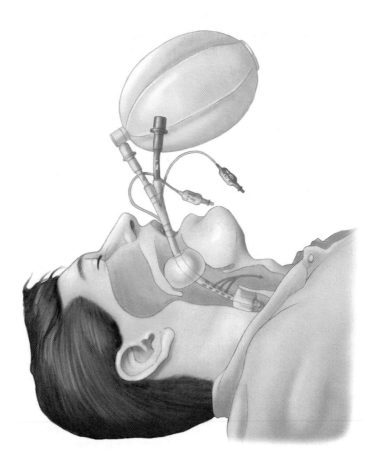

tach the bag-valve device to the shorter port. The distal cuff isolates the distal
port, and the larger proximal cuff isolates the proximal port, encouraging air
that is insufflated into the hypopharynx to enter the trachea.

Advantages of the Esophageal Tracheal CombiTube

- It provides alternative airway control when conventional intubation
  techniques are unsuccessful or unavailable.
- Insertion is rapid and easy.
- Insertion does not require visualization of the larynx or special
  equipment.
- The pharyngeal balloon anchors the airway behind the hard palate.
- The patient may be ventilated regardless of tube placement
  (esophageal or tracheal).
- It significantly diminishes gastric distention and regurgitation.
- It can be used on trauma patients, since the neck can remain in
  neutral position during insertion and use.
- If the tube is placed in the esophagus, gastric contents can be
  suctioned for decompression through the distal port.

Disadvantages of the Esophageal Tracheal CombiTube

- Maintaining adequate mask seal is difficult.
- Suctioning tracheal secretions is impossible when the airway is in the
  esophagus.

- Placing an endotracheal tube is very difficult with the ETC in place.
- It cannot be used in conscious patients or in those with a gag reflex.
- The cuffs can cause esophageal, tracheal, and hypopharyngeal ischemia.
- It does not isolate and completely protect the trachea.
- It cannot be used in patients with esophageal disease or caustic ingestions.
- It cannot be used with pediatric patients.
- Placement of the CombiTube is not foolproof—errors can be made if assessment skills are not adequate.

Inserting the Esophageal Tracheal CombiTube

To insert the Esophageal Tracheal CombiTube, follow these steps:

1. Complete basic manual and adjunctive manoeuvres, and provide supplemental oxygen and ventilatory support with a bag-valve mask and hyperventilation.
2. Place the patient supine, and kneel at the top of her head.
3. Prepare and check the equipment.
4. Place the patient's head in neutral position. Stabilize the cervical spine if cervical injury is possible.
5. Insert the ETC gently at midline through the oropharynx, using a tongue-jaw-lift manoeuvre, and advance it past the hypopharynx to the depth indicated by the markings on the tube. The black rings on the tube should be between the patient's teeth.
6. Inflate the pharyngeal cuff with 100 mL of air and the distal cuff with 10–15 mL of air.
7. Ventilate through the longer blue proximal port with a bag-valve device connected to 100-percent oxygen while auscultating over the chest and stomach. If you hear bilateral breath sounds over the chest and none over the stomach, secure the tube, and continue ventilating.
8. If you hear gastric sounds over the chest instead of breath sounds, change ports, and ventilate through the clear connector. Confirm breath sounds over the chest with no gastric sounds. Use multiple confirmation techniques as previously discussed (visualize, auscultate, use $ETCO_2$ detector, monitor clinical improvement).
9. Secure the tube and continue ventilating with 100-percent oxygen.
10. Frequently reassess the airway and adequacy of ventilation.

Laryngeal Mask Airway

The laryngeal mask airway (LMA) may assist with ventilations in the unconscious patient without laryngeal reflexes when tracheal intubation is unsuccessful. It has an inflatable distal end (similar to a face mask) that is placed in the hypopharynx and then inflated (Figure 27-48). A bag-valve device at the proximal end assists respirations (similar to an endotracheal tube). The LMA can be disposable and comes in various sizes. Its blind insertion requires less skill and training than does endotracheal intubation. The LMA's disadvantage is that it does not isolate the trachea; therefore, it does not protect the airway from regurgitation and aspiration. Also, it cannot be used in a patient who has a gag re-

FIGURE 27-48   Laryngeal mask airway.

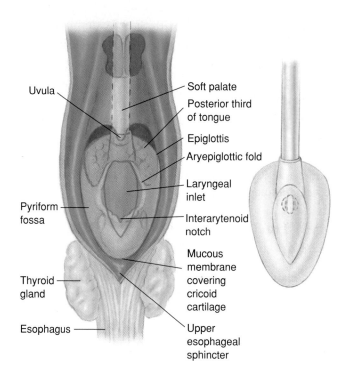

Uvula

Soft palate

Posterior third of tongue

Epiglottis

Aryepiglottic fold

Laryngeal inlet

Pyriform fossa

Interarytenoid notch

Mucous membrane covering cricoid cartilage

Thyroid gland

Esophagus

Upper esophageal sphincter

flex or is semiconscious. You must weigh these disadvantages against the benefits of establishing a patent airway.

PHARYNGO-TRACHEAL LUMEN AIRWAY

✱ pharyngo-tracheal lumen airway (PtL) is a two tube system.

The **pharyngo-tracheal lumen airway** (PtL) is a two-tube system (Figure 27-49). The first tube is short, with a large diameter; its proximal end is green. A large cuff encircles the tube's lower third. When inflated, the cuff seals the entire oropharynx. Air introduced at this tube's proximal end will enter the hypopharynx. The second tube is long, with a small diameter, and clear. It passes through and extends approximately 10 cm beyond the first tube. This second tube may be inserted blindly into either the trachea or the esophagus. A distal cuff, when inflated, seals off whichever anatomical structure the tube has entered. When the second tube enters the trachea, you will ventilate the patient through it.

Each of the PtL's tubes has a 15/22-mm connector at its proximal end, allowing the attachment of a standard ventilatory device. A semi-rigid plastic stylet in the clear plastic tube allows redirection of the oropharyngeal cuff, while the other cuff remains inflated. An adjustable, cloth neck strap holds the tube in place. When the long, clear tube is in the esophagus, deflating the cuff in the oropharynx allows you to move the device to the left side of the patient's mouth. This may permit endotracheal intubation while continuing esophageal occlusion. However, placement of an endotracheal tube with a PtL already in place is difficult at best.

Advantages of the Pharyngo-Tracheal Lumen Airway

- It can function in either the tracheal or esophageal position.
- It has no face mask to seal.
- It does not require direct visualization of the larynx and thus does not require the use of a laryngoscope or additional specialized equipment.

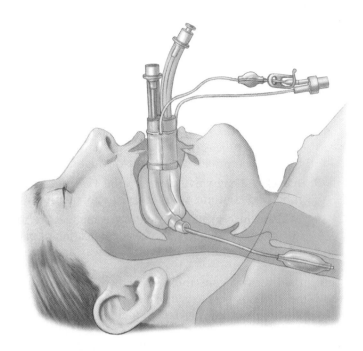

FIGURE 27-49 Pharyngo-tracheal lumen airway.

- It can be used in trauma patients, since the neck can remain in neutral position during insertion and use.
- It helps protect the trachea from upper airway bleeding and secretions.

Disdvantages of the Pharyngo-Tracheal Lumen Airway

- It does not isolate and completely protect the trachea from aspiration.
- The oropharyngeal balloon can migrate out of the mouth anteriorly, partially dislodging the airway.
- Intubation around the PtL is extremely difficult, even with the oropharyngeal balloon deflated.
- It cannot be used in conscious patients or those with a gag reflex.
- It cannot be used in pediatric patients.
- It can only be inserted orally.

Inserting the Pharyngo-Tracheal Lumen Airway

To insert the pharyngo-tracheal lumen airway, follow these steps:

1. Complete basic manual and adjunctive manoeuvres and provide supplemental oxygen and ventilatory support with a bag-valve mask and hyperoxygenation.
2. Place the patient supine, and kneel at the top of her head.
3. Prepare and check the equipment.
4. Place the patient's head in the appropriate position. Hyperextend the neck if there is no risk of cervical spine injury. Maintain neutral position with stabilization of the cervical spine if cervical spine injury is possible.
5. Insert the PtL gently, using the tongue-jaw-lift manoeuvre.

6. Inflate the distal cuffs on both PtL tubes simultaneously with a sustained breath into the inflation valve.

7. Deliver a breath into the green oropharyngeal tube. If the patient's chest rises and you auscultate bilateral breath sounds, the long clear tube is in the esophagus. Inflate the pharyngeal balloon, and continue ventilations via the green tube.

8. If the chest does not rise and you auscultate no breath sounds, the long clear tube is in the trachea. Remove the stylet from the clear tube, and ventilate the patient through that tube.

9. Attach the bag-valve device to the 15-mm connector, secure the tube, and continue ventilatory support with 100-percent oxygen.

10. Multiple placement confirmation techniques are again essential, as are good assessment skills. Misidentification of placement has been reported. Frequently reassess the airway and adequacy of ventilation.

If the patient regains consciousness or if the protective airway reflexes return, remove the PtL. It is best to remove the PtL before endotracheal intubation. Complications of PtL placement include the following:

- Pharyngeal or esophageal trauma from poor technique
- Unrecognized displacement of the long tube from the trachea into the esophagus
- Displacement of the pharyngeal balloon

FOREIGN BODY REMOVAL UNDER DIRECT LARYNGOSCOPY

Direct visualization of the larynx with a laryngoscope may enable you to remove an obstructing foreign body using Magill forceps or a suction device (Figure 27-50). Initially, you should carry out basic life support manoeuvres for airway obstruction, including the Heimlich manoeuvre, finger sweep, and chest thrust. As you recall from your basic training, the Heimlich manoeuvre involves initiating a forceful upward thrust with your fist on the choking patient's abdomen, halfway between the umbilicus and the xiphoid process. Use suction as indicated. If these fail to alleviate the obstruction, direct visualization of the airway for foreign body removal is indicated. The procedure for visualizing the airway is identical to that used for orotracheal intubation.

SURGICAL AIRWAYS

* **needle cricothyrostomy** surgical airway technique that inserts a 14-gauge needle into the trachea at the cricothyroid membrane.

* **open cricothyrotomy** surgical airway technique that places an endotracheal or tracheostomy tube directly into the trachea through a surgical incision at the cricothyroid membrane.

With proper training and frequent practice, you will be able to secure most airways in the field by endotracheal intubation. Occasionally, however, extreme circumstances prohibit successful endotracheal intubation. In such incidents, resort to the basic principles of airway management with the use of an airway adjunct and a bag-valve mask. Although not routinely used by PCPs or ACPs in Canada but rather by CCPs and in hospital emergency rooms, a surgical airway technique may be the only way to ensure a patient's survival. Two different techniques, **needle cricothyrostomy** (also called translaryngeal cannula ventilation) and **open cricothyrotomy,** both provide access to the airway through the cricothyroid membrane. A needle cricothyrostomy is generally the easier procedure but makes providing adequate ventilation more difficult; an open cricothyrotomy is the more difficult procedure but allows for more effective oxygenation and ventilation.

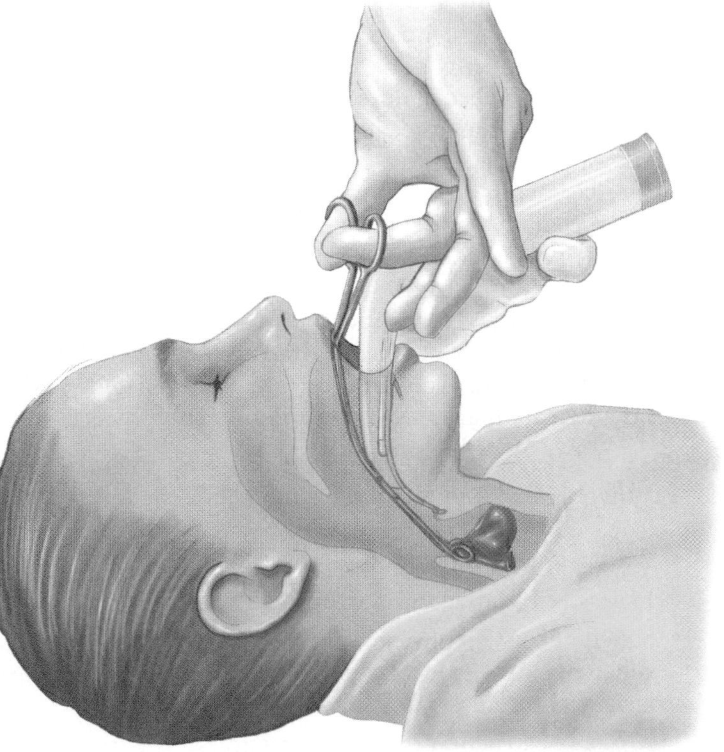

FIGURE 27-50 Foreign body removal with direct visualization and Magill forceps.

Surgical airway procedures should only be attemped after you have exhausted your other airway skills and have decided that no other means will establish an airway. Even when performed correctly, these procedures are highly invasive and prone to complications, which you must recognize and treat immediately. The major long-term complication, tracheal **stenosis,** can cause difficulty if the patient requires intubation at some point in the future. You must master the skills for performing surgical airways and continually practise them under the direct supervision of the physician medical director, who should determine that you can perform the technique and that you understand and can treat its possible complications.

Indications that warrant a surgical cricothyrotomy include problems that prevent intubating or ventilating a patient by the nasal or oral routes. Massive facial or neck trauma is the most common cause. Some cases involve so much facial or airway distortion that you cannot identify normal landmarks. Other indications of a surgical cricothyrotomy include total upper airway obstruction due to epiglottitis, severe anaphylaxis, burns to the face and respiratory tract, posterior laceration of the tongue, or the inability to open the mouth. You can perform surgical airways with the patient's head and neck in neutral position. Contraindications to performing surgical airways in the field include inability to identify anatomical landmarks (including trauma and short, thick necks), crush injury to the larynx, tracheal transection, and underlying anatomical abnormalities, such as trauma, tumour, or subglottic stenosis.

Needle Cricothyrostomy

Though it is an invasive surgical procedure that you must master before performing it in the field, a needle cricothyrostomy is technically easier to accomplish than

✱ stenosis narrowing or constriction.

The only indication for a surgical airway is the inability to establish an airway by any other method.

an open cricothyrotomy and has a lower complication rate. It can be rapidly performed, does not manipulate the cervical spine, and provides adequate ventilation when performed properly. It is a temporary airway, used until a larger diameter, definitive airway is provided. It does not interfere with subsequent intubation attempts because it uses a 14-gauge needle, which has a relatively small diameter so that an ETT can pass beside it. However, because the catheter does not fill the tracheal diameter, needle cricothyrostomy cannot protect the patient against aspiration.

This procedure requires different oxygenation and ventilation techniques than other airway manoeuvres. Transtracheal jet insufflation (ventilation) uses a high-pressure jet ventilator to force oxygen through the small-diameter catheter and provide adequate oxygenation and ventilation. Because very high pressures insufflate large volumes of oxygen, **barotrauma**, including pneumothorax, is a potential complication. This procedure is not indicated if exhalation is not possible or if adequate high-pressure ventilation equipment is not available.

Needle Cricothyrostomy Complications The potential complications of needle cricothyrostomy with jet ventilation include the following:

- Barotrauma from overinflation
- Excessive bleeding due to improper catheter placement
- Subcutaneous emphysema from improper placement into the subcutaneous tissue, excessive air leak around the catheter, or laryngeal trauma
- Airway obstruction from compression of the trachea secondary to excessive bleeding or subcutaneous air
- Hypoventilation from use of improper equipment, incorrect use of the jet ventilator, or misplacement of the catheter

Needle Cricothyrostomy Technique To perform needle cricothyrostomy with jet ventilation, follow these steps:

1. Place the patient supine, and hyperextend the head and neck (maintain neutral position if you suspect cervical spine injury). Position yourself at the patient's side. Manage the patient's airway with basic manoeuvres and supplemental oxygen, and prepare your equipment.

2. Gently palpate the inferior portion of the thyroid cartilage and the cricoid cartilage. The indention between the two is the cricothyroid membrane (Figures 27-51 and 27-52).

3. Prepare the anterior neck with povidone-iodine swabs. Firmly grasp the laryngeal cartilages, and reconfirm the site of the cricothyroid membrane.

4. Attach a large-bore IV needle, with a catheter (adults: 14- or 16-gauge; pediatrics: 18- or 20-gauge) to a 10- or 20-mL syringe. Carefully insert the needle into the cricothyroid membrane at midline, directed 45 degrees caudally (toward the feet) (Figure 27-53). Often, you will feel a pop as the needle penetrates the membrane.

5. Advance the needle no more than 1 cm, and then aspirate with the syringe. If air returns easily, the catheter is in the trachea. If blood returns or you feel resistance to return, reevaluate needle placement. After you confirm proper placement, hold the needle steady, and advance the catheter. Then, withdraw the needle (Figure 27-54).

6. Reconfirm placement by again withdrawing air from the catheter with the syringe. Secure the catheter in place (Figure 27-55).

*barotrauma injury caused by pressure within an enclosed space.

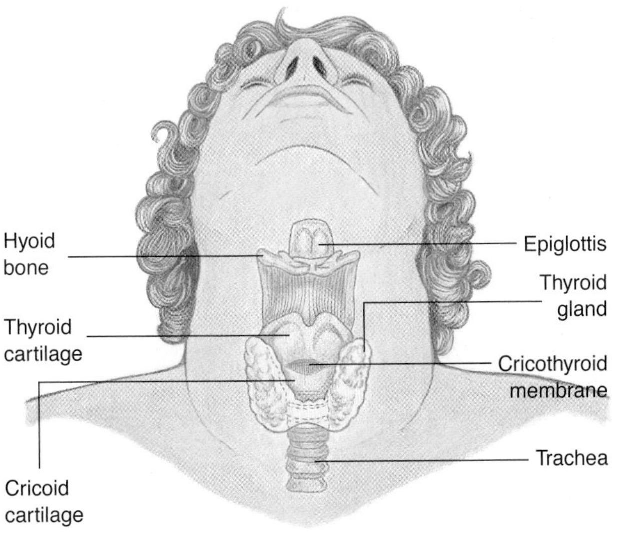

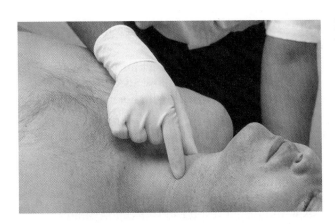

FIGURE 27-51   Anatomical landmarks for cricothyrostomy.

Hyoid bone

Thyroid cartilage

Cricoid cartilage

Epiglottis

Thyroid gland

Cricothyroid membrane

Trachea

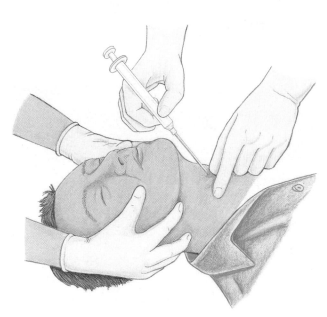

FIGURE 27-52   Locate/palpate the cricothyroid membrane.

FIGURE 27-53   Proper positioning for cricothyroid puncture.

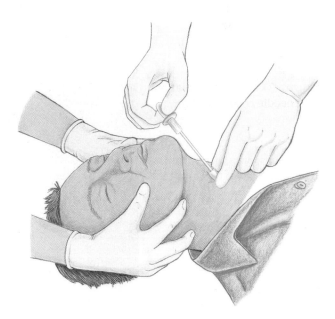

FIGURE 27-54   Advance the catheter with the needle.

FIGURE 27-55 Cannula
properly placed in the trachea.

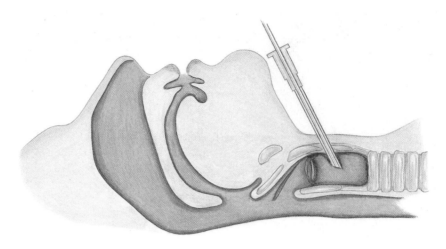

7. Check for adequacy of ventilations. Look for chest rise with each ventilation, and listen for bilateral breath sounds in the chest. If spontaneous ventilations are absent or inadequate, begin transtracheal jet ventilation.

8. Connect one end of the oxygen tubing to the catheter and the other end to the jet ventilator.

9. Open the release valve to introduce an oxygen jet into the trachea (Figure 27-56). Then adjust the pressure to allow adequate lung expansion (usually about 50 psi, compared with about 1 psi through a regulator).

10. Watch the chest carefully, turning off the release valve as soon as the chest rises. Exhalation then occurs passively through the glottis due to the elastic recoil of the lungs and chest wall. Deliver at least 20 breaths per minute to ensure adequate oxygenation and ventilation. The inflation-to-deflation time ratio should be approximately 1:2, as with normal respirations. Keep in mind that you may need to adjust this to the patient's needs, particularly in COPD and asthma patients, who often require a longer expiration time.

FIGURE 27-56 Jet ventilation with needle cricothryrotomy.

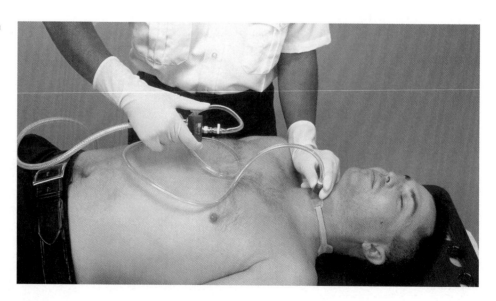

11. Continue ventilatory support, assessing for adequacy of ventilations and looking for the development of any potential complications.

Open Cricothyrotomy

An open cricothyrotomy is preferred to needle cricothyrostomy when a complete obstruction prevents a glottic route for expiration. Indications are the same as for needle cricothyrostomy. It involves obtaining an airway by placing an endotracheal or tracheostomy tube directly into the trachea through a surgical incision at the cricothyroid membrane. It can be rapidly performed and does not manipulate the cervical spine. Its greater potential complications mandate even more training and skills monitoring than with the needle method.

Contraindications are the same as for needle cricothyrostomy. Additionally, open cricothyrotomy is contraindicated in children under the age of 12 because the cricothyroid membrane is small and underdeveloped in them.

Cricothyrotomy Complications Complications that can occur with this invasive procedure include:

- Incorrect tube placement into a false passage
- Cricoid and/or thyroid cartilage damage
- Thyroid gland damage
- Severe bleeding
- Laryngeal nerve damage
- Subcutaneous emphysema
- Vocal cord damage
- Infection

Open Cricothyrotomy Technique To perform an open cricothyrotomy, follow these steps (Procedure 27-4):

1. Locate the thyroid cartilage and the cricoid cartilage. Find the cricothyroid membrane between the two cartilages.
2. Clean the area with iodine-containing solution if time permits, while your partner sets up suction, pulse oximetry, and cardiac monitor.
3. Stabilize the cartilages with one hand while using a scalpel in the other hand to make a 1- to 2-cm vertical skin incision over the membrane.
4. Find the cricothyroid membrane again, and make a 1-cm incision in the horizontal plane through the membrane, avoiding nearby veins and arteries as well as the recurrent laryngeal nerve.
5. Insert curved hemostats into the membrane incision, and spread it open.
6. Insert either a cuffed endotracheal tube (6 mm or 7 mm) or tracheostomy tube (6 or 8 Shiley), directing the tube into the trachea.
7. Inflate the cuff, and ventilate.
8. Confirm placement with auscultation, end-tidal CO_2 detector, and chest rise.
9. Secure the tube in place.

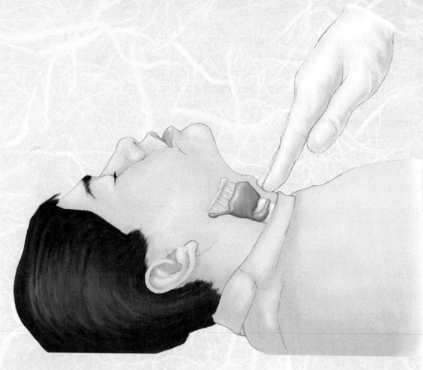

27-4a   Locate the cricothyroid membrane.

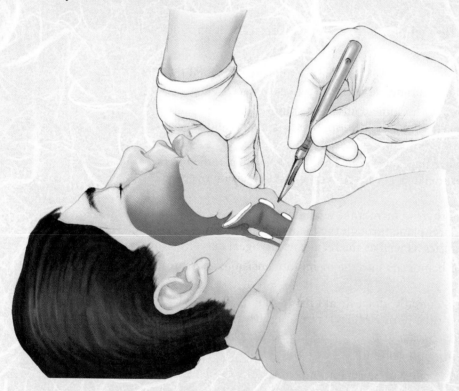

27-4b   Stabilize the larynx and make a 1- to 2-cm skin incision over cricothyroid membrane.

(continued)

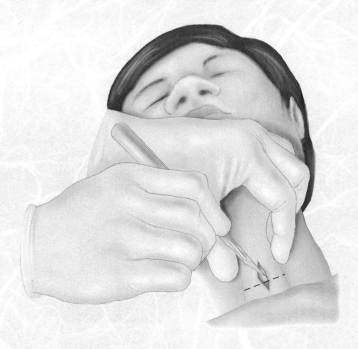

27-4c   Make a 1-cm horizontal incision through the cricothyroid membrane.

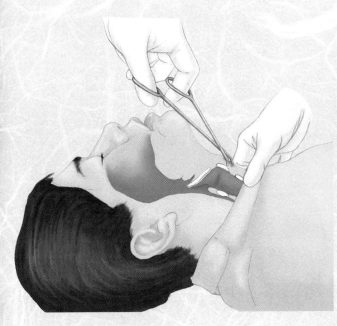

27-4d   Using a curved hemostat, spread the membrane incision open.

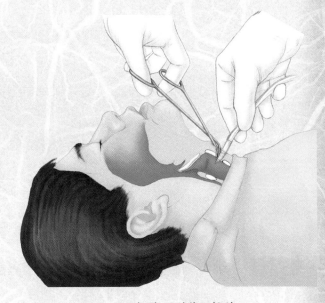

27-4e   Insert an ETT (6.0) or Shiley (6.0).

(continued)

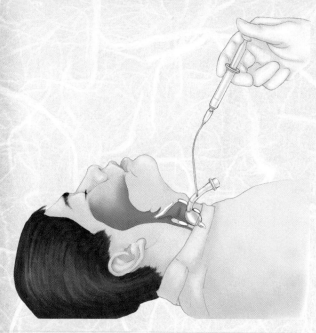

27-4f   Inflate the cuff.

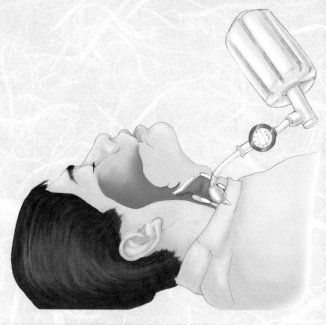

27-4g   Confirm placement.

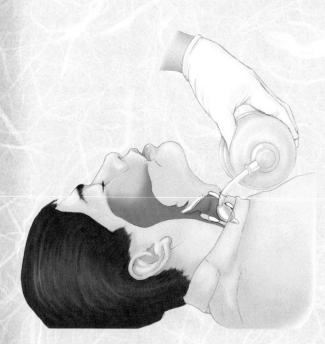

27-4h   Ventilate.

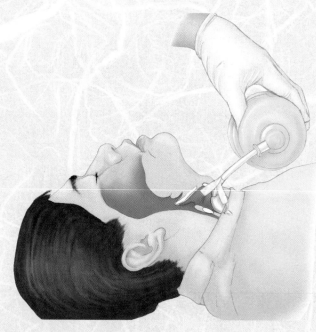

27-4i   Secure the tube, reconfirm placement, and evaluate the patient.

MANAGING PATIENTS WITH STOMA SITES

Often, patients who have had a laryngectomy (removal of the larynx) or tracheostomy (surgical opening into the trachea) breathe through a **stoma,** an opening in the anterior neck that connects the trachea with the ambient air. These patients frequently have tracheostomy tubes, which consist of inner and outer cannulae, in place to keep the soft-tissue stoma open (Figure 27-57).

A patient with a stoma often has problems with excessive secretions. A laryngectomy produces a less effective cough, making it more difficult to clear secretions. If these secretions organize, they form a mucous plug that can occlude the stoma and thus the airway. A stoma apparatus generally has a fixed outer portion and an inner cannula. The inner cannula can be easily removed and cleaned, then replaced. Timely replacement of the outer cannula is important if it must also be removed because the stoma can constrict within just a few hours to prohibit its replacement without dilation.

As the external stoma site narrows, so can the inner tracheal diameter; either can produce potentially life-threatening stenosis. Any acute inflammation that leads to soft-tissue swelling can worsen this by further reducing the stoma and tracheal diameter. Further, this stenosis may make the cannula very difficult or impossible to replace. In this case, choose the largest diameter ETT that will pass through the stoma to maintain the airway before complete obstruction occurs.

✳ **stoma** opening in the anterior neck that connects the trachea with ambient air.

Timely replacement of a stoma device's outer cannula is important because the stoma can constrict within just a few hours to prohibit its replacement without dilation.

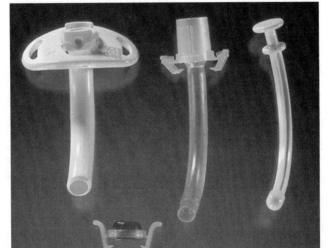

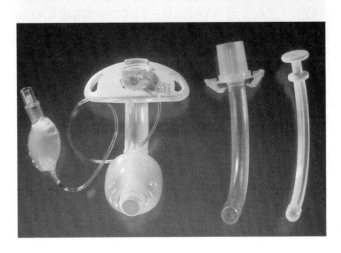

FIGURE 27-57 Tracheostomy cannulae.

Lubricate the ETT, instruct the patient to exhale, and gently insert the ETT to about 1–2 cm beyond the distal cuff. Inflate the cuff, and then confirm comfort, patency, and proper placement. Be certain to suspect and check for improper placement into the surrounding subcutaneous tissue, which will produce a false lumen. Subcutaneous emphysema, as well as the lack of clinical improvement in the patient, indicates a false lumen.

You must use extreme caution with any suctioning, as this process can itself cause soft-tissue swelling. In order to suction, begin by preoxygenating the patient with 100-percent oxygen. Inject 3 mL sterile saline down the trachea through the stoma. Instruct the patient to exhale, then gently insert the catheter until resistance is met. While the patient coughs or exhales, suction the airway during withdrawal of the catheter.

When the patient with a stoma requires ventilatory assistance, a bystander may use the mouth-to-stoma technique, while paramedics will generally use a bag-valve-mask device.

SUCTIONING

✱ **suction** to remove with a vacuum-type device.

Anticipating complications when managing airways is the key for successful outcomes. You must be prepared to **suction** all airways in order to remove blood or other secretions and for the patient to vomit. Suctioning equipment must be readily available for all patients, to prevent a simple vomiting episode from becoming a complicated aspiration episode that increases the patient's risk for greater morbidity or for mortality.

SUCTIONING EQUIPMENT

Many different suctioning devices are available. They may be handheld, oxygen-powered, battery-operated, or mounted (nonportable). To suit the prehospital environment, your equipment should be lightweight, portable, durable, generate a vacuum level of at least 300 mmHg when the distal end is occluded, and allow a flow rate of at least 30 litres per minute (Lpm) when the tube is open. In addition to a portable device, the ambulance should have a mounted, vacuum-powered suction device that can generate stronger suction and can be a backup device in case of equipment failure. The most commonly used suction catheters are either hard/rigid catheters ("Yankauer" or "tonsil tip") or soft catheters ("whistle tip"). Table 27-7 summarizes their differences.

Table 27-7 TYPES OF SUCTIONING CATHETERS	
Hard/Rigid Catheter	**Soft Catheters**
A large tube with multiple holes at the distal end	Long, flexible tube; smaller diameter than hard-tip catheters
Suctions larger volumes of fluid rapidly	Cannot remove large volumes of fluid rapidly
Standard size	Various sizes
Used in oropharyngeal airway only	Can be placed in the oropharynx, nasopharynx, or down the endotracheal tube
Removes larger particles	Suction tubing without catheter (facilitates suctioning of large debris)

Because suctioning reduces a patient's access to oxygen, you should limit each attempt to 10 seconds. If possible, hyperoxygenate the patient with 100-percent oxygen before and after each effort. Clear any fluids from the upper airway first, as assisted breathing may cause aspiration. Do not apply suction while inserting the catheter. Apply suction only as you withdraw the catheter after properly positioning it.

Complications of suctioning are related to hypoxia from prolonged suctioning attempts without proper ventilation. The decrease in myocardial oxygen supply can cause cardiac dysrhythmias. Suctioning can also stimulate the vagus nerve, causing bradycardia and hypotension, or the anxiety of being suctioned can cause hypertension and tachycardia. Stimulation of the cough reflex will cause a patient to cough, causing an increase in intracranial pressure and reducing cerebral blood flow.

SUCTIONING TECHNIQUES

You must have suction equipment ready for any patient who has airway compromise and will need airway management. To suction a patient, follow these steps:

1. Wear protective eyewear, gloves, and face mask.
2. Preoxygenate the patient.
3. Determine the depth of catheter insertion by measuring from the patient's earlobe to her lips.
4. With the suction turned off, insert the catheter into your patient's pharynx to the predetermined depth.
5. Turn on the suction unit, and place your thumb over the suction control orifice; limit suction to 10 seconds.
6. Continue to suction while withdrawing the catheter. When using a whistle-tip catheter, rotate it between your fingertips.
7. Hyperoxygenate the patient with 100-percent oxygen.

In many cases, you will suction extremely viscous, or thick, secretions, that can obstruct the flow of fluid through the tubing. To reduce this problem, suction water through the tubing between suctioning attempts. This dilutes the secretions and facilitates flow to the suction canister. Most suction units have small water canisters for this purpose.

Tracheobronchial Suctioning

You may have to suction some patients through an endotracheal tube or a tracheostomy tube to remove secretions or mucous plugs that can cause respiratory distress. Suctioning these patients poses the risk of hypoxia, and so oxygenating them before and after the procedure is essential. If possible, use sterile technique to avoid contaminating the pulmonary system. Use only the soft-tip catheter to avoid damaging any structures, and be certain to prelubricate it. Once you have preoxygentated the patient with 100-percent oxygen, lubricate the catheter tip with a water-soluble gel, and gently insert it until you feel resistance. Then, apply suction for only 10–15 seconds while extracting the catheter. Ventilation and oxygenation are mandatory immediately after each suctioning attempt. You may have to inject 3–5 mL of sterile water down the endotracheal tube to help loosen thick secretions.

GASTRIC DECOMPRESSION

A common problem with ventilating a nonintubated patient is gastric distention, which occurs when the procedure's high pressures trap air in the stomach. As the stomach expands with this trapped air, the risk of vomiting rises. The enlarged stomach also pushes against the diaphragm, inhibiting the lungs' expansion and increasing their resistance to ventilation. Once the patient has gastric distention, you should place a tube in her stomach for gastric decompression, using either the nasogastric or the orogastric approach.

Nasogastric tube placement is generally preferred in awake patients as it allows them to talk, while orogastric tube placement is recommended in patients with facial fractures to avoid placing the tube through a skull fracture into the brain. Indications for gastric tube placement include the need for decompression because of the risk of aspiration or difficulty ventilating. In addition, large-bore gastric tubes are occasionally placed for gastric lavage in hypothermia and some overdose emergencies. The possibility of esophageal bleeding dictates extreme caution in patients with esophageal disease or trauma. Avoid placing gastric tubes in the presence of an esophageal obstruction because of the increased risk of esophageal perforation. Both routes effectively accomplish gastric decompression; the orogastric route adds the advantage of allowing the use of a larger bore tube for lavage. Disadvantages of both routes include discomfort to patients and minor interference with orotracheal intubation. When no contraindication exists, nasogastric tube placement for gastric decompression is generally preferred. Both routes put the patient at risk for vomiting, misplacement into the trachea, or trauma and bleeding from poor technique.

As for any other invasive procedure, you should always wear protective eyewear, gloves, and face shield whenever you place a nasogastric or orogastric tube. To place a nasogastric or orogastric tube, follow these steps:

1. Prepare the patient's head in a neutral position while preoxygenating.

2. Determine the length of tube insertion by measuring from the epigastrium to the angle of jaw and then to the tip of the nares.

3. If the patient is awake, use a topical anesthetic to the nares or oropharynx. Suppress the gag reflex with a topical anesthetic applied into the posterior oropharynx or with IV lidocaine.

4. Lubricate the distal tip of the gastric tube, and gently insert the tube into the nares and along the nasal floor or, alternatively, into the oral cavity at midline. Advance the tube gently. If the patient is awake, encourage swallowing to facilitate the tube's passage.

5. Advance to the predetermined mark on the tube.

6. Confirm placement by injecting 30–50 mL of air while listening to the epigastric region for air sounds. Inability to speak that develops after gastric tube placement indicates malpositioning of the tube through the vocal cords and into the trachea. If this occurs, you must remove the tube.

7. Apply suction. Note gastric contents that pass through the tube.

8. Secure the tube in place.

OXYGENATION

Oxygenation is an important therapy, and you must thoroughly understand its indications and precautions. Providing supplemental oxygen to patients who are frankly hypoxic will diminish the hypoxia's secondary effects on such organs as the brain and the heart. You should provide supplemental oxygen to patients who are in shock or at risk of shock, regardless of their oxygen saturation. Although the patient may be oxygenating the arterial blood well, the oxygen may not be reaching the cells effectively. The increased oxygen levels may help improve perfusion.

Never withhold oxygen from any patient for whom it is indicated. However, use caution with COPD patients. These patients lose the impulse to breathe at normal or supranormal oxygen levels. Their normal respiratory regulatory mechanism (elevated $PaCO_2$) has failed, and their impulse to breathe is triggered by a low PaO_2, or hypoxia. This is termed hypoxic drive. As a general approach, slowly increase these patients' oxygen until their breathing is less laboured and they are more comfortable, though not necessarily back to their baseline. Watch your patient closely to be sure that the decreased breathing effort does not signal impending respiratory failure. If this occurs, be ready to support the patient's ventilations, using basic manoeuvres, adjuncts, and bag-valve mask. Oxygen toxicity is normally not a concern in the prehospital setting, since transport times are not prolonged and the patient has limited high-concentration oxygen exposure.

Never withhold oxygen from any patient for whom it is indicated.

OXYGEN SUPPLY AND REGULATORS

Oxygen is supplied either as a compressed gas or as a liquid. Compressed oxygen is stored in an aluminium or steel tank in 400-litre (D), 660-litre (E), or 3450-litre (M) volumes. Compressed oxygen is used in Canadian ambulances and usually in the form of both D and M tanks. Liquid oxygen is cooled to aqueous form and warmed back to its gaseous state for delivery. Although liquid oxygen requires less storage space than an equal amount of compressed oxygen, you must keep it upright and accommodate for other special requirements for its storage and transfer.

Regulators for oxygen tanks are either **high-pressure regulators**, which are used to transfer oxygen at high pressures from tank to tank, or **therapy regulators**, which are used for delivering oxygen to patients. The default pressure for therapy regulators is 50 psi, which is controlled within the regulator to allow adjustable low-flow oxygen delivery. Attached to each regulator is a gauge that tells how much oxygen is left in the tank. All full oxygen tanks, regardless of the size, have a total filled pressure of 2000 psi. Oxygen tanks should be changed at 500 psi to allow adequate delivery to patients and that level is called the safe residual pressure. In order to calculate how long an oxygen tank will last, you are required to know the constant for each. An M tank has a constant of 1.56, while a D tank has a constant of 0.16. Use the following formula to calculate the delivery time of oxygen in minutes:

✱ **high-pressure regulators** are used to transfer oxygen at high pressures from tank to tank.

✱ **therapy regulators** are used to deliver oxygen to patients.

$$\text{Tank life in minutes} = \frac{\text{Gauge pressure} - \text{safe residual pressure}}{\text{Oxygen delivered in litres per minute}} \times \text{Constant}$$

OXYGEN DELIVERY DEVICES

Oxygen delivery to patients is measured in litres of flow per minute (L/min). A number of delivery devices are available; the patient's condition will dictate which method you use. You must continually reassess the patient who requires oxygen

You must continually reassess the patient who requires oxygen therapy to be certain that the method of delivery and flow rate are adequate.

therapy to be certain that the method of delivery and flow rate are adequate. You should not use these devices in patients with poor respiratory effort, severe hypoxia, or apnea or in patients who exhibit mouth breathing.

Nasal Cannula The **nasal cannula** is a catheter placed at the nares. It provides an optimal oxygen supplementation of up to 40 percent when set at 6 L/min flow. At flow rates above 6 L/min, the nasal mucous membranes become very dry and easily break down. Patients generally tolerate the nasal cannula well. It is indicated for low to moderate oxygen requirements and long-term oxygen therapy.

Venturi Mask The **venturi mask** is a high-flow face mask that uses a venturi system to deliver relatively precise oxygen concentrations, regardless of the patient's rate and depth of breathing. As oxygen passes into the mask through a jet orifice in the base of the mask, it entrains room air. The device then delivers the resulting mixture to the patient. Some venturi masks have dial selectors to control the amount of ambient air taken in; others have interchangeable caps. Either type can deliver concentrations of 24-, 28-, 35-, or 40-percent oxygen. The litre flow depends on the oxygen concentration desired. The venturi mask is particularly useful in COPD patients, who benefit from careful control of inspired oxygen concentration and is usually not utilized in a prehospital setting.

Simple Face Mask The simple face mask is indicated for patients requiring moderate to high oxygen concentrations. Side ports allow room air to enter the mask and dilute the oxygen concentration during inspiration. Flow rates generally range from about 6 L/min to 10 L/min, providing 40–60 percent oxygen at the maximum rate, depending on the patient's respiratory rate and depth. Delivery of volumes beyond 10 L/min does not enhance oxygen concentration.

Partial Rebreather Mask The partial rebreather mask is indicated for patients requiring moderate to high oxygen concentrations when satisfactory clinical results are not obtained with the simple face mask. One-way discs that cover the partial rebreather mask's side ports prevent the inspiration of room air. Minimal dilution occurs with inspiration of residual expired air along with the supplemental oxygen. Maximal flow rate is 10 L/min.

Nonrebreather Mask The nonrebreather mask has one-way side ports as well but also has an attached reservoir bag to hold oxygen ready to inhale. It provides the highest oxygen concentration of all oxygen delivery devices available, 80–95 percent at 15 L/min. It is not indicated as continuing support for poor respiratory effort and severe hypoxia; however, you should place it initially to attempt to preoxygenate these patients while you prepare to intubate them unless initial ventilatory support with a bag-valve mask and 100-percent oxygen is indicated.

Small-Volume Nebulizer Nebulizer chambers containing 3–5 cc of fluid are attached to a face mask that allows for delivery of medications in aerosol form (nebulization). Pressurized oxygen or air enters the chamber to create a mist, which the patient then inspires.

Oxygen Humidifier You can provide humidified oxygen to the patient by attaching a sterile water reservoir to the oxygen outlet. Humidified oxygen benefits patients with croup, epiglottitis, or bronchiolitis, as well as those patients receiving long-term oxygen therapy.

* **nasal cannula** catheter placed at the nares.

* **venturi mask** high-flow face mask that uses a venturi system to deliver relatively precise oxygen concentrations.

The venturi mask is particularly useful for COPD patients, who benefit from careful control of inspired oxygen concentration.

Content Review

OXYGEN DELIVERY DEVICES

- Nasal cannula
- Venturi mask
- Simple face mask
- Partial rebreather mask
- Nonrebreather mask
- Small-volume nebulizer
- Oxygen humidifier

VENTILATION

Many of your cases in the field will call for ventilatory support. These situations will range from apneic patients to less obvious instances when patients are experiencing depressed respiratory function. Remember that an unconscious patient's respiratory centre may not function adequately. A significant decrease in the patient's rate or depth of breathing will lead to decreased respiratory minute volume, hypercarbia, hypoxia, and a lowered pH. If you do not correct this, respiratory or cardiac arrest may occur. Effective ventilatory support requires a tidal volume of at least 800 mL of oxygen at 12–20 breaths per minute.

When providing ventilatory support, you must generate enough force to overcome the elastic resistance of the lungs and chest wall, as well as the frictional resistance in the respiratory passageways, without overinflating the lungs. This is similar to blowing up a balloon; you must overcome the balloon's resistance in order to inflate it. Keep in mind that air will travel the path of least resistance. If you do not maintain a tight seal between the ventilation mask and your patient's face, air will flow out of the gaps, rather than through the respiratory passageways.

Effective artificial ventilation requires a patent airway, an effective seal between the mask and the patient's face, and delivery of adequate ventilatory volumes. Exercise care when you attempt to generate enough pressure to ventilate the lungs. Too much pressure may lead to gastric distention and regurgitation. Also, be certain that you allow the patient to exhale between delivered breaths.

MOUTH-TO-MOUTH/MOUTH-TO-NOSE VENTILATION

Mouth-to-mouth and mouth-to-nose ventilation methods are the most basic methods of rescue ventilation. Both are indicated in the presence of apnea when no other ventilation devices are available. They require no special equipment, and yet both allow an adequate seal between the rescuer and the patient and can provide effective ventilatory support, with adequate tidal volumes and oxygenation; however, the capacity of the person delivering the ventilations limits both methods. Also, both methods provide only limited oxygen—the rescuer's expired air will contain only 17-percent oxygen. This procedure's major drawback is its potential for exposing either the rescuer or the patient to communicable diseases through contact with blood and other body fluids. Take care not to hyperinflate the patient's lungs or to hyperventilate yourself. This ventilation technique is not utilized by paramedics in Canada.

MOUTH-TO-MASK VENTILATION

The pocket mask is a clear plastic device that you place over an apneic patient's mouth and nose. It prevents direct contact between you and your patient's mouth, thus reducing the risk of contamination and subsequent infection. It may be easier to obtain a good seal on the patient's face using a mask. However, the mask is only useful if it is readily available. Do not use it in awake patients.

A variety of pocket masks are available. Some are reusable, while others are disposable. Most are small and compact enough to fit in a pocket or purse, and you should always carry one. Because of the increasing risks of infectious diseases, you should use a disposable mask whenever you ventilate a patient. These devices usually have a one-way valve that prevents you from contacting the patient's expired air. The valve may also provide an inlet for supplemental oxygen; mouth-

If you do not correct any significant decrease in the patient's rate or depth of breathing, respiratory or cardiac arrest may occur.

Exercise care when you attempt to generate enough pressure to ventilate the lungs.

Content Review

VENTILATION METHODS

- Mouth-to-mouth/mouth-to-nose
- Mouth-to-mask
- Bag-valve device
- Demand valve device
- Automatic transport ventilator

to-mask ventilation combined with an oxygen flow rate of 10 L/min can deliver an inspired oxygen concentration of approximately 50 percent. To apply the mouth-to-mask technique, position the head to open the airway by one of the previously discussed methods, position the mask to obtain a good seal, and provide adequate ventilatory volumes. As with mouth-to-mouth and mouth-to-nose methods, hyperinflation of the patient's lungs, gastric distention in the patient, and hyperventilation in the rescuer are potential complications.

BAG-VALVE DEVICES

For patients with apnea or an unsatisfactory respiratory effort, prehospital and emergency department personnel most commonly use the bag-valve device. Used correctly, the bag-valve device assists in ventilating patients by expanding the lungs and improving alveolar ventilation, thus preventing hypoxia. When using the bag-valve device with the mask (bag-valve mask, or BVM), the paramedic must still open the airway with either the jaw-thrust or head-tilt/chin-lift manoeuvre. Do not use the BVM in awake patients who do not tolerate the procedure.

The **bag-valve mask** consists of an oblong, self-inflating, silicone or rubber bag with two one-way valves (an air/oxygen-inlet valve and a patient valve) and a transparent plastic face mask, which is available in three sizes: neonatal, child, or adult. There are many masks available for use with the bag device. Stiff rubber masks in child and adult sizes are pliable but more difficult to maintain an appropriate seal. The blob style mask or Seal Easy mask is similar to a circular blow up toy for the swimming pool. It attaches to the bag and is positioned over the nose or mouth depending on which orifice is to ventilated. The paramedic may find this mask much easier to obtain and maintain a seal. Some BVMs have a built-in colorimetric end-tidal CO_2 detector (Figure 27-58).

 bag-valve mask ventilation device consisting of a self-inflating bag with two one-way valves and a transparent plastic face mask.

Do not reuse bag-valve masks.

FIGURE 27-58 Bag-valve-mask with built-in colorimetric ETCO$_2$ detector.

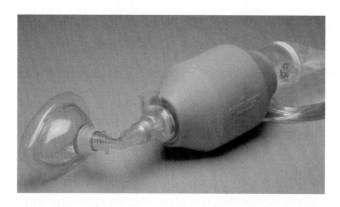

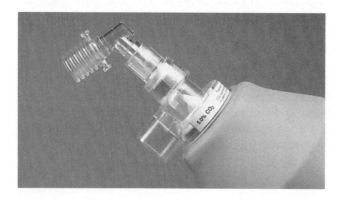

With the increasing risks of transmitting infectious diseases, BVMs should be disposable. Do not reuse them.

You can use BVMs with or without oxygen. Without oxygen they deliver only room air (21 percent oxygen) to the patient; with oxygen attached, the deliverable amount of oxygen increases to 60–70 percent. The bag-valve device also has an adjunct oxygen reservoir or corrugated tubing that can deliver 90–95 percent oxygen when coupled with an oxygen source. If possible, connect all patients who require a bag-valve device to an oxygen reservoir with oxygen at 15 L/min.

Bag-valve masks for pediatric cases may have a pop-off valve. Bag-valve masks for adults should not have pop-off valves because patients with high airway resistance and poor lung compliance will activate the pop-off valve, thus preventing effective ventilation.

One, two, or three rescuers may perform BVM ventilation. One-person BVM ventilation is the most difficult method to master because obtaining and maintaining the mask seal can be challenging. You must not only keep the airway open with a jaw-thrust or chin-lift but at the same time keep the mask sealed well and squeeze the BVM to deliver an adequate tidal volume. Two-person BVM ventilation is the most efficient method, providing superior mask seal and tidal volumes when applied correctly. It requires the availability of an adequate number of trained medical personnel. Three-person BVM ventilation also provides excellent mask seal and volume delivery, but it requires more personnel, and it crowds access to the patient's airway.

To perform the two-person BVM method, the first rescuer maintains the mask seal, while the second squeezes the bag. With the three-person BVM method, the first rescuer applies manual airway manoeuvres, the second maintains the mask seal, and the third squeezes the bag. Observe the patient for chest rise, development of gastric distention, and changes in compliance of the bag with ventilation. Complications of BVM ventilation include inadequate volume delivery if there is a poor mask seal or improper technique, barotrauma from overinflation of the lungs, and gastric distention.

Ventilation of Pediatric Patients The differences in the pediatric patient's anatomy require some variation in ventilation technique. First, her relatively flat nasal bridge makes achieving mask seal more difficult. Pressing the mask against the child's face to improve the seal can obstruct the airway, which is more compressible than an adult's. You can best achieve the mask seal with the two-person BVM technique, using jaw thrust to maintain an open airway.

For BVM ventilation, the bag size depends on the child's age. Full-term neonates and infants will require a pediatric BVM with a capacity of at least 450 mL. For children up to eight years of age, the pediatric BVM is preferred, though for patients in the upper age range you can use an adult BVM with a capacity of 1500 mL if you do not maximally inflate it. Children older than eight years require an adult BVM to achieve adequate tidal volumes. Additionally, be certain that the mask fits properly, from the bridge of the nose to the cleft of the chin. If a length-based resuscitation tape (Broselow Tape) is available, you can use it to help determine the proper size.

To achieve a proper mask seal, place the mask over the patient's mouth and nose; avoid compressing the eyes. Using one hand, place your thumb on the mask at the apex and your index finger on the mask at the chin (C-grip). Apply gentle pressure downward on the mask to establish an adequate seal. Maintain the airway by lifting the bony prominence of the chin with the remaining fingers forming an *E* under the jaw; avoid placing pressure on the soft area under the chin. You may use the one-rescuer technique, although the two-rescuer technique will be more effective.

Ventilate according to current standards, obtaining chest rise with each breath. Begin the ventilation and say "squeeze," providing just enough volume to initiate chest rise—be very careful not to overinflate the child's lungs. Allow adequate time for exhalation, saying "release, release." Continue ventilations, saying "squeeze, release, release." To assess adequacy of ventilations, look for adequate chest rise, listen for lung sounds at the third intercostal space, mid-axillary line, and assess for clinical improvement (skin colour and heart rate).

AUTOMATIC TRANSPORT VENTILATOR

Several compact mechanical ventilators are available for prehospital care. Designed for convenience and easy use during patient care and transport, these lightweight and durable portable devices offer a number of advantages. They maintain minute volume better than bag-valve devices, and they tolerate temperatures ranging from $-1°C$ to $52°C$ ($-30°F$ to $125°F$) with great dependability. In cardiac arrest, the automatic ventilator allows you to interpose chest compressions between mechanical breaths. They are mechanically simple and adapt to a portable oxygen supply.

The compact ventilator typically comes with two or three controls: one for the ventilatory rate, the other for tidal volume (Figure 27-59). It also has a standard 15/22-mm adapter so that you can attach it to a variety of airway devices. Some of these automatic units deliver controlled ventilation only. Others, such as the CAREvent ALS Resuscitator (see Figure 27-60), function as an automatic time/cycled ventilatory resuscitator, with patients who are not breathing, reverting to demand breathing capability with patients who spontaneously start to breathe. Tidal volume and rate are adjustable according to the patient's weight. The delivery of the rate ensures an inspiratory–expiratory ratio of 1:2, which allows adequate removal of CO_2 through normal chest relaxation. The inspired oxygen concentration is usually fixed at 100 percent.

Many ventilators have a pop-off valve that prevents pressure-related injury. When airway pressure exceeds a preset level (typically 60 cmH$_2$O), the valve opens, venting some of the tidal volume. This feature can hinder ventilating patients with cardiogenic pulmonary edema, adult respiratory distress syndrome (ARDS), pulmonary contusion, bronchospasm, or other disorders in which high airway pressures must be overcome. If this problem occurs, consider using a bag-valve device that allows you to feel bag compliance.

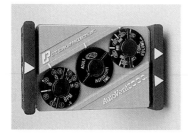

FIGURE 27-59   Portable mechanical ventilator.

FIGURE 27-60   CAREvent ALS Resuscitator.

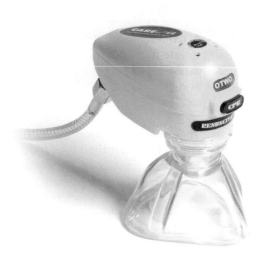

As a rule, you should not use mechanical ventilators in children less than five years old (under 20 kg), awake patients, or patients with obstructed airways or increased airway resistance, as described above. Otherwise, when indicated, the device can prove a valuable tool. In intubated patients, the mechanical ventilator allows you to perform other vital tasks.

SUMMARY

Respiratory emergencies are commonly encountered in prehospital care. It is important to recognize that all respiratory disorders may produce derangements in ventilation, perfusion, or diffusion. Recognition and treatment must be prompt. Understanding the underlying cause of the respiratory disorder can guide therapy. The primary treatment is to correct hypoxia. Necessary steps include establishing and maintaining the airway, assisting ventilations as required, and administering supplemental oxygen. Appropriate pharmacological agents may be subsequently ordered by medical direction.

No matter what the underlying cause of respiratory dysfunction, the primary treatment is to establish and maintain the airway, administer oxygen, and assist ventilations as required.

Airway assessment and maintenance are the most critical steps in managing any patient. If you do not promptly establish a definitive airway and provide proper ventilation, the patient's outcome will be poor. Frequently reassessing the airway is mandatory to ensure that the patient has not decompensated, requiring additional airway procedures. Successful management of all airways requires the paramedic to follow the proper management sequence.

Basic airway and management skills can make the difference between a successful outcome and a poor prognosis. You must maintain proficiency in all airway skills, especially the more advanced techniques, through ongoing education, physician medical direction, and testing with each EMS service. Advanced care and critical care paramedics can perform advanced airway control through intubation. As a skill set, critical thinking and assessment skills must be incorporated for the paramedic to proceed to this treatment. If you cannot do this, it is in the patient's best interest for you to focus on less sophisticated airway skills. If you anticipate that every airway will be complicated, apply basic airway skills and procedures, and perform frequent reassessments, then you will give the patient her best chance for meaningful survival.

CHAPTER 28

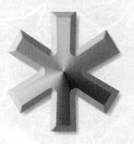

Cardiology

Objectives

Part 1: **Cardiovascular Anatomy and Physiology, ECG Monitoring, and Dysrhythmia Analysis (begins on p. 448)**

After reading Part 1 of this chapter, you should be able to:

1. Describe the incidence, morbidity, and mortality of cardiovascular disease. (p. 447)
2. Discuss prevention strategies that may reduce the morbidity and mortality of cardiovascular disease. (p. 447)
3. Identify the risk factors most predisposing to coronary artery disease. (p. 447)
4. Describe the anatomy of the heart, including the position in the thoracic cavity, the layers of the heart, the chambers of the heart, and the location and function of cardiac valves. (pp. 448–449; also see Chapter 12)
5. Identify the major structures of the vascular system, the factors affecting venous return, the components of cardiac output, and the phases of the cardiac cycle. (pp. 448–449; also see Chapter 12)
6. Define preload, afterload, and left ventricular end-diastolic pressure, and relate each to the pathophysiology of heart failure. (see Chapter 12)

Continued

7. Identify the arterial blood supply to any given area of the myocardium. (see Chapter 12)

8. Compare and contrast the coronary arterial distribution to the major portions of the cardiac conduction system. (see Chapter 12)

9. Identify the structure and course of all divisions and subdivisions of the cardiac conduction system. (see Chapter 12)

10. Identify and describe how the heart's pacemaking control, rate, and rhythm are determined. (see Chapter 12)

11. Explain the physiological basis of conduction delay in the AV node. (see Chapter 12)

12. Define the functional properties of cardiac muscle. (see Chapter 12)

13. Define the events composing electrical potential. (see Chapter 12)

14. List the most important ions involved in myocardial action potential and their primary function in this process. (see Chapter 12)

15. Describe the events involved in the steps from excitation to contraction of cardiac muscle fibres. (see Chapter 12)

16. Describe the clinical significance of Starling's law. (see Chapter 12)

17. Identify the structures of the autonomic nervous system and their effect on heart rate, rhythm, and contractility. (see Chapter 12)

18. Define and give examples of positive and negative inotropism, chronotropism, and dromotropism. (see Chapter 12)

19. Discuss the pathophysiology of cardiac disease and injury. (pp. 465–510)

20. Explain the purpose of ECG monitoring and its limitations. (p. 452)

21. Correlate the electrophysiological and hemodynamic events occurring throughout the entire cardiac cycle with the various ECG wave forms, segments, and intervals. (pp. 456–465)

22. Identify how heart rates, durations, and amplitudes may be determined from ECG recordings. (pp. 456–463)

23. Relate the cardiac surfaces or areas to the ECG leads. (p. 453)

24. Differentiate among the primary mechanisms responsible for producing cardiac dysrhythmias. (pp. 461–463, 465–510)

25. Describe a systematic approach to the analysis and interpretation of cardiac dysrhythmias. (pp. 463–465)

26. Describe the dysrhythmias originating in the sinus node, the AV junction, the atria, and the ventricles. (pp. 466–510)

27. Describe the process and pitfalls of differentiating wide QRS complex tachycardias. (pp. 499–500)

28. Describe the conditions of pulseless electrical activity. (pp. 507–508)

29. Describe the phenomena of reentry, aberration, and accessory pathways. (pp. 466, 507)

30. Identify the ECG changes characteristically produced by electrolyte imbalances and specify their clinical implications. (p. 510)

31. Identify patient situations in which ECG rhythm analysis is indicated. (pp. 465–510)

32. Recognize the ECG changes that may reflect evidence of myocardial ischemia and injury and their limitations. (pp. 461–463)

33. Correlate abnormal ECG findings with clinical interpretation. (pp. 465–510)

34. Identify the major mechanical, pharmacological, and electrical therapeutic objectives in the treatment of the patient with any dysrhythmia. (pp. 465–510)

35. Describe artifacts that may cause confusion when evaluating the ECG of a patient with a pacemaker. (pp. 452–453, 505–506)

36. List the possible complications of pacing. (pp. 505–506)

37. List the causes and implications of pacemaker failure. (pp. 505–506)

38. Identify additional hazards that interfere with artificial pacemaker function. (p. 505–506)
39. Recognize the complications of artificial pacemakers as evidenced on an ECG. (pp. 505–506)
40. Describe the characteristics of an implanted pacemaking system. (pp. 505–506)

Part 2: Assessment and Management of the Cardiovascular Patient (begins on p. 511)

After reading Part 2 of this chapter, you should be able to:

41. Identify and describe the components of the focused history as it relates to the patient with cardiovascular compromise. (pp. 512–517)
42. Identify and describe the details of inspection, auscultation, and palpation specific to the cardiovascular system. (pp. 517–520)
43. Identify and define the heart sounds and relate them to hemodynamic events in the cardiac cycle. (p. 519)
44. Describe the differences between normal and abnormal heart sounds. (p. 519)
45. Define pulse deficit, pulsus paradoxus, and pulsus alternans. (p. 548)
46. Identify the normal characteristics of the point of maximal impulse (PMI). (p. 519)
47. On the basis of field impressions, identify the need for rapid intervention for the patient in cardiovascular compromise. (pp. 511–520)
48. Describe the incidence, morbidity, and mortality associated with myocardial conduction defects. (pp. 541, 542)
49. Identify the clinical indications, components, and the function of transcutaneous cardiac pacing. (pp. 533–535)
50. Explain what each setting and indicator on a transcutaneous pacing system represents and how the settings may be adjusted. (pp. 533–535)
51. Describe the techniques of applying a transcutaneous pacing system. (pp. 533–535)
52. Describe the epidemiology, morbidity, mortality, and pathophysiology of angina pectoris. (pp. 537–538)
53. Describe the assessment and management of a patient with angina pectoris. (pp. 537–539)
54. Identify what is meant by the OPQRST of chest pain assessment. (p. 513)
55. List other clinical conditions that may mimic signs and symptoms of coronary artery disease and angina pectoris. (pp. 537–538)
56. Identify the ECG findings in patients with angina pectoris. (pp. 538–539)
57. On the basis of the pathophysiology and clinical evaluation of the patient with chest pain, list the anticipated clinical problems according to their life-threat potential. (pp. 537–539)
58. Describe the epidemiology, morbidity, mortality, and pathophysiology of myocardial infarction. (pp. 539–541)
59. List the mechanisms by which a myocardial infarction may be produced from traumatic and nontraumatic events. (p. 540)
60. Identify the primary hemodynamic changes produced in myocardial infarction. (pp. 540–541)
61. List and describe the assessment parameters to be evaluated in a patient with a suspected myocardial infarction. (pp. 540–541)
62. Identify the anticipated clinical presentation of a patient with a suspected acute myocardial infarction. (pp. 541–542)

63. Differentiate the characteristics of the pain/discomfort occurring in angina pectoris and acute myocardial infarction. (pp. 541–542)

64. Identify the ECG changes characteristically seen during evolution of an acute myocardial infarction. (p. 542)

65. Identify the most common complications of an acute myocardial infarction. (pp. 541–543)

66. List the characteristics of a patient eligible for thrombolytic therapy. (p. 542)

67. Describe the "window of opportunity" as it pertains to reperfusion of a myocardial injury or infarction. (p. 542)

68. On the basis of the pathophysiology and clinical evaluation of the patient with a suspected acute myocardial infarction, list the anticipated clinical problems according to their life-threat potential. (pp. 541–545)

69. Specify the measures that may be taken to prevent or minimize complications in the patient suspected of myocardial infarction. (p. 543)

70. Describe the most commonly used cardiac drugs in terms of therapeutic effect and dosages, routes of administration, side effects, and toxic effects. (pp. 525–526)

71. Describe the epidemiology, morbidity, mortality, and physiology associated with heart failure. (pp. 545–546)

72. Identify the factors that may precipitate or aggravate heart failure. (pp. 545–546)

73. Define acute pulmonary edema and describe its relationship to left ventricular failure. (p. 546)

74. Differentiate between early and late signs and symptoms of left ventricular failure and those of right ventricular failure. (p. 546)

75. Define and explain the clinical significance of paroxysmal nocturnal dyspnea, pulmonary edema, and dependent edema. (pp. 546–548)

76. List the interventions prescribed for the patient in acute congestive heart failure. (pp. 548–549)

77. Describe the most commonly used pharmacological agents in the management of congestive heart failure in terms of therapeutic effect, dosages, routes of administration, side effects, and toxic effects. (pp. 525–526, 548)

78. Define and describe the incidence, mortality, morbidity, pathophysiology, assessment, and management of the following cardiac-related problems (pp. 549–557):
    • Cardiac tamponade
    • Hypertensive emergency
    • Cardiogenic shock
    • Cardiac arrest

79. Identify the limiting factor of pericardial anatomy that determines intrapericardiac pressure. (p. 548)

80. Describe how to determine if pulsus paradoxus or pulsus alternans is present. (p. 548)

81. Explain the essential pathophysiological defect of hypertension in terms of Starling's law of the heart. (pp. 546, 552)

82. Rank the clinical problems of patients in hypertensive emergencies according to their levels of urgency. (pp. 550–551)

83. Identify the drugs of choice for hypertensive emergencies, cardiogenic shock, and cardiac arrest, including their indications, contraindications, side effects, route of administration, and dosages. (pp. 525–526, 551, 556)

84. Describe the major systemic effects of reduced tissue perfusion caused by cardiogenic shock. (pp. 552–553)

85. Explain the primary mechanisms by which the heart may compensate for a diminished cardiac output and describe their efficiency in cardiogenic shock. (pp. 552–553)

86. Identify the clinical criteria and progressive stages of cardiogenic shock. (pp. 552–553)

87. Describe the dysrhythmias seen in cardiac arrest. (p. 556)
88. Explain how to confirm asystole using the three-lead ECG. (p. 555)
89. Define the terms *defibrillation* and *synchronized cardioversion*. (pp. 527, 531)
90. Specify the methods of supporting the patient with a suspected ineffective implanted defibrillation device. (p. 528)
91. Describe resuscitation and identify circumstances and situations in which resuscitation efforts would not be initiated. (pp. 555–559)
92. Identify communication and documentation protocols with medical direction and law enforcement used for termination of resuscitation efforts. (p. 559)
93. Describe the incidence, morbidity, mortality, pathophysiology, assessment, and management of vascular disorders, including occlusive disease, phlebitis, aortic aneurysm, and peripheral artery occlusion. (pp. 559–562)
94. Identify the clinical significance of claudication and presence of arterial bruits in a patient with peripheral vascular disorders. (pp. 559–562)
95. Describe the clinical significance of unequal arterial blood pressure readings in the arms. (p. 563)

96. Recognize and describe the signs and symptoms of dissecting thoracic or abdominal aneurysm. (pp. 560–561)
97. Differentiate between signs and symptoms of cardiac tamponade, hypertensive emergencies, cardiogenic shock, and cardiac arrest. (pp. 549–557)
98. Utilize the results of the patient history, assessment findings, and ECG analysis to differentiate among, and provide treatment for, patients with the following conditions (pp. 511–557):
    - Cardiovascular disease
    - Chest pain
    - Need for a pacemaker
    - Angina pectoris
    - A suspected myocardial infarction
    - Heart failure
    - Cardiac tamponade
    - A hypertensive emergency
    - Cardiogenic shock
    - Cardiac arrest
99. On the basis of the pathophysiology and clinical evaluation of the patient with chest pain, characterize the clinical problems according to their life-threat potential. (pp. 537–538)
100. Given several preprogrammed patients with cardiac complaints, provide the appropriate assessment, treatment, and transport. (pp. 511–557)

INTRODUCTION

Cardiovascular disease (CVD) is defined as diseases and injuries of the cardiovascular system: the heart, the blood vessels of the heart, and the system of blood vessels (veins and arteries) throughout the body and within the brain. Stroke is the result of a blood-flow problem in the brain and is therefore considered a form of cardiovascular disease.

The exact number of Canadians who have cardiovascular disease is unknown. It is estimated that one in four Canadians has some form of heart disease—disease of the blood vessels or risk for stroke. If this estimate is accurate, approximately eight million Canadians have some form of cardiovascular disease.

Cardiovascular disease accounts for the death of more Canadians than any other disease. In 1999 (the latest year for which Statistics Canada has data), cardiovascular disease accounted for 78 942 deaths in Canada.

Thirty-five percent of all male deaths in Canada in 1999 were due to heart diseases, diseases of the blood vessels, and stroke. For women, the toll was even higher—37 percent of all female deaths in 1999 were due to cardiovascular disease.

Fifty-four percent of all cardiovascular deaths are due to coronary artery disease; 20 percent to stroke; 16 percent to other forms of heart disease, such as problems with the electrical system of the heart, viral heart infections, and heart muscle disease; and the remaining 10 percent to vascular problems, such as high blood pressure and hardening of the arteries.

Cardiovascular diseases cost the Canadian economy more than $18 billion a year, according to a 1994 study by the Heart and Stroke Foundation of Canada.

Sudden death from cardiovascular disease is often preventable. To decrease the chances of sudden death, the patient must recognize the signs and symptoms early and seek health care. Then, the health-care system must provide definitive care promptly, usually within the first hour after the onset of symptoms.

Public education about cardiovascular disease has focused on two strategies. The first is to educate the public about the risk factors for the development of cardiovascular disease. This program encourages patients to modify their lifestyle to minimize these risk factors. A variety of factors have been *proven* to increase the risk of cardiovascular disease:

- Smoking
- Older age
- Family history of cardiac disease
- Hypertension (high blood pressure)
- Hypercholesterolemia (excessive cholesterol in the blood)
- Carbohydrate intolerance (diabetes mellitus)
- Cocaine use
- Male gender

These factors that are *thought* to increase the risk of coronary heart disease:

- Diet
- Obesity
- Oral contraceptives (birth control pills)
- Sedentary lifestyle
- Type A personality (competitive, aggressive, hostile)
- Psychosocial tensions (stress)

* **cardiovascular disease (CVD)** disease affecting the heart, peripheral blood vessels, or both.

The second component of public education is recognition of the signs and symptoms of heart attack. Patients can only benefit from medical intervention if they recognize the signs and symptoms and promptly access the health-care system. Patients are encouraged to access the emergency medical service (EMS) early. As a paramedic, you will treat patients who already have developed the manifestations of cardiac disease. This will be an opportunity for you to further serve your patients by teaching them preventive strategies, including early recognition of symptoms, education, and alteration of lifestyle.

This chapter discusses the advanced prehospital care of cardiovascular emergencies. First, we will review the pertinent anatomy and physiology, and then we will use that knowledge to discuss assessing, recognizing, and treating cardiovascular disorders.

Part 1: Cardiovascular Anatomy and Physiology, ECG Monitoring, and Dysrhythmia Analysis

REVIEW OF CARDIOVASCULAR ANATOMY AND PHYSIOLOGY

Cardiac anatomy and physiology were discussed in detail in Chapter 12. The following is a brief review of that information.

CARDIOVASCULAR ANATOMY

The heart is located in the centre of the chest in the *mediastinum*. It is a muscular organ, consisting of three tissue layers: *endocardium* (the innermost layer that lines the chambers), *myocardium* (the middle layer with its unique ability to generate and conduct electrical impulses, causing the heart to contract), and *pericardium* (the protective sac surrounding the heart).

The heart (Figure 28-1) contains four chambers—two superior (the *atria*) and two inferior (the *ventricles*). Valves control the flow of blood through the heart: the *mitral valve* between the left atrium and ventricle; the *tricuspid valve* between the right atrium and ventricle; the *aortic valve* between the left ventricle and aorta; the *pulmonary valve* between the right ventricle and pulmonary artery.

The right atrium receives deoxygenated blood from the body via the *superior* and *inferior venae cavae*. The right ventricle sends the deoxygenated blood to the lungs via the *pulmonary artery*. Oxygenated blood is returned from the lungs to the *left atrium* via the *pulmonary veins*. The left ventricle pumps the oxygenated blood to the body via the *aorta*. Oxygenated blood is pumped from the heart to the tissues via the *arteries,* and deoxygenated blood is transported from the tissues back to the heart via the *veins*. The *capillaries* connect arteries and veins. The exchange of oxygen and carbon dioxide with the body tissues takes place through the very thin capillary walls.

The heart receives its nutrients from the *coronary arteries* (Figure 28-2) that originate in the aorta and spread over the heart. The *left coronary artery* supplies the left ventricle, interventricular septum, part of the right ventricle, and the conduction system. Its two main branches are the *anterior descending artery* and *circumflex artery*. The *right coronary artery* supplies a portion of the right atrium and right ventricle and part of the conduction system. Its two major branches are the *posterior descending artery* and *marginal artery*.

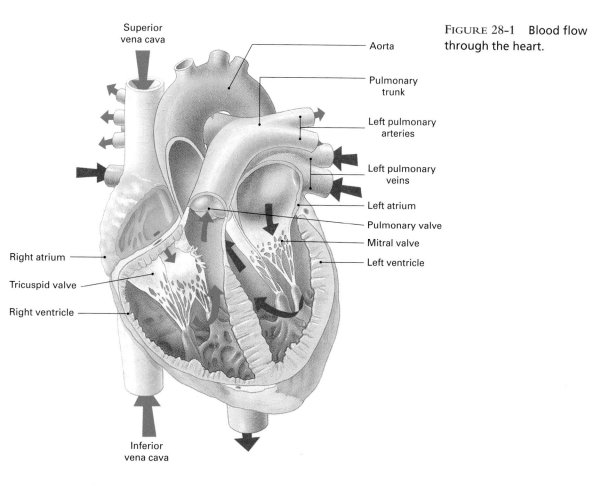

Superior
vena cava

FIGURE 28-1   Blood flow
through the heart.

Aorta

Pulmonary
trunk

Left pulmonary
arteries

Left pulmonary
veins

Left atrium

Pulmonary valve

Mitral valve

Left ventricle

Right atrium

Tricuspid valve

Right ventricle

Inferior
vena cava

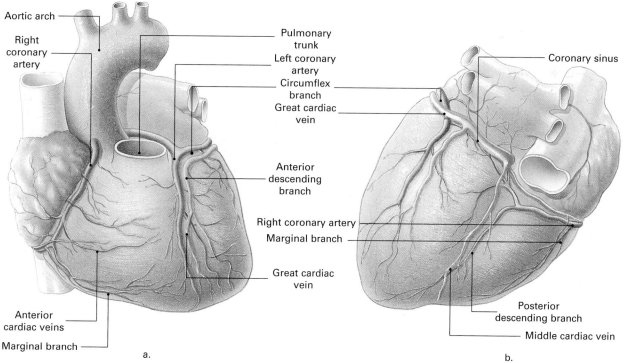

Aortic arch

Right
coronary
artery

Pulmonary
trunk

Left coronary
artery

Circumflex
branch

Great cardiac
vein

Anterior
descending
branch

Right coronary artery

Marginal branch

Great cardiac
vein

Anterior
cardiac veins

Marginal branch

a.

Coronary sinus

Posterior
descending branch

Middle cardiac vein

b.

FIGURE 28-2   The coronary circulation: (a) anterior; (b) posterior.

Cardiac Physiology

The *cardiac cycle* consists of *diastole,* the relaxation phase that takes place at the end of a cardiac contraction, and *systole,* the contraction phase. Normally, when the heart contracts, each ventricle ejects about two-thirds of the blood it contains (the *ejection fraction*). The amount of blood ejected, known as the *stroke volume,* averages 70 mL. The stroke volume depends on three factors: preload, cardiac contractility, and afterload. *Preload* is the end-diastolic volume and influences the force of the next contraction because of the stretch it exerts. (*Starling's law of the heart* states that the more the myocardial muscle is stretched, the greater its force of contraction will be.) *Afterload* is the resistance against which the heart muscle must pump. An increase in peripheral vascular resistance will decrease stroke volume; a decrease in resistance will increase stroke volume.

Cardiac output is calculated as stroke volume times heart rate. Since the normal heart rate is 60–100 beats per minute (bpm) and the average stroke volume is 70 mL, the average cardiac output is about 5 litres (5000 millilitres) per minute (70 mL $\times$ 70 bpm = 4900 mL/min).

Heart function is regulated by the sympathetic and parasympathetic nervous components of the autonomic nervous system, working in opposition to one another to maintain a balance. During stress, the sympathetic system dominates to raise the heart rate and increase contractile force. During sleep, the parasympathetic system dominates to decrease heart rate and contractile force. The terms *chronotropy* (referring to heart rate), *inotropy* (referring to contractile strength), and *dromotrophy* (referring to rate of nervous impulse conduction) describe autonomic control of the heart.

Cardiac function depends heavily on electrolyte balances. Electrolytes that affect cardiac function include sodium (Na^+), calcium (Ca^{++}), potassium (K^+), chloride (Cl^-), and magnesium (Mg^{++}). Sodium plays a major role in depolarizing the myocardium. Calcium takes part in myocardial depolarization and myocardial contraction. Potassium influences repolarization. Research into the roles of magnesium and chloride is ongoing.

Electrophysiology

Within the cardiac muscle fibres are special structures called *intercalated discs.* These discs connect cardiac muscle fibres and conduct electrical impulses quickly from one muscle fibre to the next. Thus, when one cell becomes excited, the action potential spreads rapidly across the entire group of cells, resulting in a coordinated contraction. This functional unit is a *syncytium.* The heart has two syncytia—the *atrial syncytium* and the *ventricular syncytium.* The atrial syncytium contracts from superior to inferior so that the atria express blood to the ventricles. The ventricular syncytium contracts from inferior to superior, expelling blood from the ventricles into the aorta and pulmonary arteries. An impulse can be conducted from the atria to the ventricles only through the *atrioventricular (AV) bundle.*

The cardiac muscle functions according to an "all-or-none" principle. That is, if a single muscle fibre becomes *depolarized,* the action potential will spread through the whole syncytium. Stimulating a single atrial fibre will thus completely depolarize the atria, and stimulating a single ventricular fibre will completely depolarize the ventricles.

Cardiac Depolarization

Normally, an ionic difference exists on the two sides of a cell membrane. The cell's sodium-potassium pump expels sodium (Na^+) from the cell, leaving the inside of the cell more negatively charged than the outside. This difference is called the *resting potential*. When the myocardial cell is stimulated, the membrane changes to allow positively charged sodium ions to rush into the cell, giving the inside of the cell a greater positive charge than the outside. This change of membrane polarity is the *action potential*. After the influx of sodium, a slower influx of calcium ions (Ca^{++}) increases the positive charge inside the cell.

This change from the resting potential (when the inside of the cell is more negatively charged) to a relatively more positive charge inside the cell is called *cardiac depolarization*. Once depolarization occurs in a muscle fibre, it is transmitted throughout the entire syncytium, via the intercalated discs, until the entire muscle mass is depolarized. Contraction of the muscle follows depolarization. The cell membrane remains permeable to sodium for only a fraction of a second. Thereafter, sodium influx stops and potassium escapes from inside the cell. This returns the charge inside the cell to normal (negative). In addition, sodium is actively pumped outside the cell, allowing the cell to *repolarize* and return to its normal resting state.

Understanding the process of cardiac depolarization is critical to understanding and interpreting electrocardiograms (ECGs).

The Cardiac Conductive System

The cardiac conductive system stimulates the ventricles to depolarize in the proper direction. It initiates an impulse, spreads it through the atria, transmits it to the apex of the heart, and from there stimulates the ventricles to depolarize from inferior to superior. The conduction system relies on specialized conductive fibres that transmit the depolarization potential through the heart very quickly.

To accomplish their task, the cardiac conductive cells have the following:

- *Excitability.* The cells can respond to an electrical stimulus.
- *Conductivity.* The cells can propagate the electrical impulse from cell to cell.
- *Automaticity.* Each conductive cell can depolarize without any outside impulse (called self-excitation). Generally, the cell with the fastest rate of discharge becomes the heart's pacemaker. Usually, this is the sinoatrial (SA) node; however, if one pacemaker cell fails to discharge, then the cell with the next fastest rate becomes the pacemaker.
- *Contractility.* The cells have the ability to contract.

Internodal atrial pathways connect the SA node to the atrioventricular (AV) node (Figure 28-3). These internodal pathways conduct the depolarization impulse to the atrial muscle mass and through the atria to the AV junction. The AV junction (the "gatekeeper") slows the impulse and allows the ventricles time to fill. Then, the impulse passes through the AV junction into the AV node and on to the AV fibres, which conduct the impulse from the atria to the ventricles. In the ventricles, the AV fibres form the *bundle of His*.

The bundle of His subsequently divides into the right and left bundle branches. The *right bundle branch* delivers the impulse to the apex of the right ventricle. From there, the *Purkinje system* spreads it across the myocardium. The *left bundle branch* divides into *anterior and posterior fascicles* that also ultimately terminate in the Purkinje system. At the same time that the impulse is transmitted to the right ventricle, the Purkinje system spreads it across the mass of the myocardium. Repolarization predominantly occurs in the opposite direction.

Each conductive system component has an intrinsic rate of self-excitation (SA node 60–100 bpm; AV node 40–60 bpm; Purkinje system 15–40 bpm).

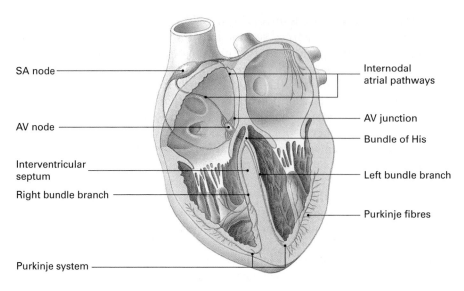

SA node —————— Internodal atrial pathways

AV node —————— AV junction

Interventricular septum —————— Bundle of His

Right bundle branch —————— Left bundle branch

—————— Purkinje fibres

Purkinje system ——————

FIGURE 28-3 The cardiac conductive system.

ELECTROCARDIOGRAPHIC MONITORING

One of your most important skills as a paramedic will be obtaining and interpreting ECG rhythm strips.

* **rhythm strip** electrocardiogram printout.

One of your most important skills as a paramedic will be obtaining and interpreting electrocardiographic (ECG) **rhythm strips.** Your patient's subsequent treatment will be based on rapid, accurate interpretation of these strips. At first, rhythm strips may seem very difficult to read, for only through classroom instruction and repeated practice can you master their interpretation. Nor will every rhythm strip you encounter be a "textbook" example; you must be comfortable with all possible variants. With practice and a systematic approach, however, you will soon become skilled in their interpretation. This section presents basic information about ECG monitoring, as well as recognizing and interpreting dysrhythmias.

THE ELECTROCARDIOGRAM

* **electrocardiogram (ECG)** the graphic recording of the heart's electrical activity. It may be displayed either on paper or on an oscilloscope.

The **electrocardiogram (ECG)** is a graphic recording of the heart's electrical activity. However, it tells you nothing about the heart's pumping ability, which you must evaluate by pulse and blood pressure readings.

The body acts as a giant conductor of electricity, and the heart is its largest generator of electrical energy. Electrodes on the skin can detect the total electrical activity within the heart at any given time. The electrical impulses on the skin surface have a very low voltage. The ECG machine amplifies these impulses and records them over time on ECG graph paper or a monitor. *Positive impulses* appear as *upward* deflections on the paper, *negative impulses* as *downward* deflections. The absence of any electrical impulse produces an *isoelectric line,* which is flat.

* **artifact** deflection on the ECG produced by factors other than the heart's electrical activity.

Artifacts are deflections on the ECG produced by factors other than the heart's electrical activity. Common causes of artifacts include the following:

- Muscle tremors
- Shivering
- Patient movement
- Loose electrodes
- 60 hertz interference
- Machine malfunction

It is important for ECGs to be free of artifacts. When an artifact is present, you must first try to eliminate it before recording the ECG. Loose electrodes should be replaced. Occasionally, patients may be quite diaphoretic, thus preventing the electrodes from adhering well to the skin. In these cases, you may need to wipe the skin and apply tincture of Benzoin before applying the electrode.

ECG Leads

You can obtain many views of the heart's electrical activity by monitoring the voltage change through *electrodes* placed at various places on the body surface. Each pair of electrodes is a *lead*. In the hospital, 12 leads are normally used. As a rule, most EMS systems use only three leads in the field. In fact, one lead alone is adequate for detecting life-threatening dysrhythmias. With the advent of thrombolytic therapy and computer interpretation, however, 12-lead ECGs are becoming more common in the field, especially in rural EMS systems.

The three types of ECG leads are bipolar, augmented, and precordial. **Bipolar leads,** the kind most frequently used, have one positive electrode and one negative electrode. Any electrical impulse moving toward the positive electrode will cause a positive (upward) deflection on the ECG paper. Any electrical impulse moving toward the negative electrode will cause a negative (downward) deflection. The absence of a positive or negative deflection means either that there is no electrical impulse or that the impulse is moving perpendicular to the lead. Leads I, II, and III, commonly called *limb leads,* are bipolar. They are the most frequently used leads in the field. Table 28-1 lists their placement sites.

These three bipolar leads form **Einthoven's triangle,** named after Willem Einthoven, who invented the ECG machine (Figure 28-4). The direction from the negative to the positive electrode is the lead's *axis.* Each lead shows a different axis of the heart. Lead I, at the top of Einthoven's triangle, has an axis of 0 degree. Lead II forms the right side of the triangle and has an axis of 60 degrees. Lead III forms the left side of the triangle and has an axis of 120 degrees.

The bipolar leads provide only three views of the heart. **Augmented,** or **unipolar, leads** provide additional views that are sometimes useful. Although these leads evaluate different axes than the bipolar leads, they utilize the same electrodes. They do this by electronically combining the negative electrodes of two of the bipolar leads to obtain an axis. These augmented leads are designated aVR, aVL, and aVF. The letter *a* indicates that the lead is augmented. The letter *V* identifies it as a unipolar lead. The *R, L,* and *F* identify the extremity on which the lead is placed (R = right arm, L = left arm, and F = left foot).

In addition, six **precordial leads** can be placed across the surface of the chest to measure electrical cardiac activity on a horizontal axis. These leads help in viewing the left ventricle and septum. They are designated V_1 through V_6, with the letter *V* identifying them as unipolar leads.

* **bipolar leads** ECG leads applied to the arms and legs that contain two electrodes of opposite (positive and negative) polarity; leads I, II, and III.

* **Einthoven's triangle** the triangle around the heart formed by the bipolar leads.

* **augmented leads** another term for unipolar leads (see definition below), reflecting the fact that the ground lead is disconnected, which increases the amplitude of deflection on the ECG tracing.

* **unipolar leads** ECG leads applied to the arms and legs, consisting of one polarized (positive) electrode and a non-polarized reference point that is created by the ECG machine combining two additional electrodes; also called augmented limb leads; leads aVR, aVL, and aVF.

* **precordial leads** ECG leads applied to the chest in a pattern that permits a view of the horizontal plane of the heart; leads V1, V2, V3, V4, V5, and V6.

Table 28-1 BIPOLAR LEAD PLACEMENT SITES

Lead	Positive Electrode	Negative Electrode
I	Left arm	Right arm
II	Left leg	Right arm
III	Left leg	Left arm

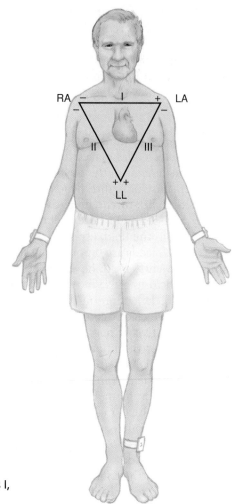

FIGURE 28-4   Einthoven's
triangle as formed by Leads I,
II, and III.

Routine ECG Monitoring

Whether in the ambulance, emergency department, or coronary care unit (CCU), routine ECG monitoring generally uses only one lead. The most common monitoring leads are either Lead II or the *modified chest lead 1* (MCL₁). Of these, Lead II is used more frequently because most of the heart's electrical current flows toward its positive axis. This gives the best view of the ECG waves and best depicts the conduction system's activity. MCL₁ is a special monitoring lead that some systems use selectively to help determine the origin of abnormal complexes, such as premature beats. To avoid confusion, we will use Lead II as the monitor lead throughout this text.

Einthoven's triangle offers a basis for placing the leads. Usually, you should place the electrodes on the chest wall instead of the extremities. This helps reduce artifacts from arm movement. (If you use the arms, place the lead as high as possible on the extremity to decrease movement.) Make certain that the skin is clean and free of hair before you place the electrodes on the chest wall. For Lead II, the positive electrode is usually placed at the apex of the heart on the chest wall (or on the left leg), the negative electrode below the right clavicle (or on the right arm). The third electrode, the ground, is placed somewhere on the left upper chest wall (or on the left arm).

Lead II gives the best view of the ECG waves and best depicts the conduction system's activity.

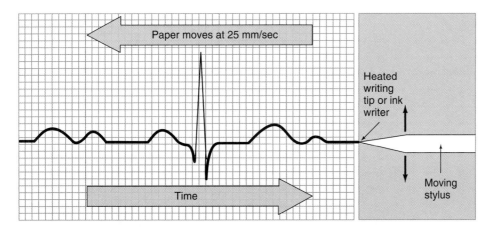

FIGURE 28-5   Recording of the ECG.

A single monitoring lead can provide considerable information:

- The rate of the heartbeat
- The regularity of the heartbeat
- The time it takes to conduct the impulse through the various parts of the heart

A single lead cannot provide the following information:

- The presence or location of an infarct
- Axis deviation or chamber enlargement
- Right-to-left differences in conduction or impulse formation
- The quality or presence of pumping action

ECG Graph Paper

ECG graph paper is standardized to allow comparative analysis of ECG patterns. The paper moves across the stylus at a standard speed of 25 mm/sec (Figure 28-5). The *amplitude* of the ECG *deflection* is also standardized. When properly calibrated, the ECG stylus should deflect two large boxes when one millivolt (mV) is present. Most machines have calibration buttons, and a calibration curve should be placed at the beginning of the first ECG strip. Many machines do this automatically when they are first turned on.

The ECG graph is divided into a grid of light and heavy lines. The light lines are 1 mm apart, and the heavy lines are 5 mm apart. The heavy lines thus enclose large squares, each containing 25 of the smaller squares formed by the lighter lines (Figure 28-6). The following relationships apply to the horizontal axis:

1 small box = 0.04 sec

1 large box = 0.20 sec (0.04 sec × 5 = 0.20 sec)

These increments measure the duration of the ECG complexes and time intervals. The vertical axis reflects the voltage amplitude in millivolts (mV). Two large boxes equal 1.0 mV.

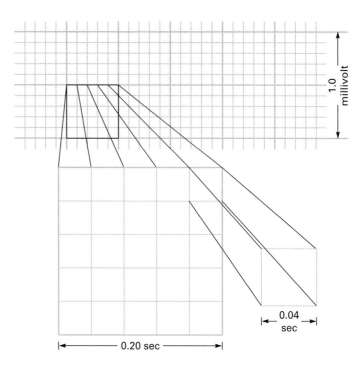

FIGURE 28-6   The ECG paper and markings.

In addition to the grid, the ECG paper has time interval markings at the top. These marks are placed at three-second intervals. Each three-second interval contains 15 large boxes (0.2 sec × 15 boxes = 3.0 sec). The time markings measure heart rate.

RELATIONSHIP OF THE ECG TO ELECTRICAL EVENTS IN THE HEART

The ECG tracing's components reflect electrical changes in the heart (Figure 28-7).

- *P wave.* The first component of the ECG, the P wave corresponds to atrial depolarization. On Lead II, it is a positive, rounded wave before the QRS complex (Figures 28-8 to 28-12).

- *QRS complex.* The QRS complex reflects ventricular depolarization. The *Q wave* is the first negative deflection after the P wave; the *R wave* is the first positive deflection after the P wave; and the *S wave* is the first negative deflection after the R wave. Not all three waves are always present, and the shape of the QRS complex can vary from individual to individual (Figure 28-13).

- *T wave.* The T wave reflects repolarization of the ventricles. Normally positive in Lead II, it is rounded and usually moves in the same direction as the QRS complex (Figure 28-14).

- *U wave.* Occasionally, a U wave appears. U waves follow T waves and are usually positive. U waves may be associated with electrolyte abnormalities, or they may be a normal finding.

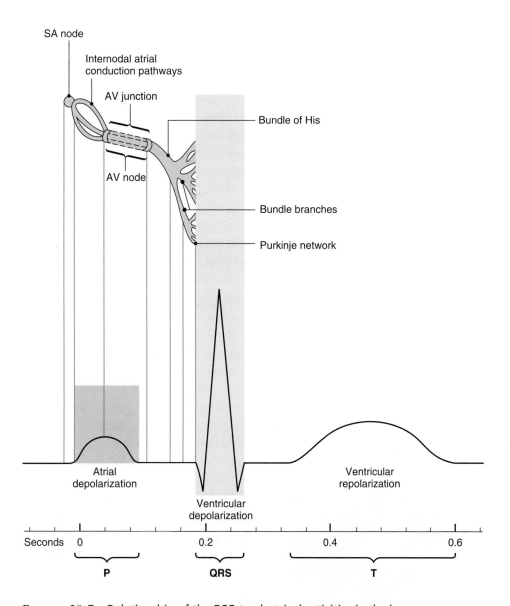

FIGURE 28-7   Relationship of the ECG to electrical activities in the heart.

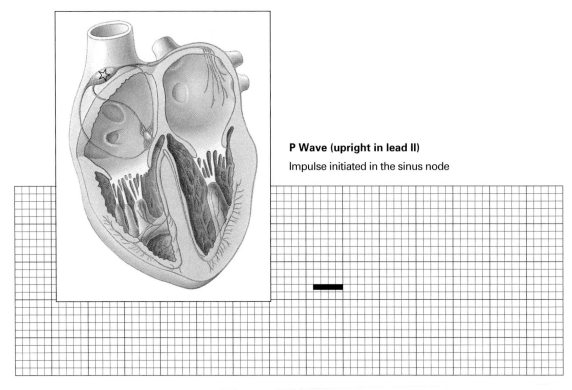

P Wave (upright in lead II)

Impulse initiated in the sinus node

FIGURE 28-8   Impulse initiation in the SA node.

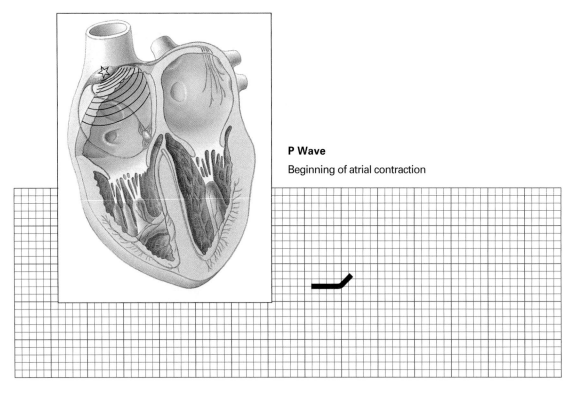

P Wave

Beginning of atrial contraction

FIGURE 28-9   Beginning of atrial contraction.

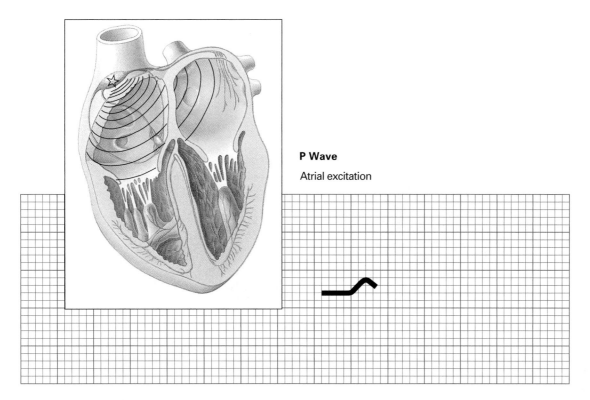

P Wave

Atrial excitation

FIGURE 28-10   Atrial excitation.

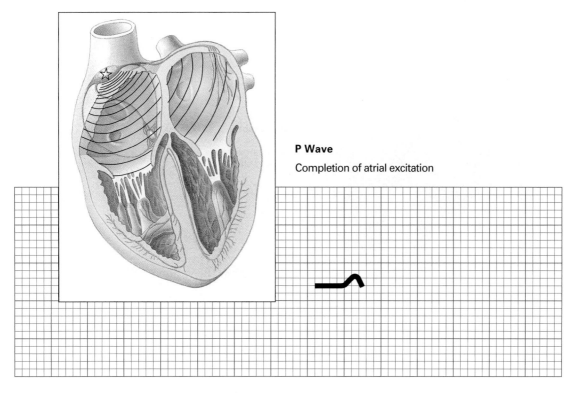

P Wave

Completion of atrial excitation

FIGURE 28-11   Completion of atrial excitation.

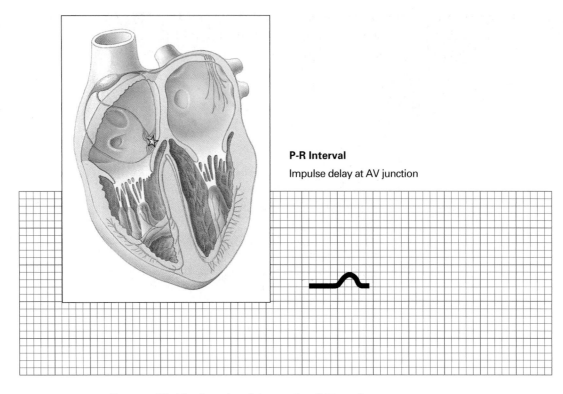

P-R Interval

Impulse delay at AV junction

FIGURE 28-12   Impulse delay at the AV junction.

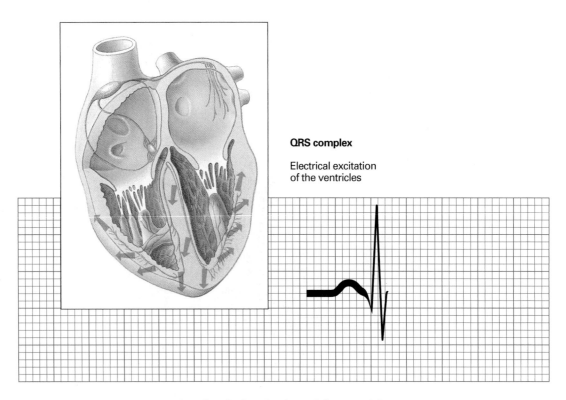

QRS complex

Electrical excitation
of the ventricles

FIGURE 28-13   Electrical excitation of the ventricles.

FIGURE 28-15 The ECG.

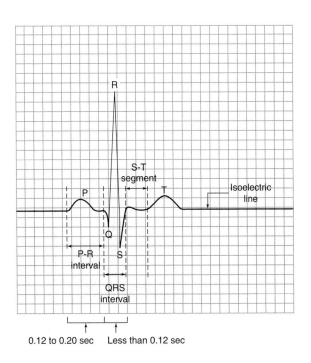

0.12 to 0.20 sec   Less than 0.12 sec

* refractory period the period of time when myocardial cells have not yet completely repolarized and cannot be stimulated again.

* absolute refractory period the period of the cardiac cycle when stimulation will not produce any depolarization whatever.

* relative refractory period the period of the cardiac cycle when a sufficiently strong stimulus may produce depolarization.

and cannot be stimulated again (Figure 28-16). This **refractory period** has two parts, an **absolute refractory period** and a **relative refractory period**. During the absolute refractory period, stimulation produces no depolarization whatsoever. This usually lasts from the beginning of the QRS complex to the apex of the T wave. During the relative refractory period, a sufficiently strong stimulus may produce depolarization. This usually corresponds to the T wave's down slope.

S-T Segment Changes The S-T segment is usually an isoelectric line. Myocardial infarctions, which are caused by lack of blood flow to a part of the heart, produce changes in this line. The affected area is then electrically dead and cannot conduct electrical impulses. Myocardial infarctions usually follow this sequence:

1. Ischemia (lack of oxygen)
2. Injury
3. Necrosis (cell death, infarction)

Each of these stages results in distinct S-T segment changes. Ischemia causes S-T segment depression or an inverted T wave. The inversion is usually symmetrical. Injury elevates the S-T segment, most often in the early phases of a myocardial infarction. As the tissue dies, a significant Q wave appears. As we noted earlier, small, insignificant Q waves may show up in normal ECG tracings. A significant Q wave is at least one small square wide, lasting 0.04 seconds, or is more than one-third the height of the QRS complex. Q waves may also indicate extensive transient ischemia.

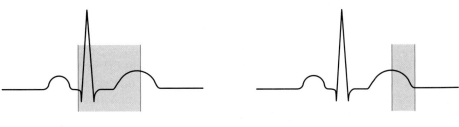

Absolute Refractory Period   Relative Refractory Period

FIGURE 28-16   Refractory periods of the cardiac cycle.

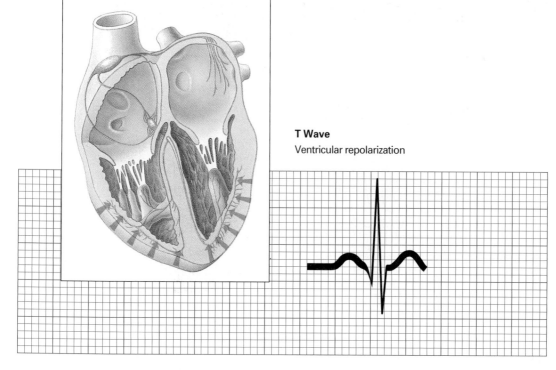

T Wave
Ventricular repolarization

FIGURE 28-14   Ventricular repolarization.

In addition to the wave forms described above, the ECG tracing reflects these important time intervals (Figure 28-15):

- *P-R interval (PRI) or P-Q interval (PQI).* The P-R interval is the distance from the beginning of the P wave to the beginning of the QRS complex. It represents the time the impulse takes to travel from the atria to the ventricles. Occasionally, the R wave is absent, in which case this interval is called the P-Q interval. The terms P-R interval and P-Q interval may be used interchangeably.

- *QRS interval.* The QRS interval is the distance from the first deflection of the QRS complex to the last. It represents the time necessary for ventricular depolarization.

- *S-T segment.* The S-T segment is the distance from the S wave to the beginning of the T wave. Usually, it is an isoelectric line; however, it may be elevated or depressed in certain disease states, such as ischemia.

A normal P-R interval is 0.12–0.20 seconds. A short PRI lasts less than 0.12 seconds; a prolonged PRI lasts longer than 0.20 seconds. A prolonged PRI indicates a delay in the AV node. A normal QRS complex lasts between 0.08 and 0.12 seconds. A value of less than 0.12 seconds means that the ventricles depolarized in a normal length of time.

The **QT interval** represents the total duration of ventricular depolarization. A normal QT interval is 0.33–0.42 seconds. QT intervals and heart rate have an inverse relationship: increases in heart rate usually decrease the QT interval, while decreases in heart rate usually prolong it. A **prolonged QT interval** is thought to be related to an increased risk of certain ventricular dysrhythmias and sudden death.

The all-or-none nature of myocardial depolarization results in an interval when the heart cannot be restimulated to depolarize. From our earlier discussion, you will recall that during this time the myocardial cells have not yet repolarized

Table 28-2   OVERVIEW OF ECG LEAD GROUPINGS

Leads	Portion of the heart examined
I and aVL	The left side of the heart in a vertical plane
II, III, and aVF	The inferior (diaphragmatic) side of the heart
aVR	The right side of the heart in a vertical plane
V_1 and V_2	The right ventricle
V_3 and V_4	The intraventricular septum and the anterior wall of the left ventricle
V_5 and V_6	The anterior and lateral walls of the left ventricle

Lead Systems and Heart Surfaces Using the various ECG leads is comparable to waiting for a train at a railroad crossing. You will want to know how long you have to wait (in other words, how long is the train), but you can only see the front of the train. If you had cameras at other viewpoints, you could see how long the train actually was. Similarly, by combining the different ECG leads you can view different parts of the heart.

Leads V_1–V_4 view the anterior surface of the heart. Leads I and aVL view the lateral surface of the heart. The inferior surface of the heart can be visualized in leads II, III, and aVF. These leads can show ischemia, injury, and necrotic changes and can provide information about the corresponding heart surface (Table 28-2). For example, significant S-T elevation in V_1–V_4 may indicate anterior involvement, while elevation in II, III, and aVF may indicate inferior involvement.

Medical procedures (angioplasty) and drugs (thrombolytics) can treat acute myocardial infarction (AMI). The earlier they are initiated, the better is the patient's potential outcome. Earlier identification in the field of patients with AMI will allow for earlier interventions, but the 12-lead ECG's role in out-of-hospital care remains unresolved. Its use may not be appropriate in many EMS settings. Individual EMS medical directors will determine the application and use of the 12-lead ECG in their specific EMS settings.

Earlier identification in the field of patients with AMI will allow for earlier intervention.

INTERPRETATION OF RHYTHM STRIPS

The key to interpreting rhythm strips is to approach each strip logically and systematically. Attempts to nonanalytically "eyeball" the strip often lead to incorrect interpretations. Your approach to rhythm strip interpretation should include the following basic criteria:

The key to interpreting rhythm strips is to approach each strip logically and systematically.

- Always be consistent and analytical.
- Memorize the rules for each dysrhythmia.
- Analyze a given rhythm strip according to a specific format.
- Compare your analysis with the description for each dysrhythmia.
- Identify the dysrhythmia by its similarity to established descriptions.

Use ECG calipers to measure ECG tracings to ensure accuracy and to avoid misinterpretation.

The health-care profession uses several standard formats for ECG analysis. We will use the following five-step procedure:

1. Analyze the rate.
2. Analyze the rhythm.
3. Analyze the P waves.
4. Analyze the P-R interval.
5. Analyze the QRS complex.

Analyzing Rate The first step in ECG strip interpretation is to analyze the heart rate. Usually, this means the ventricular rate; however, if the atrial and ventricular rates differ, you must calculate both. The normal heart rate is 60–100 beats per minute (bpm). A heart rate faster than 100 bpm is a **tachycardia**. A heart rate slower than 60 bpm is a **bradycardia**. You can use any of the following methods to calculate the rate.

* *Six-Second Method.* Count the number of complexes in a six-second interval. Mark off a six-second interval by noting two three-second marks at the top of the ECG paper. Then, multiply the number of complexes within the six-second strip by 10.

* *Heart Rate Calculator Rulers.* Commercially available heart rate calculator rulers allow you to determine heart rates rapidly. Always use them according to the accompanying directions, since variations occur among different manufacturers. Also learn a manual method so that you can still calculate rates if you forget your ruler.

* *R-R Interval.* The R-R interval is related directly to heart rate. The R-R interval method is accurate only if the heart rhythm is regular. You can calculate it in the following ways:
  – Measure the duration between R waves in seconds. Divide 60 by this number, giving the heart rate per minute.
    Example: 60 ÷ 0.65 second = 92 (heart rate)
  – Count the number of large squares within an R-R interval, and divide 300 by the number of squares.
    Example: 300 ÷ 3.5 large boxes = 86 (heart rate)
  – Count the number of small squares within an R-R interval, and divide 1500 by the number of squares.
    Example: 1500 ÷ 29 small boxes = 52 (heart rate)

* *Triplicate Method.* Another method, also useful only with regular rhythms, is to locate an R wave that falls on a dark line bordering a large box on the graph paper. Then, assign numbers corresponding to the heart rate to the next six dark lines to the right. The order is: 300, 150, 100, 75, 60, and 50. The number corresponding to the dark line closest to the peak of the next R wave is a rough estimate of the heart rate.

Pick one of the above methods, and become comfortable with it. Use it to determine the rate on all strips that you look at.

Analyzing Rhythm The next step is to analyze the rhythm. First, measure the R-R interval across the strip. Normally, the R-R rhythm is fairly regular. Some minimal variation, associated with respirations, should be expected. If the rhythm is irregular, note whether it fits one of the following patterns:

* Occasionally irregular (only one or two R-R intervals on the strip are irregular)
* Regularly irregular (patterned irregularity or group beating)
* Irregularly irregular (no relationship among R-R intervals)

Analyzing P Waves The P waves reflect atrial depolarization. Normally, the atria depolarize away from the SA node and toward the ventricles. In Lead II, this appears as a positive, rounded P wave. When analyzing the P waves, ask yourself the following questions:

* Are P waves present?
* Are the P waves regular?

---

* **tachycardia** a heart rate of more than 100 bpm.

* **bradycardia** a heart rate of fewer than 60 bpm.

- Is there one P wave for each QRS complex?
- Are the P waves upright or inverted (compared with the QRS complex)?
- Do all the P waves look alike?

Analyzing the P-R Interval The P-R interval represents the time needed for atrial depolarization and conduction of the impulse up to the AV node. Remember, the normal P-R interval is 0.12–0.20 sec (3 to 5 small boxes). Any deviation is an abnormal finding. The P-R interval should be consistent across the strip.

Analyzing the QRS Complex The QRS complex represents ventricular depolarization. When evaluating the QRS complex, ask yourself the following questions:

- Do all of the QRS complexes look alike?
- What is the QRS duration?

Remember, the QRS duration is usually 0.04–0.12 sec. Anything longer than 0.12 sec (three small boxes) is abnormal.

DYSRHYTHMIAS

On a normal ECG, the heart rate is between 60 and 100 bpm. The rhythm is regular (both P-P and R-R). The P waves are normal in shape, upright, and appear only before each QRS complex. The P-R interval lasts 0.12–0.20 sec and is constant. The QRS complex has a normal morphology, and its duration is less than 0.12 sec. All of these factors indicate a **normal sinus rhythm** (Figure 28-17A). Any deviation from the heart's normal electrical rhythm is a **dysrhythmia**. The absence of cardiac electrical activity is **arrhythmia**. The causes of dysrhythmias include the following:

- Myocardial ischemia, necrosis, or infarction
- Autonomic nervous system imbalance
- Distention of the chambers of the heart (especially in the atria, secondary to congestive heart failure)
- Blood gas abnormalities, including hypoxia and abnormal pH
- Electrolyte imbalances (Ca^{++}, K^+, Mg^{++})
- Trauma to the myocardium (cardiac contusion)
- Drug effects and drug toxicity
- Electrocution
- Hypothermia
- CNS damage
- Idiopathic events
- Normal occurrences

Dysrhythmias in the healthy heart are of little significance. No matter what the etiology or type of dysrhythmia, treat the patient and his symptoms, not the dysrhythmia. You will hear this repeated over and over: Treat the patient, not the monitor.

MECHANISM OF IMPULSE FORMATION

Several physiological mechanisms can cause cardiac dysrhythmias. The depolarization impulse is normally transmitted forward (*antegrade*) through the conductive system and the myocardium. In certain dysrhythmias, however, the depolarization impulse is conducted backward (*retrograde*).

* **normal sinus rhythm** the normal heart rhythm.

* **dysrhythmia** any deviation from the normal electrical rhythm of the heart.

* **arrhythmia** the absence of cardiac electrical activity; often used interchangeably with dysrhythmia.

Treat the patient, not the monitor.

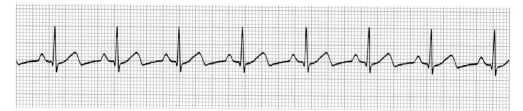

FIGURE 28-17A   Normal sinus rhythm.

Ectopic Foci   One cause of dysrhythmias is *enhanced automaticity*. This condition results when **ectopic foci** (heart cells other than the pacemaker cells) automatically depolarize, producing **ectopic** (abnormal) **beats**. Premature ventricular contractions and premature atrial contractions are examples of ectopic beats. Ectopic beats can be intermittent or sustained.

Reentry   *Reentry* may cause isolated premature beats, or *tachydysrhythmias*. It occurs when ischemia or another disease process alters two branches of a conduction pathway, slowing conduction in one branch and causing a unidirectional block in the other. An antegrade depolarization wave travels slowly through the branch with ischemia and is blocked in the branch with a unidirectional block. After the depolarization wave goes through the slowed branch, it enters the branch with the unidirectional block and is conducted in a retrograde manner back to the branch's origin. By now the tissue is no longer refractory, and stimulation occurs again. This can result in rapid rhythms, such as paroxysmal supraventricular tachycardia or atrial fibrillation.

CLASSIFICATION OF DYSRHYTHMIAS

Dysrhythmias can be classified in any number of ways. Some of the classification methods include the following:

- Nature of origin (changes in automaticity versus disturbances in conduction)
- Magnitude (major versus minor)
- Severity (life threatening versus non-life threatening)
- Site of origin

Classifying dysrhythmias by site of origin is closely related to basic physiology and thus is easy to understand. This approach divides dysrhythmias into the following categories:

- Dysrhythmias originating in the SA node
- Dysrhythmias originating in the atria
- Dysrhythmias originating within the AV junction
- Dysrhythmias sustained in or originating in the AV junction
- Dysrhythmias originating in the ventricles
- Dysrhythmias resulting from disorders of conduction

DYSRHYTHMIAS ORIGINATING IN THE SA NODE

Dysrhythmias originating in the SA node most often result from changes in autonomic tone. However, disease can exist in the SA node itself. Dysrhythmias that originate in the SA node include the following:

- Sinus bradycardia
- Sinus tachycardia
- Sinus dysrhythmia
- Sinus arrest

Sinus Bradycardia

Description: Sinus bradycardia results from slowing of the SA node.

Etiology: Sinus bradycardia may result from any of the following conditions:

- Increased parasympathetic (vagal) tone
- Intrinsic disease of the SA node
- Drug effects (digitalis, propranolol, quinidine)
- Normal finding in healthy, well-conditioned persons

Rules of Interpretation/Lead II Monitoring (Figure 28-17B):

Rate—fewer than 60
Rhythm—regular
Pacemaker site—SA node
P waves—upright and normal in morphology
P-R interval—normal (0.12–0.20 sec and constant)
QRS complex—normal (0.04–0.12 sec)

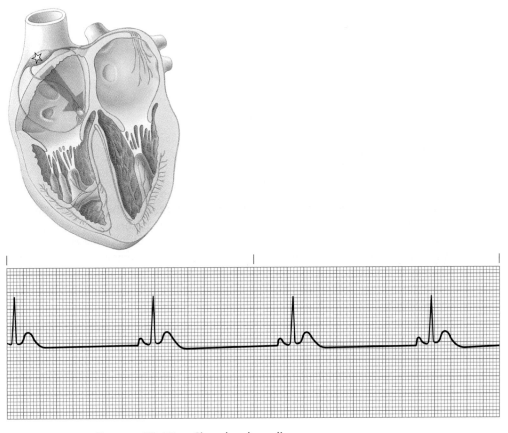

FIGURE 28-17B   Sinus bradycardia.

Clinical Significance: The decreased heart rate can cause decreased cardiac output, hypotension, angina, or CNS symptoms. This is especially true for rates slower than 50 bpm. The slow heart rate may also lead to atrial ectopic or ventricular ectopic rhythms. In a healthy athlete, sinus bradycardia may have no clinical significance.

Treatment: Treatment is generally unnecessary unless hypotension or ventricular irritability is present (Figure 28-18). Remember, treat your patient and not the monitor. If treatment is required, administer a 0.5-mg bolus of atropine sulphate. Repeat every 3–5 minutes until you have obtained a satisfactory rate or have given 0.04 mg/kg of the drug. If atropine fails, consider transcutaneous cardiac pacing (TCP) if available.

Sinus Tachycardia

Description: Sinus tachycardia results from an increased rate of SA node discharge.

Etiology: Sinus tachycardia may result from any of the following:

- Exercise
- Fever
- Anxiety
- Hypovolemia
- Anemia
- Pump failure
- Increased sympathetic tone
- Hypoxia
- Hyperthyroidism

Rules of Interpretation/Lead II Monitoring (Figure 28-19):

Rate—more than 100
Rhythm—regular
Pacemaker site—SA node
P waves—upright and normal in morphology
P-R interval—normal
QRS complex—normal

Clinical Significance: Sinus tachycardia is often benign. In some cases, it is a compensatory mechanism for decreased stroke volume. If the rate is greater than 140 bpm, cardiac output may fall because ventricular filling time is inadequate. Very rapid heart rates increase myocardial oxygen demand and can precipitate ischemia or infarct in diseased hearts. Prolonged sinus tachycardia accompanying acute myocardial infarction (AMI) is often an ominous finding suggesting cardiogenic shock.

Treatment: Treatment is directed at the underlying cause. Hypovolemia, fever, hypoxia, or other causes should be corrected.

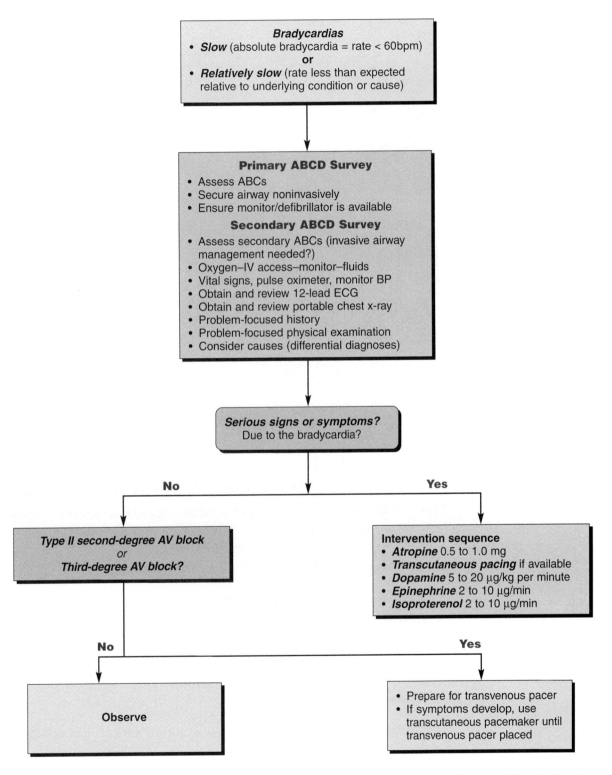

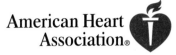

FIGURE 28-18   Management of bradycardia. Reproduced with permission from *Guidelines 2000 for Cardiopulmonary Resuscitation and Emergency Cardiovasular Care,* ©2000, Copyright American Heart Association.

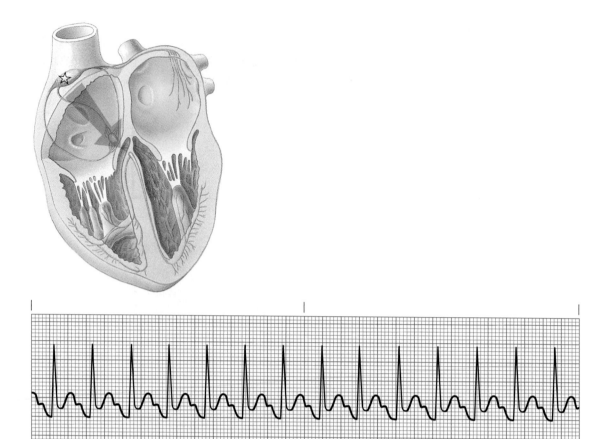

FIGURE 28-19   Sinus tachycardia.

Sinus Dysrhythmia

Description: Sinus dysrhythmia often results from a variation of the R-R interval.

Etiology: Sinus dysrhythmia is often a normal finding and is sometimes related to the respiratory cycle and changes in intrathoracic pressure. Pathologically, sinus dysrhythmia can be caused by enhanced vagal tone.

Rules of Interpretation/Lead II Monitoring (Figure 28-20):

   Rate—60–100 (varies with respirations)
   Rhythm—irregular
   Pacemaker site—SA node
   P waves—upright and normal in morphology
   P-R interval—normal
   QRS complex—normal

Clinical Significance: Sinus dysrhythmia is a normal variant, particularly in the young and the aged.

Treatment: Typically, none required.

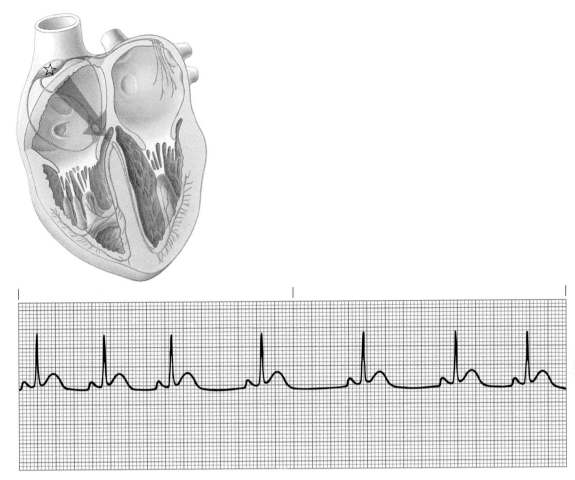

FIGURE 28-20   Sinus dysrhythmia.

Sinus Arrest

Description: Sinus arrest occurs when the sinus node fails to discharge, resulting in short periods of cardiac standstill. This standstill can persist until pacemaker cells lower in the conductive system discharge (escape beats) or until the sinus node resumes discharge.

Etiology: Sinus arrest can result from any of the following conditions:

- Ischemia of the SA node
- Digitalis toxicity
- Excessive vagal tone
- Degenerative fibrotic disease

Rules of Interpretation/Lead II Monitoring (Figure 28-21):

Rate—normal to slow, depending on the frequency and duration of the arrest

Rhythm—irregular

Pacemaker site—SA node

P waves—upright and normal in morphology

P-R interval—normal

QRS complex—normal

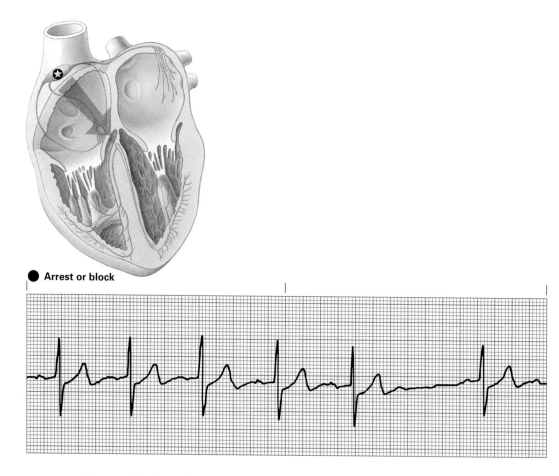

● **Arrest or block**

FIGURE 28-21   Sinus arrest.

Clinical Significance: Frequent or prolonged episodes may compromise cardiac output, resulting in syncope (fainting) and other problems. There is always the danger of complete cessation of SA node activity. Usually, an escape rhythm develops; however, cardiac standstill occasionally can result.

Treatment: If the patient is asymptomatic, observation is all that is required. If the patient is extremely bradycardic or symptomatic, administer a 0.5-mg bolus of atropine sulphate. Repeat every 3–5 minutes until you have obtained a satisfactory rate or have administered 0.04 mg/kg of the drug. If atropine fails, consider transcutaneous cardiac pacing (TCP) if available.

DYSRHYTHMIAS ORIGINATING IN THE ATRIA

Dysrhythmias can originate outside the SA node in the atrial tissue or in the internodal pathways. Ischemia, hypoxia, atrial dilation, and other factors can cause atrial dysrhythmias. Dysrhythmias originating in the atria include the following:

- Wandering atrial pacemaker
- Multifocal atrial tachycardia
- Premature atrial contractions
- Paroxysmal supraventricular tachycardia
- Atrial flutter
- Atrial fibrillation

Wandering Atrial Pacemaker

Description: *Wandering atrial pacemaker* is the passive transfer of pacemaker sites from the sinus node to other latent pacemaker sites in the atria and AV junction. Often, more than one pacemaker site will be present, causing variation in R-R interval and P wave morphology.

Etiology: Wandering atrial pacemaker can result from any of the following conditions:

- A variant of sinus dysrhythmia
- A normal phenomenon in the very young or the aged
- Ischemic heart disease
- Atrial dilation

Rules of Interpretation/Lead II Monitoring (Figure 28-22):

Rate—usually normal

Rhythm—slightly irregular

Pacemaker site—varies among the SA node, atrial tissue, and the AV junction

P waves—morphology changes from beat to beat; P waves may disappear entirely

P-R interval—varies; may be less than 0.12 sec, normal, or greater than 0.20 sec

QRS Complex—normal

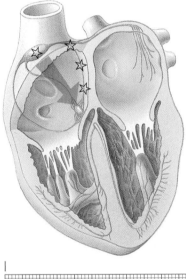

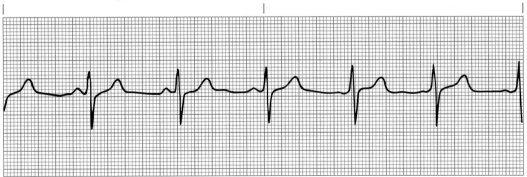

FIGURE 28-22   Wandering pacemaker.

Clinical Significance: Wandering atrial pacemaker usually has no detrimental effects. Occasionally, it can be a precursor of other atrial dysrhythmias, such as atrial fibrillation. It sometimes indicates digitalis toxicity.

Treatment: If the patient is asymptomatic, observation is all that is required.

Multifocal Atrial Tachycardia

Description: Multifocal atrial tachycardia (MAT) is usually seen in acutely ill patients. Significant pulmonary disease is seen in about 60 percent of these patients. Certain medications used to treat lung disease (such as theophylline) may worsen the dysrhythmia. Three different P waves are noted, indicating various ectopic foci.

Etiology: Multifocal atrial tachycardia can result from any of the following conditions:

- Pulmonary disease
- Metabolic disorders (hypokalemia)
- Ischemic heart disease
- Recent surgery

Rules of Interpretation/Lead II Monitoring (Figure 28-23):

Rate—more than 100

Rhythm—irregular

Pacemaker site—ectopic sites in atria

P waves—organized, discrete nonsinus P waves with at least three different forms

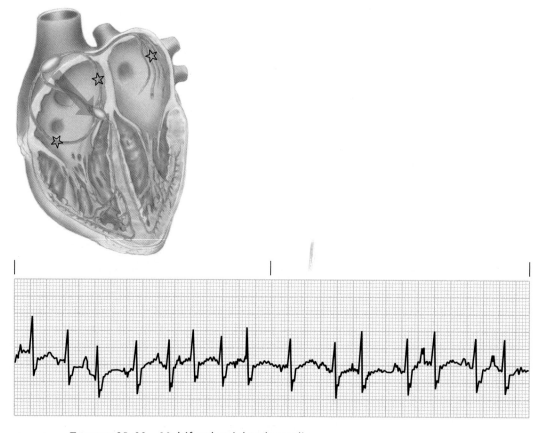

FIGURE 28-23   Multifocal atrial tachycardia.

P-R interval—varies

QRS complex—may be less than 0.12 sec, normal, or greater than 0.20 sec, depending on the AV node's refractory status when the impulse reaches it

Clinical Significance: Frequently, these patients are acutely ill; this dysrhythmia may indicate a serious underlying medical illness.

Treatment: Treatment of the underlying medical disease usually resolves the dysrhythmia. Specific antidysrhythmic therapy is frequently not needed.

Premature Atrial Contractions

Description: Premature atrial contractions (PACs) result from a single electrical impulse originating in the atria outside the SA node, which, in turn, causes a premature depolarization of the heart before the next expected sinus beat. Because it depolarizes the atrial syncytium, this impulse also depolarizes the SA node, interrupting the normal cadence. This creates a **noncompensatory pause** in the underlying rhythm.

Etiology: A premature atrial contraction can result from any of the following conditions:

* Use of caffeine, tobacco, or alcohol
* Sympathomimetic drugs
* Ischemic heart disease
* Hypoxia
* Digitalis toxicity
* No apparent cause (idiopathic)

Rules of Interpretation/Lead II Monitoring (Figure 28-24):

Rate—depends on the underlying rhythm

Rhythm—depends on the underlying rhythm; usually regular except for the PAC

Pacemaker site—ectopic focus in the atrium

P waves—the P wave of the PAC differs from the P wave of the underlying rhythm. It occurs earlier than the next expected P wave and may be hidden in the preceding T wave.

P-R interval—usually normal; can vary with the location of the ectopic focus. Ectopic foci near the SA node will have a P-R interval of 0.12 sec or greater, whereas ectopic foci near the AV node will have a P-R interval of 0.12 sec or less.

QRS complex—usually normal; may be greater than 0.12 sec if the PAC is abnormally conducted through partially refractory ventricles. In some cases, the ventricles are refractory and will not depolarize in response to the PAC. In these cases, the QRS complex is absent.

Clinical Significance: Isolated PACs are of minimal significance. Frequent PACs may indicate organic heart disease and may precede other atrial dysrhythmias.

Treatment: If the patient is asymptomatic, observation is all that is required in the field. If the patient is symptomatic, administer oxygen via a nonrebreather mask, and start an IV line. Contact medical direction.

* **noncompensatory pause** pause following an ectopic beat when the SA node is depolarized and the underlying cadence of the heart is interrupted.

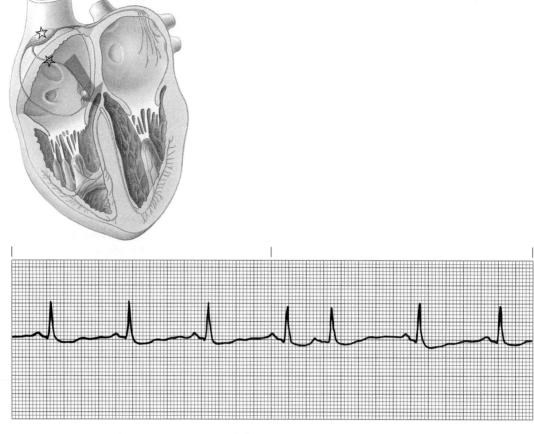

FIGURE 28-24   Premature atrial contractions.

Paroxysmal Supraventricular Tachycardia

Description: Paroxysmal supraventricular tachycardia (PSVT) occurs when rapid atrial depolarization overrides the SA node. It often occurs in paroxysm with sudden onset, may last minutes to hours, and terminates abruptly. It may be caused by increased automaticity of a single atrial focus or by reentry phenomenon at the AV node.

Etiology: Paroxysmal supraventricular tachycardia may occur at any age and often is not associated with underlying heart disease. It may be precipitated by stress, overexertion, smoking, or ingestion of caffeine. It is, however, frequently associated with underlying atherosclerotic cardiovascular disease and rheumatic heart disease. PSVT is rare in patients with myocardial infarction. It can occur with accessory pathway conduction, such as in Wolff-Parkinson-White syndrome.

Rules of Interpretation/Lead II Monitoring (Figure 28-25):

Rate—150–250 per minute

Rhythm—characteristically regular, except at onset and termination

Pacemaker site—in the atria, outside the SA node

P waves—the atrial P waves differ slightly from sinus P waves. The P wave is often buried in the preceding T wave. The P wave may be impossible to see, especially if the rate is rapid. Turning up the speed of the graph paper or oscilloscope to 50 mm/sec spreads out the complex and can help identify P waves.

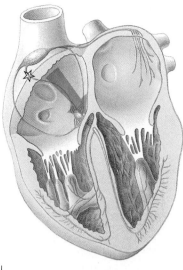

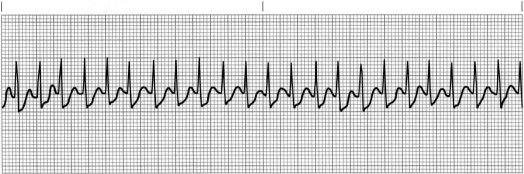

FIGURE 28-25   Paroxysmal supraventricular tachycardia.

P-R interval—usually normal; however, it can vary with the location of the ectopic pacemaker. Ectopic pacemakers near the SA node will have P-R intervals close to 0.12 sec, whereas ectopic pacemakers near the AV node will have P-R intervals of 0.12 sec or less.

QRS complex—normal

Clinical Significance: Young patients with good cardiac reserves may tolerate PSVT well for short periods. Patients often sense PSVT as palpitations. However, rapid rates can cause a marked reduction in cardiac output because of inadequate ventricular filling time. The reduced diastolic phase of the cardiac cycle can also compromise coronary artery perfusion. PSVT can precipitate angina, hypotension, or congestive heart failure.

Treatment: If the patient is not tolerating the rapid heart rate, as evidenced by hemodynamic instability, attempt the following techniques in the order given in Figure 28-26:

1. *Vagal manoeuvres.* Ask the patient to perform a Valsalva manoeuvre. This is a forced expiration against a closed glottis, or the act of "bearing down" as if to move the bowels. This results in vagal stimulation, which may slow the heart. If this is unsuccessful, attempt carotid artery massage, if it is suitable. Do not attempt carotid artery massage in patients with carotid **bruits** or known cerebrovascular or carotid artery disease.

✱ **bruit** the sound of turbulent blood flow through a vessel; usually associated with atherosclerotic disease.

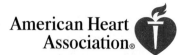

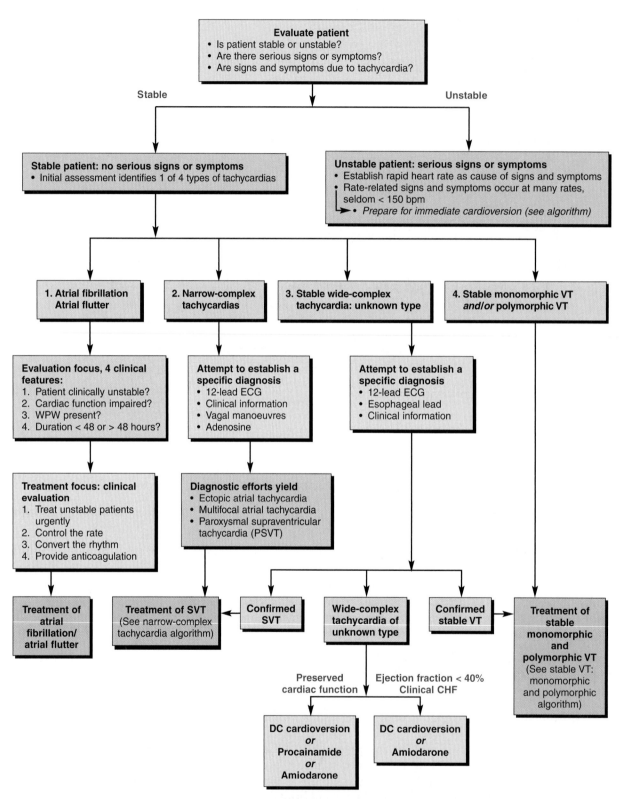

FIGURE 28-26   Management of tachycardia. Reproduced with permission from *Guidelines 2000 for Cardiopulmonary Resuscitation and Emergency Cardiovascular Care,* ©2000, Copyright American Heart Association.

2. *Pharmacological therapy.* Adenosine (Adenocard) is very safe and highly effective in terminating PSVT, especially if its etiology is reentry. Administer 6 mg of adenosine by rapid IV bolus over 1–3 sec through the medication port closest to the patient's heart or central circulation. (Adenosine has a very short half-life, and you must immediately follow administration with a bolus of normal saline to allow the medication to reach its site of action while it is still effective.) If the patient does not convert after 1–2 minutes, administer a second bolus of 12 mg over 1–3 sec in the medication port closest to the patient's heart or central circulation. If this fails and the patient has a normal blood pressure, then look again at the width of the cardiac QRS. If it appears to be a narrow complex rhythm with a normal blood pressure, medical direction may request the administration of verapamil 2.5–5.0 mg. This can be repeated once in 15–30 minutes, if needed, at a dose of 5–10 mg. Verapamil is contraindicated in patients with a history of bradycardia, hypotension, or congestive heart failure. Do not use it with intravenous beta-blockers; use it with caution in patients on chronic beta-blocker therapy. Hypotension following verapamil administration can often be reversed with 0.5–1.0 g of calcium chloride administered intravenously.

3. *Electrical therapy.* If the ventricular rate is greater than 150 bpm, or if the patient is hemodynamically unstable, use synchronized cardioversion (described later in the chapter). If time allows, sedate the patient with 5–10 mg of diazepam or 2–5 mg of midazolam (Versed) IV. Apply synchronized direct current (DC) countershock of 100 joules. If this is unsuccessful, repeat the countershock at increased energy as ordered by medical direction. DC countershock is contraindicated if you suspect digitalis toxicity as the PSVT's cause.

Atrial Flutter

Description: Atrial flutter results from a rapid atrial reentry circuit and an AV node that physiologically cannot conduct all impulses through to the ventricles. The AV junction may allow impulses in a 1:1 (rare), 2:1, 3:1, or 4:1 ratio or greater, resulting in a discrepancy between atrial and ventricular rates. The AV block may be consistent or variable.

Etiology: Atrial flutter may occur in normal hearts, but it is usually associated with organic disease. It rarely occurs as the direct result of an MI. Atrial dilation, which occurs with congestive heart failure, is a cause of atrial flutter.

Rules of Interpretation/Lead II Monitoring (Figure 28-27):

Rate—atrial rate is 250–350 per minute. Ventricular rate varies with the ratio of AV conduction.

Rhythm—atrial rhythm is regular; ventricular rhythm is usually regular but can be irregular if the block is variable

Pacemaker site—sites in the atria outside the SA node

P waves—flutter (F) waves are present, resembling a sawtooth or picket-fence pattern. This pattern is often difficult to identify in a 2:1 flutter. However, if the ventricular rate is approximately 150, suspect 2:1 flutter.

P-R interval—usually constant but may vary

QRS complex—normal

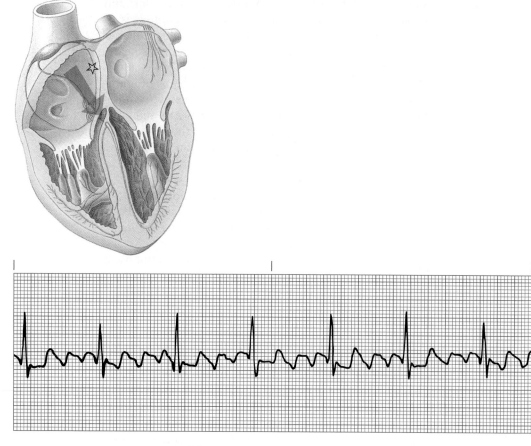

FIGURE 28-27   Atrial flutter.

Clinical Significance: Atrial flutter with normal ventricular rates is generally well tolerated. Rapid ventricular rates may compromise cardiac output and result in symptoms. Atrial flutter often occurs in conjunction with atrial fibrillation and is referred to as "atrial fib-flutter."

Treatment: Treatment is indicated only for rapid ventricular rates with hemodynamic compromise (review Figure 28-26).

1. *Electrical therapy.* Immediate cardioversion is indicated in unstable patients—those with a heart rate greater than 150 and associated chest pain, dyspnea, a decreased level of consciousness, or hypotension. If time allows, sedate the patient with 5–10 mg of diazepam (Valium) or 2–5 mg of midazolam (Versed) IV. Then, apply synchronized DC countershock of 100 joules. If this is unsuccessful, repeat the countershock at increased energy as recommended by American Heart Association (AHA) guidelines.

2. *Pharmacological therapy.* Occasionally, you may use pharmacological therapy in stable patients with atrial flutter, especially if the rapid heart rate is causing congestive heart failure. Several medications slow the ventricular rate. The most frequently used is diltiazem (Cardizem). In addition, you may use verapamil, digoxin, beta-blockers, procainamide, and quinidine. Procainamide and quinidine are often used to convert atrial flutter

back to a sinus rhythm. Consult medical direction, or refer to local protocols concerning pharmacological therapy for atrial flutter.

Atrial Fibrillation

Description: Atrial fibrillation results from multiple areas of reentry within the atria or from multiple ectopic foci bombarding an AV node that physiologically cannot handle all of the incoming impulses. AV conduction is random and highly variable.

Etiology: Atrial fibrillation may be chronic and is often associated with underlying heart disease, such as rheumatic heart disease, atherosclerotic heart disease, or congestive heart failure. Atrial dilation occurs with congestive heart failure and often causes atrial fibrillation.

Rules of Interpretation/Lead II Monitoring (Figure 28-28):

Rate—atrial rate is 350–750 per minute (cannot be counted); ventricular rate varies greatly depending on conduction through the AV node.

Rhythm—irregularly irregular

Pacemaker site—numerous ectopic foci in the atria

P waves—none discernible. Fibrillation (f) waves are present, indicating chaotic atrial activity.

P-R interval—none

QRS complex—normal

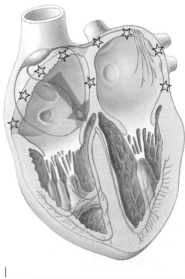

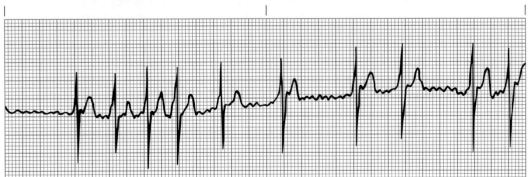

FIGURE 28-28   Atrial fibrillation.

Clinical Significance: In atrial fibrillation, the atria fail to contract and the so-called atrial kick is lost, thus reducing cardiac output by 20–25 percent. There is frequently a *pulse deficit* (a difference between the apical and peripheral pulse rates). If the rate of ventricular response is normal, as often occurs in patients on digitalis, the rhythm is usually well tolerated. If the ventricular rate is fewer than 60 bpm, cardiac output can fall. Suspect digitalis toxicity in patients taking digitalis, with atrial fibrillation and a ventricular rate slower than 60. If the ventricular response is rapid, coupled with the loss of atrial kick, cardiovascular decompensation may occur, resulting in hypotension, angina, infarct, congestive heart failure, or shock.

Treatment: Treatment is indicated only for rapid ventricular rates with hemodynamic compromise (review Figure 28-26).

1. *Electrical therapy.* Immediate cardioversion is indicated in unstable patients—those with heart rates greater than 150 and associated chest pain, dyspnea, a decreased level of consciousness, or hypotension. If time allows, sedate the patient with 5–10 mg of diazepam (Valium) or 2–5 mg of midazolam (Versed) IV. Then, apply synchronized DC countershock of 100 joules. If this is unsuccessful, repeat the countershock at increased energy, as ordered by medical direction.

2. *Pharmacological therapy.* Occasionally, you will use pharmacological therapy in stable patients with atrial fibrillation, especially if the rapid heart rate is causing congestive heart failure. Several medications slow the ventricular rate. The most frequently used is diltiazem (Cardizem). In addition, verapamil, digoxin, beta-blockers, procainamide, and quinidine can be used. Procainamide and quinidine are used to convert atrial fibrillation to a normal sinus rhythm. Atrial fibrillation is a documented risk factor for the development of stroke. As the atria fibrillate, they dilate. This allows for stagnation of blood flow within the atria and subsequent clot development. Because of this, it is sometimes prudent to administer an anticoagulant (heparin or warfarin [Coumadin]) to these patients to prevent stroke. Consult medical direction, or refer to local protocols concerning pharmacological therapy for atrial fibrillation.

Patients with accessory pathways, such as in Wolff-Parkinson-White syndrome, who develop atrial flutter or atrial fibrillation present special concerns. Usually, the electrical impulse reaches the ventricles via the accessory tract, the AV node (normal conduction pathway), or both. If the patient's refractory period is short in his accessory tract, more atrial impulses will be conducted down the accessory tract than through the AV node. This will result in a wide QRS complex. Rapid atrial rates occur with atrial fibrillation and flutter and can cause rapid ventricular rates. These rhythms, which have a wide complex, may resemble ventricular tachycardia. Excessive stimulation of the ventricles may actually precipitate ventricular fibrillation.

Verapamil will decrease conduction through the AV node and may shorten the refractory period of the accessory tract. Because of this, however, verapamil may accelerate the ventricular response rate and may precipitate ventricular tachycardia and ventricular fibrillation. Wolff-Parkinson-White and the other pre-excitation syndromes are presented in more detail later in this chapter.

DYSRHYTHMIAS ORIGINATING WITHIN THE AV JUNCTION (AV BLOCKS)

Two potential problems in the AV junction (or AV node) may result in dysrhythmias. One is an atrioventricular (AV) block, in which the electrical impulse is slowed or blocked as it passes through the AV node. The other is dysrhythmias due to a malfunction of AV junctional cells themselves.

The AV junction is an important part of the conductive system, serving two important physiological purposes (Figure 28-29). First, it effectively slows the impulse between the atria and the ventricles to allow for atrial emptying and ventricular filling. Second, it serves as a backup pacemaker if the SA node or cells higher in the conductive system fail to fire. Part of the AV tissues function as a pacemaker node and other parts serve as the junction between the atria and the ventricles.

The internodal fibres that blend to form the AV junction are called *transitional fibres*. These small fibres slow the impulse. The transitional fibres then blend into the AV junction. The lower portion of the AV node penetrates the fibrous tissue that separates the atria from the ventricles. This part of the node also slows impulse conduction. After penetrating the fibrous band, the AV node then becomes the AV bundle, which is also called the bundle of His. The bundle of His subsequently divides into the left and right bundle branches.

Atrioventricular Blocks

An *AV block* delays or interrupts impulses between the atria and the ventricles. These dysrhythmias can be caused by pathology of the AV junctional tissue or by a physiological block, such as occurs with atrial fibrillation or flutter. Their causes include AV junctional ischemia, AV junctional necrosis, degenerative disease of the conductive system, and drug toxicity (particularly from digitalis).

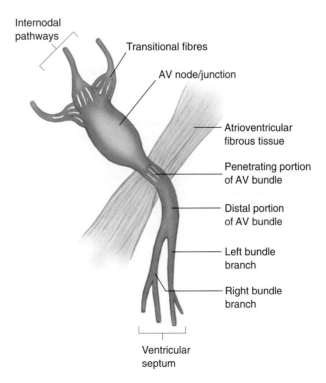

FIGURE 28-29 Organization of the AV node.

AV blocks can be classified according to the site or the degree of the block. Blocks may occur at the following sites:

- At the AV node
- At the bundle of His
- Below the bifurcation of the bundle of His

Our discussion classifies AV blocks by the following degrees (traditional classification):

- First-degree AV block
- Type I second-degree AV block
- Type II second-degree AV block (Mobitz II, or Infranodal)
- Third-degree AV block

First-Degree AV Block

Description: A *first-degree AV block* is a delay in conduction at the level of the AV node, rather than an actual block. First-degree AV block is not a rhythm in itself but a condition superimposed on another rhythm. The underlying rhythm must also be identified (for example, sinus bradycardia with first-degree AV block).

Etiology: AV block can occur in the healthy heart. However, ischemia at the AV junction is the most common cause.

Rules of Interpretation/Lead II Monitoring (Figure 28-30):

Rate—depends on underlying rhythm

Rhythm—usually regular; can be slightly irregular

Pacemaker site—SA node or atria

P waves—normal

P-R interval—greater than 0.20 sec (diagnostic)

QRS complex—usually less than 0.12 sec; may be bizarre in shape if conductive system disease exists in the ventricles

Clinical Significance: First-degree block is usually no danger in itself. However, a newly developed first-degree block may precede a more advanced block.

Treatment: Generally, no treatment is required, except observation, unless the heart rate drops significantly. If possible, avoid drugs that slow AV conduction, such as lidocaine and procainamide.

Type I Second-Degree AV Block

Description: A *type I second-degree AV block* (also called *second-degree, Mobitz I;* or *Wenckebach*) is an intermittent block at the level of the AV node. It produces a characteristic cyclic pattern in which the P-R intervals become progressively longer until an impulse is blocked (not conducted). The cycle is repetitive, and the P-P interval remains constant. The ratio of conduction (P waves to QRS complexes) is commonly 5:4, 4:3, 3:2, or 2:1. The pattern may be constant or variable.

Etiology: Low-grade AV blocks (first-degree and second-degree, Mobitz I) can occur in the healthy heart. However, ischemia at the AV junction is the most common cause. Increased parasympathetic tone and drugs are also common etiologies.

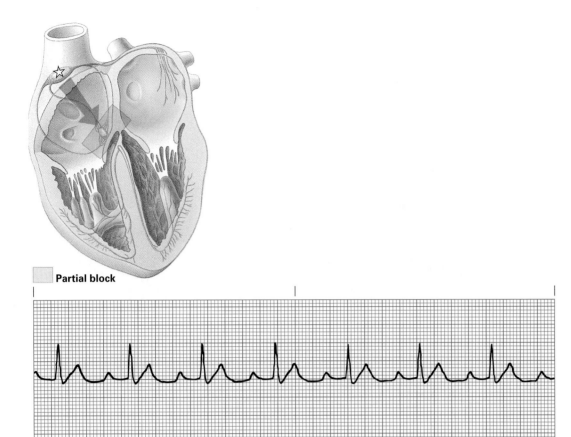

Partial block

FIGURE 28-30   First-degree AV block.

Rules of Interpretation/Lead II Monitoring (Figure 28-31):

Rate—atrial rate is unaffected; the ventricular rate may be normal or slowed

Rhythm—atrial rhythm is typically regular; ventricular rhythm is irregular because of the nonconducted beat

Pacemaker site—SA node or atria

P waves—normal; some P waves are not followed by QRS complexes

P-R interval—becomes progressively longer until the QRS complex is dropped; the cycle then repeats

QRS complex—usually less than 0.12 sec; may be bizarre in shape if conductive system disease exists in the ventricles

Clinical Significance: If beats are frequently dropped, second-degree block can compromise cardiac output by causing such problems as syncope and angina. This block is often a transient phenomenon that occurs immediately after an inferior wall myocardial infarction.

Treatment: Generally, no treatment other than observation is required. If possible, avoid drugs that slow AV conduction, such as lidocaine and procainamide. If the heart rate falls and the patient becomes symptomatic, administer 0.5 mg of atropine IV. Repeat every 3–5 minutes until you have obtained a satisfactory rate or have given 0.04 mg/kg of the drug. If atropine fails, consider transcutaneous cardiac pacing (TCP) if available.

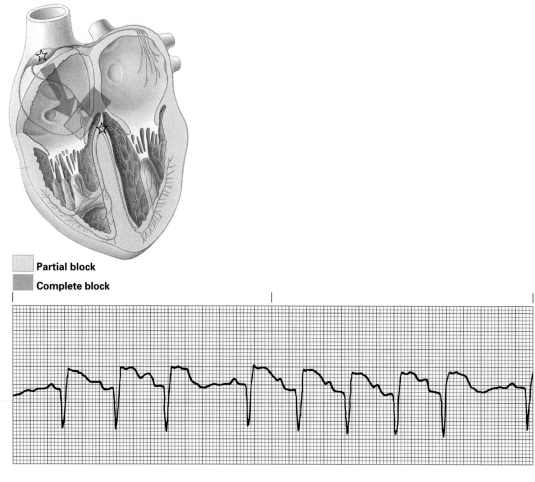

Partial block

Complete block

FIGURE 28-31   Type I second-degree AV block.

Type II Second-Degree AV Block

Description: A *type II second-degree AV block* (also called *second-degree, Mobitz II;* or *infranodal*) is an intermittent block characterized by P waves that are not conducted to the ventricles but without associated lengthening of the P-R interval before the dropped beats. The ratio of conduction (P waves to QRS complexes) is commonly 4:1, 3:1, or 2:1. The ratio may be constant or may vary. A 2:1 Mobitz II block is often indistinguishable from a 2:1 Mobitz I block.

Etiology: Second-degree AV block, Mobitz II, is usually associated with acute myocardial infarction and septal necrosis.

Rules of Interpretation/Lead II Monitoring (Figure 28-32):

Rate—atrial rate is unaffected; ventricular rate is usually bradycardic

Rhythm—regular or irregular, depending on whether the conduction ratio is constant or varied

Pacemaker site—SA node or atria

P waves—normal; some P waves are not followed by QRS complexes

P-R interval—constant for conducted beats; may be greater than 0.21 sec

QRS complex—may be normal; however, it is often greater than 0.12 sec because of abnormal ventricular depolarization sequence

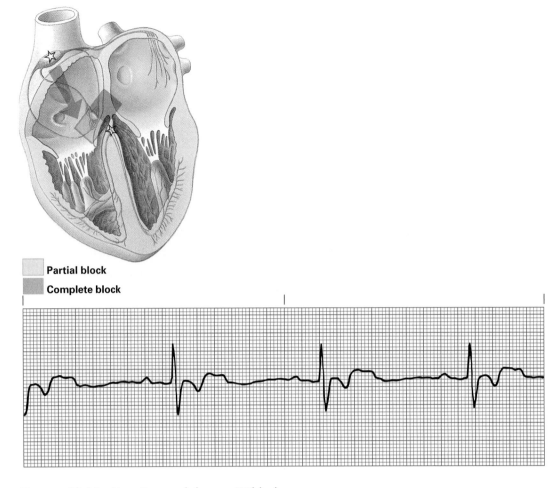

Partial block

Complete block

FIGURE 28-32   Type II second-degree AV block.

Clinical Significance: A Mobitz II block can compromise cardiac output, causing such problems as syncope and angina if beats are frequently dropped. Since this block is often associated with cell necrosis resulting from myocardial infarction, it is considered much more serious than Mobitz I. Many Mobitz II blocks develop into full AV blocks.

Treatment: Pacemaker insertion is the definitive treatment. In the field, administer medications if stabilization is required. If the heart rate falls and the patient becomes symptomatic, administer 0.5 mg of atropine IV. Repeat every 3–5 minutes until you have obtained a satisfactory rate or have given 0.04 mg/kg of the drug. Use atropine with caution in patients who have high-grade blocks (second-degree, Mobitz II, and third-degree). The atropine may accelerate the atrial rate, but it may also worsen the AV nodal block. Consider transcutaneous cardiac pacing (TCP) if available. If the patient remains symptomatic, do not delay application of TCP while waiting for IV access or for atropine to take effect.

Third-Degree AV Block

Description: A *third-degree AV block,* or *complete block,* is the absence of conduction between the atria and the ventricles resulting from complete electrical block at or below the AV node. The atria and ventricles subsequently pace the heart independently of each other. The sinus node often functions normally, depolarizing the atrial syncytium, while the escape pacemaker, located below the atria, paces the ventricular syncytium.

Etiology: Third-degree AV block can result from acute myocardial infarction, digitalis toxicity, or degeneration of the conductive system, as occurs in the elderly.

Rules of Interpretation/Lead II Monitoring (Figure 28-33):

Rate—atrial rate is unaffected. Ventricular rate is 40–60 if the escape pacemaker is junctional, slower than 40 if the escape pacemaker is lower in the ventricles.

Rhythm—both atrial and ventricular rhythms are usually regular

Pacemaker site—SA node and AV junction or ventricle

P waves—normal. P waves show no relationship to the QRS complex, often falling within the T wave and QRS complex.

P-R interval—no relationship between P waves and R waves

QRS complex—greater than 0.12 sec if pacemaker is ventricular; less than 0.12 second if pacemaker is junctional

Clinical Significance: Third-degree block can severely compromise cardiac output because of decreased heart rate and loss of coordinated atrial kick.

Treatment: Pacemaker insertion is the definitive treatment. In the field, administer medications if stabilization is required. If the heart rate falls and the patient becomes symptomatic, administer 0.5 mg of atropine IV. You can repeat this every

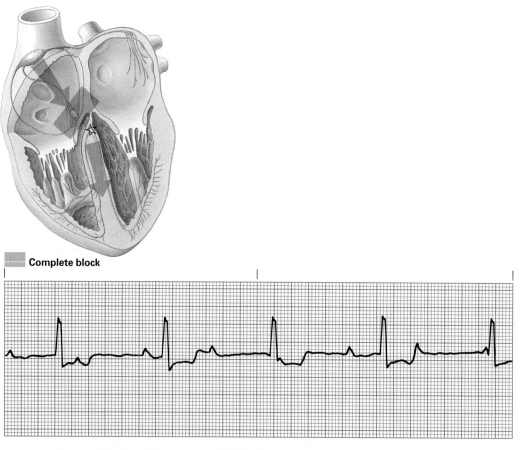

■ **Complete block**

FIGURE 28-33   Third-degree AV block.

3–5 minutes until you have obtained a satisfactory rate or have given 0.04 mg/kg of the drug. Use atropine with caution in patients with high-grade blocks (second-degree, Mobitz II, and third-degree). The atropine may accelerate the atrial rate, but it may also worsen the AV nodal block. Consider transcutaneous cardiac pacing (TCP) if available. If the patient remains symptomatic, do not delay application of TCP while waiting for IV access or for atropine to take effect. Never use lidocaine to treat third-degree heart block with ventricular escape beats.

Never use lidocaine to treat third-degree heart block with ventricular escape beats.

DYSRHYTHMIAS SUSTAINED OR ORIGINATING IN THE AV JUNCTION

Dysrhythmias can originate within the AV node. The location of the pacemaker site will dictate the morphology of the P wave. Ischemia, hypoxia, and other factors have been identified as causes. Dysrhythmias originating in the AV junction include the following:

- Premature junctional contractions
- Junctional escape complexes and rhythm
- Accelerated junctional rhythm
- Paroxysmal junctional tachycardia

All dysrhythmias that originate in the AV junction have in common the following ECG features:

- Inverted P waves in Lead II, resulting from retrograde depolarization of the atria. The P wave's relation to QRS depolarization depends on the relative timing of atrial and ventricular depolarization. The P wave can occur before the QRS complex, if the atria depolarize first; after the QRS, if the ventricles depolarize first; or during the QRS, if the atria and ventricles depolarize simultaneously. Depolarization of the atria during ventricular depolarization masks the P wave. Some atrial complexes that originate near the AV junction can also result in inverted P waves.
- P-R interval of less than 0.12 sec
- Normal QRS complex duration

Premature Junctional Contractions

Description: Premature junctional contractions (PJCs) result from a single electrical impulse originating in the AV node that occurs before the next expected sinus beat. A PJC can result in either a **compensatory pause** or noncompensatory pause, depending on whether the SA node is depolarized. A noncompensatory pause occurs if the premature beat depolarizes the SA node and interrupts the heart's normal cadence. A compensatory pause occurs only if the SA node discharges before the premature impulse reaches it.

✱ **compensatory pause** the pause following an ectopic beat where the SA node is unaffected and the cadence of the heart is uninterrupted.

Etiology: A PJC can result from any of the following conditions:

- Use of caffeine, tobacco, or alcohol
- Sympathomimetic drugs
- Ischemic heart disease
- Hypoxia
- Digitalis toxicity
- No apparent cause (idiopathic)

Rules of Interpretation/Lead II Monitoring (Figure 28-34):

Rate—depends on the underlying rhythm

Rhythm—depends on the underlying rhythm, usually regular except for the PJC

Pacemaker site—ectopic focus in the AV junction

P waves—inverted; may appear before or after the QRS complex. P waves can be masked by the QRS complex or be absent.

P-R interval—if the P wave occurs before the QRS complex, the P-R interval will be less than 0.12 sec; if the P wave occurs after the QRS complex, then technically it is an R-P interval

QRS complex—usually normal; may be greater than 0.12 sec if the PJC is abnormally conducted through partially refractory ventricles

Clinical Significance: Isolated PJCs are of minimal significance. Frequent PJCs indicate organic heart disease and may be precursors to other junctional dysrhythmias.

Treatment: If the patient is asymptomatic, only observation is required in the field.

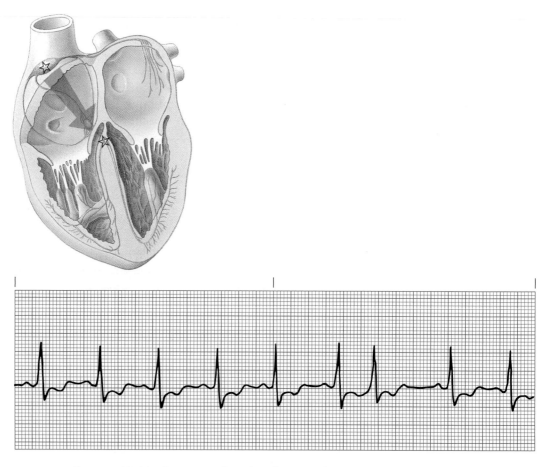

FIGURE 28-34   Premature junctional contractions.

Junctional Escape Complexes and Rhythms

Description: A *junctional escape beat,* or *junctional escape rhythm,* is a dysrhythmia that results when the rate of the primary pacemaker, usually the SA node, is slower than that of the AV node. The AV node then becomes the pacemaker. The AV node usually discharges at its intrinsic rate of 40–60 bpm. This is a safety mechanism that prevents cardiac standstill.

Etiology: Junctional escape rhythm has several etiologies, including increased vagal tone, which can result in SA node slowing; pathological slow SA node discharge; or heart block.

Rules of Interpretation/Lead II Monitoring (Figure 28-35):

Rate—40–60 per minute

Rhythm—irregular in single junctional escape complex; regular in junctional escape rhythm

Pacemaker site—AV junction

P waves—inverted; may appear before or after the QRS complex. The P waves can be masked by the QRS or be absent.

P-R interval—if the P wave occurs before the QRS complex, the P-R interval will be less than 0.12 sec. If the P wave occurs after the QRS complex, technically it is an R-P interval.

QRS complex—usually normal; may be greater than 0.12 sec

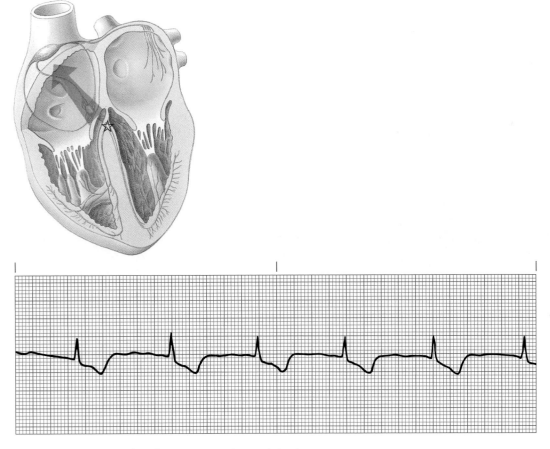

FIGURE 28-35   Junctional escape complex and rhythm.

Clinical Significance: The slow heart rate can decrease cardiac output, possibly precipitating angina and other problems. If the rate is fairly rapid, the rhythm can be well tolerated.

Treatment: If the patient is asymptomatic, only observation is required in the field. Treatment is unnecessary unless hypotension or ventricular irritability is present. If treatment is required, administer a 0.5-mg bolus of atropine sulphate. Repeat every 3–5 minutes until you have obtained a satisfactory rate or have given a total of 0.04 mg/kg of the drug. If atropine fails, consider transcutaneous cardiac pacing (TCP) if available.

Accelerated Junctional Rhythm

Description: An *accelerated junctional rhythm* results from increased automaticity in the AV junction, causing the AV junction to discharge faster than its intrinsic rate. If the rate becomes fast enough, the AV node can override the SA node. Technically, the rate associated with an accelerated junctional rhythm is not a tachycardia. However, when compared with the intrinsic rate of the AV junctional tissue (40–60 bpm), it is considered accelerated.

Etiology: Accelerated junctional rhythms often result from ischemia of the AV junction.

Rules of Interpretation/Lead II Monitoring (Figure 28-36):

Rate—60–100 per minute

Rhythm—regular

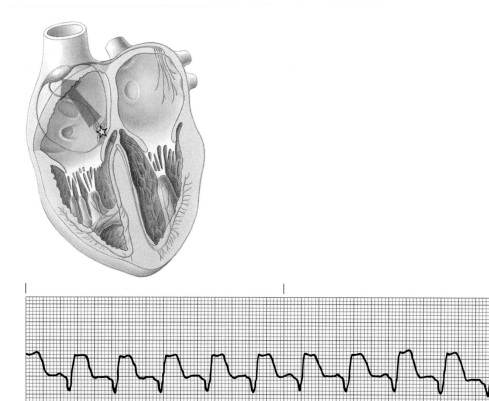

FIGURE 28-36   Accelerated junctional rhythm.

Pacemaker site—AV junction

P waves—inverted; may appear before or after the QRS complex. P waves may be masked by the QRS or be absent.

P-R interval—if the P wave occurs before the QRS complex, the P-R interval will be less than 0.12 sec. If it occurs after the QRS, technically it is an R-P interval.

QRS complex—normal

Clinical Significance: An accelerated junctional rhythm is usually well tolerated. However, since ischemia is often the etiology, the patient should be monitored for other dysrhythmias.

Treatment: Prehospital treatment generally is unnecessary.

Paroxysmal Junctional Tachycardia

Description: Paroxysmal junctional tachycardia (PJT) develops when rapid AV junctional depolarization overrides the SA node. It often occurs in *paroxysms* (attacks with sudden onset), may last minutes or hours, and terminates abruptly. It may be caused by increased automaticity of a single AV nodal focus or by a reentry phenomenon at the AV node. Paroxysmal junctional tachycardia is often more appropriately called *paroxysmal supraventricular tachycardia (PSVT),* since the rapid rate may make it indistinguishable from paroxysmal atrial tachycardia.

Etiology: Paroxysmal junctional tachycardia may occur at any age and may not be associated with underlying heart disease. Stress, overexertion, smoking, or ingestion of caffeine may precipitate it. However, it is frequently associated with underlying atherosclerotic heart disease (ASHD) and rheumatic heart disease. PJT rarely occurs with myocardial infarction. It can occur with accessory pathway conduction, as in Wolff-Parkinson-White syndrome.

Rules of Interpretation/Lead II Monitoring (Figure 28-37):

Rate—100–180 per minute

Rhythm—characteristically regular, except at onset and termination of paroxysms

Pacemaker site—AV junction

P waves—if present, P waves are inverted. They can occur before, during, or after the QRS complex. Turning up the speed of the graph paper or oscilloscope to 50 mm/sec spreads out the complex and aids in identifying P waves.

P-R interval—if the P wave occurs before the QRS complex, the P-R interval will be less than 0.12 sec. If it occurs after the QRS complex, technically it is an R-P interval.

QRS complex—normal

Clinical Significance: Young patients with good cardiac reserve may tolerate PJT well for a short time. The patient often will sense PJT as palpitations. However, rapid rates can preclude adequate ventricular filling time and markedly reduce cardiac output. The reduced diastolic phase of the cardiac cycle can also compromise coronary artery perfusion. PJT can precipitate angina, hypotension, or congestive heart failure.

Treatment: If the patient is not tolerating the rapid heart rate, as evidenced by hemodynamic instability, attempt the following techniques in the given order.

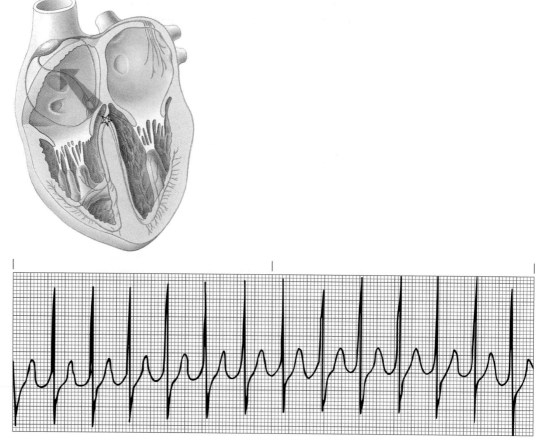

FIGURE 28-37   Paroxysmal junctional tachycardia.

1. *Vagal manoeuvres.* Ask the patient to perform a Valsalva manoeuvre. This is a forced expiration against a closed glottis, or "bearing down" as if to move the bowels. This results in vagal stimulation, which may slow the heart. If this is unsuccessful, attempt carotid artery massage if the patient is eligible. (Do not attempt carotid artery massage in patients with carotid bruits or known cerebrovascular or carotid artery disease.)

2. *Pharmacological therapy.* Adenosine (Adenocard) is relatively safe and highly effective in terminating PJT. This is especially true if its etiology is reentry. Administer 6 mg of adenosine by rapid IV bolus over 1–3 seconds through the medication port closest to the patient's heart or central circulation. If the patient does not convert after 1–2 minutes, administer a second bolus of 12 mg over 1–3 seconds in the medication port closest to the patient's heart or central circulation. If this fails, and the patient has a normal blood pressure, medical direction may request the administration of verapamil. Verapamil is contraindicated in patients with a history of bradycardia, hypotension, or congestive heart failure. Do not use it with intravenous beta-blockers; use it with caution in patients on chronic beta-blocker therapy. Hypotension that occurs following verapamil administration can often be reversed with 0.5–1.0 g of calcium chloride administered intravenously.

3. *Electrical therapy.* If the ventricular rate is greater than 150 bpm or the patient is hemodynamically unstable, use synchronized cardioversion. If time allows, sedate the patient with 5–10 mg of diazepam (Valium) or 2–5 mg of midazolam (Versed) IV. Apply synchronized DC countershock of 100 joules. If this is unsuccessful, repeat the countershock at increased energy as ordered by medical direction. DC countershock is contraindicated if you suspect digitalis toxicity as the cause of the PJT.

DYSRHYTHMIAS ORIGINATING IN THE VENTRICLES

Some dysrhythmias originate within the ventricles. The pacemaker site will dictate the morphology of the QRS complex. Many factors, including ischemia, hypoxia, and medications, have been identified as causes. Dysrhythmias originating in the ventricles include the following:

- Ventricular escape complexes and rhythms
- Accelerated idioventricular rhythm
- Premature ventricular contraction
- Ventricular tachycardia
- Related dysrhythmia
- Ventricular fibrillation
- Asystole
- Artificial pacemaker rhythm

ECG features common to all dysrhythmias that originate in the ventricles include:

- QRS complexes of 0.12 sec or greater
- Absent P waves

Ventricular Escape Complexes and Rhythms

Description: A *ventricular escape beat* (*ventricular escape rhythm* or *idioventricular rhythm*) results either when impulses from higher pacemakers fail to reach the ventricles or when the discharge rate of higher pacemakers becomes less than that of the ventricles (normally 15–40 bpm). Ventricular escape rhythms serve as safety mechanisms to prevent cardiac standstill.

Etiology: Ventricular escape complexes and ventricular rhythms have several etiologies, including slowing of supraventricular pacemaker sites or high-degree AV block. They are frequently the first organized rhythms seen following successful defibrillation.

Rules of Interpretation/Lead II Monitoring (Figure 28-38):

Rate—15–40 per minute (occasionally fewer)

Rhythm—the rhythm is irregular in a single ventricular escape complex. Ventricular escape rhythms are usually regular unless the pacemaker site is low in the ventricular conductive system. Such placement makes regularity unreliable.

Pacemaker site—ventricle

P waves—none

P-R interval—none

QRS complex—greater than 0.12 sec and bizarre in morphology

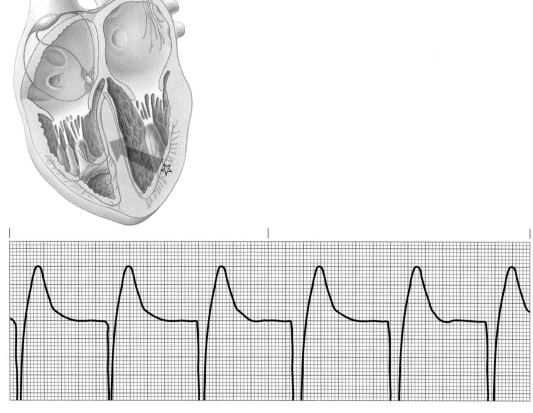

FIGURE 28-38   Ventricular escape complexes and rhythms (idioventricular rhythms).

Clinical Significance: The slow heart rate can significantly decrease cardiac output, possibly to life-threatening levels. The ventricular escape rhythm is a safety mechanism that you should not suppress. Escape rhythms can be perfusing or nonperfusing.

Treatment: Treatment depends on whether the escape rhythm is perfusing or nonperfusing. If it is perfusing, the object of treatment is to increase the heart rate. Administer a 0.5-mg bolus of atropine sulfate. Repeat every 3–5 minutes until you have obtained a satisfactory rate or have given 0.04 mg/kg of the drug. If atropine fails, consider transcutaneous cardiac pacing (TCP) if available. If the rhythm is nonperfusing, follow the pulseless electrical activity (PEA) protocol. This includes airway stabilization and cardiopulmonary resuscitation (CPR). Place an IV line, and administer 1 mg of epinephrine 1:10 000 IV. Direct treatment at correcting the primary problem (hypovolemia, hypoxia, cardiac tamponade, acidosis, or others). Consider a fluid challenge.

Accelerated Idioventricular Rhythm

Accelerated idioventricular rhythm is an abnormally wide ventricular dysrhythmia that usually occurs during an acute myocardial infarction. It is a subtype of ventricular escape rhythm. Typically the rate is 60–100 bpm. The patient does not require treatment unless he becomes hemodynamically unstable. If this occurs, treat the ventricular focus with atropine or overdrive pacing. The principal action should be aggressive treatment of the underlying myocardial infarction as indicated, including appropriate prehospital care.

Premature Ventricular Contractions

Description: A *premature ventricular contraction* (*PVC, or ventricular ectopic*) is a single ectopic impulse arising from an irritable focus in either ventricle that occurs earlier than the next expected beat. It may result from increased automaticity in the ectopic cell or a reentry mechanism. The altered sequence of ventricular depolarization results in a wide and bizarre QRS complex and may additionally cause the T wave to occur in the direction opposite the QRS complex.

A PVC does not usually depolarize the SA node and interrupt its rhythm. That is, it does not interrupt the heart's normal cadence. The pause following the PVC is fully *compensatory*. Occasionally, an **interpolated beat** occurs when a PVC falls between two sinus beats without interrupting the rhythm.

If more than one PVC occurs, each can be classified as unifocal or multifocal. Because the PVC's morphology depends on the ectopic pacemaker's location, two PVCs of different morphologies imply two different pacemaker sites (multifocal). PVCs with the same morphology imply one pacemaker site (unifocal). If the **coupling interval** (the distance between the preceding beat and the PVC) is constant, the PVCs are most likely unifocal.

PVCs often occur in patterns of group beating:

* *Bigeminy*—every other beat is a PVC

* *Trigeminy*—every third beat is a PVC

* *Quadrigeminy*—every fourth beat is a PVC

These terms can be applied to PACs and PJCs as well.

Repetitive PVCs are two consecutive PVCs without a normal complex in between. They can occur in groups of two (couplets) or three (triplets). More than three consecutive PVCs are often considered ventricular tachycardia.

PVCs can trigger lethal dysrhythmias, such as ventricular fibrillation, if they fall within the relative refractory period (the so-called R on T phenomenon). They are often classified by their relationship to the previous normal complex.

Etiologies: Etiologies for PVCs include the following:

* Myocardial ischemia
* Increased sympathetic tone
* Hypoxia
* Idiopathic causes
* Acid-base disturbances
* Electrolyte imbalances
* Normal variant

Rules of Interpretation/Lead II Monitoring (Figure 28-39):

Rate—depends on underlying rhythm and rate of PVCs

Rhythm—interrupts regularity of underlying rhythm; occasionally irregular

Pacemaker site—ventricle

P waves—none; however, a normal sinus P wave (interpolated P wave) sometimes appears before a PVC.

P-R interval—none

QRS complex—greater than 0.12 sec and bizarre in morphology

✱ **interpolated beat** a PVC that falls between two sinus beats without effectively interrupting this rhythm.

✱ **coupling interval** distance between the preceding beat and the PVC.

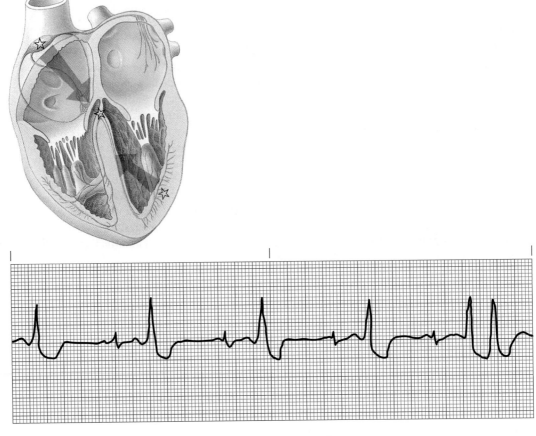

FIGURE 28-39   Premature ventricular contractions.

Clinical Significance: Patients often sense PVCs as "skipped beats." In a patient without heart disease, PVCs may be insignificant. In patients with myocardial ischemia, PVCs may indicate ventricular irritability and may trigger lethal ventricular dysrhythmias. PVCs are often classified as malignant or benign. Malignant PVCs have at least one of the following traits:

- More than six PVCs per minute
- R on T phenomenon
- Couplets or runs of ventricular tachycardia
- Multifocal
- Associated chest pain

With most PVCs, the ventricles do not fill adequately. Because of this, you will usually not feel a pulse during the PVCs themselves. Frequent PVCs may reduce cardiac output.

PVCs can be described in terms of the Lown grading system for premature beats. The higher the grade, the more serious is the ectopy:

Grade 0 = No premature beats
Grade 1 = Occasional (< 30 per hour) PVCs
Grade 2 = Frequent (> 30 per hour) PVCs
Grade 3 = Multiform (multifocal)

Grade 4 = Repetitive (couplets, salvos of three consecutive) PVCs

Grade 5 = R on T phenomenon

Treatment: If the patient has no history of cardiac disease and no symptoms, and if the PVCs are nonmalignant, no treatment is required. If the patient has a prior history of heart disease or symptoms, or if the PVCs are malignant, administer oxygen, and place an IV line. If the patient is symptomatic, administer lidocaine at a dose of 1.0–1.5 mg/kg of body weight. Give an additional lidocaine bolus of 0.5–0.75 mg/kg every 5–10 minutes if necessary until you have given a total of 3.0 mg/kg of the drug. If the PVCs are effectively suppressed, start a lidocaine drip beginning at a rate of 2–4 mg/min. Reduce the dose in patients with decreased cardiac output (those with congestive heart failure or shock, for instance), in patients who are age 70 or older, or in patients who have hepatic dysfunction. Give these patients a normal bolus dose first, followed by half the normal infusion. If the patient is allergic to lidocaine, or if you have given a maximum dose of lidocaine (3 mg/kg), consider procainamide or bretylium.

Ventricular Tachycardia

Description: Ventricular tachycardia (VT) consists of three or more ventricular complexes in succession at a rate of 100 bpm or more. This rhythm overrides the heart's normal pacemaker, and the atria and ventricles are asynchronous. Sinus P waves may occasionally be seen, dissociated from the QRS complexes. In *monomorphic VT*, the complexes all appear the same; in *polymorphic VT*, they have different sizes and shapes. One example of a polymorphic VT is *torsade de pointes.*

Etiology: As with PVCs, etiologies for ventricular tachycardia include the following:

- Myocardial ischemia
- Increased sympathetic tone
- Hypoxia
- Idiopathic causes
- Acid-base disturbances
- Electrolyte imbalances

Rules of Interpretation/Lead II Monitoring (Figure 28-40):

Rate—100–250 (approximately)

Rhythm—usually regular; can be slightly irregular

Pacemaker site—ventricle

P waves—if present, not associated with the QRS complexes

P-R interval—none

QRS complex—greater than 0.12 sec and bizarre in morphology

Clinical Significance: Ventricular tachycardia usually results in poor stroke volume, which, coupled with the rapid ventricular rate, may severely compromise cardiac output and coronary artery perfusion. Whether ventricular tachycardia is perfusing or nonperfusing dictates the type of treatment. Ventricular tachycardia may eventually deteriorate into ventricular fibrillation.

Treatment: If the patient is perfusing, as evidenced by the presence of a pulse, administer oxygen, and place an IV line. Administer lidocaine at a dose of 1.0–1.5 mg/kg body weight intravenously. Administer additional doses of 0.5–0.75 mg/kg, until you have given a total of 3 mg/kg. If this treatment is unsuccessful, attempt to administer

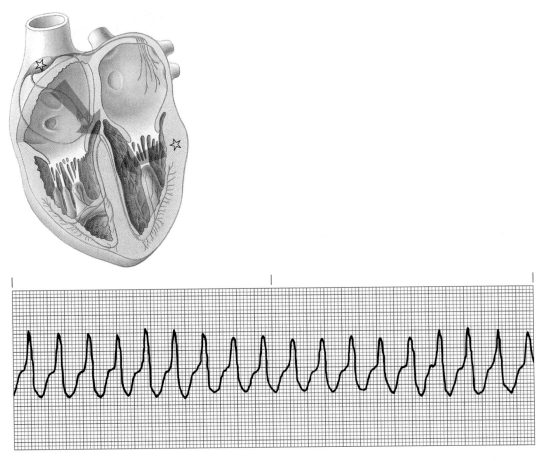

FIGURE 28-40   Ventricular tachycardia.

procainamide at 20–30 mg/minute to a maximum of 17 mg/kg. If procainamide fails, consider other second-line agents. Amiodarone (Cordarone) is becoming increasingly popular in the treatment of ventricular tachycardia. It is primarily a second-line agent to lidocaine. In several of the Commonwealth countries, amiodarone is considered first-line treatment. The dose is 150–300 mg intravenously. Use synchronized cardioversion if the patient becomes unstable, as evidenced by chest pain, dyspnea, or systolic blood pressure of less than 90 mmHg/kg.

If the patient's condition is unstable, as evidenced by an altered level of consciousness or falling blood pressure, initiate cardioversion immediately after placing an IV line and administering oxygen. If time allows, sedate the patient first. The treatment plan is illustrated in the protocol (review Figure 28-26).

If the patient is nonperfusing, follow the protocol for ventricular fibrillation.

Torsade de Pointes Torsade de pointes is a polymorphic ventricular tachycardia that differs in appearance and cause from ventricular tachycardia in general. Torsade is most commonly caused by the use of certain antidysrhythmic drugs, including quinidine, procainamide (Pronestyl), disopyramide (Norpace), sotolol (Betapace), and amiodarone (Cordarone). These agents' effects all seem to be exacerbated by the co-administration of certain nonsedating antihistamines, most notably aztemizole (Hismanol) and terfenadine (Seldane) and, in addition, the azole antifungal agents and macrolide antibiotics: erythromycin (PCE), azithromycin, (Zithromax), and clarithramycin (Biaxin). Any of these agents increase the likelihood of the patient's developing torsade de pointes.

The morphology of the QRS varies from beat to beat (hence the term torsade de pointes, which means "twisting on a point"). In addition, the QT interval is markedly increased to 600 milliseconds or more. Torsade will usually occur in bursts that are not sustained. During the "breaks" from these bursts, you should examine the rhythm strip for a prolonged QT interval. The QRS rate is usually between 166 and 300 bpm, and the R-R interval varies in an irregularly irregular pattern. The QRS complexes are wide and change in size over the span of several complexes (Figure 28-41). Attempting treatment of torsade de pointes with the antidysrhythmics usually used for the treatment of ventricular tachycardia can have disastrous consequences. Therefore, recognition of torsade de pointes as a separate dysrhythmia is essential. Treatment is 1–2 g of magnesium sulfate placed in 100 mL of D_5W and administered over 1–2 minutes. This can be repeated every four hours, with close monitoring of the deep tendon reflexes. Amiodarone (Cordarone) has proven effective in the treatment of torsade. Correct any underlying electrolyte problems, especially hyperkalemia.

Ventricular Fibrillation

Description: Ventricular fibrillation is a chaotic ventricular rhythm usually resulting from the presence of many reentry circuits within the ventricles. There is no ventricular depolarization or contraction.

Etiology: A wide variety of causes have been associated with ventricular fibrillation. Most cases result from advanced coronary artery disease.

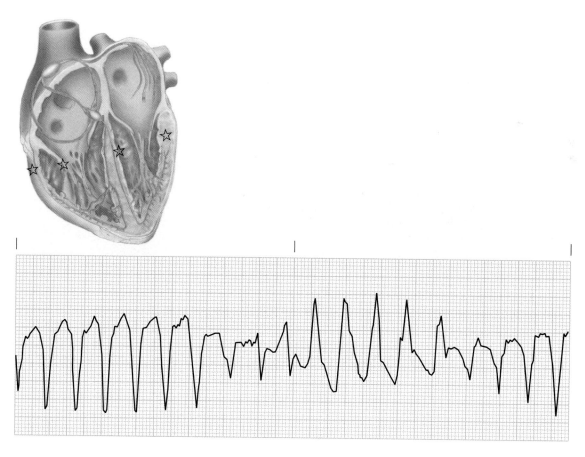

FIGURE 28-41   Torsade de pointes.

Rules of Interpretation/Lead II Monitoring (Figure 28-42):

    Rate—no organized rate

    Rhythm—no organized rhythm

    Pacemaker site—numerous ectopic foci throughout the ventricles

    P waves—usually absent

    P-R interval—absent

    QRS complex—absent

Clinical Significance: Ventricular fibrillation is a lethal dysrhythmia. The absence of cardiac output or an organized electrical pattern results in cardiac arrest.

Treatment: Ventricular fibrillation and nonperfusing ventricular tachycardia are treated identically. Initiate CPR. Follow this with DC countershock at 200 joules. If this is unsuccessful, repeat at 200–300 joules. If still unsuccessful, repeat at 360 joules. Subsequently, control the airway, and establish an IV line. Epinephrine 1:10 000 or vasopressin are the drugs of first choice; administer every 3–5 minutes as required. If unsuccessful, consider second-line agents, such as lidocaine, amiodarone, procainamide, or possibly magnesium sulphate.

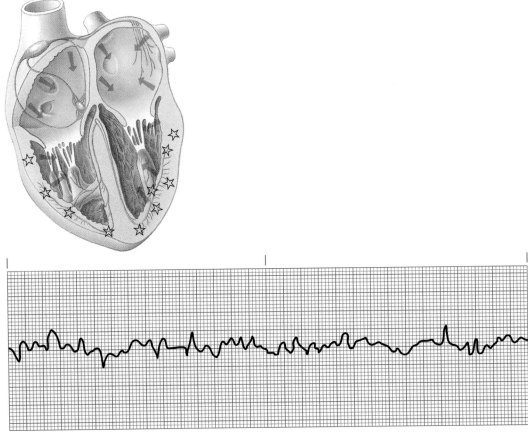

FIGURE 28-42   Ventricular fibrillation.

Asystole

Description: *Asystole (cardiac standstill)* is the absence of all cardiac electrical activity.

Etiology: Asystole may be the primary event in cardiac arrest. It is usually associated with massive myocardial infarction, ischemia, and necrosis. Resulting from heart blocks when no escape pacemaker takes over, asystole is often the final outcome of ventricular fibrillation.

Rules of Interpretation/Lead II Monitoring (Figure 28-43):

    Rate—no electrical activity

    Rhythm—no electrical activity

    Pacemaker site—no electrical activity

    P waves—absent

    P-R interval—absent

    QRS complex—absent

Clinical Significance: Asystole results in cardiac arrest. The prognosis for resuscitation is very poor.

Treatment: Treat asystole with CPR, airway management, oxygenation, and medications. If you have any doubt about the underlying rhythm, attempt defibrillation. Medications include epinephrine, atropine, and in certain situations, sodium bicarbonate (Figure 28-44).

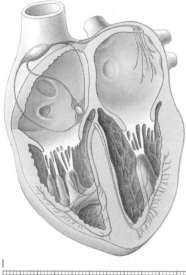

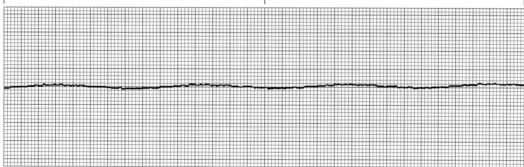

FIGURE 28-43　Asystole.

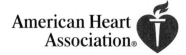

American Heart
Association.

Fighting Heart Disease and Stroke

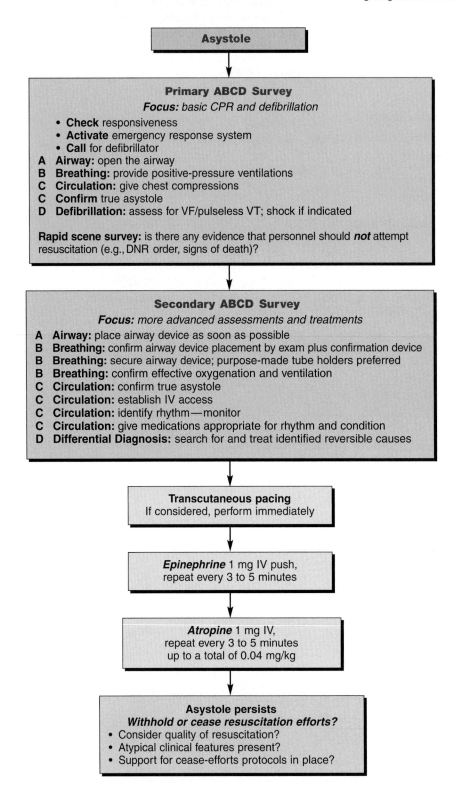

FIGURE 28-44 Management of asystole. Reproduced with permission from *Guidelines 2000 for Cardiopulmonary Resuscitation and Emergency Cardiovasular Care,* ©2000, Copyright American Heart Association.

Artificial Pacemaker Rhythm

Description: An *artificial pacemaker rhythm* results from regular cardiac stimulation by an electrode implanted in the heart and connected to a power source. The pacemaker lead may be implanted in any of several locations in the heart, although it is most often placed in the right ventricle (ventricular pacemaker) or in both the right ventricle and the right atria (dual-chambered pacemaker.)

    Fixed-rate pacemakers fire continuously at a preset rate, regardless of the heart's electrical activity. *Demand pacemakers* contain a sensing device and fire only when the natural heart rate drops below a set rate. In these cases, the pacemaker acts as an escape rhythm.

    Ventricular pacemakers stimulate only the right ventricle, resulting in a rhythm that resembles an idioventricular rhythm. *Dual-chambered pacemakers,* commonly called *AV sequential pacemakers,* stimulate the atria first and then the ventricles. They are most beneficial for patients with marginal cardiac output who need the extra atrial kick to maintain cardiac output.

    Pacemakers are usually inserted into patients who have chronic high-grade heart block or sick sinus syndrome or who have had episodes of severe symptomatic bradycardia.

Rules of Interpretation/Lead II Monitoring (Figure 28-45):

Rate—varies with the preset rate of the pacemaker

Rhythm—regular if pacing constantly; irregular if pacing on demand

Pacemaker site—depends on electrode placement

P waves—none produced by ventricular pacemakers. Sinus P waves may be seen but are unrelated to the paced QRS complexes. Dual-chambered pacemakers produce a P wave behind each atrial spike. A pacemaker spike is an upward or downward deflection from the baseline, which is an artifact created each time the pacemaker fires. The pacemaker spike tells you only that the pacemaker is firing. It reveals nothing about ventricular depolarization.

P-R interval—varies if present

QRS complex—the QRS complexes associated with pacemaker rhythms are usually longer than 0.12 sec and bizarre in morphology. They often resemble ventricular escape rhythms. A QRS complex should follow each pacemaker spike. If so, the pacemaker is said to be "capturing." With demand pacemakers, some of the patient's own QRS complexes may appear. A pacemaker spike should not be associated with these complexes.

Problems with Pacemakers: Although rare, pacemakers can have problems. One cause is battery failure. Most pacemaker batteries have relatively long lives. The cardiologist can check them and usually replaces them before problems arise. If a battery fails, however, no pacing will occur and the patient's underlying rhythm, which may be bradycardic or asystolic, may return.

    Occasionally, a pacemaker can *run away.* This condition, rarely seen with new pacemakers, results in a rapid discharge rate. Runaway pacemaker usually occurs when the battery runs low; newer models compensate for this by gradually increasing the rate as their batteries run low.

    Demand pacemakers can fail to shut down when the patient's intrinsic heart rate exceeds the rate set for the device. Thus, the pacemaker competes with the patient's natural pacemaker. Occasionally, a paced beat can fall in the absolute or relative refractory period, precipitating ventricular fibrillation.

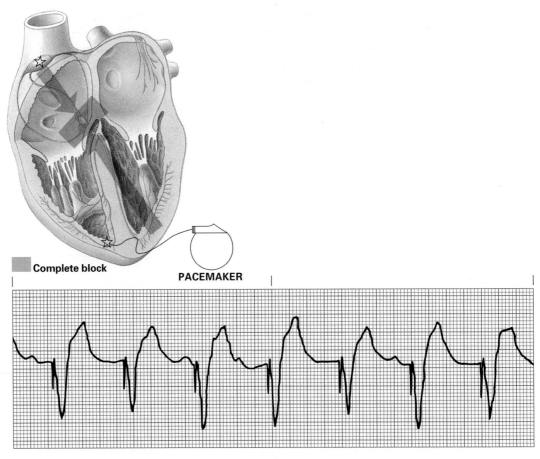

Complete block

PACEMAKER

FIGURE 28-45   Artificial pacemaker rhythm.

Finally, pacemakers can fail to capture if the leads become displaced or the battery fails. In such cases, pacemaker spikes are usually present without P waves or QRS complexes. Bradycardia often results.

Considerations for Management: Always examine any unconscious patient for a pacemaker. Battery packs are usually palpable under the skin, often in the shoulder or axillary region. Treat bradydysrhythmias, asystole, and ventricular fibrillation from pacemaker failure as in any other patient. You may use lidocaine to treat ventricular irritability without fear of suppressing ventricular response to the pacemaker. Defibrillate patients with pacemakers as usual, but do not discharge the paddles directly over the battery pack. If external cardiac pacing is available, you can use it until definitive care is available. Transport patients with pacemaker failure promptly without prolonged field stabilization. Definitive care consists of battery replacement or temporary pacemaker insertion.

Use of a Magnet: Applying a magnet over the pulse generator inhibits all sensing and sets the pacemaker to a predetermined rate (usually 70). The patient should carry a card with information about his particular pacemaker, since these rates are manufacturer and model dependent. Use the magnet only for short periods to avoid the unlikely development of a serious dysrhythmia (including ventricular fibrillation). The indicator for magnet use is a runaway pacemaker.

Pulseless Electrical Activity

Formerly termed electrical mechanical dissociation, *pulseless electrical activity (PEA)* essentially means that electrical complexes are present, but with no accompanying mechanical contractions of the heart. PEA is a perfect example of why you should treat the patient, not the monitor. Your monitor may show a textbook-perfect, normal sinus rhythm, but the patient may be pulseless.

Causes of PEA include the following:

- Hypovolemia
- Cardiac tamponade
- Tension pneumothorax
- Hypoxemia
- Acidosis
- Massive pulmonary embolism
- Ventricular wall rupture

Administer epinephrine 1 mg every 3–5 minutes, and treat the underlying cause(s). Table 28-3 shows suggested treatment for the different underlying causes. Early treatment can potentially reverse some of these conditions; therefore, prompt recognition and initiation of therapy are essential. Treatment for pulseless electrical activity is summarized in Figure 28-46.

DYSRHYTHMIAS RESULTING FROM DISORDERS OF CONDUCTION

Several dysrhythmias result from improper conduction through the heart. The three general categories of conductive disorders include:

- Atrioventricular blocks (discussed earlier in a separate section)
- Disturbances of ventricular conduction
- Preexcitation syndromes

Disturbances of Ventricular Conduction

Disturbances in conduction of the depolarization impulse are not limited to the AV node. Problems can arise within the ventricles as well. **Aberrant conduction** is a single supraventricular beat conducted through the ventricles in a delayed manner. **Bundle branch block** is a disorder in which all supraventricular beats are conducted through the ventricles in a delayed manner. Either the left or right bundle branch can be involved. If both branches are blocked, then a third-degree

✷ **aberrant conduction** conduction of the electrical impulse through the heart's conductive system in an abnormal fashion.

✷ **bundle branch block** a kind of interventricular heart block in which conduction through either the right or left bundle branch is blocked or delayed.

Table 28-3	SUGGESTED TREATMENT FOR UNDERLYING CAUSES OF PULSELESS ELECTRICAL ACTIVITY
Condition	**Treatment (if allowed by local protocols)**
Hypovolemia	Fluids
Cardiac tamponade	Pericardiocentesis
Tension pneumothorax	Needle thoracotomy
Hypoxemia	Intubation/oxygen
Acidosis	Sodium bicarbonate

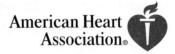

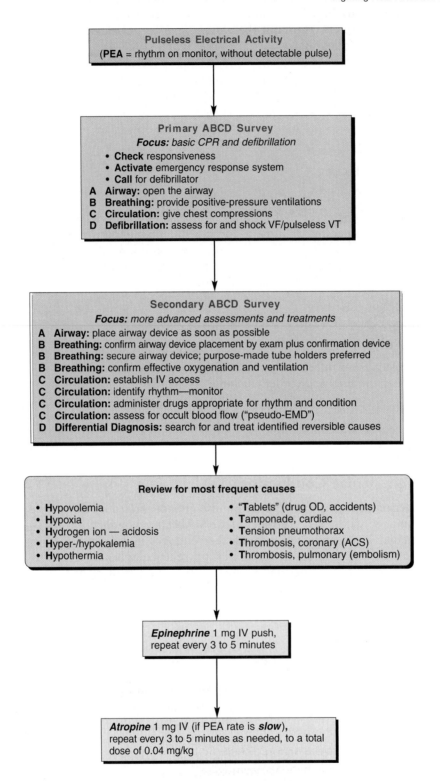

FIGURE 28-46   Management of pulseless electrical activity (PEA). Reproduced with permission from *Guidelines 2000 for Cardiopulmonary Resuscitation and Emergency Cardiovasular Care*, ©2000, Copyright American Heart Association.

AV block exists. These complexes originate above the ventricles and should be distinguished from pure ventricular rhythms, which can have a similar QRS morphology. An *incomplete bundle branch block* has a normal QRS complex; a complete block has a wide QRS complex.

One of the two known causes of ventricular conduction disturbances is ischemia or necrosis of either the right or left bundle branch, rendering it incapable of conducting the impulse to the ventricle. The second is either a premature atrial contraction or a premature junctional contraction that reaches the ventricles or one of the bundle branches, usually the right, when it is still refractory. This often happens in atrial fibrillation because of the irregular rhythm's varying speed of repolarization.

The ECG features of ventricular conduction disturbances include a QRS complex longer than 0.12 sec because the blocked side of the heart is depolarized much more slowly than the unaffected side. The impulse passes much more slowly through the myocardium than through the rapid electrical conduction pathway. The QRS morphology is often bizarre. It can be notched or slurred, reflecting rapid depolarization through the normal conductive system and slow depolarization through the myocardium on the blocked side.

Ventricular conduction disturbances sometimes complicate ECG rhythm strip interpretation. In these cases, supraventricular beats can have abnormally wide QRS complexes. If you suspect a conduction system disturbance relating to supraventricular beats, then it is prudent to inspect some of the other leads in order to determine the problems.

Although exceptions do occur, supraventricular tachycardias caused by disturbances in conduction usually differ in several ways from wide complex tachycardias originating in the ventricles:

- A changing bundle branch block suggests supraventricular tachycardia (SVT) with aberrancy.
- A trial of carotid sinus massage may slow conduction through the AV node and may terminate a reentrant SVT or slow conduction with other supraventricular tachydysrhythmias. These manoeuvres will have no effect on ventricular tachycardias.
- AV dissociation, also known as AV block, indicates a ventricular origin of the dysrhythmia.
- A full compensatory pause, usually seen after a ventricular beat, indicates ventricular tachycardia.
- Fusion beats suggest ventricular tachycardia.
- A QRS duration of longer than 0.14 sec usually indicates VT.

The patient's history may also help to differentiate the etiologies of wide complex tachycardias. In older patients with a history of myocardial infarction, congestive heart failure, or coronary artery disease, these dysrhythmias most likely have a ventricular origin.

When in doubt, treat the patient as if he has the more lethal dysrhythmia, ventricular tachycardia. In either case, use cardioversion if the patient is unstable; it is effective for both ventricular and supraventricular tachycardias.

Preexcitation Syndromes

Preexcitation syndromes involve premature ventricular excitation by an impulse that bypasses the AV node. The most common of these is *Wolff-Parkinson-White (WPW) syndrome*. WPW occurs in approximately 3 of every 1000 persons. It is characterized by a short P-R interval, generally less than 0.12 sec, and a long QRS duration, generally more than 0.12 sec. Additionally, the upstroke of the QRS often has a slur, called the *delta wave* (Figure 28-47). In WPW, conduction of the depolarization impulse from the atria to the ventricles is abnormal. The **bundle of Kent,** an extra conduction pathway between the atria and ventricles, effectively bypasses the AV node, shortening the P-R interval and prolonging the QRS complex. Most WPW patients are asymptomatic; however, the disorder is associated with a high incidence of tachydysrhythmias, usually through a reentry mechanism. WPW is also frequently associated with organic heart diseases, such as atrial septal defects or mitral valve prolapse. Base your treatment on the underlying rhythm.

ECG CHANGES DUE TO ELECTROLYTE ABNORMALITIES AND HYPOTHERMIA

Electrolyte imbalances can cause dysrhythmias that will appear on ECG rhythm strips. Suspect *hyperkalemia* (excessive potassium in the blood) in patients with a history of renal failure who are on dialysis. On an ECG, tall, peaked T waves in the precordial leads are an early sign of hyperkalemia. As the levels increase further, conduction decreases and the P-R and QT intervals increase. At very high potassium levels, an idioventricular rhythm may develop and eventually become a classic sine wave (a wave that rises to a maximum positive level and then drops to a maximal negative level). Prominent U waves appear with *hypokalemia* (deficient potassium levels in the blood). Very low levels can widen the QRS complex.

In *hypothermia,* the Osborn wave, or J wave, is apparent. It is a slow, positive deflection at the end of the QRS complex (Figure 28-48). Other ECG changes may include the following:

- T wave inversion
- P-R, QRS, QT prolongation
- Sinus bradycardia
- Atrial fibrillation or flutter
- AV block
- PVCs
- Ventricular fibrillation
- Asystole

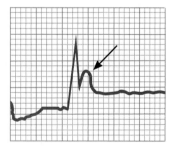

FIGURE 28-48 **The Osborn (J) wave.**

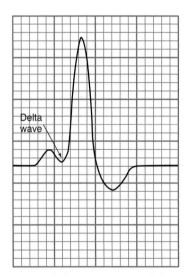

FIGURE 28-47 **The delta wave of Wolff-Parkinson-White syndrome.**

Part 2: Assessment and Management of the Cardiovascular Patient

Part 2 of this chapter will help you build on the information about cardiovascular anatomy (in Chapter 12) and cardiac physiology, electrographic monitoring, and dysrhythmias (in Part 1 of this chapter) as you develop the skills for assessing and managing a patient suffering a cardiovascular emergency.

Part 2 begins with general principles of assessment and management of cardiovascular emergencies and concludes with discussions of a variety of specific conditions and emergencies, including angina pectoris, myocardial infarction, heart failure, cardiac tamponade, hypertensive emergencies, cardiogenic shock, cardiac arrest, and cardiovascular emergencies.

ASSESSMENT OF THE CARDIOVASCULAR PATIENT

The key to providing your cardiovascular patient with the best possible medical care is to take a systematic, step-by-step approach. When you initially encounter your patient, always determine the most important problems first. Airway, breathing, and circulatory problems and shock are always the most critical issues during the first minute of patient care. What may have caused any life-threatening problems does not matter at this point. In some instances, such as cardiac arrest, your focus during prehospital care may never go beyond these four concerns.

Airway, breathing, and circulatory problems and shock are always the most critical issues during the first minute of patient care.

After you have managed any life-threatening problems, the focused history and secondary assessment will help you form your field diagnosis. Cardiovascular diseases may affect the myocardium, the electrical conductive system, the pericardium, or the blood vessels. They may also involve a combination of these problems or problems associated with other systems, such as diabetes. Diseases of the myocardium include myocardial infarction, heart failure, or cardiogenic shock. In electrical conductive illnesses, the heart rate is either too fast or too slow. Although pericardial emergencies, such as pericarditis or pericardial tamponade, are usually diagnosed clinically by the physical assessment findings, the focused history (blunt/penetrating trauma or recent infection, for example) may help you to recognize them. Vascular problems may include coronary artery occlusion, peripheral venous or arterial occlusion, or pulmonary embolism.

In the field, therapeutic treatments are generally limited to the following:

- Administering nitrates, aspirin, and analgesics for symptomatic chest pain
- Treating pulmonary edema
- Giving analgesics in peripheral vascular emergencies

In your ongoing assessment, continually reevaluate your initial management. On the basis of the patient's needs, you will transport him in the appropriate mode to the appropriate facility. As with any patient, your management of the cardiac patient should include patient advocacy as well as communication and emotional support for the patient and his family. You must also effectively communicate the details of your assessment and management to the receiving staff. Additionally, your knowledge of nontransport criteria, education and prevention, proper documentation, and ongoing quality assurance will all contribute to providing optimum care.

Your assessment of the patient with a cardiovascular emergency should vary according to the acuity of the situation. Patients with serious illnesses should have a limited, yet focused assessment. Patients who are less seriously ill should receive a more comprehensive assessment. It is important to remember that the cardiovascular system affects virtually every other body system. Signs of cardiac disease may initially be evident only in the respiratory system as dyspnea. A comprehensive assessment, however, will often reveal subtle findings that point to cardiovascular disease as the cause.

SCENE ASSESSMENT AND PRIMARY ASSESSMENT

After ascertaining that the scene is safe, begin an initial cardiovascular assessment. This allows you to identify life-threatening problems and set transport priorities. First, determine the patient's level of responsiveness. Is he speaking with you or unresponsive? Then, move on to the ABCs. Make sure the airway is patent and free of debris and blood. Suction the airway if appropriate. Next, check the patient's rate and depth of breathing. Listen for the presence or absence of breath sounds. Certain breath sounds, such as moist rales, should heighten your suspicion of cardiovascular disease. Note the effort or "work" of breathing. If the patient is not breathing, initiate manual ventilation and intubate as soon as possible. Check for the rate and quality of pulses. If no pulse is present, immediately begin cardiopulmonary resuscitation (CPR). The skin can indicate the degree of perfusion present. Look for the following:

- Colour
- Temperature
- Moisture
- Turgor
- Mobility
- Edema

Finally, check the patient's blood pressure. Is he in shock? Is this a hypertensive emergency? Treat all life-threatening conditions as you find them.

FOCUSED HISTORY

After you have completed your initial cardiovascular assessment and treated life-threatening conditions, proceed with your focused history, using the SAMPLE format (*symptoms*, *allergies*, *medications*, *past medical history*, *last oral intake*, and *events* preceding the incident).

Common Symptoms

Cardiac disease can manifest itself in several ways. Some common chief complaints and symptoms include the following:

- Chest pain or discomfort
- Dyspnea
- Cough
- Syncope
- Palpitation

Chest pain is the most common presenting symptom in cases of cardiac disease.

Chest Pain Chest pain or discomfort that may radiate to the shoulder, neck, jaw, or back is a common symptom of cardiac disease. Always remember, however, that not all patients who have cardiac disease will have chest pain. This is especially true in diabetic patients, who may have a myocardial infarction with no pain at all. Also, remember that chest pain can be benign and may have no association with cardiac disease. Differentiating between benign and life-threatening chest pain is extremely difficult; do not attempt it in the field. If a cardiac etiology is even a remote possibility, treat the patient accordingly.

Follow the OPQRST acronym to obtain the patient's description of the pain.

Not all patients who have cardiac disease will have chest pain.

O = *Onset*. Ask about the onset of the pain. When did it begin? What was the patient doing when it started? If the patient has had chest pain in the past, ask him to compare it with previous episodes. For instance, if there was a major heart attack in the past and the present pain is the same, then strongly suspect that it is also from the heart.

P = *Provocation/Palliation*. What provoked the pain? Is it exertional or nonexertional? The relationship of pain to exertion is very important. During exertion, the heart muscle needs more oxygen. If it does not receive the additional oxygen, the muscle becomes ischemic and the patient has pain (angina). The patient may tell you that he is now walking shorter distances before the pain begins, indicating reduced blood flow to the heart. Untreated, this may lead to pain at rest and, eventually, infarction. What alleviates the pain (palliation)? Is the pain related to movement or inspiration?

Q = *Quality*. Ask the patient to describe the quality of the pain. Ask open-ended questions, and allow the patient to characterize this symptom in his own words. Common descriptive words include sharp, tearing, pressure, and heaviness.

R = *Region/Radiation*. The patient may complain of pain radiating to other regions of the body, most commonly the arms, neck, jaw, and back.

S = *Severity*. Ask the patient to rate the pain on a scale of 1 to 10, with 1 being very little and 10 being the worst pain ever felt. This can also be a useful gauge of your management's effectiveness. Some systems will use a pain scale of 1 to 5. Regardless of the scale, it is important that the scale used is standardized in the system. It can be problematic if a paramedic asks a patient to rate his pain on a scale of 1 to 5, but when the patient gets to the hospital, the nurse or doctor is using a scale of 1 to 10. Although seemingly trivial, this can significantly affect patient care.

T = *Timing*. Check the timing of the pain. How long has the pain lasted? Always find out the time the pain began, and record it. The onset and duration of pain directly affect decisions about the use of thrombolytic drugs. Is the pain constant or intermittent? Is it getting worse? Better? Does it occur at rest or with activity?

Dyspnea Because of the heart's close relationship with the respiratory system, many cardiac patients have dyspnea (laboured breathing). Dyspnea is often associated with myocardial infarction and may be the only symptom in some patients. Also, patients with congestive heart failure (CHF) will experience increased dyspnea when lying down.

When confronted with a dyspneic patient, ask about the following:

- *Duration.* How long has it lasted? Is it continuous or intermittent?
- *Onset.* Was the onset sudden or rapid?
- *Provocation/palliation.* Does anything aggravate or relieve the dyspnea? Is it exertional or nonexertional?
- *Orthopnea.* Does sitting upright give relief?

Cough Frequently, patients who cough have chest pain. Is the cough dry or productive? Did the patient pull a chest muscle during coughing? Try to determine if the coughing results from CHF.

Other Related Signs and Symptoms Other related signs and symptoms to look for and ask about include the following:

- *Level of consciousness.* The level of consciousness indicates brain perfusion. An alteration in the level of consciousness can be due to problems within the cardiovascular system.
- *Diaphoresis (perspiration).* Cardiac problems significantly affect the autonomic nervous system. Stimulation of the sympathetic nervous system can result in marked diaphoresis.
- *Restlessness and anxiety.* Restlessness and anxiety are among the earliest symptoms when a patient is experiencing lowered brain perfusion, whether due to decreased oxygenation, decreased blood supply, or both.
- *Feeling of impending doom.* The significant and massive stimulation of the sympathetic nervous system associated with severe cardiovascular emergencies can cause a feeling of impending doom. This is a part of the "fight-or-flight" response. A patient with a sensation of impending doom can be experiencing a significant cardiovascular event.
- *Nausea and/or vomiting.* Nausea and vomiting are common during cardiovascular events, such as myocardial ischemia. This often results from slowed peristalsis due to sympathetic stimulation.
- *Fatigue.* Fatigue is a generalized finding associated with many diseases. In patients with cardiovascular disease, it can be caused by anemia, poor oxygenation, or poor overall functioning of the cardiovascular system.
- *Palpitations.* Palpitations are a sensation that the heart is beating fast or skipping beats. This can result from tachycardia or simply from increased awareness of the heart's normal function.
- *Edema.* Edema is the accumulation of fluid in the third (interstitial) spaces. It accompanies poor cardiac function and often indicates chronic cardiovascular disease.
  - *Extremities.* Ambulatory patients usually will develop edema in the extremities, due to the effects of gravity.
  - *Sacral.* Sacral or presacral edema is seen in bed-bound patients. Fluid collects in the lowest part of the patient's body, usually around the sacrum.
- *Headache.* Headache is a factor in cardiovascular disease for several reasons. First, decreased central nervous system (CNS) perfusion can result in headaches. These are often severe. Many patients with

established heart disease take nitroglycerine or other nitrate drugs. Excessive intake of nitrates can cause a severe headache and may indicate worsening heart disease.

- *Syncope.* Syncope is a brief loss of consciousness due to a transient decrease in cerebral blood flow. It occurs in certain cardiac dysrhythmias and in ischemic lesions where blood flow to the heart may be impaired, reducing cardiac output and interrupting CNS perfusion. Severe pain can also cause syncope as well as other forms of psychic stress.

- *Behavioural change.* A behavioural change may very subtly indicate cardiovascular disease. More common in the elderly, it may point to either an acute or chronic decrease in cerebral blood flow.

- *Anguished facial expression.* The pain that accompanies myocardial ischemia can be quite severe. This, coupled with the effects of sympathetic nervous system stimulation, may cause the patient to exhibit anguished facial expressions.

- *Activity limitations.* Decreased cardiac performance can significantly limit a patient's physical activities. These limitations may develop slowly and be considered chronic or develop quickly and be considered acute.

- *Trauma.* Trauma, especially unexplained trauma, can be due to a temporary decrease in CNS perfusion. Unexplained facial injuries or bruises may indicate a cardiovascular problem.

Many of the signs and symptoms of cardiovascular disease can be subtle. Always assess for them and look for any sign or symptom patterns that point to cardiovascular disease.

Allergies

Ask about the patient's allergies. Is he allergic to any medications? Does he have an allergy to x-ray dye (IVP dye)? Try to differentiate between true medication allergies and the undesirable side effects of a particular medication. For instance, the patient who tells you that he breaks out in hives and stops breathing when penicillin is taken is having an allergic reaction. The patient who says he gets an upset stomach from aspirin is, most likely, experiencing a side effect. If in doubt, withhold the medication, and contact medical direction.

If in doubt about a possible medication allergy, withhold the medication and contact medical direction.

Medications

The patient's current use of prescription medications is important. What medications is he currently taking? Has there been a recent change in any medications? The following drugs may be especially significant:

- Nitroglycerine (Nitrostat)
- Propranolol (Inderal) and other beta-blockers
- Digitalis (Lanoxin)
- Diuretics (Lasix, Aldactone)
- Antihypertensives (Vasotec, Capoten)
- Antidysrhythmics (Mexitil)
- Lipid-lowering agents (Mevacor, Lopid)

Also, question the patient in detail about his compliance with medications. Does the patient take his medications? Does the patient take the right amount? Does the patient take them at the right time?

The patient's use of nonprescription drugs is also important. Ask if he takes any over-the-counter medications. Numerous drugs interact, and you must be aware of all medications the patient is currently taking, prescription or otherwise. Try to bring all drug containers with you to the hospital if doing so will not adversely prolong transport time. Drug information is very important for the hospital staff. Recreational drug use is another major problem. For example, cocaine causes vasoconstriction of the blood vessels and can lead to myocardial infarction and severe hypertension, often in the absence of coronary artery disease. These effects can last up to two weeks. Even though this question may create an uncomfortable situation, you must ask it.

Try to bring all of the patient's prescription and nonprescription drug containers to the hospital with you.

Past Medical History

Avoid spending excessive time obtaining a cardiac patient's past medical history. If the patient's condition permits, however, a past medical history may help you determine if the symptoms are attributable to a cardiac condition.

- Does the patient have a history of coronary artery disease, angina, or a previous myocardial infarction? If so, chances are good that the symptoms are cardiac in origin. Comparing prior symptoms with his present ones is helpful. If the patient tells you this pain is just like a previous heart attack, then he likely is experiencing another.
- Has the patient had any prior heart problems? Ask about the following:
  - Valvular disease (rheumatic heart disease)
  - Aneurysm
  - Previous cardiac surgery
  - Congenital cardiac anomalies
  - Pericarditis or other inflammatory cardiac disease
  - Congestive heart failure (CHF)
- What other medical problems does the patient have? Ask about the following:
  - Pulmonary disease/chronic obstructive pulmonary disease (COPD)
  - Diabetes mellitus
  - Renal (kidney) disease
  - Hypertension
  - Peripheral vascular disease
- Does anyone in the patient's family have cardiac disease? At what age did it first develop? Cardiac disease before the age of 50 in a close relative should heighten your concern about heart disease. If a family member had a cardiac event at a young age, especially sudden death, your patient is also at risk earlier in life. Has anyone in his family died of heart disease? At what age? Also, ask if the family has a history of stroke, diabetes, or hypertension.
- Does the patient smoke? Does he know his cholesterol level? These are other modifiable risk factors for cardiac disease.

Last Oral Intake

When was the patient's last oral intake? If the patient ingested a meal high in saturated fats before the onset of symptoms, then gallbladder disease should be considered as a possible etiology. Also, inquire if the patient has had an increase in caffeine intake, and ask when he last drank a caffeinated beverage.

Events Preceding the Incident

What was the patient doing before the onset of symptoms? Was there emotional upset? Had he just completed a strenuous task, such as mowing the yard? Has he recently started a new exercise program? Did the symptoms begin during sexual intercourse? Does the patient take Viagra or Levitra? The development of chest pain during sexual intercourse is not uncommon. However, patients often will not volunteer this information. Asking about such intimate events may be uncomfortable, but it is necessary for optimal patient care. Be discrete, and respect your patient's privacy.

SECONDARY ASSESSMENT

After addressing any life-threatening problems you find in the primary assessment, begin the secondary assessment. Be systematic and thorough, and remember to look (inspect), listen (auscultate), and feel (palpate) while performing your detailed assessment.

Inspection

During your inspection, look for the following:

- *Tracheal Position.* The trachea should be midline. Movement toward a side may indicate a pneumothorax. Inspect the neck veins for evidence of jugular vein distention (JVD). The internal jugular veins are major vessels. Thus, JVD often evidences an increase in central venous pressure (Figure 28-49). Pump failure or cardiac tamponade can cause back pressure in the systemic circulation and jugular vein engorgement. Try to have the patient seated at a 45-degree angle, not lying flat, for this examination. Remember, however, that JVD is often difficult to assess in an obese patient.

- *Thorax.* Watch the patient breathe. To do this properly, expose the patient's chest wall, maintaining patient privacy if possible. Evidence of laboured breathing includes retractions and accessory muscle use. Retractions are visible depressions in the soft tissues between the ribs that occur with increased respiratory effort. Accessory muscle use involves the muscles of the neck, back, and abdomen. Normally, these muscles play a small role in breathing,

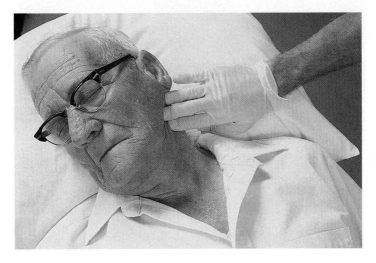

FIGURE 28–49 Look for the presence of jugular venous distension, ideally with the patient elevated at a 45-degree angle.

but patients with laboured breathing put them to greater use. A patient with COPD may have an increased anteroposterior (AP) diameter and may appear "barrel chested." Examination of the thorax can provide a great deal of information about the patient, including chronic problems, such as COPD. The presence of a sternotomy scar, especially in an older patient, is a significant indicator of heart disease.

- *Epigastrium.* While the chest wall is exposed, inspect the epigastrium. Look for abdominal distention and visible pulsations. This may mean that the patient has an aortic aneurysm with dissection or rupture.

- *Peripheral and Presacral Edema.* Chronic back pressure in the systemic venous circulation causes peripheral and presacral edema. These symptoms are most obvious in dependent parts, such as the ankles (Figure 28-50). Often, in bedridden patients, you must inspect and palpate the sacral region for edema. Edema is generally classified as either mild or pitting. To distinguish between them, press firmly on the edematous part. If the depression remains after you remove pressure, the edema is pitting; otherwise it is mild.

- *Skin.* Several changes in the skin can be associated with cardiovascular disease. Pale and diaphoretic skin indicates peripheral vasoconstriction and sympathetic stimulation. It accompanies heart disease and other problems. A mottled appearance often indicates chronic cardiac failure.

- *Subtle Signs of Cardiac Disease.* Look for indicators of cardiac disease. Observe for signs that a patient is being treated for cardiac problems. These include midsternal scars from coronary artery bypass surgeries, pacemakers, or nitroglycerine skin patches.

Auscultation

During your inspection listen for the following:

- *Breath Sounds.* Assessing breath sounds in the cardiac patient is just as important as it is in the respiratory patient. Assess the lung fields

FIGURE 28–50   Check for peripheral edema.

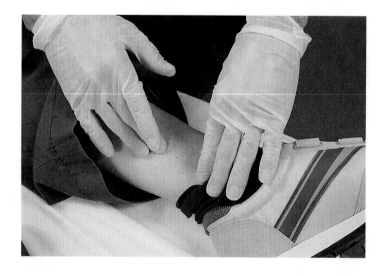

for equality. Also listen for *adventitious sounds,* those that arise or occur sporadically or in unusual locations. Such sounds as crackles (rales), wheezes, or rhonchi (whistling or snoring sounds) may indicate pulmonary congestion or edema. Patients with pulmonary edema may also have foamy, blood-tinged sputum from the mouth and nose. In severe cases, this is audible from a distance as an ominous "gurgling" sound.

- *Heart Sounds.* Avoid wasting precious time auscultating heart sounds in the field. Background noise from traffic, family members, sirens, and other sources makes it very difficult to hear heart sounds, and the information you obtain generally will not affect patient management. Nonetheless, you should be familiar with normal heart sounds and be able to distinguish abnormal from normal findings (Figure 28-51). The first heart sound (S_1) is produced by closure of the AV valves (tricuspid and mitral) during ventricular systole. The second heart sound (S_2) is produced by closure of the aortic and pulmonary valves. S_1 and S_2 are normal. Any extra heart sounds are abnormal. The third heart sound (S_3) is associated with CHF. Occasionally, the skilled listener can hear the fourth heart sound (S_4), which occurs immediately before S_1. It is associated with increased atrial contraction. Ideally, the heart should be examined from the four classic auscultatory sites: aortic, pulmonic, mitral, and tricuspid. The point on the chest wall where the heartbeat can best be heard or felt is known as the point of maximum impulse (PMI). The PMI and examination of the heart are discussed in more detail in Chapter 6, Physical Assessment Techniques.

- *Carotid Artery Bruit.* Auscultation of the carotid arteries may reveal bruits (murmurs), which are a sign of turbulent blood flow through a vessel (Figure 28-52). They are audible over all major arteries, including the abdominal aorta. A bruit indicates partial blockage of the vessel, most commonly from atherosclerosis. If you detect a bruit, do not attempt carotid sinus massage. This procedure may dislodge plaque, resulting in a stroke or other mishap.

An S_3 heart sound has a cadence like "Kentucky." An S_4 heart sound has a cadence like "Tennessee."

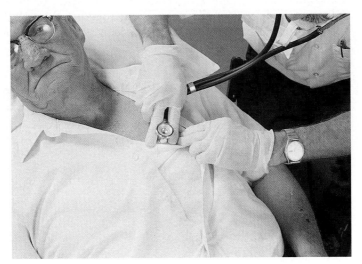

FIGURE 28–51 Auscultate the chest. Listen for heart sounds.

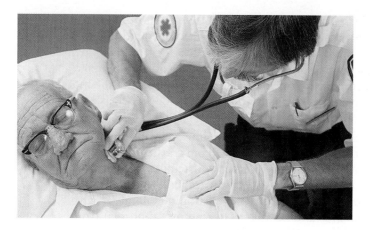

FIGURE 28–52 Listen to the carotid arteries. The presence of noisy blood flow is termed a bruit and may indicate underlying disease in the artery.

Palpation

During your examination, feel for the following:

- *Pulse.* Determine the rate and regularity of the pulse (Figure 28-53). Also, note the pulse's equality. Any pulse deficit can indicate underlying peripheral vascular disease and should be reported to medical direction.

- *Thorax.* Palpation of the thorax is extremely important as chest wall problems are quite common. These can only be elicited by palpation, which may reveal crepitus. *Crepitus* is a grating sensation that suggests the rubbing of broken bone ends or a "bubble wrap" crackling that suggests subcutaneous emphysema (air in the subcutaneous tissue). Palpation may also reveal tenderness associated with a chest wall muscle strain, costochondritis (inflammation of the joint where the rib attaches to the sternum), or even rib fractures. It is important to remember that at least 15 percent of patients with acute myocardial infarction will have associated chest wall tenderness.

- *Epigastrium.* Also, feel the abdomen for pulsations and distention, which may indicate an abdominal aortic aneurysm.

Secondary assessment of the chest is an essential aspect of comprehensive prehospital care. Employ the standard techniques of inspection, auscultation, palpation, and occasionally, percussion. Together, these skills can provide a great deal of information about chronic problems as well as the ongoing acute episode.

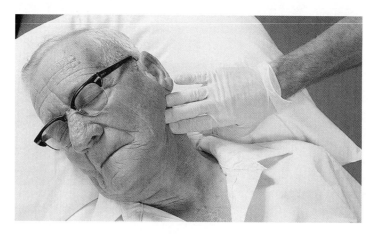

FIGURE 28–53 Check the patient's pulse for both strength and character.

MANAGEMENT OF CARDIOVASCULAR EMERGENCIES

The following section discusses management techniques frequently used in cardiac emergencies. You should also become familiar with your local protocols and procedures, since they vary from system to system.

BASIC LIFE SUPPORT

Basic life support is the primary skill for managing serious cardiovascular problems. These include basic airway manoeuvres as well as CPR. Review basic life support techniques frequently to keep your skills at their peak.

Basic life support is the primary skill for managing serious cardiovascular problems.

ADVANCED LIFE SUPPORT

Most of the procedures that paramedics employ to manage cardiovascular emergencies are considered advanced life support. The number of skills will vary from system to system. Advanced prehospital skills used in managing cardiovascular emergencies include the following:

- ECG monitoring
- Vagal manoeuvres (carotid sinus massage)
- Precordial thump
- Pharmacological management
- Defibrillation
- Synchronized cardioversion
- Transcutaneous cardiac pacing (TCP)

MONITORING ECG IN THE FIELD

Most systems' primary tool for ECG monitoring in the field is a combination ECG monitor/defibrillator that operates on a direct current (DC) battery source (Procedure 28-1). It has the following parts:

- Paddle electrodes
- Defibrillator controls
- Synchronizer switch
- Oscilloscope
- Paper strip recorder
- Patient cable and lead wires
- Controls for monitoring
- Special features (such as data recorders)

To monitor your patient's ECG, you will place the three limb electrodes on the chest (in left arm, right arm, and left leg positions). Some manufacturers require a fourth lead on the right leg. By placing the three principal electrodes, you can monitor any of the bipolar leads (I, II, or III). On certain machines, you can also monitor the three augmented leads (aVR, aVL, or aVF) through these three electrodes. As a rule, Lead II is usually monitored, as its axis is almost the same as that of the heart. Modified chest lead 1 (MCL_1) is used occasionally and is often better for determining the site of ectopic beats.

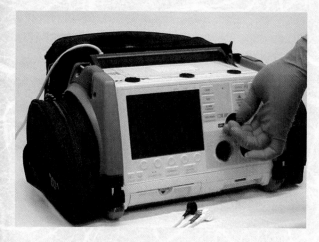

28-1a   Turn on the machine.

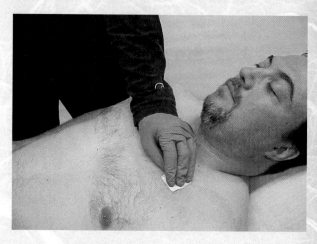

28-1b   Prepare the skin.

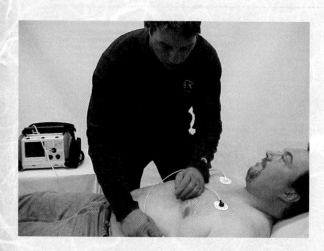

28-1c   Apply the electrodes.

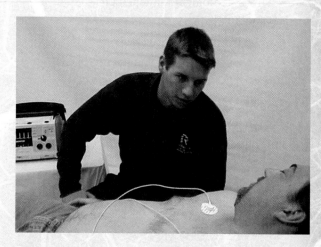

28-1d   Ask the patient to relax and remain still.

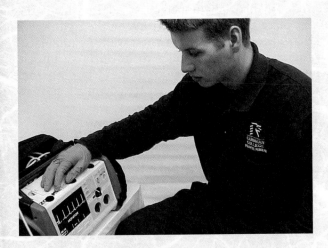

28-1e   Check the ECG.

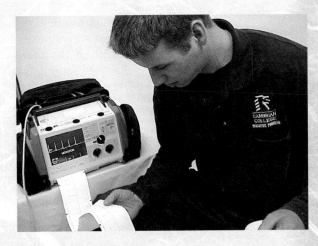

28-1f   Obtain a tracing.

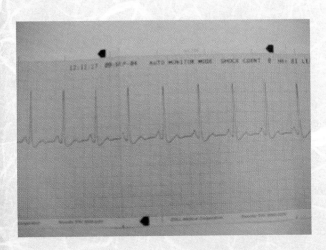

28-1g   ECG strip.

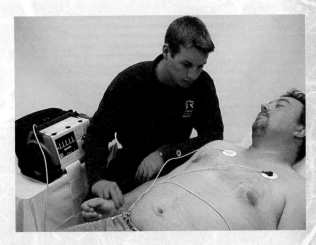

28-1h   Continue patient care and intervention.

You can also monitor your patient through the defibrillator pads. The pads are more frequently used in cases of cardiac arrest, when there is no time to place chest electrodes. You can also use this system when the patient cable is inoperative.

Chest electrodes vary from manufacturer to manufacturer. Usually, to mimic Lead II, you will place the positive electrode on the patient's left lower chest and the negative electrode on his right upper chest. Placement of the ground wire varies. For MCL_1, place the positive electrode on the right lower chest wall and the negative electrode on the left upper chest wall. Again, placement of the ground wire varies. Place the electrodes to avoid large muscle masses, large quantities of chest hair, or anything that keeps the electrodes from resting flat on the skin. Also, avoid placing electrodes where you might have to place defibrillator pads.

To place electrodes, follow these steps:

1. Cleanse the skin with alcohol or abrasive pad. This removes dirt and body oil for better skin contact. If chest hair is thick, shave a small area before placing the electrodes.
2. Apply electrodes to the skin surface.
3. Attach wires to the electrodes.
4. Plug the cable into the monitor.
5. Adjust gain or sensitivity to the proper level.
6. Adjust the QRS volume. (The continual beep of the ECG may disturb the patient.)
7. Obtain a baseline tracing.

Poor ECG signals are useless, and you should correct them. Their most common cause is faulty skin contact. Whenever you spot a poor signal, check for the following possible causes:

- Excessive hair
- Loose or dislodged electrode
- Dried conductive gel
- Poor placement
- Diaphoresis

An initially poor tracing may improve as the conductive gel breaks down skin resistance. Other causes of poor tracings include the following:

- Overhead fluorescent lighting
- Patient movement or muscle tremor
- Broken patient cable
- Broken lead wire
- Low battery
- Faulty grounding
- Faulty monitor
- Radio frequencies

Obtain a paper printout from each patient you monitor. Be sure to adjust the stylus heat properly. Calibrate each strip when you begin monitoring so that 1 mV deflects the stylus 10 mm (two large boxes).

Again, treat the patient and not the monitor. Always compare the rhythm you see on the monitor with the patient's signs and symptoms. A patient may have a perfect rhythm on the monitor but have no pulse or blood pressure.

Vagal Manoeuvres

For a stable patient with symptomatic tachycardia, vagal manoeuvres sometimes help slow the heart rate. Ask the patient to perform a Valsalva manoeuvre (bearing down as if attempting to have a bowel movement) or to cough. If these are unsuccessful and the patient is eligible, attempt carotid artery massage. Do not attempt carotid artery massage on patients with carotid bruits or known cerebrovascular or carotid artery disease, as it may precipitate a stroke. Carotid sinus massage is discussed in more detail later in this chapter.

Precordial Thump

The precordial thump, a blow to the midsternum with the heel of the fist, can stimulate depolarization within the heart. This is most effective when performed immediately after the onset of ventricular fibrillation or pulseless ventricular tachycardia. On occasion, the precordial thump can cause depolarization of enough ventricular cells to allow resumption of an organized rhythm. Additionally, conversions from ventricular tachycardia, complete AV block, and occasionally ventricular fibrillation have been reported. If no defibrillator is immediately available, you may attempt a precordial thump on a pulseless patient who has a witnessed arrest. Since the amount of energy needed to convert ventricular fibrillation increases rapidly with time, a thump is likely to succeed only if delivered early. It is not recommended in pediatric patients.

To deliver a precordial thump, strike the midsternum with the heel of your fist from a distance of 25–30 cm (Figure 28-54). To avoid rib fractures and other problems, keep your arm and wrist parallel to the sternum's long axis.

Pharmacological Management

The drugs that you will use to manage cardiovascular emergencies (Table 28-4) generally fall into the categories of antidysrhythmics, sympathomimetics, and drugs used specifically for myocardial ischemia (including thrombolytics), along with other prehospital medications, some of which are used only infrequently. For more detailed information on these types of drugs, see Chapter 14, on pharmacology.

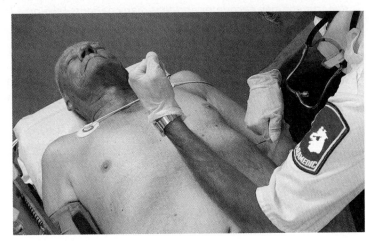

FIGURE 28–54 The precordial thump.

| Table 28-4 | DRUGS USED TO MANAGE CARDIOVASCULAR EMERGENCIES |

Antidysrhythmics

Antidysrhythmic medications control or suppress dysrhythmias.

atropine sulphate	adenosine
lidocaine	amiodarone
procainamide	verapamil

Sympathomimetic Agents

Sympathomimetic agents are similar to the naturally occurring hormones epinephrine and norepinephrine. They duplicate or mimic sympathetic nervous system stimulation.

dopamine	norepinephrine
dobutamine	
epinephrine	

Drugs Used for Myocardial Ischemia

Drugs used to treat myocardial ischemia also act to relieve its pain.

oxygen	morphine sulphate
nitrous oxide	
nitroglycerin	

Thrombolytic Agents

Thrombolytic agents act to break up blood clots blocking a blood vessel.

aspirin (not a thrombolytic but inhibits aggregation of platelets)	alteplase (Activase) (tPA)
	reteplase (Retavase)

Other Prehospital Drugs

In some situations, medical direction or local protocol may recommend the following drugs:

furosemide (diuretic)	promethazine (sedative; antihistamine; antiemetic; anticholinergic)
diazepam (sedative-hypnotic; anticonvulsive)	sodium nitroprusside (vasodilator)

Drugs Infrequently Used in the Prehospital Setting

The following are drugs that paramedics who work in the emergency department may encounter and that many patients take on a long-term basis:

digitalis (Digoxin, Lanoxin) (cardiac glycoside: increases cardiac contratile force and cardiac output)

beta-blockers (propranolol) (dysrhythmia control)

calcium channel blockers (verapamil, diltiazem, nifedipine) (control supraventricular tachydysrhythmias; help manage hypertension; increase coronary artery perfusion in angina pectoris)

alkalinizing agents (sodium bicarbonate) (occasional use in management of cardiac arrest)

Defibrillation

Defibrillation is the process of passing a current through a fibrillating heart to depolarize the cells and allow them to repolarize uniformly, thus restoring an organized cardiac rhythm. A critical mass of the myocardium must be depolarized in order to suppress all of the ectopic foci. The critical mass is related to the size of the heart, but it cannot be calculated for a given individual or situation.

The *defibrillator* is an electrical capacitor that stores energy for delivery to the patient at a desired time. It consists of an adjustable high-voltage power supply and energy storage capacitor. A current-limiting inductor connects the capacitor to the defibrillator pads. Recently, different defibrillation wave forms, most commonly biphasic wave forms, have been utilized to decrease possible tissue damage and to increase battery life. This technology evolved with the development of the compact automated external defibrillators (AEDs).

Most defibrillators use direct current (DC). Alternating current (AC) models should not be used. Direct current is more effective, more portable, and causes less muscle damage. It delivers an electrical charge of several thousand volts over a very short time, generally 4–12 milliseconds. The shock's strength is commonly expressed in energy according to the following formula:

$$energy \; (joules) = power \; (watts) \times duration \; (seconds)$$

The chest wall offers resistance to the electrical charge, which lowers the amount of energy actually delivered to the heart. Therefore, lowering the resistance pathway between the defibrillator pads and the chest is important. Factors that influence chest wall resistance include the following:

- Pad pressure
- Pad-skin interface
- Pad surface area
- Number of previous countershocks
- Inspiratory versus expiratory phase at time of countershock

The following factors influence the success of defibrillation:

- *Time until ventricular fibrillation.* In conjunction with effective CPR, defibrillation begun within four minutes after the onset of fibrillation will yield significantly improved resuscitation rates, compared with defibrillation begun within eight minutes.

- *Condition of the myocardium.* Converting ventricular fibrillation is more difficult in the presence of acidosis, hypoxia, hypothermia, electrolyte imbalance, or drug toxicity. Secondary ventricular fibrillation (ventricular fibrillation that results from another cause) is more difficult to treat than primary ventricular fibrillation.

- *Heart size and body weight.* The effects of heart size and body weight on defibrillation are controversial. Pediatric and adult energy requirements differ, but it is not clear whether size and energy level settings are related in adults.

- *Previous countershocks.* Repeated countershocks decrease transthoracic resistance, thereby allowing the defibrillator to deliver more energy to the heart at the same energy level.

- *Pad size.* Larger defibrillator pads are thought to be more effective and cause less myocardial damage. The ideal size for adults, however, has not been established.

✻ defibrillation the process of passing an electrical current through a fibrillating heart to depolarize a critical mass of myocardial cells. This allows them to depolarize uniformly, resulting in an organized rhythm.

- *Pad Placement.* For both adults and children in the emergency setting, place the pads on the chest. Position one pad to the right of the upper sternum, just below the clavicle. Place the other to the left of the left nipple in an anterior axillary line immediately over the apex of the heart. Do not place pads over the sternum. Do not place pads over the generator of an implanted automatic defibrillator or pacemaker, which can damage or disable the device. Place the pads approximately 12.5 cm from the generator. The pads may be marked as apex (positive electrode) and sternum (negative electrode). Although reversing polarity inverts the ECG tracing, it does not affect defibrillation.

- *Pad-skin interface.* Pad-skin interface should have as little electrical resistance as possible. Greater resistance decreases energy delivery to the heart and increases heat production on the skin. Many available materials decrease resistance, including prepackaged gel pads. Never use alcohol-soaked pads, as they can ignite.

- *Pad contact pressure.* The pad contact pressure is important. Firm, downward pressure decreases transthoracic resistance.

- *Properly functioning defibrillator.* The machine should deliver the amount of energy that it indicates. Therefore, frequent inspection and testing of the machine are necessary. Change and cycle the batteries according to manufacturer directions.

To perform defibrillation, use the following steps (Procedure 28-2):

1. Confirm ventricular fibrillation or pulseless ventricular tachycardia on the cardiac monitor.
2. Place the patient in a safe environment if initially in contact with some electrically conductive material, such as metal or water.
3. Place commercial defibrillation pads on the patient's exposed thorax.
4. Turn on and charge the defibrillator to 200 joules for the first shock.
5. Ensure that no one else is in contact with the patient. Verbally and visually clear everybody, including yourself, before any defibrillation attempt.
6. Deliver a defibrillatory shock by pressing the shock button on the defibrillator.
7. Reconfirm the rhythm on the monitor screen; if the patient is still in ventricular fibrillation or pulseless ventricular tachycardia, recharge the defibrillator and repeat steps 5 and 6 at higher energy levels.

Keep in mind the basic energy recommendations for defibrillation. After initially attempting defibrillation at 200 joules in an adult, increase dosage to a maximum of 360 joules in one or two repeat countershocks. The pediatric dosage is generally 2 joules/kg initially, repeated at 4 joules/kg if required.

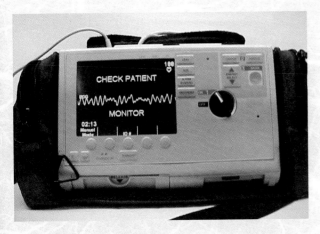

28-2a   Identify rhythm on the cardiac monitor and assess the patient as VSA (Vital Signs Absent).

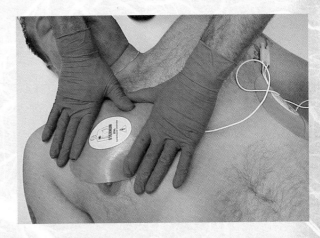

28-2b   Apply electrode gel to the pads, or place commercial defibrillation pads on the patient's exposed thorax.

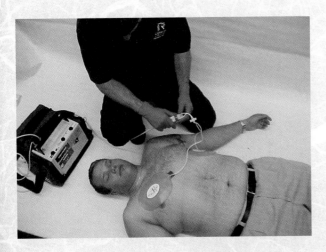

28-2c   Charge the defibrillation paddles.

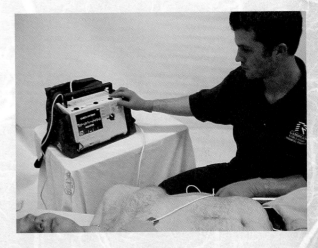

28-2d   Reconfirm the rhythm on the cardiac monitor.

(continued)

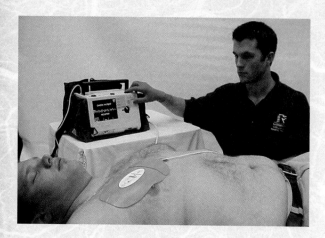

28-2e Verbally and visually clear everybody, including yourself, from the cardiac patient.

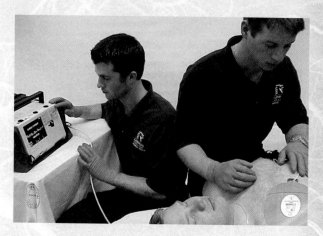

28-2f Deliver a shock by pressing both buttons simultaneously.

Emergency Synchronized Cardioversion

Synchronized cardioversion is a controlled form of defibrillation for patients who still have organized cardiac activity with a pulse. A synchronizing circuit in the defibrillator interprets the QRS cycle and delivers the electrical discharge during the R wave of the QRS complex. This reduces the likelihood of delivering the cardioversion during the vulnerable period of the QRS cycle, which can precipitate ventricular fibrillation. Synchronizing also permits the use of lower energy levels and reduces the potential for secondary dysrhythmias. Depending on the type of dysrhythmia being treated, as little as 10 joules may be adequate, especially if the origin is atrial.

Indications for emergency synchronized cardioversion in an unstable patient include the following:

- Perfusing ventricular tachycardia
- Paroxysmal supraventricular tachycardia
- Rapid atrial fibrillation
- 2:1 atrial flutter

The procedure for synchronized cardioversion is the same as for defibrillation. Sedate conscious patients if at all possible. Turn on the synchronizer switch, and verify that the machine is detecting the R waves (Figure 28-55). If not, you may need to reposition the electrodes. Press and hold the discharge buttons until the machine discharges on the next R wave. Some models automatically turn off the synchronizer after a cardioversion and return to defibrillation mode. To give a second synchronized shock, you must depress the synchronizer button again. If ventricular fibrillation occurs, you must turn off the synchronizer switch and use the machine in the defibrillation mode because the heart produces no R waves in ventricular fibrillation and the machine will not discharge. The procedure for synchronized cardioversion is summarized in Figure 28-56.

* **synchronized cardioversion** the passage of an electric current through the heart during a specific part of the cardiac cycle to terminate certain kinds of dysrhythmias.

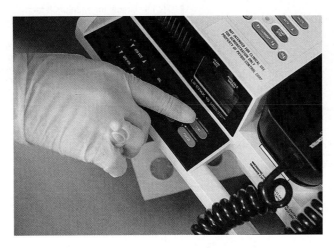

FIGURE 28–55 Activate the synchronizer.

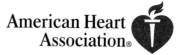

American Heart
Association®

Fighting Heart Disease and Stroke

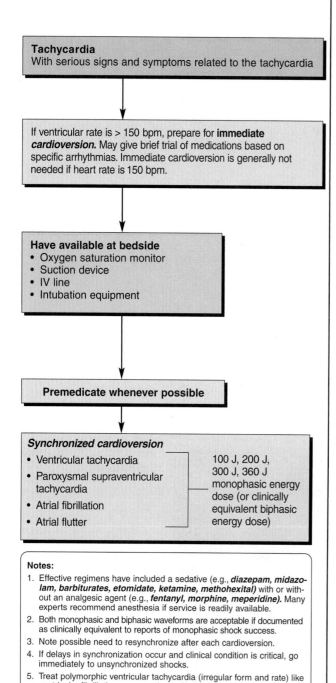

Tachycardia
With serious signs and symptoms related to the tachycardia

If ventricular rate is > 150 bpm, prepare for **immediate cardioversion.** May give brief trial of medications based on specific arrhythmias. Immediate cardioversion is generally not needed if heart rate is 150 bpm.

Have available at bedside
• Oxygen saturation monitor
• Suction device
• IV line
• Intubation equipment

Premedicate whenever possible

Synchronized cardioversion
• Ventricular tachycardia
• Paroxysmal supraventricular tachycardia
• Atrial fibrillation
• Atrial flutter

100 J, 200 J, 300 J, 360 J monophasic energy dose (or clinically equivalent biphasic energy dose)

Notes:
1. Effective regimens have included a sedative (e.g., *diazepam, midazolam, barbiturates, etomidate, ketamine, methohexital)* with or without an analgesic agent (e.g., *fentanyl, morphine, meperidine).* Many experts recommend anesthesia if service is readily available.
2. Both monophasic and biphasic waveforms are acceptable if documented as clinically equivalent to reports of monophasic shock success.
3. Note possible need to resynchronize after each cardioversion.
4. If delays in synchronization occur and clinical condition is critical, go immediately to unsynchronized shocks.
5. Treat polymorphic ventricular tachycardia (irregular form and rate) like ventricular fibrillation: see ventricular fibrillation/pulseless ventricular tachycardia algorithm.
6. Paroxysmal supraventricular tachycardia and atrial flutter often respond to lower energy levels (start with 50 J).

Steps for
Synchronized Cardioversion

1. Consider sedation.
2. Turn on defibrillator (monophasic or biphasic).
3. Attach monitor leads to the patient ("white to right, red to ribs, what's left over to the left shoulder") and ensure proper display of the patient's rhythm.
4. Engage the synchronization mode by pressing the "sync" control button.
5. Look for markers on R waves indicating sync mode.
6. If necessary, adjust monitor gain until sync markers occur with each R wave.
7. Select appropriate energy level.
8. Position conductor pads on patient (or apply gel to pads).
9. Position paddle on patient (sternum-apex).
10. Announce to team members: *"Charging defibrillator—stand clear!"*
11. Press "charge" button on apex paddle (right hand).
12. When the defibrillator is charged, begin the final clearing chant. State firmly in a forceful voice the following chant before each shock:
    • *"I am going to shock on three. One, I'm clear."* (Check to make sure you are clear of contact with the patient, the stretcher, and the equipment.)
    • *"Two, you are clear."* (Make a visual check to ensure that no one continues to touch the patient or stretcher. In particular, do not forget about the person providing ventilations. That person's hands should not be touching the ventilatory adjuncts, including the tracheal tube!)
    • *"Three, everybody's clear."* (Check yourself one more time before pressing the "shock" buttons.)
13. Apply 55 kg pressure on both paddles.
14. Press the "discharge" buttons simultaneously.
15. Check the monitor. If tachycardia persists, increase the joules according to the electrical cardioversion algorithm.
16. **Reset the sync mode after each synchronized cardioversion because most defibrillators default back to unsynchronized mode.** This default allows an immediate shock if the cardioversion produces VF.

FIGURE 28–56   Electrical (synchronized) cardioversion algorithm. Reproduced with permission from *Guidelines 2000 for Cardiopulmonary Resuscitation and Emergency Cardiovascular Care,* ©2000, Copyright American Heart Association.

Transcutaneous Cardiac Pacing

Many of the newer cardiac monitor/defibrillators have a built-in cardiac pacing device that enables paramedic units to perform *transcutaneous* (external) cardiac pacing (TCP), which allows electrical pacing of the heart through the skin via specially designed thoracic electrodes. Before the development of TCP, electrical cardiac pacing required placing an electrode through a major vein or directly into the chest. With TCP, pacing can now be provided in the prehospital setting. This is beneficial in such cases of symptomatic bradycardia as occur with high-degree AV blocks, atrial fibrillation with slow ventricular response, and other significant bradycardias (including asystole). Use TCP if pharmacological intervention has no effect and the patient is hypotensive or hypoperfusing.

To perform external cardiac pacing, follow these steps (Procedure 28-3):

1. Initiate IV, oxygen, and ECG monitoring.
2. Place the patient supine.
3. Confirm symptomatic bradycardia, and confirm medical direction order for external cardiac pacing.
4. Apply the pacing electrodes according to the manufacturer's recommendations, being sure that they interface well with the skin.
5. Connect the electrodes.
6. Set the desired heart rate on the pacemaker. This will typically range from 60 to 80 beats per minute (bpm).
7. Turn the output setting to 0.
8. Turn on the pacer.
9. Slowly increase the output until you note ventricular capture.
10. Check the pulse and blood pressure, and adjust the rate and amperage as medical direction orders.
11. Monitor the patient's response to treatment.

To manage patients in asystole, place the output on its maximum setting. Then, decrease the output if capture occurs.

Occasionally, external cardiac pacing may cause patient discomfort. If this occurs, medical direction may advise administration of an analgesic.

Overdrive pacing may deter recurrent tachycardia. This involves increasing the rate above the heart's current rate in order to suppress ventricular ectopy. This is particularly useful in torsade de pointes. Failure of TCP is similar to the failure of a permanent pacemaker, as discussed earlier in the section on artificial pacemaker rhythm.

External pacing is of benefit in bradycardias and heart blocks that are symptomatic. The electrodes are placed on the chest as shown. The desired heart rate is selected. The current is then adjusted until "capture" of the heart's conductive system is obtained.

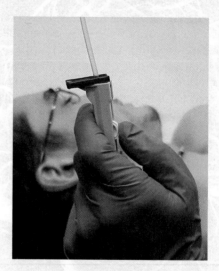

28-3a   Establish an IV line.

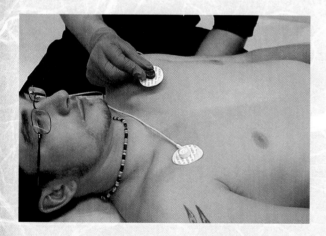

28-3b   Place ECG electrodes.

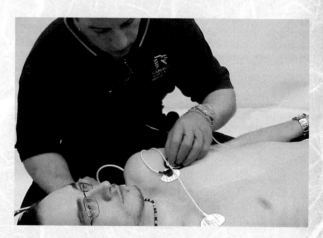

28-3c   Carefully assess vital signs, and contact medical direction.

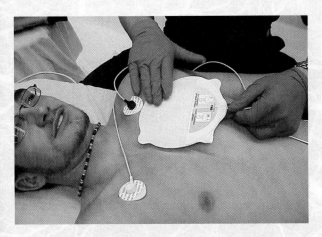

28-3d   If external pacing is ordered, apply the pacing electrodes according to the manufacturer's recommendations.

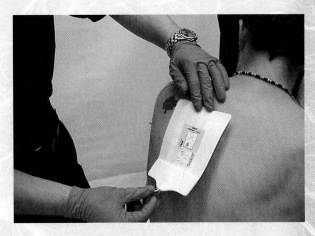

28-3e   Connect the electrodes.

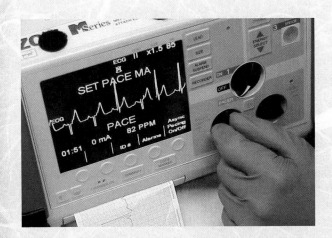

28-3f   Select the desired pacing rate and current.

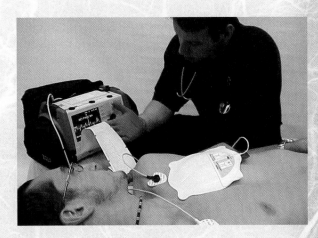

28-3g   Monitor the patient's response to treatment.

CAROTID SINUS MASSAGE

Carotid sinus massage can convert paroxysmal supraventricular tachycardia into sinus rhythm by stimulating the baroreceptors in the carotid bodies. This increases vagal tone and decreases heart rate.

To perform carotid sinus massage, have atropine sulphate readily available and use the following technique:

1. Initiate IV, oxygen, and ECG monitoring.
2. Position patient on his back, slightly hyperextending the head.
3. Gently palpate each carotid pulse separately. Auscultate each side for carotid bruits. Do not attempt carotid sinus massage if the pulse is diminished, if carotid bruits are present, or if patient is > 60 years old.
4. Tilt the patient's head to one side. Place your index and middle fingers over one artery, below the angle of the jaw and as high up on the neck as possible.
5. Firmly massage the artery by pressing it against the vertebral body and rubbing.
6. Monitor the ECG, and obtain a continuous readout. Terminate massage at the first sign of slowing or heart block.
7. Maintain pressure no longer than 15–20 seconds.
8. If the massage is ineffective, you may repeat it, preferably on the other side of the patient's neck.

Complications of carotid sinus massage include dysrhythmias, such as asystole, premature ventricular contractions (PVCs), ventricular tachycardia, or fibrillation. In addition, this procedure can interfere with cerebral circulation, causing syncope, seizure, or stroke. Increased parasympathetic tone can cause bradycardia, nausea, or vomiting.

SUPPORT AND COMMUNICATION

As with other emergencies, appropriate support and communication are an integral part of the treatment you provide for your cardiovascular patient. Time permitting, explain your treatment to the patient and his family, and offer emotional support as indicated. When rapid transport is necessary, explain why. If the patient refuses transport, you will need to clearly explain the potential consequences, and use every available means to convince him of the need for appropriate treatment. As you transfer care of your patient to the receiving facility staff, you must clearly explain your findings to the receiving nurse or physician in a formal verbal briefing. This briefing should include the patient's vital information, chief complaint and history, secondary assessment findings, and any treatments rendered. In cardiovascular emergencies, any ECG findings will be especially important to the receiving staff.

MANAGING SPECIFIC CARDIOVASCULAR EMERGENCIES

The following section details the pathophysiology of common cardiovascular emergencies. Each section covers epidemiology, morbidity and mortality, assessment, and management.

ANGINA PECTORIS

Angina pectoris literally means "pain in the chest." This condition, however, is much more complicated than simple pain. Angina occurs when the heart's blood supply is transiently exceeded by myocardial oxygen demands. In other words, during periods of increased oxygen demand, the coronary arteries cannot deliver an adequate amount of blood to the myocardium. This can cause ischemia of the myocardium and chest pain.

As a rule, the reduced blood flow through the coronary arteries results from atherosclerosis. Atherosclerotic plaques can develop throughout the coronary circulation. Some patients may have atherosclerotic lesions that are isolated to one vessel, while others will have diffuse disease involving several vessels. Fixed blockages in the coronary arteries decrease blood flow. Remember that blood flow through a vessel is related to its diameter. Reducing the diameter of a vessel by one-half, as can occur in atherosclerosis, drastically reduces the amount of blood that the vessel can transport.

In addition to atherosclerosis, angina can result from abnormal spasm of the coronary arteries. This disorder, commonly called **Prinzmetal's angina,** *vasospastic angina,* or *atypical angina,* can also lead to inadequate blood flow, causing pain. Approximately two-thirds of the people who have vasospastic angina also have atherosclerotic coronary artery disease. Spasm of the vessel on top of atherosclerotic blockage can cause ischemia. However, one-third of patients with vasospastic angina will have little or no coronary atherosclerosis.

Angina is generally classified as stable or unstable. *Stable angina* occurs during activity, when the heart's oxygen demands are increased. Attacks of stable angina are usually precipitated by physical or emotional stress. They are relatively brief and often respond readily to treatment. *Unstable angina,* conversely, occurs at rest and may not respond as readily to treatment. Because unstable angina often indicates severe atherosclerotic disease, it is also called preinfarction angina. Unstable angina usually indicates that the patient's disease process is worsening.

Angina is not a self-limiting disease. It results from underlying coronary artery disease. If it is untreated and its contributing factors are unchanged, the underlying problem remains, even after the pain has resolved. Because of the nature of the episodes, angina is usually progressive (that is, it accelerates in frequency and duration). Myocardial infarction may follow a single episode of angina.

It is important to remember that there are other causes of chest pain. While cardiac ischemia is one of its major causes, chest pain can arise from problems in the cardiovascular system, the respiratory system, the gastrointestinal system, and the musculoskeletal system. Causes of chest pain include the following:

- Cardiovascular causes
  - Cardiac ischemia
  - Pericarditis (viral or autoimmune)
  - Thoracic dissection of the aorta
- Respiratory causes
  - Pulmonary embolism
  - Pneumothorax
  - Pneumonia
  - Pleural irritation (Pleurisy)
- Gastrointestinal causes
  - Cholecystitis
  - Pancreatitis
  - Hiatal hernia
  - Esophageal disease
  - Gastroesophageal reflux (GERD)

✱ **angina pectoris** chest pain that results when the blood supply's oxygen demands exceed the heart's.

✱ **Prinzmetal's angina** variant of angina pectoris caused by vasospasm of the coronary arteries, not blockage per se; also called *vasospastic angina* or *atypical angina.*

- Peptic ulcer disease
- Dyspepsia
• Musculoskeletal causes
    - Chest wall syndrome
    - Costochondritis
    - Acromioclavicular disease
    - Herpes zoster (shingles)
    - Chest wall trauma
    - Chest wall tumours

Diagnosing the cause of a patient's chest pain can be challenging in the hospital and even more so in the prehospital setting. As frequently occurs in emergency medicine, we look for the worst and hope for the best. Always be prepared to treat patients with chest pain as if they are suffering cardiac ischemia or another major disease process. Once you have excluded these possibilities, you can consider less critical causes.

Field Assessment

When you assess an angina patient, remember that weak or absent peripheral pulses indicate potential or pending shock, which you should treat immediately. Changes in skin colour, such as paleness or cyanosis, or changes in temperature, such as cold extremities, also suggest shock.

The typical angina patient's chief complaint is a sudden onset of chest discomfort. The pain may radiate, or it may be localized to the chest. Often, epigastric pain accompanies the chest pain. The patient with angina, however, often denies having chest pain, largely because he has dealt with this type of chest pain before. Although anginal episodes are common for the patient with a cardiac history, they should be considered significant when EMS is activated.

Angina usually lasts from 3–5 minutes, sometimes as long as 15 minutes, and is relieved with rest and/or nitroglycerine. Atypical, or Prinzmetal, angina most often occurs at rest or without a precipitating cause. Prinzmetal angina is often accompanied by S-T segment elevation on the ECG, which can indicate myocardial tissue ischemia.

Laboured breathing may or may not be present. After establishing the patency of the patient's airway, auscultate the lungs for congested breath sounds, particularly in the bases. Remember, however, the lungs may be clear. The anginal patient's heart rate and rhythm may be altered. Peripheral pulses should be equal. Typically, the blood pressure will elevate during the episode and normalize later.

The contributing history may indicate that this is the patient's first recognized instance of angina, that it is a recurring event, or that the episodes are increasing in frequency or duration. A recurrence of angina or an increase in its frequency or duration is often the reason an anginal patient calls EMS. Any change in typical anginal pain is significant.

Without prolonging scene time, obtain an ECG tracing. If feasible, a 12-lead ECG is preferred for its additional diagnostic detail. Typical 12-lead findings in the patient with angina are limited to patterns of ischemia: S-T depression and/or T-wave inversion. After relief of pain, the S-T depression and T-wave inversion generally will return to normal. This can take a few minutes or several hours. Occasionally, the patterns may not return to normal.

Many 12-lead monitors have internal computerized pattern identification programs that will identify baseline, certain dysrhythmias, and anomalies that you might otherwise miss. These devices are most often accurate, but they do not always identify everything that may be pertinent. For example, patients experiencing Prinzmetal angina can have S-T segment elevation that dissipates after the pain has been relieved. Never trust the computer interpretation alone. Always double-check the tracing for accuracy. The most common ECG finding in the angina patient is S-T segment depression. S-T segment changes often are not specific, however, and dysrhythmias and ectopy may not be present when the tracing is obtained.

Management

The patient experiencing angina is often apprehensive. Place him at rest in a position of physical and emotional comfort to decrease myocardial oxygen demand. Administer oxygen, generally at a high-flow rate, to increase oxygen delivery to the myocardium. Establish an IV either on scene, without delaying transport, or en route. If possible, and again without prolonging scene time, obtain and record a 12-lead or 3-lead ECG tracing. This is important because the ECG findings may be normal once the patient is pain free. Measure any S-T segment changes and communicate them to the receiving facility. Because a single anginal episode can be a precursor to a myocardial infarction, anticipate ECG changes, such as dysrhythmias and S-T segment elevation.

Administer nitroglycerine sublingually, either as a tablet or a spray. It decreases myocardial work and, to a lesser degree, dilates coronary arteries. If the patient's symptoms persist after three doses of nitroglycerine, assume something more serious than angina, such as myocardial infarction. Consider morphine sulphate for chest pain that does not respond to nitrates as well as ASA prophylactically.

Patients with first episodes of angina or episodes that medication does not relieve are usually admitted to the hospital for evaluation. There is often a fine line between unstable angina and early myocardial infarction. Immediate transport is indicated if the patient does not feel relief after receiving oxygen and/or nitrate. The absence of relief indicates that the patient's underlying disease process may be worsening. If the event is the beginning of a myocardial infarction, *reperfusion* (restoring blood flow to the ischemic tissue) is crucial. Hypotension can occur, especially if the patient has taken nitroglycerine. Its presence calls for transport, because it may lead to hypoperfusion of myocardial tissue. S-T segment changes, especially S-T segment elevation, call for rapid transport. Transport should be efficient and fast but without lights and sirens unless clinically indicated. The lights and sirens could make the patient apprehensive and increase his pain.

Sometimes, the patient experiencing anginal chest pain will call EMS and then refuse transport after the chest pain is relieved. This may be due to a number of reasons, such as denial or the patient's having taken older nitrates, which take longer to work. In any case, strongly encourage immediate evaluation because of the potential serious complications, such as MI. Document patient refusal and be sure the patient signs the refusal and understands the potential risks. Encourage the patient to see his cardiologist or private care physician as soon as possible for followup.

Explain to the patient and family the reason and necessity for rapid transport, if indicated. Time permitting, also explain your treatment. On arrival at the emergency department, inform the physician of your findings—past history, vital signs, laboured breathing, relief of pain, no relief of pain, and ECG findings, especially S-T segment findings.

MYOCARDIAL INFARCTION

Myocardial infarction (MI) is the death of a portion of the heart muscle from prolonged deprivation of oxygenated arterial blood. MI can also occur when the heart's oxygen demand exceeds its supply over an extended time. MI is most often associated with *atherosclerotic heart disease (ASHD)*. The precipitating event is

* **myocardial infarction (MI)** death and subsequent necrosis of the heart muscle caused by inadequate blood supply; also *acute myocardial infarction (AMI)*.

commonly the formation of a *thrombus,* or blood clot, in a coronary artery already diseased from atherosclerosis. Atherosclerosis places many anginal patients at high risk for an MI, especially those suffering from persistent or unstable angina. MI can also result from coronary artery spasm, microemboli (as seen with the recreational use of cocaine), acute volume overload, hypotension (from any cause), or from acute respiratory failure (acute hypoxia). Trauma can also cause MI.

The location and size of the infarction depend on the vessel involved and the site of the obstruction (Figure 28-57). Most infarctions involve the left ventricle. Obstruction of the left coronary artery may result in anterior, lateral, or septal infarcts. Right coronary artery occlusions usually result in infarctions of the inferior wall, posterior wall, or the right ventricle. The actual infarction is often classified as either transmural or subendocardial. In a **transmural infarction,** the entire thickness of the myocardium is destroyed. This lesion is associated with Q-wave changes on the ECG and is occasionally called a pathological Q-wave infarction. A **subendocardial infarction** involves only the subendocardial layer. Because ECG Q-wave changes usually do not accompany this type of infarction, it is often called a *non-Q-wave infarction.*

Myocardial infarction causes varying degrees of tissue damage. First, following occlusion of the coronary artery, the affected tissue develops ischemia. If the blockage is not relieved and collateral circulation is inadequate, the tissue will infarct and die. In trauma, the usual cause of occlusion is plaque that has broken loose. The infarcted tissue becomes necrotic and eventually forms scar tissue. A ring of ischemic tissue that surrounds the area of infarcted myocardium survives primarily because of collateral circulation. This ischemic area is the site of many dysrhythmias' origins. Cardiogenic shock can develop, typically appearing first as ischemia on the 12-lead ECG (S-T depression or T-wave inversion), followed by injury (S-T elevation), and finally infarction (sometimes a pathological Q wave).

Dysrhythmias are the most common complications of MI. They are also the most common direct cause of death resulting from MI. Life-threatening dysrhythmias can occur almost immediately and can result in sudden death or death within one hour after the onset of symptoms. Ventricular fibrillation or ventricular tachycardia may present early with myocardial infarction.

✱ transmural infarction myocardial infarction that affects the full thickness of the myocardium and almost always results in a pathological Q wave in the affected leads.

✱ subendocardial infarction myocardial infarction that affects only the deeper levels of the myocardium; also called non-Q-wave infarction because it typically does not result in a significant Q wave in the affected lead.

Anticipate life-threatening dysrhythmias while caring for any patient you suspect to be having a myocardial infarction.

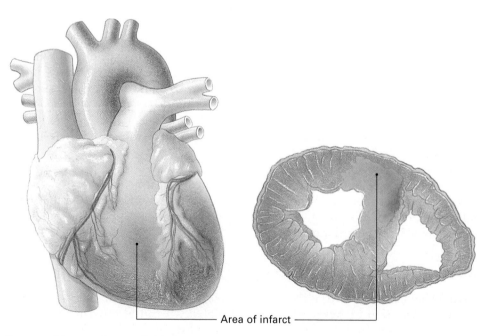

Area of infarct

FIGURE 28–57 Myocardial infarction.

In addition to dysrhythmias, the destruction of a portion of the myocardial muscle mass can cause congestive heart failure (CHF). Such patients may have right heart failure, left heart failure, or both. *Heart failure* occurs if the heart's pumping ability is impaired but the heart can still meet the demands of the body. That is, the heart is inefficient but adequate. If the heart cannot meet the body's oxygen demands, *inadequate tissue perfusion* results in cardiogenic shock. In cardiogenic shock, the heart is both inefficient and inadequate. Another cause of death from MI is *ventricular aneurysm* of the myocardial wall. The damaged portion of the wall weakens and in some cases bursts, resulting in sudden death. *Pump failure* resulting from extensive myocardial damage can also result in death.

The primary strategies in managing an MI are pain relief and reperfusion. For reperfusion to be effective, rapid and safe transport is paramount. Maximum efficiency on scene and in transit is the most important care you can provide for the patient suffering an MI.

Field Assessment

The patient's breathing may or may not be laboured. Look for evidence of shock. Check for regularity of the peripheral pulses, which should be equal in the patient experiencing cardiac ischemia. Take the blood pressure; it usually elevates during the episode and normalizes later.

The chief complaint in MI is chest pain. Use the OPQRST mnemonic (see p. 513) to determine specifics about the chest pain. Typically, the onset of the chest pain is acute, severe, constant, and unrelenting. Unlike the angina patient, the MI patient's discomfort usually lasts longer than 30 minutes. The pain can radiate to the arms (primarily left), the neck, posterior to the back, or down to the epigastric region of the abdomen. Have the patient rate the pain on a scale of 1 to 10. Patients with true myocardial ischemia can have severe pain and may rate their chest pain with high numbers, such as 8, 9, 10, or above 10. Often they will confirm an acute onset of nausea and vomiting. Neither nitroglycerine/morphine nor rest offers much pain relief.

Atypically, a patient may have mild symptoms or minimize the symptoms during your assessment. This is more common in diabetics. The patient can be vague when describing chest pain and may complain of generally not feeling well. You might easily mistake this for angina. This patient generally does not complain of vomiting and may or may not have nausea. The patient also will rate the pain low on a scale of 1 to 10. His vague, general descriptions may arise from many pathological causes. One is that MIs generally evolve over 48–72 hours. If the patient is more than 24 hours into the infarction, the pain can be different from what it was 12–24 hours after onset.

The patient experiencing chest pains tends to be very frightened, although this is not always the case. "A feeling of impending doom" describes the patient's fright and pain. This pain is so severe and intense that the patient fears death, especially if he is experiencing chest pain for the first time. Ask the patient if this is the first recognized episode of chest pain or a recurring event. A patient who has suffered infarction before or who has chronic angina may be less concerned with the current pain. If it is recurring, are the episodes increasing in frequency or duration? These patients often have angina-like pain with increasing frequency and/or duration. Denial is common among both the patient with a significant cardiac history and the first-time chest-pain sufferer.

After establishing the patient's airway, auscultate lung sounds. They may present clear or with congestion in the bases. The patient suffering an MI usually presents with pallor and diaphoresis. Temperature may vary from the norm. Cold skin or extremities indicate shock. Check the heart rate and rhythm, which may be irregular, and check the peripheral pulses for equality, which MI usually does not affect. The patient's blood pressure may be elevated, normal, or lower than normal.

Apply the ECG. First, examine the underlying rhythm and potential dysrhythmias. If you are using a 12-lead monitor, examine the S-T segment and Q waves. Check the S-T segment for height, depth, and overall contour. Note such changes as S-T depression, which suggests ischemia or reciprocal changes, or elevation, which suggests injury. A *pathological Q wave*—deeper than 5 mm or wider than 0.04 seconds—can indicate infarcted tissue (necrosis) or extensive transient ischemia.

Cardiac dysrhythmias are the greatest threat to the patient before he arrives at the emergency department. Of the many potential dysrhythmias, the most serious are asystole (confirmed in two leads), pulseless electrical activity (PEA), ventricular fibrillation, and ventricular tachycardia. Other dysrhythmias include narrow- or wide-complex tachycardia, heart block, sinus bradycardia, and sinus tachycardia with or without ectopy. Remember, life-threatening dysrhythmias are the leading cause of death among MI patients. Anticipate such dysrhythmias while caring for any patient you suspect to be having a MI.

After reviewing the patient's ECG tracing, prepare for rapid transport of the patient to the hospital for possible reperfusion. Reperfusion uses thrombolytics, such as streptokinase or tPA (Activase), to stop further injury. Used properly, thrombolytics can reperfuse all ischemic tissue and much of the injured myocardial tissue, thus reducing the total damage caused by an MI. They work by destroying blood clots—all clots—which, when lodged in arteries congested with plaque, are the most common cause of AMI. The window of time in which a thrombolytic can be given and be effective is generally considered to be six hours from the onset of symptoms. Occasionally, the window will be expanded for a particularly young patient or one who is suffering serious complications. The complications associated with giving thrombolytics include hemorrhage (which can be fatal), allergic reactions, and reperfusion dysrhythmias. Unfortunately, not all MIs are caused by blood clots. In addition, many patients have conditions that preclude them from receiving thrombolytics. These include bleeding or clotting disorders, possible blood in the stool, uncontrolled hypertension, recent trauma, recent hemorrhagic stroke, or recent surgery.

Signs of acute injury or pathological Q waves call for rapid transport of the patient for reperfusion, if symptoms began within six hours. Ascertain as near as possible the exact time when the symptoms started, the locations of the ischemia and of the infarction if evidenced on the 12-lead, and any S-T segment changes occurring on the 12-lead. This will help the physician determine quickly if the patient is a candidate for reperfusion.

After analyzing the patient's rhythm, prepare him for transport. Since reperfusion is the ultimate goal, time is of the utmost importance. Expediently treat any signs of acute ischemia, injury, or infarction. Carefully weigh treating the patient's pain while on scene against rapid transport. Whenever practical, treat the patient suffering from an MI during transit.

Many EMS systems have checklists similar to those that emergency departments use to determine if a patient qualifies for thrombolytic therapy. While these checklists vary from area to area, their use has reduced the waiting time for patients who meet the clinical criteria for thrombolytic therapy. Standard information that should be relayed to the emergency department physician or staff includes the time of the pain's onset, S-T segment elevation, and the location of ischemia and infarction on a 12-lead.

If you are not certain the patient meets local criteria for thrombolytic therapy, assume that he does.

Whenever practical, treat the patient suffering from a myocardial infarction during transit.

Management

Prehospital Management of MI Treatment of the MI patient is summarized in Figure 28-58. Keep in mind that the patient experiencing MI is often apprehensive. Place him at rest in a position of physical and emotional comfort to decrease myocardial oxygen demand. Administer oxygen, generally at a high-flow rate, to increase oxygen delivery to the myocardium. Establish at least one IV, taking great care not to miss the vein; avoid multiple misses, which could jeopardize a patient's chance of receiving thrombolytics.

Administer medications according to written protocols or on the orders of medical direction. Remember, always ask the patient if he is allergic to any medication before giving any drug. Medications that might be indicated for the patient suspected of having an MI include the following:

- Aspirin
- Morphine sulphate
- Nitroglycerine
- Atropine sulphate
- Lidocaine
- Procainamide
- Vasopressin
- Adenosine

Monitor the ECG constantly. Life-threatening dysrhythmias are possible. The patient may need rapid defibrillation or synchronized cardioversion at any moment. Plan to quickly provide defibrillation, cardioconversion, or transcutaneous cardiac pacing (TCP) if needed.

Transport without delay the patient you suspect of having an MI. Since most MI patients are extremely apprehensive and frightened, you should transport the normotensive patient without lights and sirens. Rapid transport is called for if the S-T segment has any changes, such as depression or elevation or if pathological Q waves present on the 12-lead. If a patient exhibits S-T or Q-wave anomalies, has had signs and symptoms less than three hours, or has no relief from medications, consider him a candidate for thrombolytic reperfusion. Hypotension calls for immediate transport, especially if the patient has taken nitroglycerine, because the potential hypoperfusion of myocardial tissue can compound the problem. Other factors that call for rapid transport are any rhythm abnormalities and the presentation within six hours of the pain's onset.

If the patient is in the early stages of an MI, the outcome of refusing transport is likely to have devastating consequences, ranging from extensive, unnecessary myocardial damage to death. Prevent refusal at all cost, using every means at your disposal to convince the patient to allow transport. If the patient still refuses, document the fact that the patient was repeatedly warned of the possible outcome and was also aware of the potential for severely constricted lifestyle or death. Have the patient sign to the fact that he understands the implications, and if at all possible, obtain witness signatures as well.

Explain to the patient and his family the reason and necessity for rapid transport, if indicated, and inform them of your treatment, time permitting. On arrival at the emergency department, inform the physician of your findings—past history, vital signs, laboured breathing, relief of pain, no relief of pain, and ECG readings, especially S-T segment results.

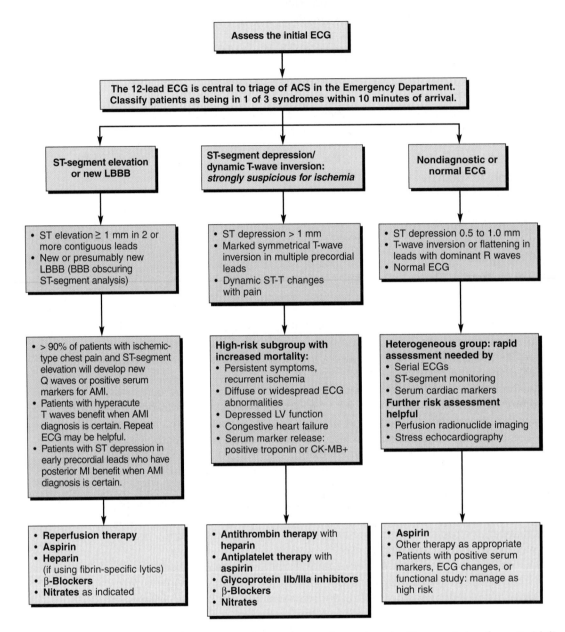

FIGURE 28–58   Management of acute coronary syndrome. Reproduced with permission from *Guidelines 2000 for Cardiopulmonary Resuscitation and Emergency Cardiovascular Care*, ©2000, Copyright American Heart Association.

In-Hospital Management of MI   Your understanding of the management of the MI patient after you have delivered him to the emergency department is important. This is especially pertinent if you belong to an EMS system whose paramedics also regularly staff emergency departments.

With the advent of thrombolytic therapy, many hospitals have opened specially designed chest-pain units. These facilities specialize in diagnosing and observing patients with chest pain. In addition to 12-lead ECGs, obtaining cardiac enzyme levels in chest pain patients is routine. Because dead or dying myocardial cells release cardiac enzymes, elevated levels of these enzymes indicate MI. The enzyme levels do not increase, however, until the infarction is several hours old, and so intervention ideally should occur before the enzymes have a chance to rise. Commonly assayed cardiac enzymes are lactate dehydrogenase (LDH) and creatine phosphokinase (CK). Several newer markers show promise in aiding earlier identification of myocardial injury. These include troponin (I, T, and C), myoglobin, and CK-MB (a type of CK specific for cardiac muscle).

In many chest-pain patients, the diagnosis will be readily evident. In many others, however, it will remain unclear. These patients are commonly stratified according to risk. Patients with a low likelihood of cardiac ischemia may be discharged with instructions for followup care, which may include diagnostic tools, such as stress tests. Patients with a higher likelihood of having myocardial ischemia are usually admitted to the hospital and are typically observed for 24 hours. During the patient's hospitalization, his cardiac enzyme levels are obtained several times, as is the ECG. If the tests all remain negative, the patient will usually see a cardiologist and have a stress test before going home. If the stress test is negative, the cardiologist will work up the problem on an outpatient basis. If the stress test is positive, additional testing is done prior to discharge. This testing includes nuclear medicine cardiac imaging and, possibly, coronary angiography. Usually, cardiology immediately sees patients who have a high likelihood of cardiac ischemia but nondiagnostic ECGs and enzymes. These patients ordinarily are not observed but are taken directly to the cardiac lab for an angiogram.

The trend in emergency cardiac care is rapid cardiac catheterization and therapeutic intervention, such as PTCA.

Several treatment options are available. Patients with isolated coronary artery lesions may be candidates for percutaneous transluminal coronary angioplasty (PTCA). In these patients, lesions are identified during coronary angiography. A balloon catheter is inserted into the coronary artery with the lesion. At the level of the lesion, the balloon is inflated, thus increasing the artery's diameter and reducing the relative size of the blockage. Often, the patient will have several lesions. If the arteries do not stay open following angioplasty, another alternative is to place a *stent* in the artery at the site of the lesion. The stent is a hollow tube that keeps the artery open. Patients with severe and diffuse coronary artery disease may not be candidates for angioplasty. The best option for these patients is surgical revascularization of their coronary arteries. The most common operation is the coronary artery bypass graft (CABG), in which grafts are sewn on from the aorta to the coronary arteries, thus effectively bypassing the blockage. In younger patients, the surgeon may use the internal mammary artery as the source. Recently, technology has evolved to the point where some bypass grafts can be performed endoscopically. These require only small "keyhole" incisions instead of the classic sternotomy, thus markedly decreasing the pain and the recovery time. Patients whose disease is either too mild or too severe may not be candidates for surgery. These patients are managed with medication alone.

HEART FAILURE

Heart failure is a clinical syndrome in which the heart's mechanical performance is compromised so that cardiac output cannot meet the body's needs. Heart failure is generally divided into left ventricle or right ventricle failure. Its many etiologies include valvular, coronary, or myocardial disease. Dysrhythmias can also cause or aggravate heart failure. Many other factors can contribute to heart failure, such as excess fluid or salt intake, fever (sepsis), hypertension, pulmonary embolism, or excessive alcohol or drug use. It can manifest due to exertion in the patient who has an underlying disease or as a progression of the underlying disease.

✱ **heart failure** clinical syndrome in which the heart's mechanical performance is compromised so that cardiac output cannot meet the body's needs.

Left Ventricular Failure Left ventricular failure occurs when the left ventricle fails as an effective forward pump, causing back pressure of blood into the pulmonary circulation, which often results in pulmonary edema. Its causes include various types of heart disease, such as MI, valvular disease, chronic hypertension, and dysrhythmias. In left ventricular failure, the left ventricle cannot eject all of the blood that the right heart delivers to it via the lungs. Left atrial pressure rises and is subsequently transmitted to the pulmonary veins and capillaries. When pulmonary capillary pressure becomes too high, it forces the blood plasma into the alveoli, resulting in pulmonary edema. Progressive fluid accumulation in the alveoli decreases the lungs' oxygenation capacity and can cause death from hypoxia. Since MI is a common cause of left ventricular failure, you should consider that all patients with pulmonary edema may have had an MI.

Right Ventricular Failure In right ventricular failure, the right ventricle fails as an effective forward pump, resulting in back pressure of blood into the systemic venous circulation and venous congestion. The most common cause of right ventricular failure is left ventricular failure. This is because MI is more common in the left ventricle than in the right and because chronic hypertension affects the left ventricle more adversely than the right. Right ventricular failure's other causes include systemic hypertension, which can affect both sides of the heart and can cause pure right ventricular failure. Pulmonary hypertension and *cor pulmonale* (heart failure due to pulmonary disease) result from the effects of chronic obstructive pulmonary disease (COPD). These problems are related to increased pressure in the pulmonary arteries, which results in right ventricular enlargement, right atrial enlargement, and if untreated, right heart failure.

* **pulmonary embolism (PE)**
blood clot in one of the
pulmonary arteries.

Pulmonary embolism (PE), a blood clot in one of the pulmonary arteries, also can cause right heart failure. If the clot is large enough to occlude a major vessel, the pressure against which the right ventricle must pump increases. This can throw the right ventricle into failure in much the same manner as pulmonary hypertension. In fact, it can be considered an acute form of pulmonary hypertension. Infarct of the right atrium or ventricle, although rare, is another cause of right ventricular failure.

Starling's law of the heart enables heart failure patients to compensate, at least for a time. Starling's law states that the more the myocardial muscle is stretched, the greater will be its force of contraction. Thus, the greater the preload (the volume of blood filling the chamber), the farther the myocardial muscle stretches and the more forceful is the cardiac contraction. This has its limits, however. If myocardial muscle is stretched too far, it will not contract properly, and the contraction will be weaker. Afterload (the resistance against which the ventricle must contract) also affects stroke volume. An increase in peripheral vascular resistance will decrease stroke volume. The reverse is also true: stroke volume will increase as peripheral vascular resistance decreases.

* **congestive heart failure (CHF)**
condition in which the heart's
reduced stroke volume causes
an overload of fluid in the
body's other tissues.

Congestive Heart Failure In **congestive heart failure (CHF)**, the heart's reduced stroke volume causes an overload of fluid in the body's other tissues. This presents as edema, which can be pulmonary, peripheral, sacral, or ascitic (peritoneal edema). CHF can manifest in an acute setting as pulmonary edema, pulmonary hypertension, or MI. In the chronic setting, it can manifest as cardiomegaly (enlargement of the heart), left ventricular failure, or right ventricular failure. Heart failure can present in a first-time event, as in MI, or in multiple events, as in left heart failure. CHF is one of the few diseases still on the rise in North America. CHF is a common and serious condition that affects 200 000 to 300 000 people in Canada. It is the leading reason for hospital admission among elderly Canadians. Furthermore, since 1970, the rate of death from CHF has increased by 60 percent, and the current survival rate is 62 percent. Survival rate is only five years in 50 percent of CHF patients. The end stage of this disease involves pulmonary edema and respiratory failure, followed by death. When the CHF patient calls EMS, one thing is clear; Starling's law is no longer allowing the patient to compensate.

Field Assessment

As in all cardiac emergencies, begin your assessment by checking the ABCs and managing any life threats. Often, patients with pulmonary edema will cough up large quantities of clear or pink-tinged sputum. Patients with profound pulmonary edema generally have laboured breathing, although this may not present until the patient begins to exert himself by simply standing or walking a few steps. Look for any changes or differences in skin colour on the patient's arms, face, chest, and back. In profound CHF, mottling is often present.

Focus on the patient's chief complaint. Use the OPQRST mnemonic (see p. 513) to elicit the patient's description of symptoms. Patients with pulmonary edema will complain of progressive or acute shortness of breath and will confirm being awakened by shortness of breath (**paroxysmal nocturnal dyspnea, or PND**). If the patient's episodes of PND are becoming more frequent, the disease process usually is worsening.

✳ **paroxysmal nocturnal dyspnea (PND)** a sudden episode of difficulty breathing that occurs after lying down; most commonly caused by left heart failure.

Often, the heart failure patient will confirm progressive accumulation of edema or weight gain over a short time. Because many heart failure patients have an underlying cardiac or prior MI history, they may complain of mild chest pain or generalized weakness. This may be due to a weakened myocardial muscle mass, myocardial ischemia, or current MI.

Determine the patient's current medications. CHF patients are generally prescribed a loop diuretic, such as Lasix and/or hypertension medication. Many are prescribed digoxin (Lanoxin), which increases the heart's contractile force; many are oxygen dependent and may be on home oxygen. Find out if the patient has been compliant in taking medications; if not, determine how long he has been off medications. Also record and report any over-the-counter medications or herbal medications that the patient is taking, as well as any prescription medications borrowed from another person.

Unconsciousness or an altered level of consciousness indicates pending respiratory failure. If the patient shows any sign of respiratory failure, immediately assist breathing with 100-percent oxygen by bag-valve mask and prepare to intubate if clinically warranted.

Next, assess the patient's breathing. Often, laboured breathing, dyspnea, and productive cough appear. Laboured breathing is the most common symptom of CHF, and it generally worsens with activity. CHF patients frequently assume the tripod position—sitting upright with both arms supporting the upper body—and confirm PND and pillow orthopnea, the inability to recline in bed without a pillow). Ask the patient how many pillows he sleeps on at night. As a rule, the more the pillows, the worse is the problem.

Laboured breathing is the most common symptom of CHF.

Check the skin. CHF patients present with changes in the skin colour, such as pallor, diaphoresis, mottling, or signs of cyanosis. Check the peripheral pulses for quality and rhythm. Also, check for edema, which is usually found in the lower extremities, localized from the ankles to the midcalf or the knees. Sometimes, the edema will be so severe that it obliterates the distal pulses. Check the edematous area for pitting, and record its severity on a scale from 0 to 4+. Edema may also be present in the sacral area of the back, especially in the bed-confined patients, or in the upper quadrants of abdominal cavity. Ascites (abdominal cavity edema or swelling) is very difficult to assess accurately without x-ray or ultrasound. Blood pressure may be elevated in the CHF patient due to the body's attempt to compensate for decreased cardiac output, but this can change quickly. A decompensating patient can have a normal blood pressure that drops quickly.

The most serious complication of heart failure is pulmonary edema. Untreated pulmonary edema can quickly lead to respiratory failure. This is because the abundant serum fluid in a large portion of the alveoli inhibits oxygen exchange in the lungs and hypoxia ensues. Respiratory failure will quickly lead to death. Patients with severe pulmonary edema present with tachypnea and adventitious lung sounds. Pulmonary edema can present as crackles (rales) at both bases. Rhonchi, which indicates fluid in the larger airways of the lungs, is a sign of severe pulmonary edema. Wheezes in the CHF patient are a sign of the lungs' protective mechanisms, since bronchioles constrict in an attempt to keep additional fluid from entering the lungs. This wheezing in pulmonary edema and CHF is often called cardiac asthma. This term is confusing, however, and you should avoid using it. Consider wheezes in a geriatric patient to be pulmonary edema until proven otherwise.

Other complications of pulmonary edema are pulsus paradoxus and pulsus alternans. *Pulsus paradoxus* occurs when systolic blood pressure drops more than 10 mmHg with inspiration. This is due to compression of the great vessels or the ventricles. In *pulsus alternans,* the pulse alternates between weak and strong. Pulses may be thready or weak, and jugular vein distention (JVD) might be present. The apical pulse may be abnormal or difficult to auscultate because of such abnormalities as bulges in the heart, a displaced apex, or severe pulmonary edema. The patient may produce frothy sputum with coughing, and cyanosis may present in the late stages of CHF.

Management

In severe CHF with pulmonary edema, obtain pertinent medical history and complete the secondary assessment while initiating treatment. Reassess all life-threatening conditions and treat them accordingly. Do not have the patient exert himself in any way, including standing up or walking. Do not have the patient lie flat at any time. Position him in the Fowler's position with extremities elevated. This will promote venous pooling, thus decreasing preload.

Administer high-flow oxygen. If necessary, provide positive-pressure assistance with either a demand valve if the patient can assist or a bag-valve-mask unit if he is unresponsive. When possible, establish an IV at a to-keep-open (TKO) rate. Consider placing a saline lock, since limiting fluids is imperative.

Place ECG electrodes. Record a baseline ECG, and keep the monitor in place throughout care.

Administer medications according to written protocols or on the order of the medical director. Some left ventricular failures result from very rapid dysrhythmias. If you suspect a dysrhythmia as a cause, treat it according to established protocols. Before giving any drug, ask the patient's family if he is allergic to any medication. Medications frequently used in left ventricular failure and pulmonary edema include the following:

- Morphine sulphate
- Nitroglycerine
- Furosemide (Lasix)
- Dopamine (Intropin)
- Dobutamine (Dobutrex)

Transport the heart-failure patient as a nonemergency unless clinical conditions indicate otherwise. Conditions that indicate emergency transport include hypertension or hypotension, severe respiratory distress or pending respiratory failure, or life-threatening dysrhythmias. Remember that transporting with lights and sirens can increase the conscious patient's anxiety and worsen his condition. If nonemergency transport might compromise the patient's condition, use lights and siren. Place the patient in a position of comfort but not supine.

If the patient who is definitely in the early stages of CHF refuses transport, the outcome is likely to be devastating, leading to worsening signs and symptoms, unnecessary myocardial damage, severe pulmonary edema, and even death. Prevent refusal at all costs, and use every means at your disposal to convince the patient to be transported. If he still refuses, document the fact that you repeatedly warned the patient of the possible outcome.

CARDIAC TAMPONADE

In **cardiac tamponade,** excess fluid accumulates inside the pericardium. The normal amount of fluid between the visceral pericardium and the parietal pericardium is approximately 25 mL. This excess fluid causes an increase in intrapericardial pressure that impairs diastolic filling and drastically decreases the amount of blood the ventricles can expel with each contraction. Chest pain or dyspnea is the chief complaint; depending on the underlying cause, the chest pain may be dull or sharp and severe.

Cardiac tamponade's onset may be gradual, as in pericarditis or as in a benign or malignant neoplasm. Or it may be acute, as in MI or trauma. All forms of cardiac tamponade involve pericardial effusion of air, pus, serum, blood, or any combination of these four. Gradual onset usually results from an underlying condition, and overlooking or misdiagnosing the tamponade is easy. Renal disease and hypothyroidism can cause cardiac tamponade, though such instances are rare. Traumatic causes can include cardiopulmonary resuscitation (CPR) and penetrating or nonpenetrating injuries. Whether onset is gradual or acute, cardiac tamponade can lead to death.

> ✱ **cardiac tamponade** accumulation of excess fluid inside the pericardium.

Field Assessment

Perform your primary assessment, including the patient's airway, breathing, and circulation. If you suspect cardiac tamponade, limit your history taking to determining the precipitating cause(s). Determine if the cause might be acute trauma, such as penetrating or blunt trauma. Has the patient sustained recent trauma, including recent CPR? If you suspect a gradual onset, determine if the patient has recently had an infection or MI. Is he currently having an MI? Does he have a history of renal disease or hypothyroidism? Has he been ill? Use the OPQRST mnemonic (see p. 513) to obtain information about the patient's symptoms.

> *Always consider the possibility of pericardial tamponade in a patient who received CPR and later deteriorated.*
>

The patient generally will present with dyspnea and orthopnea. Anterior and posterior lung sounds are usually clear. Typically, the pulse is rapid and weak. In the early stages, venous pressures are often elevated, as evidenced by jugular vein distention (JVD). Blood pressure readings show a decrease in systolic pressure, pulsus paradoxus, and narrowing pulse pressures. Heart sounds are normal early on but then become muffled or faint.

Do not use the ECG, whether monitor-quality or 12-lead, to diagnose cardiac tamponade; rather, consider it a tool to support your clinical suspicions. The ECG is generally inconclusive, but ectopy is usually a late sign of cardiac tamponade. This is because an effusion easily irritates the heart's epicardial tissue. QRS and T-wave voltages are low, and nonspecific T-wave changes occur. S-T segments may be elevated. Electrical alternans (weak voltage, then normal) may appear in the P, QRS, T, and S-T segments.

Management

While obtaining any pertinent medical history and completing the secondary assessment, initiate treatment. Management of cardiac tamponade is primarily supportive, except when you detect shock or low perfusion. Maintain a patent airway and deliver high-flow oxygen. If clinically indicated, secure the patient's airway with endotracheal intubation, and maintain the patient's circulation with IV support, pharmacological agents, or CPR. Before administering any medication, ask the patient or family if he is allergic to any medications. Medications used in the treatment of cardiac tamponade the following:

- Morphine sulphate
- Furosemide (Lasix)
- Dopamine (Intropin)
- Dobutamine (Dobutrex)

Rapid transport is indicated for patients with cardiac tamponade. Remember to be supportive of the patient and family throughout your care. On arrival at the emergency department, inform the physician of your findings—past history, medications, vital signs, laboured breathing, ECG readings, pulsus paradoxus, and shock. The therapy of choice is invasive *pericardiocentesis,* which involves aspirating fluid from the pericardium with a cardiac needle.

HYPERTENSIVE EMERGENCIES

* **hypertensive emergency** an acute elevation of blood pressure that requires the blood pressure to be lowered within one hour; characterized by end-organ changes, such as hypertensive encephalopathy, renal failure, or blindness.

* **hypertensive encephalopathy** a cerebral disorder of hypertension indicated by severe headache, nausea, vomiting, and altered mental status. Neurological symptoms may include blindness, muscle twitches, inability to speak, weakness, and paralysis.

A **hypertensive emergency** is a life-threatening elevation of blood pressure. It occurs in 1 percent or less of patients with hypertension, usually when the hypertension is poorly controlled or untreated. A hypertensive emergency is characterized by a rapid increase in diastolic blood pressure (usually > 130 mmHg) accompanied by restlessness, confusion, blurred vision, nausea, and vomiting. It often occurs with **hypertensive encephalopathy,** a condition of acute or subacute consequence of severe hypertension characterized by severe headache, vomiting, visual disturbances (including transient blindness), paralysis, seizures, stupor, and coma. On occasion, this condition may cause left ventricular failure, pulmonary edema, or stroke.

A prior history of hypertension is the precipitating cause of most hypertensive emergencies. In many cases, the patient has not complied with his hypertensive medication or other prescribed drugs. Another cause of hypertensive crisis, toxemia of pregnancy (preeclampsia), can appear at any time between the twentieth week of pregnancy and term delivery. It occurs in 5 percent of pregnancies and is defined as a blood pressure of at least 140/90 mmHg. Hypertension is a sign of the toxemia, not the cause. Preeclampsia poses a high risk of abruptio placentae and generally progresses to eclampsia (coma and seizures). Left untreated, it progresses to eclampsia and death for the mother and unborn fetus.

Many Canadians are treated for hypertension. Its prevalence increases with age, and it has a higher incidence as well as a higher mortality and morbidity among blacks. With modern medications, hypertensive encephalopathy has become rare, yet it is still seen in the prehospital setting. Ischemic and hemorrhagic stroke are more common results of severe hypertension. Both hypertensive encephalopathy and stroke (ischemic or hemorrhagic) can have devastating consequences or lead to death if left untreated.

Field Assessment

After making your primary assessment, including airway, breathing, and circulation, conduct your focused history taking and secondary assessment. Generally, hypertensive patients have a chief complaint of headache, accompanied by nausea and/or vomiting, blurred vision, shortness of breath, epistaxis (nosebleed), and vertigo (dizziness). However, any one of these symptoms might be the patient's only complaint. The patient may be semiconscious, unconscious, or seizing. In pregnancy-induced toxemia, the expectant mother usually has edema of the hands or face. Photosensitivity and headache are common complaints.

Determine if the patient has a history of hypertension and if he has been taking medications as prescribed. Often, he has been noncompliant, taking medicines only occasionally or not at all. In some situations, the patient will borrow another patient's medications or take over-the-counter medications, such as herbal medications. He may be on home oxygen.

If left ventricular failure accompanies the hypertension, the lung sounds generally present with pulmonary edema; otherwise, they are clear. Often, the pulse is strong and at times may be bounding. By definition, hypertension is a systolic pressure greater than 160 mmHg and a diastolic pressure greater than 90 mmHg. Consider signs or symptoms of hypertensive encephalopathy associated with hypertension to be a hypertensive emergency.

The hypertensive patient's level of consciousness may be normal or altered, or the patient may be unconscious. The skin may be pale, flushed, or normal, cool or warm, moist or dry. Look for edema, either pitting or nonpitting. The patient may confirm PND, orthopnea, vertigo, epistaxis, tinnitus (ringing of the ears), nausea or vomiting, or visual acuities. In addition, he may have seizures or motor/sensory deficits in parts of the body or on one side. ECG findings are generally inconclusive unless the patient has an underlying cardiac condition, such as angina or MI.

Management

Place the patient in a position of comfort, unless a risk exists for airway compromise, as in stroke. Provide airway and ventilatory support, if clinically indicated. Provide oxygen, and base your transport considerations on the patient's clinical presentation. Attempt supportive IV therapy at the scene or en route. Do not prolong on-scene time to establish an IV. Place pregnant patients on their left side, and transport them as smoothly and quietly as possible.

Some systems still use loop diuretics, such as Lasix or nitroglycerine, to reduce the patient's blood pressure by manipulating preload and afterload. These treatments' effectiveness is also being scrutinized. Follow your local protocols. In severe cases, especially if hypertensive encephalopathy is present, medical direction may order one of the following medications:

Elevated blood pressures should only be treated in the prehospital setting if these are associated with end-organ changes.

- Morphine sulphate
- Furosemide (Lasix)
- Nitroglycerine
- Sodium nitroprusside (Nipride)

Explain to the patient and family the reason and necessity for rapid transport if indicated. Advise the patient who refuses transport of the serious complications that are likely without further medical attention. Stroke, seizures, pulmonary edema, and kidney damage are but a few possible outcomes. Prevent refusal at all costs. As always, use every means at your disposal to convince the patient to be transported. Document refusals as described earlier.

On arrival at the emergency department, inform the physician of your findings—vital signs, history, laboured breathing, pulmonary edema, hand or facial edema, and neurological deficits.

CARDIOGENIC SHOCK

Cardiogenic shock is the most severe form of pump failure.

Cardiogenic shock, the most severe form of pump failure, is shock that remains after existing dysrhythmias, hypovolemia, or altered vascular tone have been corrected. It occurs when left ventricular function is so compromised that the heart cannot meet the body's metabolic demands and the compensatory mechanisms are exhausted. This usually happens after extensive myocardial infarction (MI), often involving more than 40 percent of the left ventricle, or with diffuse ischemia.

A variety of mechanisms can cause cardiogenic shock, and its onset may be acute or progressive. Among the more common mechanical causes are tension pneumothorax and cardiac tamponade. Both affect ventricular filling, or preload, and tend to manifest acutely. Interference with ventricular emptying, or afterload, as in pulmonary embolism and prosthetic valve malfunction, can also cause cardiogenic shock. Impairments in myocardial contractility, as seen in MI, myocarditis, and recreational drug use, can manifest either progressively or acutely. Trauma, too, can cause cardiogenic shock, secondary to hypovolemia or to significant underlying disease processes, such as neurological, gastroenterological, renal, or metabolic disorders.

In cardiogenic shock, the body tries to compensate either by increasing the contractile force, by improving preload, by reducing the peripheral resistance, or by all three. In the early stages, a conscious patient presents with obvious signs of shock (cold extremities, weak pulses, and low blood pressure). As Starling's law loses effect, the patient's mental status diminishes and his radial pulses are no longer palpable. Finally, when preload, afterload, and contractility fail to meet vital organ demands, unconsciousness occurs, and if left untreated, the patient will die.

Cardiogenic shock has a high mortality rate.

Cardiogenic shock can occur at any age, but it is most often seen as an end-stage event in the geriatric patient, with significant underlying disease(s). Cardiogenic shock's mortality rate is high for geriatric patients following massive MI or septic shock. This is because end-organ damage is so severe or multiple end-organ damage reaches such a point that life cannot be sustained.

Field Assessment

After conducting your primary assessment, including airway, breathing, and circulation, perform your focused history taking and secondary assessment. The chief complaint may range from acute onset of chest pain to shortness of breath, altered mental status or unconsciousness, or general weakness; onset may be acute or progressive. Ask about the patient's past medical history, and determine if he has had any recent trauma. Look for evidence of a hypovolemic cause, such as a gastrointestinal bleed, septic shock, and traumatic or nontraumatic internal hemorrhage. Has the patient recently suffered an MI? Cardiogenic shock is most often associated with large anterior infarction and/or loss of 40 percent or more of the left ventricle.

The patient's medication history is important. Large amounts of different cardiac medications may indicate the patient has significant preexisting damage or a compromised but adequate cardiac output. Also, noncompliance with prescribed medications can further insult a preexisting weakened cardiac state, and the use of borrowed or over-the-counter medications can have unpredictable effects.

The altered mental status secondary to decreased cardiac output and unconsciousness common in cardiogenic shock may begin as restlessness and progress to confusion ending in coma. Airway findings include dyspnea, productive cough, or laboured breathing. Paroxysmal nocturnal dyspnea, tripoding, adventitious lung sounds, and retractions on inspiration are also common findings. Typical ECG findings include tachycardia and atrial dysrhythmias, such as atrial tachycardias. Ectopy is also common.

MI often precedes cardiogenic shock, and symptoms are initially the same as expected with MI; however, as cardiogenic shock develops and compensatory mechanisms fail, hypotension develops. The systolic blood pressure is often less than 80 mmHg. The usual heart rhythm is sinus tachycardia, a reflection of the cardiovascular system's attempts to compensate for the decreased stroke volume. If serious dysrhythmias are present, determining whether they are the cause of the hypotension or the result of the cardiogenic shock may be difficult; therefore, you must correct any major dysrhythmias.

The patient's skin is usually cool and clammy, reflecting peripheral vasoconstriction. Tachypnea is often present, since pulmonary edema is a common complication. Pitting or nonpitting peripheral edema may be present in the lower extremities or in the sacral area and may obliterate peripheral pulses.

Management

To manage the patient in cardiogenic shock, place him in a position of comfort if hemodynamically stable. If any pulmonary edema is present, the patient may prefer sitting upright, with both legs hanging off the stretcher. Treatment of cardiogenic shock (Figure 28-59) consists mostly of treating the underlying problem (such as MI and CHF) or providing supportive treatment. Remember to always treat the rate and rhythm first. Some medications that may be used to treat cardiogenic shock include the following:

Cardiogenic shock should be aggressively treated, with rapid transport to follow.

- Vasopressors
  - Dopamine (Intropin)
  - Dobutamine (Dobutrex)
  - Norepinephrine (Levophed)

Other useful medications may include

- Morphine sulphate
- Nitroglycerine
- Furosemide (Lasix)
- Digitalis, digoxin (Lanoxin)
- Sodium bicarbonate

If the patient refuses transport, follow the general guidelines; however, remember that untreated cardiogenic shock has a grim outcome. No matter how well compensated the patient may appear, true cardiogenic shock will decompensate quickly into irreversible shock. Use every means at your disposal to convince the patient to be transported. If the patient still refuses, document accordingly.

On arrival at the emergency department, inform the physician of your findings—vital signs, laboured breathing, pulmonary edema, dysrhythmias, or severe shock that remains despite your treatment.

American Heart
Association®

Fighting Heart Disease and Stroke

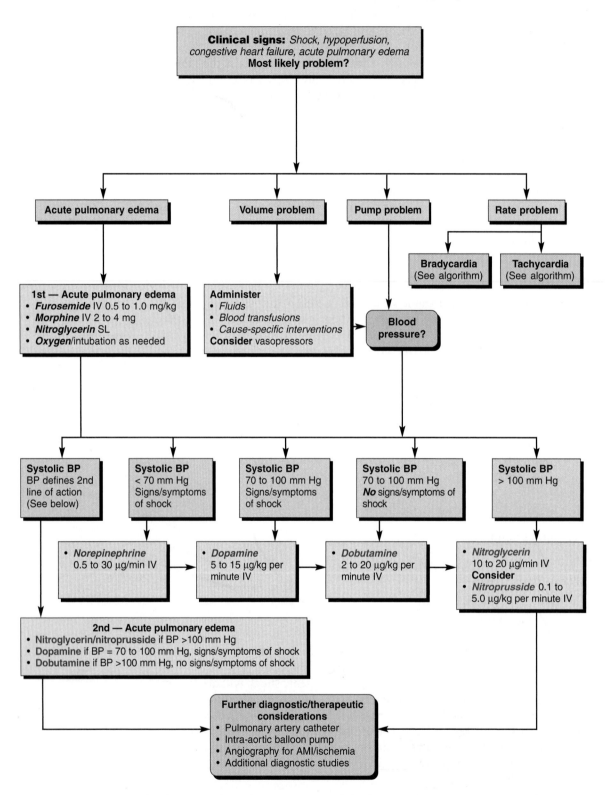

FIGURE 28–59   Management of pulmonary edema, hypotension, and shock. Reproduced with permission from *Guidelines 2000 for Cardiopulmonary Resuscitation and Emergency Cardiovascular Care,* ©2000, Copyright American Heart Association.

CARDIAC ARREST

Cardiac arrest and sudden death accounts for 60 percent of all deaths from coronary artery disease. **Cardiac arrest** is the absence of ventricular contraction that immediately results in systemic circulatory failure. **Sudden death** is any death that occurs within one hour of the symptoms' onset. At autopsy, actual infarction often is not present. Because severe atherosclerotic disease is common, authorities usually believe that a lethal dysrhythmia is the mechanism of death. The risk factors for sudden death are basically the same as those for atherosclerotic heart disease (ASHD) and coronary artery disease (CAD). In a large number of patients, cardiac arrest is the first manifestation of heart disease. Other causes of sudden death include the following:

* Drowning
* Acid-base imbalance
* Electrocution
* Drug intoxication
* Electrolyte imbalance
* Hypoxia
* Hypothermia
* Pulmonary embolism
* Stroke
* Hyperkalemia (high levels of potassium)
* Trauma
* End-stage renal disease

✱ **cardiac arrest** the absence of ventricular contraction.

✱ **sudden death** death within one hour after the onset of symptoms.

Field Assessment

In cardiac arrest, the patient is unresponsive, apneic, and pulseless. Peripheral pulses are absent. After initiating CPR, place ECG leads. Dysrhythmias found in the patient include ventricular fibrillation, ventricular tachycardia, asystole, or PEA. If you find asystole, you should confirm it in two or more leads.

Centre your questions on events prior to the arrest. Did bystanders or EMS personnel witness the cardiac arrest? Did bystanders start CPR? How much time passed from the discovery of the arrest until CPR was initiated? From discovery until EMS was activated? These questions all focus on **down time,** the duration from the beginning of the cardiac arrest until effective CPR is established. Often, physicians want to know the **total down time,** which is the time from the beginning of the cardiac arrest until you deliver the patient to the emergency department. If possible, obtain the patient's past history and medications.

✱ **down time** duration from the beginning of the cardiac arrest until effective CPR is established.

✱ **total down time** duration from the beginning of the cardiac arrest until the patient's delivery to the emergency department.

Management

To manage the patient in cardiac arrest properly, you must understand the terms *resuscitation, return of spontaneous circulation,* and *survival.*

* **Resuscitation** is the provision of efforts to return a spontaneous pulse and breathing to the patient in cardiac arrest.
* **Return of spontaneous circulation** (ROSC) occurs when resuscitation results in the patient's having a spontaneous pulse. ROSC patients may or may not have a return of breathing and may or may not survive.
* **Survival** means that the patient is resuscitated and survives to be discharged from the hospital. Many resuscitated patients reach ROSC, but not all resuscitated patients survive.

✱ **resuscitation** provision of efforts to return a spontaneous pulse and breathing.

✱ **return of spontaneous circulation** resuscitation results in the patient's having a spontaneous pulse.

✱ **survival** when a patient is resuscitated and survives to be discharged from the hospital.

Begin management of airway, breathing, and circulation simultaneously. When resuscitation is indicated, start CPR immediately. Remember that basic life support is the mainstay of treatment for cardiac arrest. Ventilate the patient with a bag-valve mask and 100-percent oxygen. Intubate or insert an alternative airway as quickly as possible. If changes in the ECG indicate defibrillation or synchronized cardioversion, perform it in conjunction with CPR, stopping CPR only to apply the pads and to deliver the shock(s). Make sure no one touches the patient when you deliver the shock. If the patient has an internal pacemaker or defibrillator, treat the cardiac arrest normally, taking care not to defibrillate over the device.

After establishing CPR and advanced airway management, establish IV access. The site of venipuncture should be as close to the heart as possible—for example, the antecubital area (bend of the forearm and humerus) or the external jugular vein. Follow all intravenous medications with a 30–45 second flush. After each flush, set the IV at a to-keep-open (TKO) drip rate.

These pharmacological agents might be used in a cardiac arrest setting:

- Atropine sulphate
- Lidocaine
- Procainamide
- Vasopressin
- Epinephrine
- Norepinephrine
- Isoproterenol
- Dopamine
- Dobutamine
- Sodium bicarbonate

Post–cardiac-arrest management of the patient generally presents an unusual situation. The patient's blood pressure can return at low, normal, or high readings because of the drugs used in resuscitation. In addition, the pulse can return at bradycardic, normal, or tachycardic rates. Ventricular ectopy is the most serious concern. If the patient presented in ventricular fibrillation or ventricular tachycardia during the cardiac arrest, or if ectopy presents following the arrest, use an antidysrhythmic agent, such as lidocaine. The blood pressure may return at low readings. The ideal range of the blood pressure is 80–100 mmHg in the postarrest period. Do not be concerned if the patient does not show any signs of response. He has endured a very harsh experience, and recovery, if any, can be slow. The postarrest setting can be unnerving, with the patient's vitals and ECG changing every minute. Approach problems one at a time, and do not be fooled by a return in pulse that fades away while the monitor still has a rhythm (PEA).

Your management of all patients in cardiac arrest should follow the American Heart Association guidelines for cardiopulmonary resuscitation and emergency cardiac care and/or local protocols. Figure 28-60 summarizes the treatment for ventricular fibrillation or ventricular tachycardia (VF/VT) and the cardiac arrest rhythms with the best prognosis for successful resuscitation. Also, review the algorithms for asystole (Figure 28-44) and pulseless electrical activity (PEA) (Figure 28-46).

Once you have established advanced life support, move the patient to the mobile intensive care unit (MICU) as quickly as possible, while taking great care to avoid disrupting IVs, endotracheal intubation, CPR, or pharmacological treatment. Transport the patient to the nearest appropriate facility as safely and as smoothly as possible using lights and siren. Offer emotional support to the patient throughout your care. On arrival at the emergency department, inform the physician of your findings, especially down time, total down time, changes in rhythm, or return of pulses.

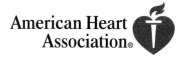

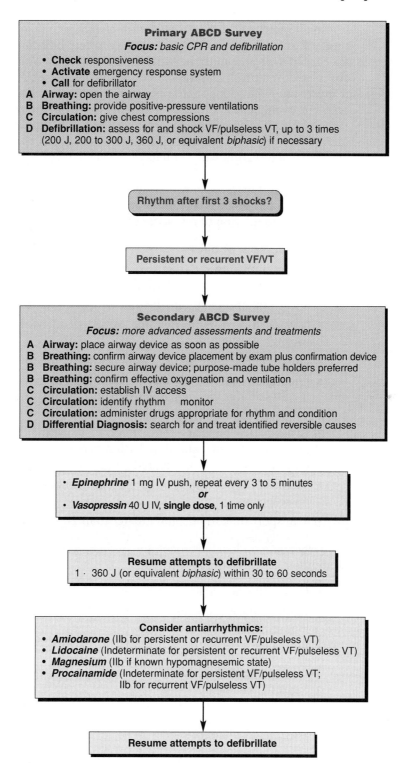

FIGURE 28–60 Management of ventricular fibrillation and pulseless ventricular tachycardia (VF/VT). Reproduced with permission from *Guidelines 2000 for Cardiopulmonary Resuscitation and Emergency Cardiovascular Care,* ©2000, Copyright American Heart Association.

Withholding and Terminating Resuscitation

In some situations, the certainty that the patient will not survive calls for not initiating resuscitation efforts. Rigor mortis, fixed dependent lividity (pooling of the blood), decapitation, decomposition, and incineration are all situations in which you should not initiate resuscitation.

In addition, withhold resuscitation efforts if the patient has an out-of-hospital advance directive. Advance directives may be completed by the patient at an earlier time and must be witnessed and dated. Alternatively, they may be completed by a proxy. A physician must sign and date the advance directive, and it must state conditions that apply to the patient at the time of the cardiac arrest. For example, the directive may state that resuscitation should be withheld if the patient has an end-stage terminal illness. Each province and territory and many local regions treat advance directives differently. Review local protocol and medical direction when you have to decide whether or not to honour an advance directive.

In other instances, poor prognosis and survivability of many cardiac arrest patients makes termination of resuscitation a consideration. Some of the *inclusion* criteria for termination of resuscitation are as follow:

- 18 years old or older
- Arrest is presumed cardiac in origin and not associated with a treatable cause, such as hypothermia, overdose, or hypovolemia
- Successful and maintained endotracheal intubation
- Advanced cardiac life support (ACLS) standards have been applied throughout the arrest
- Down time greater than 20 minutes
- On-scene advanced life support (ALS) efforts have been sustained for 20 minutes, or the patient remains in asystole through four rounds of ALS drugs
- Patient's rhythm is asystolic or agonal when the decision to terminate is made, and this rhythm persists until the resuscitation efforts are actually terminated
- Victims of blunt trauma who present in asystole or develop asystole on scene
- Transport time to hospital greater than 20 minutes

Depending on local protocol, the *exclusion* criteria for termination of resuscitation may include the following:

- Under 18 years old
- Etiology that could benefit from in-hospital treatment (such as hypothermia)
- Persistent or recurring ventricular tachycardia or fibrillation
- Transient return of a pulse
- Signs of neurological viability
- Arrest witnessed by EMS personnel
- Family or responsible party opposed to termination

These criteria should not be considered as either inclusionary or exclusionary:

- The patient's age if 18 or over (for example, geriatric)
- Down time before EMS arrival

- Presence of a nonofficial do not resuscitate (DNR) order
- Quality-of-life evaluations by EMS

Review local protocol and medical direction before attempting termination of resuscitation. Most systems use documented protocols and direct communication with an online medical director or physician to approve or deny termination of resuscitation. The medical director or physician may base his decision on the following information:

Review local protocol and medical direction before attempting termination of resuscitation.

- Medical condition of the patient
- Known etiological factors
- Therapy rendered
- Family's presence and appraisal of the situation
- Communication of any resistance or uncertainty on the part of the family
- Maintenance of continuous documentation, including the ECG

It is important to provide grief support to the family at this time. This requires EMS personnel or a community agency to be in place soon after termination of resuscitation. EMS personnel deal not only with the living or viable patients but also with the families of lost loved ones, especially when those families have witnessed the death. Many systems employ assigned personnel to support the family after termination of resuscitation. In other systems, paramedics on the scene provide support until a predetermined person from another local agency can arrive. Although this supportive role can be uncomfortable, it will be part of your job.

Law enforcement regulations require that all local, provincial or territorial, or federal laws pertaining to a death be followed. These, too, may vary from region to region, but their basic principles are the same. The officer discusses the death certificate with the attending physician. He will determine whether the event or patient requires assignment to a medical examiner if the nature of the death is suspicious in any way, or if the physician is at all hesitant to sign the death certificate. The officer also may be required to assign the patient to a medical examiner if he does not have a physician. Check with local law enforcement agencies to determine their protocol. In some regions, paramedics are presented with a terminally ill "vital signs absent" (VSA) patient who does not have to be resuscitated. Prior arrangements with the patient's physician would have resulted in a policy care directive or do not resuscitate (DNR) order for the patient. Once at the scene, after assessing the patient as VSA, obtaining such documentation and confirming it with a medical director or base hospital physician, the paramedic can officially pronounce the patient deceased. The ambulance call report serves as an interim death certificate, and the body can be taken directly to a funeral home, depending on previous arrangements.

PERIPHERAL VASCULAR AND OTHER CARDIOVASCULAR EMERGENCIES

In addition to cardiac arrest, MI, and hypertension emergencies, other common cardiovascular emergencies involve the arterial and venous systems. Such disorders are generally classified as traumatic or nontraumatic. Nontraumatic vascular emergencies typically arise from preexisting conditions or from a disease process.

Atherosclerosis

The major underlying factor in many cardiovascular emergencies is **atherosclerosis,** a progressive degenerative disease of the medium-sized and large arteries.

* atherosclerosis a progressive, degenerative disease of the medium-sized and large arteries.

Atherosclerosis affects the aorta and its branches, the coronary arteries, and the cerebral arteries, among others. It results from fats (lipids and cholesterol) deposited under the tunica intima (inner lining) of the involved vessels. The fat causes an injury response in the tunica intima, which subsequently damages the tunica media (middle layer) as well. Over time, calcium is deposited, causing plaques, where small hemorrhages can occur. These hemorrhages, in turn, lead to scarring, fibrosis, larger plaque buildup, and aneurysm. The involved arteries can become completely blocked by additional plaque, by a blood clot, or by an aneurysm that results from tearing in the arterial wall.

The results of atherosclerosis are evident in many disease processes. First, disruption of the vessel's intimal surface destroys the vessel's elasticity. This condition, **arteriosclerosis,** can cause hypertension and other related problems. Second, atherosclerosis can reduce blood flow through the affected vessel; common manifestations include angina pectoris and intermittent **claudication.** Frequently, thrombosis will develop, totally obstructing the vessel or the tissues it supplies. Myocardial infarction (MI) is a classic example of this process.

Aneurysm

Aneurysm is a nonspecific term meaning dilation of a vessel. There are several types of aneurysms:

- Atherosclerotic
- Dissecting
- Infectious
- Congenital
- Traumatic

Most aneurysms result from atherosclerosis and involve the aorta because the blood pressure there is the highest of any vessel in the body. An aneurysm occurs when blood surges into the aortic wall through a tear in the aortic tunica intima. Infectious aneurysms are most commonly associated with syphilis and are rare. Congenital aneurysms can occur with several disease states, such as Marfan's syndrome, a hereditary disease that affects the connective tissue. Aortic aneurysm occurs in people with this disease because it involves the connective tissue within the vessel wall. Those affected may experience sudden death, usually from spontaneous rupture of the aorta, often at a fairly young age.

Abdominal Aortic Aneurysm Abdominal aortic aneurysm commonly results from atherosclerosis and occurs most frequently in the aorta, below the renal arteries and above the bifurcation of the common iliac arteries (Figure 28-61). It is 10 times more common in men than in women and most prevalent between ages 60 and 70.

Signs and symptoms of an abdominal aneurysm include the following:

- Abdominal pain
- Back and flank pain
- Hypotension
- Urge to defecate, caused by the retroperitoneal leakage of blood

Dissecting Aortic Aneurysm Degenerative changes in the smooth muscle and elastic tissue of the aortic media cause most **dissecting aortic aneurysms.** This can result in hematoma and, subsequently, aneurysm. The original tear often results from **cystic medial necrosis,** a degenerative disease of connective tissue often associated with hypertension and to a certain extent, aging. Predisposing factors in-

∗ arteriosclerosis a thickening, loss of elasticity, and hardening of the walls of the arteries from calcium deposits.

∗ claudication severe pain in the calf muscle due to inadequate blood supply. It typically occurs with exertion and subsides with rest.

∗ aneurysm the ballooning of an arterial wall, resulting from a defect or weakness in the wall.

∗ dissecting aortic aneurysm aneurysm caused when blood gets between and separates the layers of the aortic wall.

∗ cystic medial necrosis death or degeneration of a part of the wall of an artery.

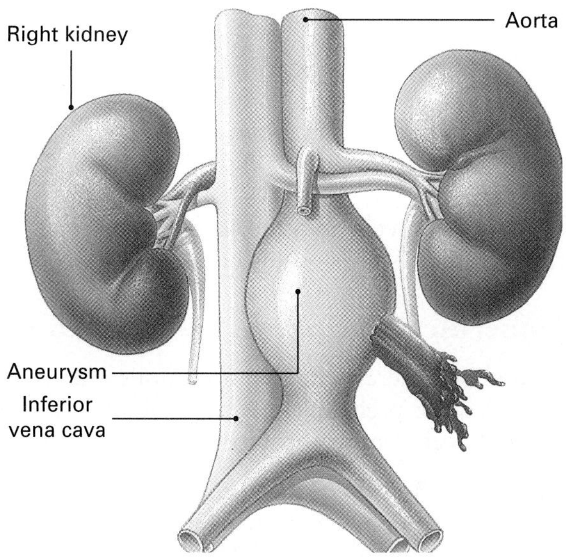

FIGURE 28–61 Rupture of an abdominal aortic aneurysm.

clude hypertension, which is present in 75–85 percent of cases. It occurs more frequently in patients older than 40–50, although it can occur in younger individuals, especially pregnant women. A tendency for this disease also runs in families.

Of dissecting aortic aneurysms, 67 percent involve the ascending aorta. Once dissection has started, it can extend to all of the abdominal aorta as well as its branches, including the coronary arteries, aortic valve, subclavian arteries, and carotid arteries. The aneurysm can rupture at any time, usually into the pericardial or pleural cavity.

Acute Pulmonary Embolism

Acute pulmonary embolism occurs when a blood clot or other particle lodges in a pulmonary artery and blocks blood flow through that vessel. Pulmonary emboli may be composed of air, fat, amniotic fluid, or blood clots. Factors that predispose a patient to blood clots include prolonged immobilization, *thrombophlebitis* (inflammation and clots in a vein), use of certain medications, and atrial fibrillation.

✷ **acute pulmonary embolism** blockage that occurs when a blood clot or other particle lodges in a pulmonary artery.

When a pulmonary embolism blocks the blood flow through a vessel, the right heart must pump against increased resistance, which, in turn, increases pulmonary capillary pressure. The area of the lung supplied by the occluded vessel then stops functioning, and gas exchange decreases.

The signs and symptoms of pulmonary embolism depend on the size of the obstruction. The patient suffering acute pulmonary embolism may report a sudden onset of severe and unexplained dyspnea that may or may not be associated with chest pain. He may have a recent history of immobilization from a hip fracture, surgery, or other debilitating illness.

Acute Arterial Occlusion

An **acute arterial occlusion** is the sudden occlusion of arterial blood flow due to trauma, thrombosis, tumour, embolus, or idiopathic means. Emboli are probably the most common cause. They can arise from within the chamber (*mural emboli*), from a thrombus in the left ventricle, from an atrial thrombus secondary to atrial fibrillation, or from a thrombus caused by abdominal aortic atherosclerosis. Arterial occlusions most commonly involve vessels in the abdomen or extremities.

✷ **acute arterial occlusion** the sudden occlusion of arterial blood flow.

Vasculitis

Vasculitis is an inflammation of blood vessels. Most vasculitis stems from a variety of rheumatic diseases and syndromes. The inflammatory process is usually segmental, and inflammation within the media of a muscular artery tends to destroy the internal elastic lamina. Necrosis and hypertrophy (enlarging) of the vessel occur, and the vessel wall has a high likelihood of breaching, leaking fibrin and red blood cells into the surrounding tissue. This potentially can lead to partial or total vascular occlusion and subsequent necrosis.

Noncritical Peripheral Vascular Conditions

Several peripheral vascular conditions are not immediately life threatening but often require prehospital care. They include peripheral arterial atherosclerotic disease, deep venous thrombosis, and varicose veins.

Peripheral Arterial Atherosclerotic Disease Peripheral arterial atherosclerotic **disease** is a progressive degenerative disease of the medium-sized and large arteries. It affects the aorta and its branches, the brachial and femoral peripheral arteries, and the cerebral arteries. For reasons unknown, it does not affect the coronary arteries. It is a gradual, progressive disease, often associated with diabetes mellitus. In extreme cases, significant arterial insufficiency may lead to ulcers and gangrene. Occlusion of the peripheral arteries causes chronic and acute ischemia.

In the chronic setting, intermittent claudication (diminished blood flow in exercising muscle) produces pain with exertion. It occurs most commonly with the calf but can affect any leg muscle. Rest initially relieves this pain. When the disease progresses, however, the pain presents even at rest. The extremity usually appears normal, but pulses will be reduced or absent. As the ischemia worsens, the extremity becomes painful, cold, and numb, and ulceration, gangrene, and necrosis may be present. There is no edema.

In the acute setting, arterial occlusion from an embolus, aneurysm, or thrombus occurs. The patient experiences a sudden onset of pain, coldness, numbness, and pallor. Pulses are absent distal to the occlusion. Acute occlusion may cause severe ischemia with motor and sensory deficits. Edema is not present.

Deep Venous Thrombosis Deep venous thrombosis is a blood clot in a vein. It most commonly occurs in the larger veins of the thigh and calf. Predisposing factors include a recent history of trauma, inactivity, pregnancy, or varicose veins.

The patient frequently complains of gradually increasing pain and calf tenderness. Often, the leg and foot are swollen because of occluded venous drainage. Leg elevation may alleviate the signs and symptoms. In some cases, the patient may be asymptomatic. Gentle palpation of the calf and thigh may reveal tenderness and, on occasion, cord-like clotted veins. Dorsiflexion of the foot may cause Homan's sign, discomfort behind the knee. This is associated with deep venous thrombosis. The skin may be warm and red.

Varicose Veins Varicose veins are dilated superficial veins, usually in the lower extremities. Predisposing factors include pregnancy, obesity, and genetics. Signs and symptoms include the visible distention of the leg veins, lower leg swelling and discomfort (especially at the end of the day), and skin colour and texture changes in the legs and ankles. If the condition is chronic, venous stasis ulcers, a noncritical condition, can develop. Venous stasis ulcers can rupture, but direct pressure usually can control the bleeding, which occasionally is significant.

General Assessment and Management of Vascular Disorders

Occlusion of any vessel can result in ischemia, injury, and necrosis of the affected tissue. Depending on the tissue or organ involved, untreated occlusion can cause severe disability or death. In pulmonary occlusion, hypotension and cardiac collapse can ensue quickly, and death can occur rapidly. In cerebral occlusion, debilitating seizures, paralysis, or death can occur. Mesenteric occlusion can cause necrosis, giving rise to sepsis. Or it can affect vital organs, causing a slow and agonizing death. Pulmonary embolus, aortic aneurysm, and some acute arterial occlusions can produce a hypoperfusion state, and death can be rapid.

Assessment Begin your assessment by checking airway, breathing, and circulation. Breathing is usually not affected, except in pulmonary embolism and a decompensated state of shock. In decompensated shock resulting from aneurysm, arterial occlusion, or pulmonary embolism, breathing may be laboured. Circulation may be compromised or absent distal to the affected area. Check circulation for the five Ps:

- Pallor
- Pain
- Pulselessness
- Paralysis
- Paresthesia

Check the skin for pallor or mottling distal to the affected area. Skin temperature may appear normal systemically but cool or cold at the affected area, or it may be systemically cool and clammy, as occurs in decompensated shock.

Determine the patient's chief complaint. Depending on the type of vascular emergency, the patient may complain of a sudden or gradual onset of discomfort, and the pain may be localized. Use the OPQRST acronym (see p. 513) to elicit the patient's description of symptoms and pain. Is the pain in the chest, abdomen, or extremity? Does it radiate, or is it localized? Was its onset gradual or sudden? If there is claudication, and is it relieved with rest?

Conduct your focused history and secondary assessment. Determine the contributing history. This may well be the patient's first recognized event, or it may be a recurrence. Patients with a prior vascular emergency are prone to recurrences. They may report an increase in the frequency or duration of events. Breath sounds may be clear to auscultation. Alterations in the heart rate and rhythm may occur with pulmonary embolism and aortic aneurysm. Unequal bilateral blood pressures may indicate a high thoracic aneurysm. Peripheral pulses may be diminished or absent in the affected extremity with arterial occlusion or peripheral arterial atherosclerotic disease. Bruits may be audible over the affected carotid artery. The skin may be cool, moist, or dry, reflecting diminished circulation to the affected area or extremity. ECG findings generally do not contribute to vascular emergency treatment. If dysrhythmias or ectopy are present, treat them accordingly.

Management Managing the patient with a vascular emergency is mostly supportive. Place the patient in a position of comfort. Give oxygen by nonrebreather mask if you suspect pulmonary embolism, aortic aneurysm, or arterial occlusion or if any hypotension or a hypoperfusion state presents.

Before administering any drug, ask the patient or the family if he is allergic to any medications. Pharmacological agents that might be used in a vascular emergency include these:

- Nitrous oxide (Nitronox)
- Morphine sulphate

Transport the patient as soon as possible. Indications for rapid transport with lights and sirens include any situation in which medications do not relieve the patient's symptoms or in which you suspect pulmonary embolism, aortic aneurysm, or arterial occlusion. Also, consider any presentation of hypotension or hypoperfusion to be an emergency, and transport the patient rapidly. Report your findings to the emergency department staff.

If the patient refuses transport, advise him that serious complications are likely to occur without further medical attention. Vascular emergencies can reach a point where the patient permanently loses a limb or quickly decompensates into irreversible shock. Some patients will attempt to refuse transport because they have received relief from pain medications. Use every means at your disposal to convince them to be transported. Document refusals according to general guidelines.

PREHOSPITAL ECG MONITORING

Technology has evolved to a point where portable 12-lead ECG monitoring is readily available. Many manufacturers now make 12-lead machines for prehospital care. Most machines have sophisticated electronics, many with ECG diagnostic packages. Some now have a defibrillator/pacer unit. The principles of 12-lead monitoring are similar to those for routine ECG monitoring described earlier in this chapter.

PREHOSPITAL 12-LEAD ECG MONITORING

The following skill sequence details 12-lead prehospital ECG monitoring (see Procedure 28-5).

1. Explain what you are going to do. Reassure the patient that the machine will not shock him.
2. Prepare all of the equipment, and ensure the cable is in good repair. Check to make sure there are adequate leads and materials for prepping the skin.
3. Prep the skin (Procedure 28-5a). Dirt, oil, sweat, and other materials on the skin can interfere with obtaining a quality tracing. The skin should be cleansed with an appropriate substance. If the patient is diaphoretic, dry the skin with a towel. On very hot days or in situations where the patient is extremely diaphoretic, tincture of Benzoin can be applied to the skin before attaching the electrode. Occasionally, it may be necessary to slightly abrade the skin to obtain a good interface. Patients with a lot of body hair may need to have the area immediately over the electrode site shaved to ensure good skin/electrode interface.
4. Place the four limb leads according to the manufacturer's recommendations (Procedure 28-5b).
5. Following placement of the limb leads, prepare for placement of the precordial leads. Procedure 28-5c illustrates proper placement of the precordial leads.
6. First, place Lead V_1 by attaching the positive electrode to the right of the sternum at the fourth intercostal space (Procedure 28-5d.)
7. Next, place Lead V_2 by attaching the positive electrode to the left of the sternum at the fourth intercostal space (Procedure 28-5e).
8. Next, place Lead V_4 by attaching the positive electrode at the midclavicular line at the fifth intercostal space (Procedure 28-5f).
9. Next, place Lead V_3 by attaching the positive electrode in a line midway between Lead V_2 and Lead V_4 (Procedure 28-5g).

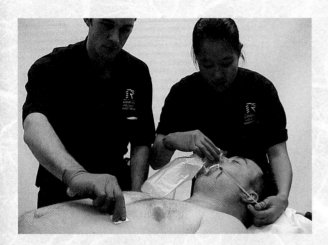

28–5a   Prep the skin.

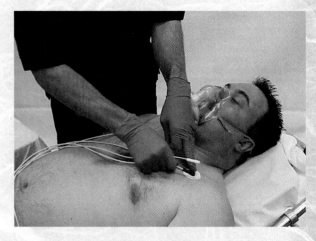

28–5b   Place the four limb leads according to the manufacturer's recommendations.

Lead V₁ The electrode is at the fourth intercostal space just to the right of the sternum.
Lead V₂ The electrode is at the fourth intercostal space just to the left of the sternum.
Lead V₃ The electrode is at the line midway between leads V₂ and V₄.
Lead V₄ The electrode is at the midclavicular line in the fifth interspace.
Lead V₅ The electrode is at the anterior axillary line at the same level as lead V₄.
Lead V₆ The electrode is at the midaxillary line at the same level as lead V₄.

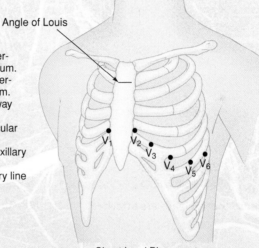

Angle of Louis

Chest Lead Placement

28–5c   Proper placement of the precordial leads.

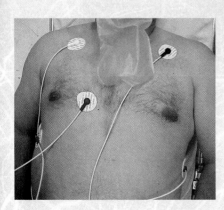

28–5d   Place lead V₁.

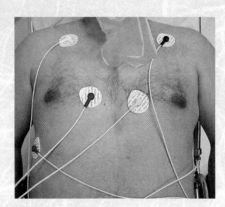

28–5e   Place lead V₂.

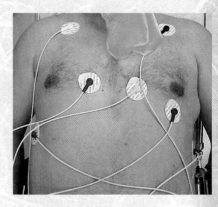

28–5f   Place lead V₄.

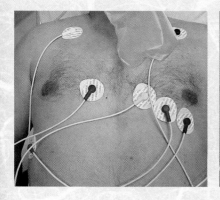

28–5g   Place lead V₃.

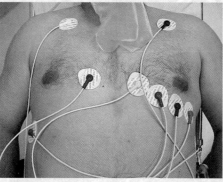

28–5h   Place lead V₅.

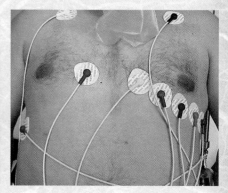

28–5i   Place lead V₆.

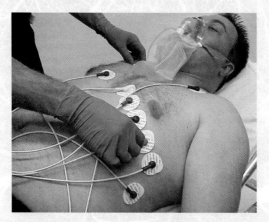

28–5j   Ensure that all leads are attached.

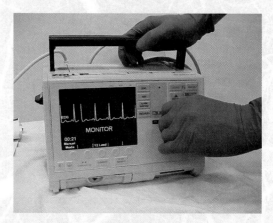

28–5k   Turn on the machine.

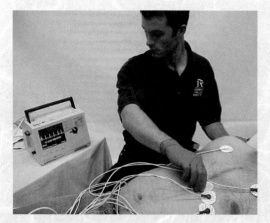

28–5l   Record the tracing.

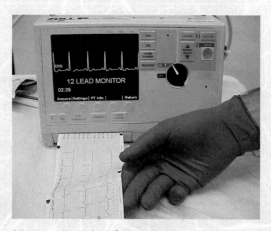

28–5m   Examine the tracing.

10. Next, place Lead V_5 by attaching the positive electrode at the anterior axillary line at the same level as V_4 (Procedure 28-5h).

11. Finally, place V_6 by attaching the positive electrode to the mid-axillary line at the same level as V_4 (Procedure 28-5i).

12. Ensure that all leads are attached (Procedure 28-5j).

13. Turn on the machine (Procedure 28-5k).

14. Check to ensure all leads are properly attached and a good tracing is being received from each channel.

15. Record the tracing (Procedure 28-5l).

16. Examine the tracing. Do not completely rely on the machine's interpretation of the tracing. If necessary, confirm with medical direction (Procedure 28-5m).

17. Perform patient handover to the hospital personnel.

18. Restock equipment for next call.

19. Compare field interpretation with emergency department and cardiology interpretations.

SUMMARY

Cardiovascular disease is the number one cause of death in Canada and the United States. Many deaths from heart attack occur within the first 24 hours—frequently within the first hour. With the advent of thrombolytic therapy, time is of the essence when managing the patient with suspected ischemic heart disease. EMS plays an ever-increasing role in the early recognition of patients suffering coronary ischemia. In certain areas, EMS provides definitive care by initiating thrombolytic therapy in the field. This is especially important in cases where transport times can be long. With cardiovascular disease, EMS can truly mean the difference between life and death.

CHAPTER 29

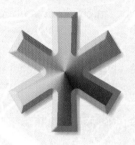

Neurology

Objectives

After reading this chapter, you should be able to:

1. Describe the incidence, morbidity, and mortality of neurological emergencies. (p. 569)
2. Identify the risk factors most predisposing to diseases of the nervous system. (pp. 585, 589–590, 594, 595, 602-603)
3. Discuss the anatomy and physiology of the nervous system. (see Chapter 12)
4. Define and discuss the epidemiology (including the morbidity/mortality and preventative strategies), pathophysiology, assessment findings, and management for the following neurological problems:

a. Coma and altered mental status (pp. 582–584)
b. Seizures (pp. 589–594)
c. Syncope (pp. 594–595)
d. Headache (pp. 595–596)
e. Neoplasms (pp. 597–598)
f. Abscess (p. 598)
g. Stroke (pp. 584–589)
h. Intracranial hemorrhage (pp. 585–586)
i. Transient ischemic attack (pp. 587–588)
j. Degenerative neurological diseases (pp. 598–602)

Continued

5. Describe and differentiate among the major types of seizures. (pp. 590–591)
6. Describe the phases of a generalized seizure. (p. 590)
7. Define the following:
   a. Muscular dystrophy (p. 599)
   b. Multiple sclerosis (p. 599)
   c. Dystonia (p. 599)
   d. Parkinson's disease (pp. 599–600)
   e. Trigeminal neuralgia (p. 600)
   f. Bell's palsy (p. 600)
   g. Amyotrophic lateral sclerosis (p. 601)
   h. Peripheral neuropathy (pp. 571–572)
   i. Myoclonus (p. 601)
   j. Spina bifida (p. 601)
   k. Poliomyelitis (p. 601)

8. Define and discuss the pathophysiology, assessment findings, and management of nontraumatic spinal injury, including the following:
   a. Low back pain (pp. 602–603)
   b. Herniated intervertebral disc (p. 603)
   c. Spinal cord tumours (p. 604)
9. Differentiate between neurological emergencies on the basis of assessment findings. (pp. 572–581)
10. Given several preprogrammed nontraumatic neurological emergency patients, provide the appropriate assessment, management, and transport. (pp. 572–605)

INTRODUCTION

Nervous conditions and diseases affect the lives of hundreds of Canadians each year. Strokes afflict about 50 000 people every year, of which 60 percent are women. Epilepsy affects 300 000 people, or just less than 1 percent of the Canadian population. An additional 100 000 Canadians have been diagnosed with Parkinson's disease. These are only a few examples of the impact of nervous system disorders. Millions of people are also affected by headache, multiple sclerosis, syncope, neoplasm, and other nervous system emergencies, all of which you will learn about in this chapter.

Many conditions, diseases, and injuries can cause nervous system disorders. Such disorders may be caused by internal or external factors. Modern advances and clinical studies continue to yield new medications and treatments for many conditions. Paramedics should maintain a solid knowledge of the nervous system and remain familiar with current trends and advancements in treating the neurological patient.

This chapter provides an overview of the common neurological conditions that may be encountered in the prehospital setting. It discusses the relevant pathophysiology of the nervous system, assessment techniques, and the recommended prehospital management. Figure 29–1 provides an overview of the central and peripheral nervous systems.

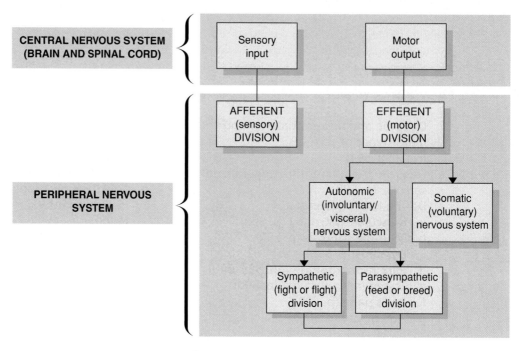

CENTRAL NERVOUS SYSTEM
(BRAIN AND SPINAL CORD)

PERIPHERAL NERVOUS
SYSTEM

Sensory input

Motor output

AFFERENT (sensory) DIVISION

EFFERENT (motor) DIVISION

Autonomic (involuntary/visceral) nervous system

Somatic (voluntary) nervous system

Sympathetic (fight or flight) division

Parasympathetic (feed or breed) division

FIGURE 29-1   Overview of the nervous system.

PATHOPHYSIOLOGY

A firm grasp of the pathophysiology of nontraumatic neurological emergencies is essential in order for the paramedic to provide appropriate and timely emergency care.

ALTERATION IN COGNITIVE SYSTEMS

Consciousness is a condition in which an individual is fully responsive to stimuli and demonstrates awareness of the environment. The ability to respond to stimuli is dependent on an intact reticular activating system (RAS). Cognition and the ability to respond to the environment rely on an intact cerebral cortex. Therefore, altered forms of consciousness can result from dysfunction or interruption of the central nervous system (CNS).

CENTRAL NERVOUS SYSTEM DISORDERS

An alteration in mental status is the hallmark sign of CNS injury or illness.

✱ **coma** a state of unconsciousness from which the patient cannot be aroused.

An alteration in mental status is the hallmark sign of CNS injury or illness. Any alteration in mental status is abnormal and warrants further examination. Alterations may vary from minor thought disturbances to unconsciousness. Unconsciousness, also called **coma,** is a state in which the patient cannot be aroused, even by powerful external stimuli. There are generally two mechanisms capable of producing alterations in mental status:

- *Structural lesions.* Structural lesions (e.g., tumours, contusions) depress consciousness by destroying or encroaching on the substance of the brain. Examples of causes of structural lesions include
  - Brain tumour (neoplasm)
  - Degenerative disease
  - Intracranial hemorrhage
  - Parasites
  - Trauma

- *Toxic-metabolic states.* Toxic-metabolic states involve either the presence of circulating toxins or metabolites or the lack of metabolic substrates (oxygen, glucose, or thiamine). These states produce diffuse depression of both sides (hemispheres) of the cerebrum, with or without depression within the brainstem. Various causes of toxic-metabolic states include
  - Anoxia (lack of oxygen)
  - Diabetic ketoacidosis
  - Hepatic failure
  - Hypoglycemia
  - Renal failure
  - Thiamine deficiency
  - Toxic exposure (e.g., cyanide, organophosphates)

Within the two general mechanisms (structural lesions and toxic metabolic states), there are many difficult-to-classify causes of altered mental status. Some of the more common causes are listed in the following four general categories:

- Drugs
  - Depressants (including alcohol)
  - Hallucinogens
  - Narcotics

- Cardiovascular
  - Anaphylaxis
  - Cardiac arrest
  - Stroke
  - Dysrhythmias
  - Hypertensive encephalopathy
  - Shock

- Respiratory
  - Chronic obstructive pulmonary disease (COPD)
  - Inhalation of toxic gas
  - Hypoxia

- Infectious
  - Acquired immune deficiency syndrome (AIDS)
  - Encephalitis
  - Meningitis

CEREBRAL HOMEOSTASIS

The autonomic nervous system (ANS) maintains cerebral homeostasis (internal balance) and regulates and coordinates the body's vital functions, such as blood pressure, temperature regulation, respiration, and metabolism. It can be strongly affected by emotional influences, resulting in blushing, palpitations, clammy hands, and dry mouth.

PERIPHERAL NERVOUS SYSTEM DISORDERS

Peripheral neuropathy is any malfunction or damage of the peripheral nerves. It can affect muscle activity, sensation, reflexes, or internal organ function. The disorder can involve a single nerve, a *mononeuropathy,* or multiple nerves, known as *polyneuropathy.*

Mononeuropathy is usually caused by localized conditions, such as trauma, compression, or infections. Fractured bones, for example, may lacerate or compress

* **peripheral neuropathy** any malfunction or damage of the peripheral nerves. Results may include muscle weakness, loss of sensation, impaired reflexes, and internal organ malfunctions.

Peripheral neuropathy can affect muscle activity, sensation, reflexes, or internal organ function.

a nerve; excessively tight tourniquets may compress and injure a nerve; and such infections as herpes zoster may affect a single segment of an afferent nerve. Another common example is carpal tunnel syndrome, a compression-type neuropathy. It is caused by compression of the median nerve that travels through the flexor tendon canal of the lower arm. Carpal tunnel syndrome can cause pain or motor dysfunction in the fingers innervated by the median nerve.

Polyneuropathy is characterized by demyelination or degeneration of peripheral nerves. It leads to sensory, motor, or mixed sensorimotor deficits. A number of conditions, such as immune disorders, toxic agents, and metabolic disorders, are known causes of polyneuropathy. One example of a polyneuropathy is Guillian-Barré syndrome, which is characterized by rapidly worsening muscle weakness of the limbs that can sometimes lead to paralysis. Diabetes is one of the major causes of peripheral neuropathy. It usually affects the distal nerves of the hands and feet in the classic "stocking and glove" distribution.

Autonomic Nervous System Disorders

Disorders affecting the ANS are frequently a result of another condition. Since the control of the body's internal environment is vested in the ANS, most conditions that affect the integrity of an individual are accompanied by some changes in ANS functioning.

GENERAL ASSESSMENT FINDINGS

Assessment of the neurological system is often difficult. Many of the signs and symptoms of nervous system dysfunction are subtle. As you conduct the scene assessment and begin the primary assessment, form a general impression of the patient, and evaluate mental status before assessing the ABCs (airway, breathing, circulation). If your primary assessment causes you to suspect nervous system dysfunction, this will prompt you to place particular emphasis on the neurological examination during the focused history and secondary assessment.

SCENE ASSESSMENT AND PRIMARY ASSESSMENT

A great deal of crucial information can be obtained while approaching the patient. Assess the scene and the surroundings as well as the patient to form a general impression. Is there evidence of toxic exposure or trauma? Look for clues that can indicate a patient's condition:

General Appearance

- Is the patient conscious?
- Alert?
- Confused?
- Sitting upright?

Speech

- Can the patient speak?
- Clear and coherent?
- Full sentences?
- Slurred speech?

During the primary assessment, be alert to any signs of nervous system dysfunction. If present, these will prompt you to place particular emphasis on the neurological evaluation during the focused history and secondary assessment.

Skin

- Colour (pink, pale, cyanotic)?
- Temperature (warm, hot, cool)?
- Moisture (diaphoretic, clammy)?

Facial drooping present?

Posture/Gait

- Upright?
- Leaning?
- Staggering?
- Steady gait?

Next, quickly check the patient's mental status through the "AVPU" method.

- **A** = The patient is *alert and aware* of the surroundings. A patient alert and orientated to time, place, person, and self, is said to be "alert and oriented times four." Remember, no patient is "oriented" unless she has answered the questions that the paramedic has to ask.
- **V** = The patient responds to *verbal stimuli*. The patient responds when talked to, perhaps in a loud voice. Note if the patient delivers the answers normally or sluggishly. Also, observe whether the patient has purposeful or uncoordinated movements.
- **P** = The patient responds to *painful stimuli*. The patient responds when tactile stimulation is used, such as a sternal rub, a squeeze of the trapezius muscle, or pinching the thenar (thumb) web space.
- **U** = The patient is *unresponsive*. The patient is not alert and does not respond to verbal or painful stimuli.

Assessment of cerebral functioning also includes assessing the patient's emotional status. If the patient is conscious, you can detect changes in the following:

Mood

- Is the patient's affect natural, or is the patient irritable, anxious, or apathetic?
- Does the patient appear depressed? Manic? Happy? Solemn? Reserved?

Thought

- What is the patient's thought pattern? Is it logical? Appropriate? Scattered?

Perception

- How does the patient perceive the surroundings? Are her interactions appropriate?

Judgment

- Is the patient using reasonable and sound judgment? Is she logical?

Memory and Attention

- Is short-term memory present? Long-term memory? Question family members or caregivers to obtain this information.
- Does the patient maintain conversation? Pay attention? Repeatedly ask or answer questions?

Any alteration from the patient's normal mental status or mood should be considered significant and warrants additional assessment.

Once a patient's level of consciousness is determined, place the greatest emphasis on maintenance of the airway. If the patient is unconscious, assume that a cervical spine injury exists, and treat it appropriately. Use the modified jaw-thrust manoeuvre to open the airway. Once opened, insert the appropriate airway adjunct. In unresponsive patients, the tongue may be occluding the airway. In such cases, you may need only to place an oropharyngeal or nasopharyngeal airway to maintain the airway. If the patient tolerates an oropharyngeal airway, consider intubation, if you are an ACP or CCP.

Vigilantly monitor the airway in any patient with CNS injury. It is essential to observe for respiratory arrest that can result from increased intracranial pressure (ICP). Remain alert for an absent gag reflex and for vomiting. In addition, blood from facial injuries and possible aspiration of gastric contents further threaten the patient's airway.

Observe the patient for any signs and symptoms of inadequate or impaired breathing or the presence of any abnormal respiratory patterns. Remember, the body's "breathing centre" is located in the brain. Certain neurological conditions can cause these areas to malfunction and limit the patient's ability to breathe.

Complete assessment of the body's circulatory status is also a crucial part of the primary assessment. Evaluation of the heart rate, rhythm, and electrocardiographic (ECG) pattern can shed light on the body's overall state of perfusion. Observe the patient's skin colour, temperature, and moisture for abnormal findings, such as cyanosis and moisture. A healthy adult's skin is usually warm, dry, and pink.

FOCUSED HISTORY AND SECONDARY ASSESSMENT

Following completion of the primary assessment and correction of any immediate threats to the patient's life, turn your attention to the focused history and secondary assessment. This assessment should include an accurate history and a secondary assessment, including vital signs. Remember that any indications of nervous system dysfunction should cause you to place particular emphasis on neurological evaluation. Neurological evaluation will be detailed under "Nervous System Status" later in this chapter.

History

A thorough, accurate history of a patient is crucial in determining the current problem and subsequent treatment of a patient. One of the first steps in obtaining a thorough history involves attempting to determine whether the neurological problem is traumatic or medical. Clarification will help determine the plan for subsequent prehospital treatment. The primary history may not be easy to obtain because of the patient's altered mental status. In these cases, it is critical for you to obtain information from family, friends, or other bystanders, if available.

If the neurological emergency is due to trauma, ask the following questions:

- When did the incident occur?
- How did the incident occur, or what is the mechanism of injury?

- Was there any loss of consciousness?
- Was there evidence of incontinence? (Incontinence suggests loss of consciousness.)
- What is the patient's chief complaint?
- Has there been any change in symptoms?
- Are there any complicating factors?

If there is no evidence of a traumatic cause of the neurological emergency, ask the following questions to determine the nature of illness:

- What is the chief complaint?
- What are the details of the present illness, or what is the nature of the illness?
- Is there a pertinent underlying medical problem, such as
  - Cardiac disease
  - Chronic seizures
  - Diabetes
  - Hypertension
- Have these symptoms occurred before?
- Are there any environmental clues? These may include
  - Evidence of current medications
  - Medic-Alert identification
  - Alcohol bottles or drug paraphernalia
  - Chemicals, hazardous materials

Secondary Assessment

The secondary assessment of a patient with a neurological emergency should include the standard head-to-toe physical assessment and a more detailed neurological assessment. Pay particular attention to the pupils, respiratory status, and spinal evaluation.

Face A patient's ability to smile, frown, and wrinkle her forehead indicates an intact facial nerve (cranial nerve VII). If the patient is conscious, test these abilities. Note any drooping or facial paralysis.

Eyes The pupils are controlled by the oculomotor nerve (cranial nerve III). This nerve follows a long course through the skull and is easily compressed by brain swelling. While slight pupillary inequality is normal, abnormal pupils can be an early indicator of increasing intracranial pressure. If both pupils are dilated and do not react to light, the patient probably has a brainstem injury or has suffered serious brain anoxia. If the pupils are dilated but still react to light, the injury may be reversible. However, the patient must be transported quickly to an emergency facility capable of treating CNS injuries. A unilaterally dilated pupil that remains reactive to light may be the earliest sign of increasing intracranial pressure. The patient with altered mental status who presents with or develops a unilaterally dilated pupil is in the "immediate transport" category. Constricted, or pinpoint, pupils suggest a toxic etiology for the altered mental status.

A common method of assessing extraocular movement is to have the patient follow finger movements. For example, ask the patient to follow your finger to the extreme left, then up, then down. Repeat the same motions to the extreme right. These positions are referred to as the *cardinal positions of gaze*. Because extraocular movements are controlled by cranial nerves III (oculomotor), IV (trochlear), and VI (abducens), inability to look in all directions with both eyes can be an early indication of a CNS problem. This is particularly important in the indication of facial trauma.

When examining a patient's pupils, it is important to check for contact lenses. Contact lenses, if present, should be removed and placed into their container or a saline solution and transported with the patient.

Nose/Mouth In the presence of facial paralysis, drooping of the patient's mouth may occur. Pay particular attention to any of these changes that may potentially compromise the patient's airway. A common way to assess for mouth droop is to ask the patient to smile. Also, ask the patient: "show your teeth." Both manoeuvres will help determine whether there is any degree of facial drooping.

Respiratory Status Respiratory derangement can occur with CNS illness or injury. Any of five abnormal respiratory patterns may commonly be observed (Figure 29-2):

- *Cheyne-Stokes respiration.* A breathing pattern characterized by a period of apnea lasting 10–60 seconds, followed by gradually increasing depth and frequency of respirations.
- *Kussmaul's Respiration.* Rapid, deep respirations caused by severe metabolic and CNS problems.
- *Central Neurogenic Hyperventilation.* Hyperventilation caused by a lesion in the CNS, often characterized by rapid, deep, noisy respirations.
- *Ataxic Respirations.* Poor respirations due to CNS damage, causing ineffective thoracic muscular coordination.
- *Apneustic Respirations.* Breathing characterized by prolonged inspiration unrelieved by expiration attempts. This is seen in patients with damage to the upper part of the pons.

Several other respiratory patterns are also possible, depending on the injury. A patient's respirations can be affected by so many factors—fear, hysteria, chest injuries, spinal cord injuries, or diabetes—that they are not as useful as other signs in monitoring the course of CNS problems. Just before death, the patient may present with central neurogenic hyperventilation.

It is important to remember that the level of carbon dioxide ($PaCO_2$) in the blood has a critical effect on cerebral vessels. The normal blood $PaCO_2$ is 40 mmHg. Increasing the $PaCO_2$ causes cerebral vasodilation, while decreasing it results in cerebral vasoconstriction. If the patient is poorly ventilated, the $PaCO_2$ will increase, causing even further vasodilatation with a subsequent increase in intracranial pressure. Hyperoxygenation can decrease the $PaCO_2$ effectively causing vasoconstriction of the cerebral vessels. This will assist in minimizing brain swelling. Therefore, hyperoxygenate any patient who is suspected of having increased intracranial pressure at a rate of 16–20 breaths per minute. It is important to avoid *excessively* hyperoxygenating a patient so as to prevent decreasing $PaCO_2$ levels to dangerously low levels. It is important to maintain adequate perfusion of the patient without compromising an increase in intracranial pressure.

Cardiovascular Status Patients suffering from a neurological event are also likely to suffer changes to the cardiovascular system. Vigilant assessment of a patient's vital signs is necessary to observe these changes. Look for these changes:

- *Heart rate.* A heart rate that is too fast (tachycardia), too slow (bradycardia), or irregular (dysrhythmias).
- *ECG/rhythm.* Development of any changes to the ECG rhythm, including S-T segment changes, the onset of bradycardia,

✱ Cheyne-Stokes respiration a breathing pattern characterized by a period of apnea lasting 10–60 seconds, followed by gradually increasing depth and frequency of respirations.

✱ Kussmaul's respiration rapid deep respirations caused by severe metabolic and CNS problems.

✱ central neurogenic hyperventilation hyperventilation caused by a lesion in the CNS, often characterized by rapid, deep, noisy respirations.

✱ ataxic respiration poor respirations due to CNS damage, causing ineffective thoracic muscular coordination.

✱ apneustic respiration breathing characterized by a prolonged inspiration unrelieved by expiration attempts, seen in patients with damage to the upper part of the pons.

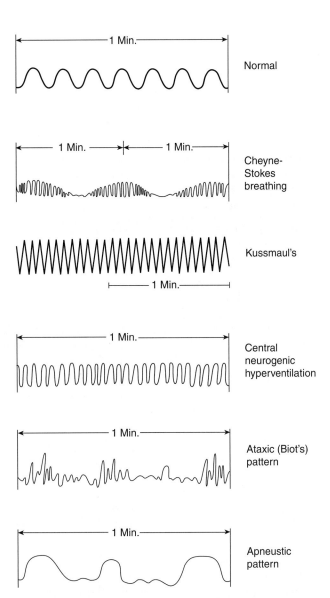

FIGURE 29-2 Respiratory patterns seen with CNS dysfunction.

Normal

Cheyne-Stokes breathing

Kussmaul's

Central neurogenic hyperventilation

Ataxic (Biot's) pattern

Apneustic pattern

tachycardia, or potentially lethal dysrhythmias, such as ventricular fibrillation or ventricular tachycardia.

- *Bruits.* The sound of turbulent blood flow through the carotid arteries, known as a *bruit,* may be indicative of atherosclerotic disease and decreased blood flow to the brain.

- *Jugular venous distention (JVD).* Increased jugular venous pressure, known as jugular venous distention, may be present, indicating that the heart is not pumping effectively.

Nervous System Status To evaluate nervous system status, take into account sensorimotor status, motor system status, and the status of the cranial nerves.

Sensorimotor Evaluation The purpose of sensorimotor evaluation is to document loss of sensation and/or motor function. To initially assess the patient with a possible spinal injury, perform these steps:

1. If the patient is unconscious, determine the response to voice, gentle tactile stimulation, and then, if necessary, pain.

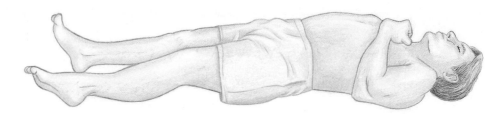

FIGURE 29-3 Patient with decorticate posturing.

2. Evaluate the spine for pain and tenderness.
3. Observe for bruises on the spine.
4. Observe for deformity of the spine.
5. Note any incontinence.
6. Check for circulation, motor function, and sensation in each extremity. Does the patient have feeling in her hands and feet? Ask the patient to wiggle her toes and push them against resistance. Compare both sides. Check bilateral grip strength. If the patient is unconscious, pain response should be observed. If the unconscious patient withdraws or localizes to the pinching of fingers and toes, there is intact sensation and motor function. This is a sign of normal or only minimally impaired cortical function.

A patient with a suspected spinal cord injury will require full spinal immobilization on a long spine board. See Chapter 24 for a discussion of traumatic spinal cord injury.

Both **decorticate posturing** (arms flexed, legs extended) and **decerebrate posturing** (arms and legs extended) are ominous signs of deep cerebral or upper brainstem injury (Figures 29-3 and 29-4). Flaccid paralysis usually indicates spinal cord injury.

Motor System Status A thorough examination of the motor system of the body includes an assessment of muscle tone, strength, flexion, extension, coordination, and balance. Assess the patient for the following:

* *Muscle Tone.* Are the patient's muscles firm? Or is atrophy present?
* *Strength.* Does the patient have adequate muscle strength? Or is weakness present? Does the patient have strong and equal grip strength?

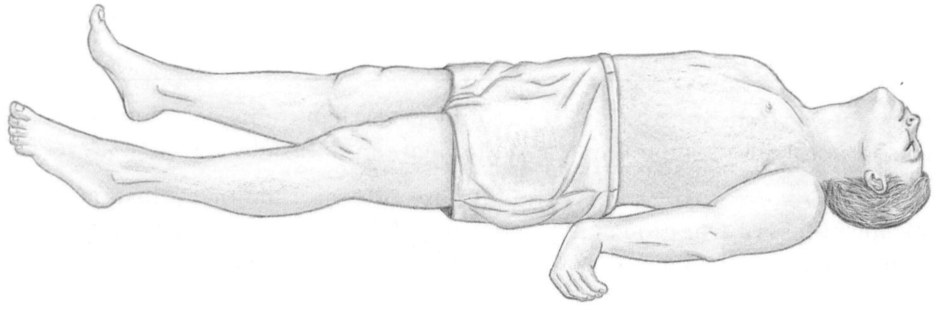

✱ **decorticate posture** characteristic posture associated with a lesion at or above the upper brainstem. The patient presents with the arms flexed, fists clenched, and legs extended.

✱ **decerebrate posture** sustained contraction of extensor muscles of the extremities resulting from a lesion in the brainstem. The patient presents with stiff and extended extremities and retracted head.

FIGURE 29-4 Patient with decerebrate posturing.

- *Flexion/Extension.* Can the patient flex, extend, and move extremities adequately?
- *Coordination.* Are the patient's gait and movements steady and smooth? Can the patient touch finger to nose?
- *Balance.* Can the patient stand or sit upright without becoming dizzy?

Cranial Nerves Status As you learned earlier, 12 pairs of cranial nerves extend from the lower surface of the brain. Each pair is designated by a Roman numeral from I to XII. Proper and intact functioning of these nerves may be assessed during a complete neurological examination as detailed in Chapter 6, "Physical Assessment Techniques." Review Figure 12-72 in Chapter 12, which outlines the cranial nerves and their functions.

Further Mental Status Assessment For patients with an altered mental status or those who are unresponsive, the **Glasgow Coma Scale (GCS)** is a simple tool that can be used to evaluate and monitor the patient's condition. While it is used most commonly in trauma situations, the scale can also be a valuable tool for monitoring a medical patient's status (Figure 29-5). The scale includes three components:

✱ **Glasgow Coma Scale (GCS)** tool used in evaluating and quantifying the degree of coma by determining the best motor, verbal, and eye-opening responses to standardized stimuli.

- Eye opening
- Verbal response
- Motor response

Glasgow Coma Scale

Eye Opening	Spontaneous	4	
	To Voice	3	
	To Pain	2	
	None	1	
Verbal Response	Oriented	5	
	Confused	4	
	Inappropriate Words	3	
	Incomprehensible Words	2	
	None	1	
Motor Response	Obeys Commands	6	
	Locailzes Pain	5	
	Withdraw (Pain)	4	
	Flexion (Pain)	3	
	Extension (Pain)	2	
	None	1	
Glasgow Coma Score Total			

TOTAL GLASGOW COMA SCALE POINTS	
13–15 = 5	Conversion = Approximately One-Third Total Value
9–12 = 4	
6–8 = 3	
4–5 = 1	

| **Neurologic Assessment** | |

FIGURE 29-5 Glasgow Coma Scale.

A number is applied to each of the components based on the patient's condition. The total score can serve as an indicator of survival. The lowest GCS score possible is 3; the highest possible score is 15. The GCS can also be used as a predictor of long-term morbidity and mortality. The following are examples of the predictive value of the GCS system:

A patient with a total score of	Has an estimated
8 or better	94% favourable outcome
5, 6, 7	50% favourable (adult), 90% (children)
3, 4	10% favourable outcome
5, 6, 7 who drop a grade	0% favourable outcome
5, 6, 7 who improve to more than 7	80% favourable outcome

Vital Signs

Vital signs are crucial in following the course of neurological problems. Such signs can indicate changes in intracranial pressure. Increased intracranial pressure is characterized by the following changes in vital signs, sometimes collectively referred to as **Cushing's reflex:**

✳ **Cushing's reflex** a collective change in vital signs (increased blood pressure and temperature and decreased pulse and respirations) associated with increasing intracranial pressure.

- Increased blood pressure
- Decreased pulse
- Decreased respirations
- Increased temperature

A patient in the early stages of increased intracranial pressure usually exhibits a decrease in pulse rate and an increase in blood pressure and temperature. Later, if the intracranial pressure continues to rise without correction, the pulse will increase, the blood pressure will fall, and the body temperature will remain elevated. Dysrhythmias may be seen with increased intracranial pressure. Continuous ECG monitoring and pulse oximetry, if available, should be utilized to spot early signs of CNS lesions. Table 29-1 compares vital signs of a patient in shock with those of a patient with head injury and increased intracranial pressure. Remember, if you suspect that a patient has a CNS injury, take and record vital signs every five minutes.

Additional Assessment Tools

Additional technological tools may be useful in assessing and monitoring the neurological patient. Such tools should be used as adjuncts to a complete patient assessment, and they should not be relied on as sole indicators of a patient's

Table 29-1	COMPARISON OF VITAL SIGNS IN SHOCK AND INCREASED INTRACRANIAL PRESSURE	
Vital Signs	**Shock**	**Increased ICP**
Blood pressure	Decreased	Increased
Pulse	Increased	Decreased
Respirations	Increased	Decreased
Level of Consciousness	Decreased	Decreased

condition. Paramedics should continue to base their clinical decisions on a patient's entire presentation. Use such instruments as the end-tidal CO_2 detector, pulse oximeter, and blood glucometer to gain further insight into a patient's condition.

End-Tidal CO_2 Detector The end-tidal CO_2 detector monitors the amount of carbon dioxide being exhaled by a patient while being ventilated. This device works on the premise that during exhalation CO_2 should be detected. In the apneic patient with a suspected neurological injury, the device can be used to monitor the effectiveness of the assisted ventilations. Monitoring the levels of CO_2 can ensure that ventilation rate and quality are appropriate for decreasing the increased intracranial pressure.

Pulse Oximeter The pulse oximeter is an effective tool for monitoring a patient's general state of perfusion. Any patient with a pulse oximetry reading of less than 90 percent is likely to be hypoxic. In a patient who has suffered a stroke, altered mental status, or syncope, the oximeter can be a useful adjunct in monitoring a patient's condition. It can also monitor the effectiveness of airway management techniques.

Blood Glucometer A common cause of an altered mental status or focal neurological deficits is hypoglycemia. Determining the blood glucose level is often a crucial step in caring for the neurological patient. Use the glucometer to obtain an accurate blood glucose level. See Chapter 30 for a discussion of this procedure. Documented hypoglycemia should be treated with a bolus of 50 percent dextrose or subcutaneous glucagon 1.0 mg.

Geriatric Considerations in Neurological Assessment

The neurological system of the geriatric patient is susceptible to systemic illness and is often affected by other body disorders. In addition, certain neurological changes, such as pupil sluggishness, loss of overall body strength, and muscle atrophy, occur naturally with the aging process. Slowing of nerve conduction is another characteristic often seen in the geriatric patient. Such slowing may indicate that a little more time is necessary to obtain a complete neurological history.

The level of consciousness and overall mental status of a geriatric patient is evaluated by assessing judgment, memory, affect, mood, orientation, speech, and grooming. Interviewing family members about the patient's normal state may reveal any change in mental status. Common neurological problems of the older patient include headache, low back pain, dizziness, weakness, loss of balance, such disorders as Parkinson's disease, and vascular emergencies, such as stroke.

ONGOING ASSESSMENT

Any patient suffering from a neurological emergency should be reassessed every five minutes during your care and during transport. Constantly reevaluate and monitor the patient's airway and neurological system.

MANAGEMENT OF SPECIFIC NERVOUS SYSTEM EMERGENCIES

The primary treatment for nervous system emergencies in the field is supportive. Most conditions will not be "cured" in the prehospital setting but symptoms may

The primary treatment for nervous system emergencies in the field is supportive.

be reduced or controlled. Make a strong effort to make the patient comfortable and to reduce any of the existing symptoms. Follow these steps:

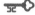

The major concerns in any CNS emergency are always airway, breathing, circulation, and, if indicated, C-spine control.

- *Airway and Breathing.* Properly position any patient that you suspect has a neurological emergency and protect the airway. If there is known or possible trauma, maintain C-spine immobilization. Administer oxygen via a nonrebreather mask. If the patient is breathing inadequately or is apneic, initiate ventilatory assistance. If an airway problem is detected, first apply basic airway manoeuvres, such as head positioning or the modified jaw-thrust manoeuvre. Intubate, if indicated.

- *Circulatory Support.* Establish an IV with a crystalloid solution, such as Ringer's Lactate or normal saline. Alternatively, consider placing a heparin or saline lock. It is important to have an accessible route for medications. Generally, running an IV at a to-keep-open rate will be sufficient.

- *Pharmacological Interventions.* Few medications are available to alleviate signs and symptoms in patients with neurological emergencies. Medications may include dextrose, naloxone, and diazepam.

- *Psychological Support.* Patients suffering a nervous system emergency, acute or chronic, are likely also to suffer anxiety. Neurological deficits of any kind are frightening experiences. Provide the patient with emotional support, and explain the treatment regimen. In most cases, it is appropriate to explain to the patient what is occurring and why. Careful explanation and emotional support will help allay anxiety and apprehension.

- *Transport Considerations.* Assess, provide emergency care, and package the patient as quickly and safely as possible. Rapidly transport any patient with a neurological deficit or altered mental status to an appropriate emergency department, equipped with a computed tomography (CT) or magnetic resonance imaging (MRI) scanner and facilities capable of managing strokes using thrombolytic therapy. Modern medicine has seen the development of new advances in pharmacological and surgical interventions that are only available in the hospital setting.

There are numerous causes of nervous system emergencies. The more common nontraumatic nervous emergencies encountered in the prehospital setting include altered mental status, stroke, transient ischemic attacks (TIA), seizures, and headache. The following discussion details the assessment and management of these frequently encountered nontraumatic nervous system emergencies.

ALTERED MENTAL STATUS

When evaluating a patient, you may find mnemonic devices useful as assessment aids. A mnemonic that may help you remember some of the common causes of altered mental status is "AEIOU-TIPS."

A = Acidosis, alcohol
E = Epilepsy
I = Infection
O = Overdose
U = Uremia (kidney failure)

T = Trauma, tumour, toxin
I = Insulin (hypoglycemia or diabetic ketoacidosis)
P = Psychosis, poison
S = Stroke, seizure

Make an effort through history taking and patient assessment to determine the underlying cause of the altered level of consciousness. Often, however, a clear cause will not be evident and cannot be determined in the prehospital setting.

Assessment

Using the AVPU method discussed earlier (see p. 573), determine the patient's level of consciousness. Unresponsive patients require vigilant monitoring and protection of the airway. Use information from family, friends, or other bystanders to try to determine the underlying cause of unconsciousness. Perform a secondary assessment to uncover any hidden injuries, signs, or symptoms.

Management

Your initial priority is to ensure that the patient's airway is open and the cervical spine is immobilized (in cases of suspected head/neck injury). Secure the patient's airway, and administer supplemental oxygen simultaneously. If the patient is breathing inadequately, support respirations. An unresponsive patient requires an appropriate airway adjunct. Then, assess the patient's circulatory status. Evaluate the patient's heart rate and blood pressure, and monitor the cardiac rhythm.

After the above are completed, perform the following steps:

- Establish an IV of normal saline or Ringer's Lactate at a to-keep-open rate, or place a heparin or saline lock.

- Determine the blood glucose level using a glucometer. A serum glucose determination will assist in determining if the altered mental status is due to hypoglycemia.

- If the blood glucose level is low, administer 50-percent dextrose. This will mediate hypoglycemia, which may be the cause of the altered mental status. Even if the patient has uncontrolled diabetes and her body is not producing enough insulin, hyperglycemia produced by administration of glucose will do limited harm in the short time before arrival at the hospital. If, however, the patient is hypoglycemic, for example, from too much insulin or missing a meal, the administration of glucose can be life saving, and the patient may respond immediately. For the alcoholic patient who is hypoglycemic, the glucose may be life saving as well. For more information on diabetic emergencies, see Chapter 30.

- Administer naloxone if a narcotic overdose is suspected. Naloxone, a narcotic antagonist, has proven effective in the management and reversal of overdose caused by narcotics or synthetic narcotic agents. For more information, see Chapter 34.

Chronic Alcoholism Chronic alcoholism interferes with the intake, absorption, and use of thiamine. A significant percentage of alcoholics have thiamine deficiency that can cause Wernicke's syndrome or Korsakoff's psychosis. **Wernicke's syndrome** is an acute but reversible encephalopathy (brain disease) characterized by ataxia, eye muscle weakness, and mental derangement. Of even greater concern is

✱ **Wernicke's syndrome** condition characterized by loss of memory and disorientation, associated with chronic alcohol intake and a diet deficient in thiamine.

Korsakoff's psychosis, characterized by memory disorder. Once established, Korsakoff's psychosis may be irreversible. Paramedics should follow local protocols. If ordered by medical direction, administer 100 mg of thiamine IV or IM.

Increased Intracranial Pressure If an increase in intracranial pressure is likely, as occurs in a closed head injury, hyperoxygenate the patient at 16–20 breaths per minute. Decreasing the carbon dioxide level will cause cerebral vasoconstriction and will help minimize brain swelling. Use caution not to overhyperoxygenate, which could decrease CO_2 levels to dangerously low levels. Medical direction may order administration of the osmotic diuretic mannitol (Osmotrol). Mannitol causes diuresis, eliminating fluid from the intravascular space through the kidneys. Many authorities feel that its oncotic effect also causes a fluid shift from the substance of the brain to the circulation, thus reducing brain edema. As with all drugs, follow local protocols.

STROKE AND INTRACRANIAL HEMORRHAGE

Stroke, also called a "brain attack," is a general term that describes injury or death of brain tissue usually due to interruption of cerebral blood flow. The term "brain attack" is used because it compares the physiology of a stroke with that of a heart attack. In both cases, oxygen deprivation causes damage to the affected tissue.

The term "brain attack" also reflects recent trends in the treatment of a stroke, which in many cases now parallels the treatment available for heart attack. Prior to 1995, prehospital care of the stroke patient was considered primarily supportive. Since then, modern medicine has discovered new therapies and has realized the importance of early intervention. Now, early recognition and rapid transport to the hospital are identified as crucial to improving the outcome for stroke patients. Transport of the patient to an emergency facility with the capability to respond to a stroke patient quickly, such as a facility equipped with computed tomography (CT) and neurological services, is highly recommended.

In addition, studies have proven that *tissue plasminogen activator (tPA)* and other thrombolytic agents used in the treatment of heart attack are also effective in treating certain occlusive strokes. Stroke patients who may be candidates for the thrombolytic therapy must receive definitive treatment within three hours of onset. Because of the possibility of intervention with thrombolytics, it is crucial to determine the exact time of the onset of symptoms as accurately as possible. In addition, it is essential that the public be aware of the signs and symptoms of stroke so that EMS can be notified. Therefore, extensive public education is necessary in achieving early recognition of symptoms and appropriate intervention and treatment. Transport to an emergency facility is crucial in achieving the best possible outcome for these patients.

Strokes are the third most common cause of death and in middle-aged and older patients are a frequent cause of disability. Therefore the public, particularly those with a history of atherosclerosis (hardening of the arteries), heart disease, or hypertension, should be educated on the signs and symptoms of stroke as well as the need to contact EMS at the outset of symptoms. Likewise, paramedics must understand stroke as a serious, potentially life-threatening condition that warrants rapid recognition and prompt transport.

Strokes can be divided into two broad categories: those caused by occlusion (blockage) of an artery and those caused by hemorrhage from a ruptured cerebral artery (Figure 29-6):

- *Occlusive Strokes.* An occlusive stroke occurs when a cerebral artery is blocked by a clot or other foreign matter. This results in *ischemia,* an inadequate blood supply to the brain tissue, and progresses to *in-*

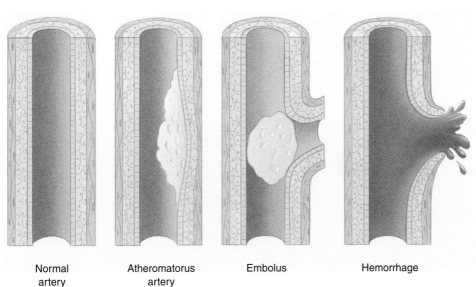

FIGURE 29-6   Etiologies of stroke.

Normal   Atheromatorus   Embolus   Hemorrhage
artery   artery

farction, the death of tissues as a result of cessation of blood supply. In infarction, the tissue that has died will swell, causing further damage to nearby tissues, which only have a marginal blood supply. If swelling is severe, *herniation* (protrusion of brain tissue from the skull through the foramen magnum, the narrow opening at the base of the skull) may result. Occlusive strokes are classified as either embolic or thrombotic, depending on the cause.

- *Embolic Strokes.* An *embolus* is a solid, liquid, or gaseous mass carried to a blood vessel from a remote site. The most common emboli are clots (thromboemboli), which usually arise from diseased blood vessels in the neck (carotid) or from abnormally contracting chambers in the heart. Atrial fibrillation often results in atrial dilation, a precursor to the formation of clots. Other types of emboli that may cause occlusion in cerebral blood vessels are air, tumour tissue, and fat. Embolic strokes occur suddenly and may be characterized by severe headaches.

- *Thrombotic Strokes.* A *cerebral thrombus* is a blood clot that gradually develops in and obstructs a cerebral artery. As a person ages, atheromatous plaque deposits can form on the inner walls of arteries. The buildup causes a narrowing of the arteries and reduces the amount of blood that can flow through them. This process is known as atherosclerosis. Once the arteries are narrowed, platelets adhere to the roughened surface and can create a blood clot that blocks the blood flow through the cerebral artery. This ultimately results in brain tissue death. Unlike the embolic stroke, the signs and symptoms of thrombotic stroke develop gradually. This type of stroke often occurs at night and is characterized by a patient awakening with altered mental status and/or loss of speech, sensory, or motor function.

• *Hemorrhagic Strokes.* Hemorrhagic strokes are usually categorized as being within the brain (intracerebral) (Figure 29-7a) or in the space around the outer surface of the brain (subarachnoid) (Figure 29-7b). Onset is often sudden and marked by a severe headache. Most intracranial hemorrhages occur in the hypertensive patient when a

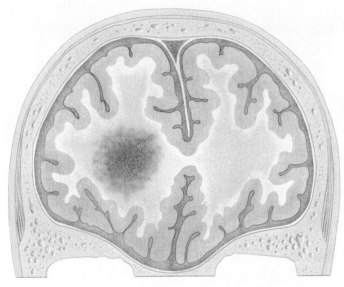

a.

b.

FIGURE 29-7   (a) Intracerebral hemorrhage; (b) Subarachnoid hemorrhage.

small vessel deep within the brain tissue ruptures. Subarachnoid hemorrhages most often result from congenital blood vessel abnormalities or from head trauma. Congenital abnormalities include aneurysms (weakened vessels) and arteriovenous malformations (collections of abnormal blood vessels). Aneurysms tend to be on the surface and may hemorrhage into the brain tissue or the subarachnoid space. Arteriovenous malformations may be within the brain, in the subarachnoid space, or both. Hemorrhage inside the brain often tears and separates normal brain tissue. The release of blood into the cavities within the brain that contain cerebrospinal fluid may paralyze vital centres. If blood in the subarachnoid space impairs drainage of cerebrospinal fluid, it may cause a rise in intracranial pressure. Herniation of brain tissue may then occur.

Assessment

Signs and symptoms of a stroke will depend on the type of stroke and the area of the brain damaged. Areas commonly affected are the motor, speech, and sensory centres. The onset of symptoms will be acute, and the patient may experience unconsciousness. There may be stertorous breathing (laborious breathing accompanied by snoring) due to paralysis of a portion of the soft palate. Respiratory expiration may be puffs of air out of the cheeks and mouth. The patient's pupils may be unequal, with the larger pupil on the side of the hemorrhage. Paralysis will usually involve one side of the face, one arm, and one leg. The eyes often will be turned away from the side of the body paralysis. The patient's skin may be cool and clammy. Speech disturbances, or aphasia, may also be noted.

Signs and symptoms of a stroke include the following:

- Facial drooping
- Headache
- Confusion and agitation
- Dysphasia (difficulty speaking)
- Aphasia (inability to speak)
- Dysarthria (impairment of the tongue and muscles essential to speech)
- Vision problems, such as monocular blindness (blindness in one eye) or double vision
- Hemiparesis (weakness on one side)
- Hemiplegia (paralysis on one side)
- Paresthesia (numbness or tingling)
- Inability to recognize by touch
- Gait disturbances or uncoordinated fine motor movements
- Dizziness
- Incontinence
- Coma

Predisposing factors that may contribute to stroke include hypertension, diabetes, abnormal blood lipid levels, oral contraceptives, sickle cell disease, and some cardiac dysrhythmias (e.g., atrial fibrillation).

Distinguishing Transient Ischemic Attacks (TIAs) Some patients may have transient stroke-like symptoms known as **TIAs,** or **transient ischemic attacks.** These indicate temporary interference with the blood supply to the brain, producing symptoms of neurological deficit. These symptoms may last for a few minutes or for several hours but usually resolve within 24 hours. After the attack, the patient will show no evidence of residual brain or neurological damage. The patient who experiences a TIA may, however, be a candidate for an eventual stroke. In fact, one-third of TIA patients suffer a stroke soon thereafter.

✱ **transient ischemic attack (TIA)** temporary interruption of blood supply to the brain.

The onset of a transient ischemic attack is usually abrupt. The specific signs and symptoms depend on the area of the brain affected. Any one or a combination of stroke symptoms may be present. In fact, it is virtually impossible to determine whether such a neurological event is due to a stroke or to a TIA in the prehospital setting.

The most common cause of a TIA is carotid artery disease. Other causes can be a small embolus, decreased cardiac output, hypotension, overmedication with antihypertensive agents, or cerebrovascular spasm.

While obtaining the history of the patient suspected of sustaining a TIA, you should try to collect information on or take note of the following factors:

- Previous neurological symptoms
- Initial symptoms and their progression
- Changes in mental status
- Precipitating factors
- Dizziness
- Palpitations
- History of hypertension, cardiac disease, sickle cell disease, or previous TIA or stroke

Management

Care for the stroke or TIA patient emphasizes early recognition, supportive measures, rapid transport, and notification of the emergency department (Figure 29-8). Aggressive airway management is a priority in caring for these patients. Field management of the stroke patient generally includes the following procedures:

- Ensure scene safety, including body substance isolation.
- Establish and maintain an adequate airway. Have suction equipment readily available. Control of the patient's airway is a priority. Brain damage can affect a patient's ability to swallow and maintain an open airway.
- If patient is apneic or if breathing is inadequate, provide positive pressure ventilations at a rate of 16–20 per minute. Hyperoxygenation of the stroke patient will eliminate excessive CO_2 levels. Avoid overzealous hyperoxygenation that may bring CO_2 levels to detrimentally low levels causing profound cerebral vasoconstriction.
- If breathing is adequate, administer oxygen via a nonrebreather mask at 15 litres per minute.
- Complete a detailed patient history.
- Keep the patient supine or in the recovery position. If the patient has congestive heart failure, she could be maintained in a semi-upright position, if necessary.
- If an altered mental status is present or there is potential for airway compromise, place the patient in the left lateral recumbent or in the recovery position.
- Determine the blood glucose level.
- Start an IV of normal saline or Ringer's Lactate at a to-keep-open rate, or place a heparin or saline lock. (Avoid dextrose solutions that may increase intracranial pressure due to increased osmotic effects.) If hypoglycemia is present, consider the administration of 50-percent dextrose by intravenous push or subcutaneous glucagon 1.0 mg.
- Monitor the cardiac rhythm.
- Protect the paralyzed extremities.
- Give the patient reassurance—all procedures should be explained. The patient may be unable to speak but still may be able to hear and understand.
- Rapidly transport the patient, without excessive movement or noise, to an appropriate medical facility.

FIGURE 29-8 Management of suspected stroke. Reproduced with permission from *Guidelines 2000 for Cardiopulmonary Resuscitation and Emergency Cardiovascular Care,* ©2000, Copyright American Heart Association.

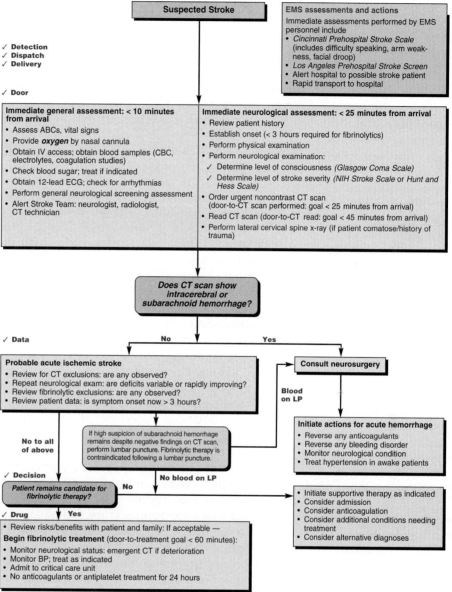

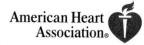

SEIZURES AND EPILEPSY

A **seizure** is a temporary alteration in behaviour due to the massive electrical discharge of one or more groups of neurons in the brain. Seizures in any individual may be caused by stresses to the body, such as hypoxia, or a rapid lowering of blood sugar. Febrile seizures can occur in young children with sudden elevations in body temperature. Structural diseases of the brain, such as tumours, head trauma, toxic eclampsia, and vascular disorders, also cause seizures. The most common cause is *idiopathic epilepsy*. The term *idiopathic* means "without a known cause."

✱ **seizure** a temporary alteration in behaviour due to the massive electrical discharge of one or more groups of neurons in the brain. Seizures can be clinically classified as generalized or partial.

Content Review

TYPES OF SEIZURES

- Generalized seizures
  - Tonic-clonic
  - Absence
- Partial seizures
  - Simple partial seizures
  - Complex partial seizures

✱ generalized seizures seizures that begin as an electrical discharge in a small area of the brain but spread to involve the entire cerebral cortex, causing widespread malfunction.

✱ partial seizures seizures that remain confined to a limited portion of the brain, causing localized malfunction. Partial seizures may spread and become generalized.

✱ tonic-clonic seizure type of generalized seizure characterized by rapid loss of consciousness and motor coordination, muscle spasms, and jerking motions.

✱ tonic phase phase of a seizure characterized by tension or contraction of muscles.

✱ clonic phase phase of a seizure characterized by alternating contraction and relaxation of muscles.

Content Review

PHASES OF A GENERALIZED SEIZURE

- Aura
- Loss of consciousness
- Tonic phase
- Hypertonic phase
- Clonic phase
- Postseizure
- Postictal

The terms *epilepsy* or *epileptic* indicate nothing more than the potential to develop seizures in circumstances that would not induce them in most individuals. Seizures can provoke a great deal of anxiety in both you and bystanders.

To assess seizures quickly under such conditions, you need to be thoroughly familiar with their various forms.

Types of Seizures

Seizures can be clinically classified as generalized or partial. **Generalized seizures** begin as an electrical discharge in a small area of the brain but spread to involve the entire cerebral cortex, causing widespread malfunction. **Partial seizures** may remain confined to a limited portion of the brain, causing localized malfunction, or may spread and become generalized.

Generalized Seizures Generalized seizures include tonic-clonic and absence seizures. Another type, pseudoseizures, may mimic generalized seizures.

- *Tonic-Clonic.* A **tonic-clonic seizure,** also known as a *grand mal seizure,* is a generalized motor seizure, producing a loss of consciousness. It typically includes a **tonic** (increased tone) **phase,** characterized by tensed, contracted muscles, and a **clonic phase,** characterized by rhythmic jerking movements of the extremities. During the seizure episode, a patient's intercostal muscles and diaphragm become temporarily paralyzed, interrupting respirations and producing cyanosis. The patient's neck, head, face, and eye muscles may also jerk. Once respirations resume, copious amounts of oral secretions (frothing) may be present. Incontinence is also common during a seizure. Agitation or confusion, drowsiness, or coma may also follow the seizure.

    Tonic-clonic seizures have a specific progression of events. It is descriptively convenient to refer to this progression as ranging from warning phase to period of recovery. However, not all seizure patients experience all of these events.
  - *Aura.* An aura is a subjective sensation preceding seizure activity. The aura may precede the attack by several hours or by only a few seconds. An aura may be of a psychic or a sensory nature, with olfactory, visual, auditory, or taste hallucinations. Some common types include hearing noise or music, seeing floating lights, smelling unpleasant odours, feeling an unpleasant sensation in the stomach, or experiencing tingling or twitching in a specific body area. Not all seizures are preceded by an aura.
  - *Loss of Consciousness.* The patient will become unconscious at some point after the aura sensations, if any.
  - *Tonic Phase.* This is a phase of continuous muscle tension, characterized by contraction of the patient's muscles.
  - *Hypertonic Phase.* The patient experiences extreme muscular rigidity, including hyperextension of the back.
  - *Clonic Phase.* The patient experiences muscle spasms marked by rhythmic movements, The patient's jaw usually remains clenched, making airway management difficult.
  - *Postseizure.* The patient remains in a coma.
  - *Postictal.* The patient may awaken confused and fatigued. She may complain of a headache and may experience some neurological deficit. In many cases, patients will be in this postictal state on the arrival of paramedic crews. There may be evidence of incontinence, which supports the likelihood that seizure activity has taken place.

- *Absence.* An **absence seizure,** also called a *petit mal seizure,* is a brief, generalized seizure that usually presents with a 10- to 30-second loss of consciousness or awareness, eye or muscle fluttering, and an occasional loss of muscle tone. Loss of consciousness may be so brief that the patient or observers may be unaware of the episode. Absence seizures are idiopathic disorders of early childhood and rarely occur after age 20. Children who suffer frequent absence seizures are often accused of day dreaming or inattentiveness. Absence seizures may not respond to normal treatment modalities.

- *Pseudoseizures.* Pseudoseizures, also called "hysterical seizures," stem from psychological disorders. The patient presents with sharp and bizarre movements that can often be interrupted with a terse command, such as "stop it!" The seizure is usually witnessed, and there will not be a postictal period. Very rarely do patients experiencing a pseudoseizure injure themselves.

Partial Seizures Partial seizures may be either simple or complex.

- *Simple Partial Seizures.* **Simple partial seizures,** also sometimes called focal motor, focal sensory, or Jacksonian seizures, are characterized by chaotic movement or dysfunction of one area of the body. When there is abnormal electrical discharge from a specific portion of the brain, only those functions served by that area will have dysfunction. Simple partial seizures involve no loss of consciousness and begin as localized tonic/clonic movements. They frequently spread and can progress to generalized tonic-clonic seizures. Therefore, it is crucial that you document how such seizures begin and the course that they subsequently take.

- *Complex Partial Seizures.* **Complex partial seizures,** sometimes called temporal lobe or psychomotor seizures, are characterized by distinctive auras. They include unusual smells, tastes, sounds, or the tendency of objects to look either very large and near or small and distant. Sometimes, a seizure patient may visualize scenes that look very familiar (*deja vu*) or very strange. A metallic taste in the mouth is a common psychomotor seizure aura. These are focal seizures, lasting approximately 1–2 minutes. The patient experiences a loss of contact with her surroundings. Additionally, the patient may act confused, stagger, perform purposeless actions, or make unintelligible sounds. She may not understand what is said. The patient may even refuse medical aid. Some patients develop automatic behaviour or show a sudden change in personality, such as abrupt explosions of rage.

* **absence seizure** type of generalized seizure with sudden onset, characterized by a brief loss of awareness and rapid recovery.

* **simple partial seizure** type of partial seizure that involves local motor, sensory, or autonomic dysfunction of one area of the body. There is no loss of consciousness.

* **complex partial seizure** type of partial seizure usually originating in the temporal lobe characterized by an aura and focal findings such as alterations in mental status or mood.

Assessment

Your initial contact with the patient and bystanders will offer a unique opportunity to obtain a history that may influence your plan of management. What an untrained observer calls a seizure may be a simple fainting spell. Therefore, you need to ascertain exactly what the patient may recall or what bystanders witnessed.

Many other problems can mimic or suggest a seizure. These include migraine headaches, cardiac dysrhythmias, hypoglycemia after exercise or drug ingestion, and the tendency to faint when rising from a supine or sitting position (orthostatic hypotension). Hyperventilation, meningitis, intracranial hemorrhage, or certain tranquilizers can cause stiffness of the extremities. Decerebrate movements, if present, may be caused by increased intracranial pressure. If you are unsure whether the patient has had a seizure, it may be more harmful than beneficial to administer an anticonvulsant medication.

A good history will be important in distinguishing a seizure from other conditions that may mimic seizure.

Syncope	Seizure
Usually begins in a standing position	May begin in any position
Patient will usually remember a warning of fainting (feeling of weakness or dizziness)	May begin without warning or may be preceded by an aura
Jerking motions usually not present	Jerking motions present during unconsciousness
Patient regains consciousness almost immediately on becoming supine	Patient remains unconscious during seizure, remains drowsy during postictal period

It is also important to try to distinguish between syncope and true seizure (Table 29-2). Syncope patients sometimes have a short initial period of seizure-like activity (usually less than one minute), but this is not followed by a postictal state. The most common cause of fainting is vasovagal syncope associated with fatigue, emotional stress, or cardiac disease. Syncope will be discussed in greater detail later in this chapter.

When obtaining a history, remember to include the following points:

- History of seizures. These data should include length of any past seizure; whether it was generalized or focal; and presence of auras, incontinence, or trauma to the tongue.
- Recent history of head trauma.
- Any alcohol and/or drug abuse.
- Recent history of fever, headache, or stiff neck.
- History of diabetes, heart disease, or stroke.
- Current medications. Most chronic seizure patients take anticonvulsant medication on a regular basis. Common anticonvulsant medications include phenytoin (Dilantin), phenobarbital, carbamazepine (Tegretol), and valproic acid (Depakene).

The secondary assessment of the seizure patient should include the following steps:

- Note any signs of head trauma or injury to the tongue.
- Note any evidence of alcohol and/or drug abuse.
- Document dysrhythmias.

Management

The prime concerns in seizure management are control of the airway and prevention of injury.

Remember that seizures tend to provoke anxiety in patients, families, and paramedics. From a medical standpoint, however, most of these situations only require managing the airway and preventing the patient from injuring herself. Because the patient may become hypo- or hyperthermic if exposed, protecting body temperature is also crucial. Field management of the seizure patient generally includes the following procedures:

- Ensure scene safety.
- Maintain the airway. Do not force objects between the patient's teeth—this includes padded tongue blades. Pushing objects into the patient's mouth may cause vomiting or aspiration. It can also cause laryngospasm.
- Administer high-flow oxygen.
- Establish intravenous access. Initiate normal saline or Ringer's Lactate solution at a to-keep-open rate.

- Determine the blood glucose level. If the patient is hypoglycemic, administer 50-percent dextrose or glucagon.
- Never attempt to restrain the patient. This may injure her. However, protect the patient from hitting objects close by (Figure 29-9). Note: If there is evidence of head trauma, C-spine immobilization must be considered as in any other head injury.
- Maintain body temperature.
- Position the patient on her left side after the clonic-tonic phase (Figure 29-10).
- Suction if required.
- Monitor cardiac rhythm.
- If seizure is prolonged (> 5 minutes), consider an anticonvulsant, such as diazepam.
- Provide a quiet, reassuring atmosphere.
- Transport the patient in the supine or lateral recumbent position.

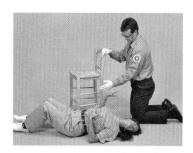

FIGURE 29-9   Protection of a seizing patient.

Status Epilepticus

Status epilepticus is a series of two or more generalized motor seizures without an intervening return of consciousness. The most common cause in adults is failure to take prescribed anticonvulsant medications. Status epilepticus is a major emergency, since it involves a prolonged period of apnea, which, in turn, can cause hypoxia of vital brain tissues. These seizures may result in respiratory arrest, severe metabolic and respiratory acidosis, extreme hypertension, increased intracranial pressure, serious elevations in body temperature, fractures of the long bones and spine, necrosis of the cardiac muscle, and severe dehydration.

The most valuable intervention is to protect the patient from airway obstruction and deliver 100-percent oxygen. Preferably this should be accomplished by bag-valve-mask assistance, since the normal ventilatory mechanisms of the patient are seriously impaired and air exchange is generally ineffective. Once the airway is maintained and ventilations are being assisted, take the following steps:

- Start an IV of normal saline at a to-keep-open rate.
- Monitor cardiac rhythm.
- Administer 25 g of 50-percent dextrose IV push, or glucagon if hypoglycemia is present.

✱ **status epilepticus** series of two or more generalized motor seizures without any intervening periods of consciousness.

Status epilepticus—two or more generalized motor seizures with no intervening return of consciousness—is a life-threatening emergency.

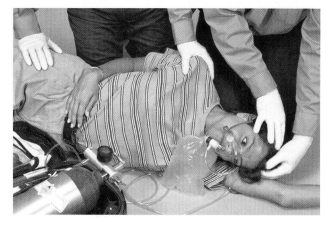

FIGURE 29-10   Place a seizing patient with no suspected spine injury on her left side.

- Administer 5–10 mg diazepam IV push for an adult. Diazepam is a sedative and anticonvulsant that depresses the spread of seizure activity across the motor cortex of the brain. (Follow local ACP/CCP protocols.)
- Continue to monitor the airway. Some patients may require large doses of diazepam.

SYNCOPE

* syncope transient loss of consciousness due to inadequate flow of blood to the brain with rapid recovery of consciousness on becoming supine; fainting.

As discussed earlier, **syncope** (fainting) is a neurological condition characterized by the sudden, temporary loss of consciousness caused by insufficient blood flow to the brain, with recovery of consciousness almost immediately on becoming supine. Nearly half of all Canadians will experience at least one episode of syncope during their lifetime.

Assessment

Focus on what caused the patient to faint, or lose consciousness. The causes of syncope can be classified into these three general categories:

- *Cardiovascular* conditions, such as dysrhythmias or mechanical problems—A heart rate that is too fast or too slow, or an abnormally functioning heart valve may trigger hypoxia in the brain and subsequent fainting.
- *Noncardiovascular* disease, such as metabolic, neurological, or psychiatric conditions—Hypoglycemia, a transient ischemic attack, or an anxiety attack can all be causes of syncope.
- *Idiopathic,* or unknown, cause—Often, the cause of a patient's syncope remains unknown despite careful assessment and diagnostic tests.

*Syncope involves rapid recovery of consciousness. If a patient does not regain consciousness within a few moments, it is **not** syncope, but something more serious.*

Syncope can occur in all ages from the very young to the very old. Symptoms may include feeling faint, dizziness, lightheadedness, or a loss of consciousness without warning. Keep in mind, however, that the definition of syncope includes rapid recovery of consciousness (usually less than a minute). If a patient does not spontaneously regain consciousness within a few moments, it is *not* syncope—it is something more serious.

Management

When caring for someone who has fainted, it is important to attempt to identify the underlying cause and treat it. If no cause can be identified, anyone who loses consciousness should be transported to an appropriate emergency department and evaluated. Field management of the syncopal patient generally includes the following procedures:

- Ensure scene safety.
- Establish and maintain an adequate airway.
- Administer high-flow oxygen and assist ventilations when required.
- Check circulatory status (heart rate, blood pressure, cardiac rhythm).
- Check and continuously monitor mental status.
- Start an IV of normal saline or Ringer's Lactate at a to-keep-open rate.
- Determine the blood glucose level.
- Monitor the cardiac rhythm.

- Reassure the patient.
- Transport the patient to an emergency department.

HEADACHE

Headache can seriously disrupt a person's life. Nearly three million Canadian suffer migraine headaches. Women tend to develop migraines more than men (3:1).

Headache pain can be acute (sudden onset) or chronic (constant or recurring), generalized (all over) or localized (in one specific area) and can range from mild to severe. In some cases, the cause is known. In others, it is not. The most common types of headache can be classified into three categories:

- *Vascular.* Vascular headaches include migraines and cluster headaches. *Migraines* can last from several minutes to several days. They can be characterized by an intense or throbbing pain, photosensitivity (sensitivity to light), nausea, vomiting, and sweats. Migraines are frequently unilateral (on one side of the head) and may be preceded by an aura. *Cluster* headaches usually occur as a series of one-sided headaches that are sudden, intense, and may continue for 15 minutes to four hours. Symptoms may include nasal congestion, drooping eyelid, and an irritated or watery eye. Migraines occur more commonly in women, while cluster headaches generally occur in men.
- *Tension.* A significant percentage of headaches are tension headaches. Most personnel in the emergency medical field have, at one time or another, suffered from a tension headache. Sometimes, such headaches occur on a daily basis. Sufferers often awake in the morning with a mild headache that gets worse during the course of the day. The tension headache produces a dull, achy pain that feels like a forceful pressure is being applied to the neck and/or head.
- *Organic.* A third, less common category includes organically caused headaches. They occur in individuals suffering from tumours, infection, or other diseases of the brain, eye, or other body system.

A continuous throbbing headache (often predominantly over the occiput) with fever, confusion, and nuchal rigidity (stiffness of the neck) are classic signs and symptoms of *meningitis*. Be alert for these features while assessing patients complaining of headache, particularly those who have also been complaining of nausea, vomiting, or rash. Chapter 6 provides further discussion on meningitis and other infectious diseases.

Assessment

In addition to pain, those suffering from a headache of any type may also complain of nausea, vomiting, blurred vision, dizziness, weakness, or watery eyes. A complete and thorough history of the patient's headache is crucial to its treatment. Determine as much as you can about the pain:

- What was the patient doing during the onset of pain?
- Does anything provoke, or worsen, the pain (light, sound, or movement)?
- What is the quality of the pain? (Is it throbbing? Crushing? Tension?)
- Does the pain radiate to the neck, arm, back, or jaw?
- What is the severity of the pain? (On a scale of 1–10, how does the patient rate the pain?)
- How long has the headache been present? (acute versus chronic)

> *When assessing a patient complaining of headache, ascertain any associated signs and symptoms, such as nausea, vomiting, blurred vision, dizziness, weakness, or watery eyes.*
>
>

Headache of acute onset or of a changing pattern demands immediate attention. A sudden onset of pain, description of the pain as "the worst headache in my life," or changes in the pattern of pain should all be considered characteristics of potential serious conditions, such as intracranial hemorrhage.

Management

Treatment for a victim of headache is supportive. Field management of the headache patient generally includes the following:

- Ensure scene safety.
- Establish and maintain an adequate airway.
- Place the patient in a position of comfort. Patients will often place themselves in a position that best alleviates the symptoms, such as lying flat in a dark room.
- Administer high-flow oxygen, and assist ventilations when required.
- Start an IV of normal saline or Ringer's Lactate at a keep-open rate.
- Determine the blood glucose level.
- Monitor the cardiac rhythm.
- Reassure the patient.
- Ensure a calm, quiet environment. Dimming the interior ambulance lights will provide comfort to the headache patient with photosensitivity.
- Transport the patient to an emergency department.

"WEAK AND DIZZY"

A frequent problem that paramedics encounter is the patient who is "weak and dizzy" or "weak all over." Generalized weakness and dizziness, although vague, can be symptoms of many diseases. Furthermore, the feeling of being weak or the feeling of being dizzy can be quite disconcerting, especially to the elderly.

Assessment

Obtain a more detailed history of the illness. Has the patient ever had symptoms like this before? Has she had vomiting and/or diarrhea? Has there been a change in medication regimen recently? Has she taken a new medication in the last 72 hours?

Patients with weakness and/or dizziness should receive a focused assessment, including a neurological examination. Be alert for the presence of nystagmus (a constant, involuntary, cyclical motion of the eyeball), which can indicate a CNS or inner ear problem. Assess the various muscle groups to determine whether the weakness reported by the patient is localized or diffuse. Be alert for potential causes. These can be neurological, respiratory, cardiovascular, endocrinological, or infectious. Many viral illnesses will cause a feeling of malaise in the early stages. Inner ear infections (labyrinthitis) often will cause dizziness, especially with sudden movements of the head. Mild volume depletion (dehydration) can cause both weakness and dizziness. Sometimes, the dizzy patient will become nauseated or may actually vomit.

Management

While assessing the patient, provide supportive care. This includes the following:

- Ensure scene safety.
- Establish and maintain an adequate airway.

- Place the patient in a position of comfort, generally with the head elevated. Avoid sudden or exaggerated movement of the head as it can exacerbate symptoms.
- Administer high-flow oxygen.
- Start an IV of normal saline or Ringer's Lactate at a to-keep-open rate. Consider a fluid bolus if the patient appears dehydrated.
- Check the blood glucose level.
- Monitor the cardiac rhythm.
- Ensure a calm, quiet environment.
- Reassure the patient.
- Transport the patient to an emergency department.

NEOPLASMS

Brain and spinal cord tumours are abnormal growths of tissue found inside the skull or the bony spinal column. The term **neoplasm** is used to describe the new growth of a tumour (as contrasted with those present at birth, known as congenital tumours). Neoplasms that affect the CNS have a mortality rate of 188 per 100 000 in Canada per year.

✱ **neoplasm** literally meaning "new form"; a new or abnormal formation; a tumour.

Neurological neoplasms can be divided into two main categories. *Benign* (noncancerous) *tumours* are those comprising cells that grow similarly to normal cells, grow relatively slowly, and are confined to one location. *Malignant* (cancerous) *tumours* are those with growth very different from that of normal cells. They grow quickly and spread easily to other sites within the body.

Benign neoplasms in most parts of the body are not particularly harmful. Such tumours within the brain or spinal cord, however, pose a greater threat. Because the nervous system is contained within the rigid confines of the skull and spinal column, abnormal growth can place pressure on tissues and impair function. Any tumour located near any of the vital structures of the brain may seriously threaten the ability to breathe, move, or regulate other bodily functions.

Malignant tumours in most parts of the body have a tendency to spread, or *metastasize*. Most brain tumours are metastases from cancers that started somewhere else in the body. For example, breast cancers often metastasize to the brain. These metastases can grow in a single area of the brain or in several areas. However, tumours that originate in the brain or spinal cord rarely spread to other sites in the body. There are numerous types of brain tumours, which must be diagnosed in a medical facility with CT or MRI scan. The causes of most tumours—and most cancers—remain incompletely known.

Assessment

Central nervous system neoplasms present with many signs and symptoms. The clinical manifestations a patient exhibits will depend on the size, type, and the location of the tumour. As a paramedic, it is not your role to diagnose such new tumours. Instead, you will likely be called to care for someone with a previously diagnosed tumour. Or perhaps you will be asked to assess a patient with one or more of these common signs and symptoms of a neoplasm:

- Headache (often severe and recurring frequently)
- New seizures in an adult with no history of a seizure disorder
- Nausea
- Vomiting
- Behavioural or cognitive changes
- Weakness or paralysis of one or more limbs or a side of the face

- Change in sensation of one or more limbs or a side of the face
- Lack of coordination
- Difficulty walking or unsteady gait
- Dizziness
- Double vision

Be alert for any of the classic signs and symptoms of a brain or spinal cord tumour. Obtain a thorough medical history. In addition to the SAMPLE questions, ask the following:

- What is the state of the patient's general health?
- Has the patient had any seizure activity, headache, or nosebleed?

Ask about the type and timing of prior treatment:

- Surgery for removal of a tumour
- Chemotherapy
- Radiation therapy
- Holistic therapy
- Experimental treatments

Management

Treatment of a patient with a neoplasm is primarily supportive.

Treatment of a patient with a neoplasm is primarily supportive. You should attempt to alleviate the patient's anxiety and to reduce her symptoms. Field management of the patient with a neoplasm generally includes the following:

- Ensure scene safety.
- Establish and maintain an adequate airway.
- Place the patient in a position of comfort, generally with head elevated.
- Administer high-flow oxygen, and assist ventilations when required.
- Start an IV of normal saline or Ringer's Lactate at a to-keep-open rate or a saline or heparin lock.
- Monitor the cardiac rhythm.
- Consider narcotic analgesia if medical direction approves.
- Consider diazepam if seizure activity is present.
- Ensure a calm, quiet environment.
- Reassure the patient.
- Transport the patient to an emergency department.

BRAIN ABSCESS

brain abscess a collection of pus localized in an area of the brain.

A **brain abscess** is a collection of pus localized in an area of the brain. Brain abscesses are uncommon, accounting for 2 percent of all intracranial masses. Signs and symptoms are similar to those of a neoplasm and include headache, lethargy, hemiparesis, seizures, nuchal rigidity, nausea, and vomiting. Frequently, there is also fever. Paramedic management of a patient with an abscess is supportive and similar to that for a neoplasm or meningitis.

DEGENERATIVE NEUROLOGICAL DISORDERS

degenerative neurological disorders a collection of diseases that selectively affect one or more functional systems of the CNS.

A collection of diseases that selectively affect one or more functional systems of the CNS are known as **degenerative neurological disorders.** They generally produce symmetrical and progressive involvement of the CNS, affect similar areas of the brain, and produce similar clinical signs and symptoms.

Types of Degenerative Neurological Disorders

Alzheimer's Disease Alzheimer's disease is perhaps the most important of all the degenerative neurological disorders because of its frequent occurrence and devastating nature. It is the most common cause of dementia in the elderly. Alzheimer's disease results from death and disappearance of nerve cells in the cerebral cortex. This causes marked atrophy of the brain. Initially, patients will have problems with short-term memory. This will usually progress to problems with thought and intellect. The patient will develop a shuffling gait and will have stiffness of the body muscles. As the disease progresses, the patient will develop aphasia (inability to speak) and psychiatric disturbances. In the final stages, the patient may become nearly decorticate, losing all ability to think, speak, and move.

✳ Alzheimer's disease a degenerative brain disorder; the most common cause of dementia in the elderly.

Muscular Dystrophy Muscular dystrophy (MD) refers to a group of genetic diseases characterized by progressive muscle weakness and degeneration of the skeletal or voluntary muscle fibres. The heart and other involuntary muscles are affected in some types of MD. There are several forms of MD, the most common of which is Duchenne. Some forms begin in childhood, while others do not appear until middle age. The prognosis of MD varies depending on the type and progression of the disorder.

✳ muscular dystrophy a group of genetic diseases characterized by progressive muscle weakness and degeneration of the skeletal or voluntary muscle fibres.

Multiple Sclerosis Multiple sclerosis (MS) refers to an unpredictable disease of the CNS. MS involves inflammation of certain nerve cells followed by demyelination, or the destruction of the myelin sheath, which is the fatty insulation surrounding nerve fibres of the brain and spinal cord. When the myelin sheath is damaged, the nerves are unable to properly conduct impulses. An estimated 50 000 Canadians are presently diagnosed with multiple sclerosis (MS). Every day, three people in Canada are diagnosed with MS. Canada has one of the highest rates of multiple sclerosis in the world, and MS is the most common neurological disease affecting young adults in Canada. Most MS sufferers are women and first experience symptoms between the ages of 20 and 40.

✳ multiple sclerosis disease that involves inflammation of certain nerve cells followed by demyelination, or the destruction of the myelin sheath, which is the fatty insulation surrounding nerve fibres.

The disease is known to involve an autoimmune on myelin. Signs and symptoms include weakness of one or more limbs, sensory loss, paresthesias, and changes in vision. Symptoms can wax and wane over years and range from mild to severe. Severe cases can be debilitating, rendering a patient unable to care for herself.

Dystonias The **dystonias** are a group of disorders characterized by muscle contractions that cause twisting and repetitive movements, abnormal postures, or freezing in the middle of an action. Such movements are involuntary and sometimes painful. They may affect a single muscle, a group of muscles, or the entire body.

✳ dystonias a group of disorders characterized by muscle contractions that cause twisting and repetitive movements, abnormal postures, or freezing in the middle of an action.

Early symptoms of dystonia include a deterioration in handwriting, foot cramps, or a tendency of one foot to drag after walking or running. These initial symptoms can be mild and may be noticeable only after prolonged exertion, stress, or fatigue. In many cases, they become more noticeable and widespread over time. In other individuals, there is little or no progression.

Parkinson's Disease **Parkinson's disease** belongs to a group of conditions known as motor system disorders. James Parkinson, a British physician who published a paper on what he called "the shaking palsy," first described the disease in 1817. In his paper, Parkinson described the major symptoms of the disease that would later bear his name. Since then, scientists have been searching diligently for a cause and subsequent cure.

✳ Parkinson's disease chronic and progressive motor system disorder characterized by tremor, rigidity, bradykinesia, and postural instability.

In the 1960s, researchers identified that a naturally occurring chemical crucial to muscle activity, dopamine, is lower in people affected by Parkinson's disease. This discovery led to the first successful treatment for the disease.

It is estimated that approximately 100 000 Canadians have Parkinson's disease. Symptoms generally appear around age 60, although it can present in much younger people as well. The number of cases increases with age. Parkinson's disease affects 1 percent of the population over age 65 and increases to 2 percent in the population aged 70 and older. Parkinson's disease affects men and women in almost equal numbers, and it knows no social, economic, or geographic boundaries. The average age of onset is 60 years, and it usually does not occur in patients less than 40 years old.

Parkinson's disease is a chronic and progressive disorder. It has four main characteristics:

- *Tremor.* Sometimes called "pill rolling," the typical tremor is a rhythmic back-and-forth motion of the thumb and forefinger. It usually begins in the hand and may progress to an arm, a foot, or the jaw.
- *Rigidity.* Most Parkinson's patients suffer rigidity, or resistance to movement. All muscles have an opposing muscle. In the healthy adult, one muscle contracts, while the opposing muscle relaxes. In Parkinson's disease, the balance of this opposition is disturbed, leading to rigidity.
- *Bradykinesia.* Normal, spontaneous, or autonomic movement is slowed and sometimes lost. Such loss of movement is unpredictable. While one moment the patient can move easily, the next moment she cannot.
- *Postural Instability.* Impaired balance and coordination cause patients to develop a forward or backward lean, stooped posture, and the tendency to fall easily.

Victims of Parkinson's disease may also be plagued with depression, a slowing or "shuffling" gait, a stiff or "stone-like" face, and dementia.

central pain syndrome condition resulting from damage or injury to the brain, brainstem, or spinal cord characterized by intense, steady pain described as burning, aching, tingling, or a "pins and needles" sensation.

Central Pain Syndrome **Central pain syndrome** is a condition that results from damage or injury to the brain, brainstem, or spinal cord. It is characterized by intense, steady pain described as burning, aching, tingling, or a "pins and needles" sensation. The syndrome may develop weeks, months, or years after an injury to the CNS. It occurs in patients who have had strokes, multiple sclerosis, limb amputations, or spinal cord injuries. Pain medications generally provide no relief for victims of central pain syndrome. Patients rely on sedation and other methods to keep the CNS free from stress.

One type of chronic pain is known as trigeminal neuralgia, or *tic douloureux.* It is caused by abnormal electrical conduction along the trigeminal nerve (cranial nerve V). The condition is characterized by episodes of facial pain that are brief, yet intense. The fear of such an episode is often debilitating. Patients are treated with such medications as the anticonvulsant carbamazepine (Tegretol). In select cases, surgical interventions may be used.

Bell's palsy one-sided facial paralysis with an unknown cause characterized by the inability to close the eye, pain, tearing of the eyes, drooling, hypersensitivity to sound, and impairment of taste.

Bell's Palsy **Bell's palsy** is the most common form of facial paralysis. It results from inflammatory reaction of the facial nerve (cranial nerve VII). The condition affects roughly 6000 Canadians every year. It is characterized by one-sided facial paralysis, the inability to close the eye, pain, tearing of the eyes, drooling, hypersensitivity to sound, and impairment of taste.

Although the specific cause is often unknown, some causes have been identified. They are head trauma, herpes simplex virus, and Lyme disease. Treatment is usually aimed at protecting the eye. Corticosteroids may be prescribed for inflammation when pain is severe. Most patients recover within three months.

Amyotrophic Lateral Sclerosis Amyotrophic lateral sclerosis (ALS), also known as Lou Gehrig's disease, is a progressive degeneration of specific nerve cells that control voluntary movement. Characterized by weakness, loss of motor control, difficulty speaking, and cramping, the disease eventually weakens the diaphragm, which leads to breathing problems. ALS belongs to a class of disorders known as motor neuron diseases. ALS affects 1500 to 2000 Canadians, with two to three deaths a day due to it.

There is currently no cure for ALS. There is also no effective therapy. However, the U.S. Food and Drug Administration (FDA) has approved riluzole, the first drug that has been shown to prolong the lives of ALS patients. The prognosis continues to be poor. Most patients die within three to five years of being diagnosed, usually as a result of pulmonary infection.

Myoclonus Myoclonus is a term that refers to the temporary, involuntary twitching or spasm of a muscle or group of muscles. It is generally considered not a diagnosis but a symptom. It is usually one of several symptoms of a variety of nervous system disorders, such as multiple sclerosis, Parkinson's disease, or Alzheimer's disease. Some simple examples of myoclonus include hiccups or muscle twitching. Pathological myoclonus can distort normal movement and limit a person's ability to eat, walk, and talk.

Treatment of myoclonus consists of medications to reduce symptoms. Many of these drugs are also used to treat epilepsy, such as barbiturates, clonazepam, phenytoin, and sodium valproate.

Spina Bifida Spina bifida (SB) is a neural defect that results from the failure of one or more of the fetal vertebrae to close properly during gestation. This leaves a portion of the spinal cord unprotected. The spinal opening can usually be repaired shortly after birth, but the nerve damage is permanent. Long-term effects include physical and mobility impairments, and most individuals also have some form of learning disability. The three most common types of SB are as follows:

- *Myelomeningocele*—the severest form and one in which the spinal cord and the meninges protrude from an opening in the spine.
- *Meningocele*—characterized by the normal development of the spinal cord, but the meninges protrude through a spinal opening.
- *Occulta*—the mildest form and one in which one or more vertebrae are malformed and covered by a layer of skin.

There is presently no cure for SB. Treatment includes surgery, medications, and physiotherapy. With proper care, many children with SB live into adulthood.

Poliomyelitis Poliomyelitis (polio) is an infectious, inflammatory viral disease of the CNS that sometimes results in permanent paralysis. It is characterized by fatigue, headache, fever, vomiting, stiffness of the neck, and pain in the hands and feet. New cases in North America are rare. A vaccine developed in the 1950s caused the number of cases to decline from 50 000 to only a few per year. Thousands of prevaccine survivors of the disease are alive today. Many of these require supportive care.

Assessment of Degenerative Neurological Disorders

When you encounter a patient with a degenerative neurological disorder, use your assessment and history-taking skills to determine the patient's chief complaint. You may be called to treat someone with an exacerbation (flare-up) of one of the degenerative diseases or someone with an unrelated complaint. In either case, it is important to conduct a primary assessment, correct any life-threatening problems, and find out exactly what prompted the call to EMS.

* **amyotrophic lateral sclerosis (ALS)** progressive degeneration of specific nerve cells that control voluntary movement characterized by weakness, loss of motor control, difficulty speaking, and cramping. Also called *Lou Gehrig's disease*.

* **myoclonus** temporary, involuntary twitching or spasm of a muscle or group of muscles.

* **spina bifida (SB)** a neural defect that results from the failure of one or more of the fetal vertebrae to close properly during the first month of gestation.

* **poliomyelitis (polio)** infectious, inflammatory viral disease of the central nervous system that sometimes results in permanent paralysis.

Management of Degenerative Neurological Disorders

When caring for a patient with a degenerative neurological disease, make treating the chief complaint a priority. Do not overlook the patient's underlying condition, but do not allow it to cloud a more serious problem. After performing a primary assessment and managing any life-threatening conditions, manage the chief complaint. While providing care, consider the following about patients who suffer from a degenerative neurological disorder:

- *Mobility.* The ability to walk and move about freely is often taken for granted by many of us. Patients with neurological problems often lack this ability and require assistance.
- *Communication.* Certain neurological disorders will affect a patient's ability to speak clearly and distinctly. Take the necessary time to ensure open communication. Speak with bystanders and family members to assist in gaining a thorough history.
- *Respiratory Compromise.* Exacerbations of ALS and other conditions may affect the patient's ability to breathe. Treat any breathing problem as a priority.
- *Anxiety.* Coping with a debilitating disease is a strenuous and taxing task. Ongoing battles with a neurological condition will cause stress—and anxiety. Approach the patient and her family with compassion and care.

The following steps may be appropriate, depending on the patient's chief complaint:

- Determine the blood glucose level. A serum glucose determination will assist in determining if an altered mental status is due to hypoglycemia.
- Establish an IV of normal saline or Ringer's Lactate at a to-keep-open rate.
- Monitor the cardiac rhythm.
- Transport the patient to an emergency department.

BACK PAIN AND NONTRAUMATIC SPINAL DISORDERS

Back pain is one of the most common reasons people seek health care. Millions and millions of health-care dollars are spent each year on the treatment of back pain. Back pain can be classified as either traumatic or nontraumatic in origin. Many people develop chronic back pain, which is a significant cause of disability and lost time from work. EMS is occasionally called to treat persons with back pain. These calls can be due to a new injury or exacerbation of chronic back pain. In addition, some patients develop back pain without any identifiable injury.

Low Back Pain

Back pain can be felt anywhere along the spinal column. However, low back pain (LBP) is the most common back-pain complaint. It is a common, yet debilitating condition. Low back pain is defined as back pain felt between the lower rib cage and the gluteal muscles, often radiating to the thighs.

Both chronic and new-onset low back pain are increasingly common. Low back pain is the cause of great amount of lost work time in Canada. Between 60 and 90 percent of the population experience some form of low back pain at some time in their lives. Men and women are equally affected, although women over 60 years of age report symptoms of low back pain more often, most likely as a result of postmenopausal osteoporosis. Occupations that involve exposure to vibrations from vehicles or machinery and those that require repetitive lifting are often implicated in low back pain. As a paramedic, you are also particularly at risk for back problems.

About 1 percent of acute low back pain results from sciatica, which causes severe pain along the path of the sciatic nerve, down the back of the thigh and inner leg. This is sometimes accompanied by motor and sensory deficits, such as muscle weakness. Sciatica may be caused by compression or trauma to the sciatic nerve or its roots, often resulting from a herniated intervertebral disc or osteoarthrosis of the lumbosacral vertebrae. It may also be caused by inflammation of the sciatic nerve from metabolic, toxic, or infectious causes.

Pain occurring at the level of L-3, L-4, L-5, and S-1 may be due to inflammation of the interspinous bursae. Low back pain may also result from inflammation, sprains, or strains of the muscles and ligaments that attach to the spine or from vertebral fractures. Additional causes of back pain include tumours, inflammation of the synovial sacs, rising venous pressure, degenerative joint disease, abnormal bone pressure, problems with spinal mobility, and inflammation caused by infection (osteomyelitis).

In fact, most low back pain is idiopathic. That is, the cause may be difficult or impossible to diagnose, even by a physician or in a hospital setting. This makes treatment of many cases of low back pain frustrating and sometimes unsuccessful.

Causes of Nontraumatic Spinal Disorders and Back Pain

Spinal problems may be caused by trauma, but many spinal disorders have nontraumatic causes. Nontraumatic spinal injuries most often result from three causes:

- Degeneration or rupture of the discs that separate the vertebrae
- Degeneration or fracture of the vertebrae
- Cyst or tumour that impinges on the spine

The type and degree of pain that results from these conditions differs from person to person.

Disc Injury The cartilaginous discs that separate the vertebrae may rupture as a result of injury or may rupture or degenerate as part of the process of aging. Degeneration may cause a narrowing of the disc that compromises spinal stability. Degenerative disc disease is more common in patients over 50 years of age.

A herniated disc occurs when the gelatinous centre of the disc (the *nucleus pulposa*) extrudes through a tear in the tough outer capsule (the *anulus fibrosa*). The pain that results from these conditions usually results from pressure on the spinal cord or muscle spasm at the site. The intervetebral discs themselves have no innervation. Herniation may be caused by degenerative disc disease, by trauma, or by improper lifting. Improper lifting is the most common cause. Men aged 30 to 50 years are more prone to disc herniation than are women. Herniation most commonly affects the discs at L-4, L-5, and S-1 but may also occur in C-5, C-6, and C-7.

Vertebral Injury The vertebrae themselves may break down (vertebral spondylolysis), especially the lamina or vertebral arch between the articulating facets (the areas where adjoining vertebrae come in contact with one another). Heredity is thought to be a significant factor in the development of spondylolysis. Rotational fractures are common at these sites. Spinal fractures are frequently associated with osteoporosis (brittle bones), which tends to develop in many elderly persons.

Cysts and Tumours A cyst or tumour along the spine or intruding into the spinal canal may cause pain by pressing on the spinal cord, by causing degenerative changes in the bone, or by interrupting blood supply. The specific manifestations depend on the location and the type of the cyst or tumour.

Other Medical Causes Back pain can also be caused by medical conditions associated with neither traumatic nor nontraumatic spinal injury. For example, back pain may manifest as referred pain from such disorders as diabetic neuropathy, renal calculus, abdominal aortic aneurysm, and many other conditions discussed in this chapter. It would be a mistake to assume that all back complaints are related to the spinal cord, the vertebrae, the intervetebral discs, or the muscles and ligaments surrounding the vertebrae.

Assessment

Assessment of back pain is based on the patient's chief complaint, the history, and the secondary assessment. When the complaint is low back pain, a precise diagnosis is likely to be difficult. Preliminary diagnosis may be based on a history of risk factors, such as an occupation requiring repetitive lifting, exposure to vibrations from vehicles or industrial machinery, or a known history of osteoporosis.

The complaint of low back pain often involves radiation of the pain from the gluteus to the thigh, leg, and foot. Usually, there is history of slow onset over several weeks to months and the patient has called for your help secondary to an increase in pain and the lack of relief from warm compresses or over-the-counter analgesics. The patient may or may not recall a particular incident that has caused this "low back pain"; direct trauma is very rarely a contributing factor in this type of pain.

Just because low back pain is a common complaint that can be hard to diagnose, do not dismiss this type of complaint as "not real pain." A complete history and secondary assessment by a physician are necessary to determine the cause of any back pain. Diagnosis will often depend on the results of a CT or MRI scan, electromyelography (EMG), or other in-hospital testing.

In the prehospital setting, the important task is to determine if the patient's pain is caused by a life-threatening or a non-life-threatening condition. A good patient history will help in this determination. A history of work or play involving lifting or twisting and a sudden onset of pain, often associated with straining, coughing, or sneezing, may point to a mechanical type of muscle or ligament injury. A gradual onset of pain may point instead to a chronic condition, such as degenerative disc disease or tumour development. The presence of associated neurological deficits may also point to a more serious underlying cause. When the complaint is back pain, be sure to inquire about prior back surgery, physical therapy, and time lost from work.

Location of the injury may be revealed by a limited range of motion in the lumbar spine, tenderness on palpation at the location of the injury, alterations in sensation, pain, and temperature at the site, pain or paresthesia below the injury (in the upper extremities with cervical injury, symptoms increasing with neck motion, with possible slight motor weakness in the biceps and triceps; similar symptoms in the lower extremities with injury to the thoracic or lumbar spine).

Keep in mind that you are very unlikely to be able to determine the cause of your patient's back pain in the field. Primarily, you need to gather information from the history and secondary assessment that you will report to the receiving physician and that will help you determine what degree of immobilization, if any, will be necessary during transport.

Management

Prehospital management of back pain is primarily aimed at decreasing any pain or discomfort caused by moving the patient and keeping a watchful eye for signs and symptoms of any serious underlying disorder.

Should cervical spine (C-spine) precautions be taken with the patient complaining of back pain? Should this patient be immobilized to a long back board or a vacuum-type stretcher? These questions are best answered: "It depends." First, you must consider trauma as a possible cause of the patient's pain. If there is no recent mechanism of injury, consider whether the patient has a possible history of osteoporosis or another disease that might lead to spinal fracture. In these cases, consider immobilizing the patient.

If trauma and possible fracture are ruled out, you may still undertake C-spine precautions and immobilization because the less movement a patient is put through, the more comfortable she will feel. Long-board or vacuum-stretcher immobilization may be the best mode of transport. If in doubt, immobilize, remembering the injunction to "do no harm."

Some patients with back pain and back spasms may require parenteral analgesics and parenteral diazepam before they can even lie on the stretcher. Contact medical direction regarding analgesic and muscle relaxant therapy.

Conduct ongoing assessment en route, with special attention to the airway, breathing, vital signs, and possible presence or development of motor and sensory deficits that may indicate a critical condition and that can adversely affect the patient's breathing effort.

Prehospital management of back pain is primarily aimed at decreasing pain and discomfort. Follow local protocols regarding immobilization of a patient with back pain.

$\int$UMMARY

Nervous system emergencies include a complex variety of illnesses and injuries. A thorough patient assessment and medical history will help guide your care and will prove invaluable for subsequent hospital management.

Primary field management is directed at ensuring an adequate airway and ventilation. The brain requires a constant supply of oxygen, glucose, and vitamins. After 10–20 seconds without blood flow, the patient becomes unconscious. Significant loss of oxygen (anoxia) or low blood sugar (hypoglycemia) can cause coma or seizures. Supply high-flow oxygen to patients with neurological disorders. Treat any neurological patient with hypoglycemia within your PCP/ACP or CCP scope of practice.

Neurological injuries and illnesses often require treatment as soon as possible to prevent progressive damage. Patients suffering an altered level of consciousness, stroke (brain attack), transient ischemic attack, seizures, or syncope require early intervention and transport to the closest appropriate facility.

You will also be called to care for patients suffering from headaches, neoplasms, degenerative neurological disorders, or back pain. These conditions may be relatively minor or indicative of a much more serious underlying condition. They, too, require a complete patient assessment, medical history, and supportive care.

Care for the neurological patient may simply be supportive. In other cases, you should provide drug therapy or other interventions to limit or reduce the presenting symptoms. Airway management remains a priority in caring for any patient with an alteration in neurological function.

CHAPTER 30

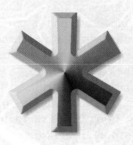

Endocrinology

Objectives

After reading this chapter, you should be able to:

1. Describe the incidence, morbidity, and mortality of endocrinological emergencies. (pp. 608–609, 611–612, 616–617)
2. Identify the risk factors that predispose a person to endocrinological disease. (pp. 611, 616–617, 619, 620)
3. Discuss the anatomy and physiology of the endocrine system. (see Chapter 12)
4. Discuss the pathophysiology, assessment findings, need for rapid intervention and transport, and management of endocrinological emergencies. (pp. 608–620)
5. Describe osmotic diuresis and its relationship to diabetes mellitus. (p. 611)
6. Describe the pathophysiology of adult- and juvenile-onset diabetes mellitus. (pp. 611–612)
7. Differentiate between normal glucose metabolism and diabetic glucose metabolism. (pp. 609–611)
8. Describe the mechanism of ketone body formation and its relationship to ketoacidosis. (pp. 610, 612–614)

Continued

Objectives Continued

9. Discuss the physiology of the excretion of potassium and ketone bodies by the kidneys. (pp. 610–611)
10. Describe the relationship of insulin to serum glucose levels. (pp. 608–616)
11. Describe the effects of decreased levels of insulin on the body. (pp. 611–615)
12. Describe the effects of increased serum glucose levels on the body. (pp. 615–616)
13. Discuss the pathophysiology, assessment findings, and management of the following endocrinological emergencies:
    a. Nonketotic hyperosmolar coma (pp. 612–613, 614–615)
    b. Diabetic ketoacidosis (pp. 612–614)
    c. Hypoglycemia (pp. 615–616)
    d. Hyperglycemia (pp. 614–615)
    e. Thyrotoxicosis (pp. 616–617)

f. Myxedema (pp. 618–619)
g. Cushing's syndrome (pp. 619–620)
h. Adrenal insufficiency, or Addison's disease (p. 620)

14. Describe the actions of epinephrine as it relates to the pathophysiology of hypoglycemia. (p. 615)
15. Describe the compensatory mechanisms utilized by the body to promote homeostasis when hypoglycemia is present. (pp. 608, 615)
16. Differentiate among different endocrine emergencies on the basis of assessment and history. (pp. 608–620)
17. Given several scenarios involving endocrinological emergency patients, provide the appropriate assessment, management, and transport. (pp. 608–620)

INTRODUCTION

The *endocrine system* is an important body system that includes eight major glands (Table 30-1). Closely linked to the nervous system, the endocrine system controls numerous physiological processes. Unlike the nervous system, which exerts its control through nervous impulses, the endocrine system controls the body through specialized chemical messengers called **hormones.** The fundamental structural units of the endocrine system are the **endocrine glands.** Each endocrine gland produces one or more hormones. (An example of an endocrine gland is the pancreas.) The endocrine glands are the chief focus of this chapter.

Endocrine glands differ from other glands in that they are ductless. Instead of releasing hormones through ducts to a local site, they secrete their hormones directly into capillaries to circulate in the blood throughout the body. In contrast, the majority of glands are **exocrine glands,** which release their chemical products through ducts and tend to have a local effect. For example, the salivary glands are a type of exocrine gland. The salivary glands are located near the pharynx and secrete digestive enzymes, such as amylase, into the pharynx.

Keep in mind these important points about endocrine glands:

- In contrast to the exocrine glands, whose effects tend to be localized, endocrine glands tend to have widespread effects.

✱ **hormone** chemical substance released by a gland that controls or affects processes in other glands or body systems.

✱ **endocrine gland** gland that secretes chemical substances directly into the blood; also called a *ductless gland.*

✱ **exocrine gland** gland that secretes chemical substances to nearby tissues through a duct; also called a *ducted gland.*

The effects of exocrine glands tend to be localized, while the effects of endocrine glands tend to be widespread.

Table 30-1	MAJOR ENDOCRINE GLANDS
Hypothalamus	Thymus
Pituitary	Pancreas
Thyroid	Adrenals
Parathyroid	Gonads

- The hormones released by endocrine glands typically act on distant tissues. They exert a very specific effect on their target tissues.
- Some hormones, such as insulin, have many target organs. Other hormones have only a few target organs.
- Through the release of hormones, the endocrine system plays an important role in regulating body function.

As noted above, the principal product of an endocrine gland is a hormone. The term *hormone* comes from the Greek for "to set in motion," and hormones keep in motion, or regulate, numerous vital cell processes. For example, the hormones insulin and glucagon enable the body to maintain a stable blood glucose level, both after and between meals. This is an example of **homeostasis,** the natural tendency of the body to maintain an appropriate internal environment in the face of changing external conditions. Such hormones as growth hormone and thyroid hormone regulate **metabolism.** Metabolism encompasses all the cellular processes that produce the energy and molecules needed for growth or repair. In addition, such hormones as estrogen and testosterone regulate the sexual development of puberty and the subsequent reproductive function of adulthood.

Many people have endocrine disorders involving excessive or deficient hormone function. Some common conditions, such as hypothyroidism, are readily controlled by hormone replacement medication. Other hormonal disorders may have a more difficult course. You will find that diabetes mellitus, a hormonal disorder, is commonly involved in medical emergencies encountered in the prehospital setting.

ENDOCRINE DISORDERS AND EMERGENCIES

The most common endocrine emergencies you should expect to treat will involve complications of diabetes mellitus. This section explains the pathophysiology of diabetes and its complications, including ketoacidosis and hypoglycemia, as a basis for discussion of field management. In addition, the section covers endocrine emergencies involving disorders of the thyroid and adrenal glands.

DISORDERS OF THE PANCREAS

Diabetes Mellitus

The disease **diabetes mellitus** is marked by inadequate insulin activity in the body. As noted earlier, insulin is critical to maintaining normal blood glucose levels. Glucose is important for all cells, but it is especially important for brain cells. In fact, glucose is the *only* substance that brain cells can readily and efficiently use as an energy source. In addition, insulin enables the body to store energy as glycogen, protein, and fat.

Diabetes mellitus, or sugar diabetes, is not only a serious disease but also a common and ancient one. About 1.2 to 1.4 million Canadians have been diagnosed with

* **homeostasis** the natural tendency of the body to keep the internal environment and metabolism steady and normal.

* **metabolism** the sum of cellular processes that produce the energy and molecules needed for growth and repair.

* **diabetes mellitus** disorder of inadequate insulin activity, due either to inadequate production of insulin or to decreased responsiveness of body cells to insulin.

diabetes, and health experts believe that nearly the same number of Canadians may be living with undiagnosed diabetes. The disease was named in ancient times by Greek physicians who noted that affected persons produced large volumes of urine that attracted bees and other insects, hence *diabetes* (meaning "to syphon," or "to pass through") for excessive urine production and *mellitus* (meaning "honey sweet") for the presence of sugar in the urine. If you remember that *mellitus* means sweet and *insipidus* means neutral, you will remember the common trait and the major distinctions in the presentations of untreated diabetes insipidus and diabetes mellitus.

Before presenting pathophysiology, we will examine in detail the normal handling of glucose by the body. The discussion of glucose metabolism will focus on events at the molecular and cellular levels, whereas the discussion on regulation of blood glucose will focus on events in the blood and in major target tissues, such as the liver, fat cells, and kidneys.

Glucose Metabolism You learned in the chapter introduction that metabolism is the sum of the processes that produce the energy and molecules needed for cell growth or repair. The word *metabolism* comes from the Greek for "to change." Two kinds of change take place within a cell. One kind builds complex molecules from simpler ones. The synthesis of glycogen from glucose is an example. The other kind breaks down complex molecules into simpler ones. The breakdown of glucose into carbon dioxide, water, and energy (in the form of adenosine triphosphate, or ATP) is an example.

The building processes within a cell are collectively called **anabolism.** The prefix *ana-* comes from the Greek for "up," and anabolic pathways build molecules of higher complexity. Breakdown processes are collectively called **catabolism.** The prefix *cata-* comes from the Greek for "down," and catabolic pathways produce molecules of lower complexity. Anabolic pathways usually require energy to drive them, and catabolic pathways often release energy as part of the process. In other words, anabolic activity uses energy, while catabolic activity produces energy.

Look at the summary of the effects of insulin and glucagon in Table 30-2. When materials are abundant after meals and blood glucose is high, insulin enables cells to use glucose directly and to store energy as glycogen, protein, and fat. Insulin stimulates anabolic pathways. In contrast, glucagon is the dominant hormone during periods of low blood glucose. It stimulates catabolic pathways to produce usable energy from the body's stores.

In order for anabolic pathways to proceed, insulin must first exert its stimulatory effects. Insulin acts by binding to receptors in the outer cell membrane. These receptors are proteins whose structure reacts specifically with insulin. When insulin is bound to a receptor, it changes the permeability of the membrane

✳ **anabolism** the constructive or "building up" phase of metabolism.

✳ **catabolism** the destructive or "breaking down" phase of metabolism.

Table 30-2 SUMMARY OF GLUCOSE METABOLISM

Hormonal Effects of Insulin and Glucagon

Insulin	Glucagon
Dominant hormone when blood glucose level is high	Dominant hormone when blood glucose level is low
Major Effects on Target Tissues	*Major Effects on Target Tissues*
all cells: ↑ uptake glucose	
liver: ↑ production of glycogen, protein, fat	liver: ↑ glycogenolysis → glucose
liver, fat: ↑ production of fats	liver: ↑ gluconeogenesis (protein, fat → glucose)

such that glucose enters the cell far more readily. The rate at which glucose can be transported into cells can be increased tenfold or more by the action of insulin. Without insulin activity, the amount of glucose that can enter cells is far too small to meet average body energy demands. Note the two requirements for insulin effectiveness:

1. There must be sufficient insulin circulating in the bloodstream to satisfy cellular needs.
2. Insulin must be able to bind to body cells in such a way that adequate levels of stimulation occur.

The importance of these two requirements will become clear when you learn about the two types of diabetes mellitus.

Sometimes, the body cannot use glucose as a primary energy source. In diabetes, this occurs when insufficient insulin activity exists for blood glucose to be taken in and used by cells. Other conditions, such as a high-fat, low-carbohydrate diet or starvation (which can occur in conjunction with some eating disorders) cause depletion of body stores of carbohydrate. Under any of these conditions, the body slowly switches from glucose to fat as the primary energy source. Adipose cells break down fats into their component free fatty acids, and the blood concentration of fatty acids rises considerably.

Most of the fatty acid is used directly by body cells as an energy source. Some of it is taken in by liver cells. In the liver, catabolism of fatty acids produces acetoacetic acid. When more acetoacetic acid is released from the liver than can be used by body cells, it accumulates in the blood along with two closely related substances, acetone and β-hydroxybutyric acid. These three substances are collectively called **ketone bodies,** and their presence in biologically significant quantity in the blood is called **ketosis.** This catabolic state is significant in the context of the emergency condition called diabetic ketoacidosis, or diabetic coma.

Regulation of Blood Glucose Homeostasis of blood glucose is remarkably effective. If you draw venous blood samples from a group of healthy persons, you will find that fasting blood glucose (generally done after an overnight fast) is usually between 4.4 to 5.0 mmol/L blood. In the first hour or so after a meal, blood glucose may increase to about 6.6 to 7.7 mmol/L before falling toward the fasting, or baseline, level. The principal tissues involved in homeostasis are the alpha and beta tissues of the islets of Langerhans (producing glucagon and insulin, respectively) and the liver—as shown in Table 30-2. Liver disease, even in the presence of normal pancreatic function, can cause significant disturbances in glucose homeostasis.

A blood glucose level lower than baseline (often defined as less than 4.0 mmol/L) reflects **hypoglycemia,** or low blood sugar. Similarly, a blood glucose level higher than that expected shortly after a meal (often defined as greater than 7.0 mmol/L when drawn in a setting other than directly following a meal) reflects **hyperglycemia,** or high blood sugar. Both terms indicate the blood glucose level only, not the cause of the abnormality.

The last factor to consider in discussing regulation of blood glucose is the role of the kidneys. When blood is filtered through the glomeruli of the kidneys, glucose, along with water and many other small molecules, passes from the blood into the proximal tubule. Water, glucose, and other useful materials are then reabsorbed, while waste products that are not reabsorbed become part of the urine, which will be excreted from the body. The amount of glucose that is reabsorbed depends on the blood level of glucose that already exists. Reabsorption of glucose is essentially complete at blood glucose levels up to about 10 mmol/L. Above that level, glucose begins to be lost in urine.

* **ketone bodies** compounds produced during the catabolism of fatty acids, including acetoacetic acid, β-hydroxybutyric acid, and acetone.

* **ketosis** the presence of significant quantities of ketone bodies in the blood.

* **hypoglycemia** deficiency of blood glucose. Sometimes called *insulin shock*. Hypoglycemia is a medical emergency.

* **hyperglycemia** excessive blood glucose.

Glucose loss in urine can lead to dehydration, which has its physiological basis in osmosis. Osmosis is the tendency of water molecules to migrate across a semipermeable membrane such that the concentrations of particles approach equivalence on both sides. Our example is the cell membranes that form the boundaries between the tubules of the kidney and the capillaries that surround them.

When glucose spills into the urine, the osmotic pressure, or concentration of particulates, rises inside the kidney tubule to a level higher than that of the blood. Water follows glucose into the urine to cause a marked water loss termed **osmotic diuresis,** which is the basis of the excessive urination characteristic of untreated diabetes. The term **diuresis** alone refers to increased formation and secretion of urine. The presence of glucose in urine, **glycosuria,** creates the sweet urine that added *mellitus* to *diabetes.*

Last, you should note that whenever the flow rate of fluid inside the kidney tubules rises, as in osmotic diuresis, an increase in excretion of potassium occurs. This leads to the potential for significant hypokalemia and its effects, including cardiac dysrhythmias.

Type I Diabetes Mellitus When we discussed the elements essential to normal insulin activity, the first was the presence of adequate amounts of insulin in the body. *Type I diabetes mellitus* is characterized by very low production of insulin by the pancreas. In many cases, no insulin is produced at all. Type I diabetes is commonly called juvenile-onset diabetes because of the average age at diagnosis. The term *insulin-dependent diabetes mellitus (IDDM)* is also used because patients require regular insulin injections to maintain glucose homeostasis. This type of diabetes is less common than is Type II diabetes, but it is more serious. Diabetes is regularly among the ten leading causes of death in Canada, and Type I diabetes accounts for most diabetes-related deaths.

Heredity is an important factor in determining which persons will be predisposed to development of Type I diabetes. The cause of Type I diabetes is often unclear. However, viral infection, production of autoantibodies directed against beta cells, and genetically determined early deterioration of beta cells are all possible. The immediate cause of the disease is destruction of beta cells.

In untreated Type I diabetes, blood glucose levels rise because, without adequate insulin, cells cannot take up the circulating sugar. Hyperglycemia in the range of 6.6 to 7.6 mmol/L is not uncommon. As glucose spills into the urine, large amounts of water are lost, too, through osmotic diuresis. Catabolism of fat becomes significant as the body switches to fatty acids as the primary energy source. Overall, this pathophysiology accounts for the constant thirst (polydipsia), excessive urination (polyuria), ravenous appetite (polyphagia), weakness, and weight loss associated with untreated Type I diabetes. Ketosis can occur as the result of fat catabolism, and it may proceed to frank diabetic ketoacidosis, a medical emergency that you will encounter in the field (discussed later in this chapter).

Type II Diabetes Mellitus The second requirement for proper insulin activity is insulin binding such that adequate stimulation of cells occurs. *Type II diabetes mellitus* is associated with a moderate decline in insulin production accompanied by a markedly deficient response to the insulin that is present in the body. Type II diabetes is also called adult-onset diabetes or *non-insulin-dependent diabetes mellitus (NIDDM).*

Heredity may play a role in predisposition. In addition, obese persons are more likely to develop Type II diabetes, and obesity probably plays a role in development of the disease. Increased weight (and increased size of fat cells) causes a relative deficiency in the number of insulin receptors per cell, which makes fat cells less responsive to insulin. This type of diabetes is far more common than is

* **osmotic diuresis** greatly increased urination and dehydration that result when high levels of glucose cannot be reabsorbed into the blood from the kidney tubules and the osmotic pressure of the glucose in the tubules also prevents water reabsorption.

* **diuresis** formation and secretion of large amounts of urine.

* **glycosuria** glucose in urine, which occurs when blood glucose levels exceed the kidney's ability to reabsorb glucose.

Content Review

SYMPTOMS OF UNTREATED DIABETES MELLITUS
Polydipsia
Polyuria
Polyphagia
Weakness
Weight loss

Type I diabetes, accounting for about 90 percent of cases of diabetes mellitus. It is also less serious.

Untreated Type II diabetes typically presents with a lower level of hyperglycemia and fewer major signs of metabolic disruption. For instance, glucose use is usually sufficient to keep the body from switching to fats as the primary energy source. Thus, diabetic ketoacidosis is uncommon in these patients. However, a complication called hyperglycemic hyperosmolar nonketotic coma can occur, and you may see it as a medical emergency. It is discussed later in this chapter.

Medical treatment of Type II diabetes is less intensive than that required for Type I diabetes. Initial therapy often consists of dietary change and increased exercise in an attempt to improve body weight. If nonpharmacological therapy is insufficient to bring blood glucose levels down to the normal range, oral hypoglycemic agents may be prescribed. These drugs stimulate insulin secretion by beta cells and promote an increase in the number of insulin receptors per cell. In some cases, however, control may eventually require use of insulin.

✱ **diabetic ketoacidosis** complication of Type I diabetes due to decreased insulin intake. Marked by high blood glucose, metabolic acidosis, and, in advanced stages, coma. Ketoacidosis is often called diabetic coma.

Diabetic Ketoacidosis (Diabetic Coma)

Diabetic ketoacidosis is a serious, potentially life-threatening complication associated with Type I diabetes. It occurs when there is profound insulin deficiency coupled with increased glucagon activity. It may occur as the initial presentation of severe diabetes, as a result of patient noncompliance with insulin injections, or as the result of physiological stress caused by surgery or serious infection. Some of the major characteristics of diabetic ketoacidosis are listed in Tables 30-3 and 30-4.

Table 30-3 DIABETIC EMERGENCIES

Diabetic Ketoacidosis	Hyperglycemic Hyperosmolar Nonketotic (HHNK) Acidosis	Hypoglycemia
Common Causes	**Common Causes**	**Common Causes**
Cessation of insulin injections	Physiological stress (from infection or stroke) producing hyperglycemia and a noncompensated diuresis, modulated by both insulin and glucagon activity	Excessive administration of insulin
Physiological stress (from infection or surgery) that causes release of catecholamines, potentiating glucagon effects and blocking insulin effects		Excess insulin for dietary intake
		Overexertion, resulting in lowered blood glucose level
Signs and Symptoms	**Signs and Symptoms**	**Signs and Symptoms**
Polyuria, polydipsia, polyphagia	Polyuria, polydipsia, polyphagia	Cold, clammy skin
Warm, dry skin and mucous membranes	Warm, dry skin and mucous membranes	Weakness, uncoordination
Nausea/vomiting	Orthostatic hypotension	Headache
Abdominal pain	Tachycardia	Irritable, agitated behaviour
Tachycardia	Decreased mental function or frank coma	Decreased mental function or bizarre behaviour
Deep, rapid respirations (Kussmaul's respirations)		Coma (severe cases)
Fruity odour on breath		
Fever (if associated with infection)		
Decreased mental function or frank coma		
Management	**Management**	**Management**
Fluids, insulin as directed	Fluids, insulin as directed	Dextrose/Glucagon

Table 30-4 DIAGNOSTIC SIGNS BY SYSTEM FOR DIABETIC EMERGENCIES

System	Diabetic Emergency		
	Diabetic Ketoacidosis	*HHNK Coma*	*Hypoglycemia*
Cardiovascular			
Pulse	Rapid	Rapid	Normal
Blood Pressure	Low	Normal to low (may be affected by position, or orthostatic)	Normal
Respiratory			
Respiration rate	Exaggerated air hunger	Normal, unlaboured	Normal or shallow
Breath odour	Acetone (sweet fruity)	None	None
Nervous			
Headache	Absent	None	Present
Mental state	Restlessness/ unconsciousness	Lethargy/ unconsciousness	Apathy, irritability/ unconsciousness
Tremors	Absent	Absent	Present
Convulsions	None	Possible	In late stages
Gastrointestinal			
Mouth	Dry	Dry	Drooling
Thirst	Intense	Excessive	Absent
Vomiting	Common	Common	Uncommon
Abdominal pain	Frequent	Common	Absent
Ocular			
Vision	Dim	Normal	Double vision (diplopia)

Pathophysiology Reread the discussion of ketosis in the prior section on Glucose Metabolism. Diabetic ketoacidosis reflects amplification of the same physiological mechanisms as ketosis.

In the initial phase of diabetic ketoacidosis, profound hyperglycemia exists because of lack of insulin. Body cells cannot take in glucose. The compensatory mechanism for low glucose levels within cells, gluconeogenesis, only contributes more blood glucose. The consequent loss of glucose in the urine, accompanied by loss of water through osmotic diuresis, produces significant dehydration.

As the body switches to fat-based metabolism, the blood level of ketones rises. The ketone load accounts for the observed acidosis. By the time the characteristic decrease in pH from about 7.4 to about 6.9 has occurred, the patient is hours from death if left untreated.

Signs and Symptoms The onset of clinically obvious diabetic ketoacidosis is slow, lasting from 12 to 24 hours. In the initial phase, signs of diuresis appear, including increased urine production and dry, warm skin and mucous membranes. The individual often has excessive hunger and thirst, coupled with a progressive sense of general malaise. Volume depletion induces tachycardia and feelings of physical weakness.

As ketoacidosis develops, a major compensatory mechanism for acidosis appears: the rapid, deep breathing pattern termed *Kussmaul's respirations*, which helps expel carbon dioxide (CO_2) from the body (Figure 30-1). The breath itself may have a fruity or acetone-like smell as some blood acetone is expelled through the lungs. The blood profile includes not only hyperglycemia and acidic pH but also electrolyte abnormalities. Low bicarbonate levels reflect loss of acid-base buffer via Kussmaul's respirations. Low potassium levels may be

The presence of a sweet, fruity odour on the patient's breath is a hallmark of diabetic ketoacidosis.

FIGURE 30-1 Kussmaul's respirations.

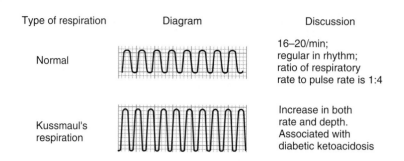

Type of respiration	Diagram	Discussion
Normal		16–20/min; regular in rhythm; ratio of respiratory rate to pulse rate is 1:4
Kussmaul's respiration		Increase in both rate and depth. Associated with diabetic ketoacidosis

found secondary to diuresis, with marked hypokalemia increasing the risk for cardiac dysrhythmias or death. Over time, mental function declines, and frank coma may occur. A fever is not characteristic of ketoacidosis. If present, it is a sign of infection.

Assessment and Management The approach used with the patient suffering from diabetic ketoacidosis is essentially the same as with any other patient who has mental impairment or is unconscious. First, complete your primary assessment of airway, breathing, and circulation. Then, complete a focused history and secondary assessment. Look for a Medic-Alert bracelet on the patient and/or insulin in the refrigerator. Obtain a history from anyone present. The sweet, fruity odour of ketones occasionally can be detected on the breath. If possible, complete the rapid test for blood glucose level. It is not uncommon for patients with ketoacidosis to have blood glucose levels well in excess of 16 mmol/L.

Focus field management on maintenance of the ABCs and fluid resuscitation to counteract dehydration. In such cases, draw a red-top tube (or the tube specified by local protocols) of blood. Following blood sampling, administer one to two litres of normal saline per protocol. If transport time is likely to be lengthy, the medical direction physician may request that a critical care paramedic (CCP) administer intravenous or subcutaneous regular insulin.

Expedite transport to an appropriate facility for definitive therapy.

Hyperglycemic Hyperosmolar Nonketotic (HHNK) Coma

* **hyperglycemic hyperosmolar nonketotic (HHNK) coma** complication of Type II diabetes due to inadequate insulin activity. Marked by high blood glucose, marked dehydration, and decreased mental function. Often mistaken for ketoacidosis.

Hyperglycemic hyperosmolar nonketotic (HHNK) coma is a serious complication associated with Type II diabetes. Typically, both insulin and glucagon activity are present. HHNK coma develops when two conditions occur: Sustained hyperglycemia causes osmotic diuresis sufficient to produce marked dehydration, and water intake is inadequate to replace lost fluids. Dialysis, high-osmolarity feeding supplements, infection, and certain drugs can also be associated with development of HHNK coma. Some characteristics of HHNK coma are listed in Tables 30-3 and 30-4.

Pathophysiology As sustained hyperglycemia develops, glucose spills into the urine, causing osmotic diuresis and resultant dehydration. The level of hyperglycemia is often much higher than the levels seen in ketoacidosis (up to 55 mmol/L). However, insulin activity in patients with HHNK coma prevents significant production of ketone bodies. Inadequate fluid replacement results in characteristic signs and symptoms.

The mortality rate for HHNK coma is higher than that for ketoacidosis, ranging from 40 to 70 percent. The higher mortality rate may be due to the lack of early signs and symptoms that bring patients with ketoacidosis to the attention of family or health-care professionals. The mortality rate of HHNK is also high because it primarily affects the elderly.

Signs and Symptoms The onset of HHNK coma is even slower than that of ketoacidosis, with development often occurring over several days. Early signs include increased urination and increased thirst. Subsequent volume depletion can result in orthostatic hypotension when the patient gets out of bed, along with other signs, such as dry skin and mucous membranes as well as tachycardia. The patient may become lethargic and confused or enter frank coma. Kussmaul's respirations are rarely seen because of the lack of acidosis.

Assessment and Management The approach used with the patient suffering from HHNK coma is essentially the same as with any other patient who has mental impairment or is unconscious. It is often difficult in the field to distinguish diabetic ketoacidosis from HHNK coma. Therefore, the prehospital treatment of both emergencies is identical (see the earlier discussion of management of ketoacidosis), and transport should be expedited.

Hypoglycemia (Insulin Shock)

Hypoglycemia, or low blood glucose, is a medical emergency. It can occur when a patient takes too much insulin, eats too little to match an insulin dose, or overexerts and uses almost all available blood glucose. As the period of hypoglycemia lengthens, there is a rise in the risk that brain cells will be permanently damaged or killed due to lack of glucose. You have learned that brain cells can adapt to use fats as an energy source. Note, however, that this adaptation requires hours to develop, and the switch to fat-based metabolism cannot correct any damage already incurred. This is why every second counts in treating hypoglycemia.

Pathophysiology Hypoglycemia, or insulin shock, reflects high insulin and low blood glucose. Regardless of the reason for low blood sugar, insulin causes almost all remaining blood glucose to be taken up by cells. Because of the high level of insulin, glucagon may be ineffective in raising blood glucose levels. In prolonged fasts, almost half the glucose normally produced through gluconeogenesis is of renal origin. This activity is stimulated by epinephrine. Diabetic patients with kidney failure may be predisposed to hypoglycemia because of lack of renal gluconeogenesis.

Signs and Symptoms The signs and symptoms of hypoglycemia are many and varied. Altered mental status is the most important. In the earliest stages of hypoglycemia, the patient may appear restless or impatient or complain of excessive hunger. As blood glucose falls lower, he may display inappropriate anger (even rage) or display a bizarre behaviour. Sometimes, the patient may be placed in police custody for such behaviour or be involved in an automobile accident.

Physical signs may include diaphoresis and tachycardia. If blood glucose falls to a critically low level, the patient may have a **hypoglycemic seizure** or become comatose.

In contrast to diabetic ketoacidosis, hypoglycemia can develop quickly. A clear change in mental status can occur without warning. Always consider hypoglycemia when encountering a patient with bizarre behaviour. Review Tables 30-3 and 30-4 for additional information.

Assessment and Management In suspected cases of hypoglycemia, perform the primary assessment quickly. Look for a Medic-Alert bracelet. If possible, determine the blood glucose level. Because of the acute nature of this emergency, all paramedic units need to have the capability to perform this task.

If the blood glucose level is less than 4.0 mmol/L start an IV of normal saline. Next, administer 50 mL (25 g) of 50-percent dextrose intravenously. If the patient is conscious and able to swallow, complete glucose administration with orange juice, sugared sodas, or commercially available glucose pastes.

✱ **hypoglycemia** deficiency of blood glucose.

Hypoglycemia is a true medical emergency that requires prompt intervention to prevent permanent brain injury.

Hypoglycemia virtually never occurs outside the context of diabetes mellitus.

✱ **hypoglycemic seizure** seizure that occurs when brain cells are not functioning normally due to low blood glucose.

All paramedics must have the capability of rapidly determining a patient's blood glucose level.

When an IV cannot be started, hypoglycemic patients may improve following the administration of glucagon. This is a much slower process and will only work if there are adequate stores of glycogen available. Glucagon must be reconstituted immediately prior to administration. An adult dose of 1.0 mg intramuscularly or subcutaneously is usually adequate.

DISORDERS OF THE THYROID GLAND

You are more likely to see thyroid dysfunction as part of the medical history than as an emergency. However, you may see patients with acute complications of thyroid disorders. The most common of these disorders are

* **Hyperthyroidism**—the presence of excess thyroid hormones in the blood.
* **Thyrotoxicosis**—a condition that reflects prolonged exposure of body organs to excess thyroid hormones, with resultant changes in structure and function. Thyrotoxicosis is generally caused by *Graves' disease.*
* **Hypothyroidism**—the presence of inadequate levels of thyroid hormones in the blood.
* **Myxedema**—a condition that reflects long-term exposure of body organs to inadequate levels of thyroid hormones, with resultant changes in structure and function.

Graves' Disease

More than 95 percent of cases of thyrotoxicosis are due to **Graves' disease.** Roughly 15 percent of Graves' disease patients have a close relative with Graves' disease, which suggests a strong hereditary role in predisposition to the disorder. In addition, Graves' disease is about six times more common in women than in men, with onset typically in young adulthood (20s and 30s).

Pathophysiology Graves' disease has an autoimmune origin. Autoantibodies are generated that stimulate thyroid tissue to produce excessive amounts of thyroid hormones. The resultant changes in organ function are either responses to excess thyroid hormones or responses to the autoantibodies themselves.

Signs and Symptoms Signs and symptoms of Graves' disease include agitation, emotional changeability, insomnia, poor heat tolerance, weight loss despite increased appetite, weakness, dyspnea, and tachycardia or new-onset atrial fibrillation in the absence of a cardiac history. Nervous system symptoms tend to be more common in younger adults, whereas serious cardiovascular symptoms tend to predominate in older individuals. Prolonged reaction of orbital tissues with the pathological thyroid-stimulating autoantibodies can cause exophthalmos (protrusion of the eyeballs), whereas interaction of autoantibodies with thyroid tissue often produces diffuse goitre (a generally enlarged thyroid gland) (Figure 30-2).

Assessment and Management Cardiac dysfunction is probably the most likely context in which an emergency call may arise from thyrotoxicosis (usually caused by Graves' disease, as noted earlier). Use of β-adrenergic blockers, such as propranolol, may temporarily reduce cardiac stress, but make sure the patient does not have heart failure before considering use. Glucocorticoid therapy (namely, dexamethasone) is sometimes helpful in quickly reducing the level of circulating T_4.

* **hyperthyroidism** excessive secretion of thyroid hormones resulting in an increased metabolic rate.

* **thyrotoxicosis** condition that reflects prolonged exposure to excess thyroid hormones with resultant changes in body structure and function.

* **hypothyroidism** inadequate secretion of thyroid hormones resulting in a decreased metabolic rate.

* **myxedema** condition that reflects long-term exposure to inadequate levels of thyroid hormones with resultant changes in body structure and function.

* **Graves' disease** endocrine disorder characterized by excess thyroid hormones resulting in body changes associated with increased metabolism; primary cause of *thyrotoxicosis.*

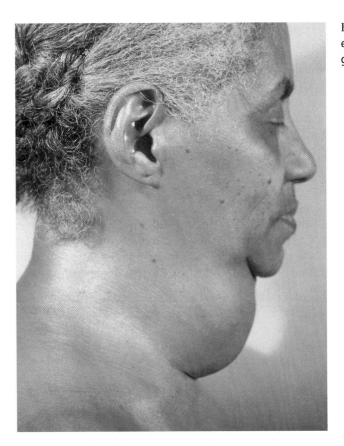

FIGURE 30-2 Generalized enlargement of the thyroid gland (goitre).

Thyrotoxic Crisis ("Thyroid Storm")

Thyrotoxic crisis, or "thyroid storm," is a life-threatening emergency that can be fatal within as few as 48 hours if untreated. It is usually associated with severe physiological stress (e.g., trauma, infection), less often with psychological stress. You may also encounter thyroid storm secondary to overdose of thyroid hormone in a hypothyroid individual.

Pathophysiology The mechanisms underlying thyrotoxic crisis are poorly understood. An acute increase in the levels of thyroid hormones does not appear to be the cause. It is more likely that thyroid storm is caused by a shift of thyroid hormone in the blood from the protein-bound (biologically inactive) state to the free (biologically active) state.

Signs and Symptoms The signs and symptoms associated with thyrotoxic crisis reflect the patient's extreme hypermetabolic state and the increased activity of the sympathetic nervous system. This syndrome is characterized by high fever 41°C (106°F) or higher, irritability, delirium or coma, tachycardia, hypotension, vomiting, and diarrhea. A less severe presentation may also occur, with slight fever and marked lethargy.

Assessment and Management In the presence of the above-mentioned signs and symptoms of thyrotoxic crisis, field management is largely focused on supportive care: oxygenation, ventilatory assistance, fluid resuscitation, and cardiac monitoring. Glucocorticoids and β-adrenergic blockers may be helpful. Transport should be expedited for definitive therapy that blocks the high blood levels of thyroid hormones.

✱ **thyrotoxic crisis** toxic condition characterized by hyperthermia, tachycardia, nervous symptoms, and rapid metabolism; also known as *thyroid storm.*

Hypothyroidism and Myxedema

Hypothyroidism can be congenital or acquired. Both sexes can be affected. The recent increase in incidence of hypothyroidism in middle-aged women may reflect better diagnostics, a true rise in incidence, or both. Advanced myxedema in middle-aged and elderly individuals is the condition you are most likely to see as part of a medical emergency, and so we will focus most attention on myxedema and the uncommon complication of myxedema coma.

Pathophysiology Hypothyroidism creates a low metabolic state, and early signs reflect poor organ function and poor response to such challenges as exercise or infection. Over time, untreated severe hypothyroidism causes the additional sign of myxedema: a thickening of connective tissue in the skin and other tissues, including the heart. Patients with myxedema may progress into a hypothermic, stuporous state called **myxedema coma**, which can be fatal if respiratory depression occurs. Triggers for progression include infection, trauma, a cold environment, or exposure to central nervous system depressants, such as alcohol or certain drugs.

Signs and Symptoms Early signs of hypothyroidism may be subtle. Symptoms may be as slight as fatigue and slowed mental function attributed falsely to aging. Typically, patients with hypothyroidism or myxedema show lethargy, cold intolerance, constipation, decreased mental function, or decreased appetite with increased weight. In addition, the relaxation stage of deep tendon reflexes (DTRs) is slowed. The classic appearance of myxedema is an unemotional, puffy face, thinned hair, enlarged tongue, and pale, cool skin that looks and feels like dough (Figure 30-3). Myxedema coma may be difficult to identify. Note if the history is consistent with hypothyroidism, and look for the physical signs of myxedema. Other signs include profound hypothermia (temperatures as low as 24°C (75°F) are not uncommon), low amplitude bradycardia, and carbon dioxide retention.

Assessment and Management The presence of the described signs and symptoms may alert you to the possible presence of myxedema. Keep in mind that heart failure due to the combination of age, atherosclerosis, and myxedematous enlargement is not uncommon, and so focus on maintenance of ABCs and close monitoring of cardiac and pulmonary status. Most patients with myxedema coma require intubation and ventilatory assistance. Active rewarming is contraindicated due to risk of cardiac dysrhythmias and cardiovascular collapse secondary to vasodilation. Although IV access is important, limit fluids because

 myxedema coma life-threatening condition associated with advanced myxedema, with profound hypothermia, bradycardia, and electrolyte imbalance.

While most patients experiencing myxedema coma require intubation and ventilatory assistance, active rewarming is contraindicated due to risk of cardiac dysrhythmias and cardiovascular collapse secondary to vasodilation.

FIGURE 30-3 Doughy, edematous skin typical of myxedema.

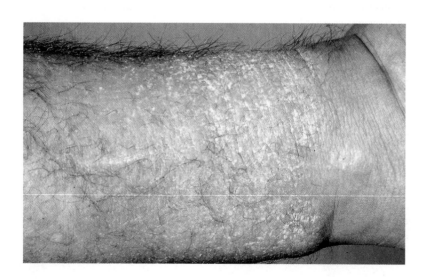

fluid and electrolyte imbalance is common. Expedite transport to an appropriate facility for definitive treatment.

DISORDERS OF THE ADRENAL GLANDS

Two disorders of the adrenal cortex can play a part in medical emergencies or complicate responses to trauma. **Cushing's syndrome** is caused by excessive adrenocortical activity. In contrast, **Addison's disease** is caused by deficient adrenocortical activity. Reread the earlier section where we discussed the anatomy and physiology of the adrenal glands to remind yourself how critical these hormones are to metabolic processes and to salt and water balance.

Hyperadrenalism (Cushing's Syndrome)

Cushing's syndrome is a relatively common disorder of the adrenals. It usually affects middle-aged persons, women being affected more often than men. Excess cortisol can be due to abnormalities in the anterior pituitary or adrenal cortex. It can also be due to treatment with glucocorticoids, such as prednisone. Check the history to note any steroid treatment for nonendocrine conditions, such as chronic obstructive pulmonary disease (COPD), asthma, and cancer or rheumatological disorders.

Pathophysiology Long-term exposure to excess glucocorticoids, primarily cortisol, produces numerous changes. Metabolically, cortisol is an antagonist to insulin. Gluconeogenesis is prominent, with profound protein catabolism. The body's handling of fats is altered, and so atherosclerosis and hypercholesterolemia are common. Over time, diabetes mellitus also may develop. Cortisol's mineralocorticoid activity causes sodium retention and increased blood volume. Increased vascular sensitivity to catecholamines occurs, and this may also be a contributor to hypertension. Potassium loss through the kidneys may cause hypokalemia. Cortisol's anti-inflammatory and immunosuppressive properties predispose the person to infection.

Signs and Symptoms Regardless of the cause, the presenting signs and symptoms are the same. The earliest sign is weight gain, particularly through the trunk of the body, face, and neck. A "moon-faced" appearance often develops (Figure 30-4). The accumulation of fat on the upper back is occasionally referred to as a "buffalo hump." Skin changes are also very common and may be an early clue

* **Cushing's syndrome** pathological condition resulting from excess adrenocortical hormones. Symptoms may include changed body habitus, hypertension, and susceptibility to infection.

* **Addison's disease** endocrine disorder characterized by adrenocortical insufficiency. Symptoms may include weakness, fatigue, weight loss, and hyperpigmentation of skin and mucous membranes.

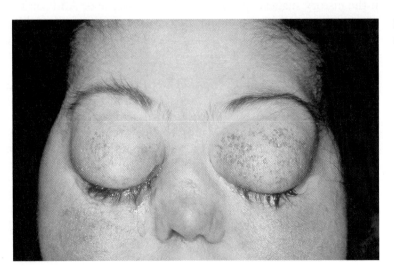

FIGURE 30-4 Facial features of Cushing's syndrome.

to potential problems. These include thinning to an almost transparent appearance, a tendency to bruise easily, delayed healing from even minor wounds, and development of facial hair in women (hirsutism). Mood swings and impaired memory or concentration are also common.

Assessment and Management Although it is unlikely you will see a patient with acute hyperadrenal crisis, you are likely to encounter patients who exhibit signs and symptoms of Cushing's syndrome. Remember that these patients have a higher incidence of cardiovascular disease, including hypertension and stroke. Pay particular attention to skin preparation when starting IV lines because of skin fragility and susceptibility to infections. Indications of Cushing's syndrome should be noted in your report and relayed to hospital staff.

Adrenal Insufficiency (Addison's Disease)

Addison's disease is due to cortical destruction. Addison's has become less common, since former leading causes of Addison's, such as tuberculosis, have been brought under control. Currently, more than 90 percent of Addison's disease cases are due to autoimmune disease. As with Graves' disease, another autoimmune disorder, heredity plays a prominent role in predisposition. In fact, patients with Addison's disease are more likely than average to have other autoimmune disorders, including Graves' disease. Persons with Addison's may be tipped into metabolic failure called **Addisonian crisis** by acute stresses, such as from infection or trauma.

Pathophysiology Destruction of the adrenal cortex results in minimal production of all three classes of hormones: glucocorticoids, mineralocorticoids, and androgens. Low mineralocorticoid activity is key to the changes of Addison's disease: It causes major disturbances in water and electrolyte balance. Increased sodium excretion in urine causes low blood volume, and potassium retention can cause hyperkalemia and ECG changes. Many cases of adrenal insufficiency are due to therapy with steroids, such as prednisone. Such therapy can completely suppress normal adrenal function. Sudden cessation of the drug may trigger symptoms of Addison's disease or even an Addisonian crisis, with cardiovascular collapse.

Signs and Symptoms Addison's disease is characterized by changes related to low corticosteroid activity: progressive weakness, fatigue, decreased appetite, and weight loss. Hyperpigmentation of the skin and mucous membranes, particularly in sun-exposed areas, is also characteristic. Include Addisonian crisis in your list of possible causes of unexplained cardiovascular collapse, particularly if the history suggests primary Addison's disease or Addison's disease secondary to drug therapy. Many patients will have gastrointestinal problems, such as vomiting or diarrhea, which will exacerbate electrolyte imbalances, low blood volume, and hypotension and increase the potential for cardiac dysrhythmias.

Assessment and Management The patient may infrom you about Addison's disease during the history, or the signs and symptoms just discussed may lead you to suspect Addison's disease. Focus emergency management on maintenance of the ABCs and close monitoring of cardiac and oxygenation status as well as blood glucose level. Hypoglycemia poses its own threat. Assess blood glucose levels and administer 25 g of 50-percent dextrose to patients with blood glucose levels less than 4.0 mmol/L and to those with altered mental status. Obtain a baseline 12-lead ECG to check for dysrhythmias related to electrolyte imbalance. Be aggressive in fluid resuscitation. Follow your local protocol or contact medical direction for specific orders based on your patient's presentation. Expedite transport to an appropriate facility.

* **Addisonian crisis** form of shock associated with adrenocortical insufficiency and characterized by profound hypotension and electrolyte imbalances.

SUMMARY

In conjunction with the nervous system, the endocrine system regulates body functions. The vast majority of endocrine emergencies involve complications of diabetes mellitus, such as hypoglycemia or ketoacidosis. Other endocrine emergencies tend to be rare and will more likely be part of the history, rather than the emergency. In the field, you should always suspect diabetes when patients present with unexplained changes in mental status. Hypoglycemia, the most urgent diabetic emergency, must be quickly treated to prevent serious nervous system damage. When the exact type of diabetic emergency is undetermined, treat for hypoglycemia. Treatment of diabetic ketoacidosis is primarily a hospital procedure.

CHAPTER 31

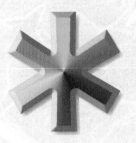

Allergies and Anaphylaxis

Objectives

After reading this chapter, you should be able to:

1. Describe the incidence, morbidity, and mortality of anaphylaxis. (p. 623–624)
2. Identify the risk factors most predisposing to anaphylaxis. (p. 623–624)
3. Discuss the anatomy and physiology of the organs and structures related to anaphylaxis. (pp. 624–626)
4. Discuss the pathophysiology of allergy and anaphylaxis. (pp. 624–627)
5. Describe the common routes of substance entry into the body. (pp. 626–627)
6. Define allergic reaction, anaphylaxis, antigen, antibody, and natural and acquired immunity.

(pp. 624–627)

7. List common antigens most frequently associated with anaphylaxis. (pp. 624–625)
8. Discuss human antibody formation. (pp. 624–626)
9. Describe the physical manifestations of anaphylaxis. (pp. 627–629, 631–632)
10. Identify and differentiate between the signs and symptoms of an allergic reaction and anaphylaxis. (pp. 631–632)
11. Explain the various treatment and pharmacological interventions used in the management of allergic

Continued

Objectives Continued

reactions and anaphylaxis.
(pp. 629–632)

12. Correlate abnormal findings in assessment with the clinical significance in the patient with an allergic reaction or anaphylaxis. (pp. 627–629, 631–632)

13. Given several preprogrammed and moulaged patients, provide the appropriate assessment, care, and transport for the patient with allergic reaction and anaphylaxis. (pp. 623–632)

INTRODUCTION

An **allergic reaction** is an exaggerated response by the immune system to a foreign substance. Allergic reactions can range from mild skin rashes to severe, life-threatening reactions that involve virtually every body system. The most severe type of allergic reaction is called **anaphylaxis**. Anaphylaxis is a life-threatening emergency that requires prompt recognition and specific treatment by paramedics. The emergency treatment of anaphylaxis is one area of prehospital care in which advanced life support measures often mean the difference between life and death. Anaphylaxis can develop within seconds and cause death just minutes after exposure to the offending agent. Fortunately, there are several emergency medications available that can reverse the adverse effects of anaphylaxis.

The first complete description of anaphylaxis was reported in 1902 by Portier and Richet. Portier and Richet were French immunologists who were attempting to immunize dogs against the toxin of the deadly sea anemone (sea flower). They were injecting small, nonlethal quantities of the toxin into the animals in hopes of stimulating immunity to the toxin. However, when the animals received secondary injections of sublethal quantities of the toxin, at a time when it might be expected that they would be immune, the dogs developed shock and died. Richet called this dramatic and unexpected phenomenon *anaphylaxis*, which means the opposite of "phylaxis" or protection.

Anaphylaxis is a serious allergic reaction that can be life threatening. Anaphylaxis results from exposure to a particular substance that sets off a biochemical chain of events that can ultimately lead to shock and death. Food is the most common cause of anaphylaxis, but insect stings, medicines, latex, or exercise can also cause a reaction.

While the exact incidence of anaphylaxis is not known, approximately 1–2 percent of Canadians live with the risk of an anaphylactic reaction. More than 50 percent of Canadians know someone who is at risk. Injected penicillin and bee and wasp (*Hymenoptera*) stings are the two most common causes of fatal anaphylaxis. Fewer than five persons die in Canada each year from *Hymenoptera* stings. Fortunately, the incidence of anaphylaxis appears to be declining. This is presumably due to earlier recognition and treatment, as well as the availability of numerous potent antihistamines.

✳ **allergic reaction** an exaggerated response by the immune system to a foreign substance.

✳ **anaphylaxis** an unusual or exaggerated allergic reaction to a foreign protein or other substance. Anaphylaxis means the opposite of "phylaxis," or protection.

Anaphylaxis is the most severe form of allergic reaction and is often life threatening.

✳ *Hymenoptera* any of an order of highly specialized insects, such as bees and wasps.

PATHOPHYSIOLOGY

The immune system is the principal body system involved in allergic reactions. However, other body systems are also affected by an allergic reaction. These include *the cardiovascular system, the respiratory system, the nervous system,* and *the gastrointestinal system,* among others. To fully appreciate the complexity of allergic and anaphylactic reactions, it is first necessary to review the anatomy and physiology of the immune system as it relates to the immune response.

THE IMMUNE SYSTEM

The **immune system** is a complicated body system responsible for combating infection. Components of the immune system can be found in the blood, the bone marrow, and the lymphatic system.

The **immune response** is a complex cascade of events that occurs following activation by an invading substance or **pathogen.** The goal of the immune response is the destruction or inactivation of pathogens, abnormal cells, or foreign molecules, such as **toxins.** The body can accomplish this through two mechanisms, cellular immunity and humoral immunity. **Cellular immunity** involves a direct attack of the foreign substance by specialized cells of the immune system. These cells physically engulf and deactivate or destroy the offending agent. **Humoral immunity** is much more complicated. Humoral immunity is basically a chemical attack on the invading substance. The principal chemical agents of this attack are **antibodies,** also called **immunoglobulins (Igs).** Antibodies are a unique class of chemicals that are manufactured by specialized cells of the immune system called *B cells.* There are five different classes of antibodies: IgA, IgD, IgE, IgG, and IgM.

The humoral immune response begins with exposure of the body to an antigen. An **antigen** is defined as any substance capable of inducing an immune response (Table 31-1). Most antigens are proteins. Following exposure to an antigen, antibodies are released from cells of the immune system. These antibodies attach themselves to the invading substance to facilitate removal of that substance from the body by other cells of the immune system.

If the body has never been exposed to a particular antigen, the response of the immune system is different from that if it has been previously exposed to the particular antigen. The initial response to an antigen is called the **primary response.**

Table 31-1 AGENTS THAT MAY CAUSE ANAPHYLAXIS

Antibiotics and other drugs

Foreign proteins (e.g., horse serum, Streptokinase)

Foods (nuts, eggs, shrimp)

Allergen extracts (allergy shots)

Hymenoptera stings (bees, wasps)

Hormones (insulin)

Blood products

Aspirin

Nonsteroidal anti-inflammatory drugs (NSAIDs)

Preservatives (sulphiting agents)

X-ray contrast media

Dextran

Following exposure to a new antigen, several days are required before both the cellular and humoral components of the immune system respond. Generalized antibodies (IgG and IgM) are first released to help fight the antigen.

At the same time, other components of the immune system begin to develop antibodies specific for the antigen. These cells also develop a *memory* of the particular antigen. If the body is exposed to the same antigen again, the immune system responds much faster. This is called the **secondary response.** As a part of the secondary response, antibodies specific for the offending antigen are released. Antigen-specific antibodies are much more effective in facilitating removal of the offending antigen than are the generalized antibodies released during the primary response.

Immunity may be either *natural* or *acquired.* **Natural immunity,** also called *innate immunity,* is genetically predetermined. It is present at birth and has no relation to previous exposure to a particular antigen. All humans are born with some innate immunity.

Acquired immunity develops over time and results from exposure to an antigen. Following exposure to a particular antigen, the immune system will produce antibodies specific for the antigen. This protects the organism as subsequent exposure to the same antigen will result in a vigorous immune response. **Naturally acquired immunity** normally begins to develop after birth and is continually enhanced by exposure to new pathogens and antigens throughout life. For example, a child contracts chicken pox (varicella) at age 18 months. Following the infection, the child's immune system creates antibodies specific for the varicella virus. Repeated exposure to the varicella virus usually will not result in another infection. In fact, it is not unusual for a patient exposed to varicella to develop lifelong immunity to the infection.

Induced active immunity, also called *artificially acquired immunity,* is designed to provide protection from exposure to an antigen at some time in the future. This is achieved through vaccination and provides relative protection against serious infectious agents. In vaccination, an antigen is injected into the body so as to generate an immune response. This results in the development of antibodies specific for the antigen and provides protection against future infection. Most vaccines contain antigenic proteins from a particular virus or bacterium. Later, when the individual is actually exposed to the pathogen, the immune response will be vigorous and will often be enough to prevent the infection from developing.

An example of a vaccine commonly used is the DPT (diphtheria/pertussis/tetanus) vaccine. This vaccine contains antigenic proteins from the bacteria that cause diphtheria, whooping cough, and tetanus. The vaccine is administered at several intervals during the first five years of life. It provides protection against infection from these bacteria. Some vaccinations will impart lifelong immunity, while others must be periodically followed with a "booster dose" to ensure continued protection.

Acquired immunity can be either *active* or *passive.* **Active immunity** occurs following exposure to an antigen and results in the production of antibodies specific for the antigen. Most vaccinations result in the development of active immunity. However, it takes some time for a patient to develop specific antibodies. In certain cases, it is necessary to administer antibodies to provide protection until the active immunity can kick in. The administration of antibodies is referred to as **passive immunity.** There are two types of passive immunity. *Natural passive immunity* occurs when antibodies cross the placental barrier from the mother to the infant so as to provide protection against embryonic or fetal infections. *Induced passive immunity* is the administration of antibodies to an individual to help fight infection or prevent diseases. An example of the clinical use of both active and passive immunity is the regimen used for the prevention of tetanus.

✱ **secondary response** response by the immune system that takes place if the body is exposed to the same antigen again; in secondary response, antibodies specific for the offending antigen are released.

✱ **natural immunity** genetically predetermined immunity that is present at birth; also called *innate immunity.*

✱ **acquired immunity** immunity that develops over time and results from exposure to an antigen.

✱ **naturally acquired immunity** immunity that begins to develop after birth and is continually enhanced by exposure to new pathogens and antigens throughout life.

✱ **induced active immunity** immunity achieved through vaccination given to generate an immune response that results in the development of antibodies specific for the injected antigen; also called *artificially acquired immunity.*

✱ **active immunity** acquired immunity that occurs following exposure to an antigen and results in the production of antibodies specific for the antigen.

✱ **passive immunity** acquired immunity that results from administration of antibodies either from the mother to the infant across the placental barrier (natural passive immunity) or through vaccination (induced passive immunity).

Most persons in the developed countries have typically received some form of tetanus vaccination during their life. These persons typically have some antibodies to tetanus and often need nothing more than a tetanus booster. However, some persons have never received any sort of tetanus vaccination. When these persons seek treatment for a tetanus-prone wound, they must receive prophylaxis for tetanus in addition to care for their wound. This is best achieved by the provision of both passive and active immunity. To provide immediate protection, the patient is administered antibodies specific for tetanus (tetanus immune globulin [TIG] BayTet®). Then, they are administered a tetanus vaccination (Td or Dt). The tetanus immune globulin (TIG) provides passive immunity until such time as the body's immune system can respond to the tetanus vaccination with the development of antibodies specific for tetanus. This should be followed by periodic tetanus boosters until such time as the patient's immunization program is complete.

ALLERGIES

The initial exposure of an individual to an antigen is referred to as **sensitization.** Sensitization results in an immune response. Subsequent exposure induces a much stronger secondary response. Some individuals can become hypersensitive (overly sensitive) to a particular antigen. **Hypersensitivity** is an unexpected and exaggerated reaction to a particular antigen. In many instances, hypersensitivity is used synonymously with the term **allergy.** There are two types of hypersensitivity reactions, delayed and immediate.

Delayed and Immediate Hypersensitivity

A **delayed hypersensitivity reaction** is a result of *cellular immunity* and therefore does not involve antibodies. Delayed hypersensitivity usually occurs in the hours and days following exposure and is the sort of allergy that occurs in normal people. Delayed hypersensitivity most commonly results in a skin rash and is often due to exposure to certain drugs and chemicals. The rash associated with poison ivy is an example of delayed hypersensitivity.

When people use the term "allergy" they are usually referring to **immediate hypersensitivity reactions.** Examples of immediate hypersensitivity reactions include hay fever, drug allergies, food allergies, eczema, and asthma. Some persons have an allergic tendency. This allergic tendency is usually genetic, meaning it is passed from parent to child and is characterized by the presence of large quantities of IgE antibodies. An antigen that causes release of the IgE antibodies is referred to as an **allergen.** Common allergens include

- Drugs
- Foods and food additives
- Animals
- Insects (*Hymenoptera* stings) and insect parts
- Fungi and moulds
- Radiology contrast materials

Allergens can enter the body through various routes. These include oral ingestion, inhalation, topically, and through injection or envenomation. The vast majority of anaphylactic reactions result from injection or envenomation.

Parenteral penicillin injections are the most common cause of fatal anaphylactic reactions. Insect stings are the second most frequent cause of fatal ana-

---

* **sensitization** initial exposure of a person to an antigen that results in an immune response.

* **hypersensitivity** an unexpected and exaggerated reaction to a particular antigen. It is used synonymously with the term *allergy.*

* **allergy** a hypersensitive state acquired through exposure to a particular allergen.

* **delayed hypersensitivity reaction** a hypersensitivity reaction that takes place after the elapse of some time following reexposure to an antigen. Delayed hypersensitivity reactions are usually less severe than immediate reactions.

* **immediate hypersensitivity reaction** a hypersensitivity reaction that occurs swiftly following reexposure to an antigen. Immediate hypersensitivity reactions are usually more severe than delayed reactions. The swiftest and most severe of such reactions is anaphylaxis.

* **allergen** a substance capable of inducing allergy of specific hypersensitivity. Allergens may be protein or nonprotein, although most are proteins.

phylactic reactions. Insects in the order *Hymenoptera* are the most frequent offending insects. There are three families in this order: fire ants *(Formicoidea)*; wasps, yellow jackets, and hornets *(Vespidae)*; and honey bees *(Apoidea)*. All produce a unique venom, although there are similar components in each. Honey bees often will leave their stinger embedded in the victim following a sting.

Following exposure to a particular allergen, large quantities of IgE antibodies are released. These antibodies attach to the membranes of **basophils** and **mast cells**—specialized cells of the immune system that contain chemicals that assist in the immune response. When the allergen binds to IgE attached to the basophils and mast cells, these cells release histamine, heparin, and other substances into the surrounding tissues. Histamine and other substances are stored in *granules* found within the basophils and mast cells. In fact, because of this feature, basophils and mast cells are often called *granulocytes*. The process of releasing these substances from the cells is called *degranulation*. This release results in what people call an *allergic reaction,* which can be very mild or very severe.

The principal chemical mediator of an allergic reaction is histamine. **Histamine** is a potent substance that causes bronchoconstriction, increased intestinal motility, vasodilation, and increased vascular permeability. Increased vascular permeability causes the leakage of fluid from the circulatory system into the surrounding tissues. A common manifestation of severe allergic reactions and anaphylaxis is angioneurotic edema. **Angioneurotic edema,** also called *angioedema,* is marked edema of the skin and usually involves the head, neck, face, and upper airway. Histamine acts by activating specialized histamine receptors present throughout the body.

There are two classes of histamine receptors. H_1 receptors, when stimulated, cause bronchoconstriction and contraction of the intestines. H_2 receptors cause peripheral vasodilation and secretion of gastric acids. The goal of histamine release is to minimize the body's exposure to the antigen. Bronchoconstriction decreases the possibility of the antigen entering through the respiratory tract. Increased gastric acid production helps destroy an ingested antigen. Increased intestinal motility serves to move the antigen quickly though the gastrointestinal system with minimal absorption of the antigen into the body. Vasodilation and capillary permeability help remove the allergen from the circulation where it has the potential to do the most harm.

ANAPHYLAXIS

Anaphylaxis usually occurs when a specific allergen is injected directly into the circulation. This is the reason anaphylaxis is more common following injections of drugs and diagnostic agents and following bee stings. When the allergen enters the circulation, it is distributed widely throughout the body. The allergen interacts with both basophils and mast cells, resulting in the massive dumping of histamine and other substances associated with anaphylaxis. The principal body systems affected by anaphylaxis are the cardiovascular system, the respiratory system, the gastrointestinal system, and the skin. Histamine causes widespread peripheral vasodilation as well as increased permeability of the capillaries. Increased capillary permeability results in marked loss of plasma from the circulation. People sustaining anaphylaxis can actually die from circulatory shock.

Also released from the basophils and mast cells is a substance called **slow-reacting substance of anaphylaxis (SRS-A)**. This causes spasm of the bronchial smooth muscle, resulting in an asthma-like attack and occasionally asphyxia. SRS-A potentiates the effects of histamine, especially on the respiratory system.

* **basophil** type of white blood cell that participates in allergic responses.

* **mast cell** specialized cell of the immune system that contains chemicals that assist in the immune response.

* **histamine** a product of mast cells and basophils that causes vasodilation, capillary permeability, bronchoconstriction, and contraction of the gut.

* **angioneurotic edema** marked edema of the skin that usually involves the head, neck, face, and upper airway; a common manifestation of severe allergic reactions and anaphylaxis.

* **slow-reacting substance of anaphylaxis (SRS-A)** substance released from basophils and mast cells that causes spasm of the bronchiole smooth muscle, resulting in an asthma-like attack and occasionally asphyxia.

ASSESSMENT FINDINGS IN ANAPHYLAXIS

The signs and symptoms of anaphylaxis begin within 30–60 seconds following exposure to the offending allergen. In a small percentage of patients, the onset of signs and symptoms may be delayed over an hour. The signs and symptoms of anaphylaxis can vary significantly. The severity of the reaction is often related to the speed of onset. Reactions that develop very quickly tend to be much more severe.

A rapid and focused assessment is crucial to the early detection and treatment of anaphylaxis. Patients suffering an anaphylactic reaction often have a sense of impending doom. This sense of impending doom is often followed by development of additional signs and symptoms.

If the patient's condition permits, a brief history should be gathered, including previous allergen exposures and reactions. If possible, try to determine how quickly symptoms started and how severe they were.

Next, quickly evaluate the patient's level of consciousness. Upper airway problems, including laryngeal edema, may result in the patient being unable to speak. As the emergency worsens, the patient will become restless. As cardiovascular collapse continues, the patient will exhibit a decreased level of consciousness. If untreated, this may continue to unresponsiveness.

As noted earlier, a common manifestation of anaphylaxis is angioneurotic edema, involving the face and neck. Laryngeal edema is also a frequent complication and can threaten the airway. Initially, laryngeal edema will cause a hoarse voice. As the edema worsens, the patient may develop stridor. Finally, this all may lead to complete airway obstruction from either massive laryngeal edema, laryngospasm, or pharyngeal edema, or a combination of any of these.

The respiratory system is significantly involved in an anaphylactic reaction. Initially, the patient will become tachypneic. Later, as lower airway edema and bronchospasm develop, respirations will become laboured as evidenced by retractions, accessory muscle usage, and prolonged expirations. Wheezing, resulting from bronchospasm and edema of the smaller airways, is a common manifestation and may be so pronounced that it can be heard without the aid of a stethoscope. Ultimately, anaphylaxis can result in markedly diminished lung sounds, which reflect decreased air movement and hypoventilation.

The skin is typically involved early in severe allergic reactions and anaphylaxis. Generally, a fine red rash will appear diffusely on the body. As histamine is released, fluid will diffuse from leaky capillaries, resulting in urticaria. **Urticaria,** also called "hives," is a weal and flare reaction characterized by red, raised bumps that may appear and disappear across the body (Figure 31-1). As cardiovascular collapse and dyspnea progress, the patient will become diaphoretic. This may, if untreated, progress to cyanosis and pallor.

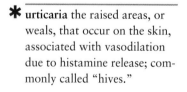

✻ urticaria the raised areas, or weals, that occur on the skin, associated with vasodilation due to histamine release; commonly called "hives."

FIGURE 31-1 Hives are red, itchy blotches, sometimes raised, that often accompany an allergic reaction.

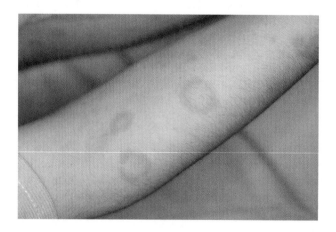

The effect of histamine on the gastrointestinal system is pronounced. Initially, the patient may note a rumbling sensation in the abdomen as gastrointestinal motility increases. On physical examination, this may be evident as hyperactive bowel sounds. Later, nausea, vomiting, and diarrhea develop as the body tries to rid itself of the offending allergen.

The vital signs will vary depending on the severity and stage of the severe allergic or anaphylactic reaction. Initially, there will be an increase in both the heart and the respiratory rates. As airway edema and dyspnea occur, the respiratory rate can fall—an ominous finding. The blood pressure will fall when significant capillary leakage and peripheral vasodilation occur. This will often result in a reflex tachycardia as the body attempts to compensate for the fall in blood pressure. Very late in anaphylaxis, the heart rate will fall. This, too, should be considered an extremely ominous sign.

State-of-the-art advanced prehospital care of anaphylaxis includes use of all available monitoring devices. These include the cardiac monitor, the pulse oximeter, and, if the patient is intubated, an end-tidal carbon dioxide detector. As anaphylaxis progresses, the end-tidal carbon dioxide level may climb due to the development of both respiratory and metabolic acidoses, which result in increased carbon dioxide elimination.

MANAGEMENT OF ANAPHYLAXIS

When responding to a patient with an anaphylactic reaction, first ensure that the scene is safe to approach. The presence of chemicals or patrolling bees can pose a risk to EMS personnel as well as to the patient and bystanders. If the patient is still in contact with the agent causing the reaction, she should be moved a safe distance away. Honey bees often leave their stinger behind after a sting. If present, the stinger should be removed by scraping the skin with a fingernail or scalpel blade.

Always consider the possibility of trauma in anaphylaxis. If there is any suspicion of coincidental trauma, stabilize the cervical spine. It is not uncommon for people to fall or otherwise injure themselves as they try to escape from wasps and bees. Signs and symptoms of trauma may be masked by those of anaphylaxis.

PROTECT THE AIRWAY

Position the patient and protect the airway. Administer oxygen via a nonrebreather mask. If the patient is hypoventilating or apneic, initiate ventilatory assistance. If an airway problem is detected, first apply basic airway manoeuvres, such as head positioning or the modified jaw-thrust manoeuvre. Use oropharyngeal and nasopharyngeal airways with caution as they can cause laryngospasm. If the patient is having severe airway problems, consider early endotracheal intubation to prevent complete occlusion of the airway. It is important to remember that the glottic opening may be smaller than expected due to laryngeal edema. Also, the larynx will be highly irritable, and any manipulation of the airway may lead to laryngospasm. Ideally, the most experienced member of the crew should perform endotracheal intubation, as only one attempt may be possible.

Establish an IV as soon as possible with a crystalloid solution, such as Ringer's Lactate or normal saline. Remember that patients suffering anaphylaxis are volume depleted due to histamine-mediated third spacing of fluid. If the patient is hypotensive, administer fluids wide open.

ADMINISTER MEDICATIONS

The primary treatment for anaphylaxis is pharmacological. If the necessary drugs cannot be administered in the field, then the patient should be transported to the emergency department immediately. Emergency treatment for anaphylaxis includes administration of oxygen, epinephrine, and vasopressors. Occasionally, inhaled beta agonists, such as salbutamol, may be required.

Oxygen Oxygen is always the first treatment to administer to a patient with an anaphylactic reaction. Administer high-concentration oxygen with a non-rebreather mask or similar device. If mechanical ventilation is required, attach supplemental oxygen to ensure as high an oxygen delivery as possible.

> *Epinephrine is the primary drug for management of anaphylaxis.*

Epinephrine The primary drug for use in treatment of severe allergic reactions and anaphylaxis is epinephrine. Epinephrine is a sympathetic agonist. It causes an increase in heart rate, an increase in the strength of the cardiac contractile force, and peripheral vasoconstriction. It can also reverse some of the bronchospasm associated with anaphylaxis. Epinephrine also reverses much of the capillary permeability caused by histamine. It acts within minutes of administration. In severe anaphylaxis, characterized by hypotension and/or severe airway obstruction, administer epinephrine 1:1000 subcutaneously. Epinephrine 1:1000 contains 1 mg of epinephrine in 1 mL of solvent. The standard adult dose is 0.3 mg; pediatric dose is 0.01 mg/kg. The effects of epinephrine wear off in 3–5 minutes, so repeat as required.

Antihistamines Antihistamines are second-line agents in the treatment of anaphylaxis. They should only be given following the administration of epinephrine. Antihistamines block the effects of histamine by blocking histamine receptors. They do not displace histamine from the receptors. They only block additional histamine from binding. They also help reduce histamine release from mast cells and basophils. Most antihistamines are nonselective and block both H_1 and H_2 receptors. Others are more selective for either H_1 or H_2 receptors.

Diphenhydramine (Benadryl) is probably the most frequently used antihistamine in the treatment of allergic reactions and anaphylaxis. It is nonselective and acts on both H_1 and H_2 receptors. The standard dose of diphenhydramine is 25–50 mg intravenously or intramuscularly. It should be administered slowly when given intravenously. The pediatric dose of diphenhydramine is 1–2 mg/kg of body weight. Other nonselective antihistamines frequently used are hydroxyzine (Atarax) and promethazine (Phenergan). Hydroxyzine is a potent antihistamine, but it can only be administered intramuscularly. Promethazine can be administered intravenously or intramuscularly but does not appear to be as potent as diphenhydramine.

Corticosteroids Corticosteroids are important in the treatment and prevention of anaphylaxis. Although they are of little benefit in the initial stages of treatment they help suppress the inflammatory response associated with these emergencies. Commonly used corticosteroids include methylprednisolone (Solu-Medrol), hydrocortisone (Solu-Cortef), and dexamethasone (Decadron).

Vasopressors Severe and prolonged anaphylactic reactions may require the use of potent vasopressors to support blood pressure. Use these medications in conjunction with first-line therapy and adequate fluid resuscitation. Commonly used agents include dopamine, norepinephrine, and epinephrine. These medications are prepared as infusions and are continuously administered to support blood pressure and cardiac output.

Beta Agonists Many patients with severe allergic reactions and anaphylaxis will develop bronchospasm, laryngeal edema, or both. In these cases, an inhaled beta agonist can be useful. The most frequently used beta agonist in prehospital care is salbutamol (Ventolin). Although usually used in the treatment of asthma, these agents will help reverse some of the bronchospasm and laryngeal edema associated with anaphylaxis. Give the adult patient 5 mg of salbutamol in 3 mL of normal saline via a handheld nebulizer. Children should receive 1.25–2.5 mg of albuterol based on their weight.

Other Agents Other drugs occasionally used in the treatment of anaphylaxis include aminophylline and cromolyn sodium. Aminophylline is a bronchodilator unrelated to the beta agonists. It can be administered by slow intravenous infusion to treat the bronchospasm associated with anaphylaxis. Although cromolyn sodium (Intal) is not used in the treatment of allergic reactions and anaphylaxis, it is used in their prevention. Cromolyn sodium helps stabilize the membranes of the mast cells, thus reducing the amount of histamine and other mediators released when these cells are stimulated.

OFFER PSYCHOLOGICAL SUPPORT

A severe allergic or anaphylactic reaction is a harrowing experience for the patient. Although it is essential to work fast, the prehospital crew should provide the patient emotional support and explain the treatment regimen. Caution patients about the potential side effects of administered medications. For example, epinephrine will often cause a rapid heart rate, anxiety, and tremulousness. Likewise, the antihistamines may cause a dry mouth, thirst, and sedation. Careful explanation and emotional support will help allay patient anxiety and apprehension.

ASSESSMENT FINDINGS IN ALLERGIC REACTION

Many patients you will be called to treat will be suffering from forms of allergic reaction less severe than anaphylaxis. An allergic reaction, as contrasted with an anaphylactic reaction, will have a more gradual onset with milder signs and symptoms and the patient will have a normal mental status (Table 31-2).

MANAGEMENT OF ALLERGIC REACTIONS

Common manifestations of mild (nonanaphylactic) allergic reactions include itching, rash, and urticaria. Patients with simple itching and nonurticarial rashes

Table 31-2 SIGNS AND SYMPTOMS OF ALLERGIC AND ANAPHYLACTIC REACTIONS

Mild Allergic Reaction	Severe Allergic Reaction or Anaphylaxis
Onset: Gradual	*Onset:* Sudden (30–60 seconds but can be more than an hour after exposure)
Skin/vascular system: Mild flushing, rash, or hives	*Skin/vascular system:* Severe flushing, rash, or hives; angioneurotic edema to the face and neck
Respiration: Mild bronchoconstriction	*Respiration:* Severe bronchoconstriction (wheezing), laryngospasm (stridor), breathing difficulty
GI system: Mild cramps, diarrhea	*GI system:* Severe cramps, abdominal rumbling, diarrhea, vomiting
Vital signs: Normal to slightly abnormal	*Vital signs:* Increased pulse early, may fall in late/severe case; increased respiratory rate early, falling respiratory rate late; falling blood pressure late
Mental status: Normal	*Mental status:* Anxiety, sense of impending doom, may decrease to confusion and to unconsciousness
	Other clues: Symptoms occur shortly after exposure to parenteral penicillin, *Hymenoptera* sting (fire ant, wasp, yellow-jacket, hornet, bee), or ingestion of foods to which patient is allergic, such as nuts or shellfish
	Ominous signs: Respiratory distress, signs of shock, falling respiratory rate, falling pulse rate, falling blood pressure

Note: Not all signs and symptoms will be present in every case.

FIGURE 31-2   Epinephrine being administered to a pediatric patient.

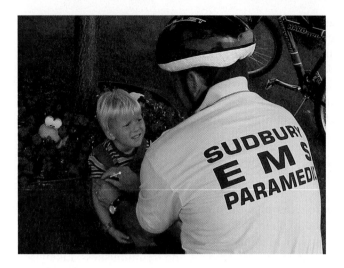

may be treated with antihistamines alone. In addition to antihistamines, epinephrine is often necessary for the treatment of urticaria.

Any patient suffering an allergic reaction who exhibits dyspnea or wheezing should receive supplemental oxygen. This should be followed by subcutaneous epinephrine 1:1000. Patients presenting with hypotension or airway problems can be adequately treated with epinephrine 1:1000 administered subcutaneously (Figure 31-2). Epinephrine 1:1000 contains 1 mg of epinephrine in 1 mL of solvent. When administered into the subcutaneous tissue, the drug is absorbed more slowly and the effect prolonged. The subcutaneous dose is the same as the intravenous dose (0.3 mL). The subcutaneous route should not be used in severe anaphylaxis. Many physicians prefer to give epinephrine 1:1000 intramuscularly because this has a faster rate of onset although a shorter duration of action.

SUMMARY

Fortunately, severe allergies and anaphylaxis are uncommon. However, when they do occur, they can progress quickly and result in death in minutes. The central physiological action in anaphylaxis is the massive release of histamine and other mediators. Histamine causes bronchospasm, airway edema, peripheral vasodilation, and increased capillary permeability. The prehospital treatment of anaphylaxis is intended to reverse the effects of these agents.

The primary, and most important, drug used in the treatment of anaphylaxis is epinephrine. Epinephrine helps reverse the effects of histamine. It also supports the blood pressure and reverses detrimental capillary leakage. Following the administration of epinephrine, potent antihistamines should be used to block the adverse effects of the massive histamine release. Inhaled beta agonists are useful in cases of severe bronchospasm and airway involvement. Intravenous fluid replacement is crucial in preventing hypovolemia and hypotension.

The key to successful prehospital management of anaphylaxis is prompt recognition and treatment.

CHAPTER 32

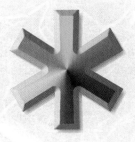

Gastroenterology

Objectives

After reading this chapter, you should be able to:

1. Describe the incidence, morbidity, and mortality of gastrointestinal emergencies. (p. 634)
2. Identify the risk factors most predisposing to gastrointestinal emergencies. (pp. 634–635)
3. Discuss the anatomy and physiology of the gastrointestinal system. (see Chapter 12)
4. Discuss the pathophysiology of abdominal inflammation and its relationship to acute pain. (pp. 635–636)
5. Define somatic, visceral, and referred pain as they relate to gastroenterology. (pp. 635–636)

6. Differentiate between hemorrhagic and nonhemorrhagic abdominal pain. (pp. 636, 638)
7. Discuss the signs and symptoms and differentiate among local, general, and peritoneal inflammations relative to acute abdominal pain. (pp. 635–636)
8. Describe the questioning technique and specific questions when gathering a focused history in a patient with abdominal pain. (pp. 636–637)
9. Describe the technique for performing a comprehensive secondary

Continued

assessment on a patient complaining of abdominal pain. (p. 638)

10. Discuss the pathophysiology, assessment findings, and management of the following gastroenterological problems:
    • Upper gastrointestinal bleeding (pp. 639–641)
    • Lower gastrointestinal bleeding (pp. 646–647)
    • Acute gastroenteritis (pp. 642–643)
    • Colitis (pp. 647–648)
    • Gastroenteritis (pp. 642–644)
    • Diverticulitis (p. 649)
    • Appendicitis (pp. 652–653)
    • Ulcer disease (pp. 644–646)

• Bowel obstruction (pp. 650–652)
• Crohn's disease (p. 648)
• Pancreatitis (pp. 654–655)
• Esophageal varices (pp. 641–642)
• Hemorrhoids (pp. 649–650)
• Cholecystitis (pp. 653–654)
• Acute hepatitis (pp. 655–656)

11. Differentiate between gastrointestinal emergencies based on assessment findings. (pp. 636–638)

12. Given several preprogrammed patients with abdominal pain and symptoms, provide the appropriate assessment, treatment, and transport. (pp. 634–656)

INTRODUCTION

Gastrointestinal (GI) emergencies account for approximately 500 000 emergency visits and hospitalizations and 5 percent of all visits to the emergency department each year in the United States. Of that number, more than 300 000 are due to GI bleeding. While statistics are not available for Canadian hospitals, we would expect a similar percentage of visits to Canadian hospitals for this reason. These figures will probably increase as more and more people treat themselves with over-the-counter medications and delay seeing a physician until their symptoms become severe. Perhaps more importantly, the numbers will rise as the general population ages. In the last few years the number of patients over 60 years of age included in these statistics has risen from approximately 3 percent to more than 45 percent.

GENERAL PATHOPHYSIOLOGY, ASSESSMENT, AND TREATMENT

Gastrointestinal emergencies usually result from an underlying pathological process that can be predicted by evaluating numerous risk factors. These risk factors are commonly known to physicians; most are self-induced by patients. They

Content Review

GASTROINTESTINAL DISEASE RISK FACTORS
• Excessive alcohol consumption
• Excessive smoking
• Increased stress
• Ingestion of caustic substances
• Poor bowel habits

include excessive alcohol consumption, excessive smoking, increased stress, ingestion of caustic substances, and poor bowel habits. The wide variety of risk factors and potential causes requires the emergency care provider to complete a thorough focused history and secondary assessment before making a field diagnosis, along with assessing the seriousness of the emergency and the need for any prevention strategy to minimize organ damage.

Gastrointestinal illnesses require the emergency care provider to complete a thorough history and secondary assessment before making a field diagnosis.

GENERAL PATHOPHYSIOLOGY

Pain is the hallmark of the acute abdominal emergency. The three main classifications of abdominal pain are visceral, somatic, and referred. **Visceral pain** originates in the walls of hollow organs, such as the gallbladder or appendix, in the capsules of solid organs, such as the kidney or liver, or in the visceral peritoneum. Three separate mechanisms can produce this pain—inflammation, distention (being stretched out or inflated), and ischemia (inadequate blood flow). Because these processes progress at varying rates, they likewise can cause varying intensities, characteristics, and locations of pain.

Inflammation, distention, and ischemia all transmit a pain signal from visceral afferent neural fibres back to the spinal column. Because the nerves enter the spinal column at various levels, visceral pain usually is not localized to any one specific area. Instead, it is often described as very vague or poorly localized, dull, or crampy. The body most often responds to this vague pain with sympathetic stimulation that causes nausea and vomiting, diaphoresis, and tachycardia.

Organs that consist of hollow viscera can frequently cause visceral pain, for example, the gallbladder (cholecystitis) and the small and large intestines. Many hollow organs first cause visceral pain when they become distended and then cause a different, more specific type of pain (somatic pain, described below) when they rupture or tear. For example, appendicitis initially presents with vague periumbilical abdominal pain that is classified as visceral. If the appendix ruptures it can spill its contents into the peritoneal cavity, causing bacterial **peritonitis** and generating somatic pain. Various microbes associated with pelvic inflammatory diseases can also cause bacterial peritonitis.

Somatic pain, as contrasted to visceral pain, is a sharp type of pain that travels along definite neural routes (determined by the dermatomes, or tissue blocks, present during embryonic development) to the spinal column. Because these routes are clearly defined, the pain can be localized to a particular region or area. As previously noted, bacterial and chemical irritations of the abdomen commonly cause somatic pain. Bacterial irritation can originate from a perforated or ruptured appendix or gallbladder. Chemical irritation of the abdomen can result from leakage of acidic juices from a perforated ulcer or from an inflamed pancreas. Whether the cause is bacterial or chemical, the resulting peritonitis can lead to sepsis and even death. The degree of pain is initially proportional to the spread of the irritant through the abdominal cavity. Somatic pain allows the examiner to locate the specific area of irritation, providing valuable information.

The third type of pain, referred pain, is not a true pain-producing mechanism. As its name implies, **referred pain** originates in a region other than where it is felt. Many neural pathways from various organs pass through or over regions where the organ was formed during embryonic development. For example, the afferent neural pathways that originate in the diaphragm enter the spinal column at the cervical enlargement at the fourth cervical vertebra. Therefore, patients who have an inflammation or injury of the diaphragm often feel pain in their necks or shoulders. One of the most significant hemorrhagic emergencies, the dissecting abdominal aortic artery, produces referred pain felt between the shoulder blades. Some common nonhemorrhagic emergencies are associated

Content Review

TYPES OF GASTROINTESTINAL PAIN
- Visceral
- Somatic
- Referred

✻ **visceral pain** dull, poorly localized pain that originates in the walls of hollow organs.

✻ **peritonitis** inflammation of the peritoneum, which lines the abdominal cavity.

✻ **somatic pain** sharp, localized pain that originates in walls of the body, such as skeletal muscles.

Pain from hollow organs tends to be vague and nondescript, whereas pain from solid organs tends to be localized.

✻ **referred pain** pain that originates in a region other than where it is felt.

with referred-pain patterns, too. Appendicitis often presents with periumbilical pain, whereas pneumonia can cause pain below the lower margin of the rib cage.

GENERAL ASSESSMENT

Your assessment of a patient who complains of abdominal discomfort or whom you suspect of having an abdominal pathology is similar to a trauma assessment with an expanded history. Do not approach the patient until you and your partner have determined the scene to be free and clear of any apparent dangers. Always take appropriate body substance isolation measures, including gloves, eyewear, mask, and disposable body gown to prevent contamination. As you approach the patient, survey the scene for potential evidence of your patient's problem. Medication bottles, alcohol containers, ashtrays, and buckets with emesis or sputum, for instance, can provide valuable information.

Scene Assessment and Primary Assessment

As you approach, look for mechanisms of injury to help determine whether the reason for the call is medical or trauma related. If you suspect trauma, always immobilize the cervical spine as you assess the adequacy of the patient's airway and his level of responsiveness. In the vast majority of medical patients you can check responsiveness and airway patency by asking the patient his name and chief complaint (why he called the ambulance today) and noting the answers. You can further evaluate the rate, depth, and quality of the patient's respirations fairly rapidly and without great difficulty. As you evaluate the respiratory functions, quickly palpate a pulse and check skin colour, temperature, and circulation, including signs of bleeding and capillary refill. If you discover a life-threatening condition during the primary assessment, treat it, and then rapidly continue the assessment to identify any other life threats.

History and Secondary Assessment

Once you have completed the primary assessment and dealt with any life threats, conduct the focused history and secondary assessment. Your ability to obtain a history from the patient will depend on his level of responsiveness. In some cases, you may detect deterioration of the patient's mental status over time as you take the history.

The history of the present illness and the past medical history will be especially helpful in piecing together a clear picture of the underlying gastrointestinal pathophysiology.

History An accurate and thorough history can provide invaluable information. After you conduct the SAMPLE history (*s*ymptoms, *a*llergies, *m*edications, *p*ast medical history, *l*ast oral intake, and *e*vents), you can take a more thorough, focused history, exploring the chief complaint, the history of the present illness, the past medical history, and the current health status. The history of the present illness and the past medical history will be especially helpful in sorting the multitude of signs and symptoms and piecing together a clear picture of the underlying pathophysiology.

History of the Present Illness Your OPQRST-ASPN history for gastrointestinal patients should address the following specific concerns:

- *Onset.* When did the pain first start? Was the onset very sudden or gradual? Sudden onsets of abdominal pain are generally caused by perforations of abdominal organs or capsules. Gradual onset of pain usually is associated with the blockage of hollow organs.

- *Provocation/Palliation.* What makes the pain worse? What makes the pain better? If the pain lessens when the patient draws his legs up to his chest or lies on his side, it usually indicates peritoneal inflammation, which is often of GI origin. If walking relieves the pain, the cause may be in the GI or urinary systems—perhaps an obstruction of the gallbladder or a stone caught in the renal pelvis or ureter.

- *Quality*. How would you describe the pain: dull, sharp, constant, intermittent? Localized, tearing pain is usually associated with the rupture of an organ. Dull, steadily increasing pain may indicate a bowel obstruction. Sharp pain, particularly in the flank, may indicate a kidney stone.

- *Region/radiation*. Does the pain travel to any other part of your body? Radiated pain, or pain that seems to change location, is common because it involves the same neural routes as referred pain. Pain referred to the shoulder or neck is usually associated with an irritation of the diaphragm, such as happens with cholecystitis.

- *Severity*. On a scale of 1 to 10, with 10 representing the worst pain possible, how would you rate the pain you are feeling now? The severity of pain usually worsens as the pathology (ischemia, inflammation, or stretching) of the organ advances.

- *Time*. When did the pain first start? Estimation of the pain's time of onset is important to determine its possible causes. Any abdominal pain lasting more than six hours is considered a surgical emergency and needs to be evaluated in the emergency department.

- *Associated Symptoms*. Have you experienced any associated nausea and or vomiting with the discomfort? If yes, try to determine the content, colour, and smell of the vomitus. Ask if the vomitus contained any bright red blood, "coffee grounds," or clots. Determining if your patient has an active gastrointestinal bleed is imperative.

  Have you experienced any changes in bowel habits—constipation or diarrhea—associated with this discomfort/pain? Question the patient further to determine if there have been any changes in feces, such as a tarry, foul-smelling stool. Changes in bowel morphology, colour, or smell can be the only indication of such conditions as a lower GI hemorrhage, gastritis, or bleeding diverticula.

  Have you had an associated loss of appetite or weight loss? Patients who have an acute abdomen usually have an associated loss of appetite.

- *Pertinent Negatives*. The absence of symptoms associated with GI function or the presence of symptoms related to urinary function may mean the problem originates in the urinary system. Pain in the lowest part of the abdomen, the pelvis, can be due to problems in the reproductive system. Last, remember that an inferior myocardial infarction (MI) can irritate the diaphragm and generate its referred-pain pattern. Be sure to check for cardiovascular history when this pain pattern (pain in shoulder and/or neck area) is present.

Keep in mind the information that your SAMPLE history gave you about your patient's last oral intake. It can help you to differentiate the possible causes of your patient's pain if the problem is in the GI system.

Not all abdominal emergencies result in abdominal pain. Some may cause chest pain. This, typically, is referred pain. Common GI emergencies that can cause chest pain include gastroesophageal reflux, gastric ulcers, duodenal ulcers, and, in some cases, gallbladder disease. When confronted by a patient with chest pain, always consider the GI system as a possible cause.

Past Medical History Have you ever experienced this same type of pain or discomfort before? If the patient answers yes, then investigate whether he saw a

Usually patients with severe abdominal pathology lie as still as possible, often in the fetal position.

Distention of the abdomen may be an ominous sign.

* **Cullen's sign** ecchymosis in the periumbilical area.

* **Grey-Turner's sign** ecchymosis in the flank.

If you auscultate the abdomen, you must do so before palpating it.

Palpating the abdomen can give you a plethora of information.

Your highest priority when treating a patient with abdominal pain is to secure and maintain his airway, breathing, and circulation.

physician for the problem and how it was diagnosed. Commonly, patients have been treated for the complaint in the past and the pain is a flare-up of an old problem.

Secondary Assessment While you are conducting the history you can also begin the secondary assessment. Your patient's general appearance and posture strongly suggest his apparent state of health and the severity of his complaint. Usually, patients with severe abdominal pathology lie as still as possible, often in the fetal position. They do not writhe around on the floor or cry out because doing so increases the pain. You also should continually monitor the patient's level of consciousness for any subtle changes that indicate early signs of shock.

Take a complete set of vital signs to establish a baseline for further evaluation and treatment. These include pulse, respiratory rate, blood pressure, and pulse oximetry. You can also ascertain additional important information, such as body temperature.

Visually inspect the abdomen before palpating it, auscultating it, or moving the patient. Remove the patient's clothing as necessary to freely visualize the entire abdomen. Distention of the abdomen may be an ominous sign. It can be caused by a buildup of free air due to an obstruction of the bowel. If the distention is caused by hemorrhage, the patient has lost a large amount of his circulating volume, for the abdomen can hold from four to six liters of fluid before any noticeable change in abdominal girth occurs. Other signs of fluid loss include periumbilical ecchymosis (**Cullen's sign**) and ecchymosis in the flank (**Grey-Turner's sign**).

Auscultating the abdomen usually provides little helpful information because bowel sounds are heard throughout this area. If you auscultate the abdomen, you must do so before palpating it. Listen for at least two minutes in each quadrant, beginning with the quadrant farthest from the affected area and auscultating the affected area last. Like auscultation, percussion requires a quiet environment and an experienced clinician. It, too, provides little or no useful information and therefore is not routinely performed in the field by paramedics.

Palpating the abdomen, conversely, can give you a plethora of information. It can define the area of pain and identify the associated organs. Before palpating, ask the patient to point to where he is experiencing the most discomfort. Then, work in reverse order, palpating that area last. Palpate the abdomen with a gentle pressure, feeling for muscle tension or its absence, as well as for masses, pulsations, and tenderness beneath the muscle. If you identify a pulsating mass, stop palpating at once; the increase in pressure may cause the affected blood vessel or organ to rupture.

GENERAL TREATMENT

Once you have completed the primary assessment and the focused history and secondary assessment, you can address treatment and transport. Your highest priority when treating a patient with abdominal pain is to secure and maintain his airway, breathing, and circulation. Be prepared to suction the airway of vomitus and blood. High-flow oxygenation and aggressive airway management may be indicated, depending on your patient's status. Monitor circulation by placing the patient on a cardiac monitor and frequently assessing his blood pressure. Measurement of the hematocrit will give an indirect measure of blood loss.

Establish a large-bore IV line in patients who complain of abdominal discomfort for use if emergency blood transfusion becomes necessary. You can use the IV for pharmacological intervention or to replace volume lost to hemorrhage or dehydration. In general, the need to avoid masking any abdominal pain for further evaluation will limit your pharmacological interventions to palliative agents, such as antiemetics. Place the patient in a comfortable position and provide emotional reassurance based on your field assessment, any information from hospital staff or family, and knowledge of estimated transport time. Keep your voice and actions quiet and collected. Calmness, as well as anxiety, is transmitted easily to patients and family. How you transport the patient will depend on his physiological status. Normally, gentle but rapid transport is sufficient. Remember that persistent abdominal pain lasting longer than six hours is classified as a surgical emergency and always requires transport. In all cases, be sure to maintain monitoring of mental status and vital signs and to give nothing by mouth. Bring vomitus to the emergency department for evaluation.

SPECIFIC ILLNESSES

The GI tract is essentially one long tube divided structurally and functionally into different parts. Three other organs, the liver, gallbladder, and pancreas, are intimately associated with it, as is the small structure called the vermiform appendix, which protrudes from the first portion of the large intestine. Collectively, these organs are called the gastrointestinal, or digestive, system. The GI system converts food into nutrient molecules that individual cells can use, and it excretes solid wastes from the body.

UPPER GASTROINTESTINAL DISEASES

For convenience, clinicians often divide the GI tract broadly into the upper and lower GI tracts. The upper GI tract consists of the mouth, esophagus, stomach, and duodenum, the last being the first part of the small intestine. Physical digestion of food and some chemical digestion take place here. As food passes through the lower GI tract, consisting of the remainder of the small intestine and the large intestine, nutrients are absorbed into the blood, and solid wastes are formed and excreted.

Upper Gastrointestinal Bleeding

Upper gastrointestinal bleeding can be defined as bleeding within the GI tract proximal to the **ligament of Treitz,** which supports the duodenojejunal junction, the point at which the first two sections of the small intestine (the duodenum and the jejunum) meet.

Upper GI bleeds account for thousands of hospitalizations in Canada per year. The mortality rate has remained fairly steady at approximately 10 percent over the past years. Many factors contribute to this high mortality. First, the number of patients who treat their symptoms with home remedies and over-the-counter medications is increasing rapidly. Many of these patients come under medical care only when their disease has caused significant damage, such as large-scale hemorrhage from an ulcerated lesion. Second, the overall age of the population is increasing. The infirmities of age and its greater likelihood of coexisting illnesses, such as hypertension, atherosclerosis, diabetes, and substance abuse (including abuse of medications), make this older population more vulnerable to the effects of upper gastrointestinal bleeds. The mortality rate is highest in those over 60 years of age. One prevention strategy for the field is to check for such coexisting problems, especially in elderly patients, and to treat accordingly. In particular, look at the history and physical for evidence of tobacco or alcohol use, or both.

The six major identifiable causes of upper GI hemorrhage, in descending order of frequency, are peptic ulcer disease, gastritis, variceal rupture, **Mallory-Weiss tear** (esophageal laceration, usually secondary to vomiting), esophagitis, and duodenitis. Peptic ulcer disease accounts for approximately 50 percent of upper GI bleeds, with gastritis accounting for an additional 25 percent. Overall, irritation or erosion of the gastric lining of the stomach causes more than 75 percent of upper

Persistent abdominal pain lasting longer than six hours always requires transport.

> **Content Review**
> ### THE GASTROINTESTINAL SYSTEM
> GI tract
> Liver
> Gallbladder
> Pancreas
> Appendix

> **Content Review**
> ### THE UPPER GI TRACT
> Mouth
> Esophagus
> Stomach
> Duodenum

* **upper gastrointestinal bleeding** bleeding within the gastrointestinal tract proximal to the ligament of Treitz.

* **ligament of Treitz** ligament that supports the duodenojejunal junction.

> **Content Review**
> ### MAJOR CAUSES OF UPPER GI HEMORRHAGE
> - Peptic ulcer disease
> - Gastritis
> - Varix rupture
> - Mallory-Weiss tear
> - Esophagitis
> - Duodenitis

* **Mallory-Weiss tear** esophageal laceration, usually secondary to vomiting.

GI bleeds. Most cases of upper GI bleeding are chronic irritations or inflammations that cause minimal discomfort and minor hemorrhage. Physicians can manage these conditions on an outpatient basis; however, if a peptic ulcer erodes through the gastric mucosa, if the esophagus is lacerated in Mallory-Weiss syndrome, or if varices (often secondary to alcoholic liver damage) rupture, an acute-onset, life-threatening, and difficult-to-control hemorrhage can result.

Upper GI bleeds may be obvious, or they may present quite subtly. Most often patients will complain of some type of abdominal discomfort ranging from a vague burning sensation to an upset stomach, gas pain, or tearing pain in the upper quadrants. Because blood severely irritates the GI system, most cases present with nausea and vomiting. If the bleeding is in the upper GI tract, the patient may experience **hematemesis** (bloody vomitus) or, if it passes through the lower GI tract, **melena**. The partially digested blood will turn the stool black and tarry. For melena to be recognizable, approximately 150 mL of blood must drain into the GI tract and remain there for from five to eight hours. Blood in emesis may be bright red (new, fresh blood) or look like coffee grounds (old, partially digested blood).

Upper GI bleeding may be light or it may be brisk and life threatening. Patients who suffer a rupture of an esophageal varix or a tear or disruption in the esophageal or gastric lining may vomit copious amounts of blood. These hemorrhages can cause the classic signs and symptoms of shock, including alteration in mental status, tachycardia, peripheral vasoconstriction, diaphoresis (sweating producing pale, cool, clammy skin), and hemodynamic instability. Besides shock, the vomitus itself can compromise the airway, resulting in impaired respirations, aspiration, and ultimately, respiratory arrest.

A frequently employed clinical indicator is the tilt test, which indicates if the patient has orthostatic hypotension (a 10-mmHg change in blood pressure or a 20-bpm change in heart rate when the patient rises from supine to standing). Hypotension suggests a decreased circulating volume. The human body can compensate for a circulating volume deficit of approximately 15 percent before clinical indicators, such as the tilt test, show positive results. Thus, those patients whose systolic blood pressure drops 10 mmHg or whose heart rate increases 20 bpm or more need aggressive fluid resuscitation.

When evaluating the patient and his laboratory values, remember that the hematocrit might be within normal ranges when the patient is in the early phase of an acute hemorrhage. The key prevention strategy is to identify subtle indicators and treat the condition before it worsens. More general complaints include malaise, weakness, syncopal (fainting) and near-syncopal (lightheaded) spells, tachycardia, and indigestion.

Your patient's general appearance may be the best indicator of his condition's severity. Because the hemorrhage is internal and histories are often misleading, you must perform a thorough secondary assessment. The patient may present doubled over in pain or lying very still. The latter is usually an ominous sign that any movement causes extreme pain. If you place the patient supine, be alert to the possibility of vomitus compromising the airway. Patients with a history of GI problems may have scars from past surgeries.

Examination in cases of suspected hemorrhage may be very helpful. Abdominal inspection may show symmetric distention or bulging in one region of the abdomen. Ecchymosis may be present if much blood has been lost into the abdominal cavity. If auscultation is subsequently performed, bowel sounds may be absent if the bleeding is severe, or they may be hyperactive if the bleeding is minimal.

Prehospital treatment of an upper GI bleed centres on maintaining a patent airway, oxygenation, and circulatory status. Place the patient in the left lateral recumbent or high semi-Fowler's position to prevent aspiration. To maximize the remaining hemoglobin molecules' carrying capability, administer high-flow oxygenation via a nonrebreather mask to all patients with a suspected GI bleed.

Establish two large-bore (14–16 gauge) IVs in any patient whom you suspect of having a GI bleed. Start one with blood tubing for possible transfusion and one with volume-replacement 0.9 percent NaCl. Base fluid resuscitation on the patient's condition and response to the treatment. In general you can administer a 20 mL/kg fluid bolus to begin treating hemorrhagic hypovolemia.

Once the patient reaches the emergency department, treatment may include gastric decompression and lavage with a nasogastric tube, further fluid/blood resuscitation, endoscopy, **Sengstaken-Blakemore tube** placement, antacid and histamine antagonist administration, or immediate surgery.

Esophageal Varices

An **esophageal varix** is a swollen vein of the esophagus. Often, these varices rupture and hemorrhage. When they do, the mortality rate is more than 35 percent.

The cause of esophageal varices usually is an increase in **portal** pressure (portal hypertension). The blood flows from the abdominal organs, through the portal vein, and into the liver, where nutrients are absorbed into liver tissue and numerous compounds are detoxified and returned to the blood. From the liver, blood courses directly into the inferior vena cava through the hepatic veins. Blood flow through the liver ordinarily encounters little, if any, resistance. Damage to that organ, however, can impede circulation, causing blood to back up into the left gastric vein and, from there, into the esophageal veins. The dramatically higher pressure in these normally low-pressure pathways causes the esophageal veins to dilate and emerge from their sheaths (to evaginate, or "outpocket"). These small evaginations are called esophageal varices (Figure 32-1). As they become engorged, the varices continue to dilate outward under extreme pressure until they rupture, causing massive hemorrhage. They may also erode through the submucosal layer and directly into the esophagus.

The primary causes of esophageal varices are the consumption of alcohol and the ingestion of caustic substances. Alcoholic liver cirrhosis accounts for two-thirds of cases of esophageal varices. Over time, alcohol consumption can cause a degenerative process known as **cirrhosis** of the liver. Cirrhosis results in fatty deposits and fibrosis in the liver parenychmal tissue, thus obstructing portal blood

✱ **Sengstaken-Blakemore tube** three-lumen tube used in treating esophageal bleeding.

✱ **esophageal varix** swollen vein of the esophagus.

When varices rupture and hemorrhage, the mortality rate is more than 35 percent.

✱ **portal** pertaining to the flow of blood into the liver.

✱ **cirrhosis** degenerative disease of the liver.

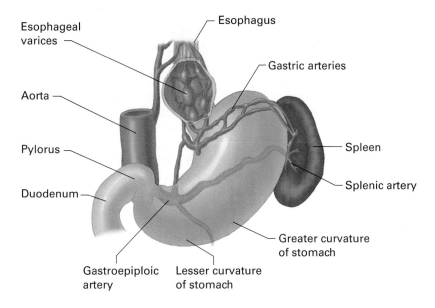

FIGURE 32-1 Esophageal varices occur when the esophageal veins dilate and emerge from their sheaths.

flow. Consequently, esophageal varices are common in the Western Hemisphere in general, where the alcohol consumption rate is high. In fact, cirrhosis is one of the leading causes of death in the Western Hemisphere. Caustic substances, such as battery acid or drain cleaners, can erode the esophagus from the inside out, causing hemorrhage of a vessel. Caustic ingestion, along with variceal formation due to viral hepatitis and erosive esophagitis accounts for the remaining one-third of cases of esophageal varices.

Patients suffering from leaking or ruptured esophageal varices often present initially with painless bleeding and signs of hemodynamic instability. They may complain of hematemesis with bright red blood, dysphagia (difficulty swallowing), and a burning or tearing sensation as the varices continue to bleed, irritating the lining of the esophagus. The hematemesis can be very forceful and copious if the hemorrhage is large. Clotting time increases because the high portal pressure backs up blood into the spleen, destroying platelets. The patient may exhibit the classic signs of shock, such as an increased pulse, increased respirations, and cool, clammy, diaphoretic skin, possibly associated with an altered level of consciousness and hypotension.

Because paramedics cannot tamponade the bleeding in the prehospital setting, your care should focus on aggressive airway management, intravenous fluid resuscitation, and rapid transport to the emergency department. Airway management is a top priority. You may need to suction emesis frequently and diligently from the airway. Orotracheal intubation also may be needed to maintain airway patency. To maximize oxygenation, administer high-flow oxygen via a nonrebreather mask. If the patient shows signs and symptoms of shock, place him in the shock position and begin fluid resuscitation. If the patient continues to hemorrhage, management in the emergency department might include the use of a Sengstaken-Blakemore tube to tamponade the bleeding, endoscopic cauterization, or sclerotherapy (injection of a thrombus-forming drug into the vein itself).

Acute Gastroenteritis

acute gastroenteritis sudden onset of inflammation of the stomach and intestines.

Acute gastroenteritis is defined as inflammation of the stomach and intestines with associated sudden onset of vomiting and/or diarrhea. It affects from three to five million people yearly worldwide and affects approximately 20 percent of all hospitalized patients. The pathological inflammation causes hemorrhage and erosion of the mucosal and submucosal layers of the GI tract. This inflammation and erosion can, in turn, damage the villi inside the intestine, which absorb water and nutrients. The water that healthy villi normally would absorb now moves through the bowel at an increased rate. Dehydration secondary to diarrhea is a common cause of death in the developing nations but is seen far less frequently in Canada. Adequate volume replacement is your major prehospital prevention strategy to minimize the likelihood of hypovolemia, or even possible hypovolemic shock.

Individuals who abuse alcohol and tobacco are at high risk for gastritis (inflammation of the stomach) and gastroenteritis (inflammation of the stomach and intestines). A wide variety of chemical agents and incidents can lead to acute gastritis. One of the most common is the use of nonsteroidal anti-inflammatory drugs (NSAIDs), such as aspirin, which break down the mucosal surfaces of the stomach and GI tract. Other causes include excessive alcohol intake and tobacco use; alcohol and nicotine have the same irritating effect on the mucosa as NSAIDs. Stress, chemotherapeutic agents, and the ingestion of acidic or alkalotic agents can also cause acute gastroenteritis. Both systemic infection (salmonellosis) and infection from ingested pathogens (*Staphylococcus*) can cause infectious acute gastroenteritis.

As the name implies, the onset of acute gastroenteritis is rapid and usually severe. The swift movement of fluid through the gastrointestinal tract causes multiple problems. First, and most obvious, diarrhea is almost always associated with this condition. Approximately 7–9 litres of fluid (secretions and ingested fluids) normally move through the GI tract every 24 hours. Of that, less then 2 percent, or approximately 100 mL, is lost in the stool. With acute gastroenteritis, the GI tract expels the fluid that normally would be absorbed. This fluid loss leads to dehydration, which can cause severe hypovolemia in pediatric, geriatric, and previously compromised patients. Besides appearing watery, the stool might show either melena or **hematochezia**; the latter is bright red blood resulting from erosion of the lining of the lower GI tract. Along with the changes in stool, patients may have bouts of hematemesis, fever, nausea and vomiting, and general malaise. Due to dehydration and hemorrhage, the patient can be hemodynamically unstable; the secondary assessment may show hypotension, tachycardia, and pale, cool, and clammy skin. The patient may appear restless or show decreased mental status. If dehydration is severe, he can develop chest pain and cardiac dysrhythmias from electrolyte disturbances. The patient may complain of widespread and diffuse abdominal pain that is not specific to any one region. Visible distention is relatively unlikely unless significant gas has built up within the intestines; palpation will probably reveal tenderness throughout the abdomen.

Treatment for acute gastroenteritis is mainly supportive and palliative. Keep the patient positioned with head forward or face to the side to minimize the risk of aspiration should vomiting occur. Be prepared to clear the airway of vomitus or secretions. Maintaining adequate oxygenation is also a high priority. When there is no significant blood loss, the circulatory system's oxygen-carrying capabilities remain intact. You can establish adequate supplemental oxygenation with a nasal cannula at 2–4 Lpm. Rehydration is the next step in treating your patient. If he is conscious and alert, oral fluid rehydration may be appropriate. The easiest and quickest route, however, is IV fluid administration. In the prehospital setting, the fluid of choice is either 0.9 percent NaCl or Ringer's Lactate solution to replace the patient's circulating volume. In-hospital treatment will switch the fluid to D_5/LR or D_5/NS to replace electrolytes. Pharmacological treatment can involve antiemetics, such as promethazine (Phenergan). Additional replacement of electrolytes, such as potassium, may be needed. Provide emotional support during transport. Exercise extreme caution, and use body substance isolation throughout patient contact to prevent the spread of any infectious disease.

Chronic Gastroenteritis

Chronic gastroenteritis is inflammation of GI mucosa marked by long-term mucosal changes or permanent mucosal damage. Unlike acute gastroenteritis, chronic gastroenteritis is primarily due to microbial infection. The most prevalent pathogen is the *Helicobacter pylori* bacillus. Other bacteria that can cause chronic gastroenteritis include *Escherichia coli, Klebsiella pneumoniae, Enterobacter, Campylobacter jejuni, Vibrio cholerae, Shigella,* and *Salmonella.* Many of these bacteria can be found as part of normal enteric flora, and effective vaccination against pathogenic strains has not been possible. *Shigella* and *Salmonella* are not part of the normal spectrum of intestinal flora. Viral pathogens include the Norwalk virus and rotavirus. Among the parasitic causes are the protozoa *Giardia lamblia, Cryptosporidium parvum,* and *Cyclosporidium cayetenis.*

All of these microbes and their associated gastric disorders are far more common in the underdeveloped countries. They are transmitted via the fecal-oral route or through infected food or water. Fecal-oral transmission can occur whenever people practise poor personal hygiene or food-handling techniques. Local water supplies can become contaminated during natural disasters that disrupt

✱ **hematochezia** bright red blood in the stool.

✱ **chronic gastroenteritis** non-acute inflammation of the gastrointestinal mucosa.

> *Most cases of gastroenteritis are viral. Patients with bacterial gastroenteritis tend to be considerably more ill than those with viral gastroenteritis.*
>

normal water distribution and sewage treatment practices. In such instances, people from outside the endemic area may be more vulnerable to infection than is the local population. *Cyclosporidium* infection reportedly can be contracted by swimming in contaminated water.

Gastroenteritis patients commonly present with nausea and vomiting, fever, diarrhea, abdominal pain, cramping, anorexia (loss of appetite), lethargy, and, in severe cases, shock. Usually, the intensity of signs and symptoms reflects the degree of microbial contamination. However, infection with *H. pylori,* the most common infectious gastroenteritis in Canada, often presents with common signs, such as heartburn, abdominal pain, and, on endoscopic examination, gastric ulcers.

When in contaminated environments, be sure to decontaminate the drinking water or use a different water source; when in doubt about the reliability of the water, drink only beverages that have been brisk boiled or disinfected. Make sure proper sanitation and preparation of foods are maintained. Handwashing and body substance isolation will protect most EMS providers and prevent transmitting the organism further. To avoid transmitting the disease to patients, health-care providers should not work when they are ill.

Prehospital treatment involves protecting yourself and the patient from further contamination, monitoring the ABCs, and transport. Medical treatment of infectious gastroenteritis will require identification of the offending organism. Some of the causative microorganisms are sensitive to antibiotics, but for most the patient will be provided supportive care while the disease takes its natural path.

Peptic Ulcers

Peptic ulcers are erosions caused by gastric acid (Figure 32-2). They can occur anywhere in the GI tract; terminology is based on the portion of the GI tract affected. Duodenal ulcers most frequently occur in the proximal portion of the duodenum; gastric ulcers occur exclusively in the stomach. Overall, peptic ulcers occur in males four times more frequently than in females, and duodenal ulcers occur from two to three times more frequently than do gastric ulcers. Current Canadian statistics place the number of peptic ulcers at 400 000, with approximately 50 000 new cases diagnosed yearly. Those patients who are more likely to have gastric ulcers are over 50 years old and work in jobs requiring physical activity. Their pain usually increases after eating or on a full stomach, and they usually have no pain at night. Duodenal ulcers are more common in patients from 25 to 50 years old who are executives or leaders under high stress. There is also some familial tendency toward duodenal ulcer, suggesting genetic predisposition. Patients with duodenal ulcers commonly have pain at night or whenever their stomach is empty. Thus, it is important in taking the focused history to get family history and a reliable estimate of the patient's last oral intake. Measurement of hematocrit may substantiate any suspicions of chronic or acute hemorrhage.

Nonsteroidal anti-inflammatory medications (aspirin, Motrin, Advil, Naprosyn), acid-stimulating products (alcohol, nicotine), or *Helicobacter pylori* bacteria are the most common causes of peptic ulcers. To help break down food boluses, the stomach secretes hydrochloric acid. One of the enzymes that controls this secretion is pepsinogen. The hydrochloric acid helps convert pepsinogen into its active form, pepsin. Between them, the pepsin and the hydrochloric acid can make the digestive enzymes highly irritating to the GI tract's mucosal lining. Ordinarily, mucous gland secretions protect the stomach's mucosal barrier from these irritants. But when NSAIDs, acid stimulators, or *H. pylori* damage the barrier, the mucosa is exposed to the highly acidic fluid, and peptic ulcers result. Prostaglandin, an important locally acting hormone, decreases the stimulation for blood flow through the gastric mucosa, thus allowing its further destruction.

Helicobacter pylori is associated with gastric and duodenal ulcers.

✱ **peptic ulcer** erosion caused by gastric acid.

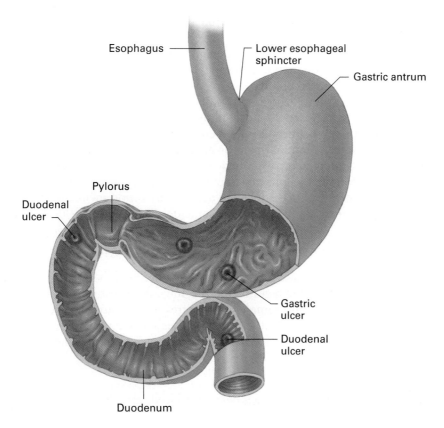

Esophagus — — ┌─ Lower esophageal
sphincter

┌─ Gastric antrum

Pylorus

Duodenal
ulcer

Gastric
ulcer

Duodenal
ulcer

Duodenum

FIGURE 32-2   Peptic ulcer.

Treatment strategies in the prehospital setting focus on antacid treatment and support of any complications, such as hemorrhage.

The recent discovery that *Helicobacter pylori* bacteria appear in more than 80 percent of gastric and duodenal ulcers has enabled physicians to treat the disease by eliminating its cause with antacids and antibiotics, rather than merely treating its symptoms. Definitive treatment includes tamponade of any bleed, possibly by surgical resection, and antibiotic therapy along with histamine blockers and antacids. If medical therapy fails and the problem persists, it may require surgical resection of the vagus nerve (vagotomy) to reduce the stimulation of acid secretion.

A blocked pancreatic duct can also contribute to duodenal ulcers. As chyme passes through the pyloric sphincter from the stomach into the duodenum, the pancreas secretes an alkalotic solution laden with bicarbonate ions that neutralize the acidic hydrogen ions in the chyme. If the pancreatic duct is blocked, however, the acidic chyme can cause ulcerations throughout the intestine. One other cause of duodenal ulcers is **Zollinger-Ellison syndrome,** in which an acid-secreting tumour provokes the ulcerations.

Findings on clinical examination of a patient with peptic ulcer can vary. Chronic ulcers can cause a slow bleed with resulting anemia. Visual inspection of the abdomen is usually helpful only if significant hemorrhage has occurred, in which case the same signs of ecchymosis and distention are found as in other causes of upper GI bleeding. On palpation, pain may be localized or diffuse. These patients often have relief of pain after eating or coating their GI tract with a liquid, such as milk.

Acute, severe pain is probably due to a rupture of the ulcer into the peritoneal cavity causing hemorrhage. Depending on the ulcer's location, the patient may have hematemesis or may have melena-coloured stool. Bouts of nausea and

✱ **Zollinger-Ellison syndrome**
condition that causes the
stomach to secrete excessive
amounts of hydrochloric acid
and pepsin.

vomiting due to the irritation of the mucosa are common. If the ulcer has eroded through a highly vascular area, massive hemorrhage can occur. Along with the signs of hemorrhage, on visual inspection, these patients will appear very ill and have signs of hemodynamic instability, such as pale, cool, and clammy skin, tachycardia, decreased blood pressure, and, possibly, altered mental status. Most patients will lie still to decrease the pain. They may have surgical scars from previous ulcer repair. Bowel sounds will usually be absent.

Treatment for peptic ulcers depends on the severity of the patient's pain. Those who have abdominal pain or hemodynamic instability may require comfortable positioning and psychological support, high-flow oxygen, IV access for fluid resuscitation and pharmacological administration, and rapid transport. Common medications to reduce the mucosal irritation include histamine blockers, such as Zantac and Pepcid, and antacids, such as Rolaids or Tums.

LOWER GASTROINTESTINAL DISEASES

The lower GI tract consists of the jejunum and ileum of the small intestine and the entire large intestine, the rectum, and the anus. As digestive fluid moves through the small intestine (approximately six metres long), nutrients are absorbed into the blood. Water is absorbed and solid wastes formed in the large intestine, also called the large bowel or colon, which is roughly 1.5 metres long.

Lower GI Bleeding

Lower gastrointestinal bleeding is defined as bleeding in the GI tract distal to the ligament of Treitz. Lower GI hemorrhages most frequently occur in conjunction with chronic disorders and anatomical changes associated with advanced age. The most common cause is diverticulosis, which is most prevalent in elderly people. Other causes are colon lesions (cancer or benign polyps), rectal lesions (hemorrhoids, anal fissures, anal fistulas), and inflammatory bowel disorders, such as ulcerative colitis and Crohn's disease. These chronic disorders and diverticulosis rarely result in a massive hemorrhage, such as that which can occur in the esophagus or stomach.

Your assessment of patients with suspected lower GI bleeds will be identical to your assessment of those with suspected upper GI bleeds. After you complete your primary assessment and treat all life-threatening conditions, you can conduct your focused history and secondary assessment. First, ask the patient whether this is a new complaint or a chronic problem. If a chronic problem, check the abdomen visually for scars from previous surgery. Frequent complaints with lower GI bleeding include cramping pain that may be described as resembling a muscle cramp or gas pain, nausea and vomiting, and changes in stool. Melenic stool usually indicates a slow GI bleed. If the stool contains bright red blood, the hemorrhage either is very large (thus passing through the intestines before melenic change can occur) or has occurred in the distal colon. In the latter case, hemorrhoids or rectal fissures are possible causes. The abdominal assessment will show findings similar to those for a bleeding peptic ulcer. If the abdomen has the distention or ecchymosis characteristic of significant hemorrhage, check for signs of early shock, such as pale, cool, and clammy skin, tachycardia, decreased blood pressure, and, possibly, altered mental status. Because most patients with lower GI bleeds have not lost significant amounts of blood, they will present with hemodynamic stability, including warm dry skin, on secondary assessment.

How you manage the patient with a lower GI bleed will depend on his physiological status. Watch his airway and oxygenation status closely. If hypoventilation or inadequate respirations develop, administer high-flow oxygenation via a nonrebreather mask or positive pressure ventilation. Establish IV access and fluid resuscitation on the basis of your patient's hemodynamic status. Place him

Content Review

LOWER GI TRACT

Jejunum
Ileum
Large intestine
Rectum
Anus

✱ **lower gastrointestinal bleeding** bleeding in the gastrointestinal tract distal to the ligament of Treitz.

Content Review

MAJOR CAUSES OF LOWER GI HEMORRHAGE

• Diverticulosis
• Colon lesions
• Rectal lesions
• Inflammatory bowel disorder

Lower gastrointestinal bleeding is usually chronic and rarely results in exsanguinating hemorrhage.

in a comfortable position, offer psychological support, and transport him for further examination.

Ulcerative Colitis

Ulcerative colitis is classified as an idiopathic inflammatory bowel disorder (IBD), that is, one of unknown origin. The inflammatory (ulcerative) process creates a continuous length of chronic ulcers in the mucosal layer of the colon; extension of the ulcers into the submucosal layer is uncommon. As ulcers heal, granular tissue replaces the ulcerations, thickening the mucosa. Approximately 75 percent of all ulcerative colitis involves the rectum or rectosigmoid portion of the large intestine. The inflammatory process usually starts in the rectum and then extends proximally into the colon, sometimes affecting the entire large intestine. If it spreads throughout the entire colon, it is called **pancolitis;** if limited to the rectum, it is called **proctitis.**

Though ulcerative colitis is relatively unusual in Africa or Asia, its occurrence in the Western Hemisphere is increasing rapidly. In Canada, many new cases are diagnosed each year. It most frequently strikes people between the ages of 20 and 40 years. Although researchers have not found a specific pathogen or cause of ulcerative colitis, they have determined many different contributing factors—psychological, allergic and other immunological, toxic, environmental, and infectious. Current research has found that the release of cytokines can cause an overwhelming inflammatory response in the submucosa, much like the release of histamines during anaphylaxis.

Acute ulcerative colitis is difficult to differentiate from other causes of lower GI bleeding. Because of its insidious presentation, diagnosing, tracking, and treating ulcerative colitis may require hematocrit and hemoglobin results, guaiac analyses of the stool, and endoscopic examinations. The severity of the signs and symptoms of ulcerative colitis is usually related directly to the extent and severity of current inflammation in the colon. In patients with mild signs and symptoms, the disease often is isolated in one distal segment of the GI tract. Severe presentations, however, normally involve the entire colon.

Typically, ulcerative colitis presents as a recurrent disorder with occasional bloody diarrhea or stool containing mucus. Accompanying the stool abnormalities are **colicky abdominal pain** (cramping), nausea and vomiting, and, occasionally, fever (suggesting infection) or weight loss (suggesting severe or longer-term colonic dysfunction). The cramping is usually limited to the lower quadrants, depending on the extent of colonic involvement, and it occurs when the hypertrophic muscles lying beneath the submucosa prevent the colon from stretching in response to pressure from its contents. These patients will typically appear restless due to abdominal discomfort but will not show signs of hemodynamic instability (that is, skin will be warm and dry, rather than cool and clammy).

More severe cases may present with bloody diarrhea and intense colicky abdominal pain, electrolyte derangements due to fluid loss through the colon, ischemic damage to the colon itself, or, eventually, perforation of the bowel. Often, these patients present with signs and symptoms of hypovolemic shock, such as pale, cool, clammy skin, hypotension, and tachycardia. Such patients with advanced disease and ongoing hemorrhage may have distention or ecchymosis on the skin and may show guarding of the lower quadrants during the secondary assessment. Significant hemorrhage is common in patients with ulcerative colitis.

Your management of the patient with ulcerative colitis will depend on his physiological status. If he presents with signs and symptoms of hypovolemic shock, administer high-flow oxygen and circulatory support, including intravenous access and fluid resuscitation. If your patient has bouts of nausea and

Content Review

LOWER GI DISEASES
Ulcerative colitis
Crohn's disease
Diverticulitis
Hemorrhoids
Bowel obstruction

✱ **pancolitis** ulcerative colitis spread throughout the entire colon.

✱ **proctitis** ulcerative colitis limited to the rectum.

✱ **colicky abdominal pain** acute pain associated with cramping or spasms in the abdominal organs.

Patients with ulcerative colitis are at increased risk of developing colon cancer.

Transport any patient who presents with lower GI bleeding or colicky pain to the emergency department for diagnostic evaluation.

vomiting, you must diligently manage his airway to prevent aspiration of vomitus. Transport any patient who presents with lower GI bleeding or colicky pain to the emergency department for diagnostic evaluation.

Crohn's Disease

✱ Crohn's disease idiopathic inflammatory bowel disorder associated with the small intestine.

Crohn's disease, along with ulcerative colitis, is the other idiopathic inflammatory bowel disorder in humans. It is more common in the Western Hemisphere, with an incidence in females of 6.5 per 100 000 and 3.1 per 100 000 in males. This disease, which strongly tends to run in families, is most prevalent among white females, those under frequent stress, and in the Jewish population.

Unlike ulcerative colitis, which affects the large intestine, Crohn's disease can occur anywhere from the mouth to the rectum. Between 35 and 45 percent of less severe cases involve the small intestine only; approximately 40 percent involve the colon itself. Severe cases of Crohn's disease may involve any portion of the GI tract, causing a variety of problems ranging from diarrhea to intestinal and perianal abscesses and fistulas (the latter are abnormal passages connecting two internal organs or different lengths of intestine). Complete intestinal obstruction, a surgical emergency, can also occur. Significant lower GI bleeding, however, is rare with Crohn's disease.

As the pathological inflammation begins, it damages the innermost layer of tissue, the mucosa. Granulomas then form and further break down the mucosal and submucosal layers. The affected section of the intestinal wall eventually becomes rubbery and nondistendable due to hypertrophy and fibrosis of the muscles underlying the submucosa. The patchwork-quilt formation of granulomas, fibrosis, and hypertrophy also decreases the intestine's internal diameter, resulting in fissures (incomplete tears) in the mucosa and possibly deeper into the submucosa as food boluses pass through. If a tear extends into the blood vessels in the submucosal layer, small bleeds result. The same pathological pattern of ulceration and scarring can lead to the creation of fistulas, most commonly between lengths of small intestine, or to obstruction of the small bowel. Increased suppressor T-lymphocyte activity suggests an immune-mediated role in the inflammatory process.

Prehospital diagnosis of Crohn's disease is next to impossible because the patient's clinical presentations can vary drastically as the disease progresses.

Crohn's patients' clinical presentations can vary drastically as the disease progresses, and prehospital diagnosis is difficult or next to impossible. Common signs and symptoms include GI bleeding, recent weight loss, intermittent abdominal cramping/pain, nausea and vomiting, diarrhea, and fever. Onset of a flare-up in disease activity is usually rapid, often requiring a visit to the emergency department or physician's office. Abdominal pain cannot be localized to any specific quadrant since the disease can affect any portion of the small intestine and often affects more than one. The secondary assessment is also nonspecific and non-localized, with diffuse tenderness the most commonly found sign. Absence of bowel sounds in a patient with Crohn's disease strongly suggests intestinal obstruction, a surgical emergency.

Because the vast majority of patients with Crohn's disease are hemodynamically stable, prehospital treatment is largely palliative. Your management depends on the patient's physiological status. If he has bouts of nausea and vomiting you must diligently manage the airway to prevent aspiration of vomitus. If he presents with signs and symptoms of obstruction or significant hemorrhage, administer high-flow oxygenation and circulatory support, including intravenous access and fluid resuscitation. As always, calmly and quietly inform the patient of all measures taken and offer psychological support en route to the emergency facility.

Diverticulitis

Diverticulitis is a relatively common complication of diverticulosis. **Diverticulosis** a condition characterized by the presence in the intestine of **diverticula**, small outpouchings of mucosal and submucosal tissue that push through the outermost layer of the intestine, the muscle. Colonic diverticula are far more common in the developed countries, such as Canada, and increase markedly in prevalence with increased age. They are present in more than half of patients over 60 years of age. Diverticulitis is an inflammation of diverticula secondary to infection. Unlike diverticulosis, it is symptomatic; patients will complain of lower left-sided pain (because most diverticula are in the sigmoid colon); exam and testing will show fever and an increased white blood cell count.

The pathogenesis of an acquired diverticulum is twofold. First, stool passes sluggishly through the colon, a condition associated with the relatively low-fibre diets common in the developed countries. The colon responds with muscle spasms that increase bulk movement by raising the pressure on the contents inside the colon and pushing the fecal material forward. Second, the outermost layer of colon tissue is made up of fibrous bands of muscle wrapped around one another. Among them are muscles called the teniae coli. Nerves and blood vessels enter the colon through small openings within the teniae coli. These openings become weakened with age, and the increased pressure of muscle spasms can cause the inner layers of tissue, the mucosa and submucosa, to herniate through the openings, forming diverticula.

These diverticula commonly trap small amounts of fecal material, including sunflower seeds, popcorn fragments, okra seeds, sesame seeds, and others. The entrapped feces may allow bacteria other then the normal flora to grow and cause an infection. The problem is compounded when the diverticula become inflamed, causing diverticulitis. Complications secondary to diverticulitis include possible hemorrhage or larger perforations of the colon wall through which the infected fecal contents can spill into the peritoneal cavity and cause peritonitis.

The most common presentation of diverticulitis is colicky pain associated with a low-grade fever, nausea and vomiting, and tenderness on palpation. The pain is usually localized to the lower left side because the sigmoid colon is involved in 95 percent of reported cases. Thus, diverticulitis is often called left-sided appendicitis. If the diverticula begin to bleed significantly, the usual signs and symptoms associated with severe lower GI bleeding may be present: cool, clammy skin, tachycardia, and diaphoresis. Bleeding diverticula can also result in bright red and bloody feces (hematochezia) because of their close proximity to the rectum. Patients may additionally complain of the perception that they cannot empty their rectums, even after defecation.

Prehospital treatment for diverticulitis is mainly supportive. Measures to counter hypovolemic shock will only be needed when significant hemorrhage has occurred. Monitor the patient's airway and oxygenation and provide supplemental oxygen if needed. Establish intravenous access and begin fluid resuscitation if the patient is hemodynamically unstable. Treatment in the hospital includes antibiotic therapy, endoscopy, and radiological tests to locate the diverticula. Long-term treatment includes implementing a high-fibre diet to stimulate daily bowel movements.

Hemorrhoids

Hemorrhoids are small masses of swollen veins that occur in the anus (external) or rectum (internal). They frequently develop during the fourth decade of life. Most hemmorhoids are idiopathic (of unknown cause), although they can result from pregnancy or protal hypertension. External hemorrhoids often result from lifting a heavy object. Other causes of hemorrhoids include straining at defecation and

---

✳ **diverticulitis** inflammation of diverticula.

✳ **diverticulosis** presence of diverticula, with or without associated bleeding.

✳ **diverticula** small outpouchings in the mucosal lining of the intestinal tract.

The most common presentation of diverticulitis is colicky pain—usually on the lower left side—associated with a low-grade fever, nausea and vomiting, and tenderness on palpation.

The presence of diverticuli in the colon is common in the elderly. Some patients with diverticuli will develop bleeding, while others will develop an infection (diverticulitis).

✳ **hemorrhoid** small mass of swollen veins in the anus or rectum.

Rarely do hemorrhoids cause a massive hemorrhage.

a diet low in fibre. Overall, hemorrhoids are very common, particularly in persons over the age of 50 years. Their morbidity is low in most cases; one marked exception is in alcoholic patients with cirrhosis of the liver.

Internal hemorrhoids most often involve the inferior hemorrhoidal plexus and vasculature. They commonly bleed during the process of defecation due to straining and then thrombose into a closed state again. External hemorrhoids result from thrombosis of a vein, often following lifting or straining, causing bright red bleeding with a bowel movement. The increased venous pressure sometimes causes the vessels to erode and bleed spontaneously, which increases the risk of infection. Rarely do hemorrhoids cause a significant hemorrhage.

Patients with hemorrhoids commonly call for emergency care because of bright red bleeding and pain on defecation. Secondary assessment usually reveals a hemodynamically stable patient with relatively normal appearance (warm, dry skin, perhaps with slight tachycardia consistent with anxiety) who bleeds with defecation. Visual examination of the stool may reveal gross bleeding. Treatment for hemorrhoids depends on the patient's condition. Most frequently, emotional reassurance and transport are all that is needed; however, you should remain alert to the possibility that the bleeding could be from a lower GI bleed, potentially resulting in uncontrolled hemorrhage. Either significant hemorrhage or bleeding hemorrhoids in an alcoholic patient warrant closer monitoring and transport for immediate followup.

Bowel Obstruction

Bowel obstructions are blockages of the hollow space, or lumen, within the small and large intestines. Obstructions can be either partial or complete. An obstructed bowel segment can be catastrophic if not rapidly diagnosed and treated. Of this malady's many different causes, **hernias, intussusception, adhesions,** and **volvulus** are the four most frequent, accounting for more than 70 percent of all reported cases (Figure 32-3). Other common causes are foreign bodies, gallstones, tumours, adhesions from previous abdominal surgery, and bowel **infarction.** The most common location for obstructions is the small intestine, due to its smaller diameter and its greater length, flexibility, and mobility.

The obstruction may be chronic, as with tumour growth or adhesion progression, or its onset may be sudden and acute, as with obstruction by a foreign body. Chronic obstruction usually results in a decreased appetite, fever, malaise, nausea and vomiting, weight loss, or, if rupture occurs, peritonitis. Acute-onset pain may follow ingestion of a foreign body. Pain might also be due to a strangulated hernia, one that has rotated through the muscle wall of the abdomen such that blood flow is suddenly cut off (the herniated tissue has been "strangulated") and ischemia, or even infarction, of tissue occurs. Patients with bowel obstruction will frequently vomit, with the vomitus often containing a significant amount of bile. Severe bowel obstructions may result in the patient's vomiting material that looks and smells like feces. All of these findings suggest a bowel obstruction.

These patients present with diffuse visceral pain, usually poorly localized to any one specific location. They may be hemodynamically unstable due to necrosis within an organ, and you may see signs and symptoms of shock (pale, cool, clammy skin, tachycardia, alterations in level of consciousness, and hypotension). Visual inspection may reveal distention, peritonitis, or free air within the abdomen secondary to rupture of a strangulated segment of intestine. Look for scars left from previous surgery, as well as for the ecchymosis indicating that significant hemorrhage has occurred into the abdominal cavity. In the earliest phase of acute obstruction, bowel sounds may be present as a high-pitched obstruction sound. In most cases, however, bowel sounds will be greatly reduced or

* **bowel obstruction** blockage of the hollow space within the intestines.

> An obstructed bowel segment can be catastrophic if not rapidly diagnosed and treated.
>

* **hernia** protrusion of an organ through its protective sheath.

* **intussusception** condition that occurs when part of an intestine slips into the part just distal to itself.

* **adhesion** union of normally separate tissue surfaces by a fibrous band of new tissue.

* **volvulus** twisting of the intestine on itself.

* **infarction** area of dead tissue caused by lack of blood.

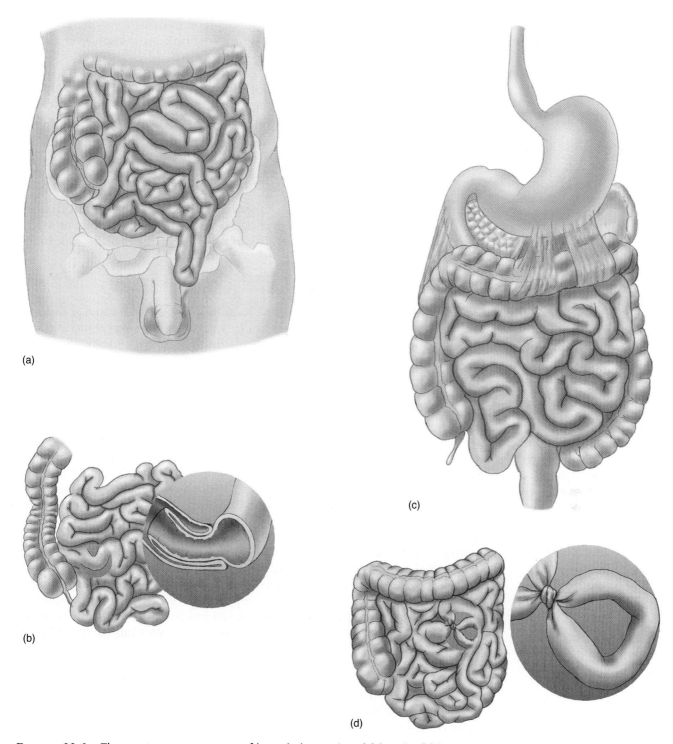

FIGURE 32-3   The most common causes of bowel obstruction: (a) hernia; (b) intussusception; (c) adhesion; (d) volvulus.

Content Review

ACCESSORY ORGAN DISEASES

• Appendicitis
• Cholecystitis
• Pancreatitis
• Hepatitis

✱ **appendicitis** inflammation of the vermiform appendix at the juncture of the large and small intestines.

Appendicitis is evaluated in the emergency department and eventually treated in the operating room more frequently than any other abdominal emergency.

🔑

✱ **McBurney's point** common site of pain from appendicitis, four to five centimetres above the anterior iliac crest in a direct line with the umbilicus.

absent. Palpation will reveal tenderness. Be careful to palpate very lightly if you suspect obstruction, as additional pressure may bring about rupture of the obstructed segment.

The treatment for a patient with an obstructed bowel is based on physiological and psychological support during expedited transport to an appropriate facility. Measures include airway management, oxygenation via a nonrebreather mask at 15 Lpm, position of comfort or shock position, and fluid resuscitation to prevent shock.

ACCESSORY ORGAN DISEASES

As you learned earlier in this chapter, the GI tract has three closely associated organs, the liver, gallbladder, and pancreas, as well as the small structure called the vermiform appendix. Accessory organ emergencies can arise in all four locations.

Appendicitis

Appendicitis is an inflammation of the vermiform appendix, located at the junction of the large and small intestines (the ileocecal junction). Appendicitis occurs in approximately 10 percent of the population in Canada, and it is most common in young adults. Acute appendicitis is the most common surgical emergency you will encounter in the field, mostly in older children and young adults. There are no particular risk factors.

The appendix has no known anatomical or physiological function; most of its tissue is lymphoid in type. It lies just inferior to the ileocecal valve and the first section of the ascending colon. Depending on the individual patient, it may be in the retroperitoneal, pelvic, or abdominal cavity. The appendix can become inflamed, and if left untreated, it can rupture, spilling its contents into the peritoneal cavity and setting up peritonitis.

The pathogenesis of appendicitis is most often due to obstruction of the appendiceal lumen by fecal material. The shape and location of the appendix make it particularly vulnerable to obstruction by feces or other material, such as food particles or tumour. This inflames the lymphoid tissue and often leads to bacterial or viral infection that ulcerates the mucosa. The inflammation also causes the appendix's internal diameter to expand, which can block the appendicular artery and cause thrombosis. With its blood supply cut off, the appendix becomes ischemic, and infarction and necrosis of tissue follows. At this point, the vessel walls often weaken to the point of rupture, spilling the appendiceal contents into the peritoneal cavity.

Appendicitis is frequently misdiagnosed due to the wide variety of signs and symptoms that can accompany it. Mild or early appendicitis causes diffuse, colicky pain often associated with nausea and vomiting and sometimes a low-grade fever. Often, the pain is initially located in the periumbilical region. Due to appendiceal blockage, the patient usually loses his appetite. As the appendix continues to dilate, the pain will localize in the right lower quadrant. A common site of pain is **McBurney's point**, 4 to 5 cm above the anterior iliac crest along a direct line from the anterior crest to the umbilicus (Figure 32-4). Once the appendix ruptures, the pain becomes diffuse due to development of peritonitis.

Secondary assessment will find the patient in apparent discomfort. The abdominal assessment will reveal tenderness or guarding around the umbilicus or right lower quadrant. Do not repeatedly palpate for rebound tenderness. The pressure that this procedure exerts can cause an inflamed appendix to rupture.

Prehospital care for appendicitis includes placing the patient in a position of comfort, giving psychological support, diligently managing his airway to prevent

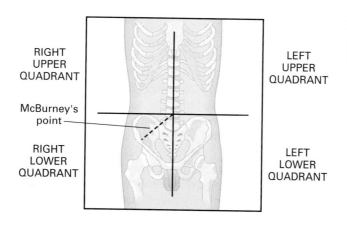

aspiration, establishing intravenous access, and transporting him. In most cases, the appendix will not have ruptured, and the patient will remain hemodynamically stable. Monitor as you would for bowel obstruction, and treat any complications, such as tachycardia or other signs of shock, as they arise.

Cholecystitis

Cholecystitis is an inflammation of the gallbladder. Cholelithiasis (the formation of gallstones), which causes 90 percent of cholecystitis cases, occurs in approximately 12–15 percent of the adult population in Canada, with more than 100 000 new cases diagnosed annually. There are two types of gallstones, cholesterol-based and bilirubin-based. Cholesterol-based stones are far more common and are associated with a specific risk profile: obese, middle-aged women who have more than one biological child.

Definitive treatment of acute cholecystitis includes antibiotic therapy, laparoscopic surgery, lithotripsy (ultrasound treatment to break up the stones), and surgery if the other, less invasive, therapies fail. With the advent of laparoscopic surgery, mortality has fallen to less then 1 percent, with an overall morbidity of approximately 6 percent.

Cholecystitis caused by gallstones can be chronic or acute. The liver produces bile, the primary vehicle for removing cholesterol from the body. The bile travels down the common bile duct to empty into the small intestine at the sphincter of Oddi. The sphincter of Oddi opens when chyme exits the stomach through the cardiac sphincter. When the sphincter of Oddi closes, the flow of bile backs up into the gallbladder via the cystic duct. The bile remains in the gallbladder until the sphincter of Oddi opens again.

The bile can become supersaturated and calculi—stone-like masses based on bilirubin, cholesterol, or both—form. These calculi travel down the cystic duct, frequently lodging in the common bile duct. When they obstruct the flow of bile, gallbladder inflammation and irritation result. The bile salts subsequently attack the mucosal membrane lining the gallbladder, leaving the underlying epithelial tissue without protection. Prostaglandins are also released, further irritating the epithelial wall. As irritation continues, the inflammation grows, increasing intraluminal pressure and ultimately reducing blood flow to the epithelium.

Other causes of cholecystitis include acalculus cholecystitis (cholecystitis without associated stones) and chronic inflammation caused by bacterial infection. Acalculus cholecystitis usually results from burns, sepsis, diabetes, and multiple organ failure. Chronic cholecystitis resulting from a bacterial infection (*Escherichia coli* and enterococci) presents with an inflammatory process similar to cholelithiasis.

Gallbladder pain is located in the right upper quadrant or epigastrium and is collicky in nature. The problem tends to recur unless surgery is performed.

An inflamed gallbladder usually causes an acute attack of upper right quadrant abdominal pain. The inflammation can cause an irritation of the diaphragm with referred pain in the right shoulder. If the gallstones are lodged in the cystic duct, the pain may be colicky, due to expansion and contraction of the duct. Often, the pain occurs after a meal that is high in fat content because of the secondary release of bile from the gallbladder. The right subcostal region may be tender because of abdominal muscle spasms. Patients may experience extreme pain as the epithelium in the gallbladder erodes away. Sympathetic stimulation because of the pain may cause pale, cool, clammy skin. If peritonitis occurs, the skin may be warm due to increased blood flow to the inflamed peritoneum. Nausea and vomiting are common, due to cystic duct spasm.

Visual inspection may reveal scars from previous gallstone surgeries, but distention and ecchymosis are rarely seen. Palpation may reveal either diffuse right-sided tenderness or point tenderness under the right costal margin, a positive **Murphy's sign.**

Prehospital treatment of the patient with acute cholecystitis is mainly palliative. Place the patient in the position of comfort, maintain his ABCs, ensuring adequate oxygenation, and finally establish intravenous access. Pain medications commonly used include meperidine (Demerol) and butorphanol (Stadol). Morphine is contraindicated because it is believed to cause spasms of the cystic duct.

Pancreatitis

Pancreatitis is an inflammation of the pancreas. Its four main categories, based on cause, are metabolic, mechanical, vascular, and infectious. Metabolic causes, specifically alcoholism, account for approximately 80 percent of all cases; consequently, pancreatitis is common in Canada, due to the high incidence of alcoholism. Mechanical obstructions caused by gallstones or elevated serum lipids account for another 9 percent. Vascular injuries caused by thromboembolisms or shock, along with infectious diseases, account for the remaining 11 percent. Overall mortality in acute pancreatitis is relatively high, approximately 30–40 percent, mainly due to accompanying sepsis and shock, which lead to multisystem organ failure. In acute pancreatitis, the rates of serious morbidity and mortality have been found to be 14 percent each in patients with fewer than three positive findings. The mortality rate exceeded 95 percent when there were three or more positive findings.

The vast bulk of the pancreatic tissue is arranged in glandular structures called *acini* (singular, *acinus*). These cells produce digestive enzymes that empty into the duodenum at the ampulla of Vater, near the junction with the stomach. The other function of the pancreas is endocrine: A small amount of tissue located in isolated islets of tissue secretes the hormones insulin and glucagon. Frequently, gallstones leaving the common bile duct become lodged at the ampulla of Vater and obstruct the pancreatic duct. These obstructions back up pancreatic digestive enzymes into the pancreatic duct and the pancreas itself. The digestive enzymes inflame the pancreas and cause edema, which reduces blood flow, as in the pathogenesis of acute appendicitis. In turn, the decreased blood flow causes ischemia and, finally, acinar destruction. This is often called acute pancreatitis based on rapidity of onset.

Acinar tissue destruction causes a second form of pancreatitis, chronic pancreatitis. Acinar tissue destruction commonly occurs due to chronic alcohol intake, drug toxicity, ischemia, or infectious diseases. Alcohol ingestion results in the deposit of platelet plugs in the acinar tissue. The plugs disrupt the enzymes' flow from the pancreas. When digestive juices back up into the pancreas from the ampulla of Vater, the digestive enzymes can become activated and begin to digest the pancreas itself. Morphologically, this autodigestion appears as lesions and fatty tissue changes on the pancreas.

As tissue digestion continues, the lesion can erode and begin to hemorrhage. This acute exacerbation of pancreatitis causes intense abdominal pain. Its intensity reflects the number of lesions affected or the degree of acinar tissue death. The pain can be localized to the left upper quadrant or may radiate to the back or the epigastric region. Most patients experience nausea followed by uncontrolled vomiting and retching that can further aggravate the hemorrhage. Visual inspection may reveal previous surgical scars for lesion removal; ecchymosis and swelling of the left upper quadrant may also be present due to hemorrhage or significant organ edema. The patient will appear acutely ill with diaphoresis, tachycardia, and possible hypotension if massive hemorrhaging is involved.

Prehospital treatment is supportive and aimed at maintaining the ABCs by providing high-flow oxygenation and establishing intravenous access. Fluid resuscitation with crystalloid solution may be warranted if the patient appears hemodynamically unstable. Definitive treatment involves gastric intubation and suctioning for emesis control, diagnostic peritoneal lavage, antibiotic therapy, fluid resuscitation, and surgery to remove the blockage.

Hepatitis

Hepatitis involves any injury to hepatocytes (liver cells) associated with an inflammation or infection. Due to its wide range of potential causes, hepatitis has a high mortality rate. Five viruses—hepatitis types A, B, C, D, and E—are the most common causes, resulting in five different kinds of hepatitis that together account for 60–70 percent of all cases. Alcoholic hepatitis, which arises from alcoholic cirrhosis, rather than an infectious agent, is responsible for another 20–30 percent. Trauma and other diseases account for the remaining 10 percent. Factors that increase the risk of contracting hepatitis include, to name a few, crowded, unsanitary living conditions, poor personal hygiene that invites oral–fecal transmission, exposure to bloodborne pathogens, and chronic alcohol intake. (Specific risk factors are associated with the different types of hepatitis—A, B, C, D, and E.)

The liver is in the upper right abdominal quadrant. A very vascular organ, it filters and detoxifies blood returning from the abdomen and certain abdominal organs. Its other important functions include synthesizing fatty acids, converting glucose to glycogen, and helping to remove toxic products, such as ammonia, from the body. Any of the viral pathogens, alcoholic exposure, or trauma can injure the hepatocytes, causing inflammation and, possibly, chronic liver disease. Whatever its cause, the results are usually similar. The changes in the liver include enlargement and hypertrophy, fatty changes, loss of architecture, and appearance of lesions and spontaneous hemorrhages. The symptoms' severity can range from mild to complete liver failure and death.

With more than 310 million carriers worldwide, HBV is epidemic.

Of the five types of viral hepatitis, hepatitis A (HAV) is probably the best known. Commonly referred to as infectious hepatitis, (HAV) spreads by the oral–fecal route. The disease is self-limiting, usually lasting between two and eight weeks. It rarely causes severe hepatic injury and thus has a very low mortality rate. Hepatitis B (HBV), known as "serum hepatitis," is transmitted as a bloodborne pathogen that can stay active in bodily fluids outside the body for days. With more than 310 million carriers worldwide, HBV is epidemic. Its effects may be only minimal, but they can also range to severe liver ischemia and necrosis. Hepatitis C (HCV) is caused by the pathogen most commonly responsible for spreading hepatitis through blood transfusions. Hepatitis C is marked by chronic and often debilitating damage to the liver. Hepatitis D (HDV) is a less common disorder because its pathogen is dormant until activated by HBV. He-

Be wary of HIV, but fear hepatitis B and C. Do not forget to use personal protective equipment (PPE) and body substance isolation (BSI) precautions.

patitis E (HEV) is a waterborne infection that has caused epidemics in Africa, Mexico, and other less-developed nations. Its mortality rate among pregnant women is high.

Patients with hepatitis commonly present with symptoms relative to the severity of their disease. Usually, they complain of upper right quadrant abdominal tenderness, not relieved by antacids, food, or positioning. They may lose their appetite and become anorexic, usually losing weight. The decrease in bile production changes their stool to a clay colour, and increased bilirubin retention causes jaundice, a yellow colouring of the skin, and scleral icterus, a yellowing of the white of the eyes. Other symptoms include severe nausea and vomiting, general malaise, photophobia, pharyngitis, and coughing.

Secondary assessment will reveal a sick patient, possibly with a jaundiced appearance. Depending on the patient's severity, his positioning can range from standing up and walking around to lying in a fetal position with his knees drawn to his chest. Pain may present in the right upper quadrant or the right shoulder (referred from diaphragmatic irritation). Fever may be secondary to infection or tissue necrosis. Inspection may yield nonspecific findings. Palpation may reveal an enlarged liver. Skin temperature can range from warm and dry (due to the infection) to cool, clammy, and diaphoretic if a hepatic lesion has ruptured and begun to bleed.

Prehospital treatment is mainly palliative. Secure the ABCs, and establish intravenous access for fluid resuscitation or antiemetic administration. You must carefully consider any pharmacological administration because the liver breaks down many active drug metabolites. Definitive treatment involves antiviral and anti-inflammatory medications and symptomatic treatment.

If you suspect hepatitis, you must consider carefully any pharmacological administration because the liver breaks down many active drug metabolites.

The key to successful treatment of gastrointestinal ailments is prompt recognition, treatment, and rapid transport to the hospital.

ЅUMMARY

Abdominal pain can originate from a wide variety of causes, either from the abdominal organs or from areas outside of the abdominal cavity. The prehospital management priorities for the abdominal patient are to establish and maintain his airway, breathing, and circulation. The differential diagnosis can include a multitude of causes that usually cannot be identified without laboratory and radiographic analysis. Airway management is of paramount importance, since patients frequently suffer from severe bouts of nausea and vomiting. Be prepared to turn the patient onto his side if necessary to clear large amounts of vomitus from the airway. Oxygenation usually can be adequately stabilized by placing the patient on high-flow oxygen via a nonrebreather mask. Fluid loss, hemorrhage, or sepsis may compromise the circulatory status. You should initiate fluid resuscitation for the hemodynamically unstable patient in the field, but never delay transport. Patients who have abdominal pain lasting more than six hours should always be evaluated by a physician.

CHAPTER 33

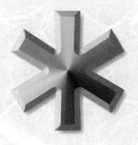

Urology and Nephrology

Objectives

After reading this chapter, you should be able to:

1. Describe the incidence, morbidity, mortality, and risk factors predisposing to urological and nephrological emergencies. (pp. 659–660, 665–666, 669–670, 675–677)

2. Discuss the anatomy and physiology of the organs and structures related to the urinary system. (see Chapter 12)

3. Define referred pain and visceral pain as they relate to urology. (p. 661)

4. Describe the questioning technique and specific questions the paramedic should use when gathering a focused history in a patient with abdominal pain. (pp. 661–663)

5. Describe the technique for performing a comprehensive secondary assessment of a patient complaining of abdominal pain. (pp. 663–665)

6. Define acute renal failure. (pp. 665–666)

7. Discuss the pathophysiology of acute renal failure. (pp. 665–668)

8. Recognize the signs and symptoms related to acute renal failure. (pp. 667–669)

9. Describe the management of acute renal failure. (pp. 668–670)

10. Integrate pathophysiological principles and assessment findings to

Continued

Objectives Continued

formulate a field impression and implement a treatment plan for the patient with acute renal failure. (pp. 665–670)

11. Define chronic renal failure. (pp. 669–670)

12. Discuss the pathophysiology of chronic renal failure. (pp. 669–670)

13. Recognize the signs and symptoms related to chronic renal failure. (pp. 670–672)

14. Describe the management of chronic renal failure. (pp. 672–675)

15. Integrate pathophysiological principles and assessment findings to formulate a field impression and implement a treatment plan for the patient with chronic renal failure. (pp. 669–675)

16. Define renal dialysis. (pp. 672–675)

17. Discuss the common complications of renal dialysis. (pp. 673–674)

18. Define renal calculi. (p. 675)

19. Discuss the pathophysiology of renal calculi. (p. 676)

20. Recognize the signs and symptoms related to renal calculi. (p. 676)

21. Describe the management of renal calculi. (p. 676)

22. Integrate pathophysiological principles and assessment findings to formulate a field impression and implement a treatment plan for the patient with renal calculi. (pp. 675–676)

23. Define urinary tract infection. (p. 677)

24. Discuss the pathophysiology of urinary tract infection. (pp. 677–678)

25. Recognize the signs and symptoms related to urinary tract infection. (pp. 678–679)

26. Describe the management of a urinary tract infection. (pp. 678–679)

27. Integrate pathophysiological principles and assessment findings to formulate a field impression and implement a treatment plan for the patient with a urinary tract infection. (pp. 677–679)

28. Apply epidemiology to develop prevention strategies for urological and nephrological emergencies. (pp. 660, 670)

29. Integrate pathophysiological principles to the assessment of a patient with abdominal pain. (pp. 660–665)

30. Synchronize assessment findings and patient history information to accurately differentiate between pain of a urological or nephrological emergency and that of another origin. (pp. 660–665)

31. Develop, execute, and evaluate a treatment plan based on the field impression made in the assessment. (pp. 659–679)

INTRODUCTION

The **urinary system** performs a number of vital functions. It maintains blood volume and the proper balance of water, electrolytes, and pH (acid-base balance). It ensures that key substances, such as glucose, remain in the bloodstream, and yet it also removes a variety of toxic wastes from the blood. It plays a major role in the regulation of arterial blood pressure. In addition, the urinary system controls the development of red blood cells, or erythrocytes.

The body eliminates water and other substances removed from blood in the form of the fluid **urine.** The kidneys' regulation of water and other important substances in blood is an example of homeostasis, the body's ability to maintain an appropriate internal environment despite changing conditions. Metabolism, the intracellular processes that generate the energy and materials necessary for cell growth and repair, also creates many waste products. For example, significant amounts of ammonia form in the liver when amino acids are broken down in gluconeogenesis, a process that produces glucose between meals. Ammonia is highly toxic to body cells, particularly brain cells. Liver cells convert the ammonia into **urea,** a less toxic compound. The kidneys remove urea efficiently from the blood and pass it into the urine. Moreover, the urinary system eliminates many foreign chemicals, such as drug metabolites.

The urinary system in women is physically distinct from the reproductive system: they share no structures. (Chapters 39 and 40 discuss medical emergencies related to the female reproductive system.) In contrast, the urinary system in men does share some structures with the reproductive system. For instance, both urine and the male reproductive fluid are excreted from the body through the opening at the tip of the penis. Consequently, the term **genitourinary system** is often used with men. The urinary and reproductive systems' proximity in women and their shared structures in men are due to the common embryonic origin of their tissues.

The most significant medical disorders involving the urinary system affect the kidneys and kidney function. **Nephrology** (from the Greek *nephros,* kidney) is the medical specialty devoted to kidney disorders. **Urology** is the surgical specialty devoted to care of the entire urinary system in women and the genitourinary system in men. We will use nephrology and nephrological (or the preferred adjective, **renal,** from the Latin *renes,* kidneys) to refer to conditions primarily affecting the kidneys. We will use urology and urological to refer to conditions that significantly affect other parts of the urinary or genitourinary systems.

Renal and urological disorders are common, affecting approximately two million Canadians. More than 4000 Canadians suffer from the most severe form of long-term kidney failure, **end-stage renal failure.** Kidney disease ranks sixth among diseases causing death in Canada and can strike anyone at any age, although people aged 65 to 74 are the fastest growing group newly diagnosed with kidney failure. The leading causes of kidney failure in new patients are diabetes mellitus, renal vascular disease (including high blood pressure), and glomerulonephritis (inflammation of the tiny filters in the kidney that clean the blood).

Every day an average of 10 Canadians learn that their kidneys have failed and that their survival depends on **dialysis** (a procedure that replaces some lost kidney functions) or a **kidney transplantation** (implantation of a kidney into a person without functioning kidneys). At the end of 2001, 3500 Canadians were on a waiting list for an organ transplantation. Of those, 80 percent were waiting for kidney transplant. In total, it is estimated that there are 25 000 Canadians with kidney failure who are living with dialysis or kidney transplants.

Among acute, or sudden-onset, disorders, **renal calculi,** or kidney stones, are very common. Infections are also common, and they may have different causes in women and men. A woman complaining of burning pain on urination probably

* **urinary system** the group of organs that produces urine, maintaining fluid and electrolyte balance for the body.

* **urine** the fluid made by the kidney and eliminated from the body.

* **urea** waste derived from ammonia produced through protein metabolism.

* **genitourinary system** the male organ system that includes reproductive and urinary structures.

* **nephrology** the medical specialty dealing with the kidneys.

* **urology** the surgical specialty dealing with the urinary/genitourinary system.

* **renal** pertaining to the kidneys.

* **end-stage renal failure** an extreme failure of kidney function due to nephron loss.

* **dialysis** a procedure that replaces some lost kidney functions.

* **kidney transplantation** implantation of a kidney into a person without functioning kidneys.

* **renal calculi** kidney stones.

has an infection in the urinary system. Men with the same chief complaint may have an infection that arose in the urinary system or as a sexually transmitted disease. Noncancerous enlargement of the prostate gland, or **benign prostatic hypertrophy,** affects about 60 percent of men by age 50 and about 80 percent by age 80. If prostatic hypertrophy obstructs urine flow, a medical emergency involving sharp pain and inability to urinate results.

All of these conditions, as well as others described later, are sufficiently common that you will see them in the field. In any case where existing kidney function may be jeopardized, prehospital care includes **preventive strategies,** or steps to minimize the likelihood of any further loss of function. Our discussion of assessment and management will cover these procedures.

GENERAL MECHANISMS OF NONTRAUMATIC TISSUE PROBLEMS

Both traumatic and nontraumatic problems can affect the urinary system, particularly the kidneys. The kidneys' retroperitoneal location protects them relatively well against injury. Nontraumatic renal and urological disorders result from four general mechanisms: inflammatory or immune-mediated disease, infectious disease, physical obstruction, or hemorrhage. Traumatic renal and urological disorders are discussed in Chapter 26. We will discuss nontraumatic disorders later in this chapter.

GENERAL PATHOPHYSIOLOGY, ASSESSMENT, AND MANAGEMENT

As you learned in Chapter 32, abdominal emergencies are common. Because of the similar presentations of many gastrointestinal (GI) and urological emergencies, you may have difficulty determining the source of an abdominal problem when pain is the sole complaint. You can often find clues to the eventual diagnosis when you take a focused history and perform the focused secondary assessment. Before reading further, you may want to review the discussion of GI pathophysiology, assessment, and management in Chapter 32.

PATHOPHYSIOLOGICAL BASIS OF PAIN

Because of the similar presentations of many gastrointestinal and urological emergencies, you may have difficulty determining the source of an abdominal problem when pain is the sole complaint.

The nerve fibres that carry pain messages to the brain are triggered by different stimuli. Some are triggered when damage to the epithelial lining of an organ exposes the underlying tissue layer, where the nerve endings are located. Others respond to stretching forces generated when an organ is inflamed or enlarged by internal hemorrhage or obstruction.

Causes of Pain

Bacterial infection damages the epithelial tissue that lines such structures as the urethra and urinary bladder. This damage causes pain that often worsens when urine flows over the affected tissue during urination. Bacteria normally found on the skin can cause infections in women. In men, the same symptom, pain on voiding, is often due to a sexually transmitted disease, such as gonorrhea. Distention of a ureter by a renal calculus (kidney stone) causes a sharp pain that may ease or worsen when the stone shifts position inside the ureter.

Types of Pain

The most common types of pain in urological emergencies are visceral and referred. **Visceral pain** usually arises in hollow structures, such as the ureters, urinary bladder, and urethra, or the vas deferens or epididymis in males. Its chief characteristic, an aching or crampy pain felt deep within the body and poorly localized, is due to the relatively low number of nerve fibres in the involved structures. Visceral pain can also be the initial presentation of urinary tract infection or of renal calculi. **Referred pain** is felt in a location other than its site of origin. This occurs when afferent nerve fibres carrying the pain message merge with other pain-carrying fibres at the junction with the spinal cord. If that junction has far more nerve fibres from one or more other locations than from the site of origin, the brain may perceive the pain as coming from those locations, rather than the affected one. Pyelonephritis, inflammation associated with kidney infection, is not only associated with pain in the flank, the skin surface closest to the kidney, but sometimes with pain in the neck or shoulder. The referred pain originates in diaphragmatic irritation due to kidney inflammation, but the brain perceives the pain as coming from the area of the neck or shoulder.

* **visceral pain** pain arising in hollow organs, such as the ureter and bladder.

* **referred pain** pain felt in a location other than that of its origin.

ASSESSMENT AND MANAGEMENT

The assessment steps are the same for all abdominal emergencies. Do not try to pinpoint the cause of abdominal pain in the field; diagnosis is often difficult even in the hospital setting. However, you do need to do an assessment to detect and manage life-threatening conditions, such as shock, and to provide historical and physical information that will be helpful in the hospital.

Do not try to pinpoint the cause of abdominal pain in the field.

Scene Assessment

During scene assessment, look for evidence of a traumatic or medical cause and for signs of a life-threatening situation, perhaps an observer performing cardiopulmonary resuscitation (CPR) or the presence of blood. Remember to employ personal protective equipment and proper handling techniques.

Blood always calls for personal protective equipment and proper sample handling on your part.

Primary Assessment

Primary assessment of the patient concentrates on the ABCs of airway, breathing, and circulation, as well as on patient disability (for example, signs of agitation and confused mental state). If the patient is conscious and responsive, ask about the chief complaint.

Focused History

Information about Pain. When the chief complaint is pain or involves pain, initial questions should elicit information about the timing, character, and associated symptoms of the pain. The OPQRST template is useful for beginning your questions.

- *Onset* When did the pain start, and what were you doing at the time? Visceral pain often arises gradually, with the patient first aware of vague discomfort and only later aware of pain.

- *Provocation/palliation* What makes the pain worse or better? Increased pain on urination, particularly in the context of a fever or history of fever, suggests urinary/genitourinary tract infection. Pain associated with the inability to urinate, particularly in elderly men, points toward urethral obstruction due to prostatic enlargement. Improvement with knees drawn up to the chest points toward peritonitis, whereas improvement with walking may indicate a kidney stone that moved into a less-pain-causing position.

- *Quality* What is the pain like? Visceral pain is frequently described as dull or crampy; because many structures of the urinary system are hollow, visceral pain is common in these emergencies. Vague discomfort followed by a change to sharp pain localized in the flank, for instance, may indicate ureteral obstruction due to a kidney stone that has moved.

- *Region/radiation* Where is the pain located, or do you feel pain in several places? Does the pain seem to move from one part of your body to another? Listen for patterns of referred pain, such as pain in the lower back and the neck or shoulder, as well as changes in perception of pain on movement of a limb or the whole body. In postpubertal women, be sure to ask for menstrual history, particularly if menstrual-like cramps are described or blood is present in the perineal area. (For more on gynecological and obstetric emergencies, see Chapters 39 and 40.)

- *Severity* Where is the pain on a scale of 1 to 10? Has the intensity changed over time, and if so, how? Sudden changes to sharp pain, particularly when associated with decreased responsiveness and early signs of shock, may indicate rupture of an internal organ, such as the appendix in appendicitis or the fallopian tube in an ectopic pregnancy. Most urological problems will not show this pattern of abrupt and significant shift in severity and type of pain.

- *Time* How long ago did the pain start? Is it constant, or does it come and go? Remember that any case of abdominal pain lasting about six hours or longer is considered a surgical emergency until proven otherwise, and the patient should be transported to an appropriate facility. Pelvic visceral pain of long duration and unchanging intensity, particularly if associated with signs suggesting urinary-tract origin, such as fever and increased pain on urination, suggests a medical case, rather than a surgical one, but you still may need to transport the patient to the hospital. When confronted with an acute abdomen (sudden onset of severe abdominal pain), always err on the side of considering it a potential surgical emergency.

- *Previous history of similar event* Some urological emergencies, such as renal calculus and infection, may recur. This makes it especially important to elicit any history of a similar event, the diagnosis at the time, and the treatment given. Because increased risk for renal calculi is genetic in some cases, listen for a history of family members similarly affected.

- *Nausea/vomiting* As you learned in Chapter 32, severe pain is often associated with autonomic nervous system discharge producing the signs of nausea, possibly with vomiting, along with profuse sweating, clammy skin, and rapid heart rate. Remember that such a presentation does not necessarily indicate that the problem is in the GI system. For instance, the severe pain of a kidney stone can cause this presentation.

- *Changes in bowel habits and stool* Frequent stools, especially if they are diarrheal or contain signs of blood (either melena or hematochezia), suggest a problem in the GI system. Recent constipation may not be relevant, except in the context of physical findings.

- *Weight loss* Significant weight loss over a very short period (hours or days) almost always reflects water loss, and signs of dehydration will be evident. Longer-term weight loss may suggest chronic illness or GI dysfunction. Be sure to ask about such conditions as diabetes, cardiovascular disease, and cancer, as well as medications and medication changes.

- *Last oral intake* The timing and content of the last meal may indicate an acute, progressive problem (a normal appetite, normal meal) or exacerbation of a longstanding one (poor appetite, small meal). Ask explicitly about fluid intake because patients may not consider beverages as food. The timing of the last oral intake is also important if the patient will be undergoing general anesthesia for a surgical procedure.

- *Chest pain* Chest pain, particularly left-sided, does not necessarily indicate a myocardial infarction (MI). Assess whether the pain pattern suggests angina (for example, chest pain associated with radiation to jaw and left arm). Also remember that patients with longstanding or severe diabetes may not show the typical pain pattern of an MI due to diabetic neuropathy (nerve damage), but signs of ischemia may appear on an electrocardiogram (ECG).

Focused Secondary Assessment

The focused assessment includes forming an overall impression as well as examining the abdomen. Remember that you will not be able to diagnose most cases of abdominal pain in the field. Your job is to gather the historical and physical evidence that can be used in the hospital and to make sure the patient is supported before and during transport.

Appearance In general, any person with significant pain, particularly pain of some duration, will appear uncomfortable. A patient may show discomfort by rigidly maintaining the position of least pain or by constantly pacing if walking helps ease the pain.

Posture Lying with knees drawn to chest suggests peritonitis, which is often of GI origin. Relief with walking suggests visceral pain; kidney stones may shift position during walking, easing the sharp pain. Check visually if the patient who is walking is upright or favouring one side. Someone who looks feverish and walks hunched up, leaning to one side, and complaining of back pain may have a pyelonephritis (kidney infection).

Level of Consciousness In the absence of fever, acute-onset decreases in responsiveness often suggest hemorrhage and evolution of hypovolemic shock. Hemorrhage is far more often tied to GI or reproductive (namely, obstetric) emergencies than to urinary system problems. You may see a decreased level of consciousness in sick patients who are undergoing dialysis, the artificial technique that replaces some vital kidney functions, including maintenance of electrolyte balance and removal of wastes. Try to determine if the change in responsiveness is acute or chronic, which may suggest a new problem or an aggravation of preexisting problems.

Apparent State of Health Patients with chronic illness, whether or not it originates in the urinary system, often look ill even without an acute problem. Extreme thinness, pale skin or mucous membranes, or the presence of home health equipment, such as a bedside toilet, dialysis machine, or an oxygen tank, all suggest chronic problems. In significant emergency states, the patient will usually

During the focused history and secondary assessment, your job is to gather the historical and physical evidence that can be used in the hospital and to make sure the patient is supported before and during transport.

not be tidy and neatly dressed. If she is, this may suggest that the emergency occurred suddenly, as with a hemorrhage or painful passage of a stone.

Skin Colour Pale, dry, cool skin and mucous membranes may suggest chronic anemia, such as that found in persons with chronic renal failure. Pale clammy skin suggests severe pain or shock, whereas flushed, dry skin may accompany fever.

Assessment of the Abdomen The four components of the abdominal assessment are inspection, auscultation, percussion, and palpation.

Always inspect the abdomen first. Note any ecchymotic discoloration or distention, as well as any surgical or traumatic scars. Most nephrological and urological emergencies will not show acute abnormalities on assessment, whereas a number of GI emergencies will. Auscultation rarely produces a positive finding because bowel sounds are almost always present. Absence of bowel sounds, however, is important and suggests a GI emergency, such as bowel obstruction.

Palpation may be more useful in the field. Pain induced by palpation of the flanks, especially when accompanied by fever, strongly suggests pyelonephritis, or kidney infection. Pain on palpation just above the pelvic rim of the abdomen, especially when accompanied by fever and an increased urge to void, suggests cystitis, or bladder infection. Constant, sharp pain increased by palpation of the affected flank may indicate where a kidney stone has lodged in a ureter.

In postpubescent girls and women, abdominal palpation may reveal pregnancy if you feel the firm, muscular mass of the gravid uterus above the pelvic rim. A ruptured ectopic pregnancy is possible when palpation increases pain in the lower quadrant, particularly when accompanied by evidence of hemorrhage or early shock. A vaginal exam is not indicated in the field; however, you should check for blood or other discharge at the urethral or vaginal openings. In all cases, find out the date of the patient's last menstrual period.

Palpation of the lower abdomen may help diagnose acute urinary obstruction in older men due to prostatic enlargement. If enough urine has been retained, you will feel a large (up to roughly the size of a two-litre bottle), painful, fluctuant mass above the pelvic rim of the abdomen. This represents the distended bladder. The male abdominal assessment should also include inspection of the penis and scrotum. Purulent discharge from the penis may indicate a sexually transmitted disease (STD). Palpation of the scrotum may detect a testicular mass (remember that testicular cancer is far more common in younger men—the opposite of the age risk for prostatic cancer). Palpable nontesticular masses may be painful (infectious epididymitis) or nonpainful (varicocele, a noninfectious swelling of the epididymis). Ask relevant questions, such as whether swelling has been present for some time (as occurs with a varicocele) or is of recent onset (epididymitis). Use discretion when palpating a patient's genitals in the field.

Vital Signs Temperature is important because fever suggests an infectious process. If you found high blood pressure, increased heart rate, or both during the ABC assessment, put those findings into context with other impressions from the assessment. For instance, both heart rate and blood pressure commonly increase in someone with severe pain. However, it is also important to find out the patient's usual readings, if either she or a bystander can tell you. Uncontrolled chronic hypertension is one of the two most common causes of nephron damage and chronic renal failure (with the other cause being diabetes mellitus).

Management and Treatment Plans

Management of the patient with abdominal pain includes general and case-specific elements.

Pain on percussion of the costovertebral angle (CVA—where the last rib meets the lumbar vertebrae) is known as Lloyd's sign and is indicative of pyelonephritis (infection of the kidney and renal pelvis).

Airway, Breathing, Circulation Field management always starts with the ABCs—airway, breathing, and circulation. Be sure to maintain an open airway, and administer high-flow oxygen via mask. Be prepared for vomiting with any patient with severe pain, whether or not it is likely of genitourinary origin. Circulatory support is also vital, especially when there is any indication of hemorrhage, dehydration, or shock or the patient appears to have any compromise of renal function. Monitor blood pressure closely, and monitor cardiac status with ECG.

Pharmacological Interventions Consider placing a large-bore IV line for volume replacement or drug administration. Where possible, use a needle of sufficiently large bore for any emergency blood transfusion. In almost all cases involving abdominal pain, the question of **analgesics**, pain-relieving medications, will arise. Analgesics may mask the problem's signs and symptoms, making it very difficult to accurately gauge progression of the pathological process. Use analgesics as sparingly as possible; local protocol or discussion with medical direction may be advisable.

Nonpharmacological Interventions Remember that patients with an acute abdominal problem are possible surgical cases. Thus, nothing should be given by mouth. Administer fluid or medication only by IV or IM routes. Monitor vital signs closely, and look for any change in level of consciousness. Be sure the patient is in a position of relative comfort, but also ensure that the position minimizes risk of aspiration if vomiting occurs.

Transport Considerations Each patient with abdominal pain of more than six hours' duration is considered a surgical emergency until hospital evaluation proves otherwise. Rapidly, yet gently, transport all such patients. During transport, talk quietly to the patient, both to calm her and to keep her informed of time until arrival or other pertinent matters. All of your actions, both with the patient and any family or friends in the ambulance, should reflect caring and competence.

RENAL AND UROLOGICAL EMERGENCIES

You must know how to respond properly and quickly to each major type of urinary or genitourinary emergency. Prevention strategies, procedures that minimize further loss of any existing kidney function, are vital. Most of this discussion focuses on renal emergencies, those affecting the kidneys. The leading causes of kidney failure are diabetes mellitus (both types) and uncontrolled or inadequately controlled hypertension. Add to that profile the fact that the number of nephrons decreases with age, and you have the general profiles of patients most at risk for significant problems affecting kidney function: older patients, those with diabetes or chronic hypertension, or those with more than one risk factor.

We will discuss three renal emergencies—acute renal failure, chronic renal failure, and renal calculi (kidney stones). We will also discuss one urological disorder, urinary tract infection, which can affect any or all parts of the urinary/genitourinary system.

ACUTE RENAL FAILURE

Acute renal failure (ARF) is a sudden (often over a period of days) drop in urine output to less than 400–500 mL per day, a condition called **oliguria**. Output may literally fall to zero, a condition called **anuria**. ARF is not uncommon among severely ill, hospitalized patients. It is less common in the field. Noting ARF in the prehospital setting is vital because the condition may be reversible, dependent on the cause and extent of damage associated with the disorder. Overall mortality is roughly 50 percent, in part because the condition usually appears in significantly injured or ill persons.

In cases of abdominal pain, use analgesics as sparingly as possible.

---

* **analgesics** pain relieving medictions.

Content Review

PATIENTS MOST AT RISK FOR SIGNIFICANT KIDNEY PROBLEMS

- Older patients
- Patients with diabetes
- Patients with chronic hypertension
- Patients with more than one risk factor

Content Review

MOST COMMON RENAL EMERGENCIES

- Acute renal failure
- Chronic renal failure
- Renal calculi

---

* **acute renal failure (ARF)** the sudden-onset of severely decreased urine production.

---

* **oliguria** decreased urine elimination to 400–500 mL or less per day.

---

* **anuria** no elimination of urine.

✱ **prerenal acute renal failure**
ARF due to decreased blood perfusion of kidneys.

Pathophysiology

The three types of ARF are prerenal, renal, and postrenal. The distinct initial pathophysiology of each type determines both the severity of ARF and the likelihood for reversal and preservation of renal function. The three types' common point is their clinical presentation: sudden-onset oliguria or anuria. You may wish to reread the summary of kidney physiology before reading about the pathophysiology for each type of ARF.

Prerenal ARF Prerenal ARF begins with dysfunction before the level of the kidney; that is, with insufficient blood supply to the kidneys, or hypoperfusion. Prerenal ARF not only accounts for the highest proportion of ARF cases—40 to 80 percent—but is also often reversible through restoration of proper perfusion. These factors make it extremely important to know conditions associated with increased risk of renal hypoperfusion and to treat the patient quickly and properly. Problems that can trigger prerenal ARF include some common field conditions: hemorrhage, heart failure, myocardial infarction, or congestive heart failure, sepsis, and shock (Table 33-1). These triggers decrease renal blood supply through a drop in blood volume, blood pressure, or both. In addition, any anomaly directly affecting blood flow into the kidneys (such as thrombosis of a renal artery or vein) can trigger prerenal ARF through an increase in renal vascular resistance. When renal vascular resistance becomes higher in the renal vessels than in systemic vessels, blood is effectively shunted away from the kidneys.

Normally, the kidneys receive about 20 to 25 percent of cardiac output. This high level of perfusion is essential to sustaining a glomerular filtration rate (GFR) sufficient to maintain blood volume and composition and to clear wastes, such as urea and creatinine, from the bloodstream. As the GFR drops, less urine forms, and the bloodstream retains water, electrolytes, and wastes, such as urea and creatinine. Because the retained electrolytes include H^+ and K^+, metabolic acidosis and hyperkalemia may appear.

If hypoperfusion is prolonged or worsens in degree, two things happen. First, the GFR decreases still further, and less filtrate means still less urine formation. Second, the nephron tubular cells become ischemic, and active reabsorption and secretion decrease or cease. All of these metabolic effects of decreased nephron function further stress the body, particularly the cardiovascular system, and increase the likelihood that tubular ischemia will advance toward tubular cell death. At this point, the process is renal ARF, not prerenal.

Table 33-1 CAUSES OF PRERENAL, RENAL, AND POSTRENAL ACUTE RENAL FAILURE (ARF)

Prerenal ARF	Renal ARF	Postrenal ARF
Hypovolemia (hemorrhage, dehydration, burns)	Small vessel/glomerular damage (vasculitis—often immune-mediated, acute glomerulonephritis, malignant hypertension)	Abrupt obstruction of both ureters (secondary to large stones, blood clots, tumour)
Cardiac failure (myocardial infarction, congestive heart failure, valvular disease)	Tubular cell damage (acute tubular necrosis—either ischemic or secondary to toxins)	Abrupt obstruction of the bladder neck (secondary to benign prostatic hypertrophy, stones, tumour, clots)
Cardiovascular collapse (shock, sepsis)	Interstitial damage (acute pyelonephritis, acute allergic interstitial reactions)	Abrupt obstruction of the urethra (secondary to inflammation, infection, stones, foreign body)
Renal vascular anomalies (renal artery stenosis, or thrombosis, embolism of renal vein)		

Note: ARF secondary to transplant rejection is considered an immune-mediated form of renal ARF.

Renal ARF In **renal ARF,** the pathological process is within the kidney tissue, or renal parenchyma, itself. Three different processes cause renal ARF. The first is injury to small blood vessels (or **microangiopathy**) or glomerular capillaries; the second is injury to tubular cells; the third is inflammation or infection in the interstitial tissue surrounding nephrons (Table 33-1).

Microangiopathy and glomerular injury both result in obstruction of these minute vessels that are a vital part of the blood vessel-tubule structure of the nephron; consequently, nephron function is lost. Microangiopathy and glomerular injury are often immune mediated and may be associated with systemic immune-mediated diseases, such as diabetes mellitus type I and systemic lupus erythematosus. In these cases, ARF involves both preexisting and ongoing (that is, chronic and acute) nephron destruction.

Tubular cell death, or **acute tubular necrosis,** can follow prerenal ARF or can develop directly due to toxin deposition. Along with heavy metals and miscellaneous inorganic and organic compounds, a number of medications (including some antibiotics and cisplatin, an anticancer agent) can cause acute tubular necrosis.

Interstitial nephritis, a chronic inflammatory process also commonly due to toxic compounds, including drugs (antibiotics, nonsteroidal anti-inflammatory drugs, diuretics), can also result in renal ARF.

Postrenal ARF The third form of ARF, **postrenal ARF,** originates in a structure distal to the kidney—the ureters, bladder, or urethra. In its earliest phase (before urine has backed up into the kidneys, shutting down further urine formation), postrenal ARF is reversible simply by removing the obstruction that is preventing elimination of urine. Urinary tract obstruction causes fewer than 5 percent of ARF cases, but like prerenal ARF, it is important to identify it because the odds of reversal are good. If the obstruction is not cleared, renal ARF may develop secondary to nephron and interstitial injury caused by renovascular obstruction.

Because both ureters must be blocked simultaneously for postrenal ARF to develop (assuming two kidneys are present), it is probably the least likely cause of the cases you will see. Far more common will be obstruction of the bladder neck or of the urethra.

Regardless of probable cause, treat ARF aggressively in the field so that the patient will have the best chance for recovery.

Assessment

The focused history will often provide clues to the severity and duration of ARF. For instance, if the patient complains of inability to void for a number of hours associated with a feeling of painful bladder fullness, the cause may simply be acute obstruction at the bladder neck or urethra. In contrast, a patient with poor mentation may be unable to give a coherent history, and a family member will tell you that the patient has felt increasingly ill for several days and has not urinated at all within the past 12 hours or so. Questions likely to provide useful information include the following:

- *When was the decrease or absence of urine first noticed, and has there been any observed change in output since the problem was first noted? What was the patient's previous output?* The last question may be useful because patients with chronic renal failure due to inadequate renal function can develop ARF as a complication.

- *Has the patient noticed development of edema (swelling) in the face, hands, feet, or torso? How about feelings of heart palpitations or irregular rhythm? Has a family member or friend noticed decreased*

* **renal ARF (renal acute renal failure)** ARF due to pathology within the kidney tissue itself.

* **microangiopathy** a disease affecting the smallest blood vessels.

* **acute tubular necrosis** a particular syndrome characterized by the sudden death of tubular cells.

* **interstitial nephritis** an inflammation within the tissue surrounding the nephrons.

* **postrenal acute renal failure** ARF due to obstruction distal to the kidney.

mental function, lethargy, or overt coma? If the patient continued to consume fluids after ARF developed, retention of water and Na^+ can lead to visible edema in a relatively short time. Retention of K^+ can lead to hyperkalemia, a condition that can be lethal, especially in a person with previously compromised heart function. Increasingly poor mentation can be a sign of metabolic acidosis.

The focused secondary assessment may be helpful in assessing the degree of ARF present, the antecedent condition, and any immediate threats to life. Impaired mentation or clear decreases in consciousness in a person with previously good mental function suggest severe ARF and a potential threat to life. In a patient without evidence of shock, cardiovascular findings may include hypertension due to fluid retention, tachycardia, and ECG evidence of hyperkalemia (Figure 33-1). If shock triggered the ARF or has developed more recently, profound hypotension may be present, accompanied by tachycardia and hyperkalemia.

General visual inspection will usually show pale, cool, moist skin; if shock is not present, these findings may still represent homeostatic shunting of blood to the internal organs, including the kidneys. Look for edema in face, hands, and feet (Figure 33-2). Examination of the abdomen will reveal very different findings dependent on the cause of ARF. As with any abdominal complaint, look for scars, ecchymosis, and distention. If the abdomen is distended, note whether the swelling is symmetrical. Palpate for pulsating masses, which may indicate an abdominal aortic aneurysm. Auscultation is rarely helpful in renal and urological emergencies, and bowel sounds may be muffled if ascites (fluid within the abdomen) is present. Palpation findings will depend on the trigger condition.

A hematocrit may be useful if either acute hemorrhage or chronic anemia is suspected (the latter is common in patients with cancer or chronic renal failure). Urinalysis can offer useful information very quickly. Proteinuria and glycosuria (urinary protein and glucose, respectively) suggest renal dysfunction. In some infections, notably pyelonephritis, the urine may contain so many white blood cells that they form a visible sediment in the specimen.

Renal function is clinically evaluated by laboratory analysis of the blood. Two frequently used indicators of renal function are the blood urea nitrogen (BUN) level and the serum creatinine. An elevation in either of these two values points toward renal insufficiency or failure. Usually, the ratio of BUN to creatinine (BUN/creatinine ratio) should be less than 20. A BUN/creatinine ratio greater than 20 indicates prerenal or postrenal problems, while a BUN/creatinine ratio of 20 or less indicates a renal problem.

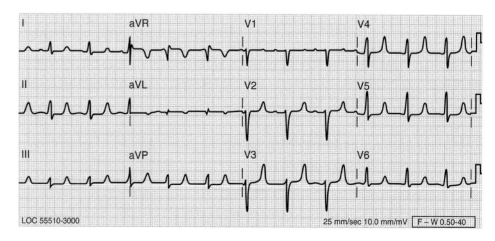

FIGURE 33-1 ECG with signs of hyperkalemia.

Management

Because ARF can lead to life-threatening metabolic derangements, monitoring and supporting the ABCs is vital. Use high-flow oxygen to maximize breathing efficiency; couple this with circulatory supports, such as positioning with head down and legs up, to assist blood flow to the brain and internal organs, and IV fluid resuscitation (bolus followed by drip) if hypovolemia is present. Monitor ECG readings closely and adjust supports as required.

The chief prevention strategies are protecting fluid volume and cardiovascular function, as indicated by some of the steps previously noted, and eliminating or reducing exposure to any nephrotoxic agents or medications. If you are unsure whether an antibiotic, analgesic, or other drug is nephrotoxic and you are not in a position to check, discontinue the medication until the patient is at the appropriate care facility.

During transport, be sure to talk quietly to the patient, both to calm her and to keep her informed of time until arrival or other pertinent matters. As always, your actions should reflect caring competence. Even if the patient is confused or comatose, you should still address her respectfully as you perform procedures and avoid saying anything you do not want her to hear.

Chronic Renal Failure

Chronic renal failure (CRF) is inadequate kidney function due to permanent loss of nephrons. Usually, at least 70 percent of the nephrons (healthy norm, one million per kidney) must be lost before significant clinical problems develop and the diagnosis is made. Metabolic instability does not occur until about 80 percent or more of nephrons are destroyed. When this point of dysfunction is reached, an individual is said to have developed *end-stage renal failure* and must have either dialysis or kidney transplantation to survive. Anuria is not necessarily present in either CRF or end-stage renal failure.

Together, diabetes mellitus and hypertension cause more than half of all cases of end-stage renal failure. The death toll from CRF is high and increasing as the population ages. More than 577 people per million in Canada have end-stage renal failure. While many are treated with dialysis, the number of donor kidneys available in years has been sufficient for only 38 percent of the persons on the waiting list.

Pathophysiology

The three pathological processes that initiate the nephron damage of CRF are the same as those underlying renal ARF: microangiopathy or glomerular capillary injury, tubular cell injury, and inflammation or infection in interstitial tissue (Table 33-2). Although the cause of initial nephron destruction is different for each of the three

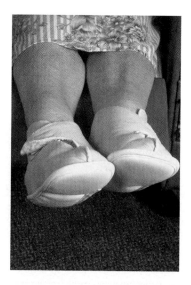

FIGURE 33-2 Edema of the feet consistent with fluid retention in acute renal failure.

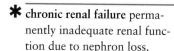
Because ARF can lead to life-threatening metabolic derangements, monitoring and supporting the ABCs is vital.

✱ **chronic renal failure** permanently inadequate renal function due to nephron loss.

Table 33-2	CAUSES OF CHRONIC RENAL FAILURE
Type of Tissue Injury	**Examples**
Microangiopathy, glomerular injury	Systemic hypertension, diabetes mellitus, atherosclerosis, glomerulonephritis, systemic lupus erythematosus
Tubular cell injury	Nephrotoxins, including analgesics and heavy metals, stones, obstruction at bladder neck or urethra
Interstitial injury	Infections including pyelonephritis, tuberculosis

Note: Congenital disorders resulting in CRF include polycystic disease and renal hypoplasia.

pathological processes, the same cycle of ongoing nephron damage becomes established: Functional nephrons adapt by increasing glomerular filtration primarily (through decreased vascular resistance in glomerular vessels and hypertrophy of capillary vessels) and by increasing tubular reabsorption and secretion secondarily (through cellular hypertrophy and functional adaptation of tubular cells). After a time, the compensatory changes damage these nephrons, leading to their destruction and initiating adaptive changes in additional, functional nephrons. Most of the damage seems to affect the glomeruli. Under the microscope, surviving nephrons often show dilated, abnormal glomeruli, and nonfunctional nephrons have heavily scarred glomeruli or no visible glomeruli, only sclerotic tissue.

This characteristic loss of nephrons, or **reduced nephron mass,** is also visible at the level of gross anatomy as shrunken, scarred kidneys, or **reduced renal mass.** Physiologically, each of the kidney's four major functions is highly disturbed or absent, depending upon the degree of renal failure:

* *Maintenance of blood volume with proper balance of water, electrolytes, and pH.* In CRF, active transport in the tubules decreases significantly or ceases. Filtrate simply passes through the tubules, leading to characteristic **isosthenuria,** the inability to concentrate or dilute urine. As the overall GFR falls over time, retention of Na^+ and water increases, causing a high-volume stress on the cardiovascular system. Retention of K^+ can lead to dangerous hyperkalemia, and retention of H^+ can lead to equally dangerous metabolic acidosis. Hypocalcemia is also common. It results from several causes, including renal retention of phosphate ions (with higher levels of serum phosphate facilitating Ca^{++} absorption into bone) and lack of renal production of vitamin D.

* *Retention of key compounds, such as glucose, with excretion of wastes, such as urea.* Glucose and other substances that normally are actively reabsorbed are also lost in urine as the filtrate flows passively through the nephron. Any hypoglycemic effect is overshadowed, however, by the significant hyperglycemic effect (**glucose intolerance**) in most patients due to cellular resistance to insulin. The wastes urea and creatinine accumulate in blood almost in direct proportion to the number of nephrons lost. In fact, the general syndrome of signs and symptoms caused by severe CRF is termed **uremia,** for this characteristic buildup of blood urea.

* *Control of arterial blood pressure.* The renin-angiotensin loop is disrupted; even small amounts of renin can lead to severe hypertension. Hypertension may also develop due to retention of Na^+ and water. Cardiac decompensation, with hypotension and tachycardia, can develop suddenly, especially if cardiac function has been independently impaired.

* *Regulation of erythrocyte development.* Because erythropoietin is no longer produced in normal quantities (or at all, in some end-stage patients), chronic anemia develops. Anemia is another cardiac stressor, and it can contribute to cardiac failure.

Assessment

During the focused history and secondary assessment, you will probably find many characteristics of uremia in patients with CRF and end-stage disease. Table 33-3 lists some of these signs and symptoms, which affect nearly every organ system. Many of the listed problems can precipitate shock or other major physiological instability; this is one reason you must always be alert when dealing with

* **reduced nephron mass** the decrease in number of functional nephrons that causes chronic renal failure.

* **reduced renal mass** the decrease in kidney size associated with chronic renal failure.

* **isosthenuria** the inability to concentrate or dilute urine relative to the osmolarity of blood.

* **glucose intolerance** the body cells' inability to take up glucose from the bloodstream.

* **uremia** the syndrome of signs and symptoms associated with chronic renal failure.

patients with CRF or end-stage disease, even when they initially appear stable. In addition, this list is by no means exhaustive. Kidney failure affects almost every organ and major function in the body.

The focused history will typically show GI symptoms, such as anorexia and nausea, sometimes with vomiting. The patient's mentation as she speaks is an important clue to central nervous system impairment. Signs may be as subtle as anxiety or mood swings or as immediately serious as seizures or coma.

Your general impression before the secondary assessment is likely to note marked abnormalities. Skin will typically be pale, moist, and cool. Scratches and ecchymoses are common skin changes associated with CRF. Mucous membranes may also be very pale, dependent on the degree of anemia. Jaundice may be present, dependent on the degree of retention of urea and other pigmented metabolic wastes. A skin condition called uremic frost appears when excessive amounts of urea are eliminated through sweat. As the sweat dries, a white "frosty" dust of urea may appear on the skin.

Always be alert for shock or other major physiological instability when dealing with CRF or end-stage disease, even when the patient initially appears stable.

Table 33-3 · COMMON ELEMENTS OF UREMIC SYNDROME

System	Pathophysiology	Clinical Sign/Symptom
Fluid/Electrolyte	Water/Na^+ retention	Edema, arterial hypertension[1]
	K^+ retention	Hyperkalemia[1]
	H^+ retention	Metabolic acidosis
	PaO_2 retention	Hyperphosphatemia/hypocalcemia[1]
Cardiovascular/Pulmonary	Fluid volume overload	Ascites, pulmonary edema
	Arterial hypertension	Congestive heart failure, accelerated atherosclerosis
	Dysfunctional fat metabolism; retention urea, other wastes	Pericarditis
Neuromuscular		
Central Nervous System	Retention urea, other wastes	Headache, sleep disorders, impaired mentation, lethargy, coma, seizures
Skeletal Muscle	Retention urea, other wastes; hypocalcemia	Muscular irritability and cramps, muscle twitching
Gastrointestinal (GI)	Retention urea, other wastes	Anorexia, nausea, vomiting
	Impaired hemostasis	Peptic ulcer, GI bleeding
Endocrine-Metabolic	Low vitamin D, other factors	Osteodystrophy
	Cellular resistance to insulin	Glucose intolerance
	Mechanisms unclear	Poor growth and development, delayed sexual maturation[2]
Dermatological	Chronic anemia	Pallor skin, mucous membranes
	Retention urea, pigments	Jaundice, uremic frost
	Clotting disorders	Ecchymoses, easy bleeding
	Secondary hyperparathyroidism	Pruritus, scratches
Hematological	Lack of renal erythropoeitin	Chronic anemia
	Impaired platelet function and prothrombin consumption	Impaired hemostasis, with easy bleeding, bruising; splenomegaly
Immunological	Lymphopenia, general leukopenia	Vulnerability to infection

[1]Although relatively uncommon, fluctuations to the other extreme (example, hypokalemia) may occur if oral intake is poor over prolonged periods or during or after dialysis treatment.

[2]Primarily seen in children, adolescents, young adults.

The major organ systems often show significant abnormalities on direct examination (see Table 33-3). Because of the failure of vital urinary system functions, cardiovascular stress can be enormous. Either hypertension or hypotension may occur, dependent on the degree of fluid retention (retention detectable as peripheral edema or pulmonary edema) and the level of cardiac function; tachycardia is common with both presentations. ECG findings may include a dysrhythmia secondary to hyperkalemia. Metabolic acidosis, when present, compounds the effects of hyperkalemia. Pericarditis is also common, and a rub may be heard on chest auscultation. Neuromuscular abnormalities, in addition to impaired mentation, include muscle cramps and "restless legs syndrome," as well as muscle twitching or tonic-clonic or other forms of seizure.

Your abdominal assessment will reveal many abnormalities. The challenge is to begin separating (by assessment and history) chronic findings from those of recent onset or aggravated by the emergency that led to your call. For instance, you know that ecchymoses on the abdomen or flank may suggest acute hemorrhage. You may find a patient with ecchymoses scattered over the body surface. Look for evidence of new abdominal ecchymoses versus older bruises or a clear history of recent onset as signs of a current problem. Be sure to note abdominal contour, including the presence of symmetric distention or localized bulges, scars, and ecchymoses before the assessment and to clearly document the preexam appearance. Findings on auscultation, percussion, and palpation will depend on the presenting problem.

The hematocrit and urinalysis generally have less value in CRF than in ARF. A hematocrit is useful only if you know the patient's baseline value, and recent changes in the amount of urinary output may be more significant than the content. The exceptions are blood (red blood cells) in urine, which is always a significant finding on dipstick analysis, and visible amounts of white blood cells, which suggest significant infection.

Management

Immediate Management As with ARF, CRF can lead to life-threatening complications, and so monitoring and supporting the ABCs is vital. Use high-flow oxygen to maximize breathing efficiency. Couple this with circulatory supports, such as positioning with the head down and the legs up, to support blood flow to the brain and internal organs. Consider a small IV bolus for fluid resuscitation if hypovolemia is evident. Indications for fluid lavage (in peritoneal dialysis patients) are the same as those for patients with ARF. Monitor the ECG readings closely and adjust supports according to your local protocol or discussion with medical direction.

The chief prevention strategies are regulation of fluid volume and cardiovascular function and major electrolyte disturbances (for example, use of a vasopressor in hypotension and administration of bicarbonate for partial correction of acidosis, respectively) and elimination or reduction of exposure to any nephrotoxic agents or medications. Although uncommon, severe swings in electrolyte levels may occur during and after dialysis, and so be cautious about replacement measures in the field in these patients. Err on the side of conservative treatment except for clearly life-threatening complications. If you are unsure whether a drug is nephrotoxic and you are not in a position to check, discontinue it until the patient is at the emergency department.

Expedite transport to an appropriate facility in the same manner appropriate for patients with ARF. Be sure to talk quietly to the patient, both to calm her and to keep her informed of the time until arrival or other pertinent matters. If the patient is confused, ask short orientation questions periodically to assess lucidity and level of consciousness.

In CRF emergencies, the challenge is to separate chronic findings from those of recent onset or aggravated by the emergency that led to your call.

In CRF, err on the side of conservative treatment except for clearly life-threatening complications.

Long-Term Management Renal dialysis, the artificial replacement of some of the kidney's most critical functions, is a fact of life for most patients with CRF and end-stage disease. Although dialysis is necessary for survival, it is not without risk. One risk that you have already learned about is the possibility of physiologically destabilizing shifts in blood volume and composition and arterial blood pressure.

Dialysis was first developed about 30 years ago. Since then, two different technologies, hemodialysis and peritoneal dialysis, have been refined. Both rely on the same physiological principles: osmosis and equalization of osmolarity across a semipermeable membrane, such as that of the renal nephron. (You may wish to reread the explanation of osmosis in this chapter's physiology section before reading further.) In dialysis, the patient's blood flows past a semipermeable membrane that has a special cleansing fluid on the other side that is hypo-osmolar to blood for a number of impurities (such as urea, creatinine) and critical substances (such as Na^+, K^+, H^+). As the blood flows over the membrane, these substances in the blood move into the hypo-osmolar solution, called the **dialysate,** and their concentrations in blood are thus reduced. The effect of dialysis is to temporarily lessen or eliminate volume overload and toxically high blood concentrations of electrolytes, urea, and other substances.

In **hemodialysis** (*hemo* = blood, *dia* = across, *lysis* = separation), the patient's blood is passed through a machine that contains an artificial membrane and the dialysate solution. Vascular access is required in order to achieve the necessary blood flow of 300 to 400 mL/min. Often, a superficial, internal fistula is created surgically by anastamosing an artery and vein in the lower forearm. If the required healthy artery and vein are not available, surgeons can insert a special vascular graft made of artificial material between an artery and vein (Figure 33-3). If creating such a fistula is not possible, an indwelling catheter may need to be placed in the internal jugular vein. Because hemodialysis can be performed in settings including outpatient clinics and at home, you may see patients both between and during hemodialysis sessions. The three most common complications relate to vascular access. Two of the three complications are bleeding from the needle puncture site and local infection. The third is the narrowing or closing of the internal fistula. Under normal flow conditions, the internal fistula will have

* **renal dialysis** artificial replacement of some critical kidney functions.

Content Review

TYPES OF DIALYSIS
• Hemodialysis
• Peritoneal dialysis

* **dialysate** the solution used in dialysis that is hypo-osmolar to many of the wastes and key electrolytes in blood.

* **hemodialysis** a dialysis procedure relying on vascular access to the blood and on an artificial membrane.

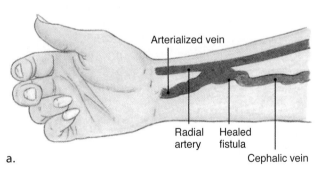

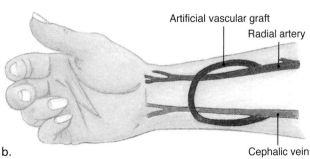

FIGURE 33-3 Vascular access for hemodialysis. (a) arteriovenous fistula; (b) artificial graft between artery and vein.

a palpable thrill (vibration), or bruit, due to the relatively high-volume turbulent flow from artery into vein. If the fistula narrows significantly or closes, however, this vibration is lost. The leading complications that require hospitalization are thrombosis, infection, and aneurysm development. They are particularly common in patients with grafts of artificial material.

Peritoneal dialysis uses the peritoneal membrane within the patient's abdomen as the semipermeable dialysis membrane, and dialysate solution is introduced and removed from the abdominal cavity via an indwelling catheter (Figure 33-4). This simpler technique, which used to be significantly less effective than hemodialysis, has been improved greatly in recent years. Currently, many patients practise either chronic peritoneal lavage (intermittent cycles in which dialysate is introduced, allowed to remain for an extended period, and then removed) or continuous peritoneal lavage (in which dialysate is introduced via a closed system that allows the patient to remain ambulatory during dialysis). Peritoneal dialysis avoids some of the risk of fluid and electrolyte shifts seen during hemodialysis, but its success requires additional physical characteristics (such as healthy vasculature around the peritoneum). The most common complication is infection in the catheter, the abdominal tunnel containing the catheter, or the peritoneum itself. The incidence of peritonitis is about one episode per year, and so you may find its signs in these patients.

Both forms of dialysis have complications not related to vascular access in common. They include hypotension, shortness of breath, chest pain, and neurologic abnormalities ranging from headache to seizure or coma. If the patient is hypotensive, check for dehydration, hemorrhage, or infection. Shortness of breath and chest pain may reflect cardiac dysrhythmias (often secondary to hyperkalemia) or may be without identifiable cause. Be aware that these patients, many of whom have cardiac compromise, are at higher risk for ischemia or MI during these periods. Neurological abnormalities may occur before, during, or after treatment. In most cases, they represent neurotoxicity of accumulated blood urea; in some cases, rapid removal of urea from blood causes an osmotic diuresis from brain tissue with a resulting increase in intracranial pressure. Benzodiazepines may be useful in patients who develop seizures.

FIGURE 33-4 Peritoneal dialysis.

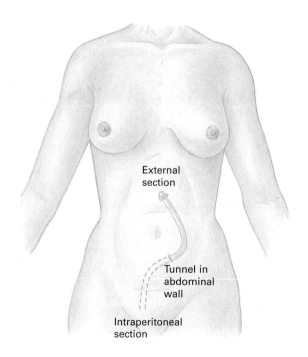

External section

Tunnel in abdominal wall

Intraperitoneal section

RENAL CALCULI

Kidney stones, or *renal calculi* (singular, *calculus*), represent crystal aggregation in the kidney's collecting system (Figure 33-5). This condition is also called nephrolithiasis (from Greek *lithos*, stone). Kidney stones affect about 5000 Canadians each year. Brief hospitalization is common due to the severity of pain as a stone travels from the renal pelvis, through the ureter, to the bladder, and is eliminated in urine. If necessary, additional treatment in hospital may include shock-wave lithotripsy, a procedure that uses sound waves to break large stones into smaller ones. Overall morbidity and mortality are low, however, unless a complication, such as hemorrhage or urinary-tract obstruction, results. Stones form more commonly in men than in women, although the ratio varies for types of stones with different compositions. Certain stones also occur in familial patterns, suggesting hereditary factors. Another risk factor for calculus formation is immobilization due to surgery or injury, with the latter including immobilization secondary to paraplegia or other paralysis syndromes that involve the absence of motor impulses, sensation, or both. The use of certain medications, including anesthetics, opiates, and psychotropic drugs, also increases the risk for stones.

Kidney stones occur more frequently in summer and fall.

Pathophysiology

Stones may form in metabolic disorders, such as gout or primary hyperparathyroidism, which produce excessive amounts of uric acid and calcium, respectively. More often, they occur when the general balance between water conservation and dissolution of relatively insoluble substances, such as mineral ions and uric acid, is lost and excessive amounts of the insolubles aggregate into stones. The problem boils down to "too much insoluble stuff" and urine being "too concentrated," a situation that may more likely arise with change in diet, climate, or physical activity.

Stones consisting of calcium salts (namely, calcium oxalate and calcium phosphate) are by far the most common. These compounds are found in 75 to 85 percent of all stones. Calcium stones are from two to three times more common in men than in women, and the average age at onset is between 20 and 30 years.

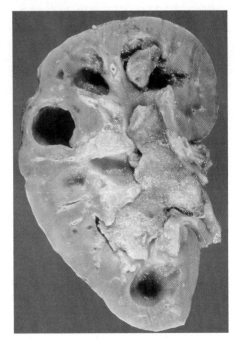

FIGURE 33-5 Sectioned kidney with kidney stones.

Their formation frequently runs in families, and anyone who has had a calcium stone is at fairly high risk to form another within two to three years.

Struvite stones (chemically denoted $MgNH_4PO_4$) are also common, representing about 10 to 15 percent of all stones. The pathophysiology of struvite stones differs from that of calcium stones. Their formation is associated with chronic urinary tract infection (UTI) or frequent bladder catheterization. The association with bacterial UTI makes struvite stones much more common in women than in men. These stones can grow to fill the renal pelvis, producing a characteristic "staghorn" appearance on x-rays.

Far less common are stones composed of uric acid or cystine. Uric acid stones form more often in men than in women and tend to occur in families; about half of all patients with uric acid stones have gout. Cystine stones are the least common. They are associated with excess levels of cystine in filtrate and are probably due, at least in part, to hereditary factors, as they often run in families.

Assessment

The focused history almost always centres on pain. (Kidney stones are generally conceded to be among the most painful of human medical conditions.) Typically, the patient first notes discomfort as a vague, visceral pain in one flank. Within 30 to 60 minutes, it progresses to an extremely sharp pain that may remain in the flank or migrate downward and anteriorly toward the groin. Migrating pain indicates that the stone has passed into the lowest third of the ureter. Stones that lodge in the lowest part of the ureter, within the bladder wall, often cause characteristic bladder symptoms, such as frequency during the day or during the night (nocturia), urgency, and painful urination. Because these latter three symptoms far more frequently suggest bladder infection, making the probable diagnosis may be difficult, particularly in women. Visible hematuria is not uncommon in urine specimens taken during passage of a stone. Fever, however, is not typical unless infection is present. Whenever kidney stones are suspected, be sure to get the patient's personal medical history and family history because both will often provide useful information.

The secondary assessment will almost always reveal someone who is very uncomfortable. The patient may be agitated or physically restless; walking sometimes reduces the pain. Vital signs will vary with level of discomfort, with highest blood pressure and heart rate associated with greatest pain. Skin will typically be pale, cool, and clammy. Abdominal examination may be difficult, depending on the patient's ability to remain still. First, inspect the abdomen for contour and symmetry. Palpation is generally useful only in ruling out GI conditions. Palpation results will vary and may depend, in part, on whether pain is so great that muscle guarding is present, making palpation of underlying structures impossible.

Management

As always, management begins with the ABCs. Positioning should centre on comfort, but be prepared for vomiting due to the severe pain, especially if the patient's last meal was within several hours. Consider analgesia en route to the hospital, according to your local protocol and your perception of the patient's condition. Use narcotics cautiously if a GI condition is at all possible or if mentation is impaired. If the pain is in the initial, intermittent, colicky phase, consider coaching pain management through breathing techniques similar to those used for women in labour. An IV line is useful for volume replacement or drug administration. The usual prevention strategy, if kidney function is adequate, is IV fluid to promote urine formation and movement through the system. Transport is the same as that for other abdominal conditions, that is, position of comfort and supportive care.

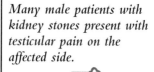

Whenever kidney stones are suspected, be sure to get the patient's personal medical history and family history.

Many male patients with kidney stones present with testicular pain on the affected side.

Parenteral narcotic analgesics or ketorolac (Toradol) should be considered for the patient with renal colic.

URINARY TRACT INFECTION

Urinary tract infection, or UTI, affects the urethra, bladder, or kidney, as well as the prostate gland in men. UTIs are extremely common, accounting for more than six million office visits yearly. Almost all UTIs start with pathogenic colonization of the bladder by bacteria that enter through the urethra. Thus, females in general are at higher risk because of their relatively short urethra. Other groups at risk for UTI are paraplegic patients or patients with nerve disruption to the bladder, including some diabetic persons. Any condition that promotes **urinary stasis** (incomplete urination with urine remaining in the bladder that may serve as nutrition for pathogens) places a person at higher risk. Pregnant women often have urinary stasis due to pressure from the gravid uterus. People with neurological impairment (some patients with spina bifida or with diabetic neuropathy, for example) also tend to have urinary stasis, which predisposes them to infection. The use of instrumentation in patients who require bladder catheterization places them at even higher risk of UTIs.

Morbidities, such as scarring, abscesses, or eventual development of CRF, are most likely in persons with anatomical abnormalities of the urinary system or chronic calculi (the latter acting as a focus for continuing infection and inflammation), those who are immunocompromised, or those who have renal disease due to diabetes mellitus or another condition.

Pathophysiology

Urinary tract infections are generally divided into those of the lower urinary tract, namely, urethritis (urethra), cystitis (bladder), and prostatitis (prostate gland), and those of the upper urinary tract, pyelonephritis (kidney).

Lower UTIs are far more common than upper UTIs, for two reasons. First, seeding of infection via the bloodstream is rare. Second, asymptomatic bacterial colonization of the urethra, especially in females, is very common and can predispose a person to infection by other, pathogenic bacteria.

In females, infection may begin when gram-negative bacteria normally found in the bowel (that is, the enteric flora) colonize the urethra and bladder. Symptomatic **urethritis,** inflammation secondary to urethral infection, is very uncommon. More often, you will see joint symptomatic infection of the urethra and bladder (urethritis and **cystitis,** respectively). Sexually active females are at higher risk, which may be attributed to use of contraceptive devices or agents, to the introduction of enteric flora during intercourse, or both. Recently, homosexually active men who engage in anal sex have also been found to be at higher risk for bacterial cystitis, possibly due to introduction of enteric bacterial flora during intercourse. In any case, sexually active persons who suffer from urinary stasis are at even higher risk for infection. Persons who urinate after intercourse might lower their risk because voiding eliminates some bacteria. The pathophysiology for persons using bladder catheterization probably differs only in that pathogenic bacteria are introduced directly into the bladder via the catheter. In general, the likelihood that active cystitis will develop, that antibiotic treatment will clear such infections, and that reinfection will occur are all determined by the interplay of the pathogen's virulence, the size of its colony, its sensitivity to antibiotic treatment, and the strength of the host's local and systemic immune functions.

Prostatitis, inflammation of the prostate gland, in our context, denotes inflammation secondary to bacterial infection, as well as any general inflammatory condition. Men with acute bacterial prostatitis, the closest parallel to acute cystitis in women, also tend to show evidence of joint urethritis, and the same bowel flora tend to be involved. The major difference between acute bacterial prostatitis and acute cystitis is the much lower incidence of prostatitis among men who do not require bladder catheterization.

* **urinary tract infection (UTI)** an infection, usually bacterial, at any site in the urinary tract.

* **urinary stasis** a condition in which the bladder empties incompletely during urination.

* **urethritis** an infection and inflammation of the urethra.

* **cystitis** an infection and inflammation of the urinary bladder.

* **prostatitis** infection and inflammation of the prostate gland.

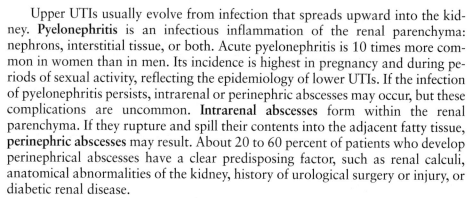

pyelonephritis an infection and inflammation of the kidney.

intrarenal abscess a pocket of infection within kidney tissue.

perinephric abscess a pocket of infection in the layer of fat surrounding the kidney.

community-acquired infection an infection occurring in a non-hospitalized patient who is not undergoing regular medical procedures, including the use of such instruments as catheters.

nosocomial infection an infection acquired in a medical setting.

Upper UTIs usually evolve from infection that spreads upward into the kidney. **Pyelonephritis** is an infectious inflammation of the renal parenchyma: nephrons, interstitial tissue, or both. Acute pyelonephritis is 10 times more common in women than in men. Its incidence is highest in pregnancy and during periods of sexual activity, reflecting the epidemiology of lower UTIs. If the infection of pyelonephritis persists, intrarenal or perinephric abscesses may occur, but these complications are uncommon. **Intrarenal abscesses** form within the renal parenchyma. If they rupture and spill their contents into the adjacent fatty tissue, **perinephric abscesses** may result. About 20 to 60 percent of patients who develop perinephrical abscesses have a clear predisposing factor, such as renal calculi, anatomical abnormalities of the kidney, history of urological surgery or injury, or diabetic renal disease.

Urinary tract infections may be community acquired or nosocomial. Among **community-acquired infections**, gram-negative enteric bacteria predominate. In fact, *E. coli* accounts for roughly 80 percent of infections in persons without the complicating factors of bladder catheterization, renal calculi, or anatomical abnormalities. In **nosocomial infections**, cases acquired in an inpatient setting or related to catheterization, *Proteus, Klebsiella,* and *Pseudomonas* are commonly identified. Less common, but still important, are sexually transmitted pathogens (among women and men), such as *Chlamydia* and *N. gonorrhoeae.* Fungi, such as *Candida,* are rarely seen except in catheterized or immunocompromised patients or patients with diabetes mellitus.

Assessment

The focused history of lower UTI typically centres on three symptoms: painful urination, frequent urge to urinate, and difficulty in beginning and continuing to void. Pain often begins as visceral discomfort that progresses to severe, burning pain, particularly during and just after urination. The evolution of pain corresponds roughly to the degree of epithelial damage caused by the pathogen. In both men and women, pain is often localized to the pelvis and perceived as in the bladder (in women) or bladder and prostate (in men). The patient may complain of a strong or foul odour in the urine. Many women will give a history of similar episodes, which may or may not have been diagnosed or treated. Patients with pyelonephritis are more likely to feel generally ill or feverish. They typically complain of constant, moderately severe or severe pain in a flank or lower back (just under the rib cage). Pain may be referred to the shoulder or neck. The triad of urgency, pain, and difficulty may or may not be present or included in the past history.

On secondary assessment, patients with UTI appear restless and uncomfortable. Typically, patients with pyelonephritis appear more ill and are far more likely to have a fever. Skin will often be pale, cool, and moist (in lower UTI) or warm and dry (in febrile upper UTI). Vital signs will vary with the degree of illness and pain, but in an otherwise healthy individual, they should not be far from the norms. Inspect and auscultate the abdomen to document findings, but neither procedure is likely to be very useful, as visible appearance and bowel sounds are usually within normal limits. Palpation will probably reveal painful tenderness over the pubis in lower UTI and at the flank in upper UTI. Lloyd's sign, tenderness to percussion of the lower back at the costovertebral angle (CVA), indicates pyelonephritis.

The patient with acute pyelonephritis will usually appear quite ill. The patient with cystitis, on the other hand, will be uncomfortable but will not appear toxic.

Management

The management of UTI should centre on the ABCs and circulatory support. If pain is severe, help the patient to a comfortable position, but consider the risk of aspiration during vomiting. Analgesics should be considered as with renal calculi; they will probably be needed only for severely painful cases of pyelonephritis. Consider nonpharmacological pain management with breathing and relaxation techniques. The best prevention technique is hydration to increase blood flow through the kidneys and to produce a more dilute urine. In many cases, this is better accomplished by IV administration, which eliminates the risk of vomiting and satisfies the guidelines for possible surgical cases. Expedite transport to an appropriate facility.

SUMMARY

The urinary system (1) maintains blood volume and the proper balance of water, electrolytes, and pH; (2) enables the blood to retain key substances, such as glucose and removes a variety of toxic wastes from the blood; (3) plays a major role in regulation of arterial blood pressure; and (4) controls maturation of red blood cells. Kidney nephrons produce urine. Homeostasis through urine production is responsible for the first two functions and assists in the third, regulating blood pressure, by producing renin, the enzyme through which blood pressure is controlled. Other kidney cells produce erythropoietin, the hormone that stimulates red blood cell maturation.

Renal and urological emergencies typically present as an acute abdomen. The most common are acute renal failure (ARF), chronic renal failure (CRF, with the subset of end-stage renal disease), and renal calculi. Both ARF and CRF may present with life-threatening complications and impaired function of other systems. Be prepared for apparently stable patients to acutely develop destabilizing complications (often, cardiovascular). Urinary tract infections, or UTIs, are divided into those of the lower urinary tract (urethra, bladder, and prostate in men) and those of the upper urinary tract (kidney). Both types of infection can present with considerable pain, but pyelonephritis is the more serious, with fever likely and complications, including abscesses, possible.

Because renal function is often lowered in the elderly and in persons with hypertension or diabetes, consider it potentially impaired in all of these patients. The best prevention strategies are to minimize the likelihood of prerenal failure by protecting blood volume and blood pressure and to investigate possible postrenal urinary tract obstruction.

CHAPTER 34

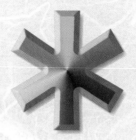

Toxicology and Substance Abuse

Objectives

After reading this chapter, you should be able to:

1. Describe the incidence, morbidity, and mortality of toxic and drug abuse emergencies. (pp. 681–682)
2. Identify the risk factors most predisposing to toxic emergencies. (pp. 681–682)
3. Discuss the anatomy and physiology of the organs and structures related to toxic emergencies. (pp. 682–684)
4. Describe the routes of entry of toxic substances into the body. (pp. 682–684)
5. Discuss the role of Poison Control Centres in Canada. (p. 682)
6. Discuss the pathophysiology, assessment findings, need for rapid intervention and transport, and management of toxic emergencies. (pp. 681–722)
7. List the most common poisonings, pathophysiology, assessment findings, and management of poisoning by ingestion, inhalation, absorption, injection, and overdose. (pp. 682–722)
8. Define the following terms:
   a. Substance or drug abuse (p. 715)
   b. Substance or drug dependence (p. 715)
   c. Tolerance (p. 715)
   d. Withdrawal (p. 715)
   e. Addiction (p. 715)
9. List the most commonly abused drugs (both by chemical name and by street names). (pp. 717–718)
10. Describe the pathophysiology, assessment findings, and management of commonly used drugs. (pp. 715–722)
11. List the clinical uses, street names, pharmacology, assessment findings, and management for patients who have taken the following drugs

Continued

Objectives Continued

or been exposed to the following substances:
  a. Cocaine (pp. 693, 716–717)
  b. Marijuana and cannabis compounds (p. 718)
  c. Amphetamines and amphetamine-like drugs (pp. 716, 718)
  d. Barbiturates (pp. 716, 718)
  e. Sedative-hypnotics (p. 718)
  f. Cyanide (p. 694)
  g. Narcotics/opiates (pp. 693, 717)
  h. Cardiac medications (p. 696)
  i. Caustics (pp. 696–698)
  j. Common household substances (p. 708)
  k. Drugs abused for sexual purposes/sexual gratification (p. 716)
  l. Carbon monoxide (p. 695)
  m. Alcohols (pp. 719–722)
  n. Hydrocarbons (p. 698)
  o. Psychiatric medications (pp. 698–701)
  p. Newer antidepressants and serotonin syndromes (pp. 700–701)
  q. Lithium (p. 701)
  r. MAO inhibitors (pp. 699–700)
  s. Nonprescription pain medications (1) nonsteroidal anti-inflammatory agents (2) salicylates (3) acetaminophen (pp. 702–703)
  t. Theophylline (p. 703)
  u. Metals (pp. 703–704)
  v. Plants and mushrooms (pp. 705–706)

12. Discuss common causative agents or offending organisms, pharmacology, assessment findings, and management for a patient with food poisoning, a bite, or a sting. (pp. 704–714)
13. Given several scenarios of poisoning or overdose, provide the appropriate assessment, treatment, and transport. (pp. 681–722)

INTRODUCTION

Toxicology is the study of **toxins** (drugs and poisons) and antidotes and their effects on living organisms. Toxicological emergencies result from the ingestion, inhalation, surface absorption, or injection of toxic substances that then exert their adverse effects on the body's tissues and metabolic mechanisms. Theoretically, all toxicological emergencies can be classified as poisoning. However, in this discussion, the term *poisoning* will be used to describe exposure to nonpharmacological substances. The term *overdose* will be used to describe exposure to pharmacological substances, whether the overdose is accidental or intentional. Substance abuse, although technically a form of poisoning, will be addressed separately.

In this chapter, we will discuss various aspects of toxicological emergencies as they apply to prehospital care. We will establish general treatment guidelines for each type of toxic exposure, and then address the specific issues surrounding some of the more common substances involved. Because the field of toxicology is rapidly changing, it is virtually impossible for a paramedic to remain up to date on treatment guidelines for each type of toxic exposure. Specific treatment should be supervised by medical direction in association with a Poison Control Centre. This plan ensures that the patient receives the most current level of care available.

* **toxicology** study of the detection, chemistry, pharmacological actions, and antidotes of toxic substances.

* **toxin** any chemical (drug, poison, or other) that causes adverse effects on an organism that is exposed to it.

EPIDEMIOLOGY

Over the years, the occurrence of toxicological emergencies has continued to increase in number and severity. The following figures reveal the high potential for toxic substance involvement on an EMS call (Table 34-1).

- Ten percent of all emergency department visits and EMS responses involve toxic exposures.
- Seventy percent of accidental poisonings occur in children under the age of six years.
- A child who has experienced an accidental ingestion has a 25-percent chance of another similar ingestion within one year.
- Eighty percent of all attempted suicides involve a drug overdose.

Although more than half of all poisonings occur in children aged 1–5, they are generally accidental and relatively mild, accounting for only 10 percent of hospital admissions for poisoning and only 5 percent of the fatalities. EMS personnel must be aware that more serious poisonings, especially in children older than five, may represent intentional poisoning by parents or caregivers. Unfortunately, poisoning due to drug experimentation and suicide attempts are also becoming a common consideration in older children.

Adult poisonings and overdoses, although less frequent, account for 90 percent of hospital admissions for toxic substance exposure. They also account for 95 percent of the fatalities in this category. Most adult poisonings and overdoses are intentional. Intentional poisonings and overdoses can be due to illicit drug use, alcohol abuse, attempted suicide, and "suicidal gesturing" in which the patient is making a cry for help but may miscalculate and take a type or amount of toxin that does actually cause injury. More rarely, intentional poisoning can result from attempted homicide or chemical warfare. Accidental poisonings are increasingly caused by exposure to chemicals and toxins on the farm or in the industrial workplace. More often, they are the result of idiosyncratic (individual hypersensitivity) reactions or dosage errors when taking prescribed medications, but these usually do not require medical attention.

POISON CONTROL CENTRES

Poison Control Centres have been set up across Canada and the United States to assist in the treatment of poison victims and to provide information on new products and new treatment recommendations. They are usually based in major medical centres and teaching hospitals and serve a large population. Almost all Poison Control Centres now have computer systems to rapidly access information.

Poison Control Centres are usually staffed by physicians, toxicologists, pharmacists, nurses, or paramedics with special training in toxicology. These experts provide information to callers 24 hours a day, seven days a week. They update information regularly and offer the most current treatment guidelines.

Memorize the number of the nearest Poison Control Centre, and access it routinely. There are several advantages to this. First, the Poison Control Centre can help you immediately determine potential toxicity based on the type of agent, amount and time of exposure, and physical condition of the patient. Second, the most current, definitive treatment can sometimes be started in the field. Finally, the Poison Control Centre can notify the receiving hospital of current treatment and recommendations even before arrival of the patient.

ROUTES OF TOXIC EXPOSURE

In order to have a destructive effect, poisons must gain entrance into the body. The four portals of entry are *ingestion, inhalation, surface absorption,* and *injection.* It is important to note that regardless of the portal of entry, toxic substances have both immediate and delayed effects.

Memorize the number of the nearest Poison Control Centre, and access it routinely for information regarding a poisoning or overdose.

Content Review

ROUTES OF TOXIC EXPOSURE
- Ingestion
- Inhalation
- Surface absorption
- Injection

Table 34-1 TEN MOST COMMON POISONS

Rank	Substance	%
All Age Groups		
1	Over-the-counter pain medication/fever medication	13.5
2	Household cleaning products	7.6
3	Personal care products and cosmetics	5.5
4	Alcohols	4.3
5	Plants	3.9
6	Antidepressants	3.9
7	Antianxiety medications and sedatives	3.5
8	Hydrocarbons	3.3
9	Fumes/gases/vapours	3.3
10	Pesticides	3.1
Preschoolers (age < 5)		
1	Over-the-counter pain medication/fever medication	12.3
2	Cough/cold preparations	9.5
3	Household cleaning products	9.2
4	Personal care products and cosmetics	8.5
5	Plants	6.7
6	Vitamins	5.1
7	Pesticides	3.0
8	Laundry cleaning products	2.8
9	Essential oils	2.6
10	Hydrocarbons	2.2
Adults		
1	Over-the-counter pain medication/fever medication	14.5
2	Antianxiety medications and sedatives	9.3
3	Antidepressants	9.0
4	Alcohols	9.0
5	Fumes/gases/vapours	6.5
6	Household cleaning products	5.8
7	Hydrocarbons	4.5
8	Pesticides	3.1
9	Chemicals	2.8
10	Laundry/cleaning products	2.6

INGESTION

Ingestion is the most common route of entry for toxic exposure. Frequently, ingested poisons include

- Household products
- Petroleum-based agents (gasoline, paint)
- Cleaning agents (alkalis and soaps)
- Cosmetics
- Drugs (prescription, nonprescription, illicit)
- Plants
- Foods

Immediate toxic effects of ingestion of corrosive substances, such as strong acids or alkalis, can involve burns to the lips, tongue, throat, and esophagus. Delayed effects result from absorption of the poison from the gastrointestinal tract. Most absorption occurs in the small intestine, with only a small amount being

> *It is important to remember that toxic substances have both immediate and delayed effects.*
>
>

✶ ingestion entry of a substance into the body through the gastrointestinal tract.

absorbed from the stomach. Some poisons may remain in the stomach for up to several hours because the intake of a large bolus of poison can retard absorption. Aspirin ingestion is a classic example of this. When a patient ingests a large number of aspirin tablets, the tablets can bind together to form a large bolus that is difficult to remove or break down.

INHALATION

Inhalation of a poison results in rapid absorption of the toxic agent through the alveolar-capillary membrane in the lungs. Inhaled toxins can irritate pulmonary passages, causing extensive edema and destroying tissue. When these toxins are absorbed, wider systemic effects can occur. Causative agents can appear as gases, vapours, fumes, or aerosols. Common inhaled poisons include

- Toxic gases
- Carbon monoxide
- Ammonia
- Chlorine
- Freon
- Toxic vapours, fumes, or aerosols
- Carbon tetrachloride
- Methyl chloride
- Tear gas
- Mustard gas
- Nitrous oxide

SURFACE ABSORPTION

Surface absorption is the entry of a toxic substance through the skin or mucous membranes. This most frequently occurs from contact with poisonous plants, such as poison ivy, poison sumac, and poison oak. Many toxic chemicals may also be absorbed through the skin. **Organophosphates,** often used as pesticides, are easily absorbed through dermal contact.

INJECTION

Injection of a toxic agent under the skin, into muscle, or into a blood vessel results in both immediate and delayed effects. The immediate reaction is usually localized to the site of the injection and appears as red, irritated, edematous skin. An allergic or anaphylactic reaction can also appear (see Chapter 31). Later, as the toxin is distributed throughout the body by the circulatory system, delayed systemic reactions can occur.

Other than intentional injection of illicit drugs, most poisonings by injection result from the bites and stings of insects and animals. Most insects that can sting and bite belong to the class *Hymenoptera*, which includes honey bees, hornets, yellow jackets, wasps, and fire ants. Only the females in this group can sting. In addition, spiders, ticks, and other arachnids, such as scorpions, are notorious for causing poisonings by injection. Higher animals that bite and sting include snakes and certain marine animals. Marine animals with venomous stings include jellyfish (especially the Portuguese man-of-war), stingrays, anemones, coral, hydras, and certain spiny fish.

GENERAL PRINCIPLES OF TOXICOLOGICAL ASSESSMENT AND MANAGEMENT

Although specific protocols for managing toxicological emergencies may vary, certain basic principles apply to most situations. Keep in mind the importance of recognizing the poisoning promptly. Have a high index of suspicion if circumstances suggest involvement of a toxin in the emergency.

SCENE ASSESSMENT

Always begin assessment with a thorough evaluation of the scene. Take note of where you are and who is around you. Be alert for any potential danger to you, the rescuer. Remember, despite your natural urge to immediately assess and treat the patient, if you are incapacitated, you will not be able to help anyone and will become a patient yourself. In toxicological emergencies, there are specific hazards to keep in mind.

- Patients who are suicidal may have the potential for violence. They are often intoxicated, may act irrationally, and will not always be cooperative or happy to see you. Therefore, look for signs of overdose, such as empty pill bottles and used needles or other drug paraphernalia. Never put your hand blindly into a patient's pocket as it may contain used needles.
- Chemical spills and hazardous material emergencies can quickly incapacitate any individuals who are nearby. Make sure you have the proper clothing and equipment needed for the particular emergency. Distribute this gear to rescuers who have been trained in their use.

PRIMARY ASSESSMENT

After the scene assessment, perform the standard primary assessment. Form a general impression, and quickly assess mental status. Assessment of the ABCs is critical in toxicological emergencies because airway and respiratory compromise are common complications. This can be due to direct airway injury, pulmonary injury, profuse secretions, or decreased respiratory effort secondary to altered mental status. After assessing the ABCs, set a transport priority for the patient.

HISTORY, SECONDARY ASSESSMENT, AND ONGOING ASSESSMENT

For responsive patients, start by obtaining a history. It is important to find out not only what toxin the patient was exposed to but also when the exposure took place, since toxic effects develop over time. Then, proceed to a focused secondary assessment with full vital signs. With unresponsive patients, start with a rapid head-to-toe assessment. Be alert for signs of trauma inconsistent with the suspected intoxication. Then, proceed to obtain a history from relatives or other bystanders. Relay this information to the local Poison Control Centre. They will advise you on the most current protocol for treatment. Be aware of your local policy, which will outline whether you can initiate this protocol or whether you must first contact online medical direction. Never delay supportive measures or immediate transport to the hospital due to a delay in contacting or obtaining information from the Poison Control Centre.

Rescuer safety takes particular priority during scene assessment for a toxicological emergency.

It is important to find out not only what toxin the patient was exposed to but also when the exposure took place, since toxic effects develop over time.

Never delay supportive measures or immediate transport due to a delay in contacting the Poison Control Centre.

A detailed secondary assessment can be performed en route if time and the patient's condition permit. Ongoing assessment is essential for these patients. Poisoned patients can deteriorate suddenly and quickly. Repeat the primary assessment and vitals and reevaluate every five minutes for critical/unstable patients and every 15 minutes for stable patients.

TREATMENT

Decontamination

Once you have initiated supportive treatment (airway control, breathing assistance, and IV fluids), proceed to a mode of treatment that is specific to toxicological emergencies: decontamination. **Decontamination** is the process of minimizing toxicity by reducing the amount of toxin absorbed into the body. There are three steps to decontamination.

✱ **decontamination** the process of minimizing toxicity by reducing the amount of toxin absorbed into the body.

1. *Reduce intake of toxin.* This means that you must remove a person from an environment in which they are inhaling toxic fumes, or you must properly remove a stinger and sac from a bee sting. A classic example involves a person who has had organophosphates spilled on him. The patient's clothes must be removed and the skin cleaned with soap and water to reduce absorption of the toxins.

2. *Reduce absorption of toxin once in the body.* This usually applies to ingested toxins, which wait in the stomach and intestines while the body absorbs them into the bloodstream.

   In the past, syrup of ipecac was used to induce vomiting in order to empty the stomach. *Use of syrup of ipecac is no longer acceptable.* Studies consistently show that the use of syrup of ipecac to induce emesis reduces absorption by only 30 percent. This still leaves 70 percent of the toxin unabsorbed and causing injury. Vomiting also limits the use of other oral agents that are more effective for decontamination (e.g., activated charcoal) or oral antidotes (e.g., N-Acetylcysteine). There is also an increased risk of aspiration with vomiting, which makes induction of vomiting a procedure with minimal usefulness and high risk. Although ipecac may have some minor role in home management of some pediatric poisonings, it has generally become an obsolete treatment.

   Gastric lavage ("pumping the stomach") has also been found to be of limited use. This process involves passing a tube into the stomach and repeatedly filling and emptying the stomach with water or saline in hopes of removing the ingested poison. Most studies have shown that gastric lavage removes almost no poisons from the stomach unless it is initiated within one hour of poison ingestion. Possible complications, such as aspiration or perforation, make this procedure a risk without much benefit. Except in limited situations involving ingestions of highly toxic substances that do not bind to charcoal and for which there is no antidote, gastric lavage has become an uncommon decontamination procedure.

   The most effective and widely used method of reducing absorption of toxins is **activated charcoal.** Because of its extremely large surface area, it can adsorb, or bind, molecules from the offending toxin and prevent their absorption into the bloodstream.

Content Review

PRINCIPLES OF DECONTAMINATION

- Reduce intake
- Reduce absorption
- Enhance elimination

✱ **gastric lavage** removing an ingested poison by repeatedly filling and emptying the stomach with water or saline via a gastric tube; also known as "pumping the stomach."

✱ **activated charcoal** a powder, usually premixed with water, that will adsorb (bind) some poisons and help prevent them from being absorbed by the body.

3. *Enhance elimination of toxin.* Cathartics, such as sorbitol (often mixed with activated charcoal), increase gastric motility, thereby shortening the amount of time toxins stay in the gastrointestinal tract to be absorbed. Cathartics must be used cautiously, since there is controversy regarding their effectiveness. Cathartics should not be used in pediatric patients because of the potential to cause severe electrolyte derangements.

    Whole bowel irrigation is another method of enhancing elimination. Using a gastric tube, polyethylene glycol electrolyte solution is administered continuously at 1–2 L/hr until the rectal effluent is clear or objects recovered. This technique seems effective with few complications and is therefore gaining popularity. Its availability, however, is limited to a few centres.

Antidotes

Finally, if indicated, the appropriate antidote should be administered. An **antidote** is a substance that will neutralize a specific toxin or counteract its effect on the body. There are not many antidotes (Table 34-2), and they will rarely be 100 percent effective. Most poisonings will not require the administration of an antidote.

    The specific actions you take when dealing with toxicological emergencies will be dictated by consultation with medical direction, by protocols obtained

* **whole bowel irrigation** administration of polyethylene glycol continuously at 1–2 L/hr through a nasogastric tube until the effluent is clear or objects are recovered.

* **antidote** a substance that will neutralize a specific toxin or counteract its effect on the body.

Specific actions in a toxicological emergency will be dictated by consultation with medical direction, protocols from the Poison Control Centre, and local policy on initiating these protocols.

Table 34-2	ANTIDOTES FOR TOXICOLOGICAL EMERGENCIES	
Toxin	**Antidote**	**Adult Dosage (Pediatric Dosage)**
Acetaminophen	N-Acetylcysteine	Initial: 140 mg/kg
Arsenic	*see* Mercury, Arsenic, Gold	
Atropine	Physostigmine	Initial: 0.5–2 mg IV
Benzodiazepines	Flumazenil	Initial: 0.2 mg q 1 min to total of 1–3 mg
Carbon monoxide	Oxygen	
Cyanide	Amyl nitrite	Inhale crushed pearl for 30 seconds, then oxygen for 30 seconds
	then sodium nitrite	10 mL of 3% sol'n over 3 min IV (Pediatric: 0.33 mL/kg)
	then sodium thiosulphate	50 mL of 25% sol'n over 10 min IV (Pediatric: 1.65 mL/kg)
Ethylene glycol	Fomepizole (or as methyl alcohol)	Initial: 15 mg/kg IV
Gold	*see* Mercury, Arsenic, Gold	
Iron	Defroxamine	Initial: 10–15 mg/kg/hr IV
Lead	Edetate calcium disodium	1 amp/250 mL D5W over 1 hr
	or Dimercaptosuccinic acid (DMSA)	250 mg PO
Mercury, Arsenic, Gold	BAL (British anti-Lewisite)	5 mg/kg IM
	DMSA	250 mg PO
Methyl alcohol	Ethyl alcohol +/− dialysis	1 mL/kg of 100% ethanol IV
Nitrates	Methylene blue	0.2 mL/kg of 1% sol'n IV over 5 min
Opiates	Naloxone	0.4–2.0 mg IV
Organophosphates	Atropine	Initial: 2–5 mg IV
	Pralidoxime (Protopam)	Initial: 1 g IV

from the Poison Control Centre, and by your local policy and procedures on initiating these protocols.

SUICIDAL PATIENTS AND PROTECTIVE CUSTODY

Before leaving a suicidal patient who claims to have been "just kidding," consider the legal ramifications. Always involve law enforcement personnel in these cases and involve them early. Only law enforcement personnel can place a patient in protective custody and ultimately consent to treatment.

INGESTED TOXINS

Poisoning by ingestion is the most common route of poisoning you will encounter in prehospital care. It is essential to initiate the following principles of assessment and treatment promptly.

Assessment

It takes time for an ingested toxin to make its way from the gastrointestinal system into the circulatory system. Therefore, you need to find out not only what was ingested but also when it was ingested. Following are some general guidelines for managing patients who have ingested toxins as well as information about specific substances.

History Begin your history by trying to find out the type of toxin ingested, the quantity of the toxin, the time elapsed since ingestion, and whether the patient took any alcohol or other potentiating substance. Also, ask the patient about drug habituation or abuse and underlying medical illnesses and allergies. Remember that in cases of poisoning, inaccuracies creep into nearly half the histories because of drug-induced confusion, patient misinformation, or deliberate patient attempts at deception.

The following questions will help you develop a relevant history.

- What did you ingest? (Obtain pill containers and any remaining contents, samples of the ingested substance, or samples of vomitus. Bring them with the patient to the emergency department.)
- When did you ingest the substance? (Time is critical for decisions regarding lab tests and the use of gastric lavage and/or antidotes.)
- How much did you ingest?
- Did you drink any alcohol?
- Have you attempted to treat yourself (including inducing vomiting)?
- Have you been under psychiatric care? If so, why? (Answers may indicate a potential for suicide.)
- What is your weight?

Secondary Assessment Because the history can be unreliable, the secondary assessment is extremely important. It has two purposes: (1) to provide physical evidence of intoxication, and (2) to find any underlying illnesses that may account for the patient's symptoms or that may affect the outcome of the poisoning. As you complete the primary assessment and rapid secondary assessment, pay attention to the following patient features:

- *Skin.* Is there evidence of cyanosis, pallor, wasting, or needle marks? Flushing of the skin may indicate poisoning with an anticholinergic

Involve law enforcement early in any possible suicide case.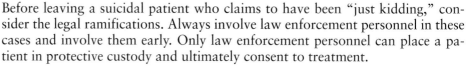

In cases of poisoning, histories are often unreliable because of drug-induced confusion, patient misinformation, or deliberate deception.

Bring pill containers and any remaining contents with the patient to the emergency department

substance. Staining of the skin may occur from chronic exposure to mercuric chloride, bromine, or similar chemicals.

- *Eyes.* Constriction or dilation of the pupils can occur with various types of poisons (e.g., marijuana, methamphetamines, narcotics). Ask about impaired vision, blurring of vision, or coloration of vision.

- *Mouth.* Look for signs of caustic ingestion, presence of the gag reflex, the amount of salivation, any breath odour, or the presence of vomitus.

- *Chest.* Breath sounds may reveal evidence of aspiration, atelectasis, or excessive pulmonary secretions.

- *Circulation.* Cardiac examination may give clues as to the type of toxin ingested. For example, the presence of tachydysrhythmias (e.g., from methamphetamine) or bradydysrhythmias (e.g., from organophosphates) may suggest specific toxins.

- *Abdomen.* Abdominal pain may result from poisoning by salicylates, methyl alcohol, caustics, or botulism toxin.

You can frequently expect to encounter patients who have ingested more than one toxin. This may be the result of a suicide attempt or of experimentation with illicit drugs. Such multiple ingestions present a diagnostic and therapeutic dilemma. Signs and symptoms may be inconsistent with a single diagnosis, and attempted treatment may produce unexpected results. A common example of this is the "speedball" (heroin mixed with cocaine). If the narcotic overdose is treated, the rescuer often encounters a patient who is now in a cocaine-induced catecholamine crisis (tachycardia, hypertension, seizures). In such cases, or if you cannot identify what the patient has ingested, consult medical direction and/or the Poison Control Centre according to your local protocols.

Management

Prevent Aspiration As previously discussed, initiation of supportive measures (maintaining airway, breathing, and circulation) is top priority in the treatment of the poisoned patient. Aspiration is a frequent complication of poisoning, resulting from an altered level of consciousness and a decreased gag reflex. Preventing aspiration must be one of your major objectives. If insertion of an endotracheal tube is necessary, nasotracheal intubation is preferred in patients who have a gag reflex.

Poisoning is a situation in which rapid sequence intubation (RSI) may be required (see Chapter 27). It is not uncommon to encounter a patient with altered mental status who is vomiting. The prevention of aspiration is a primary concern, but attempts at endotracheal intubation fail because the patient will "clamp down" his teeth. In these situations, it is often prudent to use RSI to quickly control and maintain the airway. This is far superior to waiting for the patient to deteriorate to the point at which an endotracheal tube can be placed without the aid of neuromuscular blockers. Remember, most poisoning patients will have compromised respiration or circulation, and so routinely give high-flow oxygen. RSI can only be performed by a CCP in Canada.

Administer Fluids and Drugs Once you have ensured the ABCs, establish intravenous access. An IV of Ringer's Lactate or normal saline at a to-keep-open rate is recommended for all potentially dangerous ingestions. In addition to volume replacement with a crystalloid solution, conduct cardiac monitoring and repeat assessments, including frequent monitoring of vital signs.

Maintaining airway, breathing, and circulation is top priority in treating a poisoned patient. Preventing aspiration must be one of your major objectives.

The "coma cocktail" should not be used.

Many EMS systems still utilize an empiric therapeutic regimen for comatose patients consisting of $D_{50}W$, naloxone (Narcan), and thiamine (vitamin B_1). This so-called "coma cocktail" should not be used. Instead, treatment should be guided by objective patient information obtained on scene. If immediate determination of blood glucose levels is available (glucometer and chemstrips), withhold the administration of $D_{50}W$ until determination of hypoglycemia is made. If indicated, use 25 g of $D_{50}W$ IV push. If narcotic intoxication is suspected (respiratory depression or pinpoint pupils), give 1–2 mg of naloxone IV push, only enough to have the patient control his airway and not become fully awake. Naloxone reverses the effects of narcotic intoxication. If chronic alcoholism is suspected, consider administration of 100 mg of thiamine IV to address possible encephalopathy. Do not give these medications empirically!

Follow these supportive measures with the decontamination procedures outlined earlier. Often, decontamination is performed in the emergency department, rather than on scene or during transport. This also applies to the use of most antidotes. There are exceptions, of course, and each case needs to be treated individually. Consult the Poison Control Centre and medical direction according to your local protocols.

The induction of vomiting is no longer an accepted intervention for patients who have ingested toxins.

Do Not Induce Vomiting As mentioned earlier, induction of vomiting is no longer an accepted routine intervention for patients who have ingested toxins. It is still important to contact the Poison Control Centre about this, since in rare cases of pediatric ingestion, induction of vomiting may play some role. However, for the overwhelming majority of cases, induction of vomiting is not required and may even be contraindicated.

INHALED TOXINS

Toxic inhalations can be self-induced or the result of accidental exposure from such sources as house fires or industrial accidents. Commonly abused inhaled toxins include paint (and other hydrocarbons), Freon, propellants, glue, amyl nitrite, butyl nitrite, and nitrous oxide. The general guidelines for assessment and management of toxicological emergencies apply to inhaled toxins, but the following provides some specifics.

Assessment

Inhaled toxic substances produce signs and symptoms primarily in the respiratory system. These symptoms are particularly severe in patients who have inhaled chemicals and propellants concentrated in paper or plastic bags. Patients who inhale paint or propellants are often referred to as "huffers." Look for the presence of paint on the upper or lower lip. "Huffers," who report it to be more potent, often prefer gold paint. The presence of paint on the upper or lower lips should alert you to the possibility of inhalant abuse. The sniffing of paint, propellants, or hydrocarbons has become an epidemic problem in many communities. This is particularly true in the lower socioeconomic groups as well as in isolated northern communities, including the Northwest Territories. "Huffing" can lead to serious, irreversible brain damage. As the toxins are inhaled, oxygen is gradually displaced from the respiratory system, producing a relative hypoxia. Signs and symptoms of aerosol inhalation include

- *Central nervous system:* dizziness, headache, confusion, seizures, hallucinations, coma
- *Respiratory:* tachypnea, cough, hoarseness, stridor, dyspnea, retractions, wheezing, chest pain or tightness, rales or rhonchi
- *Cardiac:* dysrhythmias

Management

Your first priority in the case of toxin inhalation is to remove the patient from the source as soon as it is safe to do so. Then, follow these guidelines:

- Safely remove the patient from the poisonous environment. In doing so, take the following essential precautions:
  - Wear protective clothing.
  - Use appropriate respiratory protection.
  - Remove the patient's contaminated clothing.
- Perform the primary assessment, history, and secondary assessment.
- Initiate supportive measures.
- Contact the Poison Control Centre and medical direction according to your local protocols.

Your first priority in any inhalation emergency is personal safety and then removal of the patient from the toxic environment.

SURFACE-ABSORBED TOXINS

Many poisons, including organophosphates, cyanide, and other toxins, can be absorbed through the skin and mucous membranes.

Assessment and Management

Signs and symptoms of absorbed poisons can vary depending on the toxin involved. See the discussion of specific toxins in the sections that follow. Whenever you suspect absorption of a toxin (especially cyanide or organophosphates), take the following steps:

- Safely remove the patient from the poisonous environment. It is essential that you follow these guidelines:
  - Wear protective clothing.
  - Use appropriate respiratory protection.
  - Remove the patient's contaminated clothing.
  - Perform the primary assessment, history, and secondary assessment.
  - Initiate supportive measures.
  - Contact the Poison Control Centre and medical direction according to your local protocols.

Your first priority in any surface-absorbed poisoning emergency is personal safety and then removal of the patient from the toxic environment.

SPECIFIC TOXINS

To recognize and implement the proper procedure in a given poisoning, you must be familiar with the signs and symptoms that a particular toxin will trigger. Often, you may not be able to identify the exact toxin a patient has been exposed to, but usually a group of toxins will have very similar manifestations and effects and will require similar interventions. Similar toxins with similar signs and symptoms are organized into **toxidromes** (toxic syndromes), which make remembering the details of their effects much simpler. Study the toxidromes listed in Table 34-3.

The following sections address specific toxins commonly encountered. While the standard toxicological emergency procedures, discussed earlier, apply to all of these toxins, pay close attention to variations in treatment. Variations include specific procedures you must perform in a particular case or a poisoning in which an antidote is available or immediately necessary. Management of injected toxins, drug overdose, and substance abuse will be covered later in the chapter.

✱ **toxidrome** a toxic syndrome; a group of typical signs and symptoms consistently associated with exposure to a particular type of toxin.

Table 34-3 TOXIC SYNDROMES

Toxidromes	Toxin			Signs and Symptoms

Anticholinergic	Belladonna alkaloids
	  Atropine (hyoscyamine)
	  Belladonna alkaloid mixtures: belladonna
	    leaf, fluid extract, tincture
	  Homatropine
	  Methscopolamine
	  Methylatropine nitrate
	  Plants: *Atropa belladonna, Datura stramonium,*
	    Hyoscyamus niger, Amanita muscaria
	    or *pantherina*
	  Scopolamine (l-hyoscine)
				Dry skin and mucous
				  membranes
				Thirst
				Dysphagia
				Vision blurred for near objects
				Fixed dilated pupils
				Tachycardia
				Sometimes hypertension
				Rash, like scarlet fever
				Hyperthermia, flushing
				Urinary urgency and retention
				Lethargy
				Confusion or restlessness,
				  excitement
				Delirium, hallucinations
				Ataxia
				Seizures
				Respiratory failure
				Cardiovascular collapse

	Synthetic anticholinergics			
	Adiphenine	Isopropamide	Pipenzolate	
	Anisotropine	Mepenzolate	Piperiodolate	
	Cyclopentolate	Methantheline	Poldine	
	Dicyclomine	Methixene	Propantheline	
	Diphemanil	Oxyphenonium	Thiphenamil	
	Eucatropine	Oxyphencyclimine	Tridihexethyl	
	Glycopyrrolate	Pentapiperide	Tropicamide	
	Hexocyclium			
	Incidential anticholinergics			
	Antihistamines	Benactyzine	Phenothiazines	
	Tricyclic antidepressants			

Acetylcholinesterase inhibition	Organophosphates
	  TEPP
	  OMPA
	  Dipterex
	  Chlorthion
	  Di-Syston
	  Co-ral
	  Phosdrin
	  Parathion
	  Methylparathion
	  Malathion
	  Systox
	  EPN
	  Diazinon
	  Guthion
	  Trithion
				Sweating, constricted pupils,
				  lacrimation, excessive
				  salivation, wheezing, cramps,
				  vomiting, diarrhea, tenesmus,
				  bradycardia *or* tachycardia,
				  hypotension *or* hypertension,
				  blurred vision, urinary
				  incontinence
				
				Striated muscle: cramps,
				  weakness, twitching, paralysis,
				  respiratory failure, cyanosis,
				  arrest
				
				Sympathetic ganglia:
				  tachycardia, elevated blood
				  pressure
				
				CNS effects: anxiety, restlessness
				  ataxia, seizures, insomnia,
				  coma, absent reflexes,
				  Cheyne-Stokes respirations,
				  respiratory and circulation
				  depression

Cholinergic	Acetylcholine	Betel nut	Methacholine	Sweating, constricted pupils,
				  lacrimation, excessive
				  salivation, wheezing, cramps,
				  vomiting, diarrhea, tenesmus,
				  bradycardia *or* tachycardia,
				  hypotension *or* hypertension,
				  blurred vision, urinary
				  incontinence

	Area catechu	Bethanechol	Muscarine	
	Carbachol	Pilocarpine		
	Clitocybe dealbata	*Pilocarpus* species		

Continued

Table 34-3 TOXIC SYNDROMES (*CONTINUED*)

Toxidromes	Toxin			Signs and Symptoms
Extrapyramidal	Acetophenazine Butaperazine Carphenazine Chlorpromazine Haloperidol	Mesoridazine Perphenazine Piperacetaxine Promazine	Thioridazine Thiothixene Trifluoperazine Triflupromazine	Parkinsonian Dysphagia, eye muscle spasm, rigidity, tremor, neck spasm, shrieking, jaw spasm, laryngospasm
Hemoglobinopathies	Carbon monoxide Methemoglobin			Headache, nausea, vomiting, dizziness, dyspnea, seizures, coma, death Cutaneous blisters, gastroenteritis Epidemic occurrence with carbon monoxide Cyanosis, chocolate blood with nonfunctional hemoglobin
Metal fume fever	Fumes of oxides of Brass Cadmium Copper	Iron Magnesium Mercury	Nickel Titanium Tungsten Zinc	Chills, fever, nausea, vomiting, muscular pain, throat dryness, headache, fatigue, weakness, leukocytosis, respiratory disease
Narcotic	Alphaprodine Anileridine Codeine Cyclazocine Dextromethorphan Dextromoramide Diacetylmorphine Dihydrocodeine Dihydrocodeinone Dipipanone Diphenoxylate (Lomotil)	Ethylmorphine Ethoheptazine (meperidene metabolite) Fentanyl Heroin Hydromorphone Levorphanol Meperidine Methadone Metopon Morphine	Normeperidene Opium Oxycodone Oxymorphone Pentazocine Phenazocine Piminodine Propoxyphene Racemorphan	CNS depression Pinpoint pupils Slowed respirations Hypotension Response to naloxone Pupils may be dilated and excitement may predominate Normeperidine: tremor, CNS excitation, seizures
Sympathomimetic	Aminophylline Amphetamines Caffeine *Catha edulus* (Khat) Cocaehylene Cocaine Dopamine	Ephedrine Epinephrine Fenfluramine Levarterenol Metaraminol Methamphetamine Methcathinone	Methylphenidate (Ritalin) Pemoline Phencyclidine Phenmetrazine Phentermine	CNS excitation Seizures Hypertension Hypotension with caffeine Tachycardia
Withdrawal	Alcohol Barbiturates Benzodiazepines Chloral hydrate	Cocaine Ethchlorvynol Glutethimide Meprobamate	Methaqualone Methyprylon Opiods Paraldehyde	Diarrhea, large pupils, piloerection, hypertension, tachycardia, insomnia, lacrimation, muscle cramps, restlessness, yawning, hallucinations Depression with cocaine

Adapted from Done, AK. *Poisoning—A Systematic Approach for the Emergency Department Physician.* Presented Aug. 6–9, 1979, at Snowmass Village, CO, Symposium sponsored by Rocky Mountain Poison Center. Used by Permission.

CYANIDE

Cyanide can enter the body by a variety of routes. It is present in many commercial and household items that can be either ingested or absorbed—rodenticides, silver polish, and fruit pits and seeds (apricots, cherries, pears, and so on). It also can be inhaled, especially in fires that release cyanide from products containing nitrogen. A roomful of burning plastics, silks, or synthetic carpeting can also be a roomful of cyanide-filled smoke. Cyanide also forms in patients on long-term sodium nitroprusside therapy. Suicidal patients have been known to take cyanide salt. Regardless of the entry route, cyanide is an extremely fast-acting toxin. Once cyanide enters the body, it acts as a *cellular asphyxiant*. It inflicts its damage by inhibiting an enzyme vital to cellular use of oxygen.

Signs and Symptoms

Signs and symptoms of cyanide poisoning include

- A burning sensation in the mouth and throat
- Headache, confusion, combative behaviour
- Hypertension and tachycardia followed by hypotension and further dysrhythmias
- Seizures and coma
- Pulmonary edema

Management

First, safely remove the patient from the source of exposure. To prevent inhalation, always wear breathing equipment when entering the scene of a fire. Initiate supportive measures immediately. Follow this with the application of the cyanide antidote kit (Figure 34-1). This kit contains amyl nitrite ampules, a sodium nitrite, and a sodium thiosulphate solution. Adding nitrites to blood converts some hemoglobin to *methemoglobin*, which allows cyanide to bind to it. Thiosulphate then binds with the cyanide to form thiocyanate, a nontoxic substance readily excreted renally. Because cyanide is rapidly toxic, you must administer the cyanide antidote kit without delay. If your unit carries this kit, familiarize yourself with its contents and use.

FIGURE 34-1 Cyanide antidote kit.

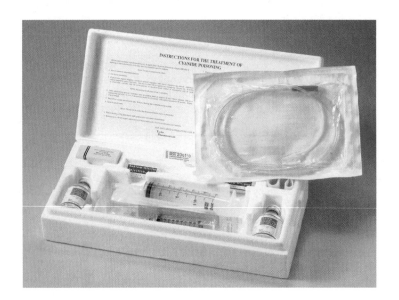

CARBON MONOXIDE

Carbon monoxide (CO) is an odourless, tasteless gas that is often the byproduct of incomplete combustion. Because of its chemical structure, it has more than 200 times the affinity of oxygen to bind with the red blood cell's hemoglobin (producing carboxyhemoglobin). Once this molecule has bound with hemoglobin, it is very resistant to removal and causes an effective hypoxia. Because of the variability of the signs and symptoms, people usually ignore CO poisoning until highly toxic levels occur. Common circumstances for CO poisoning include improperly vented heating systems or the use of a small barbecue to heat a house or camper. Symptoms of early poisoning are very similar to those of the flu. Be alert for CO poisoning in multiple patients who live together in a poorly heated and vented space and who have "flu-like" symptoms.

Signs and Symptoms

Signs and symptoms of CO poisoning include

- Headache
- Nausea, vomiting
- Confusion or other altered mental status
- Tachypnea

Management

Because of the difficulty in removing CO from hemoglobin, definitive treatment is often performed in a hyperbaric chamber (Figure 34-2). In this specially designed environment, oxygen under several atmospheres of pressure surrounds the body. This increases oxygenation of available hemoglobin. In field settings, take the following supportive steps:

- Ensure the safety of rescue personnel.
- Remove the patient from the contaminated area.
- Begin immediate ventilation of the area.
- Initiate supportive measures. High-flow oxygen via a nonrebreather mask is critical in this setting.

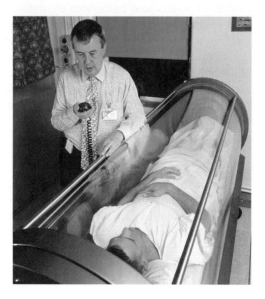

FIGURE 34-2 Hyperbaric chamber.

CARDIAC MEDICATIONS

The list of cardiac medications grows almost daily. Many classes of these drugs exist, including antidysrythmics, beta-blockers, calcium channel blockers, glycosides, ACE inhibitors, and so on. Generally, these medications regulate heart function by decreasing heart rate, suppressing automaticity, and/or reducing vascular tone. Overdoses of these drugs can be intentional but are more often due to errors in dosage.

Signs and Symptoms

In overdose quantities, signs and symptoms of cardiac medication poisoning include

- Nausea and vomiting
- Headache, dizziness, confusion
- Profound hypotension
- Cardiac dysrhythmias (usually bradycardia)
- Heart conduction blocks
- Bronchospasm and pulmonary edema (especially beta-blockers)

Management

Initiate standard toxicological emergency assessment and treatment immediately. Be aware that severe bradycardia may not respond well to atropine; therefore, you may need to use an external pacing device. Some cardiac medications do have antidotes that may help with severe adverse effects. These include calcium for calcium channel blockers, glucagon for beta-blockers, and Digoxin-specific Fab (Digibind) for digoxin. These medications are usually not used in prehospital settings.

CAUSTIC SUBSTANCES

* **acid** a substance that liberates hydrogen ions (H^+) when in solution.

* **alkali** a substance that liberates hydroxyl ions (OH^-) when in solution; a strong base.

Caustic substances are either **acids** or **alkalis** (bases) that are found in both the home and the industrial workplace. Strong caustics can produce severe burns at the site of contact and, if ingested, cause tissue destruction at the lips, mouth, esophagus, and other areas of the gastrointestinal tract.

Strong *acids* have a pH less than 2. They are found in plumbing liquids, such as drain openers and bathroom cleaners. Contact with strong acids usually produces immediate and severe pain. This is a result of tissue coagulation and necrosis. Often, this type of contact injury will produce *eschar* at the burn site, which will act like a shield and prevent further penetration or damage to deeper tissues. If ingested, acids will cause local burns to the mouth and throat. Because of the rapid transit through the esophagus, the esophagus is not usually damaged. More likely, the stomach lining will be injured. Immediate or delayed hemorrhage can occur and may be associated with perforation. Pain is severe and usually due to direct injury and spasm from irritation. Absorption of acids into the vascular system will occur quite readily, causing a significant acidemia, which will need to be managed along with the direct local effects.

Strong *alkaline* agents typically have a pH greater than 12.5. They can be in solid or liquid form (such as in drain openers) and are routinely found around the house. These agents cause injury by inducing liquefaction necrosis. Pain is often delayed, which allows for longer tissue contact and deeper tissue injury before the exposure is even recognized. Solid alkaline agents can stick to the oropharynx or esophagus. This can cause perforation, bleeding, and inflammation of central chest structures. Liquid alkalis are more likely to injure the stomach because they pass quickly through the esophagus. Within 2–3 days of exposure, complete loss of the protective mucosal tissue can occur, followed by either gradual healing and recovery or further bleeding, necrosis, and stricture formation.

Signs and Symptoms

Signs and symptoms of caustic injury include

- Facial burns
- Pain in the lips, tongue, throat, or gums
- Drooling, trouble swallowing
- Hoarseness, stridor, or shortness of breath
- Shock from bleeding, vomiting

Management

Assessment and intervention must be aggressive and rapid to minimize morbidity and mortality. Take precautions to prevent injury to rescuers. Initiate standard toxicological emergency assessment and treatment, but pay particular attention to establishing an airway. Injury to the oropharynx and larynx may make airway control and ventilation very difficult and may even require cricothyrotomy. Since caustics will not adsorb to activated charcoal, there is no indication to administer it. In the past, rescuers often gave water or milk to dilute any ingested caustics, but there is controversy as to whether this is beneficial. Rapid transport to the emergency department is essential.

HYDROFLUORIC ACID

Hydrofluoric (HF) acid deserves special attention because it is extremely toxic and can be lethal despite the appearance of only moderate burns on skin contact. HF acid penetrates deeply into tissues and is inactivated only when it comes in contact with *cations,* such as calcium. Calcium fluoride is formed by this inactivation and settles in the tissue as a salt. The removal of calcium from cells causes a total disruption of cell functioning and can even cause bone destruction as calcium is leeched out of the bones. Death has been reported from exposure of less than 2.5 percent body surface area to a highly concentrated solution.

Hydrofluoric acid is used to clean glass in lab settings and for etching glass in art.

Signs and Symptoms

Signs and symptoms of HF acid exposure include

- Burning at site of contact
- Trouble breathing
- Confusion
- Palpitations
- Muscle cramps

Management

Management includes the following steps:

- Ensure the safety of rescue personnel.
- Initiate supportive measures.
- Remove exposed clothing.
- Irrigate the affected area with water thoroughly.

- Immerse the affected limb in iced water with magnesium sulphate, calcium salts, or benzethonium chloride.
- Transport immediately for definitive care.

ALCOHOL

See the section on Alcohol Abuse later in this chapter.

HYDROCARBONS

Hydrocarbons are organic compounds composed of mostly carbon and hydrogen. They include such common recognizable names as kerosene, naphtha, turpentine, mineral oil, chloroform, toluene, and benzene. These chemicals are found in common household products, such as lighter fluid, paint, glue, lubricants, solvents, and aerosol propellants. Toxicity from hydrocarbons can occur through any route, including ingestion, inhalation, or surface absorption.

Signs and Symptoms

Signs and symptoms of hydrocarbon poisoning will vary with the type and route of exposure but may include

- Burns due to local contact
- Wheezing, dyspnea, hypoxia, and pneumonitis from aspiration/inhalation
- Headache, dizziness, slurred speech, ataxia (irregular and difficult-to-control movements), and obtundation (dulled reflexes)
- Foot and wrist drop with numbness and tingling
- Cardiac dysrhythmias

Management

Recent studies have shown that very few poisonings with hydrocarbons are serious, and less than 1 percent require physician intervention. If you know the exact chemical that the patient has been exposed to and the patient is asymptomatic, medical direction may suggest that the patient can be left at home. However, a few hydrocarbon poisonings can be very serious. Any patient who is symptomatic, who does not know what he has taken, or who has taken a hydrocarbon that requires gastrointestinal decontamination (halogenated or aromatic hydrocarbons) must be treated using standard toxicological emergency procedures. Since charcoal will not bind hydrocarbons, this may be one of the few cases in which gastric lavage can be useful.

TRICYCLIC ANTIDEPRESSANTS

* **therapeutic index** the maximum tolerated dose divided by the minimum curative dose of a drug; the range between curative and toxic dosages; also called *therapeutic window.*

Tricyclic antidepressants were once commonly used to treat depression. Close monitoring was required because these medications have a narrow **therapeutic index,** meaning that a relatively small increase in dose can quickly lead to toxic effects. The very nature of their use, treating depression, presents a dilemma because the patients most seriously in need of treatment may also be the most likely to attempt to take an overdose. Deaths due to antidepressant overdose have dropped significantly in recent years since the development and rapid acceptance of safer agents unrelated to tricyclics. However, tricyclic antidepressants are still used for various clinical problems, such as chronic pain or migraine prophylaxis, and may still be responsible for more deaths due to intentional overdose than any other medication. Common agents include amitriptyline (Elavil), amoxapine, clomipramine, doxepin, imipramine, nortriptyline.

Signs and Symptoms

Signs and symptoms of tricyclic antidepressant toxicity include

- Dry mouth
- Blurred vision
- Urinary retention
- Constipation

Late into an overdose, more severe toxicity may produce

- Confusion, hallucinations
- Hyperthermia
- Respiratory depression
- Seizures
- Tachycardia and hypotension
- Cardiac dysrhythmias (heart block, wide QRS, Torsades de pointes)

Management

Toxicity from tricyclic antidepressants requires immediate initiation of standard toxicological emergency procedures. Cardiac monitoring is critical, since dysrhythmias are the most common cause of death. If you suspect a mixed overdose with benzodiazepines, do *not* use Flumazenil, since it may precipitate seizures. If significant cardiac toxicity occurs, sodium bicarbonate can be used as an additional therapy. Contact medical direction as necessary.

If you suspect a mixed overdose with benzodiazepines, do not *use Flumazenil, since it may precipitate seizures.*

MAO INHIBITORS

Monoamine oxidase inhibitors (MAOIs) have been used, although rarely, to treat depression. Recently, they have been used, on a limited basis, to treat obsessive-compulsive disorders. They are relatively unpopular because of a narrow therapeutic index, multiple-drug interactions, serious interactions with foods containing *tyramine* (for example, red wine and cheese), and high morbidity and mortality when taken in overdose. These drugs inhibit the breakdown of neurotransmitters, such as norepinephrine and dopamine, while increasing the availability of the components needed to make even more neurotransmitters. When taken in overdose, MAOIs can be extremely dangerous, although symptoms may not appear for up to six hours.

Signs and Symptoms

Signs and symptoms of MAOI overdose include

- Headache, agitation, restlessness, tremor
- Nausea
- Palpitations
- Tachycardia
- Severe hypertension
- Hyperthermia
- Eventually bradycardia, hypotension, coma, and death occur

New MAOIs have recently entered the marketplace. The effects of these next-generation drugs are reversible and less toxic and do not cause the same reactions with food as the older MAOIs. Data are not yet available on the outcome of patients overdosing on these newer agents.

Management

No antidote exists for MAOI overdose because the inhibition is not reversible, except with newer drugs. Therefore, institute standard toxicological emergency procedures as soon as possible. If necessary, give symptomatic support for seizures and hyperthermia using benzodiazepines. If vasopressors are needed, use norepinephrine.

NEWER ANTIDEPRESSANTS

In recent years, several new agents have been developed to treat depression. Because of their high safety profile in therapeutic and overdose amounts, these drugs have been widely accepted and have virtually replaced tricyclic antidepressants.

Recently introduced drugs include trazodone (Desyrel), bupropion (Wellbutrin), and the large group of very popular *selective serotonin reuptake inhibitors,* or SSRIs, (Prozac, Luvox, Paxil, Zoloft). SSRIs prevent the reuptake of serotonin in the brain, theoretically making it more available for brain functions. The true mechanism by which these drugs treat depression is unclear.

Signs and Symptoms

When these drugs are taken in overdose, usually the signs and symptoms are mild. Occasionally, trazodone and buproprion will cause CNS depression and seizures, but deaths are very rare and have only been reported in mixed overdoses with multiple ingestions. More commonly, signs and symptoms of overdose with the newer antidepressant agents include

- Drowsiness
- Tremor
- Nausea and vomiting
- Sinus tachycardia

SSRIs are now also associated with *serotonin syndrome.* This syndrome is caused by increased serotonin levels and is often triggered by increasing the dose of SSRI or adding a second drug, such as Demerol, codeine, dextromethorphan (cough syrup), or other antidepressants. Signs and symptoms of serotonin syndrome include

- Agitation, anxiety, confusion, insomnia
- Headache, drowsiness, coma
- Nausea, salivation, diarrhea, abdominal cramps
- Cutaneous piloerection, flushed skin
- Hyperthermia, tachycardia
- Rigidity, shivering, incoordination, myoclonic jerks

Management

Overdose with these new antidepressants is not as life threatening as with previous agents unless other drugs or alcohol are taken simultaneously. Consequently, treat overdoses with the standard toxicological emergency procedures. Also, have the patient discontinue all serotonergic drugs, and implement supportive measures. Benzodiazepines or beta-blockers occasionally are used to improve patient comfort, but these are rarely given in the field.

LITHIUM

In the treatment of bipolar (manic-depressive) disorder, no other drug has been proven to be more effective than lithium. It is unclear how lithium exerts its therapeutic effect. However, like tricyclic antidepressants, lithium has a narrow therapeutic index that results in toxicity during normal use and in overdose situations.

Signs and Symptoms

Signs and symptoms of lithium toxicity include

- Thirst, dry mouth
- Tremor, muscle twitching, increased reflexes
- Confusion, stupor, seizures, coma
- Nausea, vomiting, diarrhea
- Bradycardia, dysrhythmias

Management

Treat lithium overdose with mostly supportive measures. Use the standard toxicological emergency procedures, but remember that activated charcoal will not bind lithium and need not be given. Alkalinizing the urine with sodium bicarbonate and osmotic diuresis using mannitol may increase elimination of lithium, but severe toxic cases require hemodialysis.

SALICYLATES

Salicylates are some of the more common drugs taken in overdose, largely due to the fact that they are readily available over the counter. The most recognizable forms are aspirin, oil of wintergreen, and some prescription combination medications.

Aspirin in large doses can cause serious consequences. About 300 mg/kg is required to cause toxicity. In such amounts, salicylates inhibit normal energy production and acid buffering in the body. This results in a metabolic acidosis, which further injures other organ systems.

Signs and Symptoms

Signs and symptoms of salicylate overdose include

- Rapid respirations
- Hyperthermia
- Confusion, lethargy, coma
- Cardiac failure, dysrhythmias
- Abdominal pain, vomiting
- Pulmonary edema, ARDS (adult respiratory distress syndrome)

Chronic overdose symptoms are somewhat less severe and do not tend to include abdominal complaints. It is difficult to distinguish chronic overdose from very early acute overdose or early overdose that has progressed past the abdominal irritation stage.

Management

In all cases, salicylate poisoning should be treated using standard toxicological emergency procedures. Activated charcoal definitely reduces drug absorption and should be used. If possible, find out the time of ingestion, since blood levels measured at the right time can indicate the expected degree of injury. Most symptomatic patients will require generous IV fluids and may need urine alkalinization with sodium bicarbonate. Severe cases may require dialysis.

ACETAMINOPHEN

Due to its few side effects in normal dosages, acetaminophen (e.g., paracetamol, Tylenol) is one of the most common drugs in use today. It is used to treat fever and/or pain and is a common ingredient in hundreds of over-the-counter preparations. It can be also obtained by prescription in combination with various other drugs.

In large doses, however, acetaminophen can be a very dangerous pharmaceutical. A dose of 150 mg/kg is considered toxic and may result in death due to injury to the liver. A highly reactive byproduct of acetaminophen metabolism is responsible for most adverse effects, but this is usually avoided by the body's detoxification system. When large amounts of acetaminophen enter the system, the detoxification system is overwhelmed and gradually depleted, leaving the toxic metabolite in the circulation to cause hepatic necrosis.

Signs and Symptoms

Signs and symptoms of acetaminophen toxicity appear in four stages.

Stage 1	½–24 hours	Nausea, vomiting, weakness, fatigue
Stage 2	24–48 hours	Abdominal pain, decreased urine, elevated liver enzymes
Stage 3	72–96 hours	Liver function disruption
Stage 4	4–14 days	Gradual recovery or progressive liver failure

Management

Treat acetaminophen overdose with standard toxicological emergency procedures. Find out the time of ingestion, since blood levels taken at the right time can predict the potential for injury. An antidote called N-acetylcysteine (NAC, Mucomyst) is available and highly effective. However, NAC is usually administered based on clinical and laboratory studies and is rarely given in the prehospital setting.

OTHER NONPRESCRIPTION PAIN MEDICATIONS

Nonsteroidal anti-inflammatory drugs (NSAIDs) are another group of medications that are readily available and are often overdosed. Common examples include naproxen sodium, indomethacin, ibuprofen, and ketorolac (Toradol).

Signs and Symptoms

The presentation of toxicity caused by NSAIDs varies greatly but can include

- Headache
- Ringing in the ears (tinnitus)
- Nausea, vomiting, abdominal pain
- Swelling of the extremities
- Mild drowsiness
- Dyspnea, wheezing, pulmonary edema
- Rash, itching

Management

There is no specific antidote for NSAID toxicity. Use general overdose procedures, including supportive care, as soon as possible, and transport to the emergency department for observation and any necessary symptomatic treatment.

THEOPHYLLINE

Theophylline belongs to a group of medications called xanthines. It is usually used for patients with asthma or COPD because of its moderate bronchodilation and mild anti-inflammatory effects. Like other drugs with a narrow therapeutic index and high toxicity, theophylline has become less popular recently and therefore is not implicated in as many overdose injuries as in the past.

Signs and Symptoms

Symptoms of theophylline toxicity include

- Agitation
- Tremors
- Seizures
- Cardiac dysrhythmias
- Nausea and vomiting

Management

Theophylline can cause significant morbidity and mortality. In overdose situations, it is essential that you institute toxicological emergency procedures immediately. In fact, theophylline is on the small list of drugs that have significant *entero-hepatic circulation*. This means that multiple doses of activated charcoal over time will continuously remove more and more of the drug from the body. Treat any dysrhythmias according to local protocols.

METALS

With the exception of iron, overdose of heavy metals is a rare occurrence. Other possible involved metals include lead, arsenic, and mercury. All metals affect numerous enzyme systems within the body and therefore present with a variety of symptoms. Some also have direct local effects when ingested and when accumulated in various organs.

Iron

The body only requires small amounts of iron on a daily basis to maintain a sufficient store for enzyme and hemoglobin production. Excess amounts are easily obtained from nonprescription supplements and multivitamins. Children have a tendency to accidentally overdose on iron by taking too many candy-flavoured chewable vitamins containing iron. To determine the amount of iron ingested, you must calculate the amount of elemental iron present in the type of pill ingested. Symptoms occur when more than 20 mg/kg of elemental iron are ingested.

Signs and Symptoms Excess iron will cause gastrointestinal injury and possible shock from hemorrhage, especially if it forms *concretions* (lumps of iron formed when tablets fuse together after being swallowed). Patients with significant iron ingestions will often have visible tablets or concretions in the stomach or small intestine when x-rayed. Other signs and symptoms of iron ingestion include

- Vomiting (often hematemesis), diarrhea
- Abdominal pain, shock
- Liver failure
- Metabolic acidosis with tachypnea
- Eventual bowel scarring and possible obstruction

Management It is essential to initiate standard toxicological emergency procedures immediately. Since iron tends to inhibit gastrointestinal motility, pills sit longer in the stomach and may possibly be easier to remove through gastric lavage. Because activated charcoal will not bind iron (or any metals), it should not be used. Deferoxamine, a chelating agent, may be used in iron overdose as an antidote, since it binds to iron so that less iron is moved into cells and tissues to cause damage.

Lead and Mercury

Both lead and mercury are heavy metals found in varying amounts in the environment. Lead was often used in glazes and paints before the toxic potential of such exposure became apparent. Mercury is a contaminant from industrial processing but is also found in thermometers and temperature-control switches in most homes. Chronic and acute exposures are possible with both metals.

Signs and Symptoms Signs and symptoms of heavy metal toxicity include

- Headache, irritability, confusion, coma
- Memory disturbance
- Tremor, weakness, agitation
- Abdominal pain

Management Chronic poisoning can cause permanent neurological injury, which makes it imperative that the proper agencies monitor heavy metal levels in the environment of a patient who has presented with toxicity. Learn to recognize the signs of heavy metal toxicity and institute standard toxicology emergency procedures as needed. Activated charcoal will not bind heavy metals but various chelating agents (meso-2,3-dimercapto-succinic acid [DMSA], dimercaprol or British anti-Lewisite [BAL]) are available and may be used in definitive management in the hospital.

CONTAMINATED FOOD

Food poisoning is caused by a spectrum of different factors. For example, bacteria, viruses, and toxic chemicals notoriously produce varying levels of gastrointestinal distress. The patient may present with nausea, vomiting, diarrhea, and diffuse abdominal pain.

Bacterial food poisonings range in severity. Bacterial **exotoxins** (secreted by bacteria) or **enterotoxins** (exotoxins associated with gastrointestinal diseases, including food poisoning) cause the adverse GI complaints noted previously. Food contaminated with other bacteria, such as *Shigella, Salmonella,* or *E. coli,* can produce even more severe gastrointestinal reactions, often leading to electrolyte imbalance and hypovolemia. *Clostridium botulinum,* the world's most toxic poison, presents as severe respiratory distress or arrest. The incubation of this toxin can range from four hours to eight days. Fortunately, botulism rarely occurs, except in cases of improper food storage methods, such as may occur in canning.

A variety of seafood poisonings are a result of specific toxins found in dinoflagellate-contaminated shellfish, such as clams, mussels, oysters, and scallops, and can produce a syndrome referred to as *paralytic shellfish poisoning.* This condition can lead to respiratory arrest in addition to standard gastrointestinal symptoms.

Increased fish consumption by North Americans has also increased the number of cases of poisonings from toxins found in many commonly eaten fish. *Ciguatera (bony fish) poisoning* most frequently turns up in fish caught in the Pacific Ocean or along the tropical reefs of Florida and the West Indies. Ciguatera normally takes 2–6 hours to incubate and may produce myalgia and paresthesia. *Scombroid (histamine) poisoning* results from bacterial contamination of mackerel, tuna, bonitos, and albacore. Both types of poisoning cause the common gastrointestinal symptoms. Scombroid poisoning will present with an immediate facial flushing as histamines cause vasodilation.

* **exotoxin** a soluble poisonous substance secreted during growth of a bacterium.

* **enterotoxin** an exotoxin that produces gastrointestinal symptoms and diseases such as food poisoning.

Signs and Symptoms

As mentioned above, signs and symptoms of food poisoning may include

- Nausea, vomiting, diarrhea, abdominal pain
- Facial flushing, respiratory distress (with some seafood poisonings)

Management

Except for botulism, food poisoning is rarely life threatening. Treatment, therefore, is largely supportive. In suspected cases of food poisoning, contact poison control and medical direction, and take the following steps:

- Perform the necessary assessment.
- Collect samples of the suspected contaminated food source.
- Perform the following management actions:
  – Establish and maintain the airway.
  – Administer high-flow oxygen.
  – Intubate and assist ventilations, if appropriate.
  – Establish venous access.
- Consider the administration of antihistamines (especially in seafood poisonings) and antiemetics.

POISONOUS PLANTS AND MUSHROOMS

Plants, trees, and mushrooms contribute heavily to the number of accidental toxic ingestions. While the vast majority of plants are nontoxic, many of the popular decorative houseplants can present a danger to children, who frequently ingest nonfood items. Most Poison Control Centres distribute pamphlets that identify toxic household plants. (These pamphlets will help parents "poison proof" the home.)

It is impossible to cover all the toxic plants and mushrooms. Few rescuers are trained as botanists, and they find it difficult to identify the offending material. Mushrooms are particularly difficult to identify from small pieces. Additionally, most people recognize mushrooms and other plants by common names, rather than by the nomenclature of scientific species. A general approach is to obtain a sample of the plant, if possible. Try to find a full leaf, stem, and any flowers.

Since many ornamental plants contain irritating chemicals or crystals, examine the patient's mouth and throat for redness, blistering, or edema. Identify other abnormal signs during the focused secondary assessment.

Mushroom poisoning victims generally fall into two categories: people foraging for edible mushrooms and children who ingest mushrooms accidentally. Fortunately, few of the many mushroom species possess extremely dangerous toxins. Toxic mushrooms fall into seven classes. *Amanita* and *Galerina* belong to the deadly *cyclopeptide* group (Figure 34-3). (*Amanita* accounts for more than 90 percent of all deaths.) These mushrooms produce a poison that is extremely toxic to the liver, with a mortality rate of about 50 percent.

Signs and Symptoms

Signs and symptoms of poisonous plant ingestion include

- Excessive salivation, lacrimation (secretion of tears), diaphoresis
- Abdominal cramps, nausea, vomiting, diarrhea
- Decreasing levels of consciousness, eventually progressing to coma

Management

For guidance on the treatment of plant poisonings, call the Poison Control Centre. If contact cannot be made, use the procedures outlined under treatment of food poisoning earlier.

FIGURE 34-3 Poisonous mushrooms from *Amanita* and *Galerina* classes.

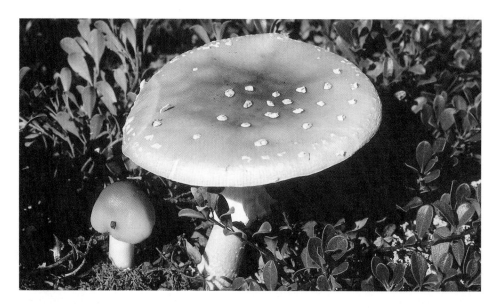

INJECTED TOXINS

Although we generally think of intentional or accidental drug overdoses as sources of injected poisons, the most common source for these poisonings is the animal kingdom. Bites and stings from a variety of insects, reptiles, and animals are among the most common injuries sustained by humans. Further injury can result from bacterial contamination or from a reaction produced by an injected substance.

GENERAL PRINCIPLES OF MANAGEMENT

The general principles of field management for bites and stings include the following:

- Protect rescue personnel—the offending organism may still be around.
- Remove the patient from danger of repeated injection, especially in the case of yellow jackets, wasps, or hornets.
- If possible, identify the insect, reptile, or animal that caused the injury, and bring it to the emergency department along with the patient (if it can be done safely).
- Perform a primary assessment and rapid secondary assessment.
- Prevent or delay further absorption of the poison.
- Initiate supportive measures as indicated.
- Watch for anaphylactic reaction (see Chapter 31).
- Transport the patient as rapidly as possible.
- Contact the Poison Control Centre and medical direction according to your local protocols.

In the case of a bite or sting, remember to protect rescue personnel. The offending organism may still be around.

INSECT BITES AND STINGS

Insect Stings

Many people die from allergic reactions to the stings from an order of insects known as *Hymenoptera*. As mentioned earlier, *Hymenoptera* includes wasps, bees, hornets, and ants. Only the common honeybee leaves a stinger. Wasps, yellow jackets, hornets, and fire ants sting repeatedly until removal from contact.

In most cases of insect bite, local treatment is all that is necessary. Unless an allergic reaction occurs, most patients will tolerate the isolated *Hymenoptera* sting.

Signs and Symptoms Signs and symptoms include

- Localized pain
- Redness
- Swelling
- Skin weal

Idiosyncratic reactions to the toxin may occur, resulting in a progressing localized swelling and edema. This is not an allergic reaction, however, if it responds well to an antihistamine, such as diphenhydramine hydrochloride. The major problem resulting from a *Hymenoptera* sting is an allergic reaction or anaphylaxis. Signs and symptoms of allergic reaction include the following:

- Localized pain, redness, swelling, and a skin weal
- Itching or flushing of the skin, rash
- Tachycardia, hypotension, bronchospasm, or laryngeal edema
- Facial edema, uvular swelling

Management For *Hymenoptera* stings, take the following supportive measures:

- Wash the area.
- Gently remove the stinger, if present, by scraping without squeezing the venom sac.
- Apply cool compresses to the injection site.
- Observe for and treat allergic reactions and/or anaphylaxis. (See Chapter 31.)

Brown Recluse Spider Bite

The brown recluse spider is not found naturally in Canada. Incidents of brown recluse spider bites are extremely rare and most often occur in those handling fruit from the southern and midwestern United States.

The brown recluse is about 15 mm in length. It generally lives in dark, dry locations and can often be found in and around the house. There is a characteristic violin-shaped marking on the back, giving the spider its nickname, "fiddleback spider" (Figure 34-4). Another identifying feature is the presence of six eyes (three pairs in a semicircle), instead of the eight eyes common to most spiders.

Signs and Symptoms Brown recluse spider bites are usually painless. Not uncommonly, bites occur at night while the person sleeps. Most victims are unaware they have been bitten until the local reaction starts. Initially, a small erythematous macule surrounded by a white ring forms at the site (Figure 34-5). This usually appears within a few minutes of the bite. Over the next eight hours, localized pain, redness, and swelling develop. Tissue necrosis at the site occurs over days to weeks (Figure 34-6). Other symptoms include chills, fever, nausea and vomiting, joint pain, and, in severe situations, bleeding disorders (disseminated intravascular coagulation).

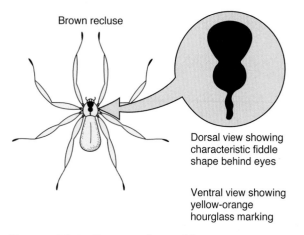

Brown recluse

Dorsal view showing characteristic fiddle shape behind eyes

Ventral view showing yellow-orange hourglass marking

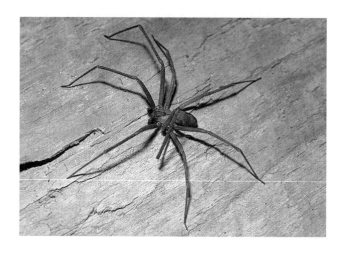

FIGURE 34-4   Brown recluse spider.

FIGURE 34-5   Brown recluse spider bite 24 hours after bite. Note the bleb and surrounding white halo. (Courtesy of Scott and White Hospital and Clinic.)

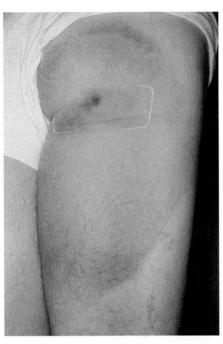

FIGURE 34-6   Brown recluse spider bite four days after the bite. Note the spread of erythema and early necrosis. (Courtesy of Scott and White Hospital and Clinic.)

Management   Treatment is mostly supportive. Since there is no antivenin, the emergency department treatment consists of antihistamines to reduce systemic reactions and possible surgical excision of necrotic tissue.

Black Widow Spider Bites

Black widow spiders live in all parts of North America. They are usually found in woodpiles or brush. The female spider is responsible for bites and can be easily identified by the characteristic orange hourglass marking on her black abdomen (Figure 34-7). The venom of the legendary black widow is very potent, causing excessive neurotransmitter release at the synaptic junctions.

Signs and Symptoms   Signs and symptoms of black widow spider bites start as immediate localized pain, redness, and swelling. Progressive muscle spasms of all large muscle groups can occur and are usually associated with severe pain. Other systemic symptoms include nausea, vomiting, sweating, seizures, paralysis, and decreased level of consciousness.

Management   Prehospital treatment is mostly supportive. It is important to reassure the patient. Intravenous muscle relaxants may be necessary for severe spasms. Diazepam (2.5–10 mg IV) or calcium gluconate (0.1–0.2/kg of 10-percent solution IV) is used in the emergency department. Note that calcium chloride is not effective and should not be used. Since hypertensive crisis is possible, monitor blood pressure carefully. Antivenin is available, so transfer the patient to the emergency department as soon as possible.

Scorpion Stings

There are many species of scorpion in the United States (Figure 34-8). All can sting, causing localized pain, but only one, the bark scorpion, has caused fatalities. These

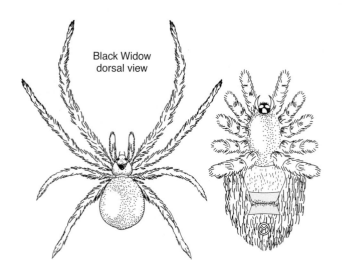

Black Widow
dorsal view

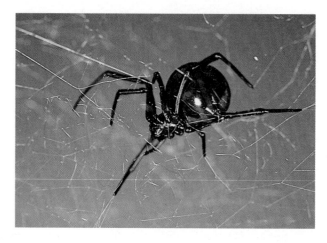

FIGURE 34-7   Black widow spider.

arthropods live mostly in Arizona and adjacent areas of California, Nevada, New Mexico, and Texas. Due to heightened interest, people now keep scorpions as pets.

Scorpions move mostly at night, hiding in the day under debris and buildings. The venom they inject is stored in a bulb at the end of the tail. If provoked, the scorpion will sting with its tail, injecting only a small amount of poison.

Signs and Symptoms   The bark scorpion's venom acts on the nervous system, producing a burning and tingling effect without much evidence of injury initially. Gradually, this progresses to numbness. Systemic effects are more pronounced with slurred speech, restlessness (hyperactivity in 80 percent of children), muscle twitching, salivation, abdominal cramping, nausea and vomiting, and seizures.

Management   Begin treatment by reassuring the patient. Apply a constricting band above the wound site no tighter than a watchband to occlude lymphatic flow only. Avoid the use of analgesics, which may increase toxicity and potentiate the venom's effect on airway control. Transport the patient to the emergency department if systemic symptoms develop. Antivenin is available but is an unlicensed goat-serum-derived product available in Arizona only. It can produce allergic or anaphylactic reactions and should be used only in severe cases.

FIGURE 34-8   Scorpion.

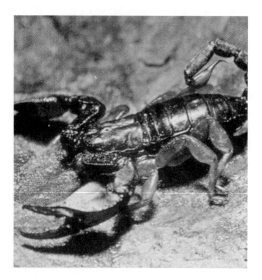

SNAKEBITES

There are hundreds of snakebites each year in North America. Fortunately, these bites result in very few deaths. The signs and symptoms of snakebite depend upon the snake, the location of the bite, and the type and amount of venom injected.

There are two families of poisonous snakes native to North America (Figure 34-9). One family (*Crotalidae*) includes the pit vipers. Common pit vipers are cottonmouths (water moccasins), rattlesnakes, and copperheads. Pit vipers are so named because of the distinctive pit between the eye and the nostril on each side of the head. These snakes have elliptical pupils, two well-developed fangs, and a triangular-shaped head. Only the rattlesnake, the most common pit viper, has rattles on the end of its tail. The Massassauga rattlesnake (*Sistrurus catenus*) is found from southwestern Ontario, along Lake Erie as far as Hamilton and north to Georgian Bay. The Western rattlesnake (*Crotalus viridis*) includes two subspecies: (1) the Prairie rattlesnake (*Crotus virdidis virdis*) found in southwestern Saskatchewan and southeastern Alberta in the arid short-grass prairie; and (2) the northern Pacific rattlesnake (*Crotalus viridis oreganos*) found in the arid valleys and their slopes in southern British Columbia.

The second family of poisonous snakes is the *Elapidae*, or coral snake, which is a distant relative of the cobra. Several varieties of coral snakes are found in North America, primarily in the southwestern United States. Because it is a small snake and has small fangs, the coral snake cannot readily attach itself to a large surface, such as an arm or leg. The coral snake has round eyes, a narrow head, and no pit. It has characteristic yellow-banded red and black rings around its body. Several nonpoisonous snakes, such as the King Snake, mimic this coloration pattern. Keep in mind a helpful mnemonic: "Red touch yellow, kill a fellow; red touch black, venom lack." This rhyme indicates the distinctive pattern of the coral snake—a pattern that signals danger.

Pit Viper Bites

Pit viper venom contains hydrolytic enzymes that are capable of destroying proteins and most other tissue components. These enzymes may produce destruction of red blood cells and other tissue components and may affect the body's blood-clotting system within the blood vessels. This will produce infarction and tissue necrosis, especially at the site of the bite.

A severe pit viper bite can result in death from shock within 30 minutes. However, most deaths from pit viper bites occur 6 to 30 hours after the bite, with 90 percent occurring within the first 48 hours.

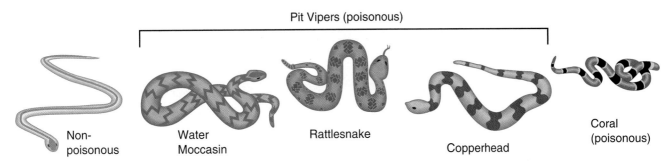

Pit Vipers (poisonous)

Non-poisonous   Water Moccasin   Rattlesnake   Copperhead   Coral (poisonous)

FIGURE 34-9   Venomous snakes in North America.

Signs and Symptoms Signs and symptoms of pit viper bite include:

- Fang marks (often little more than a scratch mark or abrasion)
- Swelling and pain at the wound site
- Continued oozing at the wound site
- Weakness, dizziness, or faintness
- Sweating and/or chills
- Thirst
- Nausea and vomiting
- Diarrhea
- Tachycardia and hypotension
- Bloody urine and gastrointestinal hemorrhage (late)
- Ecchymosis
- Necrosis
- Shallow respirations progressing to respiratory failure
- Numbness and tingling around face and head (classic)

Management In treating a person who has been bitten by a pit viper, the primary goal is to slow absorption of the venom. Remember, about 25 percent of all rattlesnake bites are "dry" and no venom is injected. The amount of venom a pit viper injects varies significantly. It is helpful to try to classify the degree of envenomation:

Degree of Envenomation	Signs and Symptoms
None	None (either local or systemic)
Minimal	Swelling
	Pain
	No systemic symptoms
Moderate	Progressive swelling
	Mild systemic symptoms
	– paresthesias
	– nausea and vomiting
	– unusual tastes
	– mild hypotension
	– mild tachycardia
	– tachypnea
Severe	Swelling (spreading rapidly)
	Severe pain
	Systemic symptoms
	– altered mental status
	– nausea and vomiting
	– hypotension (systolic < 80)
	– severe tachycardia
	– severe respiratory distress
	Blood oozes freely from puncture wounds

Antivenin is available for the various common pit vipers found in Canada and the United States. However, antivenin should only be considered for severe cases in which there is marked envenomation as evidenced by severe systemic symptoms. In some cases, people become more ill from the antivenin than they do from the snakebite itself. Routine emergency treatment of pit viper bites includes the following steps:

- Keep the patient supine.
- Immobilize the limb with a splint.
- Maintain the extremity in a neutral position. Do not apply constricting bands.

Initiate supportive care using the following guidelines:

- Apply high-flow oxygen.
- Start IV with crystalloid fluid.
- Transport the patient to the emergency department for management, which may include the administration of antivenin.
- DO NOT apply ice, cold pack, or Freon spray to the wound.
- DO NOT apply an arterial tourniquet.
- DO NOT apply electrical stimulation from any device in an attempt to retard or reverse venom spread.

Coral Snake Bites

The venom of the coral snake contains some of the enzymes found in pit viper venom. However, because of the presence of neurotoxin, coral snake venom primarily affects nervous tissue. The classic, severe coral snake bite will result in respiratory and skeletal muscle paralysis.

Signs and Symptoms After the bite of a coral snake, there may be no local manifestations or even any systemic effects for as long as 12–24 hours. Signs and symptoms of a coral snake bite include

- Localized numbness, weakness, and drowsiness
- Ataxia
- Slurred speech and excessive salivation
- Paralysis of the tongue and larynx (produces difficulty breathing and swallowing)
- Drooping of eyelids, double vision, dilated pupils
- Abdominal pain
- Nausea and vomiting
- Loss of consciousness
- Seizures
- Respiratory failure
- Hypotension

Management Treatment in cases of suspected coral snake bites includes the following steps:

- Wash the wound with copious amounts of water.
- Apply a compression bandage and keep the extremity at the level of the heart.
- Immobilize the limb with a splint.
- Start an IV using crystalloid fluid.
- Transport the patient to the emergency department for administration of antivenin.
- DO NOT apply ice, cold pack, or Freon sprays to the wound.
- DO NOT incise the wound.
- DO NOT apply electrical stimulation from any device in an attempt to retard or reverse venom spread.

MARINE ANIMAL INJECTION

Although most dangerous marine creatures prefer warm, tropical waters, some can be found in more northern waters. With the large number of people who flock to beaches and coastal recreation areas every year, the number of injuries from marine life has increased moderately. The most common encounters occur while the person is walking on the beach but can also happen while wading in shallow waters or scuba diving in deeper waters. Injection of toxins from marine creatures can result from stings of jellyfish and corals or from punctures by the bony spines of such animals as sea urchins and stingrays (Figure 34-10). All venoms of marine animals contain substances that produce pain out of proportion to the size of the injury. These poisonous toxins are unstable and heat sensitive. Heat will relieve pain and inactivate the venom.

Both fresh water and salt water contain considerable bacterial and viral pollution. Therefore, secondary infection is always a possibility in injuries caused by marine animals. Particularly severe and life-threatening infections can be inflicted by a number of organisms. In all cases of marine-acquired infections, *Vibrio* species must be considered.

Signs and Symptoms Signs and symptoms of marine animal injection include

- Intense local pain and swelling
- Weakness
- Nausea and vomiting
- Dyspnea

FIGURE 34-10 Stingray.

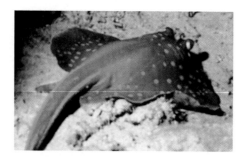

- Tachycardia
- Hypotension or shock (severe cases)

Management In suspected cases or marine animal injection, take the following steps:

- Establish and maintain the airway.
- Apply a constricting band between the wound and the heart no tighter than a watchband to occlude lymphatic flow only.
- Apply heat or hot water (43°–45°C).
- Inactivate or remove any stingers.

SUBSTANCE ABUSE AND OVERDOSE

Substance abuse, the use of a pharmacological substance for purposes other than medically defined reasons, is a very serious problem in North America. Drugs are abused because they stimulate a feeling of euphoria in the abuser. Eventually, abusers begin to crave the feeling the drug gives them and therefore develop a *dependence* on the drug, also called **addiction.** An addiction exists when a person repeatedly uses and feels an overwhelming need to obtain and continue using a particular drug. Becoming accustomed to the use of the drug is called *habituation. Physiological dependence* is the resulting condition if removal of the drug causes adverse physical reactions. There can also be *psychological dependence,* in which use of the drug is required to prevent or relieve tension or emotional stress. With continued use, **tolerance** develops, which means that the abuser must use increasingly larger doses to get the same effect.

Attempts to stop the drug can trigger a psychological or physical reaction known as **withdrawal.** Withdrawal reactions can be quite unpleasant and severe. In some cases (especially with alcohol), withdrawal can be severe enough to cause death. These reactions further strengthen the victim's dependence on the drug. At this point, the abuser may begin to withdraw from regular activities. He may have conflicts with family, friends, and coworkers as his personality and priorities change. Often, the abuser will be involved in criminal activities to support the habit. The abuser has formed an addiction at the point when the substance abuse begins to affect some part of his life. This includes the abuser's health, work, or relationships. Also, the abuser begins to act in a manner so as to seek out the drug he abuses.

The use of illicit drugs has fluctuated in recent years. Most recently, heroin has regained popularity, especially among middle to upper class teenagers and young adults. Beyond hurting themselves, substance abusers are 18 times more likely to be involved in criminal activities. These include violent crimes as well as theft to support drug habits.

In general terms, **drug overdose** refers to poisoning from a pharmacological substance, either legal or illegal. This can occur by accident, miscalculation, changes in the strength of a drug, suicide, polydrug use, or recreational drug usage. Many overdose emergencies seen in the field occur in the habitual drug abuser. It is most difficult to obtain a good history in these cases. However, if the paramedic is familiar with street-drug slang, a more accurate history may be obtained. It is imperative that the paramedic maintain a nonjudgmental attitude in these cases, even though this may be difficult.

The presentation of the drug overdose will vary based on the substance used. Management should be the same as for any ingested, inhaled, or injected poison. Poison control should be contacted for additional direction.

* **substance abuse** use of a pharmacological substance for purposes other than medically defined reasons.

* **addiction** compulsive and overwhelming dependence on a drug; an addiction may be physiological dependence, a psychological dependence, or both.

* **tolerance** the need to progressively increase the dose of a drug to reproduce the effect originally achieved by smaller doses.

* **withdrawal** referring to alcohol or drug withdrawal in which the patient's body reacts severely when deprived of the abused substance.

* **drug overdose** poisoning from a pharmacological substance in excess of that usually prescribed or that the body can tolerate.

Drugs of Abuse

Drugs Commonly Abused

Drugs of abuse are both common and dangerous. These drugs all have various signs and symptoms and require supportive treatment and general toxicological emergency management. Refer to Table 34-4 for further details on what you may find on assessment and the interventions required.

Remember these specific guidelines for patients who have taken the following drugs:

- *Alcohol*—May require thiamine and $D_{50}W$ for hypoglycemia.
- *Cocaine*—Benzodiazepines (diazepam) may be needed for sedation and to treat seizures. Beta-blockers are absolutely contraindicated because unopposed alpha receptor stimulation can cause cardiac ischemia, hypertension, and hyperthermia.
- *Narcotics/Opiates*—Naloxone is effective in reversing respiratory depression and sedation, but be careful, since it may trigger a withdrawal reaction in chronic opiate abusers.
- *Amphetamines*—Use benzodiazepines (diazepam) for seizures and in combination with haloperidol for hyperactivity.
- *Hallucinogens*—Use benzodiazepines for seizures and in combination with haloperidol for hyperactivity.
- *Benzodiazepines*—Use flumazenil to counteract adverse effects. Be careful not to trigger a withdrawal syndrome with seizures.
- *Barbiturates*—Forced diuresis and alkalinization of the urine improve elimination of barbiturates from the body.

Drugs Used for Sexual Purposes

There are a number of drugs that deserve mention as a separate category. These drugs are used to stimulate and enhance the sexual experience, but without medically approved indications for such use. *Ecstasy,* also called *MDMA,* is one such drug. Ecstasy is a modified form of methamphetamines and has similar, although milder, effects. It is very popular in today's university and nightclub environments.

Use of Ecstasy initially causes anxiety, nausea, tachycardia, and elevated blood pressure, followed by relaxation, euphoria, and feelings of enhanced emotional insight. No definitive data exist as to whether the experience of sexual intercourse is improved. Studies show that prolonged use may cause brain damage. Some deaths from MDMA ingestion have been reported. These cases present with confusion, agitation, tremor, high temperature, and diarrhea. No specific treatment exists. Standard supportive measures should be initiated.

Rohypnol (flunitrazepam) is another drug abused for sexual purposes. Illegal in Canada and the United States, it is commonly called the "date rape drug," since it can be secretly slipped into a woman's drink. This drug is a strong benzodiazepine, similar to diazepam, lorazepan, and midazolam. The resulting sedation and amnesia allow the perpetrator to rape the victim. Treatment is the same as for any benzodiazepine, but consequences of the sexual assault require attention as well.

Table 34-4 **COMMON DRUGS OF ABUSE**

Drug	Signs and Symptoms	Routes	Prehospital Management
Alcohol beer whiskey gin vodka wine tequila	CNS depression Slurred speech Disordered thought Impaired judgment Diuresis Stumbling gait Stupor Coma	Oral	ABCs Respiratory support Oxygenate Establish IV access Administer 100 mg thiamine IV ECG monitor Check glucose level Administer $D_{50}W$, if hypoglycemic
Barbiturates thiopental phenobarbital primidone	Lethargy Emotional lability Incoordination Slurred speech Nystagmus Coma Hypotension Respiratory depression	Oral IV	ABCs Respiratory support Oxygenate Establish IV access ECG monitor Contact Poison Control—may order bicarbonate
Cocaine crack rock	Euphoria Hyperactivity Dilated pupils Psychosis Twitching Anxiety Hypertension Tachycardia Dysrhythmias Seizures Chest pain	Snorting Injection Smoking (freebasing)	ABCs Respiratory support Oxygenate ECG monitor Establish IV access Treat life-threatening dysrhythmias Seizure precautions: diazepam 5–10 mg
Narcotics heroin codeine meperidine morphine hydromorphone pentazocine Darvon Darvocet methadone	CNS depression Constricted pupils Respiratory depression Hypotension Bradycardia Pulmonary edema Coma Death	Oral Injection	ABCs Respiratory support Oxygenate Establish IV access *Administer 1–2 mg naloxone IV or endotracheally as ordered by medical direction until respirations improve Larger than average doses (2–5 mg) have been used in the management of Darvon overdose and alcoholic coma ECG monitor

*With the advent of the opiate antagonist naloxone, narcotic overdosage became easier to manage. It is possible to titrate this effective medication to increase respirations to normal levels without fully awakening the patient. In the case of narcotics addicts, this prevents hostile and confrontational episodes.

Continued

Table 34-4 **COMMON DRUGS OF ABUSE** (*CONTINUED*)

Drug	Signs and Symptoms	Routes	Prehospital Management
Marijuana grass weed hashish	Euphoria Dry mouth Dilated pupils Altered sensation	Smoked Oral	ABCs Reassure the patient Speak in a quiet voice ECG monitor if indicated
Amphetamines Benzedrine Dexedrine Ritalin "speed"	Exhilaration Hyperactivity Dilated pupils Hypertension Psychosis Tremors Seizures	Oral Injection	ABCs Oxygenate ECG monitor Establish IV access Treat life-threatening dysrhythmias Seizure precautions: diazepam 5–10 mg
Hallucinogens LSD STP mescaline psilocybin PCP**	Psychosis Nausea Dilated pupils Rambling speech Headache Dizziness Suggestibility Distortion of sensory perceptions Hallucinations	Oral Smoked	ABCs Reassure the patient "Talk down" the "high" patient Protect the patient from injury Provide a dark, quiet environment Speak in a soft, quiet voice Seizure precautions: diazepam 5–10 mg

**Although PCP was originally an animal tranquilizer, it manifests hallucinogenic properties when used by humans. In addition to bizarre delusions, it can cause violent and dangerous outbursts of aggressive behaviour. The rescuer is advised to remain safe when attempting to treat this type of overdose. PCP patients have been known to have almost superhuman strength and high pain tolerance.

Drug	Signs and Symptoms	Routes	Prehospital Management
Sedatives Seconal Valium Librium Xanax Halcion Restoril Dalmane Phenobarbital	Altered mental status Hypotension Slurred speech Respiratory depression Shock Bradycardia Seizures	Oral	ABCs Respiratory support Oxygenate Establish IV access ECG monitor Medical direction may order naloxone
Benzodiazepines*** Valium Librium Xanax Halcion Restoril Dalmane Centrax Ativan Serax	Altered mental status Slurred speech Dysrhythmias Coma	Oral	ABCs Respiratory support Oxygenate Activated charcoal as ordered by medical Direction Establish IV access ECG monitor Contact poison control

***Deaths due to pure benzodiazepine are rare. Minor toxicity ranges are 500–1500 mg. A benzodiazepine antagonist (Romazicon) is available (IV dosage 1–10 mg or infusion 0.5 mg/h). It may cause seizures in a benzodiazepine-dependent patient.

ALCOHOL ABUSE

Alcohol is the most common substance of abuse in Canada and most of the world. According to a 1995 national survey by Health Canada, 72 percent of Canadians aged 15 and over said they had consumed alcohol in the past year. Consumption is highest among young adult males and those with relatively higher incomes. Canadians drink slightly more than two billion litres of beer, 231 million litres of wine, and 136 million litres of spirits each year. That amounts to about nine drinks per person per week.

Nearly 10 percent of Canadians say they have problems with their drinking. Ten percent of adult drinkers report heavy drinking which is defined as five or more drinks in a single sitting, at least once a week. In Ontario, more than 600 people die each year from alcohol-related causes. This amounts to 10 percent of all deaths in Ontario. Alcohol dependence syndrome is one of the causes of death apart from heart disease and stroke, liver disease, and cancers. Drinking is a factor in 54 percent of all assaults, murders, and attempted murders and in nearly 40 percent of all child abuse cases. Alcohol-related motor vehicle collisions remain a major cause of death, despite the considerable progress in reducing impaired driving. Among fatally injured drivers, 46 percent had some alcohol in their blood, and 39 percent were over the legal limit of 0.8 percent alcohol level. Alcoholism progresses in much the same way as does drug dependence, discussed earlier.

PHYSIOLOGICAL EFFECTS

Alcohol (ethyl alcohol, or ethanol) depresses the central nervous system (CNS), potentially to the point of stupor, coma, and death. In patients with severe liver disease, metabolism of alcohol may become impaired, which increases the course and severity of intoxication. At low doses, alcohol has excitatory and stimulating effects, thus depressing inhibitions. At higher doses alcohol's depressive effect is more obvious. Alcohol abuse and dependence is called *alcoholism*. It is a major problem, contributing to highway traffic fatalities, drownings, burns, trauma, and drug overdoses.

Alcohol is completely absorbed from the stomach and intestinal tract in approximately 30 to 120 minutes after ingestion. Once absorbed, alcohol is distributed to all body tissues and fluids, with concentrations of alcohol in the brain rapidly approaching the alcohol level in the blood.

In addition, alcohol causes a peripheral vasodilator effect on the cardiovascular system, resulting in flushing and a feeling of warmth. In cold conditions, alcohol's dilation of the blood vessels results in an increased loss of body heat. The diuretic effect seen when large amounts of alcohol are ingested is due to the inhibition of *vasopressin,* which is the hormone responsible for the conservation of body fluids. Without vasopressin, an increase in urine flow occurs. The "dry mouth syndrome" experienced after alcohol consumption may be the result of alcohol-induced cellular dehydration.

Some alcoholics will drink methanol (wood alcohol) or ethylene glycol (a component of antifreeze) if ethanol is unavailable. Ingestion of these chemicals can cause blindness or death.

In addition, methanol will also cause visual disturbances, abdominal pain, and nausea and vomiting even at low doses. In fact, death has been reported after ingestion of only 15 mL of a 40-percent solution. Occasionally, patients will complain of headache or dizziness and may even present with seizures and obtundation. Ethylene glycol ingestion has similar symptoms, but the CNS effects, such as hallucinations, coma, and seizures, are more pronounced in the early stages.

GENERAL ALCOHOLIC PROFILE

The classic alcoholic portrayed in movies is an unkempt, continually intoxicated street person who is completely nonfunctional. Although alcoholics of this type exist, it would be a grave error to consider this the typical picture of someone dependent on alcohol. More commonly, alcoholism is characterized by impaired control over drinking, preoccupation with the drug ethanol, use of ethanol despite adverse consequences, and distortions in thinking, such as denial. Obviously, this definition applies to many people, including many functional people at all levels of society who have masked their addiction well. Take note of these warning signs, which may indicate alcohol abuse:

- Drinks early in the day
- Prone to drink alone and secretly
- Periodic binges (may last for several days)
- Partial or total loss of memory ("blackouts") during period of drinking
- Unexplained history of gastrointestinal problems (especially bleeding)
- "Green tongue syndrome" (using chlorophyll-containing substances to disguise the odour of alcohol on the breath)
- Cigarette burns on clothing
- Chronically flushed face and palms
- Tremulousness
- Odour of alcohol on breath under inappropriate conditions

CONSEQUENCES OF CHRONIC ALCOHOL INGESTION

Alcohol has many deleterious effects on the body. Chronic abuse can be devastating, effecting every organ system as shown in Figure 34-11. Some of the more common effects include

- Poor nutrition
- Alcohol hepatitis
- Liver cirrhosis with subsequent esophageal varices
- Loss of sensation in hands and feet
- Loss of cerebellar function (balance and coordination)
- Pancreatitis
- Upper gastrointestinal hemorrhage (often fatal)
- Hypoglycemia
- Subdural hematoma (due to falls)
- Rib and extremity fractures (due to falls)

Keep in mind that such conditions as subdural hematomas, sepsis, and other life-threatening disease processes may mimic the signs and symptoms of alcohol intoxication. For example, diabetic ketoacidosis produces a breath odour that can easily be confused with the odour of alcohol.

Withdrawal Syndrome

The alcoholic may suffer a withdrawal reaction from either abrupt discontinuation of ingestion after prolonged use or from a rapid fall in blood-alcohol level after acute intoxication. Alcohol withdrawal can be potentially fatal. Withdrawal symp-

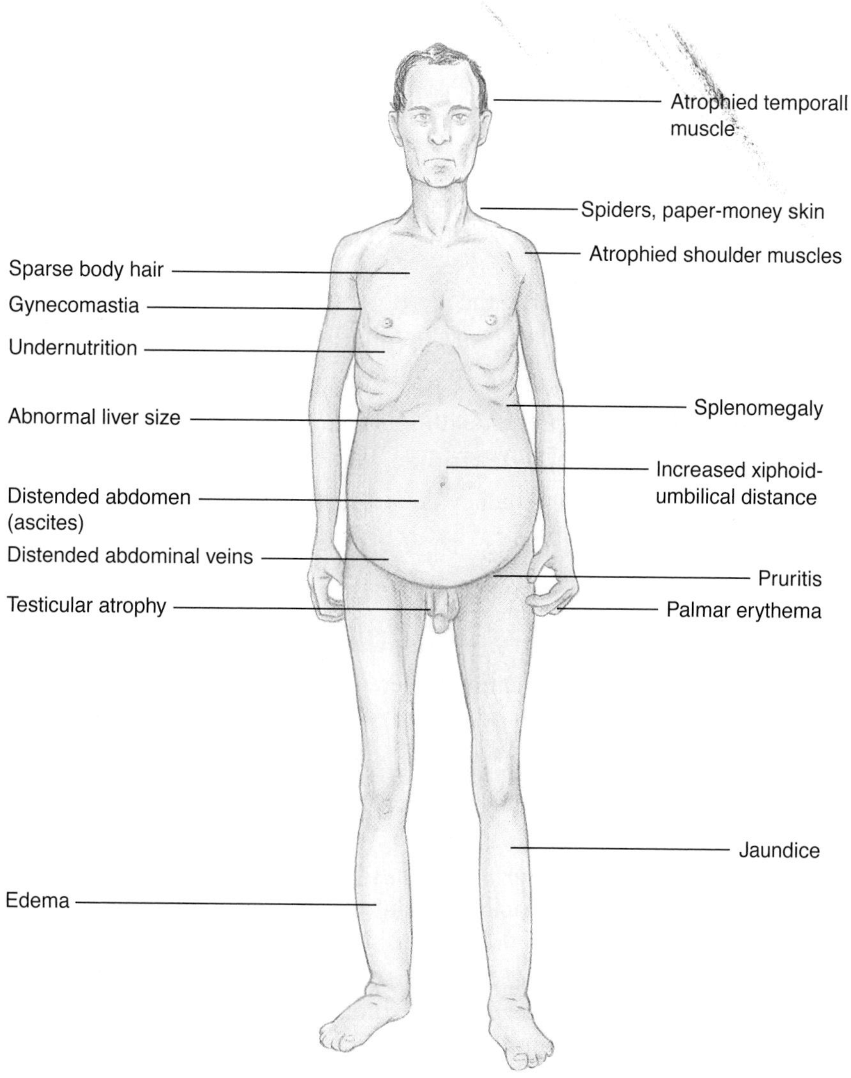

FIGURE 34-11   The chronic alcoholic.

Atrophied temporall muscle

Spiders, paper-money skin

Atrophied shoulder muscles

Sparse body hair

Gynecomastia

Undernutrition

Abnormal liver size

Splenomegaly

Distended abdomen (ascites)

Increased xiphoid-umbilical distance

Distended abdominal veins

Testicular atrophy

Pruritis

Palmar erythema

Jaundice

Edema

toms can occur several hours after sudden abstinence and can last up to 5 to 7 days. Seizures (sometimes called "rum fits") may occur within the first 24–36 hours of abstinence. **Delirium tremens (DTs)** usually develops on the second or third day of the withdrawal. Delirium tremens is characterized by a decreased level of consciousness during which the patient hallucinates and misinterprets nearby events. Seizures and delirium tremens are ominous signs. There is a significant mortality from delirium tremens. Medical direction may order diazepam in severe cases.

Signs and Symptoms Signs and symptoms of withdrawal syndrome include

- Coarse tremor of hands, tongue, and eyelids
- Nausea and vomiting
- General weakness
- Increased sympathetic tone
- Tachycardia
- Sweating
- Hypertension
- Orthostatic hypotension
- Anxiety

✱ **delirium tremens (DTs)** disorder found in habitual and excessive users of alcoholic beverages after cessation of drinking for 48–72 hours. Patients experience visual, tactile, and auditory disturbances. Death may result in severe cases.

- Irritability or a depressed mood
- Hallucinations
- Poor sleep

Do not underestimate alcohol intoxication as a toxic emergency.

Management Alcohol intoxication, whether acute or chronic, should not be underestimated as a toxic emergency problem. In cases of suspected alcohol abuse, take the following steps.

- Establish and maintain the airway.
- Determine if other drugs are involved.
- Start an IV using Ringer's Lactate or normal saline.
- Assess blood glucose, and administer 25 g of $D_{50}W$ if hypoglycemic.
- Maintain an empathetic attitude, and reassure the patient of help.
- Transport to the emergency department for further care.

Summary

Clearly, there is much to remember when dealing with toxicological emergencies. To effectively manage these situations, you must focus on three things:

1. *Recognize the poisoning promptly.* In other words, you must have a high index of suspicion when circumstances suggest a toxin may be involved.

2. *Be thorough in your primary assessment and evaluation of the patient.* This will facilitate your efforts to identify the toxin and the measures needed to control the situation.

3. *Initiate the standard treatment procedures required for all toxicological emergencies.* Beyond the usual concern for rescuer safety and rapid implementation of ABCs and supportive measures, consider the methods needed to minimize any further exposure to the toxin, decontaminate the patient from the toxins already involved, and finally administer any useful antidote if one exists for the particular toxin.

If you remember these three steps, you will be equipped to handle most toxicological emergencies promptly and efficiently.

CHAPTER 35

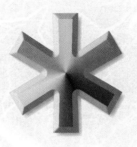

Hematology

Objectives

After reading this chapter, you should be able to:

1. Identify the anatomy and physiology of the hematopoietic system.
   (see Chapter 12)
2. Discuss the following (see Chapter 12):
   - Plasma
   - Red blood cells (erythrocytes)
   - Hemoglobin
   - Hematocrit
   - White blood cells (leukocytes)
   - Platelets, clotting, and fibrinolysis
   - Hemostasis
3. Identify the following (see Chapter 13):
   - Inflammatory process
   - Cellular and humoral immunity
   - Alterations in immunological response
4. Identify blood groups.
   (pp. 725–726)
5. List erythrocyte disorders.
   (pp. 733–735)
6. List leukocyte disorders.
   (pp. 735–737)
7. List platelet and clotting disorders.
   (pp. 737–739)

Continued

Objectives Continued

8. Describe how acquired factor deficiencies may occur. (pp. 737–739)
9. Identify the components of the physical assessment as they relate to the hematology system. (pp. 727–732)
10. Describe the pathology and clinical manifestations and prognosis associated with
    • Anemia (pp. 733–734)
    • Leukemia (pp. 736–737)
    • Lymphomas (p. 737)

    • Polycythemia (p. 735)
    • Disseminated intravascular coagulopathy (p. 739)
    • Hemophilia (pp. 738–739)
    • Sickle cell disease (pp. 734–735)
    • multiple myeloma (pp. 739–740)
11. Given several preprogrammed patients with hematological problems, provide the appropriate assessment, management, and transport. (pp. 724–740)

INTRODUCTION

✱ hematology the study of blood and the blood-forming organs.

Hematology is the study of blood and blood-forming organs. It exemplifies the way that multiple organ systems interact to maintain homeostasis, the normal balance of body functions. Hematological disorders are common and include red blood cell disorders, white blood cell disorders, platelet disorders, and coagulation problems. Although these disorders are common, they rarely are the primary cause of a medical emergency. They usually accompany other ongoing disease processes. Some hematological diseases are genetic in origin. Hemophilia A is a classic example. It is a sex-linked disease that causes abnormally low levels of an essential blood clotting protein (Factor VIII). It affects approximately 1–2 persons per 10 000 in Canada. Some hematological diseases are more common in certain ethnic groups. For example, among the population as a whole, sickle cell anemia is relatively uncommon. However, among blacks specifically, 8 percent of the population has the sickle cell trait. In addition to their primary effects, hematological disorders may predispose patients to infection and intolerance to exercise, hypoxia, acidosis, and blood loss.

Patients with hematological problems often complain of signs and symptoms that do not point directly to a specific disease process. Careful assessment and history taking may be necessary to further clarify the diagnosis. Often, however, laboratory findings will be needed to confirm the diagnosis. Thus, the final diagnosis of patients for whom you provide prehospital care is often not immediately apparent. You must use your assessment skills to recognize and treat injuries, pain, and instabilities, while formulating a field impression that enables you to anticipate further complications and thus enhance patient outcome and survivability. Because of this, it is essential that you have a good understanding of the basic pathophysiological processes of your patients' disease, including hematological disorders.

BLOOD PRODUCTS AND BLOOD TYPING

A blood transfusion is the transplantation of blood or a component of blood from one person to another. It is accomplished by IV infusion (Figure 35-1). Various types of transfusions are given for various purposes (Table 35-1).

In the 1800s, when patients received blood from others, some had a reaction that led to multiple organ failure and death. Karl Landsteiner discovered the reason for this was reaction **antigens,** proteins on the surface of the donor's red blood cells that the patient's body recognized as "not self." Following transfusion, antibodies in the patient's own blood attacked the foreign antigens present in the transfused blood. Landsteiner named the antigens A and B and the opposing antibodies anti-A and anti-B. Someone with A antigen on her red blood cells would have anti-B antibodies. Her blood type would be A. Someone with B antigens on the red blood cell surface would have anti-A antibodies; her type would be B. Some people's red blood cells have both antigens on their surface but neither antibody. Their blood type is AB. Others have neither antigen but both antibodies; their blood type is O (for zero antigens, but pronounced "Oh"). Blood type is an inherited trait. Approximately 45 percent of the Canadian population has type O, 39 percent type A, 11 percent type B, and 5 percent type AB.

Since only the antibodies recognize and attack foreign tissue, a person with no antibodies (type AB) can receive any blood type in an emergency, and the body will not attack the cells. So, a person with type AB blood is called a *universal recipient.* Conversely, blood with no antigens to any other blood group type (type O) would not trigger a reaction, as the recipient's blood recognizes nothing "foreign." So, people with type O blood are called *universal donors.*

Cross-matching blood involves checking samples from both donor and recipient to ensure the greatest compatibility. If a donor's blood does not clump together, or agglutinate, when mixed with the recipient's blood, they are compatible. Reliance on the universal donor and recipient concept is useful only in an emergency, when there is no time to check samples.

✳ **antigen** protein on the surface of a donor's red blood cells that the patient's body recognizes as "not self."

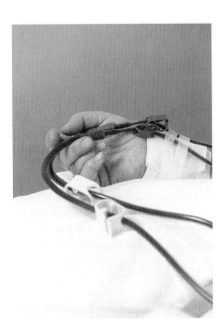

FIGURE 35-1 Blood transfusion.

Table 35-1 TYPES OF TRANSFUSIONS

Type of Transfusion	Contents	Use
Whole blood	All cells, platelets, clotting factors, and plasma	Replace blood loss from hemorrhage
Packed red blood cells (PRBCs)	Red blood cells and some plasma	Replace red blood cells in anemic patients
Platelets	Thrombocytes and some plasma	Replace platelets in a patient with thrombocytopenia
Fresh frozen plasma (FFP)	Plasma, a combination of fluids, clotting factors, and proteins	Replace volume in a burn patient or in hypovolemia secondary to low oncotic pressure
Clotting factors	Specific clotting factors needed for coagulation	Replace factors missing due to inadequate production as in hemophilia

Blood transfusion is not as simple as that, however. Approximately 40 years after the discovery of A and B antigens, Landsteiner and A.S. Weiner observed another antigen present on red blood cells. Research leading to this antigen's discovery used rhesus monkey blood, and so the antigen was called the Rh factor. If a person has the Rh factor, she is Rh positive (Rh^+); if not, she is Rh negative (Rh^-). As many as 500 other lesser antigens have since been identified but they usually do not cause the severe hemolytic reaction seen in the patients sensitized to the Rh factor. *Erythroblastosis fetalis*, more commonly called hemolytic disease of the newborn, can lead to a fatal hemolytic reaction in neonates. In this disease, the mother who is Rh^- is sensitized by previous exposure to the Rh antigen during a previous pregnancy with an Rh^+ child or from a previous blood transfusion. Therefore, if she subsequently becomes pregnant with an Rh^+ child, the mother produces antibodies that attack the fetus's red blood cells, leading to a severe and often fatal hemolytic reaction. Fortunately, the incidence of hemolytic disease of newborns has been declining due to the administration of Rh immune globulin (RhoGAM) to mothers. This inhibits formation of anti-Rh antibodies. Additionally, transfusions in utero or fetal exchange transfusions immediately after birth can diminish or eliminate the likelihood of infant death.

TRANSFUSION REACTIONS

There are many types of transfusion reactions. One of them, hemolytic transfusion reaction, occurs when a donor's and recipient's blood are not compatible. Antigens on the donor's red blood cells trigger a response from the antibodies in the recipient's blood. The antibodies attach to the red blood cells, which are then *hemolyzed*, or taken up by the fixed macrophages of the spleen's reticuloendothelial system.

If a patient receiving a blood transfusion develops what you believe to be a hemolytic reaction, stop the transfusion immediately.

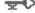

Signs and symptoms of a hemolytic transfusion reaction may include facial flushing, hyperventilation, tachycardia, and a sense of dread. Hives may appear on the skin, and the patient may develop chest pain, wheezing, fever, chills, and cyanosis. Flank pain may occur as small clots begin to clog the microvasculature of the kidneys, which can lead to kidney failure requiring dialysis. The damage can be permanent.

In caring for a hospitalized patient receiving a blood transfusion, if she develops what you believe to be a hemolytic reaction, stop the transfusion immediately. Change all associated IV tubing, and initiate IV therapy with normal saline or Ringer's Lactate solution. Administer a bolus as necessary to maintain good perfusion and blood pressure. Furosemide (Lasix) is often administered to promote diuresis. Low dose dopamine (2–5 µg/kg/minute) should be considered along with the IV fluid to help maintain adequate renal perfusion. In extreme cases of anaphylactic reaction, you may need to administer IV epinephrine if the patient is hypotensive or demonstrates severe bronchospasm.

The most common transfusion reaction is the febrile nonhemolytic reaction. It is caused by sensitization to antigens on the white blood cells, platelets, or plasma proteins. Signs and symptoms include headache, fever, and chills. As with any other transfusion reaction, always stop the transfusion before attempting to treat it. After stopping the blood product, change all tubing, and initiate normal saline IV. Patients are often given diphenhydramine (Benadryl) and an antipyretic (ibuprofen, acetaminophen) for the fever. No further treatment may be necessary, as this reaction rarely progresses to more serious complications. However, close observation is required to exclude development of a hemolytic reaction. In the event of any transfusion reaction, return all blood bags, tubing, and filters to the blood bank for analysis. Medical direction may order you to take blood and urine samples.

Because blood transfusion adds fluid to the system, a patient may experience signs and symptoms of circulatory overload. In fact, signs and symptoms are the same as those for left ventricular failure and may include pulmonary edema, dyspnea, and chest pain. Hypotension is not usually a problem, and the patient may be treated successfully by slowing the heart rate and administering diuretics.

GENERAL ASSESSMENT AND MANAGEMENT

In general, patients with disorders of the hematopoietic system may present with a variety of complaints and physical findings. Patients with infection, white blood cell abnormalities (immunocompromised and prone to infection), or transfusion reactions may present with febrile symptoms. Subsequently, these patients may develop hemodynamic instability as infection progresses to sepsis or as the transfusion reaction leads to a hemolytic reaction, renal failure, and disseminated intravascular coagulation (DIC). Acute hemodynamic compromise can also be found in patients with anemia secondary to acute blood loss, coagulation defects, or autoimmune disease. These disease processes may not be easily differentiated in the field and often require significant laboratory testing to confirm the diagnosis. In most cases, however, if you obtain a careful history, you will have a good working diagnosis.

Most hematopoietic disorders are chronic conditions that present with acute exacerbation when the patient is exposed to an additional stress, such as infection or trauma. Treatment of patients with disorders of the hematopoietic system, in most cases, is supportive. Some patients may have hemodynamic instability from blood or fluid loss. These patients may require intravenous fluids to support end-organ perfusion and prevent shock. In addition, they should receive oxygen therapy to prevent hypoxia from poor perfusion and diminished oxygen-carrying capacity of the blood. It is important to recognize the need for rapid transport in patients with hemodynamic instability who may require transfusion or other definitive care measures.

SCENE ASSESSMENT

Assessment of the patient with a possible hematopoietic abnormality begins in the same way as for any other patient. Perform a scene assessment, and take body substance isolation (BSI) precautions. During your approach, form a general impression of the patient. Is the patient a trauma or medical patient? In how much distress is the patient?

PRIMARY ASSESSMENT

Complete a primary assessment for life threats. Determine responsiveness, and assess airway, breathing, and circulation (ABCs). Alterations in the hematopoietic system may present as life-threatening bleeds or overwhelming infections with septic shock. Obtain a complete baseline set of vitals. Check the ABCs, and quickly determine your priority for transport. Critical or unstable patients should be considered candidates for expeditious transport.

FOCUSED HISTORY AND SECONDARY ASSESSMENT

Next, complete a focused history and secondary assessment. Use your general impression to choose a format for a responsive or unresponsive medical patient or trauma patient with significant or nonsignificant mechanism of injury. Each format follows a sequence of history gathering and examination designed to meet the needs of that particular patient. Trauma patients and unresponsive medical patients often present life-threatening problems that are noted in your primary assessment.

SAMPLE History

For a responsive medical patient, obtain a SAMPLE history and perform a secondary assessment. Obtain a set of vital signs and place the pulse oximeter. Keep in mind that an anemic patient will have increased heart and respiratory rates as her body attempts to compensate for less oxygen reaching the tissues. Ask for the chief complaint—why did the patient call for assistance? What signs or symptoms (SAMPLE) accompanied or preceded the complaint? Pay attention to generalized complaints, such as fatigue, lethargy, malaise, apprehension, or confusion. These may indicate inadequate oxygen delivery to the tissues. Have there been any unusual skin changes, such as colouring or bruising? Does the patient complain of itching? Inquire about lymph node enlargement (swollen glands), sore throat, or pain on swallowing. These may indicate infection.

Any change in the blood's ability to deliver oxygen to the body will appear in the cardiovascular and respiratory systems. Note dyspnea, palpitations, and dizziness with changes in the patient's position. Patients with hematological problems may suffer syncope. Did the patient have a syncopal episode, or is she just weak? Syncope can be due to several factors but is often related to a sudden change in position in a patient who has a marked anemia. Bleeding abnormalities may be disguised as gastrointestinal upset. Ask about overt bleeding with vomiting or diarrhea, but do not overlook complaints of nausea or anorexia, vomiting of "coffee ground" material, or having black tarry or cranberry, sticky, odoriferous stools. Many patients will notice bleeding of the gums when they brush their teeth. This can, on occasion, be hard to control. Atraumatic bleeding of the gums almost always points to an underlying hematological abnormality. Ask about changes in urination, hematuria (blood in the urine), and alterations in the usual menstrual pattern in females. Keep in mind that hematological disorders are often diagnosed when the patient seeks assistance for another medical condition.

Determine any allergies (SAMPLE). Be sure to ask about use of prescription or over-the-counter medications (SAMPLE). Make note of the patient's medication and dose, and the condition for which she takes the medication. Also, if time allows, note the dosing schedule of the medications. Ask about compliance. Does

Keep in mind that hematological disorders are often diagnosed when the patient seeks assistance for another medical condition.

the patient take medication as prescribed? When was the last dose taken? Medications that may indicate an alteration in the hematological system, or that might make the patient more susceptible to an alteration in the system, include pain relievers, antibiotics, anticoagulants, hormones, and medications for heart disease, arthritis, and seizures.

When asking about <u>p</u>ast medical history (SAMP<u>L</u>E), make note of surgeries, such as a splenectomy, heart-valve replacement, or placement of long-term venous-access devices. Ask about bloodborne infections, such as HIV or hepatitis B or C. Make note of liver or bone marrow disease or cancers. Include questions about family history, such as hemophilia, sickle cell disease, cancer, or death at an early age that was not trauma related. Inquire also about social habits, such as smoking, alcohol consumption, IV drug use, or long-term exposure to chemicals or radiation.

If you find a significant history, ask about the last episode of an incident or last use of a medication. Remember to include the usual questions about <u>l</u>ast oral intake (SAMP<u>L</u>E). Also, inquire about any unusual <u>e</u>vents (SAMPL<u>E</u>) that preceded the onset of the complaint, such as the start of a new medication, recent transfusion, fall, or injury.

Secondary Assessment

When performing the secondary assessment, evaluate each system methodically as you would in any other patient. If the history suggests a hematopoietic problem, look for potential pathology during the secondary assessment that may confirm your working diagnosis and be a clue to developing complications.

- *Nervous system* Always evaluate the nervous system in any patient with a suspected hematological problem. First, note the patient's level of consciousness using the AVPU system. Be alert for other nervous system disorders. Many patients with hematological problems will complain of being "weak and dizzy." Try to clarify this further. Is the patient fatigued, weak all over, or does she have focal weakness? Is she dizzy, or is she suffering true vertigo? Both can be associated with hematological problems, such as anemia. Ask if the patient has any numbness or motor deficits. Pernicious anemia can cause sensory deficits that are often unilateral. Try to determine whether the patient had a syncopal episode. What were the patient's condition and position immediately prior to the syncopal episode? Many of the hematological diseases, especially the autoimmune diseases, will affect the eye. Always examine the eyes for abnormalities. Question the patient about any visual disturbances or visual loss. In addition to the autoimmune diseases, sickle cell anemia is notorious for causing eye problems.

- *Skin* Note the patient's skin colour (Figure 35-2). Jaundice (yellow skin) may indicate liver disease or hemolysis of red blood cells, while a florid (reddish) appearance is often associated with polycythemia. Patients with anemia typically exhibit pallor. Observe for petechiae (tiny red dots in the skin), purpura (large purplish blotches related to multiple hemorrhages into the skin), and bruising. Inquire about pruritus (itching). Patients with hematological disorders often develop pruritus. Some hematological problems, such as sickle cell anemia, cause the destruction of red blood cells. This results in hemoglobin spilling into the circulatory system. Macrophages then break down the hemoglobin. The iron is removed and transported to the bones or liver. The porphyrin portion of the hemoglobin is subsequently converted into bilirubin, which is taken up by the liver.

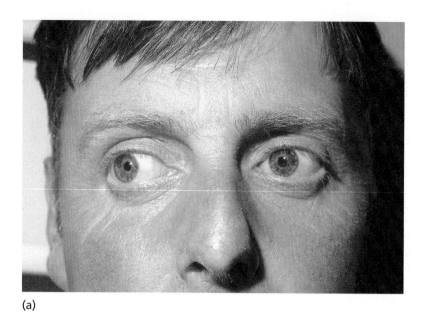

(a)

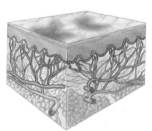

Petechiae – Reddish-purple spots, diameter less than 0.5 cm

(b)

Purpura – Reddish-purple blotches, diameter more than 0.5 cm

(c)

FIGURE 35-2   Abnormal skin colours: (a) jaundice, (b) petechiae, (c) purpura.

An excess of bilirubin, either from liver disease or from the breakdown of hemoglobin associated with the hemolytic anemias, can cause pruritis. Often, patients will develop itching over a bruise. As the hemoglobin breaks down within the bruise, the localized accumulation of bilirubin causes the itching. This is most common 1–2 weeks after the bruise occurs. When examining the skin, be alert for any evidence of prolonged bleeding. The patient may have several bandages over relatively minor wounds where she could not stop the bleeding.

- *Lymphatic* The lymphatic system is affected early in hematopoietic diseases, especially those of the immune system. During your secondary assessment, pay particular attention to the lymph nodes. Palpate the lymph nodes of the neck, clavicle, axilla, and groin. Note any enlargement. Compare sides. Splenomegaly (an enlarged spleen) is also often present, but this can be hard to examine in the field.

- *Gastrointestinal* The gastrointestinal effects of hematological problems can be quite varied. Epistaxis (nosebleed) is common. The nasal mucosa is quite vascular as it warms and humidifies the inhaled air. A slight crack in the nasal mucosa can result in brisk bleeding. This is a particular problem in people with blood clotting abnormalities, as stopping the bleeding is very difficult for them. These patients may swallow a great deal of blood and may become nauseated. Also, blood acts as a cathartic (laxative). Patients who swallow even moderate amounts of blood will often report loose stools, which are often dark (melena). Blood present in emesis may be bright red or appear like coffee grounds.

Bleeding of the gums is one of the earliest findings of hematological problems. Patients with blood clotting abnormalities and low platelet levels will often develop atraumatic bleeding of the gums. Any patient with bleeding gums requires a detailed investigation for a possible hematological disorder. Gingivitis (infection of the gums) can be due to poor hygiene, disease, or both. However, chronic gingivitis should cause increased suspicion of a hematological disorder, especially involving the immune system. Also, gingivitis increases a patient's risk of developing sepsis. Slight trauma, such as brushing the teeth, can cause the bacteria to enter the circulatory system, resulting in generalized sepsis. Always note the presence of gingivitis when examining for bleeding gums. Ulcerations of the gums and oral mucosa are typically due to viral diseases. These infections are more common in immunosuppressed patients. Thrush (yeast infection in the mouth) in adults is commonly associated with AIDS. (Thrush in children is common and not a reason for concern.)

The liver plays a major role in manufacturing many of the substances required for blood clotting. Liver disease can slow blood clotting. This is most evident in a prolonged prothrombin (PT) time. Also, as the liver fails, the bilirubin level will increase, resulting in jaundice. Thus, any patient with jaundice should be evaluated for liver disease.

Abdominal pain is not uncommon in persons with hematological disease. Two of the major organs associated with the hematopoeitic system, the liver and spleen, are in the abdomen. Problems with the spleen, liver, or both can lead to abdominal pain. Splenomegaly is common in hematological problems, as the spleen is active in the removal of abnormal or aged red cells. In some of the anemias, especially the hemolytic anemias, the spleen can become markedly enlarged. Patients with sickle cell anemia will often develop splenic infarcts as sickled cells accumulate and block blood supply to parts of the spleen. By the time children with sickle cell disease are five years of age, they are virtually asplenic (without a spleen), as the disease has completely infarcted their spleen. Because the spleen is not functional, these patients are placed at increased risk of infection, especially by encapsulated bacteria.

- *Musculoskeletal* Many hematopoietic problems are autoimmune in nature. That is, a problem develops in which the immune system has trouble determining which tissues are self and which are nonself. Autoimmune diseases, such as rheumatoid arthritis, result from the body's immune system attacking various tissues in the joints. This can cause arthralgia (pain and swelling of the joints). Autoimmune diseases tend to affect more than one joint, whereas infectious processes tend to affect only a single joint. Patients with blood clotting disorders, such as hemophilia, will often develop hemarthrosis (bleeding into a joint) with only minor trauma. This can result in an extremely swollen, discoloured, and painful joint.

Bleeding gums are often associated with a decreased platelet count.

An oral yeast infection in an adult is commonly associated with AIDS.

Always inquire about joint pain, and examine the major joints in any patient suspected of having hematopoietic disease.

- *Cardiorespiratory* The effects of hematopoietic problems on the cardiorespiratory system are varied. Patients with anemia will often develop dyspnea, tachycardia, and chest pain from the increased cardiac work caused by the anemia. In severe cases, patients can develop high-output heart failure, where the heart works excessively hard to compensate for a profound anemia. If untreated, heart failure and pulmonary edema can result. Patients with bleeding disorders may report expectorating blood with coughing. This can be due to small tears in the respiratory mucosa from the coughing. Normally, these heal quickly. Patients with bleeding disorders, however, will continue to bleed, resulting in potential airway obstruction and, in severe cases, shock. Always auscultate for breath sounds. Note crackles or rhonchi indicative of heart problems or infection.

- *Genitourinary* The genitourinary effects of hematopoietic problems are typically due to bleeding disorders or infection. Bleeding disorders can cause hematuria (blood in the urine) and blood in the scrotal sac in males. A woman who has an intact uterus may develop menorrhagia (heavy menstrual bleeding) or frank vaginal bleeding (dysfunctional uterine bleeding). Immunocompromised patients are at increased risk for developing genitourinary infections. These can range from recurrent urinary tract infections to severe sexually transmitted diseases. Sickle cell anemia, especially in the later stages, can cause priapism. This is a prolonged, painful erection due to obstruction of the blood vessels that drain the penis and allow for detumescence. Sickle cell disease is the most common cause of priapism in the emergency setting. All of these require additional evaluation in the emergency department. Detailed evaluation of the genitourinary system is not appropriate in field settings.

GENERAL MANAGEMENT OF HEMATOPOIETIC EMERGENCIES

Pay close attention to the airway and ventilation status of patients experiencing any alteration in the hematopoietic system. Place the patient on high-concentration supplemental oxygen, and monitor breathing for difficulty or fatigue. Be ready to assist ventilations with a bag-valve mask.

Assess the circulatory system. Consider fluid volume replacement, but remember that crystalloid solutions cannot carry oxygen. Too much fluid can "dilute" the blood and reduce its capacity per unit volume to carry oxygen. Be alert for dysrhythmias and treat accordingly. On the basis of your assessment and evaluation, create the optimum environment for the blood to perform its tasks of oxygen delivery and waste product removal.

Transport the patient to the appropriate facility, provide comfort measures including analgesia, and provide psychological support to both the patient and her family.

MANAGING SPECIFIC PATIENT PROBLEMS

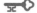
The rest of this chapter will detail the more common hematopoietic diseases that you might encounter in prehospital care. Again, it is important to remember that many hematological problems occur in conjunction with other illnesses. For ex-

ample, someone with a cancer or significant renal disease quite commonly will have coexisting anemia. In the following sections, we will first examine diseases of the red blood cells. These are the most common hematological problems encountered. Second, we will look at the white blood cell diseases. These include the leukemias, lymphomas, and similar illnesses. Finally, we will present diseases of the platelets and blood coagulation disorders.

DISEASES OF THE RED BLOOD CELLS

Red blood cell diseases result in too many red blood cells, too few red blood cells, or improperly functioning red blood cells. An excess of red blood cells is called **polycythemia**. Although uncommon, several conditions can cause polycythemia. An inadequate number of red blood cells or inadequate hemoglobin within the red blood cells is called **anemia**. Anemia is common, and several types are frequently encountered. Finally, red blood cell function can be impaired. Most commonly, this is due to problems with either hemoglobin structure and function or with the red blood cell membrane. Problems with red blood cell function include the thallasemias and sickle cell anemia.

Anemias

The most common diseases of the red blood cells are the anemias. Anemia is typically classified as a hematocrit of less than 37 percent in women or less than 40 percent in men. Most patients with anemia will remain asymptomatic until the hematocrit drops below 30 percent. The decreased hematocrit in anemia is due to a reduction in the number of red blood cells or in the amount or quality of hemoglobin in the red blood cells. Anemia is actually a sign of an underlying disease process that is either destroying red blood cells and hemoglobin or decreasing the production of red blood cells and hemoglobin. Blood loss, either acute or chronic, also can cause anemia. Anemia can be a self-limiting disease, or it can be a lifelong illness requiring periodic transfusions. Anemias that result from the destruction of red blood cells are called hemolytic anemias. These can be hereditary or acquired. Examples of hereditary hemolytic anemias include sickle cell anemia, thalassemia, and glucose-6-phosphate dehydrogenase deficiency (G6PD). Acquired hemolytic anemias can result from immune system disorders, drug effects, or environmental effects. Anemias caused by inadequate red blood cell production include such problems as iron deficiency anemia, pernicious anemia, and anemia of chronic disease. Table 35-2 shows the numerous types of anemia, all of which must be confirmed by laboratory diagnosis.

Anemia is a sign, not a disease process in itself. Since the red blood cells' primary purpose is to transport oxygen, anemia results in hypoxia. The signs and symptoms of anemia vary, depending on the rapidity of its onset and on the patient's age and underlying general health. A mild anemia may not exhibit signs or symptoms until the body is stressed, as during exercise. Then mild dyspnea, fatigue, palpitations, and syncope may be present. Chronic anemias may present signs or symptoms of pica (the craving of unusual substances, such as clay or ice), headache, dizziness, ringing in the ears, irritability or difficulty concentrating, pallor, and tachycardia. Angina pectoris can be an important indicator.

If anemia develops rapidly, the body does not have time to compensate for the change. Signs and symptoms of shock may be present, including postural hypotension and decreased cardiac output, resulting in a shunting of blood away from the periphery to the heart, lungs, and brain. Compensatory mechanisms can cause diaphoresis, pallor, cool skin, anxiety, thirst, and air hunger. If the anemia's onset is slower, the body can adjust to the oxygen's reduced availability with a right shift of the oxyhemoglobin dissociation curve and an increase in plasma volume.

* **polycythemia** an excess of red blood cells.

* **anemia** an inadequate number of red blood cells or inadequate hemoglobin within the red blood cells.

Content Review

DISEASES OF THE RED BLOOD CELLS

- Anemia
- Sickle cell disease
- Polycythemia

| Table 35-2 | TYPES OF ANEMIA |

Cause	Type	Pathophysiology
Inadequate production of red blood cells	Aplastic	Failure to produce red blood cells
	Iron deficiency	Iron is primary component of hemoglobin
	Pernicious	Vitamin B_{12} is necessary for correct red blood cell division during its development
	Sickle cell	Genetic alteration causes production of a hemoglobin that changes shape of red blood cell to a *C,* or sickle, in low-oxygen states
Increased red blood cell destruction	Hemolytic	Body destroys red blood cells at greater rate than production; red blood cell parts interfere with blood flow
Blood cell loss or dilution	Chronic disease	Bleeding leads to cell loss, while excessive fluid leads to a dilution of red blood cell concentration

Prehospital treatment of anemia is primarily symptomatic. Direct your attention at maximizing oxygenation, stemming blood loss, and transporting to a medical facility for treatment of the cause. Start volume replacement if there is evidence of dehydration, resulting in hypotension.

Sickle Cell Disease

* **sickle cell anemia** an inherited disorder of red blood cell production, so named because the red blood cells become sickle-shaped when oxygen levels are low.

Sickle cell anemia, often termed "sickle cell disease," is a disorder of red blood cell production. Normal hemoglobin is very flexible, and the red blood cell can pass easily through the tiny capillaries. Sickle hemoglobin has an abnormal chemical sequence that gives red blood cells a *C,* or sickle, shape when oxygen levels are low (Figure 35-3). Patients with sickle cell disease will have a chronic anemia that results from destruction of abnormal red blood cells (hemolytic anemia). The average life span of sickled red blood cells is 10–20 days compared with 120 days for normal red blood cells. In addition, sickled red blood cells increase the blood's viscosity, leading to sludging and obstruction of the capillaries and small blood vessels. Blockage of blood flow to various tissues and organs is common and usually occurs following a period of stress. This process, called a vaso-occlusive crisis, is characteristic of sickle cell anemia. Because of the vaso-occlusive crisis, tissues and organs are eventually damaged. Adult sickle cell patients often have multiple organ problems, including cardiopulmonary disease, renal disease, and neurological disorders.

Sickle cell disease is inherited. It primarily affects blacks although other ethnic groups can be affected. These include Puerto Ricans and people of Spanish, French, Italian, Greek, and Turkish heritage. If both parents carry a gene for sickle cell anemia, the chances are one in four that the child will have normal hemoglobin. The chances are two in four that she will have both normal hemoglobin and sickle hemoglobin, which is referred to as *sickle cell trait.* The chances

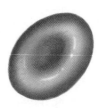 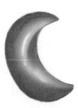

FIGURE 35-3   A normal red blood cell contrasted with a sickle cell.

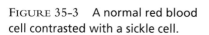

Normal red blood cell   Sickle cell

are one in four that she will have only sickle hemoglobin (no normal hemoglobin.) This condition is referred to as *sickle cell disease*.

Patients with sickle cell disease will develop three types of problems. *Vaso-occlusive crises* cause musculoskeletal pain, abdominal pain, priapisms, pulmonary problems, renal crises (renal infarctions), and central nervous system crises (cerebral infarctions). In addition, they will develop *hematological crises* that consist of a fall in the hemoglobin level, sequestration of red blood cells in the spleen, and problems with bone marrow function. In severe cases, the bone marrow can shut down, causing an aplastic crisis. These are usually self-limiting. Finally, sickle cell patients often develop *infectious crises*. They are functionally immunosuppressed, and the loss of splenic function makes them particularly vulnerable to encapsulated bacteria. Infections become common and are often the cause of death in sickle cell anemia.

Prehospital care for patients in sickle cell crisis is primarily supportive. Begin high-flow oxygen to saturate as much hemoglobin as possible. Initiate IV therapy with an isotonic crystalloid solution. These patients are often dehydrated, and hydration will sometimes help with the vaso-occlusive process. Venous access is sometimes difficult in older patients with sickle cell disease due to the large number of IV starts they have required in their lifetime. Placing a central line is occasionally necessary. Vaso-occlusive crises can be extremely painful. Start analgesic therapy in the field if possible. Always consult medical direction if there is a question regarding management. Transport is indicated.

Polycythemia

Polycythemia is an abnormally high hematocrit. It is due to excess production of red blood cells. Polycythemia is a relatively rare disorder and typically occurs in patients 50 years of age or older. It can occur secondarily to dehydration. The increased red blood cell load increases the patient's risk of thrombosis. Most deaths from polycythemia are due to thrombosis.

Polycythemia's signs and symptoms vary. The principal finding is a hematocrit of 50 percent or greater. The patient will usually have an increased number of white blood cells and platelets. However, the large number of red blood cells may cause a platelet dysfunction. This can result in bleeding abnormalities, such as epistaxis, spontaneous bruising, and gastrointestinal bleeding. Patients with polycythemia may complain of headache, dizziness, blurred vision, itching, and gastrointestinal disease. Severe cases can result in congestive heart failure.

The prehospital treatment of polycythemia is supportive. Ensure that the airway and breathing are adequate. Administer supplemental oxygen as required. Initiate an IV with an isotonic crystalloid solution. The principal treatment is phlebotomy, which removes excess red blood cells.

DISEASES OF THE WHITE BLOOD CELLS

The white blood cells are the body's principal defence system. Problems with white blood cells typically result from too few white blood cells (**leukopenia**), too many white blood cells (**leukocytosis**), or improper white blood cell function. The neutrophil is the main blood component protecting against a bacterial or fungal reaction. A reduction in the number of neutrophils (**neutropenia**) predisposes the patient to bacterial and fungal infections.

Leukopenia/Neutropenia

The status of the white blood cells is easily determined by obtaining a complete blood count. A normal white blood cell count ranges from 5000 to 9000 per cubic millimetre of blood. A decrease in the number of white blood cells indicates

* **polycythemia** an abnormally high hematocrit.

* **leukopenia** too few white blood cells.

* **leukocytosis** too many white blood cells.

* **neutropenia** a reduction in the number of neutrophils.

Content Review

DISEASES OF THE WHITE BLOOD CELLS
- Leukopenia/Neutropenia
- Leukocytosis
- Leukemia
- Lymphoma

a problem with white-blood-cell production in the marrow or destruction of white blood cells. Because bacterial infections pose a major risk to humans, an absolute neutrophil count is a better indicator of the immune system's status. The prehospital treatment of leukopenia/neutropenia is supportive. Pay special attention to preventing infection in the patient, as her immune system is overstressed or may be functioning inadequately.

Leukocytosis

Leukocytosis is an increase in the number of circulating white blood cells. This occurs when the body is exposed to an infectious agent or is particularly stressed. Following exposure, the immune system is stimulated and the marrow and spleen start releasing white blood cells to help the body fight infection. A white blood cell count between 10 800 and 23 000 per cubic millimetre of blood is characteristic of a bacterial infection. During periods of stress, immature neutrophils may be released into the circulation. These differ from mature neutrophils in that they have a segmented nucleus. These cells are referred to as "bands" or "segs." An increase in the number of bands is indicative of a significant bacterial infection. Causes of leukocytosis include bacterial infection, rheumatoid arthritis, diabetic ketoacidosis (DKA), leukemia, pain, and exercise. Viral infections tend to have little effect on the white blood cell count or, in some cases, actually cause a decrease in the white blood cell count. A white blood cell count greater than 30 000 per cubic millimetre is called a *leukemoid reaction.* A white blood cell count this high indicates a problem with excess white blood cell production. Any patient with a significantly elevated white blood cell count should be evaluated for possible leukemia.

Leukemia

✱ leukemia a cancer of the hematopoietic cells.

Leukemias are cancers of hematopoietic cells. Precursors of white blood cells in the bone marrow begin to replicate abnormally. The cells proliferate initially in the bone marrow and then spread to the peripheral blood. Leukemias affect approximately 13 in 100 000 persons. They are classified by the type of cell or cells involved. The most common types of leukemia are

- Acute lymphocytic leukemia (ALL)
- Acute myeologenous leukemia (AML)
- Chronic lymphocytic leukemia (CLL)
- Chronic myelogenous leukemia (CML)
- Hairy cell leukemia

Discussion of the pathology of the various leukemias is not within the scope of this text. ALL is primarily a disease of children and young adults. CML occurs in both children and adults. AML, CLL, and hairy cell leukemia tend to occur in the sixth and seventh decades of life. Medicine has made significant advances in the treatment of leukemia. Treatments, such as chemotherapy, radiation therapy, and bone marrow transplantation, have resulted in cures of certain types of leukemias. The treatment of pediatric leukemia is one of the great successes of modern medicine. More than 50 percent of pediatric patients with ALL live a normal life with the disease in remission or cured. Infections are a common complication of leukemia, primarily due to the low number of circulating neutrophils. Deaths from leukemias are typically secondary to infection or bleeding.

The signs and symptoms of leukemia vary. Most patients will have a moderate to severe anemia as the cancerous cell production overwhelms the bone marrow. Thrombocytopenia (an abnormal decrease in platelets) is common for the same reason. Many leukemia patients will present with bleeding, usually due to the thrombocytopenia. With the initial presentation, leukemia patients will appear acutely ill. They will be febrile and weak, usually due to a secondary infection. Various lymph nodes may be enlarged. Patients often have a history of weight loss and anorexia. In addition, liver and spleen enlargement are typical, resulting in a sensation of abdominal fullness or abdominal pain. The sternum may be tender, secondary to the increased bone marrow activity. Fatigue is a common complaint.

The prehospital treatment of the patient with leukemia is primarily supportive. Place the patient in a position of comfort. Administer supplemental oxygen via a nonrebreather mask. Initiate an IV with an isotonic crystalloid solution, such as Ringer's Lactate or normal saline. Consider a fluid bolus if the patient is hypotensive. If the patient is having pain secondary to the leukemia, consider administration of an analgesic. Remember, leukemia patients are at increased risk of developing infection. Employ proper isolation techniques.

Employ proper isolation techniques for leukemia patients, who are at increased risk of developing infection.

Lymphomas

Lymphomas are cancers of the lymphatic system. Malignant lymphoma is typically classified as follows:

* **lymphoma** a cancer of the lymphatic system.

- Hodgkin's lymphoma
- Non-Hodgkin's lymphoma

Malignant lymphoma is classified by the cell type involved, which indicates the stem cell from which the malignancy arises. In 2003, there were 6400 diagnosed cases of non-Hodgkins lymphoma diagnosed in Canada and 2800 deaths attributed to the disease. The long-term survival rate is much better with Hodgkin's lymphoma. In fact, many patients with Hodgkin's lymphoma who have been treated with radiation, chemotherapy, or both are considered cured.

The most common presenting sign of non-Hodgkin's lymphoma is painless swelling of the lymph nodes. The majority of patients with Hodgkin's lymphoma typically have no related symptoms. Patients with lymphoma may report fever, night sweats, anorexia, weight loss, fatigue, and pruritis. Treat patients with lymphomas symptomatically. Place the patient in a position of comfort. Administer supplemental oxygen via a nonrebreather mask. Initiate an IV with an isotonic crystalloid solution, such as Ringer's Lactate or normal saline. Consider a fluid bolus if the patient is hypotensive. If the patient is having pain secondary to the lymphoma, consider administration of an analgesic. As with leukemia patients, lymphoma patients are at increased risk of developing infection. Employ proper isolation techniques.

Lymphoma patients are at increased risk of developing infection. Use proper isolation techniques.

DISEASES OF THE PLATELETS/ BLOOD CLOTTING ABNORMALITIES

Various disorders can affect the platelets or the body's blood clotting system. Some of these are hereditary, while others may be acquired. Examples of platelet abnormalities include thrombocytosis (increased platelets) and thrombocytopenia (reduced platelets). Various disorders can affect the coagulation system. These include hemophilia A, hemophilia B (Christmas disease), and others.

Thrombocytosis

Thrombocytosis is an increase in the number of platelets, usually due to increased platelet production (essential thrombocytosis). It is also seen in polycythemia vera

* **thrombocytosis** an abnormal increase in the number of platelets.

where both red blood cells and platelets are increased. Thrombocytosis often complicates chronic myelogenous leukemia. Thrombcytosis can be secondary to other disorders, such as malignant diseases, hemolytic anemias, acute hemorrhage, and autoinflammatory diseases. Most patients with thrombocytosis are asymptomatic. Prehospital treatment is supportive.

Thrombocytopenia

Thrombocytopenia is an abnormal decrease in the number of platelets. It is due to decreased platelet production, sequestration of platelets in the spleen, destruction of platelets, or any combination of the three. Many drugs can induce thrombocytopenia. Acute *idiopathic thrombocytopenia purpura (ITP)* results from destruction of platelets by the immune system. It is most commonly seen in children following a viral infection. ITP is characterized by easy bruising, bleeding, and a falling platelet count. Chronic ITP usually occurs in adult women and is often associated with autoimmune disease. Prehospital treatment is supportive.

Hemophilia

Hemophilia is a blood disorder in which one of the proteins necessary for blood clotting is missing or defective. A deficiency of factor VIII is called hemophilia A. A deficiency of factor IX is known as hemophilia B (Christmas disease). Hemophilia A is the most common inherited disorder of hemostasis. The severity of the disease is directly related to the amount of circulating factor VIII available. Patients are classified as mild, moderate, or severe, based on the amount of circulating factor VIII. Hemophilia B is more rare but also more severe than hemophilia A.

When a person with hemophilia is injured, the bleeding will take longer to stop because the body cannot form stable fibrin clots. Simple trauma, such as nosebleeds or tooth extractions, can lead to prolonged, occasionally life-threatening bleeds. In extensive trauma, such as pelvic fractures, blood loss can be overwhelming. A common problem with hemophilia is hemarthrosis (bleeding into the joint space). This can result from even the most minor trauma. Eventually, repeated bleeding episodes will lead to permanent joint damage.

Hemophilia is a sex-linked, inherited bleeding disorder. The gene with the defective information is carried on the X chromosome. Females have two X chromosomes, one from the mother and one from the father. If one chromosome has the defective gene and the other does not, the disease is not expressed. Females who have one X chromosome containing the defective gene are referred to as carriers. Males, however, have an X chromosome from the mother and a Y chromosome from the father. If that X chromosome carries the defective gene, males will express the disease. Hemophilia A affects approximately 1 in 10 000 males. A female, conversely, can inherit hemophilia only if she receives two X chromosomes that express the disease. That is, she must be the offspring of a carrier mother and a father with hemophilia.

The signs and symptoms of hemophilia include numerous bruises, deep muscle bleeding characterized as pain or a "pulled muscle," and the joint bleeding called hemarthrosis. Most patients will be aware of their diagnosis and will tell you. Some may wear Medic-Alert bracelets or similar devices.

Hemophiliacs can be treated in the hospital with infusions of factor VIII. In addition to factor VIII, some hemophiliacs will require blood transfusions following bleeding due to trauma. Unfortunately, before blood and blood products were routinely tested, transfusions infected many hemophiliacs with the human immunodeficiency virus (HIV), hepatitis B, and/or hepatitis C.

Prehospital treatment of the patient with hemophilia should be comprehensive. The normal hemostatic mechanisms of vasoconstriction and platelet aggregation will still occur, but the platelet plug will not be stable, due to the deficiency of factor VIII. Thus, you should be attentive to prolonged bleeding or possible rebleeds. The hemophiliac is at risk of both. Administer supplemental oxygen via a nonrebreather mask, and initiate IV therapy with an isotonic crystalloid, such as normal saline. Be careful to help prevent additional trauma, which can result in further hemorrhage. If the patient sustained a joint injury with resultant hemarthrosis, splinting the extremity will sometimes help control pain. Occasionally, analgesics will be required.

If your patient has hemophilia, be especially careful to help prevent additional trauma, which can result in further hemorrhage.

Von Willebrand's Disease

Factor VIII actually consists of several components. One of these components is factor VIII:vWF, also called von Willebrand's factor. In **von Willebrand's disease,** this component of factor VIII is deficient. It is produced by the endothelial cells and is necessary for normal platelet adhesion. Thus, in addition to the clotting problem, platelet function is abnormal in patients with von Willebrand's disease. While the disease is inherited, it is not sex linked, equally affecting both females and males. A sign of this disease is excessive bleeding, primarily after surgery or injury. It is not associated with the deep muscle or joint bleeding of hemophilia, nor is it usually as serious, although nosebleeds, excessive menstruation, and gastrointestinal bleeds can occur. Prehospital treatment is supportive. Aspirin is generally contraindicated as it further inhibits platelet aggregation, thus exacerbating the disease. Definitive treatment is the administration of von Willebrand factor.

✳ **von Willebrand's disease** condition in which the vWF component of factor VIII is deficient.

OTHER HEMATOPOIETIC DISORDERS

Disseminated Intravascular Coagulation

Disseminated intravascular coagulation (DIC), also called consumption coagulopathy, is a disorder of coagulation caused by systemic activation of the coagulation cascade. Normally, inhibitory mechanisms localize coagulation to the affected area. A combination of protein inhibitors, rapid blood flow, and absorption of the fibrin clot restricts circulating free thrombin to the site of coagulation. In DIC, circulating thrombin cleaves fibrinogen to form fibrin clots throughout the circulation. This can cause widespread thrombosis and, occasionally, end-organ ischemia. Bleeding is the most frequent sign of DIC and is due to the reduced fibrinogen level, consumption of coagulation factors, and thrombocytopenia. DIC most commonly results from sepsis, hypotension, obstetric complications, severe tissue injury, brain injury, cancer, and major hemolytic transfusion reactions. The disease is quite grave. Its signs include oozing blood at venipuncture and wound sites. The patient may exhibit a purpuric rash, often over the chest and abdomen. Minute hemorrhages may be noted just under the skin. Prehospital care is symptomatic. The DIC patient may be hemodynamically unstable and may require IV fluids. Definitive treatment includes the administration of fresh frozen plasma and platelets.

✳ **disseminated intravascular coagulation (DIC)** a disorder of coagulation caused by systemic activation of the coagulation cascade.

Multiple Myeloma

Multiple myeloma is a cancerous disorder of plasma cells. Plasma cells are a type of B cell responsible for producing immunoglobulins (antibodies). The disease is rarely found in persons under the age of 40. Approximately 14 000 new cases are diagnosed each year. Usually, multiple myeloma begins with a change or mutation in a plasma cell in the bone marrow. These cancerous plasma cells crowd out healthy cells and lead to a reduction in blood cell production. The patient then becomes anemic and prone to infection.

✳ **multiple myeloma** a cancerous disorder of plasma cells.

The first sign of multiple myeloma often is pain in the back or ribs. The diseased marrow weakens the bones, and *pathological fractures* (those occurring with minimal or no trauma) may occur. The resulting anemia leads to fatigue, and reduced platelet production places the patient at risk for bleeding. Laboratory evaluation will reveal an elevation in the level of a circulating antibody or part of an antibody (light chain). This is due to the proliferation of plasma cells. Despite this, the patient is at increased risk of infection, as the plasma cells do not secrete specific antibodies in response to infection. In addition, the calcium level is often elevated due to bone destruction. This can lead to renal failure.

Treatment of multiple myeloma includes chemotherapy, radiation, and bone marrow transplantation. Prehospital care is supportive. Establish an IV of isotonic crystalloid solution. Consider a fluid bolus if there are symptoms of dehydration. Multiple myeloma can be very painful due to the proliferation of the plasma cells and destruction of the marrow. Consider analgesics if pain is severe. A pathological fracture in a patient with multiple myeloma is very painful, and you should start analgesic therapy if so indicated.

SUMMARY

Hematology is the study of the blood and blood-forming organs. Hematological disorders include red blood cell disorders, white blood cell disorders, platelet disorders, and coagulation problems. Problems can also be caused when the body has an immunological response to antigens present on red blood cells from a foreign donor. Although hematological disorders are common, they are seldom the primary reason for an emergency call. Rather, they are likely to accompany another ongoing disease process.

The signs and symptoms that accompany hematological problems seldom point directly to the underlying disease. Generally, lab findings are necessary to clarify the diagnosis. However, an understanding of hematological pathophysiology is important to understanding the disease process your patient may be undergoing and to helping you form a field impression and make appropriate decisions about emergency care.

CHAPTER 36

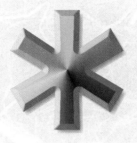

Environmental Emergencies

Objectives

After reading this chapter, you should be able to:

1. Define "environmental emergency." (p. 743)
2. Describe the incidence, morbidity, and mortality associated with environmental emergencies. (p. 743)
3. Identify the risk factors most predisposing to environmental emergencies. (p. 743)
4. Identify environmental factors that may cause illness or exacerbate a preexisting illness or complicate treatment or transport decisions. (p. 743)
5. Define "homeostasis" and relate the concept to environmental influences. (pp. 743–744)
6. Identify normal, critically high, and critically low body temperatures. (pp. 745–746, 747)
7. Describe several methods of temperature monitoring. (p. 746)
8. Describe human thermal regulation, including system components, substances used, and wastes generated. (pp. 744–747, 753)
9. List the common forms of heat and cold disorders. (pp. 747–760)

Continued

Objectives Continued

10. List the common predisposing factors and preventive measures associated with heat and cold disorders. (pp. 748–749, 754)
11. Define heat illness, hypothermia, frostbite, near-drowning, decompression illness, and altitude illness. (pp. 747, 753, 759, 761, 766, 771)
12. Describe the pathophysiology, signs and symptoms, and predisposing factors, preventive actions, and treatment for heat cramps, heat exhaustion, heatstroke, and fever. (pp. 749–753)
13. Describe the contribution of dehydration to the development of heat disorders. (p. 752)
14. Describe the differences between classical and exertional heatstroke. (p. 751)
15. Identify the fundamental thermoregulatory difference between fever and heatstroke. (p. 752)
16. Discuss the role of fluid therapy in the treatment of heat disorders. (p. 752)
17. Describe the pathophysiology, predisposing factors, signs, symptoms, and management of the following:
    a. Hypothermia (pp. 753–759)
    b. Superficial and deep frostbite (pp. 759–760)
    c. Near-drowning (pp. 761–764)
    d. Decompression illness (pp. 766, 767–769)
    e. Diving emergency (pp. 764–771)
    f. Altitude illness (pp. 771–775)
18. Identify differences among mild, severe, chronic, and acute hypothermia. (p. 754)
19. Discuss the impact of severe hypothermia on standard BCLS and ACLS algorithms and transport considerations. (pp. 755–759)

20. Differentiate between fresh-water and saltwater immersion as they relate to near-drowning. (pp. 762–763)
21. Discuss the incidence of "wet" versus "dry" drownings and the differences in their management. (pp. 761–762)
22. Discuss the complications and protective role of hypothermia in the context of near-drowning. (pp. 761, 763–764)
23. Define self-contained underwater breathing apparatus (scuba). (p. 764)
24. Describe the laws of gases and relate them to diving emergencies. (pp. 764–765)
25. Differentiate among the various diving emergencies. (pp. 764–771)
26. Identify the various conditions that may result from pulmonary overpressure accidents. (pp. 776–777, 769)
27. Describe the function of the Divers Alert Network (DAN) and how its members may aid in the management of diving-related illnesses. (p. 771)
28. Describe the specific function and benefit of hyperbaric oxygen therapy for the management of diving accidents. (p. 768)
29. Define acute mountain sickness (AMS), high-altitude pulmonary edema (HAPE), and high-altitude cerebral edema (HACE). (pp. 773–775)
30. Discuss the symptomatic variations presented in progressive altitude illnesses. (pp. 773–775)
31. Discuss the pharmacology appropriate for the treatment of altitude illnesses. (p. 773)
32. Given several preprogrammed simulated environmental emergency patients, provide the appropriate assessment, management, and transport. (pp. 743–779)

INTRODUCTION

The *environment* can be defined as all of the surrounding external factors that affect the development and functioning of a living organism. Human beings obviously depend on the environment for life. But they also must be protected from its extremes. When such factors as temperature, weather, terrain, and atmospheric pressure act on the body, they can create stresses that the body is unable to compensate for. A medical condition caused or exacerbated by such environmental factors is known as an **environmental emergency.**

Environmental emergencies include a variety of conditions, such as heatstroke, hypothermia, drowning or near-drowning, altitude sickness, nuclear radiation, and diving accidents or barotraumas, among others. Such emergencies often call for special rescue resources.

Although environmental emergencies can affect anyone, several risk factors predispose certain individuals to developing environmental illnesses. These factors include

- Age—very young children and older adults do not tolerate environmental extremes very well
- Poor general health
- Fatigue
- Predisposing medical conditions
- Certain medications—either prescription or over-the-counter

Environmental factors must also be considered when determining the risk for environmental emergencies. For example, climate in a particular place may vary greatly from moment to moment. Areas in which change in temperature can be drastic over the course of the day may catch unwary individuals off guard. For example, desert areas can have temperatures of 40.6°C during the day but drop below freezing at night, placing unprepared travellers in a difficult situation. Temperatures in parts of southern Alberta can change drastically when the Chinook winds kick up. Other considerations include the current season, local weather patterns, atmospheric pressures (high altitude or underwater), and the type of terrain, which can cause injury or hinder rescue efforts.

As a paramedic, you will frequently be called on to treat medical emergencies related to environmental conditions. It is critical that you understand the particular conditions that prevail in your region. If you live in a mountainous area, near large caves, in an area with swift-moving water, or in a resort area where diving is frequent, you need to be familiar with the specialized rescue resources these situations may require and the particular environmental emergencies they may cause. Understanding their causes and underlying pathophysiologies can help you recognize these emergencies promptly and manage them effectively.

Although many environmental factors can result in medical emergencies, this chapter will focus primarily on problems related to temperature extremes, drowning or near-drowning, diving emergencies, high altitude illness, and nuclear radiation.

* **environmental emergency** a medical condition caused or exacerbated by the weather, terrain, atmospheric pressure, or other local factors.

HOMEOSTASIS

In order for the human body to function properly, it must interact with the environment to obtain oxygen, nutrients, and other necessities, but it must also avoid being damaged by extreme external environmental conditions. The process of maintaining constant suitable conditions within the body is called **homeostasis.** Various body systems respond in an effort to maintain the correct core and peripheral temperature, oxygen level, and energy supply to maintain life.

* **homeostasis** the natural tendency of the body to maintain a steady and normal internal environment.

The following sections address how the body attempts to maintain these normal settings and what happens when certain environmental conditions exceed the ability of the body to compensate.

PATHOPHYSIOLOGY OF HEAT AND COLD DISORDERS

MECHANISMS OF HEAT GAIN AND LOSS

The body gains and loses heat in two ways, from within the body itself and by contact with the external environment.

The body receives heat from or loses it to the environment via the thermal gradient. The **thermal gradient** is the difference in temperature between the environment (the ambient temperature) and the body. The ambient temperature is usually different from body temperature. If the environment is warmer than the body, heat flows from the environment to the body. If the body is warmer than the environment, heat flows from the body to the environment. Other environmental factors, including wind and relative humidity (the percentage of water vapour in the air), also affect heat gain and loss.

The mechanisms by which heat is generated within the body and by which heat is gained or lost to the environment are discussed in more detail in the following sections.

THERMOGENESIS (HEAT GENERATION)

The amount of heat in the body continually fluctuates as a result of the heat generated or gained and the heat lost. The body gains heat from both external and internal sources. In addition to the heat the body absorbs from the environment, the body also generates heat through energy-producing chemical reactions (metabolism).

The creation of heat is called **thermogenesis.** There are several types of thermogenesis. One is *work-induced thermogenesis* that results from exercise. Our muscles need to create heat because warm muscles work more effectively than cold ones. One way muscles can produce heat is by shivering. Another type, *thermoregulatory thermogenesis,* is controlled by the endocrine system. The hormones norepinephrine and epinephrine can cause an immediate increase in the rate of cellular metabolism, which, in turn, increases heat production. The last type, metabolic thermogenesis, or *diet-induced thermogenesis,* is caused by the processing of food and nutrients. When a meal is eaten, digested, absorbed, and metabolized, heat is produced as a byproduct of these activities.

THERMOLYSIS (HEAT LOSS)

The heat generated by the body is constantly lost to the environment. This occurs because the body is usually warmer than the surrounding environment. The transfer of heat into the environment occurs through the following mechanisms (Figure 36-1):

- **Conduction.** Direct contact of the body's surface to another, cooler object causes the body to lose heat by conduction. Heat flows from higher temperature matter to lower temperature matter.
- **Convection.** Heat loss to air currents passing over the body is called convection. Heat, however, must first be conducted to the air before being carried away by convection currents.
- **Radiation.** An unclothed person will lose approximately 60 percent of total body heat by radiation at normal room temperature. This

* thermal gradient the difference in temperature between the environment and the body.

* thermogenesis the production of heat, especially within the body.

* conduction moving electrons, ions, heat, or sound waves through a conductor or conducting medium.

* convection transfer of heat via currents in liquids or gases.

* radiation transfer of energy through space or matter.

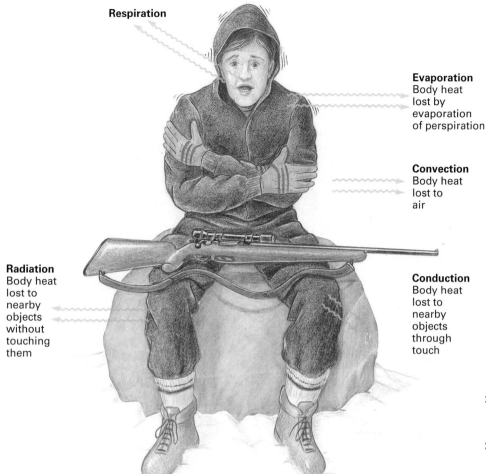

Respiration

Evaporation
Body heat
lost by
evaporation
of perspiration

Convection
Body heat
lost to
air

Radiation
Body heat
lost to
nearby
objects
without
touching
them

Conduction
Body heat
lost to
nearby
objects
through
touch

FIGURE 36-1   Heat loss by the body.

heat loss is in the form of infrared rays. All objects not at absolute zero temperature will radiate heat into the atmosphere.

- **Evaporation.** Evaporation is the change of a liquid to vapour. Evaporative heat loss occurs as water evaporates from the skin. Additionally, a great deal of heat loss occurs through evaporation of fluids in the lungs. Water evaporates from the skin and lungs at approximately 600 mL/day.

- **Respiration.** Respiration combines the mechanisms of convection, radiation, and evaporation. It accounts for a large proportion of the body's heat loss. Heat is transferred from the lungs to inspired air by convection and radiation. Evaporation in the lungs humidifies the inspired air (adds water vapour to it). During expiration, this warm, humidified air is released into the environment, creating heat loss.

THERMOREGULATION

Thermoregulation is the maintenance or regulation of temperature. The body temperature of the deep tissues, commonly called the **core temperature,** usually does not vary more than a degree or so from its normal 37°C. A naked person can be exposed to an external environment ranging anywhere from 3°C to 62°C and

✳ **evaporation** change from liquid to a gaseous state.

✳ **respiration** the exchange of gases between a living organism and its environment.

✳ **thermoregulation** the maintenance or regulation of a particular temperature of the body.

✳ **core temperature** the body temperature of the deep tissues, which usually does not vary more than a degree or so from its normal 37°C.

Content Review

COMPARATIVE BODY TEMPERATURES

Celsius	Fahrenheit
40.6°	105°
37.8°	100°
37°	98.6°
35°	95°
32°	89.6°
30°	86°
20°	68°

✱ **hypothalamus** portion of the diencephalon producing neurosecretions important in the control of certain metabolic activities, including body temperature regulation.

✱ **negative feedback** homeostatic mechanism in which a change in a variable (here, core temperature) ultimately inhibits the process that led to the shift.

still maintain a fairly constant internal body temperature. This characteristic of warm-blooded animals is called *steady-state metabolism*. The various biochemical reactions occurring within the cell are most efficient when the body temperature is within this narrow temperature range.

Evaluation of peripheral body temperature can be measured by touch or by taking the temperature by oral or axillary means. Core body temperatures can be measured using tympanic or rectal thermometers.

The body maintains a balance between the production and loss of heat almost entirely through the nervous system and negative feedback mechanisms. The **hypothalamus,** located at the base of the brain, is responsible for temperature regulation. It functions as a thermostat, controlling temperature through the release of neurosecretions (secretions produced by nerve cells). When the hypothalamus senses an increased body temperature, it shuts off the mechanisms designed to create heat, for example, shivering. When it senses a decrease in body temperature, the hypothalamus shuts off mechanisms designed to cool the body, for example, sweating. Because the action involved requires stopping, or negating, a process, it is called a **negative feedback** system.

When the heat regulating function of the hypothalamus is disrupted, the result can be an abnormally high or low body temperature. At the extremes, such abnormal temperatures can result in death (Figure 36-2).

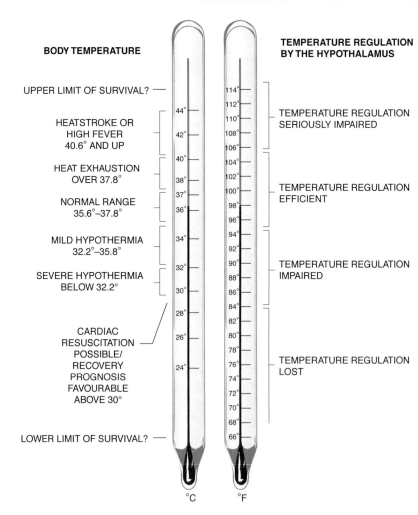

FIGURE 36-2   Temperature regulation by the hypothalamus.

Thermoreceptors

Although the hypothalamus plays a key role in body temperature regulation, temperature receptors in other parts of the body also help moderate temperatures. There are thermoreceptors in the skin and certain mucous membranes (peripheral thermoreceptors) as well as in certain deep tissues of the body (central thermoreceptors). The skin has both cold and warm receptors. Because cold receptors outnumber warm receptors, peripheral detection of temperature consists mainly of detecting cold, rather than warmth. Deep body temperature receptors lie mostly in the spinal cord, abdominal viscera, and in or around the great veins. These receptors are exposed to the body's core temperature, rather than the peripheral temperature. They also respond mainly to cold, rather than warmth. Both peripheral and central thermoreceptors act to prevent lowering of the body temperature.

Metabolic Rate

The **basal metabolic rate (BMR)** is the metabolism that occurs when the body is completely at rest. It is the rate at which the body consumes energy just to maintain itself—the rate of metabolism that maintains brain function, circulation, and cell stability. Any additional activity that the body performs demands energy consumption beyond that supported by the basal rate, metabolizing more nutrients and releasing more calories (units of heat). The rate of metabolism that supports this additional activity is called an **exertional metabolic rate.**

The body continually adjusts the metabolic rate in order to maintain the temperature of the core (where the crucial structures like the heart and brain are located). The body also achieves temperature maintenance by dilating some blood vessels and constricting others so that the blood carries the excess heat from the core to the periphery where it is close to the skin. This allows heat to dissipate through the skin into the environment.

Conversely, when the environment is too cold, *countercurrent heat exchange* is used to shunt warm blood away from the superficial veins near the skin and back into the deep veins near the core to keep vital structures warm. Another body response that counters a cold environment is shivering, a physical activity that increases metabolism and generates heat.

It is important to note that these various mechanisms can create a difference between the core body temperature and the peripheral body temperature. Core temperature is the crucial measurement since, as noted, the core is where the major organs are located. Therefore, it is important in any heat-related or cold-related emergency to obtain a core temperature reading, such as from the rectum. Oral and axillary temperatures may provide convenient approximations in some situations but may lead to incorrect interventions if relied on for treatment of the patient with an environmental illness.

* **basal metabolic rate (BMR)** rate at which the body consumes energy just to maintain stability; the basic metabolic rate (measured by the rate of oxygen consumption) of an awake, relaxed person 12 to 14 hours after eating and at a comfortable temperature.

* **exertional metabolic rate** rate at which the body consumes energy during activity. It is faster than the basal metabolic rate.

HEAT DISORDERS

Disruption of the body's normal thermoregulatory mechanisms can produce a number of heat illnesses, such as hyperthermia and fever. **Heat illness** is increased *core body temperature (CBT)* due to inadequate thermolysis.

HYPERTHERMIA

Hyperthermia is a state of unusually high body temperature, specifically the core body temperature. Hyperthermia is usually caused by heat transfer from

* **heat illness** increased core body temperature due to inadequate thermolysis.

* **hyperthermia** unusually high core body temperature.

Content Review

HEAT DISORDERS

Hyperthermia
Heat cramps
Heat exhaustion
Heatstroke

the external environment that the body cannot compensate for. Occasionally, it is caused by excessive generation of heat within the body.

As the body attempts to eliminate this excessive heat, you will see the general signs of thermolysis (heat loss). These signs are caused by the body's two chief methods of heat dissipation, sweating (which leads to evaporative heat loss) and vasodilation (which allows the blood to carry heat to the periphery for dissipation through the skin). These include

- Diaphoresis (sweating)
- Increased skin temperature
- Flushing

As heat illness progresses, you will also note signs of thermolytic inadequacy (the failure of the body's thermoregulatory mechanisms to compensate adequately):

- Altered mentation
- Altered level of consciousness

Hyperthermia can manifest as heat cramps, heat exhaustion, or heatstroke, which will be discussed in following sections.

PREDISPOSING FACTORS

Age, general health, and medications are predisposing factors in hyperthermia. Factors that may contribute to a susceptibility to hyperthermia include

- *Age of the patient*—Pediatric and geriatric populations are less tolerant of variations in temperature, and their heat-regulating mechanisms are not as responsive as those of young adult and adult populations.

* **autonomic neuropathy** condition that damages the autonomic nervous system, which usually senses changes in core temperature and controls vasodilation and perspiration to dissipate heat.

- *Health of the patient*—Diabetics can become hyperthermic more easily because they develop **autonomic neuropathy.** This condition damages the autonomic nervous system, which may interfere with thermoregulatory input and with vasodilation and perspiration, which normally dissipate heat.
- *Medications*—Various medications can affect body temperature in the following ways:
  - *Diuretics* predispose to dehydration, which worsens hyperthermia.
  - *Beta-blockers* interfere with vasodilation and reduce the capacity to increase heart rate in response to volume loss and may also interfere with thermoregulatory input.
  - *Psychotropics and antihistamines,* such as antipsychotics and phenothiazines, interfere with central thermoregulation.

* **acclimatization** the reversible changes in body structure and function by which the body becomes adjusted to a change in environment.

- *Level of acclimatization*—**Acclimatization** is the process of becoming adjusted to a change in environment. In response to an environmental change, reversible changes in body structure and function take place that help to maintain homeostasis.
- *Length of exposure.*
- *Intensity of exposure.*
- *Environmental factors,* such as humidity and wind.

PREVENTIVE MEASURES

Ideally, prevention of heat disorders is preferable to treating an illness already in progress. Measures to prevent hyperthermia include the following:

- Maintain adequate fluid intake, remembering that thirst is an inadequate indicator of dehydration.
- Allow time for gradual acclimatization to being out in the heat. Acclimatization results in more perspiration with lower salt concentration and increases body-fluid volume.
- Limit exposure to hot environments.

SPECIFIC HEAT DISORDERS

Inevitably, you will be required to respond to heat-related emergencies: heat cramps, heat exhaustion, or heatstroke. Heat cramps and heat exhaustion result from dehydration and depletion of sodium and other electrolytes. Heatstroke, a far more serious and potentially life-threatening condition, results from the failure of the body's thermoregulatory mechanisms.

Signs and symptoms and emergency care procedures for heat cramps, heat exhaustion, and heatstroke are discussed in the following sections.

Heat (Muscle) Cramps

Heat cramps are muscle cramps caused by overexertion and dehydration in the presence of high atmospheric temperatures. Sweating occurs as sodium (salt) is transported to the skin. Because "water follows sodium," water is deposited on the skin surface where evaporation occurs, aiding in the cooling process. Since sweating involves not only the loss of water but also the loss of electrolytes (such as sodium), intermittent cramping of skeletal muscles may occur. Heat cramps are painful but are not considered to be an actual heat illness.

✱ heat cramps acute painful spasms of the voluntary muscles following strenuous activity in a hot environment without adequate fluid or salt intake.

Signs and Symptoms The patient with heat cramps will present with cramps in the fingers, arms, legs, or abdominal muscles. He will generally be mentally alert with a feeling of weakness. He may feel dizzy or faint. Vital signs will be stable. Body temperature may be normal or slightly elevated. The skin is likely to be moist and warm.

Treatment Treatment of the patient with heat cramps is usually easily accomplished:

1. *Remove the patient from the environment.* Place the patient in a cool environment, such as a shaded area or the air-conditioned back of the ambulance.

In the case of severe cramps:

2. *Administer an oral saline solution* (approximately four teaspoons of salt to one litre of water) or a sports drink. Do NOT administer salt tablets, which are not absorbed as readily and may cause stomach irritation and ulceration or hypernatremia. *If the patient is unable to take fluids orally, an IV of normal saline may be needed.*

Some EMS systems recommend massaging the painful muscles. Application of moist towels to the patient's forehead and over the cramped muscles may also be helpful.

Heat Exhaustion

Heat exhaustion, which is considered to be a mild heat illness, is an acute reaction to heat exposure. It is the most common heat-related illness seen by prehospital personnel. An individual performing work in a hot environment will lose

✱ heat exhaustion a mild heat illness; an acute reaction to heat exposure.

1 to 2 litres of water an hour. Each litre lost contains 20 to 50 milliequivalents of sodium. The resulting loss of water and sodium, combined with general vasodilation, leads to a decreased circulating blood volume, venous pooling, and reduced cardiac output.

Dehydration and sodium loss due to sweating account for the presenting symptoms. However, these signs and symptoms are not exclusive to heat exhaustion. Instead, they mimic those of an individual suffering from fluid and sodium loss from any of a number of other causes. A history of exposure to high environmental temperatures is needed to obtain an accurate assessment.

If not treated, heat exhaustion may progress to heatstroke.

Signs and Symptoms Signs and symptoms that you may encounter include increased body temperature (37.8°C), skin that is cool and clammy with heavy perspiration, breathing that is rapid and shallow, and a weak pulse. There may be signs of active thermolysis, such as diarrhea and muscle cramps. The patient will feel weak and, in some cases, may lose consciousness. There may be central nervous system (CNS) symptoms, such as headache, anxiety, paresthesia, and impaired judgment or even psychosis.

Treatment Prehospital management of the patient with heat exhaustion is aimed at immediate cooling and fluid replacement. Steps include

1. *Remove the patient from the environment.* Place the patient in a cool environment, such as a shaded area or the air-conditioned ambulance.

2. *Place the patient in a supine position.*

3. *Administer an oral saline solution* (approximately four teaspoons of salt to a litre of water) or a sports drink. Do NOT administer salt tablets, which are not absorbed as readily and may cause stomach irritation and ulceration or hypernatremia. *If the patient is unable to take fluids orally, an IV of normal saline may be needed.*

4. *Remove some of the patient's clothing, and fan the patient.* Remove enough clothing to cool the patient without chilling him. Fanning increases evaporation and cooling. Again, be careful not to cool the patient to the point of chilling him. If the patient begins to shiver, stop fanning, and cover the patient lightly if necessary.

5. *Treat for shock, if shock is suspected.* However, be careful not to cover the patient to the point of overheating him.

Symptoms should resolve with fluids, rest, and supine posturing with knees elevated. If they do not, consider that the symptoms may be due to an increased core body temperature, which is predictive of impending heatstroke and should be treated aggressively, as outlined in the following section.

Heatstroke

Heatstroke is a true environmental emergency that occurs when the body's hypothalamic temperature regulation is lost, causing uncompensated hyperthermia. This in turn causes cell death and damage to the brain, liver, and kidneys. There is no arbitrary core temperature at which heatstroke begins. However, heatstroke is generally characterized by a body temperature of at least 40.6°C, central nervous system disturbances, and usually the cessation of sweating.

Signs and Symptoms Sweating is thought to stop due to destruction of the sweat glands or when sensory overload causes them to temporarily dysfunction. However, the patient's skin may be either dry or covered with sweat that is still present on the skin from earlier exertion. In either case, the skin will be hot.

✱ **heatstroke** acute, dangerous reaction to heat exposure, characterized by a body temperature usually above 40.6°C and central nervous system disturbances. The body usually ceases to perspire.

Heatstroke is a true environmental emergency.
🗝

The patient may present with the following signs and symptoms:

- Cessation of sweating
- Hot skin that is dry or moist
- Very high core temperature
- Deep respirations that become shallow, rapid at first but may later slow down
- Rapid, full pulse, may slow down later
- Hypotension with low or absent diastolic reading
- Confusion or disorientation or unconsciousness
- Possible seizures

Classic heatstroke commonly presents in those with chronic illnesses, with the increased core body temperature due to deficient thermoregulatory function. Predisposing conditions include age, diabetes, and other medical conditions. In this type of heatstroke hot, red, dry skin is common.

Exertional heatstroke commonly presents in those who are in good general health, with the increased core body temperature due to overwhelming heat stress. There is excessive ambient temperature as well as excessive exertion with prolonged exposure and poor acclimatization. In this type of heatstroke you will find that, although sweating has ceased and the skin is hot, moisture from prior sweating may still be present.

If the patient develops heatstroke due to exertion, he may go into severe metabolic acidosis caused by lactic acid accumulation. Hyperkalemia (excessive potassium in blood) may also develop because of the release of potassium from injured muscle cells, renal failure, or metabolic acidosis.

Treatment   Prehospital management of the heatstroke patient is aimed at immediate cooling and replacement of fluids. Steps include

The heatstroke patient should be cooled immediately and given fluids.

1. *Remove the patient from the environment.* This first step is essential. If you do not remove the patient from the hot environment, any other measures will be only minimally useful. Move the patient to a cool environment, such as the air-conditioned ambulance.

2. *Initiate rapid active cooling.* Body temperature must be lowered to 39°C. A target of 39°C is used to avoid an overshoot. This cooling can be accomplished en route to the hospital. Remove the patient's clothing, and cover the patient with sheets soaked in tepid water. Fanning and misting may also be used if necessary. Refrain from overcooling, as this may cause reflex hypothermia (low body temperature). This results in shivering, which can raise the core temperature again. Place ice packs in the patient's groin, neck, and axillary regions.

3. *Administer oxygen.* Administer high-flow oxygen via a nonrebreather mask. If respirations are shallow, assist with a bag-valve-mask unit supplied with 100-percent oxygen. Utilize pulse oximetry, if available.

4. *Administer fluid therapy if the patient is alert and able to swallow.*
   - *Oral fluids.* In many cases, oral fluid therapy will be all that is needed. Some salt additive is beneficial, but salt tablets should be avoided as they may cause gastrointestinal irritation and ulceration or hypernatremia. There is a very limited need for other electrolytes in oral rehydration.
   - *Intravenous fluids.* Begin 1 to 2 IVs, using normal saline. Initially, infuse them wide open.

5. *Monitor the ECG.* Cardiac dysrhythmias may occur at any time. S-T segment depression, nonspecific T-wave changes with occasional PVCs, and supraventricular tachycardias are common.

6. *Avoid vasopressors and anticholinergic drugs.* These agents may potentiate heatstroke by inhibiting sweating. They can also produce a hypermetabolic state in the presence of high environmental temperatures and relatively high humidity.

7. *Monitor body temperature.* EMS systems operating in extremely warm climates should carry some device to record the body temperature, whether a simple rectal thermometer or a sophisticated electronic device. Simple glass thermometers generally do not measure above 41°C or below 35°C. This may become significant during long transport when it is essential to detect changes in the patient's condition.

ROLE OF DEHYDRATION IN HEAT DISORDERS

Dehydration often goes hand in hand with heat disorders.

Dehydration often goes hand in hand with heat disorders because it inhibits vasodilation and therefore thermolysis. Dehydration leads to orthostatic hypotension (increased pulse and decreased blood pressure on rising from a supine position) and the following symptoms, which may occur along with the signs and symptoms of heatstroke:

Thirst is a poor indication of the degree of dehydration present.

- Nausea, vomiting, and abdominal distress
- Vision disturbances
- Decreased urine output
- Poor skin turgor
- Signs of hypovolemic shock

When these signs and symptoms are present, rehydration of the patient is critical. Oral fluids may be administered if the patient is alert and not nauseated. Administration of IV fluids may be necessary, especially if the patient has an altered mental status or is nauseated. It is not uncommon for the adult patient with moderate to severe dehydration to require 2–3 litres of IV fluids (occasionally more!).

FEVER (PYREXIA)

✳ **pyrexia** fever, or above-normal body temperature.

✳ **pyrogen** any substance causing a fever, such as viruses and bacteria or substances produced within the body in response to infection or inflammation.

A fever (**pyrexia**) is the elevation of the body temperature above the normal temperature for that person. (An individual person's normal temperature may be one or two degrees above or below 37°C.) The body develops a fever when pathogens enter and cause infection, which, in turn, stimulates the production of pyrogens.

Pyrogens are any substances that cause fever, such as viruses and bacteria or substances produced within the body in response to infection or inflammation. They reset the hypothalamic thermostat to a higher level. Metabolism is increased, which produces the elevation of temperature. The increased body temperature fights infection by making the body a less hospitable environment for the invading organism. The hypothalamic thermostat will reset to normal when pyrogen production stops or when pathogens end their attack on the body.

Fever is sometimes difficult to differentiate from heatstroke, and neurological symptoms may present with either, but there is usually a history of infection or illness with a fever. While the heatstroke patient usually has a history of exertion and exposure to high ambient temperatures, this is not always the case. In some cases, heatstroke can be caused by impaired functioning of the hypothalamus without exertion or exposure to ambient heat. Treat for heatstroke if you are unsure which it is.

When unsure if the problem is heatstroke or fever, treat for heatstroke.

Although fever may be beneficial, it can be disconcerting to the parents of children with fever. In addition, fever can be uncomfortable for the patient. If the patient is uncomfortable, measures should be taken to treat the fever. Also, if a child has a history of febrile seizures, the fever should be treated. Parents will often have their febrile children wrapped in several layers of clothing or blankets because the child is "cold." These should be removed, leaving only the diaper or underclothes, exposing the child to the ambient air. This will allow a controlled cooling.

Sponge baths and cool-water immersion should not be used. These cause a rapid drop in the body core temperature and result in shivering. This again elevates the core temperature, which complicates the process. Several medications are good antipyretics (that is, they lower body temperature in fever). These include acetaminophen (Tylenol) and ibuprofen (Motrin). Liquid acetaminophen and ibuprofen are easy to administer and effective. Acetaminophen is also available in a suppository form for patients with active vomiting. These antipyretics are typically dosed on the basis of the patient's weight:

Do not use sponge baths to cool febrile children.

- *Acetaminophen*—15 mg/kg for pediatric patients; adult dose is typically 650 mg
- *Ibuprofen*—10 mg/kg for pediatric patients; adult dose is typically 600–800 mg

These liquid medications should be dosed with syringes as teaspoons are inaccurate measuring devices.

COLD DISORDERS

Disruption of the body's normal thermoregulation may produce cold-related disorders, such as hypothermia, frostbite, and trench foot.

HYPOTHERMIA

Hypothermia is a state of low body temperature, specifically low core temperature. When the core temperature of the body drops below 35°C, an individual is considered to be hypothermic. Hypothermia can be attributed to inadequate thermogenesis, excessive cold stress, or a combination of both.

MECHANISMS OF HEAT CONSERVATION AND LOSS

Exposure to cold normally triggers compensatory mechanisms designed to conserve and generate heat in order to maintain a normal body temperature. One such mechanism is piloerection (hair standing on end, "goose bumps") to impede air flow across the skin. Shivering and increased muscle tone occur, resulting in increased metabolism. There is peripheral vasoconstriction with an increase in cardiac output and respiratory rate. When these mechanisms can no longer adequately compensate for heat lost from the body surface, the body temperature falls. As the body temperature falls, so do the metabolic rate and cardiac output.

As discussed, major mechanisms of body heat loss are conduction, convection, radiation, evaporation, and respiration. Heat loss can be increased by the removal of clothing (decreased insulation, increased radiation), the wetting of clothing by rain or snow (increased conduction and evaporation), air movement around the body (increased convection), or contact with a cold surface or cold-water immersion (increased conduction).

* **hypothermia** state of low body temperature, particularly low core body temperature.

PREDISPOSING FACTORS

Several factors can contribute to the risk of developing hypothermia. They also contribute to the severity of damage if cold injury occurs. Risk factors that increase the danger of developing hypothermia include

- *Age of the patient*—Pediatric or geriatric patients cannot tolerate cold environments and have less responsive heat-generating mechanisms to combat cold exposure. Elderly persons often become hypothermic in environments that seem only mildly cool to others.
- *Health of the patient*—Hypothyroidism suppresses metabolism, preventing patients from responding appropriately to cold stress. Malnutrition, hypoglycemia, Parkinson's disease, fatigue, and other medical conditions can interfere with the body's ability to combat cold exposure.
- *Medications*—Some drugs interfere with proper heat generating mechanisms. These include narcotics, alcohol, phenothiazines, barbiturates, antiseizure medications, antihistamines and other allergy medications, antipsychotics, sedatives, antidepressants, and various pain medications, such as aspirin, acetaminophen, and NSAIDs.
- *Prolonged or intense exposure*—The length and severity of cold exposure have a direct effect on morbidity and mortality.
- *Coexisting weather conditions*—High humidity, brisk winds, or accompanying rain can all magnify the effect of cold exposure on the human body by accelerating the loss of heat from skin surfaces.

PREVENTIVE MEASURES

Certain precautions can decrease the risk of morbidity related to cold injury.

- Dress warmly.
- Get plenty of rest to maximize the ability of heat-generating mechanisms to replenish energy supplies.
- Eat appropriately and at regular intervals to support metabolism.
- Limit exposure to cold environments.

DEGREES OF HYPOTHERMIA

Hypothermia can be classified as mild or severe, as follows:

- *Mild*—a core temperature greater than 32°C with signs and symptoms of hypothermia
- *Severe*—a core temperature less than 32°C with signs and symptoms of hypothermia

Initially, some patients may exhibit *compensated* hypothermia. In this case, signs and symptoms of hypothermia will be present but with a normal core body temperature, temporarily maintained by thermogenesis. As energy stores from the liver and muscle glycogen are exhausted, the core body temperature will drop.

The onset of symptoms may be *acute,* as occurs when a person suddenly falls through ice into a frigid lake. *Subacute* exposure can occur in such situations as when mountain climbers are trapped in a snowy, cold environment. Finally, *chronic* exposure to cold is a growing problem in inner cities where homeless people endure frequent and prolonged cold stress without shelter.

In some cases, cold exposure is the primary cause of hypothermia, but in others, hypothermia may develop secondary to other problems, such as medical problems. For example, hypothyroidism depresses the body's heat-producing mechanisms. Brain tumours or head trauma can depress the hypothalamic temperature control centre, causing hypothermia. Other conditions, such as myocardial infarction, diabetes, hypoglycemia, drugs, poor nutrition, sepsis, or old age, can also contribute to metabolic and circulatory disorders that predispose to hypothermia. Any patient thought to have hypothermia but who has no history of exposure to a cold environment should be assessed for any predisposing factors. Evaluate the patient for level of consciousness, cool skin, and shivering. Also, evaluate the rectal temperature. A rectal temperature of less than 35°C indicates hypothermia. Key findings at different degrees of hypothermia are summarized in Table 36-1.

Patients who experience body temperatures above 30°C will usually have a favourable prognosis. Those with temperatures below 30°C show a significant increase in mortality rate. Remember that most thermometers used in medicine do not register below 95°F (35°C). EMS systems in colder areas should carry special thermometers for recording subnormal temperature readings as there is no reliable correlation between signs and symptoms and actual core body temperature.

> *Services operating in colder environments should carry special hypothermia thermometers for cold exposure victims.*
>

Signs and Symptoms

Signs and symptoms of hypothermia are summarized in Table 36-2. Patients experiencing mild hypothermia (core temperature > 32°C will generally exhibit shivering. The patient may be lethargic and somewhat dulled mentally. (In some cases, however, they may be fully oriented.) Muscles may be stiff and uncoordinated, causing the patient to walk with a stumbling, staggering gait.

Patients experiencing severe hypothermia (core temperature < 32°C) may be disoriented and confused. As their temperatures continue to fall, they will proceed into stupor and complete coma. Shivering will usually stop, and physical activity will become uncoordinated. Muscles may be stiff and rigid. Continuous cardiac monitoring is indicated for anyone experiencing hypothermia. The ECG will frequently show pathognomonic (indicative of a disease) **J waves,** also called Osborn waves, associated with the QRS complexes (Figure 36-3), but these are not useful diagnostically. Atrial fibrillation is the most common presenting dysrhythmia seen in hypothermia. As the body cools, however, the myocardium becomes progressively more irritable and may develop a variety of dysrhythmias. In severe hypothermia, bradycardia is inevitable.

Ventricular fibrillation becomes more probable as the body's core temperature falls below 30°C. The severely hypothermic patient requires assessment of pulse and respirations for at least 30 seconds every 1 to 2 minutes.

> ✱ **J wave** ECG deflection found at the junction of the QRS complex and the ST segment. It is associated with hypothermia and seen at core temperatures below 32°C, most commonly in leads II and V₆; also called an *Osborn wave.*

Treatment for Hypothermia

All victims of hypothermia should have the following care (see also Figure 36-4):

1. *Remove the patient's wet garments.*
2. *Provide protection against further heat loss and wind chill.* Use *passive external warming* methods, such as application of blankets, insulating materials, and moisture barriers.
3. *Maintain the patient in a horizontal position.*
4. *Avoid rough handling,* which can trigger dysrhythmias.
5. *Monitor the core temperature.*
6. *Monitor the cardiac rhythm.*

Table 36-1		KEY FINDINGS AT DIFFERENT DEGREES OF HYPOTHERMIA
°C	°F	Clinical Findings
37.6	99.6	Normal rectal temperature
37	98.6	Normal oral temperature
36	96.8	Metabolic rate increased
35	95	Maximum shivering seen
		Impaired judgment
34	93.2	Amnesia
		Slurred speech
33	91.4	Severe clouding of consciousness/apathy
		Uncoordinated movement
32	89.6	Most shivering ceases
		Pupils dilate
31	87.8	Blood pressure may no longer be obtainable
30	86	Atrial fibrillation/other dysrhythmias develop
		Pulse and cardiac output decrease by 33%
29	84.2	Progressive decrease in pulse and breathing
		Progressive decrease in level of consciousness
28	82.4	Pulse and oxygen consumption decrease by 50%
		Severe slowing of respiration
		Increased muscle rigidity
		Loss of consciousness
		High risk of ventricular fibrillation
27	80.6	Loss of reflexes and voluntary movement
		Patients appear clinically dead
26	78.8	No reflexes or response to painful stimuli
25	77	Cerebral blood flow decreased by 66%
24	75.2	Marked hypotension
22	71.6	Maximum risk for ventricular fibrillation
19	66.2	Flat electroencephalogram (EEG)
18	64.4	Asystole
16	60.8	Lowest reported adult survival from accidental exposure
15.2	59.2	Lowest reported infant survival from accidental exposure
10	50	Oxygen consumption 8% of normal
9	48.2	Lowest reported survivor from therapeutic exposure

Table 36-2	HYPOTHERMIA: SIGNS AND SYMPTOMS
Mild	Severe
Lethargy	No shivering
Shivering	Dysrhythmias, asystole
Lack of coordination	Loss of voluntary muscle control
Pale, cold, dry skin	Hypotension
Early rise in blood pressure, heart, and respiratory rates	Undetectable pulse and respirations

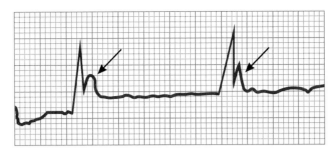

FIGURE 36-3 ECG tracing showing J wave following the QRS complex as seen in hypothermia.

Active Rewarming Victims of mild hypothermia may also be rewarmed using *active external methods.* This includes the use of warmed blankets and/or heat packs placed over areas of high heat transfer with the core: the base of the neck, the axilla, and the groin. Be sure to insulate between the heat packs and the skin to prevent burning. Intravenous fluid heaters (i.e., Hot I.V.) can be used to warm the IV fluid to 35° to 38°C. Warmed IV fluids are helpful in treating mild to moderate hypothermia. Heat guns and lights may also be used, but this will most likely take place in the emergency department. Warm water immersion in water between 39° to 40°C may be used but can induce rewarming shock (see below), and so this method also has little application in an out-of-hospital setting.

Active rewarming of the severely hypothermic patient is best carried out in the hospital using a prearranged protocol. Most patients who die during rewarming die from ventricular fibrillation, the risk of which is related to both the depth and the duration of hypothermia. Rough handling of the hypothermic patient may also induce ventricular fibrillation. Active rewarming should not be attempted in the field unless travel to the emergency department will take more than 15 minutes.

If such is the case, active internal means may also be used, including the use of warmed (38° to 40°C) humidified oxygen, and administration of warmed IV fluids (also warmed to 38° to 40°C). This is crucial to prevent further heat loss, but actual heat transferred is minimal, and so there is limited contribution to the rewarming effort.

Rewarming Shock While application of warmed blankets is a safe and effective means of rewarming the hypothermic patient, application of external heat, as with heat packs, is usually not recommended in the prehospital setting. For effective rewarming, more heat transference is generally required than is possible with out-of-hospital methods. Additionally, application of external heat may result in *rewarming shock* by causing reflex peripheral vasodilation. This reflex vasodilation causes the return of cool blood and acids from the extremities to the core. This may cause a paradoxical "afterdrop" core temperature decrease and further worsen core hypothermia. This, in turn, may cause the blood pressure to fall, especially when there is also volume depletion.

If active rewarming is necessary in the prehospital setting, for example, when transport is delayed, administration of warmed IV fluids during rewarming can prevent the onset of rewarming shock.

Cold Diuresis Volume depletion can occur as a result of *cold diuresis.* Core vasoconstriction causes increased blood volume and blood pressure, and so the kidneys remove excess fluid to reduce the pressure, thus causing diuresis. A warmed IV volume expander (e.g., normal saline) should be used both to prevent rewarming shock and to replace fluid lost from cold diuresis.

The conscious patient who is able to manage his airway may be given warmed, sweetened fluids. Alcohol and caffeine should be avoided.

Rewarming is not the mirror image of the cooling process.

Active rewarming of the severely hypothermic patient should be deferred until the patient is at the hospital unless transport time is long and rewarming is ordered by medical direction.

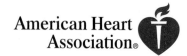

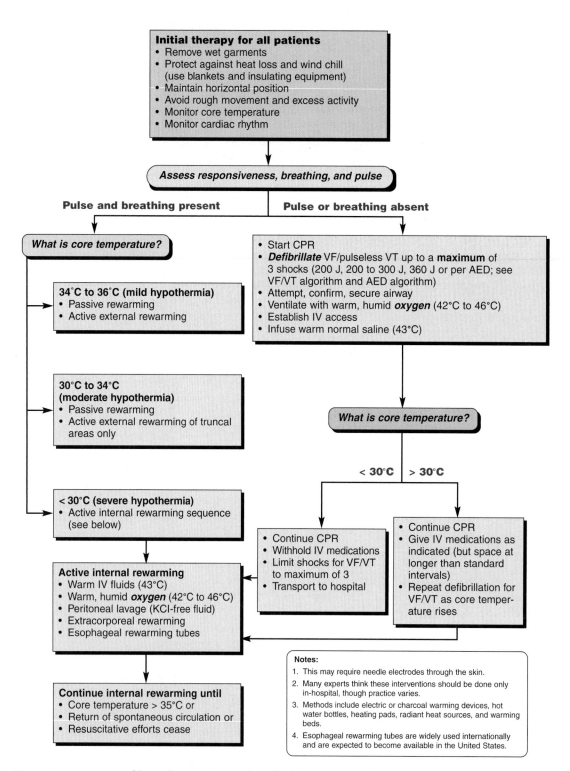

FIGURE 36-4   Management of hypothermia. Reproduced with permission from *Guidelines 2000 for Cardiopulmonary Resuscitation and Emergency Cardiovascular Care,* ©2000, Copyright American Heart Association.

Resuscitation

There are certain resuscitation considerations when handling cardiac arrest victims with core temperatures below 30°C.

Primary Care Paramedic Basic life support (BLS) providers should start cardiopulmonary resuscitation (CPR) immediately, although pulse and respirations may need to be checked for longer periods to detect minimal cardiopulmonary efforts. Use normal chest compression and ventilation rates, and ventilate with warmed, humidified oxygen. If an automated external defibrillator (AED) is available and ventricular fibrillation is detected, three shocks may be given. Further shocks should be avoided until after rewarming to above 30°C. CPR, rewarming, and rapid transport should immediately follow the three defibrillation attempts.

Advanced Care Paramedics/Critical Care Paramedics Since there is no increased risk of inducing ventricular fibrillation from orotracheal or nasotracheal intubation, advanced life support (ALS) providers may intubate the patient and ventilate with warmed, humidified oxygen. Drug metabolism is reduced, however, so administered medications, such as epinephrine, lidocaine, and atropine, may accumulate to toxic levels if used repeatedly in the severely hypothermic victim. In addition, administered drugs may remain in the peripheral circulation. When the patient is rewarmed and perfusion resumes, large, toxic boluses of these medications may be delivered to the central circulation and target tissues. Lidocaine may also paradoxically lower the fibrillatory threshold in a hypothermic heart and increase resistance to defibrillation.

The American Heart Association recommends that if the patient fails to respond to initial defibrillation attempts or initial drug therapy, subsequent defibrillations or boluses of medication should be avoided until the core temperature is about 30°C. This is because it is generally impossible to electrically defibrillate a heart that is colder than 30°C. Active core rewarming techniques are the primary modality in hypothermia victims who are either in cardiac arrest or unconscious with a slow heart rate.

Techniques that may be used include the administration of heated, humidified oxygen and warmed intravenous fluids, preferably normal saline, infused centrally at rates of 150 to 200 mL an hour to avoid overhydration. Peritoneal lavage with warmed potassium-free fluid administered two litres at a time may be used, as may extracorporeal blood warming with partial cardiac bypass. Obviously, some of these techniques may only be carried out in a hospital setting.

If the hypothermic cardiac arrest patient fails to respond to initial defibrillation attempts or drug therapy, avoid subsequent defibrillations or medication until the core temperature is about 30°C. It is generally impossible to defibrillate a heart that is colder than 30°C.

Transport

When transporting a hypothermic patient, remember that gentle transportation is necessary due to myocardial irritability and that the patient should be kept level or slightly inclined with head down. Contact the receiving hospital for general rewarming options. When determining your destination, consider the availability of cardiac bypass rewarming.

FROSTBITE

Frostbite is environmentally induced freezing of body tissues (Figure 36-5). As the tissues freeze, ice crystals form within and water is drawn out of the cells into the extracellular space. These ice crystals expand, causing the destruction of cells. During this process, intracellular electrolyte concentrations increase, further destroying cells. Damage to blood vessels from ice crystal formation causes loss of vascular integrity, resulting in tissue swelling and loss of distal nutritional flow.

✱ **frostbite** environmentally induced freezing of body tissues causing destruction of cells.

FIGURE 36-5 Frostbite.

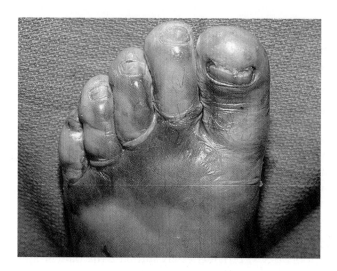

Superficial and Deep Frostbite

★ **superficial frostbite** freezing involving only epidermal tissues resulting in redness followed by blanching and diminished sensation; also called *frostnip*.

★ **deep frostbite** freezing involving epidermal and subcutaneous tissues resulting in a white appearance, hard (frozen) feeling on palpation, and loss of sensation.

Generally, there are two types of frostbite: superficial and deep. **Superficial frostbite** (frostnip) exhibits some freezing of epidermal tissue, resulting in initial redness, followed by blanching. There will also be diminished sensation. **Deep frostbite** affects the epidermal and subcutaneous layers. There is a white appearance and the area feels hard (frozen) to palpation. There is also loss of sensation in deep frostbite.

Frostbite mainly occurs in the extremities and in areas of the head and face exposed to the environment. Subfreezing temperatures are required for frostbite to occur, although they are not necessary to produce hypothermia. Many patients who have frostbite will also have hypothermia.

There can be tremendous variation in how an individual can present with frostbite. For example, some patients feel little pain at onset. Others will report severe pain. A certain degree of compliance may be felt beneath the frozen layer in superficial frostbite, but in deep frostbite, the frozen part will be hard and noncompliant.

Treatment for Frostbite

Do not thaw frozen flesh if there is any possibility of refreezing. Do not massage the frozen area or rub it with snow.

In treating frostbite, take the following recommended steps:

- Do not thaw the affected area if there is any possibility of refreezing.
- Do not massage the frozen area or rub with snow. Rubbing the affected area may cause ice crystals within the tissues to damage the already injured tissues more seriously.
- Transport to the hospital for rewarming by immersion. If transport will be delayed, thaw the frozen part by immersion in a 39°–40°C water bath. Water temperature will fall rapidly, requiring additions of warm water throughout the process.
- Cover the thawed part with loosely applied dry, sterile dressings.
- Elevate and immobilize the thawed part.
- Do not puncture or drain blisters.
- Do not rewarm frozen feet if they are required for walking out of a hazardous situation.

NEAR-DROWNING AND DROWNING

Drowning is asphyxiation resulting from submersion in liquid. There has been an attempt made to differentiate between the terms drowning and near-drowning. The term *drowning* means that death occurred within 24 hours of submersion, while the term **near-drowning** indicates that death either did not occur or occurred more than 24 hours after submersion.

It is estimated that in Canada, approximately 6000 persons die annually due to drowning. Many more sustain serious injury due to near-drowning. Drowning is the second-leading cause of unintentional death among Canadian children between the ages of one and four (motor-vehicle collisions are the leading cause). Approximately 40 percent of these deaths are of children under five years of age. There is a second peak incidence in teenagers and a final third peak in the elderly as a result of accidental bathtub drownings. Approximately 85 percent of near-drowning victims are male, and two-thirds of these do not know how to swim. Most commonly, these situations are due to fresh-water submersion, especially in swimming pools. Unfortunately, alcohol use by the victim or the supervising adult is frequently associated with this type of accident.

It is important to note that other emergency conditions are often associated with near-drowning. If the cause of the submersion is unknown, you must consider the possibility of trauma and treat the patient accordingly.

Frequently, the submersion occurs in cold water, causing hypothermia. Hypothermia slows the body's metabolic processes thereby decreasing the need for oxygen. This can have a protective effect on organs and tissues, which become hypoxic (low in oxygen) in submersion situations. However, it is important to treat the hypoxia first, once you have initiated rescue.

PATHOPHYSIOLOGY OF DROWNING AND NEAR-DROWNING

As a paramedic, you need to understand the sequence of events in drowning or near-drowning. Following submersion, if the victim is conscious, he will undergo a period of complete apnea for up to three minutes. This apnea is an involuntary reflex as the victim strives to keep his head above water. During this time, blood is shunted to the heart and brain because of the mammalian diving reflex, which is described later in this chapter.

When the victim is apneic, the $PaCO_2$ (partial pressure of CO_2) in the blood rises to greater than 50 mmHg. Meanwhile, the PaO_2 of the blood falls below 50 mmHg. The stimulus from the hypoxia ultimately overrides the sedative effects of the hypercarbia, resulting in central nervous system stimulation.

Dry versus Wet Drowning

Until unconscious, the victim experiences a great deal of panic. During this stage the victim makes violent inspiratory and swallowing efforts. At this point, copious amounts of water enter the mouth, posterior oropharynx, and stomach, stimulating severe laryngospasm (airway obstruction due to aspirated water) and bronchospasm. In approximately 10 percent of drowning victims, and in a much greater percentage of near-drowning victims, this laryngospasm prevents the influx of water into the lungs. If a significant amount of water does not enter the lungs, it is referred to as a *dry drowning*. Conversely, if a laryngospasm does not occur, and a significant quantity of water does enter the lungs, it is referred to as a *wet drowning*.

* **drowning** asphyxiation resulting from submersion in liquid with death occurring within 24 hours of submersion.

* **near-drowning** an incident of potentially fatal submersion in liquid that did not result in death or in which death occurred more than 24 hours after submersion.

The laryngospasm further aggravates the hypoxia, with coma ultimately ensuing. Persistent anoxia (absence of oxygen) results in a deeper coma. Following unconsciousness, reflex swallowing continues, resulting in gastric distention and increased risk of vomiting and aspiration. If untreated, hypotension, bradycardia, and death result in a short period.

Drowning and near-drowning are primarily due to asphyxia from airway obstruction in the lung secondary to the aspirated water or the laryngospasm. If, in a near-drowning episode, this process does not end in death, any fluid that has entered the lungs may cause lower-airway disease.

Fresh-Water versus Saltwater Drowning

Although the physiology of fresh-water and saltwater drownings differ, there is no difference in the end result or in prehospital management.

You should expect different physiological reactions in cases of fresh-water and saltwater drownings or near-drownings. However, these mechanistic differences do not make any difference in the end metabolic result or in the prehospital management.

Fresh-Water Drowning In fresh-water drowning or near-drowning, the large surface area of the alveoli and small airways allow a massive amount of hypotonic water to diffuse across the alveolar/capillary membrane and into the vascular space. This results in hemodilution, an expansion in blood plasma volume and relative reduction in red blood cell concentration. *Hemodilution* produces a thickening of the alveolar walls with inflammatory cells, hemorrhagic pneumonitis (bleeding lung inflammation), and destruction of surfactant.

✱ surfactant a compound secreted by cells in the lungs that regulates the surface tension of the fluid that lines the alveoli, important in keeping the alveoli open for gas exchange.

Surfactant is a substance in the alveoli responsible for keeping the alveoli open. In drowning, some surfactant is lost when the capillaries of the alveoli are damaged. Plasma proteins then leak back into the alveoli, resulting in the accumulation of fluid in the small airways. This, in turn, leads to multiple areas of atelectasis—areas of alveolar collapse. Atelectasis causes shunting, which is the return of unoxygenated blood from the damaged alveoli to the bloodstream. In other words, blood is travelling through the lungs without being oxygenated. The result is hypoxemia (inadequate oxygenation of the blood) (Figure 36-6).

Saltwater Drowning In saltwater drowning or near-drowning, the hypertonic nature of sea water, which is 3 to 4 times more hypertonic than plasma, draws water

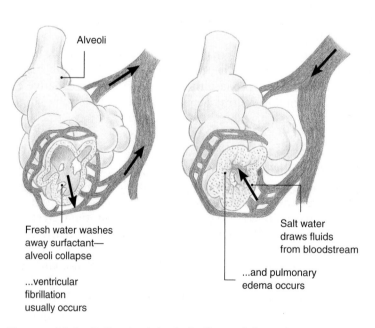

FIGURE 36-6   Pathophysiological effects of drowning.

from the bloodstream into the alveoli (see Figure 36-6). This produces pulmonary edema, leading to profound shunting. The result is failure of oxygenation, producing hypoxemia. Additionally, respiratory and metabolic acidosis develop due to the retention of CO_2 and developing anaerobic (without-oxygen) metabolism.

Factors Affecting Survival

A number of factors have an impact on drowning and near-drowning survival rates. These include the cleanliness of the water, the length of time submerged, and the age and general health of the victim. Children have a longer survival time and a greater probability of a successful resuscitation. Even more significant is the water temperature. The concept of developing brain death after four to six minutes without oxygen is not applicable in cases of near-drowning in cold water. Some patients in cold water (below 21°C) can be resuscitated after 30 minutes or more in cardiac arrest. However, persons under water 60 minutes or longer usually cannot be resuscitated.

A possible contribution to survival may be the **mammalian diving reflex.** When a person dives into cold water, he reacts to the submersion of the face. Breathing is inhibited, the heart rate becomes bradycardic, and vasoconstriction develops in tissues relatively resistant to asphyxia. Meanwhile, cerebral and cardiac blood flow is maintained. In this way, oxygen is sent and used only where it is immediately needed to sustain life. The colder the water, the more oxygen is diverted to the heart and brain. A common saying in emergency medicine states: "The cold-water drowning victim is not dead until he is warm and dead." In other words, a person who has been submerged in cold water may only seem to be dead, but due to the continued supply of oxygen to the heart and brain may, indeed, still be alive.

TREATMENT FOR NEAR-DROWNING

Since fresh-water and saltwater near-drownings both involve factors that disrupt normal pulmonary function, initial field treatment must be directed toward correcting the profound hypoxia. Take the following steps:

- Remove the patient from the water as soon as possible. This should be done by a trained rescue swimmer.
- Initiate ventilation while the patient is still in the water. Rescue personnel should wear protective clothing if water temperature is less than 22°C. In addition, attach a safety line to the rescue swimmer. In fast water, it is essential to use personnel specifically trained for this type of rescue.
- Suspect head and neck injury if the patient experienced a fall or was diving. Rapidly place the victim on a long backboard and remove him from the water. Use cervical spine precautions throughout care.
- Protect the patient from heat loss. Avoid laying the patient on a cold surface. Remove wet clothing and cover the body to the extent possible.
- Examine the patient for airway patency, breathing, and pulse. If indicated, begin CPR and defibrillation.
- Manage the airway using proper suctioning and airway adjuncts.
- Administer oxygen at a 100-percent concentration.
- Establish an IV of Ringer's Lactate or normal saline for venous access and run at 75 mL/h. If indicated, carry out defibrillation.
- Follow advanced cardiac life support (ACLS) protocols if the patient is normothermic. If the patient is hypothermic, treat him according to the hypothermia protocol presented earlier in the chapter.

✳ **mammalian diving reflex** a complex cardiovascular reflex, resulting from submersion of the face and nose in water, that constricts blood flow everywhere except to the brain.

The cold-water drowning victim is not dead until he is warm and dead.

Never attempt to rescue a drowning victim unless you have been trained and have the necessary safety equipment.

Resuscitation is not indicated if immersion has been extremely prolonged (unless hypothermia is present) or if there is evidence of putrefaction (decomposition).

Adult Respiratory Distress Syndrome

More than 90 percent of near-drowning patients survive without *sequelae* (after effects). However, all near-drowning patients should be admitted to the hospital for observation, since complications may not appear for 24 hours.

Adult respiratory distress syndrome (ARDS) is one of the more severe post-resuscitation complications, with a high rate of mortality. The physiological stress of near-drowning causes the lungs to leak fluid into the alveoli. This fluid is loaded with various chemical factors that cause severe inflammation of the tissues and failure of the respiratory system. In addition, some of these patients have problems with pulmonary parenchymal injury, destruction of surfactant, aspiration pneumonitis, or pneumothorax. A number require an extended hospital stay due to renal failure, hypoxia, hypercarbia, and mixed metabolic and respiratory acidosis. The effects of cerebral hypoxia occasionally require treatment throughout hospitalization and beyond.

DIVING EMERGENCIES

* **scuba** acronym for *self-contained underwater breathing apparatus*. Portable apparatus that contains compressed air, which allows the diver to breathe underwater.

Scuba diving has become an extremely popular recreational sport. Divers wear portable equipment containing compressed air, which allows the diver to breathe underwater. Although scuba diving accidents are fairly uncommon, inexperienced divers have a higher rate of injury. Scuba diving emergencies can occur on the surface, in one metre of water, or at any depth. The more serious emergencies usually occur following a dive. To better assess and care for diving injuries, you need to understand a few principles of pressure.

THE EFFECTS OF AIR PRESSURE ON GASES

Water is an incompressible liquid. Fresh water has a density, or weight per unit of volume, of 62.4 pounds per cubic foot. Saltwater has a density of 64.0 pounds per cubic foot. This density can be equated to pressure, which is defined as the weight or force acting on a unit area. Thus, a cubic foot of fresh water exerts a pressure ("weight") of 62.4 pounds over an area of one square foot. This measurement is typically stated in pounds per square inch (psi).

Humans at sea level live in an atmosphere of air, which is a mixture of gases. These gases weigh and exert a pressure of 14.7 pounds per square inch (760 mmHg). This pressure, however, may vary within the environment. For example, ascending to an altitude of one mile will decrease the atmospheric pressure by 17 percent to approximately 12.2 pounds.

To understand how air pressure affects diving accidents, you need to look at three physical laws: Boyle's Law, Dalton's Law, and Henry's Law.

Boyle's Law

Boyle's law states that the volume of a gas is inversely proportional to its pressure if the temperature is kept constant. As you increase pressure, the gas is compressed into a smaller space. For example, doubling the pressure of a gas mixture will decrease its volume by one-half. The pressure of air at sea level is 14.7 psi. or 760 mmHg. This pressure is called one "atmosphere absolute" or one "ata." Two ata occur at a depth of 11 metres of water, three ata occur at a depth of 22 metres of water, and so on. Therefore, one litre of air at the surface is compressed to 500 mL at 11 metres. At 22 metres, one litre of air would be compressed to 250 mL.

Dalton's Law

Dalton's Law states that the total pressure of a mixture of gases is equal to the sum of the partial pressures of the individual gases. The air we breathe is a mixture of nitrogen (about 78 percent), oxygen (about 21 percent), and carbon dioxide plus traces of argon, helium, and other rare gases (about 1 percent). Since the pressure of air at sea level is 760 mmHg, the pressure of nitrogen is about 593 mmHg, the pressure of oxygen is about 160 mmHg, and the pressure of carbon dioxide is somewhat less than 4 mmHg—each gas exerting its proportion of the total pressure of the mixture.

At different altitudes above sea level or depths below sea level, the pressure of air will change (less at higher altitudes, more at greater depths), but the component gases will still account for the same proportion of whatever the total pressure is at that level: nitrogen 78 percent, oxygen 21 percent, and carbon dioxide less than 1 percent.

Henry's Law

Henry's Law states that the amount of gas dissolved in a given volume of fluid is proportional to the pressure of the gas above it. When we descend below sea level, and the pressure bearing down on us increases, the gases that make up the air we breathe tend to dissolve in the liquids (mainly blood plasma) and tissues of the body.

Let us compare what happens to the two chief components of the air we breathe—oxygen and nitrogen—when a person descends to greater and greater depths below sea level. Much of the oxygen is used up in the normal metabolism of the cells, leaving only a small amount to be dissolved in the blood and tissues. Nitrogen, however, is an inert gas and, as such, is not used by the body. Therefore, a far greater quantity of nitrogen is available to dissolve in the blood and tissues as a person descends below sea level. In brief, at depths below sea level, oxygen metabolizes but nitrogen dissolves.

When the person ascends toward sea level again, the gases that are dissolved in the blood and tissues, being under less and less pressure, come out of the blood and tissues and, if the ascent is too rapid, form bubbles. To understand this phenomenon, compare the human body to a bottled carbonated soft drink—that is, a liquid in which carbon dioxide gas is dissolved. The gas is kept dissolved in the liquid by the cap on the bottle and a high-pressure gas under the cap, on top of the liquid. When the cap is removed and the pressure is released, the gas bubbles out of the liquid, causing a fizz that will sometimes rise completely out of the bottle.

In the following sections, we will discuss how the phenomena of gases and pressure can cause serious problems for divers.

PATHOPHYSIOLOGY OF DIVING EMERGENCIES

As noted above, gases are dissolved in the diver's blood and tissues under pressure. As the diver goes deeper into the water, pressure increases, causing more gas to dissolve in the blood (Henry's Law). According to Boyle's Law, these gases will have a smaller volume due to the increased ambient pressure. During *controlled* ascent, with decreasing pressure, dissolved gases come out of the blood and tissues slowly, escaping gradually through respiration.

If ascent is *too rapid*, however, the dissolved gases, mostly nitrogen, come out of solution and expand quickly, forming bubbles in the blood, brain, spinal cord, skin, inner ear, muscles, and joints. Once bubbles of nitrogen have formed in various tissues, it is difficult for the body to remove them. The ascending diver who comes to the surface too rapidly, not adhering to safety measures, is at risk of becoming a veritable living bottle of soda.

CLASSIFICATION OF DIVING INJURIES

Scuba diving injuries are due to barotrauma, pulmonary overpressure, arterial gas embolism, decompression illness, cold, panic, or a combination of these. Accidents generally occur at one of the following four stages of a dive:

- On the surface
- During descent
- On the bottom
- During ascent

Injuries on the Surface

Surface injuries can involve any of several factors. One such factor can be entanglement of lines or entanglement in kelp fields while swimming to the area of the dive. Divers in these situations may panic, become fatigued, and even drown. Another factor may be cold water that produces shivering and blackout. Boats in the area are another potential source of injury to the diver. To prevent such accidents, divers will usually mark the area of their dive with a flag. Maritime rules require boat operators to stay clear of a flagged area.

Injuries during Descent

✱ **barotrauma** injuries caused by changes in pressure. Barotrauma that occurs from increasing pressure during a diving descent is commonly called "the squeeze."

Barotrauma means injuries caused by changes in pressure. Barotrauma during descent is commonly called "the squeeze." It can occur if the diver cannot equalize the pressure between the nasopharynx and the middle ear through the eustachian tube. The diver can experience middle ear pain, ringing in the ears, dizziness, and hearing loss. In severe cases, rupture of the eardrum can occur. A diver who has an upper respiratory infection and who therefore cannot clear the middle ear through the eustachian tube should not dive. A similar lack of equilibrium can occur in the sinuses, producing severe frontal headaches or pain beneath the eye in the maxillary sinuses.

Injuries on the Bottom

✱ **nitrogen narcosis** a state of stupor that develops during deep dives due to nitrogen's effect on cerebral function; also called "raptures of the deep."

Major diving emergencies while at the bottom of the dive often involve **nitrogen narcosis** (a state of stupor), commonly called "raptures of the deep." This is due to nitrogen's effect on cerebral function. The diver may appear to be intoxicated and may take unnecessary risks. Other emergencies occur when a diver runs low on or out of air. The diver who panics will exacerbate this situation by consuming even more oxygen and producing even more carbon dioxide.

✱ **decompression illness** development of nitrogen bubbles within the tissues due to a rapid reduction of air pressure when a diver returns to the surface; also called "the bends."

Injuries during Ascent

Serious and life-threatening emergencies, many involving barotrauma, can occur during the ascent. For example, as during descent, an ascending diver may be unable to equalize inner ear and nasopharyngeal pressure.

✱ **pulmonary overpressure** expansion of air held in the lungs during ascent. If not exhaled, the expanded air may cause injury to the lungs and surrounding structures.

Dives below 12 metres require staged ascent to prevent **decompression illness,** also called "the bends." This condition develops in divers subjected to rapid reduction of air pressure while ascending to the surface following exposure to compressed air, with formation of nitrogen bubbles causing severe pain, especially in the abdomen and the joints.

The most serious barotrauma that occurs during ascent is injury to the lung from **pulmonary overpressure.** This can occur with a deep dive, or it can occur with a dive of as little as one metre below the surface. The injury results from the diver holding his breath during the ascent. As the diver ascends, the air in the lung, which has been compressed, expands. If it is not exhaled, the alveoli may rupture. If this occurs, the result will be structural damage to the lung and, possibly, **arterial gas embolism (AGE),** an air bubble, or air embolism, that enters the circulatory system from the damaged lung. Another result may be **pneumomediastinum,** the release of gas (air) through the visceral pleura into the mediastinum and pericardial sac around the heart as well as into the tissues of the neck. **Pneumothorax** is possible if the alveoli rupture into the pleural cavity. Air embolism can occur if the air ruptures into the pulmonary veins or arteries and returns to the left atrium and finally into the left ventricle and out into the systemic circulation.

GENERAL ASSESSMENT OF DIVING EMERGENCIES

In the early assessment of diving accidents, all symptoms of air embolism and decompression illness are considered together. Early assessment and treatment of a diving injury is of more importance than trying to distinguish the exact problem. One of your most important tasks in a diving-related injury is elicitation of a diving history or profile. There are several essential factors to consider. These include

- Time at which the signs and symptoms occurred
- Type of breathing apparatus utilized
- Type of hypothermia protective garment worn
- Parameters of the dive:
  - Depth of dive(s)
  - Number of dives(s)
  - Duration of dive(s)
- Aircraft travel following a dive (in a pressurized cabin?)
- Rate of ascent
- Associated panic forcing rapid ascent
- Experience of the diver, for example, student, inexperienced, or "pro"
- Properly functioning depth gauge
- Previous medical diseases
- Old injuries
- Previous episodes of decompression illness
- Use of medications
- Use of alcohol

From a quick assessment of the patient's diving profile, you can rapidly determine if the diver is a likely candidate for a pressure disorder.

PRESSURE DISORDERS

Injuries caused by pressure, as noted earlier, are known as *barotrauma*. In the case of diving accidents, most barotrauma results from a pressure imbalance between the external environment and gases within the body. The following sections describe some of the most common forms of barotrauma involved in diving accidents.

Decompression Illness

Decompression illness develops in divers subjected to rapid reduction of air pressure after ascending to the surface following exposure to compressed air. A

✳ arterial gas embolism (AGE) an air bubble, or air embolism, that enters the circulatory system from a damaged lung.

✳ pneumomediastinum the presence of air in the mediastinum.

✳ pneumothorax a collection of air in the pleural space. Air may enter the pleural space through an injury to the chest wall or through an injury to the lungs. In a *tension pneumothorax,* pressure builds because there is no way for the air to escape, causing lung collapse.

In a diving emergency, consider all symptoms of air embolism and decompression illness together. Early assessment and treatment are more important than identifying the exact problem.

number of general and individual factors can contribute to the development of decompression illness, or the bends (Table 36-3). Decompression illness results as nitrogen bubbles come out of solution in the blood and tissues, causing increased pressure in various body structures and occluding circulation in the small blood vessels. This occurs in joints, tendons, the spinal cord, skin, brain, and inner ear. Symptoms develop when a diver rapidly ascends after being exposed to a depth of 10 metres or more for a time sufficient to allow the body's tissues to be saturated with nitrogen.

Signs and Symptoms The principal signs and symptoms of decompression illnesses are joint and abdominal pain, fatigue, paresthesias, and central nervous system disturbances. The nitrogen bubbles produced by rapid decompression are thought to produce obstruction of blood flow and lead to local ischemia, subjecting tissues to anoxic stress. In some cases, this stress may lead to tissue damage.

Treatment Patients with decompression illness usually seek medical treatment within 12 hours of ascent from a dive. Some patients may not seek treatment for as long as 24 hours after the last dive. It is generally safe to assume that signs or symptoms developing more than 36 hours after a dive cannot reasonably be attributed to decompression illness.

Decompression illness may require urgent definitive care through **recompression.** This can be accomplished by placing the patient in a **hyperbaric oxygen chamber** (Figure 36-7). There the patient is subjected to oxygen under greater-than-atmospheric pressure to force the nitrogen in the body to redissolve, then gradually decompressed to allow the nitrogen to escape without forming bubbles. However, prompt stabilization at the nearest emergency department should be accomplished before transport to a recompression chamber.

Early oxygen therapy may reduce symptoms of decompression illness substantially. Divers who are administered high concentrations of oxygen have a considerably better treatment outcome. The following list outlines some of the steps in the prehospital management of decompression illnesses.

- Assess the ABCs.
- Administer CPR, if required.
- Administer oxygen at 100-percent concentration via a nonrebreather mask. An unconscious diver should be intubated.

✱ **recompression** resubmission of a person to a greater pressure so that gradual decompression can be achieved; often used in the treatment of diving emergencies.

✱ **hyperbaric oxygen chamber** recompression chamber used to treat patients suffering from barotrauma.

Recompression in a hyperbaric oxygen chamber may be required for the patient suspected of suffering decompression illness or an air embolism.

Table 36-3 FACTORS RELATED TO THE DEVELOPMENT OF DECOMPRESSION ILLNESS

General Factors	Individual Factors
Cold water dives	Age—older individuals
Diving in rough water	Obesity
Strenuous diving conditions	Fatigue—lack of sleep prior to dive
History of previous decompression dive incident	Alcohol—consumption before or after dive
Overstaying time at given dive depth	History of medical problems
Dive at 24 metres or greater	
Rapid ascent—panic, inexperience, unfamiliarity with equipment	
Heavy exercise before or after dive to the point of muscle soreness	
Flying after diving (24 hour wait is recommended)	
Driving to high altitude after dive	

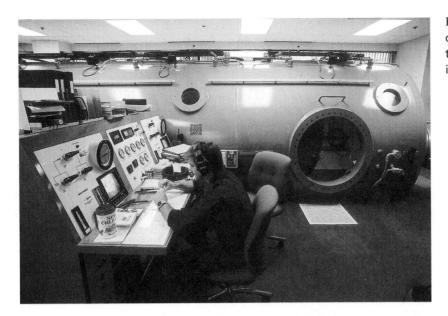

FIGURE 36-7 Hyperbaric oxygen chamber used in the treatment of decompression illness.

- Keep the patient in the supine position.
- Protect the patient from excessive heat, cold, wetness, or noxious fumes.
- Give the conscious, alert patient nonalcoholic liquids, such as fruit juices or oral balanced salt solutions.
- Evaluate and stabilize the patient at the nearest emergency department prior to transport to a recompression chamber. Begin IV fluid replacement with electrolyte solutions for unconscious or seriously injured patients. You may use Ringer's Lactate or normal saline. Do not use 5-percent dextrose in water.
- If air evacuation is used, do not expose the patient to decreased barometric pressure. Cabin pressure must be maintained at sea level, or fly at the lowest possible safe altitude.
- Send the patient's diving equipment with the patient for examination. If that is impossible, arrange for local examination and gas analysis.

Pulmonary Overpressure Accidents

Lung overinflation due to rapid ascent is the common cause of a number of emergencies, particularly at shallow depths of less than 180 m. Air can become trapped in the lungs due to mucous plugs, bronchospasm, or simple breath holding. With rapid ascent, ambient pressure drops quickly, causing the trapped air to expand. Air expansion can rupture the alveolar membranes. This can result in hemorrhage, reduced oxygen and carbon dioxide transport, and capillary and alveolar inflammation. Air can also escape from the lung into other nearby tissues and cause pneumothorax and tension pneumothorax, subcutaneous emphysema, or pneumomediastinum.

Signs and Symptoms Divers with this type of condition will complain of substernal chest pain. Respiratory distress and diminished breath sounds are common findings on examination.

Treatment Treatment for this condition is the same as for pneumothorax caused by any other mechanism (see Chapter 27). Rest and supplemental oxygen are important but hyperbaric oxygen is not usually necessary.

Arterial Gas Embolism (AGE)

As described above, a pressure buildup in the lung can damage and rupture alveoli. This can allow air in the form of a large bubble to escape into the circulation. This air embolism, or arterial gas embolism, can travel to the left atrium and ventricle of the heart and out into various parts of the body where it may lodge and obstruct blood flow, causing ischemia and possibly infarct. Such obstruction of blood flow can have devastating effects triggered by cardiac, pulmonary, and cerebral compromise.

Signs and Symptoms Signs and symptoms of air embolism include onset within 2 to 10 minutes of ascent, a rapid and dramatic onset of sharp, tearing pain, and other symptoms related to the organ system affected by blocked blood flow. The most common presentation mimics a stroke, with confusion, vertigo, visual disturbances, and loss of consciousness. Although rare, you may also encounter paralysis on one side of the body (hemiplegia), as well as cardiac and pulmonary collapse. If any person using scuba equipment presents with neurological deficits during or immediately after ascent, an air embolism should be suspected. As death or serious disability can result, prompt medical treatment is crucial.

Treatment Management of air embolism includes the following steps:

- Assess the ABCs.
- Administer oxygen via a nonrebreather mask at 100 percent.
- Place the patient in a supine position.
- Monitor vital signs frequently.
- Administer IV fluids at a to-keep-open rate.
- Transport to a recompression chamber as rapidly as possible. If air transport is utilized, it is very important to use a pressurized aircraft or to fly at a low altitude.

Pneumomediastinum

As noted earlier, a pneumomediastinum is the release of gas (air) through the visceral pleura into the mediastinum and pericardial sac around the heart. It can result from a pulmonary overpressure accident during rapid ascent from a dive.

Signs and Symptoms Signs and symptoms of a pneumomediastinum include substernal chest pain, irregular pulse, abnormal heart sounds, reduced blood pressure and narrow pulse pressure, and a change in voice. There may or may not be evidence of cyanosis.

Treatment The field management of pneumomediastinum includes

- Administer high-concentration oxygen via a nonrebreather mask.
- Start IV Ringer's Lactate solution or normal saline on medical direction.
- Transport to the emergency department.

Treatment generally ranges from observation to recompression for relief of acute symptoms. The patient should be observed for 24 hours for any other signs of lung overpressure. He should not be recompressed unless air embolism or decompression illness is also present.

Nitrogen Narcosis

Nitrogen narcosis develops during deep dives and contributes to major diving emergencies while the diver is at the bottom. With an elevated partial pressure, more nitrogen dissolves in the bloodstream. With higher concentrations of nitrogen in the body, including the brain, the result is intoxication and altered levels of consciousness very similar to the effects of alcohol or narcotic use. Between 21 and 30 metres, these effects become apparent in most divers, but at 61 metres, most divers become so impaired that they cannot do any useful work. At 91 to 106 metres, unconsciousness occurs. The main concern with nitrogen narcosis is the same as with any person who is intoxicated while in a situation requiring alertness and common sense. Impaired judgment during a deep dive can cause accidents and unnecessary risk taking.

Signs and Symptoms These include altered levels of consciousness and impaired judgment.

Treatment Treatment simply requires return to a shallow depth since this condition is self-resolving on ascent. To avoid this problem altogether in deep dives, oxygen mixed with helium is used, since helium does not have the anesthetic effect of nitrogen.

OTHER DIVING-RELATED ILLNESSES

There are less frequent problems that can occur as a result of scuba diving. For example, oxygen toxicity caused by prolonged exposure to high partial pressures of oxygen can cause lung damage or even convulsions. Hyperventilation due to excitement or panic may lead to a decreased level of consciousness or muscle cramps and spasm. This will impair the diver's ability to function properly, possibly leading to injury. Inadequate breathing or faulty equipment may lead to increased CO_2 levels, or *hypercapnia*. This also may cause unconsciousness. Finally, poorly prepared air tanks may be contaminated with other gases, which can increase the risk of hypoxia, narcosis, and accidental injury.

DIVERS ALERT NETWORK (DAN)

Clearly, scuba diving has a unique set of potential problems. With the popularity of this activity rising so dramatically, it is important for EMS personnel in popular diving areas to become familiar with recognition and treatment of these problems. If assistance is needed, the Divers Alert Network (DAN) operates a nonprofit consultation and referral service in affiliation with Duke University Medical Center. In an emergency, contact (919) 684-8111. For nonemergency situations call (919) 684-2948.

HIGH-ALTITUDE ILLNESS

In contrast to illnesses related to diving and high atmospheric pressure, high-altitude illnesses are caused by a decrease in ambient pressure. Essentially, high altitude is a low-oxygen environment. As noted in the discussion of Dalton's law, earlier, oxygen concentration in the atmosphere remains constant at 21 percent. Therefore, as you go higher and barometric pressure decreases, the partial pressure of oxygen also decreases (is 21 percent of a lower total pressure). Oxygen becomes less available, triggering a number of related illnesses as well as aggravating preexisting conditions, such as angina, congestive heart failure, chronic obstructive pulmonary disease, and hypertension.

Even in healthy individuals, ascent to high altitude, especially if it is very rapid, can cause illness. It is difficult to predict who will be affected and to what degree. The only predictor is the hypoxic ventilatory response.

Every year, millions of visitors to mountains expose themselves to altitudes greater than 2400 m, the altitude at which high-altitude illnesses start to become

High-altitude illnesses start to become manifest at altitudes greater than 2400 metres.

manifest. For reference purposes, Banff, Alberta, is at 1200 m where there is 17 percent less oxygen than at sea level. Aspen, Colorado, at 2438 m has 26 percent less oxygen, and at the top of Mount Everest (8848 m) there is 66 percent less oxygen than at sea level. At *high altitude* (1700–3500 m) the hypoxic environment causes decreased exercise performance, although without major disruption of normal oxygen transport in the body. However, if ascent is very rapid, altitude illness will commonly occur at 2400 m and beyond. *Very high altitude* (3500–6000 m) will result in extreme hypoxia during exercise or sleep. It is important to ascend to these altitudes slowly, allowing for acclimatization to the environment. *Extreme altitude* beyond 6000 m will cause severe illness in almost everyone.

Some of the signs and symptoms of altitude illness are malaise, anorexia, headache, sleep disturbances, and respiratory distress that increases with exertion.

PREVENTION

Acclimatization, exertion, sleep, diet, and medication are key considerations in preventing or limiting high-altitude medical emergencies. A description of each follows.

Gradual Ascent

To avoid developing high-altitude medical problems, it is important to allow a period of acclimatization. Slow, gradual ascent over days to weeks gives the body a chance to adjust to the hypoxic state caused by high altitudes. A person who would normally become short of breath, dizzy, and confused by a rapid drop in oxygen can function quite well if the oxygen level is decreased to the same level gradually over a long period of time. Acclimatization occurs through several mechanisms. They are

- *Ventilatory Changes.* The *hypoxic ventilatory response (HVR)* is triggered by decreased oxygen. When oxygen is decreased, ventilation increases. This hyperventilation causes a decrease in CO_2, but the kidneys compensate by eliminating more bicarbonate from the body. In essence, the body resets its normal ventilation and operating level of CO_2. The process takes 4 to 7 days at a given altitude.

- *Cardiovascular Changes.* The heart rate increases at high altitude, allowing more oxygen to be delivered to the tissues. In addition, peripheral veins constrict, increasing the central blood volume. In response, the central receptors, which sense blood volume, induce a diuresis, which causes concentration of the blood. Unfortunately, pulmonary circulation also constricts in a hypoxic environment. This causes or exacerbates preexisting hypertension and predisposes people to developing high-altitude pulmonary edema.

- *Blood Changes.* Within two hours of ascent to high altitude, the body begins making more red blood cells to carry oxygen. Over time, this mechanism will significantly compensate for the hypoxic environment. It is this mechanism that fostered the idea of "blood-doping" during athletic competition, especially at high altitudes. Athletes donate their own blood long in advance of a competition at high altitude. This allows them time to rebuild their red blood cells. Just before the competition they receive a transfusion of their own blood to increase their oxygen-carrying capacity. This practice is, however, frowned on by most athletic governing bodies.

Limited Exertion

Clearly, one of the easiest ways to avoid some effects of high altitude is to limit the amount of exertion. By limiting the body's need for oxygen, the effect of oxygen deprivation will be minimized.

Sleeping Altitude

Sleep is often disrupted by high altitude. Hypoxia causes abnormal breathing patterns and frequent awakenings in the middle of the night. Descending to a lower altitude for sleep improves rest and allows the body to recover from hypoxia. This practice will, however, interfere with the process of acclimatization.

High-Carbohydrate Diet

Carbohydrates are converted by the body into glucose and rapidly released into the bloodstream, providing quick energy. The theory that this is helpful in acclimatizing to high altitude is controversial.

Medications

Two medications will limit or prevent the development of medical conditions related to high altitude. They are

- *Acetazolamide.* Acetazolamide (Diamox) acts as a diuretic. It forces bicarbonate out of the body, which greatly enhances the process of acclimatization as discussed above. The hypoxic ventilatory response reaches a new set point more quickly. This improves ventilation and oxygen transport with less alkalosis. In addition, the periodic breathing that occurs at high altitude is resolved, thereby preventing sudden drops in oxygen.
- *Nifedipine.* Nifedipine (Procardia, Adalat) is a medication usually used to treat high blood pressure. It causes blood vessels to dilate, preventing the increase in pulmonary pressure that often causes pulmonary edema.

Other treatments are currently under evaluation. Phenytoin (Dilantin), for example, is being studied because of its membrane stabilization effects. Steroids are commonly used but their efficacy is still controversial.

TYPES OF HIGH-ALTITUDE ILLNESS

A variety of symptoms occur when the average person ascends rapidly to high altitude. These may range from fatigue and decreased exercise tolerance to headache, sleep disturbance, and respiratory distress. The following section will deal with some of the specific syndromes that will occur.

Acute Mountain Sickness (AMS)

Acute mountain sickness usually manifests in an unacclimatized person who ascends rapidly to an altitude of 2000 m or greater.

Signs and Symptoms The mild form of acute mountain sickness presents with the following symptoms:

- Lightheadedness
- Breathlessness

- Weakness
- Headache
- Nausea and vomiting

These symptoms can develop in 6 to 24 hours after ascent. More severe cases can develop, especially if the person continues to ascend to higher altitudes. These symptoms include

- Weakness (requiring assistance to eat and dress)
- Severe vomiting
- Decreased urine output
- Shortness of breath
- Altered level of consciousness

Mild AMS is self-limiting and will often improve within 1 to 2 days if no further ascent occurs.

Treatment Treatment of AMS consists of halting ascent, possibly returning to lower altitude, using acetazolamide (Diamox), and antinauseants, such as dimenhydrinate (Gravol) as necessary. It is not usually necessary to descend to sea level. Supplemental oxygen will relieve symptoms but is usually used only in severe cases. In severe cases, oxygen, if available, will help. In addition, immediate descent is the definitive treatment. For very severe cases, hyperbaric oxygen may be necessary.

Definitive treatment of all high-altitude illnesses is descent to a lower altitude. Administration of supplemental oxygen is also important.

High-Altitude Pulmonary Edema (HAPE)

HAPE develops as a result of increased pulmonary pressure and hypertension caused by changes in blood flow at high altitude. Children are most susceptible, and men are more susceptible than women.

Signs and Symptoms Initially, symptoms include dry cough, mild shortness of breath on exertion, and slight crackles in the lungs. As the condition progresses, so will the symptoms. Dyspnea can become quite severe and cause cyanosis. Coughing may be productive of frothy sputum, and weakness may progress to coma and death.

Treatment In the early stages, HAPE is completely and easily reversible with descent and the administration of oxygen. It is therefore critical to recognize the illness early and initiate appropriate treatment. If immediate descent is not possible, supplemental oxygen can completely reverse HAPE but requires 36 to 72 hours. Such a supply of oxygen is rarely available to mountain climbers. In this situation, the portable hyperbaric bag can be very useful. This is a sealed bag that can be inflated to 2 psi, which simulates a descent of 1524 metres. Acetazolamide can be used to decrease symptoms. Such medications as morphine, nifedipine (Procardia), and furosemide (Lasix) have been used with some success, but they carry complications, such as hypotension and dehydration, and therefore should be used with caution.

High-Altitude Cerebral Edema (HACE)

The exact cause of HACE is not known. It usually manifests as progressive neurological deterioration in a patient with AMS or HAPE. The increased fluid in the brain tissue causes a rise in intracranial pressure.

Signs and Symptoms The symptoms of HACE include

- Altered mental status
- Ataxia (poor coordination)

- Decreased level of consciousness
- Coma

Headache, nausea, and vomiting are less common. Occasionally, actual focal neurological changes may occur.

Treatment As in all altitude illnesses, definitive treatment is descent to lower altitude. Oxygen and steroids may also help improve recovery. If descent is not possible, the use of oxygen with steroids and a hyperbaric bag may be sufficient, although often unavailable. If coma develops, it may persist for days after descent to sea level but usually resolves, although sometimes leaving residual disability.

NUCLEAR RADIATION

Injury due to exposure to ionizing radiation occurs infrequently. However, the incidence of radiation emergencies has increased in recent years due to the expansion of nuclear medicine procedures and commercial nuclear facilities.

Keep in mind that radiation emergencies should be handled only by those with proper protective equipment and adequate training.

> *Radiation emergencies should be handled only by those with proper protective equipment and adequate training.*

BASIC NUCLEAR PHYSICS

Radiation is a general term applied to the transmission of electromagnetic or particle energy. This energy can include nuclear energy, ultraviolet light, visible light, infrared, and x-ray. A radioactive substance emits ionizing radiation. Such a substance is referred to as a *radionuclide* or *radioisotope*.

To understand nuclear radiation, you might begin by taking a look at the structure of an atom and by becoming familiar with some of the basic terms associated with nuclear physics. The atom consists of various subatomic particles. These include

- *Protons.* Positively charged particles that form the nucleus of hydrogen and that are present in the nuclei of all elements. The atomic number of the element indicates the number of protons present.
- *Neutrons.* Subatomic particles that are approximately equal in mass to a proton but lack an electrical charge. As a free particle, a neutron has an average life of less than 17 minutes.
- *Electrons.* Minute particles with negative electrical charges that revolve around the nucleus of an atom. When emitted from radioactive substances, electrons are called beta particles.

You should also be familiar with the following two basic terms associated with nuclear medicine:

- *Isotopes (radioisotope).* Atoms in which the nuclear composition is unstable. That is, they give off **ionizing radiation.**
- *Half-life.* **Half-life** is the time required for half the nuclei of a radioactive substance to lose its activity due to radioactive decay.

A radioactive substance is one that emits ionizing radiation. There are four types of ionizing radiation:

- *Alpha Particles.* Alpha particles are slow-moving, low-energy particles that usually can be stopped by such things as clothing and

* **ionizing radiation** electromagnetic radiation (e.g., x-ray) or particulate radiation (e.g., alpha particles, beta particles, and neutrons) that, by direct or secondary processes, ionizes materials that absorb the radiation. Ionizing radiation can penetrate the cells of living organisms, depositing an electrical charge within them. When sufficiently intense, this form of energy kills cells.

* **half-life** time required for half of the nuclei of a radioactive substance to lose activity by undergoing radioactive decay. In biology and pharmacology, the time required by the body to metabolize and inactivate half the amount of a substance taken in.

paper. When they contact the skin, they only penetrate a few cells deep. Because they can be absorbed (stopped) by a layer of clothing, a few centimetres of air, or the outer layer of skin, alpha particles usually constitute a minor hazard. However, they can produce serious effects if taken internally by ingestion or inhalation.

- *Beta Particles.* Smaller than alpha particles, beta particles are higher in energy. Although beta particles can penetrate air, they can be stopped by aluminum and similar materials. Beta particles generally cause less local damage than alpha particles, but they can be harmful if inhaled or ingested.

- *Gamma Rays.* Gamma rays are more highly energized and penetrating than alpha and beta particles. The origin of gamma rays is related to that of x-rays. Gamma radiation is extremely dangerous, carrying high levels of energy capable of penetrating thick shielding. Gamma rays easily pass through clothing and the entire body, inflicting extensive cell damage. They also create indirect damage by causing internal tissue to emit alpha and beta particles. Protection from gamma radiation can be provided by lead shielding.

- *Neutrons.* Neutrons are more penetrating than the other types of radiation. The penetrating power of neutrons is estimated to be 3 to 10 times greater than gamma rays, but less than the internal hazard associated with ingestion of alpha and beta particles. Exposure to neutrons causes direct tissue damage. However, in nuclear accidents, neutron exposure is not normally a problem for paramedics because neutrons tend to be present only near a reactor core.

EFFECTS OF RADIATION ON THE BODY

Ionizing radiation cannot be seen, felt, or heard. Therefore, a detection instrument is required to measure the radiation given off by the radiation source. The most commonly used device is the *Geiger counter*. The rate of radiation is measured in roentgens per hour (R/hr) or milliroentgens per hour (mR/hr) (1000 mR = 1R).

The unit of local tissue energy deposition is called *radiation absorbed dose (RAD)*. *Roentgen equivalent in man (REM)* provides a gauge of the likely injury to the irradiated part of an organism. For all practical purposes, RAD and REM are equal in clinical value. When neutrons or other high-energy radiation sources are used, a *quality factor (QF)* is applied to determine the equivalent dose.

Simply stated, ionizing radiation causes alterations in the body's cell, primarily the genetic material (DNA). Depending on the dosage received, the changes can be in cell division, cell structure, and cellular biochemical activities. Cell damage due to ionizing radiation is cumulative over a lifetime. If a person is exposed to ionizing radiation long enough, there will be a decreased number of white blood cells. Additionally, there may be defects in offspring, an increased incidence of cancer, and various degrees of bone marrow damage.

Detection of the first biological effects of exposure to ionizing radiation occurs at varying times (Table 36-4). Biological effects include

- *Acute.* Effects appearing in a matter of minutes or weeks.

- *Long-term.* Effects appearing years or decades later.

Table 36-4 | DOSE-EFFECT RELATIONSHIPS TO IONIZING RADIATION

Whole Body Exposure

Dose (RAD)	Effect
5–25	Asymptomatic. Blood studies are normal.
50–75	Asymptomatic. Minor depressions of white blood cells and platelets in a few patients.
75–125	May produce anorexia, nausea, and vomiting, and fatigue in approximately 10–20 percent of patients within two days.
125–200	Possible nausea and vomiting. Diarrhea, anxiety, tachycardia. Fatal to less than 5 percent of patients.
200–600	Nausea and vomiting, diarrhea in the first several hours, weakness, fatigue. Fatal to approximately 50 percent of patients within six weeks without prompt medical attention.
600–1000	Severe nausea and vomiting, diarrhea in the first several hours. Fatal to 100 percent of patients within two weeks without prompt medical attention.
1000 or more	"Burning sensation" within minutes, nausea and vomiting within 10 minutes, confusion ataxia, and prostration within one hour, watery diarrhea within 1–2 hours. Fatal to 100 percent within short time without prompt medical attention.

Localized Exposure

Dose (RAD)	Effect
50	Asymptomatic.
500	Asymptomatic (usually). May have risk of altered function of exposed area.
2500	Atrophy, vascular lesion, and altered pigmentation.
5000	Chronic ulcer, risk of carcinogenesis.
50 000	Permanent destruction of exposed tissue.

PRINCIPLES OF SAFETY

There are three basic principles that allow rescue personnel and patients to limit exposure to ionizing radiation. These are *time, distance,* and *shielding.* Determining exposure, absorption, and damage done by radiation requires specialized training. The amount of radiation received by a person depends on the source of radiation, the length of time exposed, the distance from the source, and the shielding between the exposed person and the source. For example, the amount of radiation at the patient's initial location may be 300 R/hr. If exposure is for 20 minutes, this is the same radiation equivalent as working for one hour at a 100 R/hr scene.

The amount of radiation may drop off rapidly as the patient is decontaminated and moved away from the exposure. The distance from an ionizing radiation source is crucial since exposure is determined by the inverse square relationship. Doubling the distance away from a radiation source reduces the exposure by a factor of four. Conversely, halving the distance to a radiation source increases exposure by a factor of four.

There are basically two types of ionizing radiation accidents—clean and dirty. In a *clean accident,* the patient is exposed to radiation but is not contaminated by the radioactive substance, particles of radioactive dust, or radioactive liquids, gases, or smoke. If he is properly decontaminated before the arrival of rescue personnel, there will be little danger, provided the source of the radiation is no longer exposed at the scene. After exposure to ionizing radiation, the patient is not radioactive. Therefore, he poses no hazard to rescue personnel.

Limiting radiation exposure is based on three principles: time, distance, and shielding.

Content Review

"CLEAN" RADIATION ACCIDENTS

Patient is exposed to radiation but not contaminated by radioactive particles, liquids, gases, or smoke.

"DIRTY" RADIATION ACCIDENTS

Patient is contaminated by radioactive particles, liquids, gases, or smoke.

In contrast, the *dirty* accident, often associated with fire at the scene of a radiation accident, exposes the patient to radiation and contaminates him with radioactive particles or liquids. The scene may be highly contaminated, although the primary source of radiation is shielded when rescue personnel arrive. Unless you are properly trained in dealing with this type of emergency, you may have to delay rescue procedures until properly trained technical assistance arrives.

MANAGEMENT

If you find yourself involved in a radioactive emergency, take the following precautionary steps:

- Park the rescue vehicle upwind to minimize contamination.
- Look for signs of radiation exposure. Radioactive packages are marked by clearly identifiable colour-coded labels (Figure 36-8).
- Use portable instruments to measure the level of radioactivity. If dose estimates are significant, rotate rescue personnel.
- Normal principles of emergency care should be applied, for example, ABCs, shock management, and trauma care.
- Externally radiated patients pose little danger to rescue personnel. Initiate normal care procedures for injuries other than radiation.
- Internally contaminated patients (who have ingested or inhaled radioactive particles) pose little danger to rescue personnel. Normal care procedures should be undertaken. Collect body wastes. If assisted ventilation is required, use a bag-valve-mask unit or demand valve. If radioactive particles are inhaled, swab the nasal passages, and save the swabs.
- Externally contaminated patients (liquids, dirt, smoke) require decontamination. Following decontamination, initiate normal emergency care procedures. Decontamination of paramedic personnel and equipment is required after the call is completed.
- Patients with open, contaminated wounds require normal emergency care procedures. Avoid cross-contamination of wounds.

In a radiation accident, **externally radiated** *and* **internally contaminated** *patients pose little danger to rescue personnel. Provide normal emergency care.* **Externally contaminated** *patients must be decontaminated before normal emergency care is initiated. Paramedic personnel and equipment must be decontaminated after the call.*

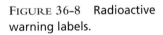

FIGURE 36-8   Radioactive warning labels.

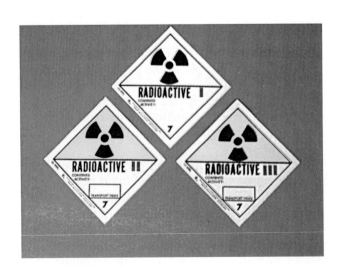

Summary

Our environment provides us with all that we need to survive and prosper. The extremes of our environment, however, can have significant impact on human metabolism. Our bodies will, of course, compensate for these extremes, but sometimes it is not enough. Sometimes, the heat gain or loss is too much. Sometimes the pressure change is too much. As a result, medical illnesses and emergencies arise. These can range from abnormal core body temperatures to decompensation, shock, and even death.

Basic knowledge of common environmental, recreational, and exposure emergencies is necessary in order for you to administer prompt and proper treatment in the prehospital setting. It is not easy to remember this type of information since these problems are not usually encountered on a daily basis. Remember the general principles involved. Remove the environmental influence causing the problem. Support the patient's own attempt to compensate. Finally, select a definitive care location, and transport the patient as rapidly as possible.

In every case, remember that you must maintain your own safety. There are too many cases in which paramedics have lost their lives as a result of attempting a rescue for which they were not properly trained. Rapid action is always necessary when performing an environmental rescue. However, common sense must prevail.

CHAPTER 37

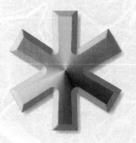

Infectious Disease

Objectives

After reading this chapter, you should be able to:

1. Describe the specific anatomy and physiology pertinent to infectious and communicable diseases. (pp. 782–787; also see Chapter 13)
2. Define specific terminology identified with infectious/communicable diseases. (pp. 782–830)
3. Discuss public health principles relevant to infectious/communicable diseases. (pp. 782–783)
4. Identify public health agencies involved in the prevention and management of disease outbreaks. (p. 783)
5. List and describe the steps of an infectious process. (p. 790)
6. Discuss the risks associated with infection. (pp. 782, 787–790)
7. List and describe the stages of infectious diseases. (pp. 787–790)
8. List and describe infectious agents, including bacteria, viruses, fungi, protozoans, and helminths (worms). (pp. 783–787)

Continued

9. Describe characteristics of the immune system. (see Chapters 13 and 31)
10. Describe the processes of the immune system defences, including humoral and cell-mediated immunity. (see Chapters 13 and 31)
11. In specific diseases, identify and discuss the issues of personal isolation. (p. 800)
12. Describe and discuss the rationale for the various types of personal protection equipment. (pp. 790–795)
13. Discuss what constitutes a significant exposure to an infectious agent. (p. 795)
14. Describe the assessment of a patient suspected of, or identified as having, an infectious/communicable disease. (pp. 795–797)
15. Discuss the proper disposal of contaminated supplies, such as sharps, gauze, sponges, and tourniquets. (pp. 790–795)
16. Discuss disinfection of patient care equipment and areas where patient care occurred. (p. 794)
17. Discuss the seroconversion rate after direct significant HIV exposure. (p. 798)
18. Discuss the causative agent, body systems affected and potential secondary complications, routes of transmission, susceptibility and resistance, signs and symptoms, patient management and protective measures, and immunization for each of the following:
    • HIV (pp. 798–801)
    • Hepatitis A (pp. 801–802)
    • Hepatitis B (pp. 802–803)
    • Hepatitis C (p. 803)
    • Hepatitis D (p. 803)
    • Hepatitis E (pp. 803–804)
    • Tuberculosis (pp. 804–807)
    • Meningococcal meningitis (pp. 811–812)
    • Pneumonia (pp. 807–808)
    • SARS (pp. 808–809)
    • West Nile Virus (pp. 809–810)
    • Tetanus (pp. 823–824)
    • Rabies (pp. 821–823)
    • Hantavirus (pp. 818–819)
    • Chickenpox (pp. 810–811)
    • Mumps (pp. 814–815)
    • Rubella (p. 815)
    • Measles (p. 814)
    • Pertussis (whooping cough) (p. 816)
    • Influenza (pp. 813–814)
    • Mononucleosis (p. 817)
    • Herpes simplex 1 and 2 (pp. 817, 827)
    • Syphilis (pp. 826–827)
    • Gonorrhea (p. 825)
    • Chlamydia (pp. 827–828)
    • Scabies (p. 830)
    • Lice (pp. 829–830)
    • Lyme disease (pp. 824–825)
    • Gastroenteritis (pp. 819–820)
19. Discuss other infectious agents known to cause meningitis, including *Streptococcus pneumoniae, Haemophilus influenzae* type B, and various varieties of viruses. (p. 811)
20. Identify common pediatric viral diseases. (pp. 810–811, 814–815, 817–818)
21. Discuss the characteristics of and organisms associated with febrile and afebrile diseases, including bronchiolitis, bronchitis, laryngitis, croup, epiglottitis, and the common cold. (pp. 817–819)
22. Articulate the pathophysiological principles of an infectious process given a case study of a patient with an infectious/communicable disease. (pp. 782–830)
23. Given several preprogrammed infectious disease patients, provide the appropriate body substance isolation procedure, assessment, management, and transport. (pp. 782–832)

INTRODUCTION

✱ **infectious disease** illness caused by infestation of the body by biological organisms.

Infectious diseases are illnesses caused by infestation of the body by biological organisms, such as bacteria, viruses, fungi, protozoans, and helminths (worms). Most infectious disease states are not life threatening, and the patient recovers completely. Some types of infection, however, such as human immunodeficiency virus (HIV), hepatitis B virus (HBV), and acute bacterial meningitis, are particularly dangerous and may result in death or permanent disability.

All health-care professionals must maintain a strong working knowledge of public health principles and infectious diseases. This is especially true for paramedics, who are often the first to encounter patients with communicable diseases. Early recognition and management of these patients may make a difference in how the patient is treated and may also ensure that care providers take necessary precautions to prevent the spread of the disease to others.

This chapter discusses infectious diseases, including the types of disease-causing organisms, functions of the immune system, and general pathophysiology of infectious diseases. It emphasizes the specific diseases, discussing those that you may encounter during interhospital transports or out-of-hospital care, especially those that you are most likely to encounter in the field.

PUBLIC HEALTH PRINCIPLES

When dealing with infectious diseases, you must consider the impact of the disease process on the community as well as on the infected patient. An infectious agent is a "hazardous material" that can affect large numbers of people.

Epidemiologists, health professionals who study how infectious diseases affect populations, attempt to describe and predict how diseases move from individuals to populations. Through various clinical studies and statistical techniques, they try to determine how effectively an infectious agent can travel through a population. Using the population of infected individuals as a standard, they attempt to predict those individuals in the larger population who may be most at risk for contracting the infectious agent. Recognizing that risk may be predictable, and not just random, is important. The characteristics of the host, the infectious agent, and the environment may yield clues as to how the infectious agent is transmitted and reveal individuals or populations susceptible to infection.

How a population is identified is important. It may be defined by such parameters as geographic boundary, workplace, school, correctional institution, age group, income level, or ethnic group. All of the characteristics of a certain population are known as its demographics. The population's tendency to expand, decline, or move is important as well. Besides stimulating social and economic progress, the movement of people and animals within and among other societies also provides a vehicle for infectious agents.

✱ **index case** the individual who first introduced an infectious agent to a population.

To track the progress of infection within a population, epidemiologists work backward through the chain of infection to determine the **index case,** that individual who first introduced the infectious agent to the population. From the index case, they then retrace the chain forward to verify their reconstruction of the infection's pattern.

To gauge a disease's potential impact on the community, paramedics must evaluate the host (patient), what they believe to be the infectious agent, and the environment. On the basis of that assessment, they may use more aggressive personal protective equipment. They must also consider the patient, those in the patient's immediate environment, and those in the environment where the patient is being transported all to be at risk for infection. On a more personal level, paramedics must appreciate that they and their families could also be at risk.

PUBLIC HEALTH AGENCIES

Local agencies are the first line of defence in disease surveillance and outbreak. Municipal, city, and county agencies, including fire departments, ambulance services, and health departments, must cooperate to monitor and report the incidence and prevalence of disease.

Local agencies are the first line of defence in disease surveillance and outbreak.

At the provincial and territorial level, a designated agency (health department or board of health, for instance) generally monitors infectious diseases. These agencies may set policies requiring vaccinations and regulate or implement control programs in vector and animal control, food preparation, water, sewer, and other sanitation control programs. Provincial and territorial and local laws sometimes require these agencies to meet or exceed federal guidelines and recommendations.

On a national level, Health Canada has a Population and Public Health Branch (PPHB) that is responsible for policies, programs, and research relating to disease surveillances, prevention and control, health promotion, and community action.

The PPHB is made up of five centres—three directorates and two laboratories—located across the country as well as within the national capital region.

Within the umbrella of the PPHB, the centres that may be of particular interest to emergency responders are the Centre for Infectious Disease Prevention and Control (CIDPC), the Centre for Emergency Preparedness and Response (CEPR), and the Centre for Surveillance Coordination (CSC).

Provinces and territories exercise responsibility for health-care delivery and, in an outbreak, will provide first-line response through provincial or territorial and local medical officers of health, augmented by the federal level as necessary, and at the request of provinces or territories. Provincial laboratories contribute to the public health response and coordinate efforts with federal laboratories and the Canadian Public Health Laboratory Network.

The Council of Chief Medical Officers of Health is the primary mechanism for strategy and protocol development in advance of disease outbreak and for information sharing in the midst of a disease outbreak. Provincial and territorial chief medical officers of health operate under the authority of ministers of health. Health Canada works with the Council to develop public health policies and strategies.

Additional information about provincial and territorial public health measures can be found on the websites of the respective ministries of health.

MICROORGANISMS

The vast majority of disease-causing organisms are microscopic (visible only under a microscope). These microorganisms surround us. They are on our skin and in the air we breathe, and they colonize virtually every orifice of our bodies. Some can even live in the highly acidic environment of our stomachs, which destroys other disease-producing microorganisms or deactivates their toxic products. Microorganisms that reside in our bodies without ordinarily causing disease are part of the *host defences* known as **normal flora.** Normal flora help keep us disease-free by creating environmental conditions that are not conducive to disease-producing microorganisms, or **pathogens.** Competition between colonies of normal flora and pathogens also discourages the survival of pathogens. Common bacterial pathogens include *Staphylococci, Streptococci,* and *Enterobacteriaceae.* Certain viruses, rickettsiae, fungi, and protozoans are also pathogenic.

✱ **normal flora** organisms that live inside our bodies without ordinarily causing disease.

✱ **pathogen** organism capable of causing disease.

Opportunistic pathogens are ordinarily nonharmful bacteria that cause disease only under unusual circumstances. Most opportunistic pathogens are normal flora. Patients who have a weakened immune system or who are under unusual stress become susceptible to diseases caused by opportunistic organisms. For example, the fungus *Pneumocystis carinii* is usually harmless but can cause a deadly form of pneumonia in patients with HIV. The fungus overwhelms the weakened immune system and begins to reproduce rapidly in the lungs. Left untreated, *Pneumocystis carinii* pneumonia may be fatal. Organ transplant recipients are also at increased risk for infectious diseases because they must take immunosuppressant medications to prevent organ rejection. A more common (and less harmful) opportunistic infection is thrush (oral candidiasis), often seen in patients who take broad-spectrum antibiotics. As the antibiotic kills normal bacterial flora in the mouth, the fungus *Candida albicans* grows almost uninhibited on the tongue and in the pharynx, producing a white coating on the mucosa.

BACTERIA

Bacteria are microscopic single-celled organisms that range in length from 1 to 20 micrometres (Figure 37-1). They are living cells that are classified as *prokaryotes* because they do not have a distinct nuclear membrane and possess only one chromosome in the cytoplasm. Bacteria reproduce independently, but they require a host to supply food and a supportive environment. Some common diseases caused by pathogenic bacteria include sinusitis, otitis media, bacterial pneumonia, pharyngitis (strep throat), tuberculosis, and most urinary tract infections.

Most bacteria are easily identifiable with stains or by their appearance under a microscope. Similar colourfastness indicates similarities in cell wall structure and other anatomical features. The **Gram stain** is the most common method of differentiating bacteria. The bacteria that this process turns purple are known as gram-positive bacteria; those it turns red are gram-negative. Because of the similarities in their cell walls, bacteria that stain alike may respond to similar treatments.

Bacteria are further categorized into groups based on their general appearance: cocci, or spheres (*Staphylococcus, Streptococcus*), are round; rods (*Enterobacter* sp., *E. coli*) are elongated; and spirals (spirochetes, vibrio) are coiled. *Enterobacter* sp. and *E. coli* are gram-negative rods. *Staphylococci* and *streptococci* are gram-positive cocci (see Figure 37-1). Regardless of how bacteria stain

FIGURE 37-1 Bacteria are single-celled organisms that range in length from 1 to 20 micrometres.

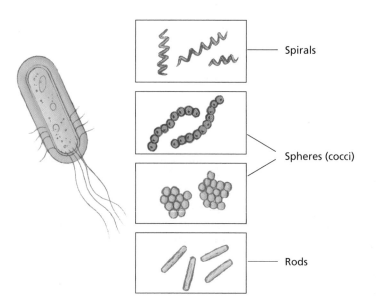

Spirals

Spheres (cocci)

Rods

or appear under a microscope, it is the specific tissues and organs that are infected that chiefly determine the patient's signs and symptoms.

Pathogenic bacteria may harm their human hosts in a number of ways. Heavy colonization may result in direct damage to tissues as the bacteria feed. Bacteria may also cause indirect damage by releasing toxic chemicals that can have localized or systemic effects. The two general categories of toxins are exotoxins and endotoxins. This classification is no longer based primarily on where they originate, as their names imply, but by their chemical structures. **Exotoxins** are poisonous proteins shed by bacteria during bacterial growth. They stimulate the immune system to form antibodies to these proteins, and they may also be deactivated by chemicals, light, or heat. Exotoxins are more toxic than endotoxins. The infectious agent of toxic shock syndrome, *Staphylococcus aureus,* releases an exotoxin, as does anthrax, which can be delivered as a biological weapon of mass destruction.

Endotoxins are composed of proteins, polysaccharides (large sugar molecules), and lipids. The immune system cannot form antibodies specific to a particular endotoxin unless both the protein and the polysaccharide portions are present. Endotoxins come from the bacterial cell wall and are released when the bacterial cell is destroyed. They are more stable in heat than are exotoxins. Only gram-negative bacteria make endotoxins. The skin lesions of meningococcemia and the signs of shock that sometimes accompany it are due to large amounts of endotoxin released by the infectious agent, *Neisseria meningitidis.*

Most bacterial infections respond to treatment with antibiotics that are either **bactericidal** (kill bacteria) or **bacteriostatic** (inhibit bacterial growth or reproduction). Antibiotics are prescribed on the basis of bacterial sensitivity; different antibiotics are required to treat different bacteria. Their administration usually decreases bacterial presence and reduces symptoms. Some types of bacterial infections respond quickly to antibiotics; others take longer. In recent years, a number of bacterial strains have developed resistance to antibiotic therapy, making treatment more difficult. The more a type of bacterium is exposed to an antibiotic, the greater the likelihood of its developing resistance. The overuse of antibiotics in both medical and veterinary settings has contributed to this serious problem. Resistant forms of tuberculosis (*Mycobacterium*) are of particular concern. Antibiotics may now be ineffective against this disease, and its mortality rate is high. The willingness of some physicians to prescribe the newest antibiotics for relatively minor infections and the widespread addition of antibiotics to animal feed have only added to the problem.

Antimicrobial treatment alters the normal flora of the skin, mouth, mucosa, and gastrointestinal tract and often results in colonization of those areas by new microorganisms that resist antibiotics. In some cases, an antibiotic may kill normal flora and allow more virulent and dangerous opportunistic pathogens to multiply freely. This can lead to a secondary infection that is more severe than the original infection being treated. For all of these reasons, antibiotics should be prescribed cautiously.

VIRUSES

Viruses are much smaller than bacteria and can be seen only with an electron microscope (Figure 37-2). Viruses cannot reproduce and carry on metabolism by themselves. Therefore, they are considered to be neither prokaryotes nor eukaryotes. Instead, viruses are **obligate intracellular parasites**; that is, they can grow and reproduce only within a host cell. Once inside, the virus takes control of the host cell's protein synthesis mechanism and directs it to begin reproducing the virus. The cell then releases new virus particles, which infect nearby cells.

Since viruses "hide" inside the host's cells, they resist antibiotic treatment. Once a virus enters a host cell, it becomes part of that host cell, making selective eradication of the virus virtually impossible, as any treatment capable of killing

Content Review

TYPES OF BACTERIA
- Spheres (cocci)
- Rods
- Spirals

✳ **exotoxin** toxic waste products released by living bacteria.

✳ **endotoxin** toxic products released when bacteria die and decompose.

✳ **bactericidal** capable of killing bacteria.

✳ **bacteriostatic** capable of inhibiting bacterial growth or reproduction.

✳ **virus** disease-causing organism that can be seen only with an electron microscope.

✳ **obligate intracellular parasite** organism that can grow and reproduce only within a host cell.

FIGURE 37-2 Viruses are much smaller than bacteria and can be seen only with an electron microscope. They grow and reproduce only within a host cell.

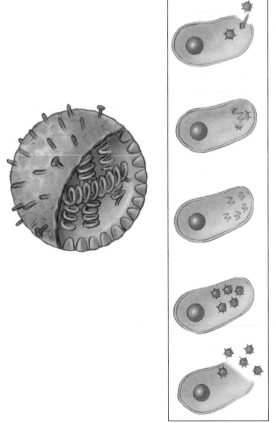

the virus will generally kill the host cell as well. This is the major obstacle facing researchers as they work to find cures for HIV and other viruses.

Approximately 400 types of viruses have been identified. One frequently encountered viral disorder, the common cold, is caused by a number of different viruses (nearly 200) that all produce similar symptoms. Fortunately, most viral diseases are mild and self-limiting. They run their course until the patient's immune system eventually fights them off. A host is generally susceptible to any particular virus only once. Once a person's immune system develops active immunity against a particular type of virus, it becomes attuned to similar attacking viruses and will destroy them.

OTHER MICROORGANISMS

✱ **prions** particles of protein folded in such a way that protease enzymes cannot act on them.

Prions are a new classification of disease-producing agents that microbiologists used to refer to as "slow viruses." They are neither prokaryotes nor eukaryotes but particles of protein folded in such a way that proteases (enzymes that break down proteins) cannot act on them. These protein particles accumulate in nervous system and brain tissue, destroying them and giving them a spongy appearance on gross examination. Prions are known to cause progressive, untreatable dementia in Kuru, Creutzfeldt-Jakob disease, bovine spongiform encephalitis (BSE, or "mad cow disease"), and fatal familial insomnia. Although EMS providers will rarely need to respond to patients with diseases caused by prions, a general discussion of infectious agents must acknowledge their existence.

✱ **fungus** plant-like microorganism.

Fungi are plant-like microorganisms, most of which are not pathogenic. Yeasts, moulds, and mushrooms are types of fungi. Some fungi have a capsule around the cell wall that provides additional protection against phagocytes.

While fungi compose a large part of the body's normal flora, they may become pathogenic in patients with compromised immune function, such as those with HIV. Fungi may also lead to disease states in patients taking broad-spectrum antibiotics. As the antibiotics kill off bacteria, the fungi are able to grow uninhibited. Fungi are a common cause of vaginal infections and often cause pneumonia in patients with weakened immune systems.

Protozoa are single-celled parasitic organisms with flexible membranes and the ability to move. Most protozoa live in the soil and ingest decaying organic matter. Although rarely a cause of disease in humans, they are considered opportunistic pathogens in patients with compromised immune function. These organisms may enter the body by the fecal-oral route or through a mosquito bite. Common diseases caused by protozoa include malaria and forms of gastroenteritis. Protozoa also cause vaginal infections (trichomoniasis) in women with normal immune function.

Parasites are common causes of disease where sanitation is poor (generally in the developing countries). Occasional cases are seen in North America. Roundworms (*Ascaris lumbricoides*) live in the intestinal mucosa and may reach 30–50 cm in length. Symptoms include abdominal cramping, fever, and cough. Diagnosis usually depends on finding eggs in the patient's stool.

Pinworms (*Enterobius vermicularis*) are common even in developed countries. It is estimated that 20 percent of children living in temperate climates harbour this disease. These tiny worms (3–10 mm long) live in the distal colon and crawl onto the anal mucosa to lay their eggs, usually when the host is asleep. Although the disease may remain asymptomatic, it is a common cause of anal pruritus (itching) and infection and is easily spread among children, especially in daycare centres. Children may carry the disease home and infect their entire family. This disease is often endemic among institutionalized children. Treatment involves a single dose of an antibiotic (mebendazole); all family members must be treated simultaneously to avoid reinfection.

Hookworms (*Ancylostoma duodenale, Necator americanus*) are found in warm, moist climates. This parasite infects an estimated 25 percent of the world's population, although it is relatively rare in North America. The larvae are passed in the stool of infected animals. The disease is most commonly contracted when a child walks barefoot in a contaminated area. The larvae enter through the skin and migrate to the intestines, where they grip and irritate the intestinal wall and feed on blood. Epigastric pain and anemia are possible. Prevention involves wearing shoes; treatment is similar to that for pinworms.

Trichinosis (*Trichinella spiralis*) may be contracted by eating raw or inadequately cooked pork products, most commonly sausage. Females burrow into the intestinal wall and produce thousands of living larvae that migrate to skeletal muscle, where each forms a cyst and remains. Symptoms include gastrointestinal disturbances, edema (especially of the eyelids), fever, and a variety of other diffuse and secondary symptoms. If the worms invade the heart, lungs, or brain in large numbers, death may result. Diagnosis is made by finding encysted worms during examination of muscle biopsy. Mebendazole is the antibiotic of choice.

Other types of worms, such as tapeworms and flukes, are rarely encountered in North America.

* **protozoan** single-celled parasitic organism with flexible membranes and the ability to move.

* **parasite** organism that lives in or on another organism.

* **pinworm** parasite that is 3–10 mm long and lives in the distal colon.

* **hookworm** parasite that attaches to the host's intestinal lining.

* **trichinosis** disease resulting from an infestation of *Trichinella spriralis*.

CONTRACTION, TRANSMISSION, AND STAGES OF DISEASE

As a paramedic you must understand the relationship between the pathophysiology and the assessment and management of patients with infections or diseases resulting from infections. This knowledge will prepare you for leadership in recognizing infectious diseases and curbing their transmission.

reservoir any living creature or environment (water, soil, etc.) that can harbour an infectious agent.

bloodborne transmitted by contact with blood or body fluids.

airborne transmitted through the air by droplets or particles.

fecal-oral route transmission of organisms picked up from the gastrointestinal tract (e.g., feces) into the mouth.

Generally, the risk of disease transmission rises if a patient has open wounds, increased secretions, active coughing, or any ongoing invasive treatment where exposure to an infectious body fluid is likely.

The interactions of host, infectious agent, and environment are the elements of disease transmission. Studying each of these factors individually and then looking for relationships among them often reveals how an infectious agent has been effectively transmitted. Infectious agents exist in all types of **reservoirs**—animals, humans, insects, and the environment. While inhabiting animal or insect reservoirs, they do not cause disease. Their presence at any time in a given environment is affected by their life cycle, by the presence of stressors that may force them outside of their normal reservoirs, and by the climate. The initiation of therapy can sometimes disrupt the life cycle of the infectious agent and may eradicate the infection. When a host and infectious agent come together at the right time and under the right conditions, disease transmission takes place.

Infectious agents may invade hosts through one of two basic mechanisms. The more common is direct transmission from person to person through a cough, sneeze, kiss, or sexual contact. The other mechanism, indirect transmission, can spread organisms in a number of ways. Infected persons often shed organisms into the environment. These organisms come to rest on doorknobs, handrails, computer keyboards, and so on. Other people who contact those surfaces are at risk for contracting the disease. Similarly, microorganisms may be transmitted via food products, water, or even through the soil.

Bloodborne diseases are transmitted by contact with the blood or body fluids of an infected person. They include AIDS, hepatitis B, hepatitis C, hepatitis D, and syphilis. The risk of transmission of bloodborne diseases increases if a patient has open wounds, active bleeding, or increased secretions. Assume that every patient has an infectious bloodborne disease and take precautions to avoid contact with blood and other body fluids.

Some infectious diseases may be transmitted through the air on droplets expelled during a productive cough or sneeze. They include tuberculosis, meningitis, mumps, measles, rubella, and chicken pox (varicella). Other, more common diseases, such as the common cold, influenza, and respiratory syncytial virus (RSV), may also be transmitted by the **airborne** route.

Some infectious diseases are transmitted orally (primarily by eating) or by the **fecal-oral route,** in which enteric microorganisms (normally found in the gastrointestinal system and the feces) are transmitted between potential hosts, as in shaking hands or other social customs, and then having the recipient somehow introduce the infectious agent into her mouth by scratching or eating with her hands. Fecal-oral diseases are prevalent in the less developed countries and in areas with unsanitary conditions. Hepatitis A, hepatitis E, and other viruses can be transmitted by this route. Foodborne illnesses include food poisoning, certain parasitic infections, and trichinosis.

The risk of infection is considered *theoretical* if transmission is acknowledged to be possible but has not actually been reported. It is considered *measurable* if factors in the infectious agent's transmission and their associated risks have been identified or deduced from reported data. Generally, the risk of disease transmission rises if a patient has open wounds, increased secretions, active coughing, or any ongoing invasive treatment where exposure to an infectious body fluid is likely (Table 37-1). In the prehospital setting, the unpredictable environment and behaviour of patients increase the risk of exposure. For example, a patient with a closed head injury and multiple lacerations may be combative, thereby contaminating EMS personnel with blood or other body fluids. Broken windshield glass contaminated with blood may easily penetrate examination gloves and skin. Patients who are violent and aggressive may deliberately bite, scratch, or spit at rescuers. Many EMS patient care activities occur in a closed, poorly ventilated environment, such as the interior of an ambulance. Thus, you must have available, and routinely use, protective clothing and other barrier devices, as indicated.

Table 37-1 MODES OF TRANSMISSION OF INFECTIOUS DISEASES

Disease	Bloodborne	Airborne	Sexual	Indirect	Opportunist	Oral-Fecal
Hepatitis A						✔
Hepatitis B	✔					
Hepatitis C						
HIV	✔		✔			
Influenza		✔	✔	✔		
Syphilis			✔			
Gonorrhea			✔			
Measles		✔				
Mumps		✔				
Strep throat		✔			✔	
Herpes virus	✔		✔	✔		
Food poisoning		✔		✔		✔
Lyme disease	✔					
Pneumonia		✔			✔	

Not all exposures to microorganisms from body fluids or infected patients will result in transmission of those agents. Nor are all infectious agents and diseases **communicable** (capable of being transmitted to another host). Communicability depends on several factors. Exposure to an infectious agent may just result in **contamination,** in which the agent exists only on the surface of the host without penetrating it. Penetration of the host implies that **infection** has occurred, but infection should never be equated with disease. Factors that affect the likelihood that an exposed individual will become infected and then actually develop disease include the following:

- *Correct Mode of Entry* Certain external barriers in hosts, particularly the skin, make it impossible for infectious agents to establish themselves. Mucous membranes, however, often present an effective point of entry.
- *Virulence* **Virulence** is an organism's strength or ability to infect or overcome the body's defences. Some organisms, such as the hepatitis B virus (HBV), are very virulent and can remain infectious on a surface for weeks. Others, such as HIV and syphilis, die when exposed to air and light. Some bacteria (*Clostridium*) may remain dormant in the soil for months and be capable of causing disease if contracted. Infection generally occurs either when a highly virulent microorganism interacts with a normal, intact host or when a less virulent microorganism enters a host with impaired defences (immunosuppression).
- *Number of Organisms Transmitted (Dose)* For most diseases, a minimum number of organisms must enter the host to cause infection. As a rule, the higher the number, the greater the likelihood of contracting the disease.
- *Host Resistance* **Resistance** is the host's ability to fight off infection. Several factors affect the host's resistance. They include general health and fitness, genetic predisposition or resistance to infection, nutrition status, recent exposure to stressors, hygiene, and the

✱ **communicable** capable of being transmitted to another host.

✱ **contamination** presence of an agent only on the surface of the host without penetrating it.

✱ **infection** presence of an agent within the host, without necessarily causing disease.

Content Review

FACTORS AFFECTING DISEASE TRANSMISSION
- Mode of entry
- Virulence
- Number of organisms transmitted
- Host resistance

✱ **virulence** an organism's strength or ability to infect or overcome the body's defences.

✱ **resistance** a host's ability to fight off infection.

presence of underlying disease processes. Persons with decreased immune function are at significantly increased risk for contracting infectious diseases. Cigarette smokers and those regularly exposed to secondhand cigarette smoke are also at increased risk.

- *Other Host Factors* The tendency of the host to travel or be in contact with other potential hosts, the age and socioeconomic status of the host, the characteristics of other hosts within the population of which the infected host is a member all effect the likelihood of contracting disease.

PHASES OF THE INFECTIOUS PROCESS

Disease progression varies greatly, depending on the infectious agent and the host. Conditions can manifest themselves in various ways. Once infected with an infectious agent, the host goes through a **latent period** when she cannot transmit the agent to someone else. Following the latent period is a **communicable period** when the host may exhibit signs of clinical disease and can transmit the infectious agent to another host.

The appearance of symptoms often lags after exposure to an infectious disease. The time between exposure and presentation, known as the **incubation period,** may range from a few days, as in the common cold, to months or years, as in HIV/AIDS or hepatitis. Thus, prehospital personnel must be notified if any patient for whom they provide care subsequently develops a life-threatening infectious disease.

Most viruses and bacteria have surface proteins, or **antigens,** that stimulate the body to produce **antibodies.** These antibodies react to or unite with the antigens. The antibodies' presence in the blood indicates exposure to the particular disease that they fight. Although testing for the presence of a specific disease antigen is difficult, laboratory tests can often spot antibodies that are specific for the disease or antigen. For example, they detect the human immunodeficiency virus (HIV) through the presence of antibodies specific to HIV. When a person develops antibodies after exposure to a disease, her previously negative test will be positive and **seroconversion** will have occurred. The time between exposure to disease and seroconversion is referred to as the **window phase.** A person in the window phase may test negative even though she is infected. From the standpoint of the immune system response, the window phase is the period when the antigen is present but antibody production has not reached detectable levels. The **disease period** is the duration from the onset of signs and symptoms of disease until the resolution of symptoms or death. Keep in mind that the resolution of symptoms does not necessarily imply that the infectious agent has been eradicated.

INFECTION CONTROL

The body protects itself from disease in many ways. At the basic level, skin defends against invading pathogens. Turbulent airflow through the airway and nasal hair assist in capturing foreign bodies. Mucus can trap and kill foreign materials. Coughing and sneezing expel foreign materials. Further, as you learned in Chapter 13 on pathophysiology, the body has a very sophisiticated immune system. The complement and lymphatic systems also assist in fighting infection through inflammatory responses and filtering of body fluids.

To supplement the body's natural defences against disease, EMS providers must protect themselves from infectious exposures (Figure 37-3). The four phases of infection control in prehospital care include preparation for response, response, patient contact, and recovery.

* **latent period** time when a host cannot transmit an infectious agent to someone else.

* **communicable period** time when a host can transmit an infectious agent to someone else.

* **incubation period** time between a host's exposure to an infectious agent and the appearance of symptoms.

* **antigen** surface protein on most viruses and bacteria.

* **antibody** protein that attacks a disease antigen.

* **seroconversion** creation of antibodies after exposure to a disease.

* **window phase** time between exposure to a disease and seroconversion.

* **disease period** the duration from the onset of signs and symptoms of disease until the resolution of symptoms or death.

To supplement the body's natural defences against disease, EMS providers must protect themselves from infectious exposures.

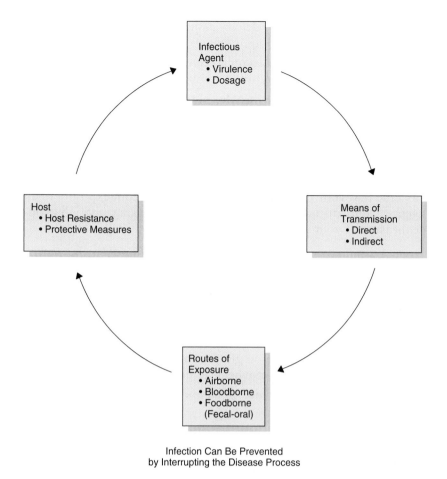

Infection Can Be Prevented
by Interrupting the Disease Process

FIGURE 37-3 Interruption of infectious disease transmission is a role of prehospital personnel.

PREPARATION FOR RESPONSE

Infection control begins long before an emergency call. To ensure proper protection, the EMS agency should implement the following procedures:

- Establish and maintain written standard operating procedures (SOPs) for infection control, and monitor employee compliance.

- Prepare an infection control plan that includes a schedule of when and how to implement Health Canada standards and guidelines.

- Provide adequate original and ongoing infection control training to all personnel, including engineering and work practice controls.

- Ensure that all employees are provided with personal protective equipment (PPE) and that it is fitted appropriately, checked regularly, maintained properly, and can be located easily.

- Ensure that all EMS personnel treat and bandage all personal wounds (e.g., open sores, cuts, or skin breaks) before any emergency response.

- Use disposable supplies and equipment whenever possible. The risk of transmitting disease is generally much lower than when reusing items, even though they have been cleaned or disinfected.

- Ensure that all EMS personnel have access to the facilities and supplies needed to maintain a high level of personal hygiene.

- Do not allow EMS personnel to deliver patient care if they exhibit signs or symptoms of an infectious disease.
- Monitor all EMS personnel for compliance with vaccinations and appropriate diagnostic tests (e.g., **PPD,** antibody titres).
- Appoint a designated infectious disease control officer (IDCO) to serve as a contact person for personnel exposed to an infectious disease and monitor the infection control program.
- Identify specific job classifications and work processes in which the possibility of exposure exists.

Do not assume that your EMS agency can protect you from exposure to all infectious agents. Your attitude toward protecting yourself against infectious agents is one measure of your professionalism.

RESPONSE

When responding to an EMS call, take the following infection control measures:

- Obtain as much information as possible from dispatch regarding the nature of the patient's illness or injury.
- Prepare for patient contact. Put on gloves, and don eye and face protection before patient contact whenever practical.
- Prepare mentally for the call. Think *infection control!*

PATIENT CONTACT

Your contact with a patient, especially at an emergency scene, poses your highest risk for acquiring an infectious disease. Have all personal protective equipment with you before leaving the emergency vehicle, and follow these guidelines:

- Isolate all body substances, and avoid any contact with them.
- Wear appropriate personal protective equipment, such as gowns, gloves, face shields, masks, protective eyewear, aprons, and similar items.
- Allow only necessary personnel to make patient contact. Limit the risk to as few people as possible, thus minimizing exposure.
- Use airway adjuncts, such as a pocket mask or bag-valve-mask unit, to minimize exposure. Disposable items are preferable.
- Properly dispose of biohazardous waste.
- Use extreme caution with sharp instruments. Utilize retractable IV needles and needleless injection systems when possible. Never bend, recap, or remove contaminated needles. Dispose of all contaminated sharps in properly labelled puncture-resistant containers.
- Never smoke, eat, or drink in the patient compartment of the ambulance. Each service should have strict guidelines regarding the presence of food and drink in the driver compartment during down times. Strictly adhere to infection control guidelines.
- Do not apply cosmetics or lip balm, or handle contact lenses when a likelihood of exposure exists.

Table 37-2 details specific measures for protection against HIV (human immunodeficiency virus) and HBV (hepatitis B virus) infections.

Table 37-2

GUIDELINES FOR PREVENTION OF TRANSMISSION OF HIV AND HBV TO PREHOSPITAL PERSONNEL

Task or Activity	Disposable Gloves	Gown	Mask	Protective Eyewear
Bleeding control with active bleeding	Yes	Yes	Yes	Yes
Bleeding control with minimal bleeding	Yes	No	No	No
Emergency childbirth	Yes	Yes	Yes	Yes
Blood drawing	Yes	No	No	No
IV insertion	Yes	No	No	No
Endotracheal intubation	Yes	No	Yes	Yes
EOA insertion	Yes	No	Yes	Yes
Oral/nasal suctioning; manually clearing airway	Yes	Yes	Yes	Yes
Handling/cleaning instruments with possible contamination	Yes	Yes	Yes	Yes
Measuring blood pressure	Yes	No	No	No
Giving an injection	Yes	No	No	No
Measuring temperature	Yes	No	No	No
Rescuing from a building fire	Yes	No	No	No
Cleaning back of ambulance after a medical call	Yes	No	No	No

RECOVERY

Infection control does not end when you deliver the patient to the emergency department. Decontaminating the ambulance and equipment is essential. Take the following steps at the completion of each response:

- Wash hands immediately after patient contact. Ample data substantiate that *effective, vigorous* hand washing is superior to some disinfectants. On scene, you can wipe your hands with a waterless hand-cleansing solution. However, this constitutes only partial cleansing because it cannot grossly remove the particles to which microorganisms adhere. Only soap and water can do that. On returning to quarters, or at the earliest opportunity, thoroughly wash your hands with soap and warm water, paying attention to the webs between fingers. Overlooking this important habit may result in the inadvertent contamination of personal clothing or anything else that you contact. Such oversight can result in transmitting the disease to family and friends.

- If you sustain a wound and are exposed to the body fluids of others, vigorously wash the wound with soap and warm water immediately, *before* contacting your employer.

- Dispose of all biohazardous wastes in accordance with local laws and regulations.

- Place potentially infectious wastes in leak-proof biohazard bags. Bag any soiled linen, and label for laundry personnel (Figure 37-4).

- Decontaminate all contaminated clothing and reusable equipment.

- Handle uniforms in accordance with the agency's standard procedures for personal protective equipment.

Infection control does not end when you deliver the patient to the emergency department.

FIGURE 37-4   Bag all linen, and label it infectious.

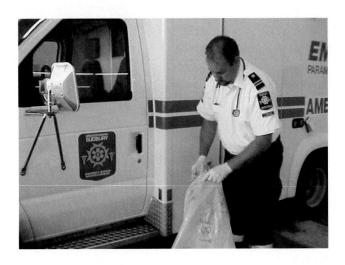

Decontamination Methods and Procedures

* decontaminate to destroy or remove pathogens.

Content Review

DECONTAMINATION LEVELS
- Low-level disinfection
- Intermediate-level disinfection
- High-level disinfection
- Sterilization

* disinfection destroying certain forms of microorganisms, but not all.

* sterilization destroying all microorganisms.

Decontaminate infected equipment according to local protocol and standard operating procedures (SOPs) established by the EMS agency. Perform decontamination in a designated area that is properly marked and secured. The room should have a suitable ventilation system and adequate drainage. Be sure to wear gloves, gowns, boots, protective eyewear, and a face mask. To begin decontamination, remove surface dirt and debris with soap and water. Then, disinfect and if required sterilize all items. The four levels of decontamination are low-level disinfection, intermediate-level disinfection, high-level disinfection, and sterilization.

Low-Level Disinfection Low-level **disinfection** destroys most bacteria and some viruses and fungi. It does not destroy *Mycobacterium tuberculosis* or bacterial spores. Use low-level disinfection for routine housekeeping and cleaning, as well as for removing visible body fluids. All EPA-registered disinfectants are suitable for low-level disinfection.

Intermediate-Level Disinfection Intermediate-level disinfection destroys *Mycobacterium tuberculosis* and most viruses and fungi. It does not, however, destroy bacterial spores. Use it for all equipment, such as stethoscopes, splints, and blood pressure cuffs, that has come into contact with intact skin. A 1:10 to 1:100 dilution of water and chlorine bleach is acceptable for intermediate-level disinfection. Hard-surface germicides and EPA-registered disinfectants/chemical germicides are also effective.

High-Level Disinfection High-level disinfection destroys all forms of microorganisms, except certain bacterial spores. High-level disinfection is required for all reusable devices, including laryngoscopes, Magill forceps, and airway adjuncts, that have come into contact with mucous membranes. For high-level disinfection, immerse objects in an EPA-approved chemical-sterilizing agent for 10 to 45 seconds (depending on the manufacturer's instructions). Alternatively, immerse the device in hot water (80°C–100°C) for 30 minutes.

Sterilization **Sterilization** destroys all microorganisms and is required for all contaminated invasive instruments. An autoclave that uses pressurized steam or ethylene-oxide gas effectively sterilizes equipment. These methods, however, are rarely available outside of a hospital setting. Alternatively, prolonged immersion (6–10 hours, depending on the manufacturer's instructions) in an EPA-approved chemical-sterilizing agent is usually adequate. Whenever possible, use disposable instruments for invasive procedures.

INFECTIOUS DISEASE EXPOSURES

Infectious disease exposures occur during all hours of a work shift. Since you may not always be able to contact an agency administrator, you need a working knowledge of your agency's SOPs, as well as of the laws and regulations applicable to exposures. The following recommendations will help ensure that exposure management will protect you, other EMS personnel and health-care professionals, the agency, and the confidentiality of the patient's information.

Reporting an Infectious Disease Exposure Immediately report exposures of EMS personnel to the designated infectious disease control officer (IDCO), according to local protocol. Report all exposures to blood, blood products, or any potentially infectious material, regardless of their perceived severity. This will permit immediate medical followup, including counselling for the EMS provider and identification of the infectious agent. It also enables the IDCO to evaluate the circumstances of the exposure and implement changes to prevent future exposures, if needed. Finally, it facilitates followup testing if the source individual consents.

Report all exposures to blood, blood products, or any potentially infectious material, regardless of their perceived severity.

Provincial and territorial laws outline the rights and responsibilities of agencies and health-care workers when an infectious disease exposure occurs. In some provinces and territories, the exposed employee has the right to ask the source patient's infection status. Political action continues to try to implement legislation requiring patients to submit to testing if an emergency worker has been exposed.

Postexposure Employers are required to provide a medical evaluation and treatment for any paramedic or other EMS provider exposed to an infectious disease. The nature of the exposure is assessed on the basis of the route, dose, and nature of the infectious agent. As part of the medical evaluation, employees are entitled to receive counselling about alternatives for treatment, risks of treatment, signs, symptoms, possibilities of developing disease, and preventing further spread of the potential infection. This includes the available medications, their potential side effects, and their contraindications. Treatment must be in line with current Health Canada recommendations.

After a paramedic is exposed to an infectious disease, she has the option to submit a blood sample for baseline testing.

The IDCO or other health-care professional who specializes in occupational infectious diseases should counsel the exposed employee and obtain informed consent for postexposure prophylaxis (PEP) based on Health Canada guidelines. All records related to employee counselling and PEP are forwarded to the IDCO. Vaccines may be made available to the employee if deemed appropriate by an occupational medicine physician.

Confidentiality The IDCO will maintain records of all exposures. All of these exposure records (like any medical records) are confidential. They must not be released to anyone without express written permission from the employee.

ASSESSMENT OF THE PATIENT WITH INFECTIOUS DISEASE

When assessing a patient, always maintain a high index of suspicion that an infectious agent may be involved. Consider the dispatch information, evaluate the environment for its suitability for transmitting infectious agents, and maintain appropriate body substance isolation (BSI). Gloves are the mandatory minimum level of personal protective equipment (PPE) required on every patient contact.

Approach every scene with a high index of suspicion that a patient may have an infectious disease.

When approaching a patient with a possible infectious disease, look for general indicators of infection, such as unusual skin signs, fever, weakness, profuse sweating, malaise, anorexia, and unexplained worsening of existing disease states. If an infection is localized, signs of inflammation may include redness, swelling, tenderness to palpation, capillary streaking, and warmth in the affected area. A rash or other diagnostic skin signs may make identifying an infectious disease much easier.

PAST MEDICAL HISTORY

The patient's past medical history (PMH) may provide valuable clues to her illness. Patients who have AIDS or who are taking immunosuppressant medications, such as steroids, are particularly susceptible to infection. Chronic obstructive pulmonary disease (COPD) patients, patients with autoimmune diseases, and transplant recipients frequently take steroids and immunosuppressants. Persons with diabetes and other endocrine disorders are also more likely to get infections due to additional stressors on their immune systems. Other conditions that increase the risk for developing infectious diseases include alcoholism, malnutrition, IV drug abuse, malignancy (cancer), and splenectomy (removal of the spleen), as well as artificial heart valves (aortic or mitral) or joints (hip or knee). Any significant increase in emotional stress may also increase a person's risk of significant illness, including infectious diseases.

A patient with a PMH of numerous untreated throat infections who suddenly develops a heart murmur, fever, and malaise may have rheumatic fever, an outcome of streptococcal infection that can affect the heart. Such patients are often found in medically underserved areas where access to primary care is difficult or nonexistent. Patients with cancer are at increased risk for acquiring numerous opportunistic infectious diseases. A recently transmitted sexual disease may precede systemic infection. Recent unfinished antibiotic treatment may lead to the proliferation of drug-resistant infectious agents, causing recurrent, persistent bacterial infections or development of other opportunistic infections.

In addition to determining past or current illnesses or diseases, thoroughly investigate the patient's chief complaint and any history of the present illness, including the following:

- When did signs and symptoms begin?
- Is fever present? How has the temperature changed over time?
- Has the patient taken any aspirin, acetaminophen, or other medications?
- Does the patient have any neck pain or stiffness when her head is moved, especially during flexion?
- Has the patient had any difficulty swallowing?
- Has the patient had any previous symptoms or illnesses similar to this one?

THE SECONDARY ASSESSMENT

Every EMS unit should have the capability of measuring and monitoring body temperature (e.g., a tympanic thermometer).

Secondary assessment of the patient whom you suspect of having an infectious disease follows the standard format for assessing a medical patient. Determine the patient's level of consciousness and vital signs early on. Increased temperature commonly indicates infection. Significant increases in pulse may occur due to the infection and as a result of elevated body temperature. As a consequence, metabolic needs will increase. The patient will require more oxygen and more nutrients to maintain normal physiological function. This may be a serious problem for elderly, very young, or debilitated patients with concurrent illnesses that limit their cardiovascular and respiratory reserve.

Hypotension in the patient with an infectious disease may result from dehydration, vasodilation, or both, as in septic shock. In rare cases, infections of the heart muscle (endocarditis) may result in decreased cardiac output (cardiogenic shock). In any case, assess the cause of hypotension, and treat it promptly. If the lungs are clear, the judicious use of fluids may be beneficial; if fluid status is not a problem, vasopressors, such as dopamine, may be necessary.

Dehydration is a common consequence of infectious diseases. Increased body temperature is often accompanied by increased respiratory rate and concomitant fluid loss, of which the patient is often unaware (insensible fluid loss). Vomiting or diarrhea can quickly cause life-threatening dehydration, especially in pediatric patients who have large body surface areas relative to their volume. Electrolyte imbalances often occur with fluid loss. Advances in technology that may soon make the prehospital evaluation of electrolytes cost effective may be indicated in the setting of significant dehydration. Clinically significant dehydration will usually cause tachycardia and hypotension, but you should be vigilant for more subtle signs that include thirst, poor skin turgor, and a shrunken and furrowed tongue. A history of decreased fluid intake, fever, vomiting, and/or diarrhea should trigger a thorough assessment of fluid status. While performing a secondary assessment similar to that for any patient with a medical emergency, assess the following:

- Skin for temperature, hydration, colour, or rash
- Sclera for icterus
- Reaction to neck flexion (Is nuchal rigidity [neck stiffness] present?)
- Lymph nodes for swelling or tenderness (lymphadenopathy)
- Breath sounds (for adventitious sounds and evidence of consolidation)
- Hepatomegaly (enlargement of the liver)
- Purulent (pus-filled) lesions

SELECTED INFECTIOUS DISEASES

The following section profiles infectious diseases that either may be encountered in the prehospital setting or are commonly known by emergency health-care practitioners. The first major category includes diseases of immediate concern to EMS. General profiles of other diseases follow. You should be familiar with the terminology of these profiles, realize which diseases you will more commonly encounter in patients, and know which BSI precautions to employ.

DISEASES OF IMMEDIATE CONCERN TO EMS PROVIDERS

The diseases of immediate concern to EMS providers include HIV/AIDS, hepatitis, tuberculosis, pneumonia, chickenpox, and bacterial meningitis. They are infectious diseases that have gained notoriety, pose a high risk for communicability and debilitating conditions, or are relevant to direct patient care. While most attention focuses on reducing transmission from patient to health-care worker, the profiles also consider reverse transmission because responsible health-care workers protect both themselves and their patients. The inclusion of chickenpox may surprise some EMS personnel, but the disease is highly communicable and poses a serious occupational risk for unvaccinated or previously unexposed health-care workers.

Content Review

DISEASES OF IMMEDIATE CONCERN TO EMS PROVIDERS
- HIV/AIDS
- Hepatitis
- Tuberculosis
- Pneumonia
- Chickenpox
- Meningitis

Human Immunodeficiency Virus

* human immunodeficiency virus (HIV) organism responsible for acquired immune deficiency syndrome (AIDS).

The **human immunodeficiency virus** (**HIV**) is the most discussed and feared infectious agent of the modern era, especially of the last two decades. The clinical condition that it causes, acquired immune deficiency syndrome (AIDS), is not a disease *per se*, but a collection of signs and symptoms that share common anatomical, physiological, and biochemical derangements in the immune system. Like other viruses, HIV utilizes the host cell's reproductive apparatus to copy itself. HIV is a retrovirus, that is, it normally carries its genetic material in RNA (instead of DNA) and utilizes an enzyme called *reverse transcriptase* (hence the designation "*retro*virus") to use RNA to synthesize DNA. This is the reverse of the usual process of transcription of DNA into RNA. The action of reverse transcriptase enables genetic material from a retrovirus to become permanently incorporated into the DNA of an infected cell. Two types of HIV have been identified, HIV-1 and HIV-2. Most research targets the HIV-1 variant, which has proven much more pathogenic than HIV-2.

The emergence of HIV infection and AIDS, more than any other infectious process, has increased emergency and health-care workers' awareness of the dangers of infectious diseases. The worldwide research and educational activities resulting from concern about HIV and AIDS are effective models for teaching health-care workers and laypersons about how other infectious diseases are transmitted and for providing personal and community action plans to prevent the spread of infectious agents. Although it is a worldwide epidemic, with an especially high mortality rate in sub-Saharan Africa, AIDS poses a significantly lower *occupational* risk to health-care workers in the developed countries than do other infectious agents.

Pathogenesis In the past five years, we have learned about the dynamics of HIV infection and the development of AIDS. It was first assumed that the virus caused a cellular immune system response and then remained in a dormant phase. The humoral response was known to produce antibodies within 1 to 3 months after infection, with clinical disease developing in from 1 to 10 years. For unexplained reasons, the virus would become active, and the worsening clinical signs were attributed to an increasing viral population. The extent of immune cell activity during the incubation phase, reported to be from months to 10 years, was not immediately understood.

Research in the mid-1980s and early 1990s determined that HIV specifically targets T-lymphocytes with the CD4 marker, a surface molecule that attaches the virus to the cell, and a better understanding of the cellular immune response and CD4 markers emerged. A reasonably reliable correlation between disease progression and the decrease in CD4 T-lymphocyte count was developed. Physicians could predict the development of specific clinical events as the CD4 count decreased. For example, *Pneumocystis carinii* pneumonia (PCP), an opportunistic AIDS infection, frequently develops when CD4 counts drop to a certain level. The CD4 count thus became a guide to diagnosis and treatment. Its usefulness, however, was limited because it only reflected the immune system's destruction.

Recent advances in molecular biology and more reliable and cost-effective assays of proteins and other biochemical molecules have revealed a tremendous increase in virus production immediately after infection and have shown that the immune system increases its activity to counter it. Eventually, the number of immune system cells (T-lymphocytes) offsets the viral load, reflected by the HIV RNA. This equilibrium, or "set point," may take years to establish. Even during the dynamic phase when the equilibrium has not yet been set, measurement of viral load is still the best available indicator of response to therapy and long-term clinical outcome.

Risk to the General Public HIV is transmitted through contact with blood, blood products, and body fluids. The virus has been noted in blood, semen, vaginal secretions, and breast milk. Although not yet reported, tears, amniotic fluid, urine, saliva, and bronchial secretions theoretically may transmit the disease.

The virus can enter the body through breaks in the skin, mucous membranes, the eyes, or by placental transmission. Reports of the transmission rate from mother to infant range from 13 to 30 percent. The virus is most commonly contracted through sexual contact or sharing contaminated needles. Before the initiation of stringent controls in screening donor blood and blood products, hemophiliacs and individuals needing frequent blood transfusions were at increased risk. Other groups initially identified as high risk included IV drug abusers and homosexual or bisexual males. The morbidity of heterosexual transmission of HIV has been steadily increasing, with vaginal and anal sex the primary concerns. The risk of oral sex has not been quantified but is believed to be low. Vector transmission by mosquitoes has been postulated but not yet reported. Coexisting sexually transmitted disease, especially with ulceration, appears to increase the risk of infection in sexual transmission. Ethnicity and gender are not established risk factors, and the period of maximum infectiousness cannot be effectively determined. No recovery from AIDS has ever been reported, although postexposure prophylaxis has been demonstrated to decrease the severity of disease and delay mortality.

Risk to Health-Care Workers Although contact with contaminated blood or body secretions potentially places health-care workers at risk, infection from HIV-positive patients has been exceedingly rare, with an estimated probability of from 0.2 to 0.44 percent after exposure to virus-containing blood. Accidental needle-stick injuries are the most frequent source of infection in health-care workers.

The risk for effective transmission of HIV to health-care workers initially depends on whether the exposure to HIV was percutaneous, mucosal, or cutaneous (to intact skin). Within each of those categories, the risk depends on fluid type. Blood is the most dangerous, followed by fluids that may or may not contain blood: semen, vaginal secretions, and cerebrospinal, synovial, pleural, peritoneal, pericardial, and amniotic fluids. Urine and saliva, unlikely to contain blood, pose a very low risk. Source patients (those possibly infecting health-care workers) who are HIV positive or die within two months after the health-care worker's exposure are considered to increase the risk. The highest risk exposure involves a large volume of blood, high antibody titre against a retrovirus in the source patient, deep percutaneous injury, or actual intramuscular injection.

Clinical Presentation The Centers for Disease Control in the Unites States first established the case definition of what constituted AIDS in 1982. Since then, it has expanded the definition of the syndrome to include other diseases, such as extrapulmonary and pulmonary tuberculosis, recurrent pneumonia, wasting syndrome, HIV dementia, and sensory neuropathy. The AIDS patient may first develop a mononucleosis-like syndrome, with nonspecific signs and symptoms, such as fatigue, fever, sore throat, lymphadenopathy (lymph node disease), splenomegaly (enlarged spleen), rash, and diarrhea. Since not all of those signs are present, the situation may seem so trivial that the patient does not seek health care. Many patients develop purplish skin lesions known as Kaposi's sarcoma. Kaposi's sarcoma is a cancerous lesion that was quite rare until the HIV virus appeared. As the disease progresses, many patients develop life-threatening opportunistic infections, such as *Pneumocystis carinii* pneumonia. Secondary infections caused by *Mycobacterium tuberculosis* may also be present. As AIDS progresses, it involves the central nervous system; dementia, psychosis, encephalopathy, and peripheral neurological disorders may develop.

Postexposure Prophylaxis There is no cure or vaccine for AIDS as yet. After an exposure to a confirmed HIV-positive source patient, the health-care worker should immediately seek evaluation and possible initiation of treatment by an occupational medicine or infectious disease physician. Current Centers for Disease Control (CDC) recommendations establish two hours as the optimum time within which to start postexposure prophylaxis with triple therapy (two reverse transcriptase inhibitors [AZT and 3TC] and one protease inhibitor [IDV]) as the current standard for comparison. This is because early, aggressive treatment may decrease the viral load and alter the set point. Counselling by the IDCO or a trained occupational infectious disease specialist must supplement the postexposure evaluation as part of the agency's exposure control plan. EMS personnel should not attempt to determine their own risk and need for postexposure prophylaxis. Health-care workers have significantly underestimated their own risk and need for medical intervention regarding other infections, and the element of denial in HIV increases that tendency.

Summary of HIV HIV-positive patients generally do not present life-threatening situations to EMS; however, they pose substantial psychosocial challenges. Despite changes in societal attitudes and increased tolerance of differences, HIV-positive individuals are often marginalized and shunned. Their subsequent feeling of social isolation is often worsened by depression. In spite of this, these patients are usually forthcoming about their infection status when dealing with health-care workers. Although a paramedic generally has little to offer in terms of treatment, it is vitally important that care be given in a compassionate, understanding, and nonjudgmental manner. Take appropriate precautions to prevent disease transmission, but if you truly understand the risk as it applies to you as a health-care worker, it should not be a barrier to your providing professional and emotionally supportive care, including a caring touch. In the EMS environment, physical isolation of the HIV-positive patient is unjustified.

Universal (Standard) Precautions Health Canada recommends universal (standard) precautions for health-care workers at increased risk for exposure to HIV and other bloodborne pathogens. Since reliably determining which patients have bloodborne infections is impossible, the following precautions are recommended for all patients.

- All health-care workers should routinely use appropriate barrier precautions to prevent exposure of the skin and mucous membranes to any contact with blood, or other body fluids, from any patient. Wear disposable gloves whenever touching blood and body fluids, mucous membranes, or broken skin; handling items or surfaces soiled with blood or body fluids; and performing venipuncture or other vascular access procedures. Change and discard gloves after contact with each patient. To prevent exposure of the mucous membranes of the mouth, nose, and eyes, wear masks and protective eyewear or protective face shields during procedures likely to aerosolize blood or other body fluids. If a glove is torn or a needle-stick occurs, remove the glove and replace it as soon as possible. Discard the needle or instrument and obtain another. Wear gowns or aprons during any procedure likely to generate splashing of bloods or other body fluids.
- Wash your hands (including the webs between your fingers) and other skin surfaces thoroughly with soap and warm water after removal of gloves and especially after contamination with blood or other body fluids.
- Take precautions to prevent injuries caused by needles, scalpels, or other sharp instruments or devices whenever performing procedures,

cleaning instruments, or disposing of instruments. To prevent needle-stick injuries, needles should not be recapped, purposely bent, broken by hand, removed from disposable syringes, or otherwise manipulated by hand. Position puncture-resistant containers as close as possible to work areas, and place disposable syringes and needles, scalpel blades, and other sharp items in them for disposal.

- Although saliva has not been directly implicated in HIV transmission, use mouthpieces with one way valves or filters, bag-valve-mask devices, and other ventilation devices to avoid mouth-to-mouth contact. Place these resuscitation items where the need for resuscitation is predictable.

- Do not put gloved hands close to your mouth, and avoid wiping your face with your forearms or the backs of your gloved hands. Use clean towels to deal with perspiration.

- If you have exudative or weeping skin lesions, refrain from direct patient care and from handling patient care equipment until the condition resolves.

- Pregnant health-care workers are not believed to be at greater risk of HIV infection than health-care workers who are not pregnant. If a health-care worker develops HIV infection during pregnancy, however, the infant is at risk for transplacental transmission. Therefore, pregnant health-care workers should be especially familiar with, and strictly adhere to, precautions to minimize the risk of HIV transmission.

- Disinfection and sterilization of diagnostic or therapeutic equipment and supplies are mandatory.

Hepatitis

Hepatitis is an inflammation of the liver caused by viruses, bacteria, fungi, parasites, excessive alcohol consumption, or medications. Viruses are by far the most common cause of hepatitis. The clinical signs and symptoms of hepatitis secondary to viral infection are the same, regardless of the type of virus. Initially, they include headache, fever, weakness, joint pain, anorexia, nausea and vomiting, and, in some cases, right upper quadrant abdominal pain. As the disease progresses, the patient may become jaundiced, with fever often resolving at the onset of jaundice. This stage is sometimes marked by a darkened urine and the development of clay-coloured stools. The various types of hepatitis are transmitted in specific ways. Hepatitis A, B, C, D, and E represent the greatest potential for communicable disease. Paramedics who practise universal precautions against bloodborne and fecal-oral transmission will drastically reduce their risk of contracting hepatitis through occupational exposure.

✱ **hepatitis** inflammation of the liver characterized by diffuse or patchy tissue necrosis.

Hepatitis A Hepatitis A (infectious or viral hepatitis) is transmitted by the fecal-oral route. The causative agent, hepatitis A virus, is usually found in the stool of infected persons, who may not exercise suitable personal hygiene. After these individuals handle food or contact another individual even as casually as shaking hands, the virus can then be transmitted via contaminated hands, food, water, ice, and eating utensils. Furthermore, the virus can exist on unwashed hands for as long as four hours. Many hepatitis A infections are asymptomatic. They do not present with obvious signs, such as jaundice, and are recognizable only through liver function studies. This is especially true of children, who represent most cases of infection and often transmit the virus to others by close social contact. Sexual contact can also spread the virus. Transmission by needle-stick injury is unlikely and has not been reported.

Diaper changing, especially in daycare centres with an infected child, is known to increase risk. Travellers to areas with poor sanitary conditions are also at risk. Two inactivated hepatitis A vaccines (Havrix and Vaqta) provide effective active immunization. Health-care workers serving on disaster medical teams to Africa, the Middle East, Central and South America, and Asia should be immunized. Immunization is not generally recommended for health-care workers in Canada but may be advised in some areas where hepatitis A prevalence is unusually high. Passive preexposure immunization with immune globulin (gamma globulin) is therefore falling out of favour, but immunization may be used after exposure in selected incidents.

The hepatitis A virus's incubation period averages from 3 to 5 weeks, with the greatest probability of transmission in the latter half of that period. Afflicted individuals are most infectious during the first week of symptoms. The disease follows a mild course, is rarely serious, and lasts from 2 to 6 weeks.

Hepatitis B The hepatitis B (serum hepatitis) virus is transmitted through direct contact with contaminated body fluids (blood, semen, vaginal fluids, and saliva) and therefore represents a substantial risk to EMS providers. Hepatitis B is much more contagious than HIV. The potential for transmitting hepatitis B following exposure to infected blood ranges from 1.9 to 40 percent and by needle stick from 5 to 35 percent. The incidence of antibodies in hepatitis B in health-care workers has been reported to be two to four times greater than in the community at large. Health-care workers infected by hepatitis B can develop acute hepatitis, cirrhosis, and liver cancer. From 5 to 10 percent of infected health-care workers may become asymptomatic chronic carriers and pose an infection risk to family and other intimate contacts. The effectiveness of the three series of immunizations has been reported to be close to 90 percent in adults and higher in children, but low rates of health-care worker compliance with immunization are distressingly common. No clearly identifiable populations are at risk, except for those individuals who are exposed to high-risk body fluids in the course of their employment.

In the general populace, sexual transmission of hepatitis B is common. Transmission has also been known to occur with transfusion, dialysis, needle and syringe sharing in IV drug use, tattooing, acupuncture, and communally used razors and toothbrushes. The virus is stable on surfaces with dried, visible blood for more than seven days. Infection of toddlers from household contacts with family member carriers has been reported. Transmission by insect vectors or the fecal-oral route has not been reported.

Serum markers that reflect amounts of antigen or antibody from surface or core molecules of the virus reliably reflect active infection, communicability, the window phase of infection, and peak virus replication levels. A detailed discussion of the clinical significance of these markers and how they guide therapy is beyond the scope of this text.

All EMS workers should receive the hepatitis B vaccination series.

Considering what is known about hepatitis B's disease process and its consequences, and the fact that effective vaccines exist, the number of health-care workers who have not been immunized or are unaware of their immune status is alarming. Two vaccines, Recombivax HB and Engerix B, both products of genetic recombinant technology, are available. They are reported to be as effective as the previously available Heptavax, derived from blood plasma, without the risk of HIV transmission or other viral infections. The immunization regimen is a series of three intramuscular injections. Following the initial dose, booster doses are administered at 1 and 6 months. After the immunization regimen, antibody assays are obtained to confirm active immunity.

The target antibody titre is 10 milli-international units per mL (10 mLU/mL), with a recommendation to draw for antibody titre from 4 to 6 weeks after the series is completed. An additional booster may be necessary if the individual does not develop adequate antibody levels. The duration of protection is thought to be five years, perhaps longer. The vaccine is safe in pregnancy. Its side effects include local redness, occasional low-grade fever, rash, nausea, joint pain, or mild fatigue.

Hepatitis B's incubation period lasts from 8 to 24 weeks. Joint pain and rash are more common with hepatitis B infection than with other types of hepatitis, but 60 to 80 percent of hepatitis B infections are asymptomatic.

Hepatitis C Health Canada estimates that 210 000 to 275 000 Canadians are infected with hepatitis C; however, only 30 percent of them know they are infected. Hepatitis C will infect more males than females and people aged 30–39 have the highest rate of infection. It is estimated that 4000 new cases of hepatitis C will occur in Canada each year and that about 63 percent of new infections are related to injection/intravenous drug use. The virus is transmitted primarily by IV drug abuse and sexual contact. Sexual contact, however, does not appear to transmit hepatitis C as effectively as it does hepatitis B. After 1989, effective blood donor screening for hepatitis C practically eliminated the risk of transfusion-associated infection. Fecal-oral transmission and household contact have not been reported as factors in transmission, and no specific groups have been identified to be at greater risk for hepatitis C infection.

Hepatitis C is a chronic condition in about 85 percent of infected people. Because of its chronic nature and its ability to cause active disease years later, it poses a great international public health problem. Antibodies can be produced against hepatitis C and provide the laboratory method for determining infection. However, the antibodies are not effective in eliminating the virus, and their presence does not indicate immunity. The ineffectiveness of antibodies is attributed to the virus's high mutation rate. Consequently, the cellular immune response, which results in the immune system's elimination of infected cells, is very aggressive and is believed, ironically, to cause most of the associated liver injury.

Hepatitis C infection, formerly called non-A, non-B hepatitis, often causes liver fibrosis, which progresses over decades to cirrhosis and is estimated to develop in about 20 percent of infected individuals. This progression is known to be accelerated in persons older than 50 at the time of initial infection, in those consuming more than 50 grams of alcohol per day, and in men. Cirrhosis has also been known to occur in those who have not consumed alcohol and can worsen to end-stage liver disease with jaundice, ascites, and esophageal varices.

No effective vaccination for hepatitis C exists. Treatment with alpha interferon has had limited success, with about 15–20 percent of patients responding positively, as defined by the liver enzymes' return to normal levels. Another drug, ribavirin (an antiviral), administered orally, is known to potentiate interferon's immune system effects, and researchers are now focusing their efforts on improving the results of combination therapy with ribavirin and alpha interferon.

Hepatitis D The hepatitis D virus (HDV), formerly called delta hepatitis, depends on a surface antigen of the hepatitis B virus (HBV) to produce its structural protein shell. Thus, HDV infection seems to exist only with a coexisting HBV infection. Immunization against HBV therefore confers immunity to HDV. When a patient who has HBV infection with liver disease develops an overlying HDV infection, mortality rates are very high.

Hepatitis D seems only to coexist with hepatitis B infection.

Parenteral HDV transmission occurs similarly to HBV in western Europe and North America. Fortunately, cases in health-care workers are extremely rare. Frequent epidemics of nonparenteral transmission occur in central Africa, the Middle East, and the Mediterranean countries. HDV's incubation period has not been determined.

Hepatitis E Hepatitis E (HEV) is transmitted like hepatitis A virus (HAV), through the fecal-oral route, and seems to be associated with contaminated drinking water more commonly than in HAV. It occurs primarily in young adults, with highest rates in pregnant women. First described in India, outbreaks have occurred in Russia, Nepal, Southeast Asia, the Middle East, Pakistan, and China.

Tuberculosis

Tuberculosis (TB) is the most common preventable adult infectious disease in the world. TB is caused by bacteria known collectively as the *Mycobacterium tuberculosis* complex, which includes *M. tuberculosis, M. bovis,* and *M. africanum.* Other bacteria in the *Mycobacterium* family can cause tuberculosis, particularly in immunocompromised patients. These other types of *Mycobacterium* are referred to as atypicals. It primarily affects the respiratory system, including a highly contagious form in the larynx. Untreated or undertreated, it may spread to other organ systems, causing extrapulmonary TB and other complications. The disease appeared about 7000 years ago and peaked in the eighteenth century. The number of new cases in North America has increased steadily since 1985, in large part because of TB in AIDS patients and in recently arrived immigrants from countries where the disease is prevalent and because of other globilization factors.

The development of multidrug-resistant tuberculosis (MDR-TB) has been known since the late 1940s. Drug resistance occurs when drug-resistant bacteria outgrow drug-susceptible bacteria. These bacteria acquire resistance either because of patient noncompliance with therapy or inadequate treatment regimens. Drug resistance occurs early in therapy, especially when only one drug is used. For this reason, most current CDC recommendations for the initiation of therapy in North America involve several options for treatment, each calling for multiple medications, including isoniazid (INH), rifampin, pyrazinamide, ethambutol, and streptomycin, among others.

M. tuberculosis is most commonly transmitted through airborne respiratory droplets but may also be contracted by direct inoculation through mucous membranes and broken skin or by drinking contaminated milk. Animal reservoirs for the bacteria include cattle, swine, badgers, and primates. Coughing and other expiratory actions (sneezing, speaking, singing) create bacteria-containing droplets from 5 to 10 microns in size, which susceptible individuals inhale into the alveoli.

The risk of transmitting tuberculosis is not as high as measles. Although the average case infects only about a third of close contacts, prolonged exposure to a person with active TB is always listed as a risk factor. Communicability varies from case to case. Although a single occupational exposure to a patient with active TB is highly unlikely to transmit the disease to a paramedic, universal precautions against TB should still be employed.

Skin Testing The commonly used purified protein derivative (PPD) skin test effectively identifies candidates for prophylactic drug therapy (to prevent active TB) in large groups of health-care workers. It has limited value in guiding individual therapy in those with active TB because a positive PPD indicates previous infection but does not distinguish active from dormant disease. Another health-care worker experienced in interpreting the results should read the skin test, rather than the worker tested, because health-care workers are known to underinterpret positive results. In addition, the skin test must be interpreted on the basis of the disease's prevalence in the community. A negative test does not rule out active disease, particularly in immunosuppressed individuals or in those who were infected so recently that their immune systems have not yet had time to mount the cellular-mediated response that causes a positive PPD.

Most EMS agencies require skin testing at least annually. This may be sufficient, but again, decisions about the frequency of testing should be based on the disease's prevalence in the community. For individuals who have not been previously skin tested or who have no documentation of a negative PPD in the last 12 months, two-step testing may be reasonable. In these individuals, an initial negative test may be due to weak reactivity to the PPD. A second skin test is administered from 1 to 3 weeks later. A positive reaction to the second test probably represents a boosted reaction, which means that the individual has been previously infected and should be evaluated for possible prophylaxis. If the second test is negative, that individual is classified as uninfected. A positive reaction to any subsequent test would represent a new infection by *M. tuberculosis*.

Pathogenesis TB's incubation period is 4–12 weeks. In most people with subclinical infections, immediate disease (primary TB) does not develop because of a cell-mediated immune response. Development of disease normally occurs 6–12 months after infection. Susceptibility to primary infection is increased in persons who are malnourished and those persons whose immune systems are suppressed, such as the elderly, HIV patients, and people taking immunosuppressant drugs. Children less than three years old are at risk because of underdeveloped immune systems, with older children identified at lowest risk. As expected, the aged are at high risk, and the reactivation of latent infections in this age group implies that the immune system has difficulty dealing with the complex nature of the *M. tuberculosis* infection. Once the bacteria enter the lungs, alveolar macrophages attack them and attempt to "wall them off" (forming granulomas) in a localized immune response. For this reason, most TB infections do not produce disease. Healed sites leave lesions of calcified areas known as Ghon foci. When Ghon foci combine with lymph nodes, they form a Ghon complex, which creates small, sharply defined shadows on a chest x-ray.

If the macrophages cannot destroy them, the bacteria lie dormant within the macrophages and are then distributed to other sites within the body. They remain dormant until some event, usually a depression of the immune system, triggers their reactivation into secondary TB. The sites of reactivation are greatest in areas of the lung with the highest oxygen tension, the apices or upper lobes. Reactivation in extrapulmonary sites, such as lymph nodes, pleura, and pericardium, are much more common in HIV-infected persons. In AIDS patients, the disease may spread to the thoracic and lumbar spine, destroying intervertebral discs and adjacent vertebral bodies. TB is also known to lead to subacute meningitis and granulomas in the brain.

Clinical Presentation The signs and symptoms of active TB can be highly nonspecific and can be manifestations of other clinical conditions. However, a typical list would include chills, fever, fatigue, productive or nonproductive chronic cough, and weight loss. Many patients report night sweats, leaving their bed linens drenched with perspiration. Hemoptysis (expectorating blood) is very suggestive of active TB. Reactivation of dormant TB manifests as signs and symptoms specific to the organ systems involved.

EMS Response Your acceptance of responsibility for protecting yourself from *M. tuberculosis* is the most important step in preventing disease transmission. A proactive response driven by a high index of suspicion is essential. The factors that increase a paramedic's risk of transmission are close and sometimes prolonged contact with the patient. Care and transport are provided in a very small, often ineffectively ventilated space, and the patient may affect various expiratory actions while in contact with EMS personnel. Placing a mask over the patient, when it does not create undue anxiety or dyspnea, effectively decreases the number of expectorated droplet nuclei. Also, nebulized medications may be administered more safely with a nebulization mask. Use appropriate respiratory precautions while performing cardiopulmonary resuscitation (CPR) and intubation.

You should don a protective respirator on contact with a patient you suspect may have TB. Your knowledge of the prevalence of TB and the most susceptible populations in your jurisdiction should reinforce your index of suspicion. The most current Health Canada standards for protecting health-care workers from TB call for N95 **respirators,** which are designed to prevent contaminated air from reaching the health-care workers wearing them (Figure 37-5a). High efficiency particulate aspirator (HEPA) respirators (Figure 37-5b) are no longer required for TB, but EMS agencies may opt to continue their use. They are more expensive, bulky, and sometimes difficult to breathe through.

Masks, as opposed to respirators, work primarily as barriers against larger particles and are not certified to prevent contaminated air from reaching the paramedic. However, they effectively prevent the transmission of many airborne pathogens, especially when both provider and patient wear them. They also provide a more comfortable and cost-effective alternative to the routine use of respirators. The extensive terminology and guidelines relative to the design, construction, and classification of various respirators is beyond the scope of this text. EMS agencies and their IDCOs are responsible for educating their personnel in the proper use and application of respirators and for ensuring proper fit and easy access. According to the National Institute for Occupational Safety and Health (NIOSH) classification, N series respirators provide protection against non-oil-based aerosols, including the droplet nuclei from TB patients. These N-type respirators must filter 95 percent of particles that are no larger than 0.3 microns in diameter, hence the designation N95. This is a very safe standard, since the diameter of TB aerosol droplets ranges from 5 to 10 microns. Health-care workers' noncompliance causes most respirator failures.

Ventilation systems currently being marketed in selected ambulances claim to effectively recycle and filter enough air to ensure the expulsion of infected droplet nuclei. Such ventilation systems should include HEPA (high-efficiency particulate aspirator) filtration in addition to recycling the patient compartment air volume according to Occupational Safety and Health Administration (OSHA) standards. Do not open patient compartment windows to increase ventilation and dilute the concentration of droplet nuclei. The moving ambulance may create a Bernoulli effect that draws engine exhaust, including carbon monoxide, into the patient compartment.

Postexposure Identification and Management Early identification of exposure and drug prophylaxis, if deemed necessary, are the keys to effectively preventing active TB from developing in health-care workers. An occupational medicine physician should assess TB skin test results and determine the appropriateness of chest x-rays, sputum cultures, and a myriad of other diagnostic pro-

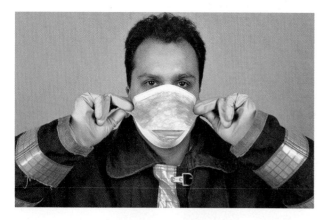

FIGURE 37-5A   NIOSH/OSHA standards call for N95 respirators when caring for patients with tuberculosis.

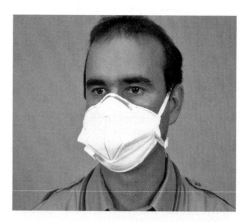

FIGURE 37-5B   EMS agencies may opt to use high-efficiency particulate aspirator (HEPA) respirators for TB.

cedures to confirm infection or the presence of frank disease. The polymerase chain reaction (PCR) test, which eliminates the need to wait for cultures and provides a diagnosis in six hours, may soon become the gold standard for identifying the presence of *M. tuberculosis.*

Pneumonia

Patients with difficulty breathing often challenge paramedics with the enigma of differentiating pneumonia from mild exacerbations of congestive heart failure (CHF) and its more severe form, acute pulmonary edema. The mistaken assumption that a patient has CHF may lead to aggressive treatment that reduces the patient's respiratory drive, dries protective mucous secretions, and contributes to hypotension.

Pneumonia, an acute lung inflammation, is not a single disease but a family of diseases that result from respiratory infection by viruses, bacteria, or fungi. The infectious agent most often associated with pneumonia, and against which the pneumococcal vaccine is targeted, is *Streptococcus pneumoniae*, which are spheres found in pairs or chains. Other microorganisms known to cause pneumonia are *Mycoplasma pneumoniae* (primary atypical pneumonia), *Haemophilus influenzae, Klebsiella pneumoniae, Moraxella catarrhalis, Legionella, Staphylococcus aureus* in nosocomial infections, and *P. carinii.* These agents are also known to cause meningitis, ear infections, and pharyngitis. In addition to droplet nuclei, the infectious agents are also spread by direct contact and through linens soiled with respiratory secretions.

✽ **pneumonia** acute infection of the lung, including alveolar spaces and interstitial tissue.

Those at highest risk for pneumonia are the immunocompromised; patients with sickle cell disease, transplanted organs, cardiovascular disease, diabetes mellitus, kidney disease, multiple myeloma, lymphoma, and Hodgkin's disease; those without functioning spleens; and the elderly, particularly those in common residential situations. Low-birth-weight neonates and malnourished infants are highly susceptible. In otherwise healthy individuals, susceptibility is increased by a previous respiratory infection, such as influenza, exposure to inhaled toxins, chronic lung disease, and aspiration (postalcohol ingestion, near drowning, ingested toxins, or gastric distention from bag-valve-mask ventilation). When patients contract infectious agents of pneumonia outside of a hospital or other health-care institution, they are referred to as cases of community-acquired pneumonia.

History and Assessment Always consider the possibility of community-acquired pneumonia. In geriatric communities where residents live in their own homes but may share common social facilities, ask if neighbours recently have been diagnosed with pneumonia or other respiratory infections. Signs and symptoms in previously healthy individuals include an acute onset of chills, high-grade fever, dyspnea, pleuritic chest pain worsened by deep inspiration, and cough, which may be productive with phlegm of various colours. The absence of fever does not rule out pneumonia. Breath sounds may include adventitious lung sounds (crackles, wheezes) and signs of consolidation. When purulent fluids accumulate in many lobes of the lung because of inflammation, alveoli collapse and their acoustic properties change to those of solid tissue, hence the name *consolidation*. Consolidation causes the expiratory sounds in the peripheral lung fields to develop the same duration as inspiration and to be just as loud. Assessment with pulse oximetry may be useful. In geriatric patients, the only presenting sign may be an altered mental status; fever is often absent, and headache, aches and pain, nausea, diarrhea, and nonproductive cough, if present, do not allow you to rule out pneumonia. In children, fever, tachypnea, and retractions are ominous signs but are not specific to pneumonia; this triad of signs, however, reliably indicates respiratory distress secondary to an infectious process in pediatric patients.

Patient Management and PPE Management of the pneumonia patient aims at supporting adequate ventilation and oxygenation, with supplemental oxygen often providing relief. Always consider TB a possibility in any patient with pneumonia and place a mask either on yourself or on your patient.

Immunization and Postexposure Management An effective vaccination exists against most serotypes of *S. pneumoniae* known to cause disease. It is highly recommended for children two years old or younger, for adults over 65 years old, and for those without spleens. Routine vaccination of EMS workers is not necessary. In health-care settings, health-care workers who routinely treat elderly, immunocompromised, or other at-risk patients may be required to be immunized because they pose the risk of transmission to patients. Because EMS workers are predominantly healthy, exposure to a single patient with pneumonia generally will not result in infection or disease. A number of antimicrobial agents are effective against the infectious agents known to cause pneumonia. However, multidrug-resistant strains have been reported.

SARS

Severe acute respiratory syndrome (SARS) is described as an atypical pneumonia because the symptoms differ from typical pneumonia, which is characterized by severe coughing and inflammation of the lungs as well as fever. The virus that causes SARS is believed to have mutated and crossed over from the avian population to humans.

In March 2003, the first Canadian SARS patient died in Toronto. As the virus spread, Ontario declared a public health emergency and ordered anyone who had set foot in a Toronto hospital to go into immediate quarantine. Many health-care workers were under forced quarantine at home. By April 2003, the number of Canadians with SARS had grown to 187, and the worldwide count was 2484, with 81 deaths.

The signs and symptoms of SARS are those of a respiratory illness of unknown etiology, a temperature of greater than 38°C, and one or more of the following symptoms or signs: cough, shortness of breath, difficulty breathing, hypoxia, or x-ray findings of either pneumonia or acute respiratory distress syndrome (ARDS). The incubation period for SARS is typically 2–7 days, although reports indicate as long as 10 days for some patients. The illness usually begins with a fever that is associated with chills, and rigors and may also be accompanied by headache, malaise, and myalgia. At onset, some people have mild respiratory symptoms. Usually rash and neurological or gastrointestinal findings are absent, although some patients have reported diarrhea.

It appears that SARS is spread from person to person mainly through contact with secretions from the nose, mouth, and throat of an infected person. In addition, contact with articles that may have been in recent contact with infected fluids can result in the spread of the virus. Concern over airborne transmission of the agent has also been raised on the basis of its spread through some apartment buildings in Hong Kong.

Treatment for SARS has included several antibiotics to treat bacterial agents of atypical pneumonia. Some therapy with antiviral agents, such as ribavirin, has been used with some success.

The U.S. Centers for Disease Control (CDC) in Atlanta, Georgia, and Health Canada recommend standard, contact, and airborne precautions when in contact with potential cases. This means that health-care workers must wear eye protection, gowns, gloves, and masks when treating patients. Patients must be kept isolated in negative-pressure rooms in hospitals. For those quarantined at home, it is recommended that they and other members of their family wear filtering masks when around the patient.

Potential SARS patients arriving in hospital or clinic settings should be assessed in a separate area from the rest of the public and should be immediately provided with a mask. Handwashing after every contact with patients or patient articles is essential. Equipment used on potential SARS patients should be disposed of after single-patient use.

Patients should be questioned as to their travel history and potential contact with SARS patients. Any suspected patients should be wearing masks prior to transport and the receiving facility should be notified prior to arrival so that isolation precautions can be initiated immediately.

West Nile Virus

Although first discovered in 1937 in Uganda, West Nile virus did not appear in North America until the summer of 1999, when an outbreak occurred in New York City. During that outbreak, 62 confirmed cases and 7 deaths were attributed to the disease. By 2002, there were 148 probable and 77 confirmed cases in Canada and 3 deaths due to the virus. Four years after its first appearance in 1999, more than 4000 North Americans have contracted the infection.

The disease occurs first in the bird population, commonly in crows and related species. A few species of mosquitoes are then able to transmit the disease from birds to humans by transmitting infected bird blood to the human bloodstream during the mosquito biting process. Although the infection is most commonly transmitted from birds to humans by the mosquito vector, there is a risk of person-to-person transmission through blood transfusions and organ/tissue transplants.

Many people who are infected with West Nile virus show no signs or symptoms of the disease. Those experiencing symptoms typically develop them 3–15 days after the mosquito bite and report mild flu-like symptoms, such as fever, headache, body aches, and fatigue. Some people develop a mild rash or swollen lymph glands. The virus exerts its severe and sometimes fatal effects due to its ability to cross the blood–brain barrier. The infection can then progress to meningitis or encephalitis. Symptoms include rapid onset of severe headache, stiff neck, vomiting, drowsiness, confusion, and muscle weakness and can progress quickly to loss of consciousness. People with weaker immune systems or chronic diseases are at the greatest risk for developing severe symptoms.

Evidence suggests that outbreaks of West Nile virus infections are often preceded by crow die-offs, approximately 2–6 weeks before the virus appears in the human population. The detection of the disease in birds thus becomes a priority for predicting and preventing the occurrence in humans. Citizens are encouraged to be alert to the presence of dead wild birds and report such incidences to their local fish and wildlife agency, which will then remove the birds for testing. While there is no evidence of disease transmission from dead birds to humans, people should not pick up birds without wearing proper protection, such as gloves and a mask.

Human surveillance occurs within the Health Canada reportable disease structure. A blood sample can detect the presence of the virus in humans. Physicians in areas where the virus is present should order this test for anyone who exhibits the signs and symptoms and has a likely history of exposure as well as anyone who experiences signs and symptoms of encephalitis. Health services should make sure that they are notified of the presence of West Nile virus in their communities. Knowing when the disease exists in the bird population can alert EMS personnel to consider the possibility of the infection in patients.

While patients themselves do not pose an infection risk to EMS workers, the environment in which patients are found may be dangerous. EMS personnel should therefore take steps to protect themselves from contracting the infection: EMS should consider uniform issue, including long-sleeved shirts or light jackets and the distribution of appropriate insect repellents or other protection methods effective against mosquito bites.

Chickenpox

Chickenpox is caused by varicella zoster virus (VZV). Varicella zoster virus is in the herpesvirus family. Although chickenpox (**varicella**) in pediatrics is considered a self-limiting disease that rarely causes severe complications, it is much more lethal in adults. It results in fewer than 100 deaths per year in the United States, but while adults represent only 2 percent of the morbidity, they account for 50 percent of the mortality. Thus, health-care workers who have not been immunized against VZV or been exposed to it as children must increase their awareness of this infection and its consequences. It is estimated that 10 percent of adults have not contracted VZV during childhood. VZV is also the infectious agent of shingles (herpes zoster), a painful condition that causes skin lesions along the course of peripheral nerves and dermatome bands. Approximately 15 percent of patients with chickenpox will eventually develop shingles.

Clinical Presentation Chickenpox usually occurs in clusters during winter and spring and presents with respiratory symptoms, malaise, and low-grade fever, followed by a rash that starts on the face and trunk and progresses to the rest of the body, including mucous membranes. The rash may be the first sign of illness, and infected persons may have anywhere from a few to 500 lesions. It is more profuse on the trunk, with less distribution to the extremities and scalp. The fluid-filled vesicles that form the rash soon rupture, forming small ulcers that eventually scab over within one week, at which point the patient is no longer contagious. Transmission occurs through inhalation of airborne droplets and direct contact with weeping lesions and tainted linen. The incubation period is from 10 to 21 days.

In adults, varicella's most common complication is a VZV pneumonia. A large percentage of adult deaths from VZV occur in immunocompromised patients. The most alarming aspect of adult epidemiology, however, is a significant death rate in previously healthy patients. Therefore, it is important for unexposed or unvaccinated paramedics to be immunized.

Assessing Immunity Most people develop immunity for life after recovery from childhood chickenpox infections. Thus, a history of chickenpox is considered adequate evidence of immunity. An available blood test can determine immunity in those who are unsure about their history or who have not had chickenpox.

Immunization A chickenpox vaccine, Varivax, has been available in Canada since 1998. Health Canada recommends that all children entering daycare facilities and elementary schools be vaccinated or have some other evidence of immunity. Such evidence would include a primary care provider's diagnosis of chickenpox, a reliable history of the disease, or blood test confirming immunity. Vaccination is also routinely recommended for all susceptible health-care workers and all other susceptible persons 13 years old or younger, including any adolescents living in the same household with younger children.

The vaccine is administered as one subcutaneous dose in children under age 12 and as two doses in susceptible adolescents and adults. Among vaccinated people 13 years old or older, 78 percent developed protective antibodies, with 99 percent seroconverting after the second dose. Health-care workers who receive the vaccination should have their antibody level checked six weeks after the second vaccination.

Patients with active TB or malignant conditions, or those being treated with immunosuppressants, should not receive the varicella vaccine. Its use in those taking steroids depends on a variety of factors that are beyond the scope of this discussion. Few adverse effects have been reported. The most frequent was rash, with some cases of herpes zoster. No incidents of chickenpox have been reported. Although a few serious adverse effects were reported, no cause-and-effect relationship was clearly established with the vaccination. The vaccine manufacturer discourages taking aspirin within six weeks after receiving the vaccination.

EMS Response and Postexposure Observe universal precautions and place masks on patients. If a patient only has chickenpox, she should remain at home until the lesions are crusted and dry. If a susceptible paramedic is exposed to chickenpox, postexposure vaccination may be warranted. Recent data indicate that if used within three days, and possibly up to five days, Varivax may be effective in preventing chickenpox or lessening its severity. Varicella–zoster immune globulin (VZIG) is an alternative postexposure prophylaxis. Unlike Varivax, it provides passive immunity, and the most current recommendation for its use is in immunocompromised patients. The use of Acyclovir within 24 hours of the onset of rash, which inhibits replication of the virus, may decrease the disease's severity in adults and adolescents.

EMS transport of a patient with chickenpox should be followed by extensive decontamination of the ambulance and any equipment used.

Meningitis

Meningitis is an inflammation of the meninges (the membranes protecting the brain and spinal cord) and cerebrospinal fluid, caused by bacterial and viral infections. Meningococcal meningitis (spinal meningitis), caused by *Neisseria meningitidis*, is the disease variant of greatest concern to EMS personnel.

✱ **meningitis** inflammation of the meninges, usually caused by an infection.

Other agents are, or have been, known to cause meningitis. *Streptococcus pneumoniae*, the primary infectious agent of concern in pneumonia, is the second most common cause of pneumonia in adults and the most common cause of otitis media in children. Vaccines have proven very effective, especially in children. *Haemophilus influenzae* type B, a gram-negative rod, was once the leading cause of meningitis in children aged six months to three years. However, with the implementation of effective childhood vaccination against *H. influenzae* since 1981, *Neisseria meningitidis* has become the bacterium most commonly implicated in serious meningitis cases. Viruses and other microorganisms are known to cause meningitis, with similar disease profiles. Enteroviruses are implicated in 90 percent of patients with viral (aseptic) meningitis. In healthy individuals, viral meningitis is a self-limiting disease that lasts about 7 to 10 days.

Transmission Factors *N. meningitidis* asymptomatically colonizes the upper respiratory tract of healthy individuals and is then transmitted by respiratory droplets. Up to 35 percent of the general population may be infected with the bacterium, which is prevented from gaining access to the cerebrospinal fluid (CSF) by the epithelial lining of the pharynx. Almost every human has probably been a carrier at some point in her life. Conversion from carrier to clinical disease is rare in the developed countries and occurs in clusters in the developing nations. The disease appears to peak in midwinter months with low temperature and humidity. This has been validated by observations of epidemic seasonal variations in the "meningitis belt" of sub-Saharan Africa. Epidemiologists have hypothesized that this pattern may represent a herd immunity, in which host resistance factors may be more a function of the population's general immunity than of the immunity of individuals within that population. One theory that could explain the phenomenon of herd immunity holds that another species within the genus *Neisseria* may be "mistaken" for *N. meningitidis* (a cross-reaction), resulting in effective antibody production against the pathogen. Meningococcal meningitis occurs more commonly in some areas of North America, and the world, for reasons not yet understood. Other factors that have been implicated in the transmission of *N. meningitidis* include contacting oral secretions of the index case (kissing, sharing food or drink), crowding, close contact, smoking, and lower socioeconomic status. For the EMS worker, contact with secretions during mouth-to-mask ventilation, intubation, or suctioning would increase the probability of transmission.

Clinical Presentation The incubation period most commonly ranges from 2 to 4 days but may last as long as 10 days. As with most bacterial infections, signs and symptoms develop rapidly within a few hours or 1–2 days of exposure and include fever, chills, headache, nuchal rigidity with flexion, arthralgia, lethargy, malaise, altered mental status, vomiting, and seizures. An upper respiratory or ear infection may precede the disease. A characteristic rash may appear and develop into hemorrhagic spots, or petechiae. Roughly 10 percent of patients may develop septic shock. Acute adrenal insufficiency, disseminated intravascular coagulation (DIC), and coma are other consequences. Death can ensue in 6–8 hours.

Newborns and infants may seem slow or inactive, vomit, appear irritable, or feed poorly. Fever in newborns should be evaluated with a high index of suspicion for meningococcemia. Rarely, bulging of an open anterior fontanelle is seen. In older children, assessment techniques that stretch the inflamed meninges and cause pain may reveal positive Brudzinski's and Kernig's signs. **Brudzinski's sign** is a secondary assessment finding suggestive of meningitis. Due to irritation of the meninges, flexion of the neck causes flexion of the hips and knees. To test for Brudzinski's sign, have the patient lie supine without a pillow. Flex the neck while observing the hips and knees. Flexion of the hips or knees when the neck is flexed is considered a positive Brudzinski's sign. **Kernig's sign** is likewise suggestive of meningitis. To elicit Kernig's sign, have the patient sit or lie and flex the hips. With the hips flexed, attempt to extend (straighten) the knee. Inability to fully extend the knee is due to meningeal irritation and is considered a positive Kernig's sign. Maternal antibodies protect newborns from meningitis and other infections until up to six months of age (slightly longer in breast-fed children). Infants from six months to two years are especially susceptible to meningitis because they no longer have circulating maternal antibodies and their immune systems are immature and incompetent.

Immunization *N. meningitidis* has several serotypes (A, B, C, X, Y, Z, 29-E, W-135), with B and C causing most disease outbreaks in North America. The A serotype is the most common cause of epidemics in Africa and Asia. An effective vaccine has been developed against the A, C, Y, and W-135 serotypes. Attempts to develop one against the B serotype have so far resulted in weak immune responses. The meningococcal vaccine is not presently recommended for routine immunization of health-care workers. Travellers to endemic areas and children younger than two years who are asplenic (without a spleen) or have a certain deficiency in their complement system are candidates for vaccination.

EMS Response and Postexposure Observing universal precautions and using masks on yourself and/or your patients with suspected meningococcal meningitis will adequately protect you against all the infectious agents of meningitis. Postexposure prophylaxis with rifampin, ciprofloxacin (Cipro), or ceftriaxone (Rocephin) is the primary means of preventing meningococcal disease. Prophylaxis should be started within 24 hours after exposure because the rate of effective transmission in close contacts (EMS personnel) with the index-case patient has been estimated to be 500–800 times that of the general population. Initiation of chemoprophylaxis 14 days or more after the onset of illness in the index case is of limited or no value. All postexposure medications are easily complied with and have few side effects.

* **Brudzinki's sign** physical exam finding in which flexion of the neck causes flexion of the hips and knees.

* **Kernig's sign** inability to fully extend the knees with hips flexed.

Other Job-Related Airborne Diseases

Influenza and colds, rubella, measles, mumps, and respiratory syncytial virus (RSV) are viral infections that may be contracted in the EMS environment. Pertussis, a highly contagious bacterial disease, also poses a risk. These diseases are transmitted by direct inhalation of infected droplets or through exposed mucosal surfaces. Handling contaminated surfaces or objects and subsequently introducing the virus by scratching, wiping, or other activities with unwashed hands (autoinoculation) is another route of transmission. Masks and ventilation are recommended for measles. Precautions against autoinoculation with RSV infections, influenza, and colds include masks, more practically placed on patients, and possibly gloves, gowns, and goggles. Avoid touching your face and areas of broken skin while in contact with the patient. Effective, vigorous handwashing with soap and warm water after patient contact is the most important personal precaution against disease transmission.

Influenza and the Common Cold Influenza is caused by viruses designated types A, B, and C. Within these types are various subtypes that mutate so often that they are identified on the basis of where they were isolated, the culture number, and year of isolation—for instance, A/Japan/305/57. Two glycoproteins, hemagglutinin and neuraminidase, on the outer membrane of an influenza virus determine its virulence. The letters H and N, which denote these two glycoproteins, are often seen in parentheses along with a number, as in A (H1N1). This method of classification helps epidemiologists to more specifically identify a flu virus, since it is based on the immune responses to hemagglutinin and neuraminidase.

Influenza is a leading cause of respiratory disease worldwide, and various strains cause epidemics, mainly during the winter months. It is easily transmittable in crowded spaces, such as public transportation vehicles, and can be spread by direct contact. The virus can persist on environmental surfaces for hours, especially in low humidity and cold temperatures. Thus, it has a high potential for transmission by autoinoculation. It is much more serious than the common cold and has caused worldwide epidemics with high mortality rates. The last great epidemic was in 1918. Health Canada, the CDC, and the World Health Organization (WHO) closely monitor worldwide disease outbreaks.

Influenza is characterized by the sudden onset of fever, chills, malaise, muscle aches, nasal discharge, and cough. The disease is more serious in the very young, the very old, and those with underlying disease. Its incubation period is from 1 to 3 days. Fever generally lasts 3 to 5 days. Signs include mild sore throat, nonproductive cough, and nasal discharge. The cough may be severe and of long duration. Secondary infections may occur as the virus damages respiratory epithelial cells, thereby decreasing resistance to other, primarily bacterial, disorders. Severe cases may result in pneumonia, hemorrhagic bronchitis, and death. The uncomplicated disease usually lasts 2 to 7 days and full recovery is the norm.

Management is primarily supportive. Fever may increase body temperature to as high as 40.6°C. Begin cooling measures for patients with temperatures of 40°C or greater. Increased body temperature may lead to significant insensible fluid loss and dehydration. Determine hydration status early and begin fluid replacement if indicated.

Everyone is susceptible to influenza. Although infection confers resistance after recovery, the influenza viruses mutate so rapidly that protection is effective only against the particular strain or variant from which the person has just recovered. Immunization is available and is recommended for the elderly, those who live or work in correctional institutions, and military recruits. Patients should be immunized between early September and mid-November for maximum effectiveness. Health Canada recommends vaccination for EMS personnel

Content Review

OTHER JOB-RELATED AIRBORNE DISEASES
- Influenza and the common cold
- Measles
- Mumps
- Rubella
- Respiratory syncytial virus
- Pertussis

Effective, vigorous handwashing with soap and warm water after patient contact is the most important personal precaution against disease transmission.

✷ **influenza** disease caused by a group of viruses.

to reduce transmission of influenza to patients and to decrease worker absenteeism. EMS responders who are diabetics, especially those requiring frequent medical followup, are strongly urged to be immunized. Three antiviral drugs—amantadine (Symmetrel), oseltamivir (Tambiflu), and rimantadine (Flumadine)—are available for the prevention and treatment of influenza; however, they only work against the type A influenza virus. They are as effective as vaccines when used preventively, and they shorten the illness's duration when used as a treatment. A new agent, zanamavir (Relenza), which is effective against type B, has been released. However, its use is limited because only 35 percent of influenza cases are type B and because it must be delivered by aerosol nebulizer.

The common cold, or viral rhinitis, is caused by the rhinoviruses, of which there are more than 100 serotypes. Its incidence in Canada rises in fall, winter, and spring, is highest in children younger than five years old, and declines in older adults, displaced by more serious diseases. Transmission is by direct contact, airborne droplets, or more importantly, by hands and linen soiled with discharges from infected individuals. The incubation period ranges from 12 hours to 5 days and averages 48 hours. The disease's course is mild, often without fever and generally without muscle aching. Aside from severity, it is often difficult to differentiate from influenza. Mortality has not been reported, but a cold may lead to more serious complications, such as otitis media and sinusitis.

* **measles** highly contagious, acute viral disease characterized by a reddish rash that appears on the fourth or fifth day of illness.

Measles Measles (rubeola, hard measles), a systemic disease caused by the measles virus of the genus *Morbilli*, is highly communicable. It is most common in children but may affect older persons who have not had it. Immunity following disease is usually lifelong. Maternal antibodies protect neonates for about 4 to 5 months after birth.

Measles is transmitted by inhalation of infective droplets and direct contact. The incubation period ranges from 7 to 14 days, averaging 10. The infection presents prodromally like a severe cold, with fever, conjunctivitis, swelling of the eyelids, photophobia, malaise, cough, and nasopharyngeal congestion. The fever increases, rising to as high as 40.6°–41.1°C, when the rash reaches its maximum. A day or two before the rash develops, Koplik's spots (bluish-white specks with a red halo approximately 1 mm in diameter) appear on the oral mucosa. The red, bumpy (maculopapular) rash normally lasts about six days and spreads from head to feet by the third day. At that point, it appears to thicken on the head and shoulders and then disappear in the same direction as its progression.

Measles is so highly communicable that the slightest contact with an active case may infect a susceptible person. Infectivity is greatest before the prodrome and subsides about four days after the rash appears or as it fades. Everyone should be immunized. Immunization is 99 percent effective in children, for whom vaccination is mandatory, since there is no specific treatment. Unimmunized or previously unexposed paramedics should put masks on their measles patients and be vigilant about handling linens and not touching their faces during and after the call. Postexposure handwashing is critical.

In otherwise healthy children or adults, uncomplicated measles has a low mortality rate. Potential complications include bacterial pneumonia, eye damage, and myocarditis. The most life-threatening sequela is encephalitis in children and adolescents that causes gradual decreases in mental capacity and muscle coordination.

* **mumps** acute viral disease characterized by painful enlargement of the salivary glands.

Mumps The **mumps** virus, a member of the genus *Paramyxovirus*, is transmitted through respiratory droplets and direct contact with the saliva of infected patients. It is characterized by painful enlargement of the salivary glands. Most cases occur in the 5- to 15-year age group. After a 12–25-day incubation period, mumps presents as a feverish cold that is soon followed by swelling and stiffening of the parotid salivary gland in front of the ear. The condition is often found bilaterally. The patient may also experience earache and difficulty chewing and swallowing.

In most cases, the submaxillary and sublingual glands are very tender to palpation. Most cases resolve spontaneously within one week without intervention.

Mumps occurs in epidemics, with danger of transmission beginning one week before the infected person feels sick and lasting about two weeks. Lifelong immunity is generally conferred after infection, even in the absence of disease (subclinical infection).

Mumps is generally benign and self-limiting; however, complications may occur. In postpubescent patients, inflammation of the testicles (orchitis), breasts (mastitis), or ovaries (oophoritis) may occur but is of short duration and of no serious consequence. Meningoencephalitis is fairly common but resolves without residual neurological sequelae.

A mumps live-virus vaccine is available and should be administered with measles and rubella vaccines to all children over one year old. Mumps is not easily transmitted, and with standard body substance isolation (BSI) precautions, the risk of contracting the disease is minimal. For the benefit of their patients, EMS workers should not work without an established mumps/measles/rubella (MMR) immunity.

Rubella Rubella (German measles) is a systemic viral disease caused by the rubella virus, of the genus *Rubivirus*, transmitted by inhalation of infective droplets. Generally milder than measles, it is characterized by sore throat and low-grade fever, accompanied by a fine pink rash on the face, trunk, and extremities that lasts about three days. The incubation period is 12–19 days, with natural infection conferring lifelong immunity, as does immunization. Transfer of maternal antibodies does not confer lifelong immunity but does protect the neonate. There is no specific treatment for rubella. More serious complications that occur in measles do not occur in rubella, but young females sometimes develop a short course of arthritis.

Rubella is devastating to a developing fetus. Mothers infected during the first trimester are at risk for abnormal fetal development, with offspring often developing congenital rubella syndrome and shedding large quantities of virus in their secretions. An infant acquiring this infection *in utero* (in the uterus) is likely to have mental retardation and suffer eye inflammation, deafness, and congenital heart defects. All women, therefore, should be immunized against rubella before becoming pregnant.

Vaccines for measles, mumps, and rubella are commonly combined in an MMR vaccination, which can be given safely with the varicella vaccine. Immunization is 98–99 percent effective but is not recommended for pregnant women because of a theoretical possibility of birth defects. Health-care workers have been identified as the source in numerous outbreaks. For this reason, and for their own protection, all EMS providers should be required to receive the MMR vaccination before they are allowed to work. Immunizations, along with placing a mask on the patient, are an effective method of preventing these diseases.

Respiratory Syncytial Virus Respiratory syncytial virus (RSV) is one of the most common causes of pneumonia and bronchiolitis in infants and young children. In this age group, RSV may be fatal. In older children and adults, RSV is less common, and its symptoms are generally milder. RSV is often associated with outbreaks of lower respiratory infections from November to April. If a patient with pneumonia or bronchitis simultaneously contracts this virus, the disease becomes more severe. RSV commonly begins as an upper respiratory infection and is often misdiagnosed as a simple cold. Children with RSV infection will initially develop a runny nose and nasal congestion. Later, this will spread to lower airway involvement evidenced by wheezing, tachypnea, and signs of respiratory distress. It is a common infection that can be diagnosed by a rapid assay using nasal washings. In winter months, wheezing in children under a year of age should be presumed to be due to RSV until proven otherwise. High-risk children (those

* rubella (German measles) systemic viral disease characterized by a fine pink rash that appears on the face, trunk, and extremities and fades quickly.

> *Paramedics should not be allowed to work until they have received the MMR vaccination.*
>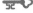

* respiratory syncytial virus (RSV) common cause of pneumonia and bronchiolitis in children.

with congenital heart conditions, prematurity, or cancers, for instance) can be treated with the antiviral agent ribavirin (Virazole). However, this treatment is quite expensive and poses a significant risk to the fetuses of pregnant health-care workers. Postexposure prophylaxis with RSV immune globulin is also an option.

Pertussis The word *pertussis* means "violent cough." **Pertussis** (whooping cough) is caused by the bacterium *Bordetella pertussis,* affecting the oropharynx in three clinical phases after an incubation period of from 6 to 20 days. The *catarrhal phase,* characterized by symptoms similar to those of the common cold, lasts from 1 to 2 weeks. The *paroxysmal phase,* during which the fever subsides, can last a month or longer. The patient develops a mild cough that quickly becomes severe and violent. Rapid consecutive coughs are followed by a deep, high-pitched inspiration. (This characteristic "whoop" often is not present in infants and adults.) The cough often produces large amounts of thick mucus, and vomiting may also occur. Sustained coughing may lead to increased intracranial pressure and intracerebral hemorrhage. Continually high intrapulmonary pressure and vigorous chest movement may cause pneumothorax. During the *convalescent phase,* the frequency and severity of coughing attacks decrease, and the patient is not contagious.

The widespread vaccination of children in a combination diphtheria-pertussis-tetanus (DTP) vaccine caused a dramatic decrease in the incidence of pertussis until the early 1980s. Over the past 20 years, however, its incidence has steadily grown, with the greatest increase in persons aged five years or older. This has occurred in spite of unprecedented pertussis vaccination coverage. One factor in the increase may be a waning effectiveness of the vaccine among adolescents and adults vaccinated during childhood. Although disease is likely to confer immunity against pertussis, the duration of that immunity is unknown. Previously immunized and exposed adolescents and adults therefore may be at risk of infection. Thus, booster doses are recommended.

For patients with pertussis, emergency medical service is most likely to be requested during the paroxysmal phase, when the primary treatment will be calming and oxygenating the patient. Anticipate the need to intubate patients with respiratory failure and to perform chest decompression for those whose coughing paroxysms might have caused a pneumothorax. During the response, remember that pertussis is highly contagious. Fortunately, the communicable period is thought to be greatest before the paroxysmal phase. Transmission occurs via respiratory secretions or in an aerosolized form. Put a mask on the patient, and observe standard BSI precautions, including postexposure hand washing.

Everyone is susceptible to *B. pertussis* infection. Routine immunization of EMS workers against pertussis is not yet recommended. Evaluation of pertussis vaccination is ongoing, however; and considering the unknown duration of immunity with past immunization or exposure, adolescent and adult immunization may be recommended in the future. Erythromycin is known to decrease the period of communicability but can reduce symptoms only if administered before the onset of violent coughing.

Viral Diseases Transmitted by Contact

Mononucleosis and herpex simplex type 1 infections pose little risk to EMS providers who observe BSI precautions and wash their hands after patient contact. Since these diseases cause relatively minor symptoms, patients may not even be aware of their infection status. The public is highly aware of these two diseases, however, and so as health-care providers, paramedics should be familiar with them.

Content Review

PHASES OF PERTUSSIS
• Catarrhal
• Paroxysmal
• Convalescent

Content Review

VIRAL DISEASES TRANSMITTED BY CONTACT
• Mononucleosis
• Herpes simplex virus Type 1

Mononucleosis Mononucleosis is caused by Epstein-Barr virus (EBV). It affects the oropharynx, tonsils, and the reticuloendothelial system (the phagocytes). A 4- to 6-week incubation period precedes the development of symptoms, which characteristically begin with fatigue. Fever, severe sore throat, oral discharges, and enlarged, tender lymph nodes generally follow several days to weeks later. Splenomegaly (enlargement of the spleen) is present in approximately one-half of patients. The disease is common; more than 95 percent of the general population has antibodies to the virus. One-half of all children will have contracted it before the age of five years. Infection by EBV generally confers immunity for life.

Mononucleosis is most commonly transmitted through oropharyngeal contact involving the exchange of saliva between an uninfected person and one who has the disease but who is asymptomatic. Kissing is implicated in adolescents and adults, and transmission from caregivers to young children is common. Blood transfusions can be a mode of transmission, with only a few cases of disease attributed to it. Active disease is most common in those between 15 and 25 years of age. The risk of contracting the disease without close facial contact is minimal. Symptoms generally dissipate within a few weeks, but full recuperation may take several months. There is no specific treatment for mononucleosis, and immunization is unavailable. Corticosteroids are occasionally administered to help minimize tonsillar swelling. Nonsteroidal anti-inflammatory drugs (NSAIDs) may provide symptomatic relief.

Herpes Simplex Virus Type 1 There are two types of **herpes simplex virus,** herpes simplex virus type 1 (HSV-1) and herpes simplex virus type 2 (HSV-2). HSV-2 will be discussed in the section on sexually transmitted diseases. HSV-1 is transmitted in the saliva of carriers and commonly infects the oropharynx, face, lips, skin, fingers, and toes. Everyone is susceptible. Infections of health-care workers' hands and fingers can result in herpetic whitlow, weeping inflammations at the distal fingers and toes. The incubation period following exposure ranges from 2 to 12 days. In the oral cavity, fluid-filled vesicles develop into cold sores or fever blisters that soon deteriorate into small ulcers. Fever, malaise, and dehydration may accompany these primary lesions. The lesions usually disappear in 2 to 3 weeks. They may recur spontaneously, especially following periods of stress or other illness. Recurrent HSV labialis (lip lesions) may cause problems for many years in some adults.

Although primarily recognized for causing skin and mucous membrane disorders, HSV-1 can cause meningoencephalitis in newborns and aseptic meningitis in adults. A high index of suspicion for HSV-1 in these situations may result in timely treatment with antiviral agents, such as acyclovir, which is somewhat effective against HSV-1.

Universal precautions, primarily gloves, are absolutely essential, especially if an intimate contact or family member of the EMS worker is afflicted. Breaks in the skin place everyone at greater risk and may not be visible to the naked eye. Treatment with acylovir (Zovirax) provides relief when used topically or orally. Immunization is not available.

OTHER INFECTIOUS CONDITIONS OF THE RESPIRATORY SYSTEM

The majority of profiles in this section discuss pathological conditions of the airway caused by a variety of infectious agents. They are not diseases, per se. Chapter 42 on pediatrics discusses croup and epiglottitis in greater detail. Hantavirus is included here, although its sites of pathology extend beyond the airways.

Epiglottitis Epiglottitis is an inflammation of the epiglottis and may also involve the areas just above and below it. In children, it is a true emergency, usually caused

✱ **mononucleosis** acute disease caused by the Epstein-Barr virus.

✱ **herpes simplex virus** organism that causes infections characterized by fluid-filled vesicles, usually in the oral cavity or on the genitals.

Content Review

OTHER INFECTIOUS RESPIRATORY CONDITIONS
- Epiglottitis
- Croup
- Pharyngitis
- Sinusitis
- Hantavirus

✱ **epiglottitis** infection and inflammation of the epiglottis.

✱ **croup** viral illness characterized by inspiratory and expiratory stridor and a seal-bark-like cough.

✱ **pharyngitis** infection of the pharynx and tonsils.

✱ **sinusitis** inflammation of the paranasal sinuses.

✱ **hantavirus** family of viruses that are carried by the deer mouse and transmitted by ticks and other arthropods.

by *H. influenzae*, with an abrupt onset over several hours and without any immediate history of upper respiratory disease. Patients present with one or more of the "four Ds:" dysphonia, drooling, dysphagia, or distress. Epiglottitis can also occur in teenagers and adults. In the older age groups, stridor, sore throat, fever, and drooling usually develop over days, not hours. Due to natural immunity from initial infection, epiglottitis is not known to recur in any age group. Increased immunization against *H. influenzae* has reduced the incidence of epiglottitis caused by this bacterium. However, *S. pneumoniae* and *S. aureus* have been implicated as causative agents of epiglottitis.

Croup Croup (laryngotracheobronchitis) is a common cause of acute upper airway obstruction in children. A viral illness characterized by inspiratory and expiratory stridor and a seal-bark-like cough, it is most common in children under the age of three. Although generally not life threatening, croup may create panic in parents and children alike. Viruses implicated in croup include the parainfluenza viruses, rhinoviruses, and RSV. Croup is often preceded by an upper respiratory infection. The child commonly awakens during the night with acute respiratory distress, tachypnea, and retractions. Seasonal outbreaks of this disease are common. Total airway obstruction is rare.

Pharyngitis Pharyngitis is a common infection of the pharynx and tonsils. It may be caused by a virus or bacterium and is characterized by a sudden onset of sore throat and fever. The tonsils and palate become red and swollen, and the cervical lymph nodes enlarge. Headache, neck pain, nausea, and vomiting may also be present. Most cases occur in late winter and early spring. Although this disease may occur in any age group, most cases are seen in five- to eleven-year-olds.

Group A *Streptococcus* (strep throat) causes a particularly serious pharyngitis that, if left untreated, in certain cases, can progress to rheumatic fever. There are several subtypes of Group A *Streptococcus*. One strain causes rheumatic fever. Another strain is responsible for scarlet fever (scarletina). Patients infected with this bacterium may present with a scarlet-coloured rash. Because strep throat is very contagious, you should wear a mask when assessing and managing these patients. Although laboratory tests can easily determine which cases of pharyngitis are caused by *Streptococcus*, it is virtually impossible to tell clinically. Assume that all cases of pharyngitis are serious and contagious until proven otherwise. Antibiotics (penicillin, amoxicillin, erythromycin, azithromycin) effectively treat "strep throat."

Sinusitis Sinusitis is an inflammation of the paranasal (ethmoid, frontal, maxillary, or sphenoid) sinuses. It occurs when mucus and pus cannot drain and become trapped in the sinus. Sinusitis is usually preceded by a viral upper respiratory infection or exposure to allergens, either of which may cause nasal congestion and blocked sinus passages. Postnasal drip may develop and nasal drainage may be blood tinged and purulent. As fluids collect in the sinus, a sensation of pressure or fullness generally develops. If left untreated, the condition may become painful, and the infection can cause an abscess or spread into the cranium and attack the brain. Discomfort often worsens when the patient bends forward or when pressure is applied over the affected sinus. Sinusitis is occasionally a causative factor of meningitis. Management includes antibiotics, decongestants, and supportive care. Apply a heat pack directly over the affected sinus to help relieve pain and facilitate drainage.

Hantavirus Hantavirus is a family of viruses carried by rodents, such as the deer mouse. Other known carriers are the rice rats and cotton rats in the southeastern United States and the white-footed mouse of the northeastern states and western Canada. The common house mouse is not known to carry the virus. The first known case of hantavirus infection occurred in the southwestern United States, particularly the Four Corners region, in 1993. Transmission is primarily by inhalation of aerosols created by stirring up the dried urine, saliva, and fecal droppings of these rodents. Contamination of food and autoinoculation after handling objects tainted by rodent droppings may also cause transmission. Direct bites are possible routes but are thought to be rare. Person-to-person transmission is not possible.

The virus causes hantavirus pulmonary syndrome (HPS), to which anyone is susceptible. The initial symptoms are fatigue, fever, and muscle aches, especially of the large muscle groups. Headaches, nausea, vomiting, diarrhea, and abdominal pain are also common. Earache, sore throat, and rash are uncommon. Approximately 4 to 10 days later, symptoms of pulmonary edema occur. Patients with fatal infections appear to have severe myocardial depression, which can progress to sinus bradycardia and subsequent electromechanical dissociation, ventricular tachycardia, or fibrillation. Hemodynamic compromise occurs a median of five days after onset of symptoms—usually dramatically within the first day of hospitalization. The only specific treatment is intensive supportive care. No immunization is available.

EMS workers who find themselves in dusty, unoccupied buildings for extended times should wear face masks to prevent inhaling aerosolized rodent droppings.

GI SYSTEM INFECTIONS

You may, on occasion, respond to scenes with single or multiple cases of foodborne illness. Although you cannot determine the causative agent outside of the hospital, you must have a basic knowledge of the infectious process and guidelines for assessment, management, and safe handling of these patients. Many EMS personnel are being recruited and volunteering for domestic and international disaster medical teams. In these situations, when the sanitation infrastructure (water treatment and distribution, sewer, animal control, and so forth) are disrupted, GI system infections increase significantly.

Gastroenteritis

Gastroenteritis is a gastrointestinal disorder manifested by nausea, vomiting, gastrointestinal cramping or discomfort, anorexia, and diarrhea. In more advanced cases, which are rare, it can cause lassitude and shock. It is a common disease that many of us have experienced. The reference to "stomach flu" in these situations is incorrect, since an influenza of the GI system has not yet been identified. What this distressing and uncomfortable condition usually represents, at least in the developed countries, is a viral gastroenteritis. The causative agents may be viruses (Norwalk virus, Rotavirus, and others), bacteria (*Escherichia coli, Klebsiella pneumoniae, Campylobacter jejuni, Enterobacter aerogenes, Vibrio cholerae, Shigella,* and *Salmonella*), and parasites (*Giardia lamblia, Cryptosporidium parvum, Cyclospora cayetansis*). Gastroenteritis is highly contagious via the fecal-oral route, including the ingestion of contaminated food and water. It is especially contagious during natural disasters in epidemic proportions. International travellers into endemic areas are highly susceptible, while native populations are generally resistant.

In otherwise healthy persons, gastroenteritis is generally self-limiting and benign; however, in the very young, the very old, or those with preexisting disease, it can be serious and often fatal. Prolonged vomiting and/or diarrhea may result in dehydration and electrolyte disturbances. Patients generally experience painful and severe abdominal cramping, and some develop hypovolemic shock. Always consider dehydration in any patient who presents with signs of gastroenteritis. If a patient has vomited many times or is actively vomiting, has multiple medical

* **gastroenteritis** generalized disorder involving nausea, vomiting, gastrointestinal cramping or discomfort, and diarrhea.

problems, is debilitated, or at risk by virtue of age and general health, start an IV with isotonic saline. Pay careful attention to hydration status. If the patient is in shock, the management objectives are no different from those for hemorrhagic shock. If the patient is not in shock, the judicious use of fluids is warranted. A good rule of thumb is to replace fluids at approximately the rate they are lost. The WHO and other international disaster-response agencies have found oral rehydration very effective in treating fluid loss, even with cholera. Do not feel compelled to pour in IV fluids. If prolonged vomiting or retching is present, administer an antiemetic, such as droperidol, prochlorperazine, or promethazine (Phenergan). Remember that vehicle movements often aggravate symptoms and increase the probability of vomiting.

With isolated cases of gastroenteritis, compliance with universal precautions and postexposure handwashing are critical to avoiding infection. In times of disaster, EMS workers must be more focused on environmental health and sanitation issues: preparing food, identifying clean sources of water, using mosquito netting while sleeping, and maintaining general sanitation. Eat hot foods only and drink hot beverages that have been brisk boiled. Be careful to avoid personal habits that facilitate fecal-oral transmission. Prevention is important because even though antimicrobials may be available to treat isolated cases, resources for treating gastroenteritis during disasters or in the developing countries may be limited. In those situations, many people receive symptomatic treatment.

Food Poisoning

✻ food poisoning nonspecific term often applied to gastroenteritis that occurs suddenly and that is caused by the ingestion of food containing preformed toxins.

Food poisoning is a nonspecific term often applied to gastroenteritis. Food poisoning occurs suddenly and is caused by eating contaminated food. Diarrhea, vomiting, and gastrointestinal discomfort characterize its more benign presentation. Most cases are caused by bacteria and their toxic products. In the majority of cases, only the GI system is affected, but other systems may be affected in some cases, as with botulism or *Escherichia coli* O157:H7, causing debilitating illness or death. *Clostridium botulinum* produces a very potent neurotoxin that causes flaccid paralysis by blocking the release of acetylcholine at motor end plates and preganglionic autonomic synapses.

E. coli O157:H7, transmitted by the ingestion of uncooked or undercooked ground beef, often causes severe bloody diarrhea and abdominal cramps; sometimes the infection causes nonbloody diarrhea or no symptoms. Drinking unpasteurized milk and swimming in or drinking sewage-contaminated water can also cause infection. Little or no fever is usually present, and the illness resolves in 5 to 10 days. In some persons, particularly children under five years of age and the elderly, the infection can cause a complication called hemolytic uremic syndrome, in which the red blood cells are destroyed and the kidneys fail. About 2–7 percent of infections lead to this complication.

Other bacteria implicated in food poisoning include *Campylobacter, Salmonella, Shigella,* and *Vibrio cholerae.* Microorganisms may be transmitted in meats that are insufficiently cooked. *Salmonella* is commonly transmitted through incompletely cooked poultry. It may also be spread through contaminated cookware and utensils used in preparation of poultry. Hepatitis A and Norwalk virus are known to have been ingested in undercooked seafood. Bacterial gastrointestinal infections tend to be much more severe than viral gastrointestinal infections. With bacterial infections, the patient will appear more toxic. There is often a history of bloody, foul-smelling diarrhea (especially with shigellosis). The presence of leukocytes in a fecal smear is suggestive of bacterial disease. Ultimately, stool cultures are required to confirm a bacterial cause of gastroenteritis.

Initiate standard advanced life support (ALS) protocols, including assessment of airway and ventilatory status, oxygenation, initiation of an IV, and cardiac monitoring. Fluid resuscitation with isotonic crystalloids is often required. It is not uncommon for an adult with severe gastroenteritis to require 2–3 litres of fluid. In patients with significant vomiting or diarrhea, also consider antiemetics. Constant reassessment of ventilatory status is essential since the neurotoxin in *C. botulinum* ingestion may cause respiratory arrest. Observing universal precautions should protect against foodborne transmission of infectious agents. No immunization against these agents or their toxins exists.

Prevention efforts are the primary means of reducing foodborne illness. Advances in technology may provide better alternatives for food supply surveillance, an aspect of foodborne disease prevention that could be improved. Lawrence Berkeley National Laboratory has developed plastic strips that turn from blue to red in the presence of toxic strains of *E. coli*. This technology's basis could become a prototype for other simple reagent strips that can detect foodborne pathogens.

NERVOUS SYSTEM INFECTIONS

Encephalitis, rabies, tetanus, and Lyme disease all have significant effects on the nervous system. These infectious conditions or diseases do not necessarily pose occupational risks to EMS providers. They are well known to the general public, however, and are very much associated with recreational activities in which context EMS personnel are called for.

Encephalitis

Encephalitis is an inflammation caused by infection of the brain and its structures, usually by such viruses as equine viruses, arboviruses, the rubella virus, or the mumps virus. These viral infections usually result in one of the following:

1. They cause no pathology until they are transported to the cerebral neurons, which they invade, and then replicate (the rabies and arthropod-borne viruses, for instance).
2. They first injure nonnervous tissues and then, rarely, invade the cerebral neurons (for example, herpes simplex 1 and varicella-zoster virus).

Bacteria, fungi, or parasites may also cause encephalitis, but the viruses are the predominant infectious agents.

The clinical presentation of encephalitis is similar to that of meningitis, since they often coexist. Signs and symptoms include decreased level of consciousness, fever, headache, drowsiness, coma, tremors, and stiff neck and back. Seizures may occur in patients of any age but are most common in infants. Characteristic neurological signs include uncoordinated and involuntary movements, weakness of the arms, legs, or other portions of the body, or unusual sensitivity of the skin to various types of stimuli.

Treatment is difficult, even when the virus has been identified. Despite the severity of illness, many patients suffer no long-term neurological deficits; however, as many as 50 percent of children younger than one year may suffer irreversible brain damage after contracting eastern or western equine encephalitis, which are diseases of horses and mules transmitted to humans by mosquitoes.

Rabies

Rabies is transmitted by the rabies virus, a member of the Rhabdovirus family and *Lyssavirus* genus, which affects the nervous system. It exists in two epidemiological forms: *urban*, propagated chiefly through unimmunized domestic dogs and

---

Content Review

NERVOUS SYSTEM INFECTIONS
- Encephalitis
- Rabies
- Tetanus
- Lyme disease

✳ **encephalitis** acute infection of the brain, usually caused by a virus.

✳ **rabies** viral disorder that affects the nervous system.

cats, and *sylvatic,* propagated by skunks, foxes, raccoons, mongooses, coyotes, wolves, and bats. Humans are especially susceptible when bitten by infected animals. The virus is transmitted in the saliva of infected mammals by bites, an opening in the skin, or direct contact with a mucous membrane. It passes along motor and sensory fibres to the spinal ganglia corresponding to the site of invasion, and then to the brain, creating an *encephalomyelitis* that is almost always fatal. Although rare, transmission is also known to occur by inhalation of aerosolized virus, through nasal nerve fibres and mucosa, along the olfactory nerve, and then to the brain. Mammals are highly susceptible to infection. Transmission is known to be affected by the severity of the wound, abundance of the nerve supply close to the wound, the distance to the CNS, the amount and strain of virus, protective clothing, and other undetermined factors. The highly variable incubation period is usually from 3 to 8 weeks but can be as short as 9 days (rare) or as long as 10 years. It is believed to be dependent on the bite site, with bites to the head and neck generally followed by shorter incubation periods.

Rabies is characterized by a nonspecific *prodrome* (symptoms that precede the appearance of a disease) of malaise, headache, fever, chills, sore throat, myalgias, anorexia, nausea, vomiting, and diarrhea. The prodrome typically lasts from 1 to 4 days. The next phase, the *encephalitic phase,* begins with periods of excessive motor activity, excitation, and agitation. This is soon followed by confusion, hallucinations, combativeness, bizarre aberrations of thought, muscle twitches and tetany, and seizures. Soon, focal paralysis appears. When left untreated, it can cause death within 2 to 6 days. Attempts to drink water may produce laryngospasm, causing the characteristic profuse drooling commonly known as hydrophobia (fear of water).

Rabies is prevalent in Canadian wildlife but still rare in humans with only 22 cases reported between 1956 and 2000. Wild animals are identified as the most important potential source of infection for humans and domestic animals. In Africa, Asia, and Latin America, dogs remain the major source. Bat rabies is found in all regions across Canada, and bats have been implicated as important wildlife reservoirs for rabies virus transmission to humans, particularly in the United States. The CDC estimates that up to one-third of persons who have contracted rabies cannot accurately recollect having been bitten by an animal. Thus, epidemiologists now believe that the inhalation route, once thought to be theoretical, may be more common than previously believed. Human-to-human transmission of rabies is not known to occur; however, paramedics should take body substance isolation (BSI) precautions to protect themselves from contact with infectious saliva. The use of masks in an environment where a patient has been exposed may be prudent, judging from the recent epidemiological evidence in the United States with bats. Currently the National Advisory Committee on Immunization recommends postexposure prophylaxis in persons who slept in a room where a bat was present and they cannot reasonably exclude the possibility of a bite with any certainty.

When caring for a bite patient, first inspect the site of the wound for bite pattern and the presence of saliva. Then, rinse the wound with copious amounts of normal saline to remove saliva and blood. Do not bandage or dress the wound, but allow it to drain freely during transport. Irrigation en route from a 10- or 15-drop/mL IV administration set may be beneficial. If the patient refuses transport to the emergency department, you must inform her of the consequences of the bite and the importance of medical followup. If time and circumstances permit, ensure that the suspect animal has been secured and contained for transport to the hospital or animal control shelter for subsequent postmortem examination of cerebral tissue.

If you are bitten or exposed to an animal you believe is rabid, take the following measures:

1. Vigorously wash the wound with soap and warm water.

2. Débride and irrigate the wound, and allow it to drain freely on the way to the emergency department.

3. Discuss postexposure prophylaxis with the physician. Consultation with public health officials may be necessary. Unless you have an actual bite from an animal whose behaviour is consistent with rabies infection, exposure is a medical urgency, not emergency.

4. Consider the need for tetanus and other antibiotic therapy as the attending physician deems appropriate.

Several alternatives now exist for rabies immunization. Individuals who should be immunized include animal care workers and shelter personnel, and those who work outdoors and have frequent contact with wild animals known to transmit rabies.

Tetanus

Tetanus is an acute bacterial infection of the central nervous system. It presents with musculoskeletal signs and symptoms caused by tetanospasmin, an exotoxin of the *Clostridium tetani* bacillus. *C. tetani* is present as extremely durable spores in the soil, street dust, and feces and is in the same genus as *C. perfringens*, the causative organism of gas gangrene. Since the *Clostridium* species favour an anaerobic environment, the bacteria are particularly suited to colonizing dead or necrotic tissue. Infection has been contracted through wounds considered too minor to warrant medical attention and through burns. Although puncture wounds are classically associated with *C. tetani* infection, deep lacerations can also be suitable environments. Transmission can even occur by injection of contaminated drugs and surgical procedures, leading to the conclusion that *C. tetani* spores are found everywhere. The incubation period is variable (usually from 3 to 21 days, sometimes from one day to several months) and depends on the wound's severity and location. Generally, a shorter incubation period leads to a more severe illness. The mortality rate increases in direct proportion to age. The general population is susceptible, but incidence is highest in agricultural areas where unimmunized people are in frequent contact with animal feces. The disease is rare in Canada, with fewer than 10 cases reported each year.

Localized tetanus symptoms include rigidity of muscles in close proximity to the injury site. Subsequent generalized symptoms may include pain and stiffness in the jaw muscles and may progress to cause muscle spasm and rigidity of the entire body. Respiratory arrest may result. In children, abdominal rigidity may be the first sign. Rigidity occurs after the toxin is taken up at the myoneural junction and transported to the CNS. The toxin then acts on inhibitory neurons, which normally suppress unnecessary efferent impulses and muscle movements. The reduction in inhibitory action results in the muscles' receiving more nervous impulses and tetany. Sometimes, a sardonic grin, *risus sardonicus*, accompanies the lock jaw and conjures memories of the Cheshire Cat in *Alice in Wonderland*.

EMS personnel will rarely encounter this disease, much less recognize its signs and symptoms until they are advanced to the point of tetany. A possible EMS scenario would be the transfer of a patient from a rural community hospital to an urban medical centre for intensive care. Universal precautions should provide adequate protection. Masks probably are not necessary unless the infectious agent is unknown. Respiratory arrest is a possibility, and so you should consider wearing masks while performing endotracheal intubation. If you incur a wound in the course of treating a patient, wash the wound thoroughly or, if warranted, have it inspected and débrided in the emergency department. Wounds that are cared for within six hours pose a lower risk for growth of anaerobic microorganisms. Consideration should be given to postexposure prophylaxis

✳ **tetanus** acute bacterial infection of the central nervous system.

with tetanus immune globulin (TIG), diphtheria-tetanus toxoid (Td), or diphtheria-tetanus toxoid-pertussis (DTP).

Immunizations, which generally begin in childhood as DTP vaccinations, include boosters before entering elementary school and every 10 years thereafter. A booster administered every 10 years is believed to confer effective active immunity. Previous documented infection is not known to confer lifelong immunity.

Lyme Disease

❋ Lyme disease recurrent inflammatory disorder caused by a tick-borne spirochete.

Lyme disease is a recurrent inflammatory disorder accompanied by skin lesions, polyarthritis, and involvement of the heart and nervous system. Caused by the tick-borne spirochete *Borrelia burgdorferi,* similar in shape to the causative organism of syphilis, it is the most commonly reported vector-borne disease in North America. The tick that carries Lyme disease is very common in the northeast, the upper midwest, and along the Pacific Coast of the United States. Deer and mice are both reservoirs of the tick, and the disease is common in people living and recreating near wooded areas with high deer populations. Most infections occur in spring and summer, when tick exposure is most likely. Everyone is susceptible, and natural infection does not appear to confer immunity. The incubation period ranges from 3 to 32 days.

Lyme disease progresses in three stages:

> **Content Review**
>
> ### STAGES OF LYME DISEASE
> • Early localized
> • Early disseminated
> • Late

- *Early Localized Stage* A painless, flat, red lesion appears at the bite site. In some patients, a ring-like rash, *erythema migrans (EM),* develops and spreads outward. The outer border remains bright red, with the centre becoming clear, blue, or even necrotic. The rash—often called a "bull's eye" rash—usually disappears in time, whether treated or not. At this stage, patients also may complain of headache, malaise, and muscle aches. Although uncommon, the patient's neck may be stiff.

- *Early Disseminated Stage* The spirochete spreads to the skin, nervous system, heart, and joints. More EM lesions develop. CNS sequelae include meningitis, seventh-cranial-nerve Bell's palsy, and peripheral neuropathy. Cardiac abnormalities include conduction defects and myopathy. Arthritis and myalgia are common months after infection. Approximately 8 percent of patients will have some cardiac involvement. The most common manifestations are varying degrees of atrioventricular block (first degree, Wenckebach, and complete heart block). Less commonly, myocarditis and left ventricular dysfunction are seen. Cardiac involvement typically lasts only a few weeks but can recur.

- *Late Stage (persistent infection)* The late stage can occur months or years after the initial exposure. Although the incidence of cardiac problems is lower, it involves the same neurological complications as second stage, plus encephalopathy with cognitive deficits, depression, and sleep disorders. Monoarthritis of large joints and more than one joint concurrently (polyarthritis) is common.

Development of erythema migrans, the bull's eye rash, usually 3 to 30 days after tick exposure, is presumptive for the diagnosis.

The EMS response to Lyme disease will probably be to treat its clinical consequences, especially those of the disseminated and late stages. Advanced life support (ALS) treatment is directed toward those consequences, not the infection. Adhere to universal precautions. After responding to calls in heavily wooded areas infested by ticks, always check both your and the patient's clothing, shoes, socks, and body for ticks. Spray the ambulance compartment with an insecticide effective against arthropods. Available antibiotic therapies are effective for the stages of the disease progression. Protection against Lyme disease is now available as a series of three vaccinations, with the second dose given at one month and the third at 12. It is recommended for persons aged 15–70 years whose activities result in frequent exposure to tick habitats and for selected travellers to endemic areas where exposure to tick habitats is anticipated.

SEXUALLY TRANSMITTED DISEASES

Infectious diseases transmitted through sexual contact are known as **sexually transmitted diseases,** or STDs. They represent some of the most prevalent communicable diseases. A variety of bacterial (gonorrhea, syphilis, chancroid, chlamydia), viral (HIV, herpes), and parasitic (pediculosis, trichomoniasis) infections are spread by this route. Other illnesses that are generally not considered STDs, including hepatitis A, B, C, D, salmonellosis, and shigellosis, may also be transmitted through sexual contact. STDs affect the genital organs, often resulting in pathology to reproductive structures. Although EMS personnel do not treat these diseases, other emergency health-care personnel commonly have the information in the following profiles. Your knowledge of these diseases will put you on a level playing field with other health-care workers and bolster your credibility. When you treat or transport patients with STDs, observe universal precautions, avoid contact with lesions and exudates, and wash your hands vigorously after exposure.

✳ **sexually transmitted disease (STD)** illness most commonly transmitted through sexual contact.

Gonorrhea

Gonorrhea—caused by *Neisseria gonorrhoeae,* a gram-negative bacterium—is one of the most commonly diagnosed communicable diseases in Canada. More than 5000 cases are treated annually. Everyone is susceptible to infection, and although antibodies develop after exposure and confer immunity, they do so only for the specific serotype that caused the infection. Thus, persons contracting gonorrhea would not be immune to penicillinase-producing *N. gonorrhoeae* (PPNG), a strain of *N. gonorrhoeae* known by military personnel during the Vietnam War as "black clap." Most commonly seen in males in their early twenties, gonorrhea is transmitted by direct contact with exudates of mucous membranes, primarily from direct sexual contact. In men, the disease presents as painful urination and a purulent urethral discharge. Untreated, it can lead to epididymitis, prostatitis, and urethral strictures. The majority of women contracting the disease have no pain and minimal discharge. In some cases, symptoms include urinary frequency, vaginal discharge, fever, and abdominal pain. Pelvic inflammatory disease (PID) often results after menstruation when bacteria spread from the cervix to the upper genital tract. Affected females are at increased risk for sterility, ectopic pregnancy, abscesses within reproductive structures, and peritonitis.

✳ **gonorrhea** sexually transmitted disease caused by a gram-negative bacterium.

Gonorrhea may occasionally become systemic, causing sepsis or meningitis. Septic arthritis may result, presenting with fever, pain, swelling, and limited range of motion in one or two joints, sometimes leading to progressive deterioration. In North America, single dosing is often effective in treating localized gonorrhea (genitourinary only). Treating systemic gonorrhea often involves additional chemotherapy. When gonorrhea infection coexists with chlamydial infections (as is estimated to occur in about 50 percent of gonorrhea patients), two-drug therapy is routinely advised. No immunization is available.

Syphilis

Syphilis is a disease caused by the spirochete *Treponema pallidum.* It is transmitted by direct contact with exudates from other syphilitic lesions of skin and mucous membranes, semen, blood, saliva, and vaginal discharges. It is therefore most commonly contracted through sexual intercourse but also may be transmitted by kissing or close contact with an open lesion. An estimated 30 percent of exposures result in infection. In congenital syphilis, infants contract the disease before birth from an infected mother. Everyone is susceptible to infection. Although the risk of transmission by blood transfusion or needle-stick injury is low, health-care workers have been infected after secondary assessment involving manual contact with a lesion. A gradual immunity does develop after infection, but aggressive antimicrobial therapy may interfere with this natural antibody formation, especially during the primary and secondary stages.

Syphilis is characterized by lesions that may involve virtually any organ or tissue. It usually has cutaneous manifestations with frequent relapses, and it may remain latent for years. The incubation period is three weeks. Syphilis may occur in four stages, depending on how early and aggressively treatment is initiated:

- *Primary syphilis (first stage)* presents as a painless lesion or chancre. In heterosexual men, the chancre is usually on the penis. In homosexual men, the chancre is often found on the anal canal, rectum, tongue, lips, or other point of entry. The chancre typically occurs 3 to 6 weeks after exposure. Nontender enlargement of regional lymph nodes may also occur.

- *Secondary syphilis (second stage),* or the bacteremic stage, begins 5 to 6 weeks after the chancre has healed. It is characterized by a maculopapular skin rash (small, red, flat lesions) on the palms and soles, condyloma latum (painless, wart-like lesions on warm, moist skin areas, which are very infectious), and cutaneous infection in areas of hair growth causing loss of hair and/or eyebrows. These skin signs last for about six weeks. CNS disease (syphilitic meningitis) and arthritis may occur, as can infections of the eyes and kidneys.

- *Latent syphilis (third stage),* a period when symptoms improve or disappear completely, may last from months to many years. Twenty-five percent of cases may relapse with secondary stage symptoms; however, relapses usually do not occur after four years. Thirty-three percent of cases will progress to tertiary syphilis, and the rest will remain asymptomatic.

- *Tertiary syphilis (fourth stage)* is the stage of syphilis that justifies its reputation as a "great imitator." Lesions with sharp borders, called gummas, may appear on skin and bones, causing a deep, gnawing pain. Cardiovascular syphilis may appear, usually 10 years after the primary infection, resulting in aortic aneurysms that antibiotic therapy does not reverse. Neurosyphilis is diagnosed when there are neurological signs in seropositive patients. Meningitis may result, with possible spinal cord disease causing loss of reflexes and reduced sensation of pain and temperature. The spirochetes can also invade the cerebral vessels, causing a stroke. A progressive dementia can also occur during this stage.

EMS personnel may treat a variety of clinical complications of syphilis, often without being aware of infection as the primary etiology. ALS is directed toward treating the clinical presentation, which may include seizures, an acute onset of dementia, signs of a stroke, aortic aneurysm, or acute myocardial infarction. Avoid frequent contact with lesions on any part of the patient's body, and pay attention to handwashing technique after patient contact, since *T. pallidum* is easily killed by heat, soap, and water.

For presumptive screening after exposure, rapid plasmin reagin (RPR) and venereal disease research labs (VDRL) tests are available. Because RPR or VDRL have fairly high rates of false-positive reactions, more specific tests should always follow. Treatment of primary syphilis is benzathine penicillin, with erythromycin and doxycycline (Vibramycin) as alternatives for patients allergic to penicillin. No immunization is available.

Genital Warts

Genital warts (condyloma acuminatum) are caused by the human papillomavirus (HPV), a DNA virus. To date, research has identified 70 HPV types, with most known to cause specific clinical manifestations. Some of the types known to cause genital warts are associated with cervical cancer. Genital warts are contagious and easily spread. In males, they generally appear as cauliflower-like, fleshy growths on the penis, anus, and mucosa of the anal canal. In females, they usually appear on the labial surfaces. Genital warts are sometimes difficult to distinguish from the condyloma latum seen in the secondary stage of syphilis. HPV has been implicated as a causative factor of cervical cancer in females.

Herpes Simplex Type 2

HSV-2 causes 70–90 percent of all genital herpes cases. Transmission is usually by sexual contact. Everyone is susceptible, but adolescents and young adults are most commonly afflicted. Neonates are often infected during passage down the birth canal. The prevalence of HSV-2 antibody, which does not confer immunity, is greater in lower socioeconomic groups and persons with multiple sex partners. The disease presents as vesicular lesions on the penis, anus, rectum, and mouth of the male depending on sexual activity. Females are sometimes asymptomatic but can display lesions of the vagina, vulva, perineum, rectum, mouth, and cervix. Recurrent infections in females are often found on the vulva, buttocks, legs, and the perineum. Patients may present with fever and enlarged lymph nodes during the initial infection. Lesions may last up to several weeks before eventually crusting over and healing. The most serious consequence of HSV-2 infection is that painful lesions may recur periodically during the patient's lifetime, significantly diminishing quality of life. Recent evidence suggests that symptomatic treatment with the antiviral agent acyclovir orally, intravenously, or topically, may decrease the incidence of recurrences and lessen the severity of their symptoms. Other treatment alternatives include CO_2 laser removal, cryotherapy (freezing and removal) with liquid nitrogen, electrical cauterization, and interferon. Immunization is not currently available.

Chlamydia

Chlamydia is a genus of intracellular parasites most like gram-negative bacteria. Once thought to be viruses, the chlamydiae are now known to have inner and outer membranes, to contain both DNA and RNA, and to be susceptible to numerous antibiotics. However, they lack peptidoglycan, a net of polysaccharides found in all true bacterial walls.

From the standpoint of STDs, *Chlamydia trachomatis* is the most clinically significant species, affecting the genital area, eyes, and respiratory system. Everyone is susceptible, and up to 25 percent of men may be carriers. *C. trachomatis* is responsible for roughly 50 percent of all cases of nongonococcal urethritis (NGU)

✳ **chlamydia** group of intracellular parasites that cause sexually transmitted diseases.

in men, usually with dysuria and penile discharge. It is transmitted by sexual activity and by hand-to-hand transfer of eye secretions, causing conjunctivitis. Internationally, this is the leading preventable cause of blindness. Because children are the major reservoir and the common use of infected linen can transmit chlamydia, childcare centre and school workers should exercise caution in handling blankets, sheets, and towels.

The symptoms are similar to gonorrhea's but less severe, often making the clinical differentiation difficult. In addition, the progression of disease in women is identical, with both causing a mucopurulent discharge that often accompanies cervicitis. Some women may have retrograde infections of the reproductive tract, causing pelvic inflammatory disease. Sterility may result. Newborns may be infected during passage through an infected birth canal, resulting in infant pneumonia or blindness.

No immunization is available, but *C. trachomatis* infection responds to a variety of antimicrobial agents, such as tetracycline, doxycycline (Vibramycin), erythromycin (PCE), and orally administered azithromycin (Zithromax). Natural infection is not known to confer immunity.

Another species of *Chlamydia*, *C. pneumoniae*, has been found in atherosclerotic lesions of patients who have died of myocardial infarction. This has led to speculation about the relationship between *C. pneumoniae* infection and atherosclerosis as an inflammatory process.

Trichomoniasis

✳ **trichomoniasis** sexually transmitted disease caused by the protozoan *Trichomonas vaginalis*.

Trichomonas vaginalis, a protozoan parasite, is a common cause of vaginitis. In women, the symptoms of **trichomoniasis** include a greenish-yellow vaginal discharge, irritation of the perineum and thighs, and dysuria. This disease is frequently present with gonorrhea. Men are generally asymptomatic carriers of the disease. When present, symptoms include dysuria, urethral discharge, and discomfort in the perineum. The infection is currently treated with metronidazole (Flagyl).

Chancroid

✳ **chancroid** highly contagious sexually transmitted ulcer.

Chancroid is a highly contagious ulcer caused by *Haemophilus ducreyi*, a gram-negative bacterium. It is more frequently diagnosed in men, particularly those who have sex with prostitutes. Uncircumcised men are at higher risk. It is spread by direct contact, mostly sexual, with open lesions and pus. Autoinoculation has occurred in infected persons. Its incubation period is typically 3–5 days but may be as long as 14 days.

The disease begins with a painful, inflamed pustule or ulcer that may appear on the penis, anus, urethra, or vulva. It spreads easily to other sites, such as breasts, fingers, and thighs. Lymph nodes may become swollen and tender, and fever may be present. Chancroid ulcer is linked with increased risk of HIV infection. Chancroid lesions in children beyond the neonatal period should alert EMS providers to the possibility of reportable child sexual abuse.

Health-care workers have contracted the disease by coming in contact with patients' ulcers. Immunization is not available, and infection does not appear to confer immunity. Several effective antimicrobials (for example, erythromycin) are available.

Content Review

DISEASES OF THE SKIN
- Impetigo
- Lice
- Scabies

DISEASES OF THE SKIN

EMS providers interactions with patients or the general public may expose them to contagious skin infections, such as impetigo, or to the ectoparasites lice and scabies. Because the public frequently attempts to consult paramedics about general topics in personal and community health, your knowledge of ectoparasites may enable you to provide education and information. As always, use universal precautions and effective postexposure handwashing.

Impetigo

Impetigo is a very contagious infection of the skin caused by staphylococci or streptococci. The disease begins as a single vesicle that ruptures and forms a thick, honey-coloured crust with a yellowish-red centre. Lesions most commonly occur on the extremities and joints. Although few patients call an ambulance for this condition, it often appears on patients who seek EMS for other reasons. EMS responders who develop impetigo should not report for work until cleared by their physician. It is easily transmitted by direct skin-to-skin contact, and so universal precautions should provide ample protection.

* impetigo infection of the skin caused by staphylococci or streptococci.

Lice

Lice (pediculosis) is a parasitic **infestation** of the skin of the scalp, trunk, or pubic area. Lice infest hosts, rather than infect them, because they do not break the skin. The three different varieties of infestations are *Pediculus humanus var. capitis* (head lice), *Pediculus humanus var. corporis* (body lice), and *Pthirus pubis* (pubic lice, or crabs). Historically, head lice have been involved in outbreaks of typhus, trench fever in World War I, and relapsing fever. Head and body lice appear similar, both being 3–4 mm long. Head lice are transmitted by sharing of combs or hats and are fairly common among young school-aged children, regardless of socioeconomic status. Outbreaks in daycare centres and schools are common. Head lice are easily diagnosed by the presence of small, white, oval-shaped eggs (nits) attached to the hair shafts. Nits can be seen with the naked eye but are more easily found with a magnifying glass. Lice themselves are rarely seen. They tend to leave febrile hosts, and so high environmental temperatures and crowding favour transmission. Lice have a three-stage life cycle of eggs, nymphs, and adults. Eggs hatch in 7–10 days but cannot hatch below 22.2°C. The nymph stage lasts about 7–13 days, again depending on temperature, with a total egg-to-egg cycle of three weeks.

* lice parasitic infestation of the skin of the scalp, trunk, or pubic area.

* infestation presence of parasites that do not break the host's skin.

Anyone can be infested, and repeated infestations may cause an allergic response. Infestation often occurs on eyebrows and eyelashes, hair, mustaches, and beards. Symptoms are generally limited to severe itching. Body lice often infest clothing along seams close to skin surfaces and attach to the skin only to feed. They can be vectors of bacteria. Red macules, papules, and urticaria commonly appear on the shoulders, buttocks, and abdomen. Pubic lice infest through sexual contact by attaching to hair in the genital and anal regions but can also infest facial hair.

Any EMS worker exposed to a patient with lice may be treated with one of several nonprescription agents. Pyrethrin preparations, such as RID, are commonly used but require two applications one week apart because they do not kill the eggs. Permethrin agents, such as Nix or Elimite, theoretically require only a single application because they kill adults and eggs. Lindane 1 percent shampoo (Kwell) may be used, but it is available only by prescription and is more toxic than the other treatments. Eliminating the eggs by combing the hair is essential. Nits are more easily removed (nit picking) after soaking combs in a white vinegar solution or using a commercial preparation, such as the Step 2 Nit Removal System. Separately bagging linen in an occupational setting is unnecessary. At home, however, isolating infested linen and clothing is advisable to avoid exposing uninfested laundry for extended periods. Lice are not known to jump great distances like fleas, and so spraying the ambulance's interior close to the cot and the area by the patient's head with an insecticide, preferably one containing premethrin, should be sufficient after a call. Clean and wipe all sprayed areas to remove insecticide residues.

Scabies

Scabies is caused by infestation of a mite (*Sarcoptes scabiei*) that is barely visible without magnification. Exposure to the mite is through close personal contact, from handholding to sexual relations. The mite can remain viable on clothing or in bedding for up to 48 hours.

On attaching to a new host, the female tunnels into the skin within 2.5 minutes and lays up to three eggs a day along the "burrow" in the epidermis. The larvae hatch shortly thereafter, leading to a full-grown adult 10 to 20 days later. The adults remain near hair follicles and forage for nourishment with their jaws and the claws of their forelegs.

The primary symptom is intense itching (hence the name "seven-year itch"), usually at night. It generally occurs from 2 to 6 weeks after infestation. The irritation results from sensitization to the mite and its droppings. Inflammatory lesions appear as fine, wavy, dark lines, usually not more than 1 cm long. In males, they most commonly occur on the webs of the fingers, wrists, elbows, armpits, belt line, thighs, and external genitalia. In females, they most often involve the areolae and nipples, abdomen, and lower portions of the buttocks. In infants, the head, neck, palms, and soles are frequently involved. Older children exhibit patterns similar to adults. Complications are generally due to infections of lesions that are broken by scratching.

Although everyone is susceptible to infection, immunocompromised patients sometimes develop Norwegian scabies, a more severe form of scabies. Persons with previous exposure appear to have fewer mites on subsequent exposures and develop symptoms much sooner (in from 1 to 4 days), suggesting an amnestic (remembered) immune system response. Outbreaks of scabies resistant to lindane (Kwell) have been reported in several nursing homes across North America.

Scabies remains communicable until all mites and eggs are destroyed. Because of the long incubation period, all household members and/or close contacts of infested EMS workers should be treated simultaneously. Although some experts recommend that clothing and uniforms worn within two days of treatment, along with towels and bed linen, should be washed in hot water or dry cleaned, this requirement is questionable for most infestations. It is essential, however, for articles that came in contact with patients with Norwegian scabies. Bag and remove all linens from the ambulance immediately after you hand over the patient. To prevent spread of the mite, clean the stretcher and patient compartment as recommended for lice. Remove and decontaminate any clothing that may have touched the patient.

The scabicides of choice are premethrin cream (Elimite) or lindane (Kwell), which is applied to the skin from the neck down, left on for 8 to 14 hours, and then washed off. This should be repeated within one week. If premethrin is ineffective, 10 percent crotamiton (Eurax) and ivermectin (Stromectol) are also available.

NOSOCOMIAL INFECTIONS

Hospitalized patients, especially those with compromised immune function, often acquire new infectious diseases. Especially virulent strains of microorganisms may cause these **nosocomial** (hospital acquired) diseases. Bacteria that resist antibiotics are of particular concern. Recently, vancomycin-resistant enterococcus (VRE) and methicillin-resistant *Staphylococcus aureus* (MRSA) have become especially alarming. Both of these organisms can cause severe host damage, and both are difficult to treat. They rapidly colonize patients in whom broad-spectrum antibiotics have eliminated normal flora. Hospitalized patients may also contract resistant strains of tuberculosis that spread easily from patient to patient if protective clothing and handwashing precautions are not strictly observed.

PREVENTING DISEASE TRANSMISSION

Preventing or limiting exposure to infectious or communicable diseases cannot be overemphasized. While some infectious diseases are relatively minor with no long-term effects, others can be very serious and even life threatening. As a paramedic, you must be extremely vigilant during patient contact and take every step possible to ensure your health and safety. Personal accountability is important. Do not go to work if you

- Have diarrhea
- Have a draining wound or any type of wet lesions (allow them to dry and crust over before returning to work)
- Are jaundiced
- Have mononucleosis
- Have been exposed to lice or scabies and have not yet been treated
- Have "strep throat" and have not been taking antibiotics for at least 24 hours
- Have a cold

Keep the following immunizations current: MMR, hepatitis A (if deemed appropriate in your jurisdiction), hepatitis B, DPT, polio, varicella, influenza (seasonal), and rabies (if appropriate).

Always approach the scene cautiously with a high index of suspicion. On arrival, control the scene to decrease the likelihood of body fluid exposure for everyone present. Observe BSI. Always wear gloves. If there is the remotest possibility of splashing or aerosolization of body fluids, wear protective eyewear or a mask with a face shield. If large volumes of blood or other fluids may result from the response, don a gown. When dealing with a patient who has or may have active TB, wear the appropriate N95 respirator.

Patients who have coughs, fever, headache, general weakness, recent weight loss, or nuchal rigidity or who are taking certain medications may raise your awareness of the potential for contracting an infectious agent. With experience, you will develop your intuition and associate certain symptoms with infectious patients you have treated. Bolster your experience by increasing your knowledge, particularly your clinical acumen in recognizing the immunocompromised patient.

After a call, wash your hands first. Decontaminate and disinfect your equipment and the interior of the ambulance. Using commercially available disinfectants that certify bactericidal activity against *M. tuberculosis* should provide ample disinfection of those infectious agents that pose your greatest occupational risk. Remember that HIV is a fragile virus that any vigorous application of soap and water will kill it. Utilize high-level disinfection on airway equipment. If the patient or the situation surrounding the response presents the possibility of lice, scabies, or ticks, spray the gurney and interior of the ambulance with the appropriate insecticide, and wipe or mop up any residue. Ensure that linen will not be taken home. If practical, do not go home in your uniform. To discourage that practice, some EMS agencies consider uniforms as PPE. Report any infectious exposure to the IDCO, human resources director, or appropriate designated official.

Proactive EMS agencies offer their personnel continuing education in infectious diseases that have high incidence or prevalence in the communities they

As a paramedic, you must be extremely vigilant during your patient contact to take every step possible to ensure your health and safety.

serve. Continuing education sessions should include identification of causative agents, modes of transmission, epidemiological patterns within the community, signs and symptoms, methods to avoid infection, and special postexposure considerations, including postexposure prophylaxis, if appropriate.

To maintain a perspective on personal risk, always consider the interaction of three major factors: infectious agent, host, and environment. Are you aware of the infectious agent's virulence? Do you have some idea of the dose of the organism involved? For example, was a large volume of body fluid involved? How healthy are you? Do you have any chronic medical conditions or take any medications that would classify you as immunocompromised? What was the nature of the exposure? Is it significantly high? The probability of risk is sometimes just a measure of exposure. Not all infections are communicable. If they are communicable, they may not necessarily pose a high probability of progressing to the disease. The risk and potential for HIV transmission to health-care workers may be high, but the probability of transmission, which averages approximately 0.3 percent, is very low.

As you are promoted within your organization, your first additional responsibility may be as a preceptor for a new paramedic or student. You therefore assume responsibility for her well being. Are you familiar with your local protocols and procedures for reporting and recording an exposure? Can you adequately document the circumstances surrounding the exposure to facilitate review by the IDCO, physician, or agency administrator? If you cannot, what kind of a role model are you for that new employee or student?

Paramedics cannot allow their personal prejudices to interfere with providing optimum care for their patients. Patients should not be treated differently because they have an infectious disease that might reflect on their ethnicity, culture, sexual preference, or social status. You should not avoid certain procedures because you find a disease process or its consequences personally repulsive. It is sometimes helpful to think in terms of doing things *for* patients, as opposed to doing things *to* them.

Summary

Over the past few decades, medical science has made tremendous progress in diagnosing and treating infectious diseases. New vaccines and antibiotics are continually being developed. Advances in laboratory technology, notably the polymerase chain reaction (PCR), have made the presence and identification of microorganisms easier, quicker, and more accurate. Despite these tremendous advances, many infectious diseases cannot be effectively treated. Specific treatments for most viral diseases remain elusive, and each year countless people die from AIDS, hepatitis, pneumonia, sexually transmitted diseases, and other infectious diseases.

EMS can have a significant impact on the incidence of infectious diseases if providers remain knowledgeable, are leaders in public education, and are consistently alert in protecting themselves and their patients. The title of the International Association of Fire Fighters (IAFF) hepatitis B curriculum, *The Silent War*, provides a metaphor for the dilemma of infectious diseases in EMS: EMS personnel deal with few infectious disease emergencies; however, when they do respond to such emergencies, they often are unaware of the disease's presence until after the call. Standard (universal) precautions, often written for clinical and research facilities with more predictable hazards and risks, are increased to body substance isolation (BSI) for emergency health-care providers because of the uncertainties of the profession. Constant vigilance and personal accountability are the keys to reducing those risks.

All body fluids are possibly infectious. Universal precautions should be followed at all times.

CHAPTER 38

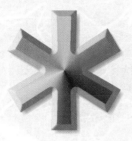

Psychiatric and Behavioural Disorders

Objectives

After reading this chapter, you should be able to:

1. Define behaviour and distinguish among normal behaviour, abnormal behaviour, and the behavioural emergency. (pp. 834–835)
2. Discuss the prevalence of behavioural and psychiatric disorders. (p. 835)
3. Discuss the pathophysiology of behavioural and psychiatric disorders. (pp. 835–836)
4. Discuss the factors that may alter the behavioural or emotional status of an ill or injured individual. (pp. 835–836)
5. Describe the medical-legal considerations for management of emotionally disturbed patients. (pp. 836–840)

6. Describe the overt behaviours associated with behavioural and psychiatric disorders. (pp. 840–851)
7. Define the following terms:
   - Affect (p. 837)
   - Anger (p. 843)
   - Anxiety (pp. 842–843)
   - Confusion (p. 837)
   - Depression (p. 843)
   - Fear (p. 837)
   - Mental status (p. 837)
   - Open-ended question (p. 837)
   - Posture (p. 837)
8. Describe verbal techniques useful in managing the emotionally disturbed patient. (pp. 838–839)

Continued

9. List the appropriate measures to ensure the safety of the paramedic, the patient, and others. (pp. 836–840, 851–853)
10. Describe the circumstances when relatives, bystanders, and others should be removed from the scene. (p. 837)
11. Describe techniques to systematically gather information from the disturbed patient. (pp. 839, 853)
12. Identify techniques for secondary assessment in a patient with behavioural problems. (pp. 837–839)
13. List situations in which you are expected to transport a patient forcibly and against his will. (pp. 853–854)
14. Describe restraint methods necessary in managing the emotionally disturbed patient. (pp. 854–856)
15. List the risk factors and behaviours that indicate a patient is at risk for suicide. (p. 850)
16. Use the assessment and patient history to differentiate among the various behavioural and psychiatric disorders. (pp. 840–851)
17. Given several preprogrammed behavioural emergency patients, provide the appropriate scene assessment, primary assessment, focused assessment, and secondary assessment, and then provide the appropriate care and patient transport. (pp. 834–856)

INTRODUCTION

A significant difference between behavioural and psychiatric conditions and other types of medical emergencies is that most of your assessment and care will depend on your people skills. You can evaluate a bradycardia with a cardiac monitor and treat it with atropine or a pacing unit. You evaluate the psychiatric patient, however, by observing his behaviour, by gathering information from his family and bystanders, and by interviewing him. Your care, which includes support, calming reassurance, and occasionally restraint, requires interpersonal skills more than diagnostic equipment.

BEHAVIOURAL EMERGENCIES

* **behaviour** a person's observable conduct and activity.

* **behavioural emergency** situation in which a patient's behaviour becomes so unusual that it alarms the patient or another person and requires intervention.

Behaviour is a person's observable conduct and activity. A **behavioural emergency** is a situation in which a patient's behaviour becomes so unusual, bizarre, threatening, or dangerous that it alarms the patient or another person, such as a family member or bystander, and requires the intervention of emergency service and/or mental health personnel.

Note that the definition of behavioural emergency does not use the word *abnormal*. The differentiation between normal and abnormal is largely subjective. What is normal varies depending on culture, ethnic group, socioeconomic class, and personal interpretation and opinion. What one person considers normal, another might consider highly abnormal. Generally, however, normal behaviour can be defined as behaviour that is readily acceptable in a society.

Indications of a behavioural or psychological condition include actions that

- Interfere with core life functions (eating, sleeping, ability to maintain housing, interpersonal or sexual relations)
- Pose a threat to the life or well-being of the patient or others
- Significantly deviate from society's expectations or norms

PATHOPHYSIOLOGY OF PSYCHIATRIC DISORDERS

Experts estimate that up to 20 percent of the population has some type of mental health problem and that as many as one person in seven will actually require treatment for an emotional disturbance. These problems may be severely disabling and require inpatient care, or the patient may quietly tolerate them with no outward symptoms. That all people with psychiatric conditions exhibit bizarre or unusual behaviour is a misconception. The small percentage of patients with psychiatric disorders who publicly exhibit bizarre behaviour tends to create this misconception among laypeople. In reality, most patients who suffer from such disorders as anxiety, depression, eating disorders, or mild personality disorders function normally on a daily basis, going unnoticed in society. Nonetheless, behavioural and psychiatric disorders incapacitate more people than all other health problems combined. Most patients with mental illness are cared for in outpatient settings, such as public mental health centres. Only those with severe psychiatric illnesses remain institutionalized. Because of this, EMS providers are increasingly being called to care for patients with behavioural complaints. A common reason for EMS intervention in psychiatric illness is patients' failure to take their psychiatric medications. When mental health patients, such as those with schizophrenia, begin to deteriorate and develop bizarre behaviour, more often than not they have not been adhering to their psychiatric medication regimen.

Another common misconception is that all mental health patients are unstable and dangerous and that their conditions are incurable. This is simply not true. Research in psychiatry, like other areas in medicine, has made great strides in determining causes and treatments for many psychiatric conditions. Having a mental disorder is not reason for embarrassment or shame, although society often stigmatizes these patients unfairly. The general causes of behavioural emergencies are biological (or organic), psychosocial, and sociocultural. Each of these three possible causes should guide your questioning during the patient interview. Keep in mind, however, that a patient's condition may result from more than one pathological process.

> *Most patients who suffer from such disorders as anxiety, depression, eating disorders, or mild personality disorders function normally on a daily basis, going unnoticed in society.*
>
>

Content Review

GENERAL CAUSES OF BEHAVIOURAL EMERGENCIES
Biological (organic)
Psychosocial (personal)
Sociocultural (situational)

BIOLOGICAL

For many years, medical practitioners have used the terms *biological* and *organic* interchangeably when discussing certain types of psychiatric disorders whose causes are physical, rather than purely psychological. These disorders result from disease processes, such as infections and tumours, or from structural changes in the brain, such as those brought on by the abuse of alcohol or drugs (including over-the-counter and prescription medications). It could be argued, however, that even purely psychological conditions originate in the brain and for that very reason are organic. Indeed, many psychiatric conditions do originate from alterations in brain chemistry.

Behavioural emergencies frequently involve biological conditions. Never assume a patient with an altered mental status or unusual behaviour is suffering from a purely psychological condition or disease until you have completely ruled out medical conditions and substance abuse.

* **biological/organic** related to disease processes or structural changes.

> *Never assume a patient with an altered mental status or unusual behaviour is suffering from a purely psychological condition or disease until you have completely ruled out medical conditions and substance abuse.*
>
>

PSYCHOSOCIAL

Psychosocial (personal) conditions are related to a patient's personality style, dynamics of unresolved conflict, or crisis management methods. These disorders are not attributable to substance abuse or medical conditions.

Environment plays a large part in psychosocial development. Traumatic childhood incidents may affect a person throughout life. Parents or other persons in positions of authority can have a tremendous impact on a child's development. Dysfunctional families, abusive parents, alcohol or drug abuse by parents, or neglect can cause behavioural problems from childhood through adulthood. Such conditions, in addition to—or in combination with genetic predisposition and brain chemistry—form the basis for psychosocial conditions.

SOCIOCULTURAL

Sociocultural (situational) causes of behavioural disorders are related to the patient's actions and interactions within society and to such factors as socioeconomic status, social habits, social skills, and values. These problems are usually attributable to events that change the patient's social space (relationships, support systems), social isolation, or otherwise have an impact on socialization.

Some events in the lives of children and adults that may cause a profound psychological change are rape, assault, witnessing the victimization of another, death of a loved one, and acts of violence, such as war or riots. Events that occur over time may also have an impact on the individual. These include the loss of a job, economic problems, such as poverty, and ongoing prejudice or discrimination. Sometimes, simply doing anything outside the norms of society can lead to stress and psychological changes.

ASSESSMENT OF BEHAVIOURAL EMERGENCY PATIENTS

The assessment and care of behavioural emergency patients is similar to that for other medical conditions. The order of assessment (scene assessment, primary assessment, focused history, and secondary assessment) remains unchanged. Potential medical conditions that mimic behavioural emergencies require you to perform a thorough medical assessment.

Among the differences between your assessment and care of a patient with a medical condition and one with a behavioural emergency is that, as already noted, you actually begin your care at the same time you begin your assessment by developing a rapport with the patient. Interpersonal skills are important for all patients, but perhaps never more than for one who is experiencing a behavioural emergency. Additionally, the focused history and secondary assessment for a behavioural emergency includes a mental status examination.

SCENE ASSESSMENT

Approach every patient cautiously to protect yourself and your crew from injury.
⚷

As with any call, determining scene safety is of the utmost importance. Approach the scene carefully. If a patient is experiencing a behavioural emergency that is significant enough to warrant EMS, it is most likely significant enough to have law enforcement authorities respond. Most patients experiencing behavioural emergencies or crises will not attack you; however, those who are behaving unusually, experiencing hallucinations or delusions, or are under the effect of a substance may become violent. Approach every patient cautiously to protect yourself and your crew from injury (Figure 38-1).

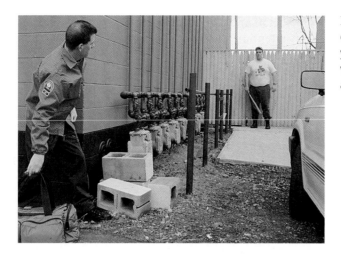

FIGURE 38-1 Approach every patient cautiously. If you determine a potential for violence, request police assistance.

The scene assessment also includes making observations that relate to patient care. Look for evidence of substance use or abuse, for therapeutic medications that may indicate an underlying medical condition (or abuse of that medication), and for signs of violence or destruction of property. Examine the general environmental condition, and when possible, observe the patient from a distance to note any visible behaviour patterns or violent behaviour.

PRIMARY ASSESSMENT

Because many behavioural emergencies are caused by or concurrent with medical conditions, you should be acutely suspicious of life-threatening emergencies. As with any other injury or condition, assess the ABCs, and intervene when necessary. Continue to observe the patient for any clues to his underlying condition. Be cautious of any overt behaviour, such as **posture** or hand gestures. Note any emotional response, such as rage, **fear**, anxiety, **confusion**, or anger. Early in the evaluation, try to determine the patient's **mental status**, the state of his cerebral functioning. Continue assessing mental status throughout the patient encounter by evaluating his awareness, orientation, cognitive abilities, and **affect** (visible indicators of mood).

Control the scene as soon as possible. Remove anyone who agitates the patient or adds confusion to the scene. Generally, a limited number of people around the patient is best. At times, performing an effective assessment and care may necessitate totally clearing a room or moving the patient to a quiet area. Finally, observe the patient's affect in greater detail. To avoid being grabbed or struck by the patient, stay alert for signs of aggression.

FOCUSED HISTORY AND SECONDARY ASSESSMENT

Your examination of a patient experiencing a behavioural emergency is largely conversational. This makes your interpersonal technique very important. Just as starting an IV with poor technique most likely will not establish a patent IV line, interviewing with poor interpersonal skills most likely will not obtain significant information. Remove the patient from the crisis area and limit interruptions. Focus your questioning and assessment on the immediate problem and follow these guidelines:

- *Listen.* Ask **open-ended questions** (those that require more than a yes or no response). These will encourage your patient to respond in

* **posture** position, attitude, or bearing of the body.

* **fear** feeling of alarm and discontentment in the expectation of danger.

* **confusion** state of being unclear or unable to make a decision easily.

* **mental status** the state of the patient's cerebral functioning.

* **affect** visible indicators of mood.

Stay alert for signs of aggression.

* **open-ended questions** those questions that require more than a yes or no response.

detail and share important information. Listen to the answer. Pay attention. No one likes being ignored. When you need information from a patient, listen.

- *Spend time.* Rushing the patient's answers, cutting him off, or appearing hurried will cause him to "shut down" and stop answering questions.
- *Be assured.* Communicate self-confidence, honesty, and professionalism.
- *Do not threaten.* Avoid rapid or sudden movements or questions that the patient might interpret as threats. Approach him slowly and confidently.
- *Do not fear silence.* Silence can be appropriate. Encourage the patient to tell his story, but do not be forceful or antagonizing.
- *Place yourself at the patient's level.* Standing over the patient may be intimidating. Unless you are intentionally attempting to gain a position of authority, crouch, kneel, or sit near the patient. Do not position yourself where you cannot respond appropriately to danger or attack.
- *Keep a safe and proper distance.* The surest way to make a behavioural emergency patient violent is to invade his "personal space" (Figure 38-2). This is an area within an approximately 1 m radius around every person; encroaching on it causes anxiety. If appropriate, however, you may touch the patient's shoulder or use another consoling touch when he allows.
- *Appear comfortable.* Do not appear uncomfortable—even if you are. Talking to patients about suicide, self-mutilation, or other psychological conditions is difficult. If the patient sees that you are uncomfortable, however, he is unlikely to open up to you. Would you expect a patient to tell you his reasons for attempting suicide when you appear uncomfortable even saying the word? To help, use terms the patient has used. If he says he wanted to "end it all," begin with that. Caregivers sometimes hesitate to use the word *suicide* because it might give the patient ideas of suicide. If you are there to care for a suicidal or potentially suicidal patient, however, he has already had those thoughts.
- *Avoid appearing judgmental.* Patients who are experiencing behavioural emergencies may feel strong emotions toward their caregivers. The patient should believe that you are interested in his condition and welfare. Be supportive and empathetic, and avoid

FIGURE 38-2   Avoid invading the patient's personal space, the area within about one metre of the patient.

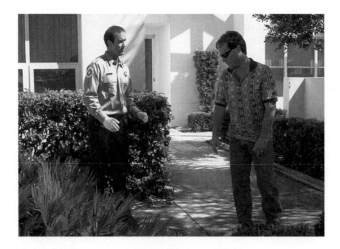

judgments, pity, anger, or any other emotions that may damage your relationship with the patient.

- *Never lie to the patient.* Honesty is the best policy. Do not reinforce false beliefs or hallucinations or mislead the patient in any way.

MENTAL STATUS EXAMINATION

As part of the focused history and secondary assessment for behavioural emergencies, do not overlook any physical or medical complaint. In addition to the medical evaluation, which is covered in depth throughout this and the other volumes of this program, your examination of the patient with psychiatric or behavioural disorders should include a psychological evaluation, also known as a **mental status examination** (MSE). The components of the MSE include

* **mental status examination** (MSE), a structured exam designed to quickly evaluate a patient's level of mental functioning.

- *General Appearance.* The patient's appearance can provide important information when looking at his "big picture." Observe hygiene, clothing, and overall appearance.
- *Behavioural Observations.* Observe verbal or nonverbal behaviour, strange or threatening appearance, or facial expressions. Note tone of voice, rate, volume, and quality.
- *Orientation.* Does the patient know who he is and who others are? Is he oriented to current events? Can he concentrate on simple questions and answer them?
- *Memory.* Is the patient's memory intact for recent and long-term events?
- *Sensorium.* Is the patient focused? Paying attention? What is his level of awareness?
- *Perceptual Processes.* Are the patient's thought patterns ordered? Does he appear to have any hallucinations, delusions, or phobias?
- *Mood and Affect.* Observe for indicators of the patient's mood. Is it appropriate? What is his prevailing emotion? Depression, elation, anxiety, or agitation? Other?
- *Intelligence.* Evaluate the patient's speech. What is his level of vocabulary? His ability to formulate an idea?
- *Thought Processes.* What is the patient's apparent form of thought? Are his thoughts logical and coherent?
- *Insight.* Does the patient have insight into his own problem? Does he recognize that a problem exists? Does he deny or blame others for his problem?
- *Judgment.* Does the patient base his life decisions on sound, reasonable judgments? Does he approach problems thoughtfully, carefully, and rationally?
- *Psychomotor.* Does the patient exhibit an unusual posture, or is he making unusual movements? Patients with hallucinations may react to them. For example, a patient who believes he is covered with insects may be picking at his skin to remove the "bugs."

PSYCHIATRIC MEDICATIONS

Many patients who suffer from psychiatric or behavioural disorders are under the care of a mental health professional and may be taking prescription medications. During the interview and history-taking process, determine whether the patient is taking medications and, if so, what type. The patient's use of such medications can provide clues to his underlying condition. Additionally, if a patient is not taking a medication as directed, his condition may deteriorate. Some schizophrenic patients may receive periodic injections of extremely long-acting antipsychotics (for example, haloperidol deconoate) because of poor compliance. They will often carry an identification card or may report that they "go to the clinic every three weeks for a shot." Types of psychiatric medications are discussed in the pharmacology chapter, Chapter 14.

SPECIFIC PSYCHIATRIC DISORDERS

Almost all psychiatric disorders have two diagnostic elements: symptoms of the disease or disorder and indications that the disease or disorder has impaired major life functions resulting in loss of relationships, a job, or housing or in another significant social problem. To define specific conditions, mental health professionals use the *Diagnostic and Statistical Manual of Mental Disorders,* Fourth Edition (*DSM-IV*). Published by the American Psychiatric Association (APA), the *DSM-IV* details diagnostic criteria for all currently defined psychiatric disorders, which are grouped according to the patient's signs and symptoms. The recognized types of behavioural and psychiatric disorders include

- Cognitive disorders
- Schizophrenia
- Anxiety disorders
- Mood disorders
- Substance-related disorders
- Somatoform disorders
- Factitious disorders
- Dissociative disorders
- Eating disorders
- Personality disorders
- Impulse control disorders

The following summaries of these illnesses' major criteria do not imply that you should diagnose behavioural disorders. Even for skilled psychologists and psychiatrists, diagnosis is complicated by the considerable overlap in symptoms from one disease to another. A patient may actually fit into several categories. You should use the information here only as a guide to better understanding the science of psychiatry and the criteria applied to patients with behavioural emergencies. Knowledge of these terms and conditions will also allow you to communicate better with psychiatric care providers.

COGNITIVE DISORDERS

Psychiatric disorders with organic causes, such as brain injury or disease, are known as cognitive disorders. This family of disorders includes conditions caused by metabolic disease, infections, neoplasm, endocrine disease, degenerative neurological disease, and cardiovascular disease. They might also be caused by physical or chemical injuries due to trauma, drug abuse, or reactions to prescribed drugs. The specific brain pathology will differ depending on the type of disease. Two types of cognitive disorders are delirium and dementia.

Delirium Delirium is characterized by a relatively rapid onset of widespread disorganized thought. These patients suffer from inattention, memory impairment, dis-

✱ **delirium** condition characterized by relatively rapid onset of widespread disorganized thought.

orientation, and a general clouding of consciousness. In some cases, individuals may experience vivid visual hallucinations. Delirium is characterized by a fairly acute onset (hours or days) and may be reversible. Delirium may be due to a medical condition, substance intoxication, substance withdrawal, or multiple etiologies. Confusion is a hallmark of delirium.

Dementia **Dementia** may be due to several medical problems. Included among the more common causes of dementia are Alzheimer's disease (both early and late onset), vascular problems, AIDS, head trauma, Parkinson's disease, substance abuse, and other chronic problems. Regardless of its cause, dementia involves memory impairment, cognitive disturbance, and pervasive impairment of abstract thinking and judgment. Unlike delirium, dementia usually develops over months and, in many cases, is irreversible.

Dementia involves cognitive deficits manifested by both memory impairment (diminished ability to learn new information or to recall previously learned information) and one or more of the following cognitive disturbances:

* *Aphasia.* Impaired ability to communicate.
* *Apraxia.* Impaired ability to carry out motor activities despite intact sensory function.
* *Agnosia.* Failure to recognize objects or stimuli despite intact sensory function.
* *Disturbance in executive functioning.* Impaired ability to plan, organize, or sequence.

These conditions must significantly impair social or occupational functioning and represent a significant decline from a previous level of functioning. Your approach to patients with either of these conditions should be supportive. Assess and manage any medical complaints or conditions, and transport to an appropriate medical facility.

SCHIZOPHRENIA

Schizophrenia is a common mental health problem, and its hallmark is a significant change in behaviour and a loss of contact with reality. Signs and symptoms often include hallucinations, delusions, and depression. The patient with schizophrenia may live in his "own world" and be preoccupied with inner fantasies. Although several biological and psychosocial theories attempt to explain the condition and its manifestations, its definitive cause is unknown.

The symptoms of schizophrenia include

* **Delusions.** Fixed, false beliefs that are not widely held within the context of the individual's cultural or religious group.
* **Hallucinations.** Sensory perceptions with no basis in reality. These are often auditory ("hearing voices").
* *Disorganized speech.* Frequent derailment or incoherence.
* **Catatonia** *or grossly disorganized behaviour.*
* *Negative symptoms* (**flat affect**).

A diagnosis of schizophrenia requires that two or more symptoms each be present for a significant portion of each month over the course of six months. The symptoms must cause a social or occupational dysfunction (decline in social relations or work from the predisease state). Most schizophrenics are diagnosed in early adulthood.

* **dementia** condition involving gradual development of memory impairment and cognitive disturbance.

* **schizophrenia** common disorder involving significant change in behaviour often including hallucinations, delusions, and depression.

* **delusions** fixed, false beliefs not widely held within the individual's cultural or religious group.

* **hallucinations** sensory perceptions with no basis in reality.

* **catatonia** condition characterized by immobility and stupor, often a sign of schizophrenia.

* **flat affect** appearance of being disinterested, often lacking facial expression.

The *DSM-IV* defines several major types of schizophrenia:

Content Review

MAJOR TYPES OF SCHIZOPHRENIA

Paranoid
Disorganized
Catatonic
Undifferentiated

- *Paranoid.* The patient is preoccupied with a feeling of persecution and may suffer delusions or auditory hallucinations.
- *Disorganized.* The patient often displays disorganized behaviour, dress, or speech.
- *Catatonic.* The patient exhibits catatonic rigidity, immobility, stupor, or peculiar voluntary movements. Catatonic schizophrenia is exceedingly rare.
- *Undifferentiated.* The patient does not readily fit into one of the categories above.

Your approach to the schizophrenic patient should be supportive and nonjudgmental. Do not reinforce the patient's hallucinations, but understand that he considers them real. Speak openly and honestly with him. Be encouraging yet realistic. Remain alert for aggressive behaviour, and restrain the patient if he becomes violent or presents a danger to you, to himself, or to others.

ANXIETY AND RELATED DISORDERS

* **anxiety disorder** condition characterized by dominating apprehension and fear.

* **anxiety** state of uneasiness, discomfort, apprehension, and restlessness.

* **panic attack** extreme period of anxiety resulting in great emotional distress.

Content Review

ANXIETY-RELATED DISORDERS

Panic attack
Phobia
Posttraumatic stress
  syndrome

The group of illnesses known as **anxiety disorders** is characterized by dominating apprehension and fear. These disorders affect approximately 2 to 4 percent of the population. Broadly defined, **anxiety** is a state of uneasiness, discomfort, apprehension, and restlessness. More specifically, anxiety disorders fall into three categories: panic disorder, phobia, and posttraumatic stress syndrome.

Panic Attack The *DSM-IV* does not list **panic attacks** in themselves as a disease. Characterized by recurrent, extreme periods of anxiety resulting in great emotional distress, they are symptoms of disease and are included among the criteria for other disorders (panic disorder, agoraphobia). Panic attacks differ from generalized feelings of anxiety in their acute nature. They are usually unprovoked, peaking within 10 minutes of their onset and dissipating in less than one hour.

The presentation of panic and anxiety may resemble a cardiac or respiratory condition. This presents a dilemma for EMS personnel. Ruling out those conditions is difficult in the prehospital setting; psychiatrists usually diagnose anxiety or panic disorders by excluding known medical conditions. Keys to identifying panic or anxiety in the field are the patient's having a history of the condition and being outside the expected age range for certain cardiac or respiratory illnesses. This, of course, is not to say that young people cannot have myocardial infarction. Many symptoms of panic resemble those of hyperventilation, and some do appear to be correlated, such as the paresthesia from panic being due largely to hyperventilation.

The diagnostic criteria for a panic attack require a discrete period of intense fear or discomfort, during which four or more of the following symptoms develop abruptly and reach a peak within 10 minutes:

- Palpitations, pounding heart, or accelerated heart rate
- Sweating
- Trembling or shaking
- Sensations of shortness of breath or smothering
- Feeling of choking
- Chest pain or discomfort
- Nausea or abdominal distress

- Feeling dizzy, unsteady, lightheaded, or faint
- Derealization (feelings of unreality) or depersonalization (being detached from oneself)
- Fear of losing control or going crazy
- Fear of dying
- Paresthesia (numbness or tingling sensations)
- Chills or hot flashes

Management for anxiety disorders is generally simple and supportive. Show empathy. Assess any medical complaints, and manage them appropriately. If the patient experiences hyperventilation, calm and reassure him in order to decrease his respiratory rate to normal. Patients with severe or incapacitating symptoms may benefit from the administration of a sedative. Benzodiazepines, such as diazepam (Valium) and lorazepam (Ativan), can be administered in the hospital setting.

Phobias Everyone has some source of fear or anxiety that they consciously avoid. When this fear becomes excessive and interferes with functioning, it is a **phobia**. A phobia, generally considered an intense, irrational fear, may be due to animals, the sight of blood (or injection or injury), situational factors (elevators, enclosed spaces), or environmental conditions (heights or water). Exposure to the situation or item will induce anxiety or a panic attack. Some patients experience extreme phobias that prevent or limit their normal daily activities. For example, a patient suffering from agoraphobia (fear of crowds) may confine himself to his home and avoid ever venturing outdoors. In most patients, however, the phobia is less severe; the patient realizes that his fear is unreasonable, and the anxiety dissipates.

✱ **phobia** excessive fear that interferes with functioning.

Management for a patient with a phobia is supportive. Understand that the patient's fear is very real to him. Do not force him to do anything that he objects to. Manage any underlying problems, and transport the patient for evaluation.

Posttraumatic Stress Syndrome EMS providers often are particularly interested in **posttraumatic stress syndrome** because their responsibilities may make them susceptible to it. Originally recognized on the battlefields of war, posttraumatic stress syndrome is a reaction to an extreme, usually life-threatening, stressor, such as a natural disaster, victimization (rape, for instance), or other emotionally taxing situation. It is characterized by a desire to avoid similar situations, recurrent intrusive thoughts, depression, sleep disturbances, nightmares, and persistent symptoms of increased arousal. The patient may feel guilty for having survived the incident, and substance abuse may frequently complicate his condition.

✱ **posttraumatic stress syndrome** reaction to an extreme stressor.

Treat any posttraumatic stress syndrome patient with respect, empathy, and support, and transport him to an appropriate facility for evaluation.

MOOD DISORDERS

The *DSM-IV* defines mood as "a pervasive and sustained emotion that colours a person's perception of the world." Common examples of mood alterations include depression, elation, **anger,** and anxiety. The main **mood disorders** are depression and bipolar disorder.

✱ **anger** hostility or rage to compensate for an underlying feeling of anxiety.

✱ **mood disorder** pervasive and sustained emotion that colours a person's perception of the world.

Depression Depression is characterized by a profound sadness or feeling of melancholy. It is common in everyday life and is to be expected following the breakup of a relationship or the loss of a loved one. Most of us have experienced some sort of depression, at least in its mildest form. It is one of the most prevalent psychiatric conditions, affecting from 10 to 15 percent of the population.

✱ **depression** profound sadness or feeling of melancholy.

When depression becomes prolonged or severe, however, it is diagnosed as a *major depressive episode.*

The symptoms of major depressive disorder include

- Depressed mood most of the day, nearly every day, as indicated by subjective report or observation by others.
- Markedly diminished interest in pleasure in all, or almost all, activities most of the day nearly every day.
- Significant weight loss (without dieting) or weight gain. A five-percent change in body weight is considered significant.
- Insomnia or hypersomnia nearly every day.
- Psychomotor agitation or retardation every day (observable by others, not just the subjective feeling of the patient).
- Feelings of worthlessness or excessive inappropriate guilt (may be delusional) nearly every day.
- Diminished ability to think or concentrate, or indecisiveness nearly every day.
- Recurrent thoughts of death (not just fear of dying), recurrent suicidal ideation without a specific plan, or a suicide attempt or a specific plan for committing suicide. (Depression greatly increases the risk of suicide.)

The diagnostic criteria for major depressive disorder require that five or more of the symptoms have been present during the same two-week period and represent a change from previous functioning; at least one of the symptoms must be either a depressed mood or loss of interest in pleasure. The condition must cause clinically significant distress or impairment in social, occupational, or other important functions. Further, it must not meet the criteria for a mixed episode (mixtures of mania and depression); it must not be due to the direct physiological effects of a substance, such as drug abuse or a medication, or to a general medical condition, such as hypothyroidism; finally, it must not be better accounted for by **bereavement**. The acronym *IN SAD CAGES* provides a screening mnemonic for major depression:

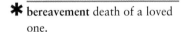

* **bereavement** death of a loved one.

- *In*terest
- *S*leep
- *A*ppetite
- *D*epressed mood
- *C*oncentration
- *A*ctivity
- *G*uilt
- *E*nergy
- *S*uicide

Depression may occur as an isolated condition, but it is often accompanied by other such disorders as substance abuse, anxiety disorders, and schizophrenia. Depression can also affect a patient who does not meet all of the identified clinical criteria. It can affect different people in different ways and is often atypical. Bereavement is one of the situations in which depression is expected. If the depression lasts longer than two months or is accompanied by suicidal ideation or marked functional impairment, it could be classified as a major depressive episode. Depression is more prevalent in females and is spread evenly throughout the life span.

Bipolar Disorder Bipolar disorder is characterized by one or more **manic** episodes (periods of elation), with or without subsequent or alternating periods of depression. In the past, the term *manic-depressive* was used to describe this condition. Bipolar disorder is not particularly common, affecting approximately less than 1 percent of the population.

Manic-depressive episodes are not the "Jeckyl and Hyde" transformations that television and the movies often portray. However, they often begin suddenly and escalate rapidly over a few days. In contrast to major depressive disorders, bipolar disorders usually develop in adolescence or early adulthood and occur as often in males as in females. Some patients with major depressive episodes will eventually develop a bipolar disorder and experience manic episodes. Commonly patients have several depressive episodes before having a manic episode.

The diagnostic criteria for a manic episode require a distinct period of abnormally and persistently elevated, expansive, or irritable mood lasting for at least one week (or for any duration when hospitalization is necessary). Three or more (four or more if the mood is only irritable) of the following symptoms must have been present to a certain degree and must have persisted during that time:

- Inflated self-esteem or grandiosity
- Decreased need for sleep
- More talkative than usual or pressure to keep talking
- Flight of ideas or subjective experience that thoughts are racing
- Distractibility
- Increase in goal-directed activity (socially, at work or school, or sexually) or psychomotor agitation
- Excessive involvement in pleasurable activities that have a high potential for painful consequences (buying sprees, sexual indiscretions, foolish business investments)
- Delusional thoughts (grandiose ideas or unrealistic plans)

The symptoms must not meet the criteria for a mixed episode. The mood disturbance must be severe enough to markedly impair occupational or social functioning, to require hospitalizing the patient to prevent harm to himself or others, or present with psychotic features. As with depression, the symptoms must not be due to the direct physiological effects of a substance or a general medical condition. Patients with bipolar illness are often prescribed lithium (Carbolith) for treatment.

Management of these patients includes maintaining a calm, protective environment. Avoid confronting the manic patient. Never leave a depressed or suicidal patient alone. Assess and manage any other coexisting medical problems, and transport to an appropriate medical facility. Bipolar patients in an extreme manic phase may be overtly psychotic. In these cases, medication with an antipsychotic medication, such as haloperidol, may be indicated.

SUBSTANCE-RELATED DISORDERS

Substance abuse is a common disorder. Any patient exhibiting symptoms of a psychiatric or behavioural disorder should be screened for substance use and/or abuse. Substance abuse patients may present as being depressed, psychotic, or delirious, and their signs and symptoms may mimic those of many behavioural disorders. The *DSM-IV* lists substance abuse as a psychiatric disorder; you should consider it a serious condition. Any mood-altering chemical has the potential for abuse. Alcohol is a common part of our culture but can be abused. The user of a substance may be intoxicated from the effects of the chemical or may

✱ **bipolar disorder** condition characterized by one or more manic episodes, with or without periods of depression.

✱ **manic** characterized by excessive excitement or activity (mania).

Many patients with bipolar disorder are treated with lithium. Lithium has a very narrow therapeutic index, making lithium toxicity a significant complicating factor.

be ill from addiction or withdrawal of the chemical. Intoxication, in and of itself, may cause behavioural problems.

Repetitive use of a mood-altering chemical may lead to dependence or addiction. Dependence on a substance is characterized by repeated use of the substance. Dependence may be either psychological, physical, or both. Psychological dependence is a compelling desire to use the substance, inability to reduce or stop use, and repeated efforts to quit. Physical dependence is characterized by the need for increased amounts of the chemical to obtain the desired effect. Also, the presence of withdrawal symptoms when the substance is reduced or stopped is characteristic of physical dependence. All drugs have the potential to cause psychological dependence; many have the potential to cause physical dependence as well.

SOMATOFORM DISORDERS

Somatoform disorders are characterized by physical symptoms that have no apparent physiological cause. They are believed to be attributable to psychological factors. People who suffer from somatoform disorders believe their symptoms are serious and real. The major types of somatoform disorder are

* *Somatization disorder.* The patient is preoccupied with physical symptoms.
* *Conversion disorder.* The patient sustains a loss of function, usually involving the nervous system (for instance, blindness or paralysis), unexplained by any medical illness.
* *Hypochondriasis.* Exaggerated interpretation of physical symptoms as a serious illness.
* *Body dysmorphic disorder.* A person believes he has a defect in physical appearance.
* *Pain disorder.* The patient suffers from pain, usually severe, that is unexplained by a physical ailment.

Somatoform disorders are often difficult to identify and diagnose. They can mimic and be confused with various bona fide physical conditions. Never attribute physical symptoms to a behavioural disorder until medical conditions have been ruled out.

FACTITIOUS DISORDERS

Factitious disorders are sometimes confused with somatoform disorders. They are characterized by the following three criteria:

* An intentional production of physical or psychological signs or symptoms
* Motivation for the behaviour is to assume the "sick role"
* External incentives for the behaviour (e.g., economic gain, avoiding work, avoiding police) are absent

While patients suffering from factitious disorders essentially feign their illnesses, that does not preclude the possibility of true physical or psychological symptoms. The disorder is apparently more common in males than in females. In severe cases, patients will go to great length to obtain medical or psychological treatment. Patients with factitious disorders often will voluntarily produce symptoms and will present with a very plausible history. They often have an extensive knowledge of medical terminology and can be very demanding and disruptive.

✱ **somatoform disorder** condition characterized by physical symptoms that have no apparent physiological cause and are attributable to psychological factors.

Content Review

SOMATOFORM DISORDERS
Somatization disorder
Conversion disorder
Hypochondriasis
Body dysmorphic disorder
Pain disorder

✱ **factitious disorder** condition in which the patient feigns illness in order to assume the sick role.

In severe cases (Munchausen syndrome), patients will undergo multiple surgical operations and other painful procedures.

DISSOCIATIVE DISORDERS

Like somatoform disorders, **dissociative disorders** are attempts to avoid stressful situations while still gratifying needs. In a manner, they permit the person to deny personal responsibility for unacceptable behaviour. The individual avoids stress by *dissociating* from his core personality. These behaviour patterns can be complex but are quite rare. The disorders include

Psychogenic Amnesia Although amnesia is a partial or total *inability* to recall or identify past events, **psychogenic amnesia** is a *failure* to recall. The "forgotten" material is present but "hidden" beneath the level of consciousness.

Fugue State An amnesic individual may withdraw even further by retreating in what is known as a **fugue state**. A patient in a fugue state actually flees as a defence mechanism and may travel hundreds of kilometres from home.

Multiple Personality Disorder In **multiple personality disorder** the patient reacts to an identifiable stress by manifesting two or more complete systems of personality. While such disorders have received a great deal of attention in television, film, and novels, they are actually quite rare.

Depersonalization Depersonalization is a relatively more frequent dissociative disorder that occurs predominantly in young adults. Patients experience a loss of the sense of their self. Such individuals suddenly feel "different"—that they are someone else or that their body has taken on a different form. The disorder is often precipitated by acute stress.

EATING DISORDERS

The two classifications of eating disorders are anorexia nervosa and bulimia nervosa. Both generally occur between adolescence and the age of 25. The condition afflicts women more than men at a rate of 20:1.

Anorexia Nervosa Anorexia is the loss of appetite. **Anorexia nervosa** is a disorder marked by excessive fasting. Individuals with this disorder have an intense fear of obesity and often complain of being fat even though their body weight is low. They suffer from weight loss (25 percent of body weight or more), refusal to maintain body weight, and often a cessation of menstruation from severe malnutrition.

Bulimia Nervosa Recurrent episodes of seemingly uncontrollable binge eating with compensatory self-induced vomiting or diarrhea, excessive exercise, or dieting and with a full awareness of the behaviour's abnormality characterize **bulimia nervosa**. Individuals often display personality traits of perfectionism, low self-esteem, and social withdrawal.

 The weight loss and body changes experienced by anorexic and bulimic patients can lead to serious physical problems. Starvation and attempts to purge can have drastic consequences, such as anemia, dehydration, vitamin deficiencies, hypoglycemia, and cardiovascular problems. In addition to psychological support, prehospital care is likely to include treatment for dehydration and physical problems. Both disorders have a high potential morbidity and mortality.

PERSONALITY DISORDERS

Most adults' personalities are attuned to social demands. Some individuals, however, often seem ill-equipped to function adequately in society. These people

---

* dissociative disorder condition in which the individual avoids stress by separating from his core personality.

Content Review

DISSOCIATIVE DISORDERS
Psychogenic amnesia
Fugue state
Multiple personality disorder
Depersonalization

* psychogenic amnesia failure to recall, as opposed to inability to recall.

* fugue state condition in which an amnesiac patient physically flees.

* multiple personality disorder manifestation of two or more complete systems of personality.

* depersonalization feeling detached from yourself.

Content Review

EATING DISORDERS
Anorexia nervosa
Bulimia nervosa

* anorexia nervosa psychological disorder characterized by voluntary refusal to eat.

* bulimia nervosa recurrent episodes of binge eating.

might be suffering from a **personality disorder.** Stemming largely from immature and distorted personality development, these personality, or character, disorders result in persistently maladaptive ways of perceiving, thinking, and relating to the world.

The broad category of personality disorder includes problems that vary greatly in form and severity. Although others might describe them as "eccentric" or "troublesome," some patients with personality disorders function adequately. In extreme cases, patients act out against or attempt to manipulate society.

Personality Disorder Clusters

The *DSM-IV* groups similar personality disorders into three broad types, Cluster A, Cluster B, and Cluster C.

Cluster A These individuals often act odd or eccentric. Their unusual behaviour can take drastically different forms. This cluster includes the following:

- *Paranoid personality disorder.* Pattern of distrust and suspiciousness.
- *Schizoid personality disorder.* Pattern of detachment from social relationships.
- *Schizotypal personality disorder.* Pattern of acute discomfort in close relationships, cognitive distortions, and eccentric behaviour.

Cluster B Individuals often appear dramatic, emotional, or fearful. This cluster includes the following:

- *Antisocial personality disorder.* Pattern of disregard for the rights of others.
- *Borderline personality disorder.* Pattern of instability in interpersonal relationships, self-image, and impulsivity.
- *Histrionic personality disorder.* Pattern of excessive emotions and attention seeking.
- *Narcissistic personality disorder.* Pattern of grandiosity, need for admiration, and lack of empathy.

Cluster C Individuals often appear anxious or fearful. This cluster includes the following:

- *Avoidant personality disorder.* Pattern of social inhibition, feelings of inadequacy, and hypersensitivity to criticism.
- *Dependent personality disorder.* Pattern of submissive and clinging behaviour related to an excessive need to be cared for.
- *Obsessive-compulsive disorder.* Pattern of preoccupation with orderliness, perfectionism, and control.

Diagnosing a personality disorder requires evaluating the individual's long-term functioning and behaviour. In many cases, the individual suffers from multiple disorders. A complete interview, history, and assessment will assist you in determining your approach. Your prehospital care will vary depending on the patient's chief complaint and overall presentation.

IMPULSE CONTROL DISORDERS

Related to the personality disorders are the **impulse control disorders.** Recurrent impulses and the patient's failure to control them characterize these disorders. Examples of impulse control disorders include

- *Kleptomania.* A recurrent failure to resist impulses to steal objects not for immediate use or for their monetary value
- *Pyromania.* A recurrent failure to resist impulses to set fires
- *Pathological gambling.* A chronic and progressive preoccupation with gambling and the urge to gamble
- *Trichotillomania.* A recurrent impulse to pull out one's own hair
- *Intermittent explosive disorder.* Recurrent and paroxysmal episodes of significant loss of control of aggressive responses

Disorders of impulse control may be harmful to the patient and others. Prior to committing the act, the patient will have an increasing sense of tension. After the act, he will either have pleasure gratification or release.

* impulse control disorder condition characterized by the patient's failure to control recurrent impulses.

SUICIDE

Suicide, simply stated, is when a person intentionally takes his own life. Suicide is alarmingly common. It is the ninth-leading cause of death overall, and it is the third-leading cause in the 15–24-year age group. Suicide rates have risen dramatically in the younger age groups and have also increased significantly in the elderly population. Women attempt suicide more than men, but men—especially those over 55 years of age—are more likely to succeed. Statistically, suicide successes and methods vary widely by race, sex, and culture. The most common methods of suicide (1992) are

1. Gunshot (60 percent)
2. Poisoning (18 percent)
3. Strangulation (15 percent)
4. Cutting (1 percent)
5. Other or unspecified (6 percent)

Assessing Potentially Suicidal Patients

In cases of attempted suicide, many focus on whether the patient really wanted to kill himself. Indeed, this question will be at the heart of the patient's future psychiatric care, and information from the paramedic will be crucial to making that determination. But never lose sight of patient care while probing the psychological nature of attempted suicide.

Perform an appropriate focused history and secondary assessment concurrently with providing sound psychological care. Mental health professionals are rarely on the scene. It is up to you to document observations at the scene, especially any detailed suicide plans, any suicide notes, and any statements of the patient and bystanders. This information may not be available after the event when the patient receives psychiatric screening at the hospital. Such care and observations at the scene, combined with detailed documentation, are critical to the patient's long-term psychiatric care.

Document observations at the scene of an attempted suicide, especially any detailed suicide plans, suicide notes, and statements by the patient and bystanders.

Risk Factors for Suicide

The risk factors for suicide are numerous. When assessing a patient who has indicated suicidal intentions, screen for any of these risk factors:

- Previous attempts (Eighty percent of persons who successfully commit suicide have made a previous attempt.)
- Depression (Suicide is 500 times more common among patients who are severely depressed than among those who are not.)
- Age (Incidence is high between the ages of 15 and 24 years and over the age of 40.)
- Alcohol or drug abuse
- Divorced or widowed (The rate is five times higher than among other groups.)
- Giving away personal belongings, especially cherished possessions
- Living alone or in increased isolation
- The presence of **psychosis** with depression (for example, suicidal or destructive thoughts or hallucinations about killing or death)
- Homosexuality (especially homosexuals who are depressed, aging, alcoholic, or HIV-infected)
- Major separation trauma (loss of mate, loved one, job, money)
- Major physical stresses (surgery, childbirth, sleep deprivation)
- Loss of independence (disabling illness)
- Lack of goals and plans for the future
- Suicide of same-sex parent
- Expression of a plan for committing suicide
- Possession of the mechanism for suicide (gun, pills, rope)

* **psychosis** extreme response to stress characterized by impaired ability to deal with reality.

Patients who have attempted suicide must be evaluated in a hospital or psychiatric facility. Many people assume that "they were just looking for attention." Applied to the wrong patient, that presumption may contribute to his death.

AGE-RELATED CONDITIONS

Some behavioural disorders are particularly common among patients at the ends of the age spectrum—the young and the elderly. Your awareness of age-related conditions will help you assess and interact with these patients.

Crisis in the Geriatric Patient

Common physical problems among the elderly include dementia, chronic illness, and diminished eyesight and hearing. The elderly also experience depression that is often mistaken for dementia. When confronted with an elderly person in a crisis, take the following steps:

- Assess the patient's ability to communicate.
- Provide continual reassurance.
- Compensate for the patient's loss of sight and hearing with reassuring physical contact.
- Treat the patient with respect. Call the patient by name and title, such as "Mrs. Jones." Avoid such terms as "dear," "honey," and "babe."

- Avoid administering medication.
- Describe what you are going to do before you do it.
- Take your time. Do not convey the impression that you are in a hurry.
- Allow family members and friends to remain with the patient if possible.

Crisis in the Pediatric Patient

Behavioural emergencies are not limited to adults. Children also have behavioural crises. While the child's developmental stage will affect his behaviour, these general guidelines will assist you when confronting an emotionally distraught or disruptive child.

- Avoid separating a young child from his parent.
- Attempt to prevent the child from seeing things that will increase his distress.
- Make all explanations brief and simple, and repeat them often.
- Be calm and speak slowly.
- Identify yourself by giving both your name and your function.
- Be truthful with the child. Telling the truth will develop trust.
- Encourage the child to help with his care.
- Reassure the child by carrying out all interventions gently.
- Do not discourage the child from crying or showing emotion.
- If you must be separated from the child, introduce the person who will assume responsibility for his care.
- Allow the child to keep a favourite blanket or toy.
- Do not leave the child alone, even for a short period.

Always be mindful of every young or elderly patient's uniqueness. Treat him equally and fairly, as you would any other patient.

MANAGEMENT OF BEHAVIOURAL EMERGENCIES

Patients who are experiencing behavioural emergencies require both medical and psychological care. In general, take the following measures when you treat a patient who is experiencing a behavioural emergency:

1. Ensure scene safety and body substance isolation (BSI) precautions.
2. Provide a supportive and calm environment.
3. Treat any existing medical conditions.
4. Do not allow the suicidal patient to be alone.
5. Do not confront or argue with the patient.
6. Provide realistic reassurance.
7. Respond to the patient in a direct, simple manner.
8. Transport the patient to an appropriate receiving facility.

Remember to treat the whole patient. Never overlook any serious, or potentially serious, medical complaints while focusing on the psychiatric assessment.

Never overlook any serious, or potentially serious, medical complaints while focusing on the psychiatric assessment.

MEDICAL

Patients who are experiencing apparent behavioural emergencies often have concurrent medical conditions—some of which may be responsible for the behavioural problem. Current literature indicates that medical conditions and/or substance abuse cause a much higher proportion of behavioural emergencies than previously believed. Medical care may include treatment for overdose, lacerations, toxic inhalation, hypoxia, or metabolic conditions. Many patients with chronic psychiatric conditions take medications for their illnesses; when abused, those medications have extremely toxic side effects. (See the pharmacology chapter, Chapter 14.) Additionally, these patients often live in conditions ranging from substandard housing to the street. This existence may predispose them to other medical problems, such as exposure, infections, and untreated illnesses.

PSYCHOLOGICAL

The time you spend developing a rapport with the patient in a behavioural emergency—before, during, and after assessment—is actually a part of the care you provide.

Patients who present with an apparent behavioural emergency also require psychological care. The time you spend developing a rapport with the patient—before, during, and after assessment—is actually a part of the care you provide. In effect, when you begin an assessment, you are also beginning your care, and you will continue to perform psychological assessment and care concurrently with medical assessment and care. Be calm and reassuring while you interview your patient.

Since much of your care will be aimed at the psychological problem, you should steer your conversation and actions in that direction. Visualize your patients on a continuum ranging from agitated and out-of-control to introverted and depressed (Figure 38-3). As a paramedic, you will need to defuse the agitated patient and attempt to communicate with the withdrawn patient. These situations especially will require the interviewing skills you learned earlier in this chapter.

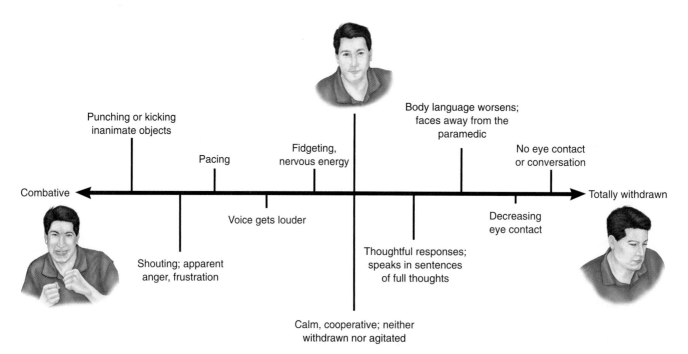

FIGURE 38-3 Continuum of patient responses during behavioural emergency. Whether dealing with an agitated or withdrawn patient, you will use your interpersonal skills to bring him to the calm, cooperative state in the middle of the continuum.

As you approach the patient, introduce yourself, and state that you want to help, since this might not be intuitively clear to a person with distorted perceptions. As you begin to converse, note how the patient reacts to you. Generally, if he responds appropriately to your actions, you should continue what you are doing. If the patient becomes more agitated or further withdrawn, rethink. Perhaps you are getting too close, talking too fast, or addressing difficult topics too early. Be sure your exit path is not blocked.

Your approach to these patients requires excellent people skills—especially listening and observing. If you do not use these skills, or if you rush or seem disinterested, your care will likely fail. Therapeutic communication, as this interaction has been called, is an art. "Talking down" the patient with a behavioural emergency requires effort and skill. Some patients, however, will not react favourably even to the best people skills. Extremely withdrawn patients or those with severe psychotic symptoms may never fully respond during the time you spend with them out of the hospital. These patients still deserve quality care and compassion, even when they are uncommunicative or restrained.

Just as we must observe the patient, the patient observes us. Patients may actually be able to "read" us as accurately as (or more accurately than) we read them. Perform your assessment and care confidently and competently. If patients sense uneasiness or indecision, they are more likely to act out. Never play along with a patient's hallucinations or delusions. It may seem to be the easiest route, but ultimately it may be harmful. Often, the patient will recognize that you are patronizing him. Or the patient may talk of hallucinations or appear delusional, but not fully believe what he says. If you play along, you will lose credibility.

VIOLENT PATIENTS AND RESTRAINT

Who should be responsible for restraining a patient at an emergency scene is sometimes controversial. Many argue that physical restraint is clearly a police responsibility and EMS should not be involved. Others point out the grey areas, such as when the police are 30 minutes away, when only one officer is available, or when a patient is in imminent danger and paramedics must choose to act. One thing is certain: You should know how to control violent situations and restrain patients safely and effectively. Your agency's policies, your safety, and your patient's safety and needs will dictate how you handle individual emergencies. No EMS personnel should ever perform an unsafe act.

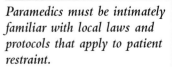

Most patients will respond to your care and therefore consent to treatment. Still, you will have patients whom the best interpersonal techniques cannot calm or reassure. If a patient must be legally transported against his will or if he becomes violent en route, restraint may be necessary.

The laws of consent state that no competent person may be transported against his will. A person who is in imminent danger of harming himself or others is not considered competent to refuse transport. Most provinces and territories have laws that allow persons fitting this criterion to be transported against their will to a hospital or approved psychiatric facility. Who has the authority to determine this varies across provinces and territories. In some areas, it is the police, in others a physician.

Patients who are suicidal or homicidal clearly meet this criterion. No one will dispute that the patient with a knife to his wrist or the patient standing on a high ledge about to jump are both potential dangers to themselves. The many others who are on the border require careful evaluation. The patient who stripped off all his clothes in subzero weather or the patient who is not oriented enough to stay on the sidewalk and wanders into traffic may also meet the criterion.

Follow medical direction or local protocol when determining who can order a patient transported against his will. Protocols or agency rules may also state whether you should be involved in restraining violent patients. Finally, scene assessment may uncover dangers that you will decide to leave for the police to defuse before providing care. In general, be guided by what is best for the patient.

METHODS OF RESTRAINT

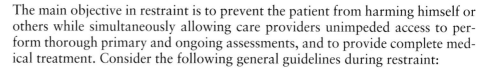

The main objective in restraint is to restrict the patient's movement in order to stop dangerous behaviours and prevent him from harming himself.

The main objective in restraint is to prevent the patient from harming himself or others while simultaneously allowing care providers unimpeded access to perform thorough primary and ongoing assessments, and to provide complete medical treatment. Consider the following general guidelines during restraint:

- Use the minimum force needed to restrain the patient. When verbal techniques will work, physical restraint may not be necessary.
- Use appropriate devices to perform restraint. Metal handcuffs may cause injury and should not be used. Thick roller bandages (Kling™, Kerlex™) are considered safer.
- Restraint is not punitive. Patients who are agitated frequently insult you, your partner, even your mother. This is not personal. The patient would make the same comments to anyone else in your position. Remain calm.
- Patients who have been restrained require careful monitoring. Assessment and care are not over when the patient is restrained; they are just beginning.

There are many techniques and devices for restraining the violent patient. Before restraining a person, consider the normal range of motion for the major joints. The arms cannot flail backward, the legs cannot kick backward, and the spinal column cannot double over backward. Also, consider the power of each major muscle group. For example, the flexor muscles of the arm are much stronger than the extensor muscles. Whenever possible, position the patient to limit his strength and range of motion.

Become familiar with the restraint devices your service employs, and periodically refresh your training in their application. Whether using gauze bandages or some form of commercial restraint, you must maintain proficiency in using restraint devices in an effective and safe manner. Many devices must be appropriately decontaminated after each use. Some devices, such as leather restraints, require monthly maintenance to ensure their continued effectiveness. Restraints can also be improvised from common materials as noted below:

- Cravats or triangular bandages are effective. Tie one cravat around the wrist or ankle and securely knot it into a "bracelet" that will not slip off the limb. Use another cravat to anchor the bracelet to the cot.
- Roller bandages (Kling™, Kerlex™) are safe and effective. Ensure that you use thick (six-ply), wide, nonstretch gauze bandages.

When you must restrain a patient, do not attempt to hold him for a long period. This sets up a confrontation and aggravates the situation. It also limits care because you will be too busy holding the patient to treat him. Continuous restraint also requires more than one paramedic or assistant per patient. Following this sequence of actions will help you restrain an unarmed patient:

1. Make certain you have adequate assistance; this will reduce the likelihood of injury both to you and to the patient. Prepare your stretcher and restraint equipment in advance. Keep restraints out of the patient's view until you need them.

2. Offer the patient one final opportunity to cooperate.

3. If the patient does not respond to this request, at least two persons, preferably three or four, should move swiftly toward him. He cannot simultaneously focus on multiple paramedics. When four rescuers are present, one person can control each extremity. This prevents the patient from striking and kicking. Keep away from the patient's mouth to avoid being bitten. Your swiftness will minimize the accuracy of a patient's kick or blow. Attempting to restrain a patient with too many rescuers can be confusing and inefficient. Someone should continue talking with the patient throughout the restraining process.

4. When the patient's extremities are physically restrained, move him to a laterally recumbent position on the stretcher, where he can be secured. This prevents him from using his strong abdominal and leg muscles to break free from restraint. If your agency uses the Reeves stretcher to secure patients, be sure that the circumferential wrapping does not restrict the patient's respiratory efforts.

5. Generally, once a patient is restrained, keeping him restrained is best. The thought of regaining control of a patient in a moving ambulance by yourself is not pleasant. If the patient calms down, you may try to reduce the discomforts caused by the restraints, but you must keep adequate restraints in place.

6. Monitor the patient carefully during transport.

POSITIONING AND RESTRAINING PATIENTS FOR TRANSPORT

Once the patient is successfully restrained, position him on his side. This dramatically reduces resistance and allows continued airway assessment and maintenance. Adjust the cot to its lowest position to improve stability, avoid lifting, and shorten the distance to the ground in case the patient falls. Do not allow the patient's large muscle groups to work together. For example, restrain one arm at the patient's side and the other above his head. Place a webbed strap across the patient's lumbar region, but do not cinch it too tightly. After applying restraints to the ankles and securing the cot, tie the ankle restraints to one another. Do not remove the restraints until enough personnel are present to control the patient. Always check the distal pulses after placing restraints.

Restraint is not without risk either to the paramedic or to the patient. Improper restraint threatens injury to everyone involved. Occasionally, a restrained patient dies. The term for this phenomenon is **restraint asphyxia**. The most common scenario in these cases involves a patient who has struggled violently, either during the restraint process or during a foot pursuit or struggle with police. The patient is eventually captured, restrained, and placed in a hog-tie or hobble restraint. He struggles for a time and then becomes quiet. While police and EMS crews think he is calming down, he is actually in cardiac arrest. Resuscitation attempts are usually unsuccessful. Some experts believe the restraint itself causes the patient's death. Others believe the combination of restraint, exertion, hyperthermia, and drug or alcohol abuse causes it. To prevent these deaths (and the liability they will bring), never use hog-tie or hobble restraints. Monitor all restrained patients carefully, as noted earlier. Be alert for mental status changes from agitated to calm or sleepy—they may mean hypoxia. Monitor respiratory rate and depth frequently.

Patients who are physically restrained must receive frequent and close monitoring. Ideally, this should include continuous ECG monitoring and pulse oximetry. Vital signs should be taken at least every 15 minutes, or every 5 minutes if the patient's condition is critical.

* **restaint asphyxia** death from positioning that prevents sufficient intake of oxygen.

Never use hog-tie or hobble restraints.

CHEMICAL RESTRAINT

Some EMS systems allow the use of antipsychotic medications for controlling acutely psychotic and combative patients. This is especially important for long transports or for aeromedical operations. The most commonly used antipsychotics include haloperidol (Haldol), chlorpromazine (Thorazine), and others. These medications can be very effective in sedating patients who are agitated or hostile. Remember that medications in this class may cause an extrapyramidal system (EPS) reaction. Be prepared for EPS reactions and, if indicated, administer diphenhydramine (Benadryl) or a similar agent. Always consult and follow local protocol regarding use of antipsychotic agents or chemical restraint. Versed is also used to control violent patients, once hypovolemia, hypoglycemia, and hypoxia are ruled out.

SUMMARY

Calls involving psychiatric and behavioural emergencies will challenge your skills as a paramedic. Differentiating physiological and psychological conditions will try your diagnostic skills, and developing the interview abilities that form the basis of psychiatric assessment and care will test your people skills. Ultimately, you will be called upon to help patients in a time of great need—the time of crisis. Once you determine that the patient is experiencing a purely behavioural emergency, your compassion and communication skills, rather than medications and procedures, will benefit him most.

Situations involving crises can drain your emotions. Observing a suicide or attempted suicide or struggling with or restraining a patient can take its toll. Take care of yourself before, during, and after these calls.

CHAPTER 39

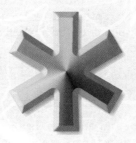

Gynecology

Objectives

After reading this chapter, you should be able to:

1. Review the anatomical structures and physiology of the female reproductive system. (see Chapter 12)
2. Identify the normal events of the menstrual cycle. (see Chapter 12)
3. Describe how to assess a patient with a gynecological complaint. (pp. 858–860)
4. Explain how to recognize a gynecological emergency. (pp. 858–860)
5. Describe the general care for any patient experiencing a gynecological emergency. (pp. 860–861)
6. Describe the pathophysiology, assessment, and management of the following gynecological emergencies:

   a. Pelvic inflammatory disease (pp. 861–862)
   b. Ruptured ovarian cyst (p. 862)
   c. Cystitis (p. 862)
   d. Mittelschmerz (p. 862)
   e. Endometritis (p. 862)
   f. Endometriosis (pp. 862–863)
   g. Ectopic pregnancy (p. 863)
   h. Vaginal hemorrhage (p. 863)
7. Describe the assessment, care, and emotional support of the sexual assault patient. (pp. 864–866)
8. Given several preprogrammed gynecological patients, provide the appropriate assessment, management, and transport. (pp. 858–866)

INTRODUCTION

✱ gynecology the branch of medicine that deals with the health maintenance and the diseases of women, primarily of the reproductive organs.

✱ obstetrics the branch of medicine that deals with the care of women throughout pregnancy.

The term **gynecology** is derived from Greek, *gynaik*, meaning "woman." Gynecology is the branch of medicine that deals with the health maintenance and the diseases of women and primarily of their reproductive organs. **Obstetrics** is the branch of medicine that deals with the care of women throughout pregnancy. This chapter focuses on the assessment and care of nonpregnant patients with problems of the reproductive system. The assessment and care of the obstetrical patient is the subject of the next chapter.

ASSESSMENT OF THE GYNECOLOGICAL PATIENT

Beyond labour and delivery, the most common emergency complaints of women in the childbearing years are abdominal pain and vaginal bleeding. Abdominal pain is often due to problems of the reproductive organs. In addition to the usual history and secondary assessment activities, you will need to ask specific questions pertinent to reproductive function and dysfunction. However, do not allow yourself to get distracted from getting complete past medical histories including chronic medical problems, medications, and allergies.

You may feel uncomfortable asking a patient about her reproductive history, but remember that you are a health-care professional who is trying to obtain pertinent information in order to provide the best possible care for your patient. If you conduct yourself in this manner, it should not be uncomfortable for you or your patient. Assess your patient's emotional state. If she is reluctant to discuss her complaint in detail, respect her wishes, and transport her to the emergency department where a more thorough assessment can be done.

> **Content Review**
>
> **MOST COMMON EMERGENCY GYNECOLOGICAL COMPLAINTS**
> Abdominal pain
> Vaginal bleeding

HISTORY

Use the SAMPLE approach for obtaining additional information about the history of the present illness. If the chief complaint is pain, then use the mnemonic OPQRST to gather more information. Is the patient's pain in the abdominal or pelvic region? Is it localized in a specific quadrant of the pelvis? Is she having her menstrual period? If so, how does the pain she is having now compare with how she usually feels? Some women have severe discomfort during their menstrual periods. This is called **dysmenorrhea**. Others may experience **dyspareunia**, painful sexual intercourse. Does walking or defecation aggravate her pain? What, if anything, alleviates her pain? Does positioning herself on her back or side with her knees bent relieve her discomfort?

✱ dysmenorrhea painful menstruation.

✱ dyspareunia painful sexual intercourse.

You need to determine if there are any associated signs or symptoms that will be helpful in determining what is wrong with your patient. For instance, does your patient report a fever or chills? Is she reporting signs of gastrointestinal problems, such as nausea, vomiting, diarrhea, or constipation? Or perhaps she is complaining of urinary problems, such as frequency, painful urination, or "colicky" urinary cramping. Does she report a vaginal discharge or bleeding? If so, you should obtain information about the colour, amount, frequency, or odour associated with either vaginal bleeding or discharge. If she reports vaginal bleeding, how does the amount compare with the volume of her usual menstrual period? Does she report dizziness with changes in position (orthostatic hypotension), syncope, or diaphoresis?

You will need to obtain specific information about her obstetric history. Has she ever been pregnant? *Gravida (G)* is the term used to describe the number of times a woman has been pregnant, including this one if she is pregnant. How many of those pregnancies ended in the delivery of a viable infant? *Term* (T) refers to the number of deliveries that progressed to a full term pregnancy of 37–42 weeks. *Para* or *parity* (P) refers to the number of deliveries. *Abortion* (A) refers to any pregnancy that was terminated before 20 weeks gestation, regardless of cause. *Living* (L) refers to the number of living children born to the mother. You may see this information recorded in "shorthand," for example, G4 T2 P1 A1 L3. This means that she has been pregnant 4 times, had 2 deliveries progress to full term, while 1 delivery was premature. She has had 1 abortion, whether therapeutic or spontaneous, and she has 3 living children. It is important to note the number of children living as this number may differ if complications arose to the infant after delivery. These terms refer to the number of pregnancies and deliveries, not the number of infants delivered, and so even twins or triplets counts only as one pregnancy and one delivery.

You will also need to obtain a gynecological history. Question the patient about previous ectopic pregnancies, infections, cesarean sections, pelvic surgeries, such as tubal ligation, abortions (either elective or therapeutic), and dilation and curettage (D&C) procedures. Also, ask the patient about any prior history of trauma to the reproductive tract. It is often helpful to find out whether the patient, if sexually active, has had pain or bleeding during or after sexual intercourse.

It is important to document the date of the patient's last menstrual period, commonly abbreviated LMP (or LNMP for "last normal menstrual period"). Ask whether the period was of a normal length and whether the flow was heavier or lighter than usual. An easy way for women to estimate menstrual flow is by the number of pads or tampons used. She can easily compare this number to her routine usage. It is also important to inquire how regular the patient's periods tend to be. Ask her what form of birth control, if any, she uses. Also, find out if she uses it regularly. Such direct questions as "Could you be pregnant?" are generally unlikely to get an accurate response. Indirect questioning is often more helpful in determining the likelihood of pregnancy, such as "When did your last menstrual period start?" If you suspect pregnancy, inquire about other signs, including a late or missed period, breast tenderness, bloating, urinary frequency, or nausea and vomiting. Until proven otherwise, you should assume that any missed or late period is due to pregnancy, even though your patient may deny it.

Contraception, or the prevention of pregnancy, takes many forms. Remember that many contraceptives are medications, and so do not forget to ask about their use. With the exception of oral contraceptives ("the pill") and intrauterine devices (IUDs), side effects caused by contraceptives are relatively rare. Oral contraceptives have been associated with hypertension, rare incidents of stroke and heart attack, and possibly pulmonary embolism. IUDs can cause perforation of the uterus, uterine infection, or irregular uterine bleeding. This is especially true for IUDs that have remained in place longer than the time recommended by the manufacturer, which rarely exceeds two years.

SECONDARY ASSESSMENT

Secondary assessment of the gynecological patient is limited in the field. More than at any other time, the patient's comfort level should guide your actions. Respect your patient's modesty, and maintain her privacy. This may mean that you need to exclude parents from the room when assessing adolescent patients or that you need to exclude spouses of married patients. Recognizing that most people are not comfortable discussing matters related to sexuality or reproductive organs, take your cues from the patient. Maintain a professional demeanour. Explain all procedures thoroughly so that your patient can understand them prior to initiating any care. Some women may feel more comfortable if they can be cared for by a female paramedic.

In the female patient of childbearing age, always document the LMP.

Any patient of reproductive age who still has her uterus should be considered to be pregnant until proven otherwise.

As always, the level of consciousness is the best indicator of your patient's status. Assess your patient's general appearance, paying particular attention to the colour of her skin and mucous membranes. Cyanosis and pallor may indicate shock or a gas-exchange problem, while a flushed appearance is more indicative of fever.

Remember that vital signs are useful clues to the nature of your patient's problem. Pain and fever tend to cause an increase in pulse and respiratory rates along with a slight increase in blood pressure. Significant bleeding will cause increased pulse and respiratory rates as well as narrowing pulse pressures (the difference between systolic and diastolic pressures). Perform a tilt test to assess for orthostatic changes in her vital signs (a decrease in blood pressure and an increase in pulse rate when the patient rises from a supine or seated position), which again points to significant blood loss.

Assess your patient for evidence of vaginal bleeding or discharge. If possible, estimate blood loss. The use of more than two sanitary pads per hour is considered significant bleeding. If serious bleeding is reported or evident, it may be necessary to inspect the patient's perineum. Document the colour and character of the discharge, as well as the amount, and the presence or absence of clots. *Do not perform an internal vaginal exam in the field.*

Pay particular attention to the abdominal examination. Gently palpate the abdomen. Document and report any masses, distention, guarding, localized tenderness, or rebound tenderness. In thin patients, a palpable mass in the lower abdomen may be an intrauterine pregnancy. At three months, the uterus is barely palpable above the symphysis pubis. At four months, the uterus is palpable midway between the umbilicus and the symphysis pubis. At five months (approximately 20 weeks), the uterus is palpable at the level of the umbilicus.

Do not perform an internal vaginal exam in the field.

MANAGEMENT OF GYNECOLOGICAL EMERGENCIES

General management of gynecological emergencies is focused on supportive care.

In general, the management of the patient experiencing a gynecological emergency is focused on supportive care. Rely on your primary assessment to guide your decision making about the need for oxygen therapy or intravenous access. If your patient's status warrants it, administer oxygen, or assist ventilation as necessary. As a rule, intravenous access and fluid replacement is usually not indicated. However, if your patient has excessive bleeding or demonstrates signs of shock, then establish at least one large bore IV, and administer normal saline at a rate indicated by the patient's presentation. You may also want to initiate cardiac monitoring if your patient is unstable.

Do not pack dressings in the vagina.

Continue to monitor and evaluate serious bleeding. *Do not pack dressings in the vagina.* Discourage the use of tampons to absorb blood flow. If your patient is bleeding heavily, count and document the number of sanitary pads used. If your patient demonstrates signs of impending shock, you may elect to place her in the Trendelenburg position (head lower than feet). If shock is not a consideration, then position your patient for comfort in the left lateral recumbent position or supine with her knees bent, as this decreases tension on the peritoneum. Analgesics (pain-control medications) are not usually given in the field for gynecological complaints because these drugs tend to mask signs and symptoms of a deteriorating condition and make assessment and diagnosis difficult.

Since it is not appropriate to perform an internal vaginal exam in the field, most patients with gynecological complaints will be transported to be evaluated by a physician. Some problems may require surgical intervention, and so you should consider emergency transport to the appropriate facility on the basis of your local protocols.

Psychological support is particularly important when caring for patients with gynecological complaints. Keep calm. Maintain your patient's modesty and privacy. Remember that this is likely to be a very stressful situation for your patient, and she will appreciate your gentle, considerate care.

SPECIFIC GYNECOLOGICAL EMERGENCIES

Gynecological emergencies can be generally divided into two categories—medical and traumatic.

MEDICAL GYNECOLOGICAL EMERGENCIES

Gynecological emergencies of a medical nature are often hard to diagnose in the field. The most common symptoms of a medical gynecological emergency are abdominal pain and/or vaginal bleeding.

Gynecological Abdominal Pain

Pelvic Inflammatory Disease Probably the most common cause of non-traumatic abdominal pain is **pelvic inflammatory disease (PID)**, an infection of the female reproductive tract that can be caused by a bacterium, virus, or fungus. The organs most commonly involved are the uterus, fallopian tubes, and ovaries. Occasionally, the adjoining structures, such as the peritoneum and intestines, also become involved. PID is the most common cause of abdominal pain in women in the childbearing years, occurring in 1 percent of that population. The highest rate of infection occurs in sexually active women ages 15 to 24. The most common causes of PID are gonorrhea *(Neisseria gonorrhoeae)* or chlamydia *(Chlamydia trachomatis),* although rarely streptococcal or staphylococcal bacteria may cause it. Commonly, gonorrhea or chlamydia progresses undetected in a female until frank PID develops.

* **pelvic inflammatory disease (PID)** an acute infection of the reproductive organs that can be caused by a bacteria, virus, or fungus.

Predisposing factors include multiple sexual partners, prior history of PID, recent gynecological procedure, or an IUD. Postinfection damage to the fallopian tubes is a common cause for infertility. PID may be either acute or chronic. If it is allowed to progress untreated, sepsis may develop. Additionally, PID may cause adhesions, in which the pelvic organs "stick together." Adhesions are a common cause of chronic pelvic pain and increase the frequency of infertility and ectopic pregnancies.

PID is a major risk factor for pelvic adhesions.

While it is possible for a patient with PID to be asymptomatic, most of these patients complain of abdominal pain. It is often diffuse and located in the lower abdomen. It may be moderate to severe, which occasionally makes it difficult to distinguish it from appendicitis. Pain may intensify either before or after the menstrual period. It may also worsen during sexual intercourse, as movement of the cervix tends to cause increased discomfort. Patients with PID tend to walk with a shuffling gait, since walking often intensifies their pain. In severe cases, fever, chills, nausea, vomiting, or even sepsis may accompany PID. Occasionally, patients have a foul-smelling vaginal discharge, often yellow in colour, as well as irregular menses. It is common also to have mid-cycle bleeding.

Generally, on secondary assessment, the patient with PID appears acutely ill or toxic. The blood pressure is normal, although the pulse rate may be slightly increased. Fever may or may not be present. Palpation of the lower abdomen generally elicits moderate to severe pain. Occasionally, in severe cases, the abdomen will be tense with obvious rebound tenderness. Such cases may be impossible to distinguish from appendicitis in the prehospital setting.

The primary treatment for PID is antibiotics, often administered intravenously over an extended period. Once the causative organism is determined, the sexual partner may also require treatment. In the field, the primary goal is to make the patient as comfortable as possible. Place the patient on the ambulance stretcher in the position in which she is most comfortable. She may wish to draw her knees up toward her chest, as this decreases tension on the peritoneum. *Do not perform a vaginal examination.* If your patient has signs of sepsis, administer oxygen, and establish intravenous access.

Ruptured Ovarian Cyst *Cysts* are fluid-filled pockets. When they develop in the ovary, they can rupture and be a source of abdominal pain. When an egg is released from the ovary, a cyst, known as a corpus luteum cyst, is often left in its place. Occasionally, cysts develop independent of ovulation. When the cysts rupture, a small amount of blood is spilled into the abdomen. Because blood irritates the peritoneum, it can cause abdominal pain and rebound tenderness. Ovarian cysts may be found during a routine pelvic examination. However, in the field setting, your patient is likely to complain of moderate to severe unilateral abdominal pain, which may radiate to her back. She may also give a history of dyspareunia, irregular bleeding, or a delayed menstrual period. It is not uncommon for patients to have ruptured ovarian cysts during intercourse or physical activity. This often results in immediate, severe abdominal pain causing the patient to immediately stop intercourse or other physical activity. Ruptured ovarian cysts may be associated with vaginal bleeding.

* **cystitis** infection of the urinary bladder.

Cystitis Urinary bladder infection, or **cystitis,** is a common cause of abdominal pain. Bacteria usually enter the urinary tract via the urethra, ascending into the bladder and ureters. The bladder lies anterior to the reproductive organs and, when inflamed, causes pain, generally immediately above the symphysis pubis. If untreated, the infection can progress to the kidneys. In addition to abdominal pain, your patient may report urinary frequency, pain or burning with urination (**dysuria**), and a low-grade fever. Occasionally, the urine may be blood tinged.

* **dysuria** painful urination often associated with cystitis.

* **mittelschmerz** abdominal pain associated with ovulation.

Mittelschmerz Occasionally, ovulation is accompanied by midcycle abdominal pain known as **mittelschmerz.** It is thought that the pain is related to peritoneal irritation due to follicle rupture or bleeding at the time of ovulation. The unilateral lower quadrant pain is usually self-limiting and may be accompanied by midcycle spotting. While some women may report a low-grade fever, it should be noted that body temperature normally increases at the time of ovulation and remains elevated until the day prior to the onset of the menstrual period. Treatment is symptomatic.

* **endometritis** infection of the endometrium.

* **miscarriage** commonly used term to describe a pregnancy that ends before 20 weeks gestation; may also be called spontaneous abortion.

Endometritis An infection of the uterine lining called **endometritis** is an occasional complication of **miscarriage,** childbirth, or gynecological procedures, such as dilatation and curettage (D&C). Commonly reported signs and symptoms include mild to severe lower abdominal pain, a bloody, foul-smelling discharge, and fever (38.3° to 40° C). The onset of symptoms is usually 48 to 72 hours after the gynecological procedure or miscarriage. These infections often mimic the presentation of PID and can be quite serious if not quickly treated with the appropriate antibiotics. Complications of endometritis may include sterility, sepsis, or even death.

* **endometriosis** condition in which endometrial tissue grows outside of the uterus.

Endometriosis Endometriosis is a condition in which endometrial tissue is found outside the uterus. Most commonly, it is found in the abdomen and pelvis, although it has been found virtually everywhere in the body, including the central nervous system and lungs. Regardless of its site, the tissue responds to the hormonal changes associated with the menstrual cycle and thus bleeds in a cyclical manner. This bleeding causes inflammation, scarring of adjacent tissues, and the subsequent development of adhesions, particularly in the pelvic cavity.

Endometriosis is usually seen in women between the ages of 30 to 40 and is rarely seen in postmenopausal women. The exact cause is unknown. The most common symptom is dull, cramping pelvic pain that is usually related to menstruation. Dyspareunia and abnormal uterine bleeding is also commonly reported. Painful bowel movements have been reported when the endometrial tissue has invaded the gastrointestinal tract. It is not uncommon for endometriosis to be diagnosed when the patient is being evaluated for infertility. Definitive treatment may include medical management with hormones, analgesics, and anti-inflammatory drugs, and/or surgery to remove the excessive endometrial tissue or adhesions from other organs.

Ectopic Pregnancy An **ectopic pregnancy** is the implantation of a fetus outside of the uterus. The most common site is within the fallopian tubes. This is a surgical emergency because the tube can rupture, triggering a massive hemorrhage. Patients with ectopic pregnancy often have severe unilateral abdominal pain which may radiate to the shoulder on the affected side, a late or missed menstrual period, and, occasionally, vaginal bleeding. Additional discussion of ectopic pregnancy is presented in the next chapter.

 ectopic pregnancy the implantation of a developing fetus outside of the uterus, often in a fallopian tube.

Ectopic pregnancy is a life-threatening condition.

Management of Gynecological Abdominal Pain

Any woman with significant abdominal pain should be treated and transported to the hospital for evaluation. Administer oxygen and establish intravenous access if indicated. Refer to the earlier section on management of gynecological emergencies for additional information.

Nontraumatic Vaginal Bleeding

Nontraumatic vaginal bleeding is rarely seen in the field unless it is severe. Refer to the earlier section in this chapter on completing a patient history. You should not presume that vaginal bleeding is due to normal menstruation. Occasionally, a woman will experience **menorrhagia,** or excessive menstrual flow, but rarely is it the cause for a 911 call. Hemorrhage, regardless of cause, is always potentially life threatening, and so be alert for signs of impending shock.

The most common cause of nontraumatic vaginal bleeding is a spontaneous abortion (miscarriage). If it has been more than 60 days since your patient's LMP, you should assume that this is the cause. Vaginal bleeding due to miscarriage is often associated with cramping abdominal pain and the passage of clots and tissue. The loss of a pregnancy, even at a very early phase, is a significant emotional event for your patient, and so your kind and considerate care is important. Spontaneous abortion and other causes of bleeding in the obstetric patient will be discussed further in the next chapter. Other potential causes of vaginal bleeding include cancerous lesions, PID, or the onset of labour.

 menorrhagia excessive menstrual flow.

The most common cause of nontraumatic vaginal bleeding is spontaneous abortion (miscarriage).

Management of Nontraumatic Vaginal Bleeding

Your field management of patients suffering nontraumatic vaginal bleeding will depend on the severity of the situation and your assessment of the patient's status. Use dressings or pads to absorb the blood flow. *Do not pack the vagina.* If your patient is passing clots or tissue, save these for evaluation by a physician. Transport your patient in a position of comfort. The initiation of oxygen therapy and intravenous access should be guided by the patient's condition.

TRAUMATIC GYNECOLOGICAL EMERGENCIES

Most cases of vaginal bleeding result from obstetrical problems or are related to the menstrual period. However, trauma to the vagina and perineum can also cause bleeding and abdominal pain.

Causes of Gynecological Trauma

The incidence of genital trauma is increasing, with vaginal injury occurring far more commonly than male genital injury. Gynecological trauma may occur at any age. Blunt trauma occurs more frequently than penetrating trauma. Straddle injury (such as may occur with riding a bicycle) is the most common form of blunt trauma. Vaginal injuries are most often lacerations due to sexual assault. Other causes of gynecological trauma include blunt force to the lower abdomen due to assault or seat-belt injuries, direct blows to the perineal area, foreign bodies inserted into the vagina, self-attempts at abortion, and lacerations following childbirth.

Management of Gynecological Trauma

Injuries to the external genitalia should be managed by direct pressure over the laceration or a chemical cold pack applied to a hematoma. In most cases of vaginal bleeding, the source is not readily apparent. If bleeding is severe or your patient demonstrates signs of shock, establish IV access to maintain intravascular volume, and monitor vital signs closely. Blunt force may cause organ rupture leading to the development of peritonitis or sepsis. *Never* pack the vagina with any material or dressing, regardless of the severity of the bleeding. Expedite transport to the emergency department, since surgical intervention is often required.

Sexual Assault

Sexual assault continues to represent the most rapidly growing violent crime in North America. In Canada, in 1999, 27 872 sexual assaults were reported to police. Unfortunately, it is estimated that only 6 percent of all sexual assaults and only 1 percent of date rapes are reported to authorities. Male victims represent 5 percent of reported sexual assaults. Sexual abuse of children is reported even less frequently. There is no "typical victim" of sexual assault. Nobody, from small children to aged adults, is immune.

Most victims of sexual assault know their assailants. Friends, acquaintances, intimates, and family members commit the vast majority (80 percent) of sexual assaults against women. Acquaintance rape is particularly common among adolescent victims. Sexual assault is a crime of violence, not passion, that is motivated by aggression and a need to control, humiliate, or inflict pain. There are very few predictors of who is capable of committing sexual assault, as age, economic status, and ethnic origins vary widely. Common behavioural characteristics found among rapists include poor impulse control, the need to achieve sexual satisfaction within the context of violence, and immaturity.

The definition of sexual assault varies across provinces and territories. The common element of any definition is sexual contact without consent. Generally, rape is defined as penetration of the vagina or rectum of an unwilling female or the rectum in an unwilling male. In most provinces and territories, penetration must occur for an act to be classified as rape. Sexual assault also includes oral-genital sex. Regardless of the legal definition, sexual assault is a crime of violence with serious physical and psychological implications.

Assessment The victim of sexual assault is a unique patient with unique needs. Your patient needs emergency medical treatment and psychological support. Your patient also needs to have legal evidence gathered. *Your* objectivity is essential, as your attitude may affect long-term psychological recovery. As a rule, victims of sexual abuse *should not* be questioned about the incident in the field. Do not ask questions about specific details of the assault. It is not important, from the

Do not ask about specific details of a sexual assault.

standpoint of prehospital care, to determine whether penetration took place. Do not inquire about the patient's sexual practices. Confine your questions to the physical injuries the patient received. Even well-intentioned questions may lead to guilt feelings in the patient. Do not ask such questions as "Why did you go with him or get in his car?"

The psychological response of sexual assault victims varies widely. The victim of sexual assault may be withdrawn or hysterical. Some use denial, anger, or fear as defence mechanisms. Approach the patient calmly and professionally. Allay the patient's fear and anxiety. Respond to the patient's feelings, but be aware of your own. If the patient is incompletely dressed, a cover should be offered. Respect the patient's modesty. Explain all procedures, and obtain the patient's permission before beginning them. Avoid touching the patient other than to take vital signs or examine other physical injuries. *Do not* examine the genitalia unless there is life-threatening hemorrhage.

Management In most situations, psychological and emotional support is the most important help you can offer. Maintain a nonjudgmental attitude, and assure the patient of confidentiality. If the patient is female, allow her to be cared for by a female paramedic (if available). If the patient desires, have a female accompany her to the hospital (Figure 39-1). Provide a safe environment, such as the back of a well-lit ambulance. Respond to the patient's feelings, and respect the patient's wishes. Unless your patient is unconscious, do not touch the patient unless given permission. Even when your patient appears to have an altered level of consciousness, explain what is going to be done before initiating any treatment.

Preservation of physical evidence is important. When the patient arrives at the hospital, a physician or sexual assault nurse examiner will complete a sexual assault examination to gather physical evidence. To protect this evidence, it is important that you adhere to the following guidelines:

- Consider the patient a crime scene, and protect that scene.
- Handle clothing as little as possible, if at all.
- If you must remove clothing, bag separately each item that must be bagged.
- Do not cut through any tears or holes in the clothing.
- Place bloody articles in brown paper bags.
- Do not examine the perineal area.

Do not examine the external genitalia of a sexual assault victim unless there is a life-threatening hemorrhage.

Psychological and emotional support are the most important elements of care for the sexual assault victim.

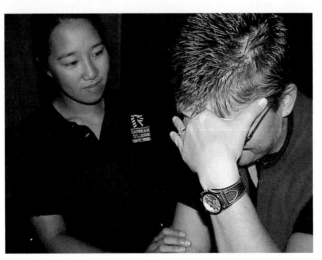

FIGURE 39-1 If possible, have a female paramedic accompany the sexual assault victim to the hospital.

- If the assault took place within the hour or the patient is bleeding, put an absorbent underpad (e.g., Chux) under the patient's hips to collect that evidence.
- If you cover the patient with a sheet or blanket, turn that over to the hospital as evidence.
- Do not allow the patient to change clothes, bathe, or douche (if female) before the medical examination.
- Do not allow the patients to comb hair, brush teeth, or clean fingernails.
- Do not clean wounds, if at all possible.
- If you must initiate care on scene, avoid disturbing of the crime scene.

Documentation When completing your patient care report, keep the following documentation guidelines in mind:

- State patient remarks accurately.
- Objectively state your observations of the patient's physical condition and environment, and the patient's appearance.
- Document any evidence (e.g., clothing, sheets) turned over to the hospital staff and the name of the individual to whom you gave it.
- Do *not* include your opinions as to whether rape occurred.

SUMMARY

Most gynecological emergency patients have either abdominal pain or vaginal bleeding. The patient with abdominal pain should be made comfortable and transported to the emergency department. The management of vaginal bleeding depends on the severity. Minor bleeding should be simply monitored. Severe bleeding should be treated with IV fluids, if indicated.

In the case of sexual assault, you should first determine if any life-threatening physical injuries exist. Second, respect the patient's wishes, and offer emotional support. Third, in treating victims of sexual assault, make every effort to preserve physical evidence. As with any type of emergency care, the primary concern is the patient.

CHAPTER 40

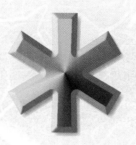

Obstetrics

Objectives

After reading this chapter, you should be able to:

1. Describe the anatomical structures and physiology of the reproductive system during pregnancy. (pp. 868–872)
2. Identify the normal events of pregnancy. (pp. 872–875)
3. Describe how to assess an obstetrical patient. (pp. 875–878)
4. Identify the stages of labour and the paramedic's role in each stage. (pp. 889–890)
5. Differentiate between normal and abnormal deliveries. (pp. 889–901)
6. Identify and describe complications associated with pregnancy and delivery. (pp. 878–889, 901–903)
7. Identify predelivery emergencies. (pp. 878–889)
8. State indications of an imminent delivery. (p. 889)
9. Differentiate the management of a patient with a predelivery emergency from that of a normal delivery. (pp. 878–889)
10. State the steps in the predelivery preparation of the mother. (pp. 891–892)
11. Establish the relationship between body substance isolation and childbirth. (p. 891)
12. State the steps to assist in the delivery of a baby. (pp. 891–894)

Continued

Objectives Continued

13. Describe how to care for the newborn. (pp. 893, 894–896)
14. Describe how and when to cut the umbilical cord. (pp. 891, 894)
15. Discuss the steps in the delivery of the placenta. (pp. 893, 894)
16. Describe the postdelivery management of the mother. (pp. 894, 901–903)
17. Summarize neonatal resuscitation procedures. (p. 896)
18. Describe the procedures for handling abnormal deliveries, complications of pregnancy, and maternal complications of labour. (pp. 878–889, 896–903)
19. Describe special considerations when meconium is present in amniotic fluid or during delivery. (p. 901)
20. Describe special considerations of a premature baby. (pp. 887–889)
21. Given several simulated delivery situations, provide the appropriate assessment, management, and transport for the mother and child. (pp. 868–903)

INTRODUCTION

Pregnancy, childbirth, and the potential complications of each are the focus of this chapter. Pregnancy is a normal, natural process of life that results from ovulation and fertilization. Complications of pregnancy are uncommon, but when they do occur, you must be prepared to recognize them quickly and manage them. Childbirth occurs daily, usually requiring only the most basic assistance. This chapter will prepare you to assess and care for the patient throughout her pregnancy and delivery of her child.

THE PRENATAL PERIOD

The *prenatal period* (literally "prebirth period") is the time from conception until delivery of the fetus. During this period, fetal development takes place. In addition, significant physiological changes occur in the mother.

ANATOMY AND PHYSIOLOGY OF THE OBSTETRIC PATIENT

As you learned in the previous chapter, the first two weeks of the menstrual cycle are dominated by the hormone estrogen, which causes the endometrium (the inner lining of the uterus) to thicken and become engorged with blood. In response to a surge of luteinizing hormone (LH) and follicle stimulating hormone (FSH), **ovulation,** or release of an egg (ovum) from the ovary, takes place. The egg travels down the fallopian tube to the uterus. If the egg has been fertilized, it becomes implanted in the uterus and pregnancy begins. If the egg has not been fertilized, menstruation (discharge of blood, mucus, and cellular debris from the endometrium) takes place 14 days after ovulation. (The time from ovulation to menstruation is always exactly 14 days. However, the time from menstruation to

* **ovulation** the release of an egg from the ovary.

the next ovulation may vary by several days from the average of 14 days, which is why it can be difficult for couples to find the optimum time of the month to conceive, or to avoid conceiving, a baby.)

If the woman has had intercourse within 24 to 48 hours before ovulation, fertilization may occur. The male's seminal fluid, which carries numerous spermatozoa or male sex cells, enters the vagina and uterus and travels toward the fallopian tubes. Fertilization, which usually takes place in the distal third of the fallopian tube, occurs when a male spermatozoon fuses with the female ovum (Figure 40-1). After fertilization, the ovum begins cellular division immediately, which continues as it moves through the fallopian tube to the uterus. The ovum then becomes a *blastocyst* (a hollow ball of cells). The blastocyst normally implants in the thickened uterine lining, which has been prepared for implantation by the hormone progesterone, where the fetus and placenta subsequently develop.

Approximately three weeks after fertilization, the placenta develops on the uterine wall at the site where the blastocyst attached (Figure 40-2). The **placenta,** known as the "organ of pregnancy," is a temporary, blood-rich structure that serves as the lifeline for the developing fetus. It transfers heat while exchanging oxygen and carbon dioxide, delivering nutrients (such as glucose, potassium, sodium, and chloride), and carrying away wastes (such as urea, uric acid, and creatinine). The placenta also serves as an endocrine gland throughout pregnancy, secreting hormones necessary for fetal survival as well as the estrogen and progesterone required to maintain the pregnancy. Additionally, the placenta serves as a protective barrier against harmful substances. (However, some drugs, such as narcotics, steroids, and some antibiotics, are able to cross the placental membrane from the mother to the fetus.) When expelled from the uterus following birth of the child, the placenta and accompanying membranes are called the **afterbirth.**

The placenta is connected to the fetus by the **umbilical cord,** a flexible, rope-like structure approximately 60 centimetres long and two centimetres in diameter.

✱ **placenta** the organ that serves as a lifeline for the developing fetus. The placenta is attached to the wall of the uterus and the umbilical cord.

✱ **afterbirth** the placenta and accompanying membranes that are expelled from the uterus after the birth of a child.

✱ **umbilical cord** structure containing two arteries and one vein that connects the placenta and the fetus.

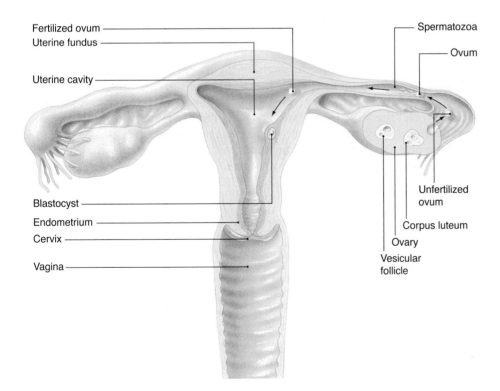

FIGURE 40-1   Fertilization and implantation of the ovum.

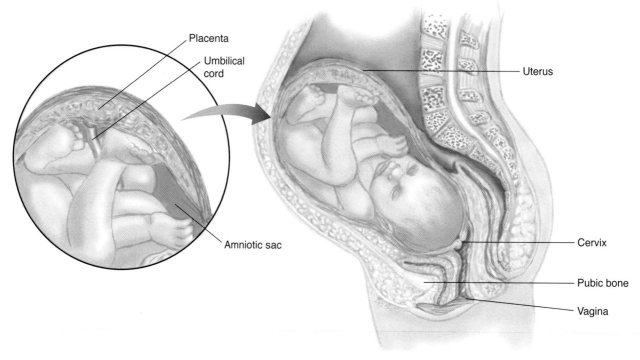

Placenta

Umbilical cord

Uterus

Amniotic sac

Cervix

Pubic bone

Vagina

Figure 40-2   Anatomy of the placenta.

Normally, the umbilical cord contains two arteries and one vein. The umbilical vein transports oxygenated blood to the fetus, while the umbilical arteries return relatively deoxygenated blood to the placenta.

The fetus develops within the **amniotic sac,** sometimes called the "bag of waters" (BOW). This thin-walled membranous covering holds the **amniotic fluid** that surrounds and protects the fetus during intrauterine development. The amniotic fluid increases in volume throughout the course of the pregnancy. After the 20th week of gestation, the volume varies from 500 to 1000 mL. The presence of amniotic fluid allows for fetal movement within the uterus and serves to cushion and protect the fetus from trauma. The volume changes constantly as amniotic fluid moves back and forth across the placental membrane. During the latter part of the pregnancy, the fetus contributes to the volume by secretions from the lungs and urination. Although it may rupture earlier, the amniotic sac usually breaks during labour, and the amniotic fluid or "water" flows out of the vagina. This is called *rupture of the membranes (ROM).* It is what has happened when the pregnant woman says, "My water has broken."

Physiological Changes of Pregnancy

The physiological changes associated with pregnancy are due to an altered hormonal state, the mechanical effects of the enlarging uterus and its significant vascularity, and the increasing metabolic demands on the maternal system. It is important for you to understand the physiological changes associated with pregnancy so that you can better assess your pregnant patients.

Reproductive System It is understandable that the most significant pregnancy-related changes occur in the uterus. In its nonpregnant state, the uterus is a small

✱ **amniotic sac** the membranes that surround and protect the developing fetus throughout the period of intrauterine development.

✱ **amniotic fluid** clear, watery fluid that surrounds and protects the developing fetus.

pear-shaped organ weighing about 60 g with a capacity of approximately 10 mL. By the end of pregnancy, its weight has increased to 1000 g, while its capacity is now approximately 5000 mL (Figure 40-3). Another notable change is that during pregnancy, the vascular system of the uterus contains about one-sixth (16 percent) of the mother's total blood volume.

Other changes include the formation of a mucous plug in the cervix that protects the developing fetus and helps prevent infection. This plug will be expelled when cervical dilation begins prior to delivery. Estrogen causes the vaginal mucosa to thicken, vaginal secretions to increase, and the connective tissue to loosen to allow for delivery. The breasts enlarge and become more nodular as the mammary glands increase in number and size in preparation for lactation.

Respiratory System As maternal oxygen demands increase, progesterone causes a decrease in airway resistance. This results in a 20-percent increase in oxygen consumption and a 40-percent increase in tidal volume. There is only a slight increase in respiratory rate. The diaphragm is pushed up by the enlarging uterus, resulting in flaring of the rib margins to maintain intrathoracic volume.

Cardiovascular System Various changes take place in the cardiovascular system during pregnancy. Cardiac output increases throughout pregnancy, peaking at 6–7 litres/minute by the time the fetus is fully developed. The maternal blood volume increases by 45 percent, and although both red blood cells and plasma increase, there is slightly more plasma, resulting in a relative anemia. To combat this anemia, pregnant women receive supplemental iron to increase the oxygen-carrying capacity of their red blood cells. Due to the increase in blood volume, the pregnant female may suffer a blood loss of 30–35 percent without a significant change in vital signs. The maternal heart rate increases by 10–15 bpm (beats per minute). Blood pressure decreases slightly during the first two trimesters, then rises to near nonpregnant levels during the third trimester.

Supine hypotensive syndrome occurs when the gravid uterus compresses the inferior vena cava when the mother lies in a supine position, causing decreased

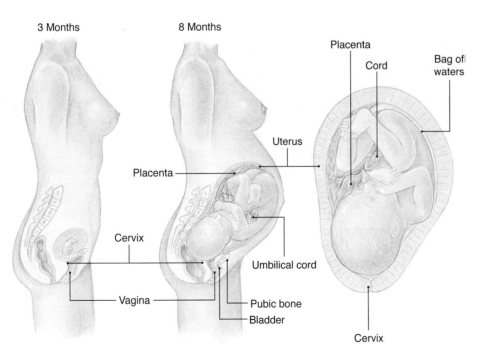

FIGURE 40-3 Uterine changes associated with pregnancy.

venous return to the right atrium, which lowers blood pressure. Current research suggests that the abdominal aorta may also be compressed. The enlarging uterus also may press on the pelvic and femoral vessels, causing impaired venous return from the legs and venous stasis. This may lead to the development of varicose veins, dependent edema, and postural hypotension. Some patients are predisposed to this problem because of an overall decrease in circulating blood volume or because of anemia. Assessment and management of supine hypotensive syndrome will be discussed later in this chapter.

Gastrointestinal System Nausea and vomiting are common in the first trimester as a result of hormone levels and changed carbohydrate needs. Peristalsis is slowed, and so delayed gastric emptying is likely, and bloating or constipation is common. As the uterus enlarges, abdominal organs are compressed, and the resulting compartmentalization of abdominal organs makes assessment difficult.

Urinary System Renal blood flow increases during pregnancy. The glomerular filtration rate increases by nearly 50 percent in the second trimester and remains elevated throughout the remainder of the pregnancy. As a result, the renal tubular absorption also increases. Occasionally, glucosuria (large amounts of sugar in the urine) may result from the kidney's inability to reabsorb all of the glucose being filtered. Glucosuria may be normal or may indicate the development of gestational diabetes. The urinary bladder gets displaced anteriorly and superiorly increasing the potential for rupture. As a result, urinary frequency is common, particularly in the first and third trimesters.

Musculoskeletal System Loosened pelvic joints caused by hormonal influences account for the waddling gait that is often associated with pregnancy. As the uterus enlarges and the mother's centre of gravity changes, postural changes take place to compensate for anterior growth, causing low back pain.

FETAL DEVELOPMENT

Fetal development begins immediately after fertilization and is quite complex. The time at which fertilization occurs is called *conception*. Since conception occurs approximately 14 days after the first day of the last menstrual period, it is possible to calculate, with fair accuracy, the approximate date the baby should be born. This estimate is usually made during the mother's first prenatal visit. The normal duration of pregnancy is 40 weeks from the first day of the mother's last menstrual period. This is equal to 280 days, which is 10 lunar months or, roughly, 9 calendar months. This estimated birth date is commonly called the *due date*. Medically, it is known as the **estimated date of confinement (EDC)**. Generally, pregnancy is divided into *trimesters*. Each trimester is approximately 13 weeks, or 3 calendar months, long.

Several different terms are used to describe the stages of development. The *preembryonic stage* covers the first 14 days following conception. The *embryonic stage* begins at day 15 and ends at approximately 8 weeks. The period from 8 weeks until delivery is known as the *fetal stage*. As a paramedic, you should be familiar with some of the significant developmental milestones that occur during these three periods (Table 40-1). During normal fetal development, the sex of the infant can usually be determined by 16 weeks gestation. By the 20th week, *fetal heart tones (FHTs)* can be detected by stethoscope. The mother also has generally felt fetal movement. By 24 weeks, the baby may be able to survive if born prematurely. Babies born after 28 weeks have an excellent chance of survival. By the 38th week, the fetus is considered *term*, or fully developed.

✱ **estimated date of confinement (EDC)** the approximate day the infant will be born. This date is usually set at 40 weeks after the date of the mother's last menstrual period (LMP).

Table 40-1 SIGNIFICANT FETAL DEVELOPMENTAL MILESTONES

	Preembryonic Stage
2 weeks	Rapid cellular multiplication and differentiation
	Embryonic Stage
4 weeks	Fetal heart begins to beat
8 weeks	All body systems and external structures are formed
	Size: approximately 3 centimetres
	Fetal Stage
8–12 weeks	Fetal heart tones audible with Doppler
	Kidneys begin to produce urine
	Size: 8 centimetres, weight about 45 g
	Fetus most vulnerable to toxins
16 weeks	Sex can be determined visually
	Swallowing amniotic fluid and producing meconium
	Looks like a baby, although thin
20 weeks	Fetal heart tones audible with stethoscope
	Mother able to feel fetal movement
	Baby develops schedule of sucking, kicking, and sleeping
	Hair, eyebrows, and eyelashes present
	Size: 19 centimetres, weight approximately 450 g
24 weeks	Increased activity
	Begins respiratory movement
	Size: 28 centimetres, weight 730 g.
28 weeks	Surfactant necessary for lung function is formed
	Eyes begin to open and close
	Weighs 900–1350 g
32 weeks	Bones are fully developed but soft and flexible
	Subcutaneous fat being deposited
	Fingernails and toenails present
38–40 weeks	Considered to be full-term
	Baby fills uterine cavity
	Baby receives maternal antibodies

Most of the fetus's organ systems develop during the first trimester. Therefore, this is when the fetus is most vulnerable to the development of birth defects.

FETAL CIRCULATION

The fetus receives its oxygen and nutrients from its mother through the placenta. Thus, while in the uterus, the fetus does not need to use its respiratory system or its gastrointestinal tract. Because of this, the fetal circulation shunts blood around the lungs and gastrointestinal tract.

The infant receives its blood from the placenta by means of the umbilical vein (Figure 40-4). The umbilical vein connects directly to the inferior vena cava by a

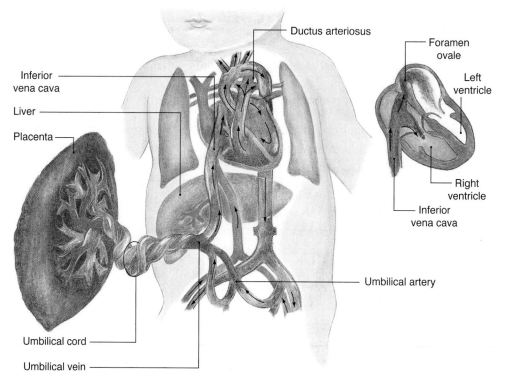

FIGURE 40-4   The maternal–fetal circulation.

specialized structure called the *ductus venosus.* Blood then travels through the inferior vena cava to the heart. The blood enters the right atrium and passes through the tricuspid valve into the right ventricle. It then exits the right ventricle, through the pulmonic valve, into the pulmonary artery. The fetus's heart has a hole between the right and left atria, termed the *foramen ovale,* which allows mixing of the oxygenated blood in the right atrium with that leaving the left ventricle bound for the aorta.

At this time, the blood is still oxygenated. Once in the pulmonary artery, the blood enters the *ductus arteriosus,* which connects the pulmonary artery with the aorta. The ductus arteriosus causes blood to bypass the uninflated lungs. Once in the aorta, blood flow is basically the same as in extrauterine life. Deoxygenated blood containing waste products exits the fetus, after passage through the liver, via the umbilical arteries.

The fetal circulation changes immediately at birth. As soon as the baby takes its first breath, the lungs inflate, greatly decreasing pulmonary vascular resistance to blood flow. Also, the ductus arteriosus closes, diverting blood to the lungs. In addition, the ductus venosus closes, stopping blood flow from the placenta. The foramen ovale also closes as a result of pressure changes in the heart, which stops blood flow from the right artium to the left atrium.

OBSTETRIC TERMINOLOGY

The field of obstetrics has its own unique terminology. You should be familiar with this terminology, since patient documentation and communications with other health-care workers and physicians often require it.

antepartum	the time interval prior to delivery of the fetus
postpartum	the time interval after delivery of the fetus
prenatal	the time interval prior to birth, synonymous with antepartum
natal	relating to birth or the date of birth
*gravidity**	the number of times a woman has been pregnant
*parity**	number of pregnancies carried to full term
primigravida	a woman who is pregnant for the first time
primipara	a woman who has given birth to her first child
multigravida	a woman who has been pregnant more than once
nulligravida	a woman who has not been pregnant
multipara	a woman who has delivered more than one baby
nullipara	a woman who has yet to deliver her first child
grand multiparity	a woman who has delivered at least seven babies
gestation	period of time for intrauterine fetal development

*The gravidity and parity of a woman is expressed in the following "shorthand": G4P2. "G" refers to the gravidity, and "P" refers to the parity. The woman in this example would have had 4 pregnancies and 2 births.

GENERAL ASSESSMENT OF THE OBSTETRIC PATIENT

PRIMARY ASSESSMENT

The primary approach to the obstetrical patient should be the same as for the nonobstetrical patient, with special attention paid to the developing fetus. Complete the primary assessment quickly. Next, obtain essential obstetric information.

HISTORY

The SAMPLE history will allow you to gain specific information about the mother's situation as well as her pertinent medical history.

General Information

You will want to obtain information about the pregnancy, such as the mother's gravidity and parity, the length of gestation, and the estimated date of confinement (EDC) if known. In addition, you should determine whether the patient has had any cesarean sections or any gynecological or obstetrical complications in the past. It is also important to ascertain whether the patient has had any prenatal care. Determine what type of health-care professional (physician or nurse midwife) is providing her care and when she was last evaluated. Ask the patient whether an ultrasonographic examination was done. An ultrasonogram reveals the age of the fetus, the presence of more than one fetus, abnormal presentations, and certain birth defects. A general overview of the patient's current state of health is important. Pay particular attention to current medications and drug and/or medication allergies.

Obtain information about the pregnancy. Ask about gravidity, parity, length of gestation, and EDC. Ask about past gynecological or obstetrical complications and prenatal care. Determine current medications and any drug allergies.

Preexisting or Aggravated Medical Conditions

Pregnancy aggravates many preexisting medical conditions and may trigger new ones.

Pregnancy can aggravate preexisting medical conditions, such as diabetes, heart disease, hypertension, seizure disorders, and neuromuscular disorders, and may trigger new ones. (However, a remission of neurological disorder symptoms during pregnancy is not unusual.)

Diabetes Previously diagnosed diabetes can become unstable during pregnancy due to altered insulin requirements. Diabetics are at increased risk of developing preeclampsia and hypertension (discussed later in this chapter). Pregnancy may also accelerate the progression of vascular disease complications of diabetes. It is not uncommon for pregnant diabetics to have problems with fluctuating blood sugar levels, causing hypoglycemic or hyperglycemic episodes. Also, many patients develop diabetes during pregnancy *(gestational diabetes)*. Pregnant diabetics cannot be managed with oral hypoglycemic agents because these drugs tend to cross the placenta and affect the fetus. Therefore, all pregnant diabetics are placed on insulin, if their blood sugar levels cannot be controlled by diet alone. It has been shown that maintaining careful control of the mother's blood sugar between 3.8 and 6.8 mmol reduces risks to mother and fetus.

Diabetes also affects the infant. Infants of diabetic mothers, especially those with poorly controlled blood sugar levels, tend to be large. This complicates delivery. Such infants also may have trouble maintaining body temperature after birth and may be subject to hypoglycemia. Babies born to diabetic mothers are also at increased risk for congenital anomalies (birth defects).

Heart Disease During pregnancy, cardiac output increases up to 30 percent. Patients who have serious preexisting heart disease may develop congestive heart failure in pregnancy. When confronted by a pregnant patient in obvious or suspected heart failure, inquire about preexisting heart disease or murmurs. It is important to be aware, however, that most patients develop a quiet systolic flow murmur during pregnancy. This is caused by increased cardiac output and is rarely a source of concern.

Hypertension Hypertension is also aggravated by pregnancy. Generally, blood pressure is lower in pregnancy than in the nonpregnant state. However, women who were borderline hypertensive before becoming pregnant may become dangerously hypertensive when pregnant. Also, many common blood pressure medications cannot be used during pregnancy. In addition, preeclampsia (discussed later in this chapter) may contribute to maternal hypertension. Persistent hypertension may adversely affect the placenta, thus compromising the fetus as well as placing the mother at increased risk for stroke, seizure, or renal failure.

Seizure Disorders Most women with a history of seizure disorders controlled by medication have uneventful pregnancies and deliver healthy babies. However, women who have poorly controlled seizure disorders are likely to have increased seizure activity during pregnancy. Medications to control seizures are commonly administered throughout the pregnancy.

Neuromuscular Disorders Disabilities associated with neuromuscular disorders, such as multiple sclerosis, may be aggravated by pregnancy. However, it is more common that pregnant women enjoy remission of symptoms during pregnancy and experience a slight increase in relapse rate during the postpartum period. The strength of uterine contractions is not diminished in these patients. Also, their subjective sensation of pain is often less than seen in other patients.

Pain

When the patient complains of pain, determine onset, character, and especially the regularity of occurrence.

If the patient is in pain, try to determine when the pain started and whether its onset was sudden or slow. Also, attempt to define the character of the pain—its duration, location, and radiation, if any. It is especially important to determine whether the pain is occurring on a regular basis.

Vaginal Bleeding

The presence of vaginal bleeding or spotting is a major concern in an obstetrical patient. Ask about events immediately prior to the start of bleeding. You also need to gain information about the colour, amount, and duration. To assess the amount of bleeding, count the number of sanitary pads used. If your patient is passing clots or tissue, save this material for evaluation. In addition, question the patient about the presence of other vaginal discharges, as well as the colour, amount, and duration.

If there is vaginal bleeding, determine events prior to its start. Assess the amount by the number of sanitary pads used and save any clots or passed tissue.

Active Labour

In the case of a patient in active labour, assess whether the mother feels the need to push or has the urge to move her bowels. Determine whether the patient thinks her membranes have ruptured. Patients often sense this as a dribbling of water or, in some cases, a true gush of water.

For a patient in labour, determine if she feels the need to push or move her bowels or if her membranes have ruptured (her "water broke")—all signs of possible imminent delivery.

Secondary Assessment

Secondary assessment of the obstetric patient is essentially the same as for any emergency patient. However, you should be particularly careful to protect the patient's modesty as well as maintain her dignity and privacy.

Always protect the patient's modesty.

When examining a pregnant patient, first estimate the date of the pregnancy by measuring the *fundal height*. The fundal height is the distance from the symphysis pubis to the top of the uterine fundus. Each centimetre of fundal height roughly corresponds to a week of gestation. For example, a woman with a fundal height of 24 cm has a gestational age of approximately 24 weeks. If the fundus is just palpable above the symphysis pubis, the pregnancy is about 12–16 weeks gestation. When the uterine fundus reaches the umbilicus, the pregnancy is about 20 weeks. As pregnancy reaches term, the fundus is palpable near the xiphoid process. If fetal movement is felt when the abdomen is palpated, the pregnancy is at least 20 weeks. Fetal heart tones can be heard by stethoscope at approximately 18–20 weeks. The normal fetal heart rate ranges from 140 to 160 beats per minute (bpm).

Generally, vital signs in the pregnant patient should be taken with the patient lying on her left side. As noted earlier, as pregnancy progresses, the uterus increases in size. Ultimately, when the patient is supine, the weight of the uterus compresses the inferior vena cava, severely compromising venous blood return from the lower extremities. Turning the patient to her left side alleviates this problem. Occasionally, it may be helpful to perform orthostatic vital signs. First, obtain the blood pressure and pulse rate after the patient has rested for five minutes in the left lateral recumbent position. Then, repeat the vital signs with the patient sitting up or standing. A drop in the blood pressure level of 15 mmHg or more, or an increase in the pulse rate of 20 bpm or more, is considered significant and should be reported and documented. When performing this manoeuvre, it is always important to be alert for syncope. This procedure should *not* be performed if the patient is in obvious shock.

You may need to examine the genitals to evaluate any vaginal discharge, the progression of labour, or the presence of a *prolapsed cord*, an umbilical cord that comes out of the uterus ahead of the fetus. This can be accomplished simply by looking at the perineum. If, during the secondary assessment, the patient reports

crowning the bulging of the fetal head past the opening of the vagina during a contraction. Crowning is an indication of impending delivery.

Do not perform an internal vaginal examination in the field.

Always remember that you are caring for two patients, the mother and the fetus.

Focus on airway, breathing, and circulation. Monitor for shock. As needed, administer oxygen, initiate IV access, consider fluid resuscitation, and monitor the heart. Place the patient in a position of comfort. The left lateral recumbent position is preferred after the 24th week.

that she feels the need to push, or if she feels as though she must move her bowels, examine her for crowning. **Crowning** is the bulging of the fetal head past the opening of the vagina during a contraction. Crowning is an indication of impending delivery. Examine for crowning only during a contraction. *Do not perform an internal vaginal examination in the field.*

GENERAL MANAGEMENT OF THE OBSTETRIC PATIENT

The first consideration for managing emergencies in obstetric patients is to remember that you are, in fact, caring for two patients, the mother and the fetus. Fetal well-being is dependent on maternal well-being. Also, keep in mind that your calm, professional demeanour and caring attitude will go a long way in reducing the emotional stress during any obstetric emergency. Remember to protect your patient's privacy and maintain her modesty.

The physiological priorities for obstetric emergencies are identical to those for any other emergency situation. Focus your efforts on maintaining the airway, breathing, and circulation. Administer high-flow, high-concentration oxygen as needed depending on the patient's condition. Initiate intravenous access by using a large-bore catheter in a large vein, and consider fluid resuscitation based on your local protocols. If your patient is bleeding or showing signs of shock, establish two IV lines. Cardiac monitoring is also appropriate. Place your patient in a position of comfort, but remember that left lateral recumbent is preferred after the 24th week.

Analgesics should be used with caution, since they can alter your ability to assess a deteriorating condition as well as other changes in patient status and may negatively affect the fetus. Nitrous oxide is the preferred analgesic in pregnancy, but narcotics are acceptable.

When transport is indicated, transport immediately to a hospital that is capable of managing emergency obstetric and neonatal care. Report the situation to the receiving hospital prior to your arrival, as emergency department personnel may want to summon obstetrics department staff to assist with patient care.

COMPLICATIONS OF PREGNANCY

Pregnancy is a normal process. However, women who are pregnant are not immune from injury or other health problems. There may also be complications associated with the pregnancy itself.

TRAUMA

Paramedics frequently receive calls to help a pregnant woman who has been in a motor-vehicle collision or who has sustained a fall. In pregnancy, syncope occurs frequently. The syncope of pregnancy often results from compression of the inferior vena cava, as described earlier, or from normal changes in the cardiovascular system associated with pregnancy. Also, the weight of the gravid uterus alters the patient's balance, making her more susceptible to falls.

Pregnant victims of major trauma are more susceptible to life-threatening injury than are nonpregnant victims because of the increased vascularity of the gravid uterus. Trauma is the most frequent, nonobstetric cause of death in pregnant women. Some form of trauma, usually a motor-vehicle collision or a fall but sometimes physical abuse, occurs in 6–7 percent of all pregnancies. Since the primary cause for fetal mortality is maternal mortality, the pregnant trauma patient presents a unique challenge. The later stage of the pregnancy, the larger is the uterus and the greater is the likelihood of injury. All patients of 20 weeks (or more) gestation with a history of direct or indirect injury should be transported for evaluation by a physician.

Paramedics should *anticipate* the development of shock on the basis of the mechanism of injury, rather than waiting for overt signs and symptoms. Due to the cardiovascular changes of pregnancy, overt signs of shock are late and inconsistent. Trauma significant enough to cause maternal shock is associated with a 70–80 percent fetal mortality. In the face of acute blood loss, significant vasoconstriction will occur in response to catecholamine release, resulting in maintenance of a normotensive state for the mother. However, this causes significant uterine hypoperfusion (20–30 percent decrease in cardiac output) and fetal bradycardia.

Generally, the amniotic fluid cushions the fetus from blunt trauma fairly well. However, in direct abdominal trauma, the pregnant patient may suffer premature separation of the placenta from the uterine wall, premature labour, abortion, uterine rupture, and possibly fetal death. The presence of vaginal bleeding or a tender abdomen in a pregnant patient should increase your suspicion of serious injury. Fetal death may result from death of the mother, separation of the placenta from the uterine wall, maternal shock, uterine rupture, or fetal head injury. Any pregnant patient who has suffered trauma should be immediately transported to the emergency department and evaluated by a physician. Trauma management essentials include the following:

- Apply a cervical collar to provide cervical stabilization, and immobilize on a long backboard.
- Administer high-flow, high-concentration oxygen.
- Initiate two large-bore IVs for crystalloid administration per protocol.
- Transport, with patient tilted to the left to minimize supine hypotension.
- Reassess frequently.
- Monitor the fetus.

Transport all trauma patients of 20 weeks or more gestation. Anticipate the development of shock.

MEDICAL CONDITIONS

The pregnant patient is subject to all of the medical problems that occur in the nonpregnant state. Abdominal pain is a common complaint. It is often caused by the stretching of the ligaments that support the uterus. However, appendicitis and cholecystitis can also occur. Pregnant women are at increased risk of developing gallstones as a result of hormonal influences that delay emptying of the gallbladder. In pregnancy, the abdominal organs are displaced because of the increased mass of the gravid uterus in the abdomen, which makes assessment more difficult. The pregnant patient with appendicitis may complain of right upper quadrant pain or even back pain. The symptoms of acute cholecystitis may also differ from those in nonpregnant patients. Any pregnant patient with abdominal pain should be evaluated by a physician.

Any pregnant patient with abdominal pain should be evaluated by a physician.

BLEEDING IN PREGNANCY

Vaginal bleeding may occur at any time during pregnancy. Bleeding is usually due to abortion, ectopic pregnancy, placenta previa, or abruptio placentae. Generally, the exact etiology of vaginal bleeding during pregnancy cannot be determined in the field. Refer to the earlier discussion in this chapter and your own local protocols for management of obstetric emergencies. Vaginal bleeding

Content Review

CAUSES OF BLEEDING DURING PREGNANCY
Abortion
Ectopic pregnancy
Placenta previa
Abruptio placentae

is associated with potential fetal loss. Keep in mind that this is a very emotionally stressful situation for your patient, and so a professional, caring demeanour is imperative.

Abortion

Abortion, the expulsion of the fetus prior to 20 weeks gestation, is the most common cause of bleeding in the first and second trimesters of pregnancy. The terms "abortion" and "miscarriage" can be used interchangeably. Generally, the lay public think of abortion as termination of pregnancy at maternal request and of miscarriage as an accident of nature. Medically, the term abortion applies to both kinds of fetal loss. Spontaneous abortion, the naturally occurring termination of pregnancy that is often called miscarriage, is most commonly seen between the 12th and 14th weeks of gestation. It is estimated that 10 to 20 percent of all pregnancies end in spontaneous abortion. If the pregnancy has not yet been confirmed, the mother often assumes she is merely having a period with unusually heavy flow.

About half of all abortions are due to fetal chromosomal anomalies. Other causes include maternal reproductive system abnormalities, maternal use of drugs, placental defects, or maternal infections. Although many people believe that trauma and psychological stress can cause abortion, research does not support that belief.

Assessment The patient experiencing an abortion is likely to report cramping abdominal pain and a backache. She is also likely to report vaginal bleeding, which is often accompanied by the passage of clots and tissue. If the abortion was not recent, then frank signs and symptoms of infection may be present. In addition to your routine emergency assessments, assess for orthostatic vital sign changes, and ascertain the amount of vaginal bleeding.

Signs and symptoms of an abortion include cramping abdominal pain, backache, and vaginal bleeding, often accompanied by passage of clots and tissue.

Management Place the patient who is experiencing an abortion in a position of comfort. Treat for shock with oxygen therapy and IV access for fluid resuscitation. As mentioned earlier, any tissue or large clots should be retained and given to emergency department personnel. If the abortion occurs during the late first trimester or later, a fetus may be passed. Often, the placenta does not detach, and the fetus is suspended by the umbilical cord. In such a case, place the umbilical clamps from the OB kit on the cord, and cut the cord. Carefully wrap the fetus in linen or other suitable material, and transport it to the hospital with the mother.

Treat the patient suffering an abortion as you would any patient at risk for hypovolemic shock. Provide emotional support to the parents.

An abortion is generally a tragic occurrence. Provide emotional support to the parents. This can be a devastating psychological experience for the mother, and so avoid saying trite, inaccurate phrases meant to provide comfort. Inappropriate remarks include "You can always get pregnant again" or "This is nature's way of dealing with a defective fetus." Parents who wish to view the fetus should be allowed to do so. Occasionally, Roman Catholic parents may request baptism of the fetus. You can perform this by making the sign of a cross and stating, "I baptize you in the name of the father, the son, and the holy spirit. Amen."

Ectopic Pregnancy

As you learned earlier, the fertilized egg normally is implanted in the endometrial lining of the uterine wall. The term *ectopic pregnancy* refers to the abnormal implantation of the fertilized egg outside of the uterus. Approximately 95 percent are implanted in the fallopian tube. Occasionally (< 1 percent), the egg is implanted in the abdominal cavity. Current research indicates that the incidence of ectopic pregnancy is 1 for every 44 live births. Improved diagnostic technology is credited with an increased incidence, as most are detected between the 2nd and

12th weeks. Ectopic pregnancy accounts for approximately 10 percent of maternal mortality.

Predisposing factors in the development of ectopic pregnancy include scarring of the fallopian tubes due to pelvic inflammatory disease (PID), a previous ectopic pregnancy, or previous pelvic or tubal surgery, such as a tubal ligation. Other factors include endometriosis or use of an intrauterine device (IUD) for birth control.

Assessment Ectopic pregnancy most often presents as abdominal pain, which starts out as diffuse tenderness and then localizes as a sharp pain in the lower abdominal quadrant on the affected side. This pain is due to rupture of the fallopian tube when the fetus outgrows the available space. The woman often reports that she missed a period or that her LMP occurred 4 to 6 weeks ago, but with decreased menstrual flow that was brownish in colour and of shorter duration than usual. As the intra-abdominal bleeding continues, the abdomen becomes rigid and the pain intensifies and is often referred to the shoulder on the affected side. The pain is often accompanied by syncope, vaginal bleeding, and shock.

Assume that any female of childbearing age with lower abdominal pain is experiencing an ectopic pregnancy.

Assume that any female of childbearing age with lower abdominal pain is experiencing an ectopic pregnancy.

Management Ectopic pregnancy poses a significant life threat to the mother. Transport this patient immediately, since surgery is often required to resolve the situation. Interim care measures should include oxygen therapy and IV access for fluid resuscitation. Trendelenburg position may be indicated by your local protocols.

Ectopic pregnancy is life-threatening. Transport the patient immediately.

Placenta Previa

Placenta previa occurs as a result of abnormal implantation of the placenta on the lower half of the uterine wall, resulting in partial or complete coverage of the cervical opening (Figure 40-5). Vaginal bleeding, which may initially be intermittent, occurs after the seventh month of the pregnancy as the lower uterus begins to contract and dilate in preparation for the onset of labour. This process pulls the placenta away from the uterine wall, causing bright red vaginal bleeding. Placenta previa occurs in about 1 of every 250 live births. It is classified as complete, partial, or marginal, depending on whether the placenta covers all or part of the cervical opening or is merely in close proximity to the opening.

Although the exact cause of placenta previa is unknown, certain predisposing factors are commonly seen. These factors include a previous history of placenta previa, multiparity, or increased maternal age. Other factors include the

Third-trimester bleeding should be attributed to either placenta previa or abruptio placentae until proven otherwise. Placenta previa usually presents with painless bleeding. Abruptio placentae usually presents with sharp pain, with or without bleeding.

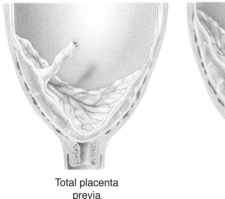
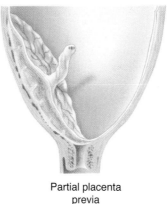

Total placenta previa   Partial placenta previa

FIGURE 40-5   Placenta previa (abnormal implantation).

presence of uterine scars from cesarean sections, a large placenta, or defective development of blood vessels in the uterine wall.

Assessment The patient with placenta previa is usually a multigravida in her third trimester of pregnancy. She may have a history of prior placenta previa or of bleeding early in the current pregnancy. She may report a recent episode of sexual intercourse or vaginal examination just before vaginal bleeding began, or she may not bleed until the onset of labour. The onset of painless bright red vaginal bleeding, which may occur as spotting or recurrent hemorrhage, is the hallmark of placenta previa. In fact, any painless bleeding in pregnancy is considered placenta previa until proven otherwise. The bleeding may or may not be associated with uterine contractions. The uterus is usually soft, and the fetus may be in an unusual presentation. *Vaginal examination should never be attempted, as an examining finger can puncture the placenta, causing fatal hemorrhage.*

The presence of placenta previa may already have been diagnosed by ultrasonography during prenatal care, in which case the mother is anticipating the onset of symptoms. The prognosis for the fetus is dependent on the extent of the previa. Obviously, in profuse hemorrhage, the fetus is at risk of severe hypoxia and the viability of the placenta is compromised. You should perform your secondary assessment as discussed earlier in this chapter.

Management If the placenta previa was previously diagnosed, the condition may already have been managed by placing the patient on bed rest. Because of the potential for profuse hemorrhage, you should treat for shock. Administer oxygen, and initiate intravenous access. Additionally, continue to monitor the maternal vital signs and fetal heart tones (FHTs). Since the definitive treatment is delivery of the fetus by cesarean section, it is imperative to transport the patient to a hospital with obstetric surgical capability.

Abruptio Placentae

Abruptio placentae, or the premature separation (abruption) of a normally implanted placenta from the uterine wall, poses a potential life threat for both mother and fetus (Figure 40-6). The incidence of abruptio placentae is 1 in 120 live births. It is associated with 20 to 30 percent fetal mortality, which rises to 100 percent in cases where the majority of the placenta has separated. Maternal

Never attempt vaginal examination since an examining finger can puncture the placenta and cause fatal hemorrhage.

Because of the potential for profuse hemorrhage, always treat the patient with suspected placenta previa for shock. Transport immediately since definitive treatment is delivery by cesarean section.

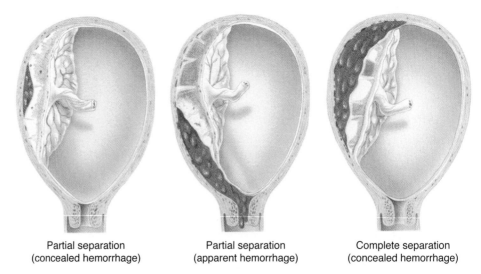

Partial separation (concealed hemorrhage) Partial separation (apparent hemorrhage) Complete separation (concealed hemorrhage)

FIGURE 40-6 Abruptio placentae (premature separation).

mortality is relatively uncommon, although it rises markedly if shock is inadequately treated. Abruptio placentae is classified as marginal (or partial), central (severe), or complete, as explained below.

Although the cause of abruptio placentae is unknown, predisposing factors include multiparity, maternal hypertension, trauma, cocaine use, increasing maternal age, and history of abruption in previous pregnancy.

Assessment The presenting signs and symptoms of abruptio placentae vary depending on the extent and character of the abruption. Partial abruptions can be marginal or central. Marginal abruptio is characterized by vaginal bleeding but no increase in pain. In central abruptio, the placenta separates centrally, and the bleeding is trapped between the placenta and the uterine wall, or "concealed," so there is no vaginal bleeding. However, there is a sudden sharp, tearing pain and development of a stiff, board-like abdomen. In complete abruptio placentae there is massive vaginal bleeding and profound maternal hypotension. If the patient is in labour at the time of the abruptio, separation of the placenta from the uterine wall will progress rapidly, with fetal distress or fetal demise dependent on percentage of separation.

Management Abruptio placentae is a life-threatening obstetrical emergency. Immediate intervention to maintain maternal oxygenation and perfusion is imperative. Immediately place two large bore intravenous lines, and begin fluid resuscitation. Position your patient in the left lateral recumbent position. Transport immediately to a hospital with available surgical obstetric and high-risk neonatal care.

MEDICAL COMPLICATIONS OF PREGNANCY

As discussed earlier, pregnancy can exacerbate preexisting medical conditions, such as diabetes, heart disease, hypertension, and seizure or neuromuscular disorder.

Hypertensive Disorders

The American College of Obstetricians and Gynecologists has identified four classifications of *hypertensive disorders of pregnancy* (formerly called "toxemia of pregnancy"):

- *Preeclampsia and eclampsia.* Pregnancy-induced hypertension (PIH), which includes preeclampsia and eclampsia, occurs in approximately 5 percent of all pregnancies. Preeclampsia is the most common hypertensive disorder seen in pregnancy. There is a higher incidence among primigravidas, particularly if they are teenagers or over the age of 35. Others at increased risk are diabetics, women with a history of preeclampsia, and those who are carrying multiple fetuses.

  Preeclampsia is a progressive disorder that is usually categorized as mild or severe. Seizures (or coma) develop in its most severe form, known as eclampsia. Preeclampsia is defined as an increase in systolic blood pressure by 30 mmHg and/or a diastolic increase of 15 mmHg over baseline on at least two occasions at least six hours apart. Remember that maternal blood pressure normally drops during pregnancy, so a woman may be hypertensive at 120/80 if her baseline in early pregnancy was 90/66. If there is no baseline blood pressure available, then a reading ≥ 140/90 is considered to be hypertensive.

  Preeclampsia is most commonly seen in the last 10 weeks of gestation, during labour, or in the first 48 hours postpartum. The

Content Review

MEDICAL COMPLICATIONS OF PREGNANCY
Hypertensive disorders
Supine hypotensive syndrome
Gestational diabetes

exact cause of preeclampsia is unknown. It is thought to be caused by abnormal vasospasm, which results in increased maternal blood pressure and other associated symptoms. Additionally, the vasospasm causes decreased placental perfusion, contributing to fetal growth retardation and chronic fetal hypoxia.

Mild preeclampsia is characterized by hypertension, edema, and protein in the urine. Severe preeclampsia progresses rapidly with maternal blood pressures reaching 160/110 or higher, while the edema becomes generalized and the amount of protein in the urine increases significantly. Other commonly seen signs and symptoms in the severe state include headache, visual disturbances, hyperactive reflexes, and the development of pulmonary edema, along with a dramatic decrease in urine output.

Patients who are preeclamptic have intravascular volume depletion, since a great deal of their body fluid is in the third space. Those who develop severe preeclampsia and eclampsia are at increased risk for cerebral hemorrhage, pulmonary embolism, abruptio placentae, disseminated intravascular coagulopathy (DIC), and the development of renal failure.

Eclampsia, the most serious manifestation of pregnancy-induced hypertension, is characterized by grand mal (major motor) seizure activity. Eclampsia is often preceded by visual disturbances, such as flashing lights or spots before the eyes. Also, the development of epigastric pain or pain in the right upper abdominal quadrant often indicates impending seizure. Eclampsia can often be distinguished from epilepsy by the history and physical appearance of the patient. Patients who become eclamptic are usually grossly edematous and have markedly elevated blood pressure, while epileptics usually have a prior history of seizures and are usually taking anticonvulsant medications. If eclampsia develops, death of the mother as well as that of the fetus frequently results. The risk of fetal mortality increases by 10 percent with each maternal seizure.

- *Chronic hypertension.* Hypertension is considered chronic when the blood pressure is $\geq$ 140/90 before pregnancy or prior to the 20th week of gestation, or if it persists for more than 42 days postpartum. As a general rule, if the diastolic pressure exceeds 80 mmHg during the second trimester, chronic hypertension is likely. The cause of chronic hypertension is unknown. The goal of management is to prevent the development of preeclampsia.

- *Chronic hypertension superimposed with preeclampsia.* It is not uncommon for the chronic hypertensive who develops preeclampsia to progress rapidly to eclampsia even prior to the 30th week of gestation. The same diagnostic criteria for preeclampsia are used (systolic blood pressure increases > 30 mmHg over baseline, edema, and protein in the urine).

- *Transient hypertension.* Transient hypertension is defined as a temporary rise in blood pressure that occurs during labour or early in postpartum and that normalizes within 10 days.

With suspected hypertensive disorder, it is critical to obtain an accurate history, including information about weight gain, headaches, visual problems, epigastric or right upper quadrant abdominal pain, apprehension, or seizures.

Assessment Obtaining an accurate history is extremely important whenever you suspect any of the hypertensive disorders of pregnancy. Question the patient about excessive weight gain, headaches, visual problems, epigastric or right upper quadrant abdominal pain, apprehension, or seizures. On secondary assessment, patients with PIH or preeclampsia are usually markedly edematous. They are often pale and apprehensive. The reflexes are hyperactive. The blood pressure, which is usually elevated, should be taken after the patient has rested for five minutes in the left lateral recumbent position.

Management Definitive treatment of the hypertensive disorders of pregnancy is delivery of the fetus. However, in the field, use the following management tactics to prevent dangerously high blood pressures or seizure activity.

- *Hypertension.* Closely monitor the patient who is pregnant and has elevated blood pressure without edema or other signs of preeclampsia. Record the fetal heart tones and the mother's blood pressure level.
- *Preeclampsia.* The patient who is hypertensive and shows other signs and symptoms of preeclampsia, such as edema, headaches, and visual disturbances, should be treated quickly. Keep the patient calm, and dim the lights. Place the patient in the left lateral recumbent position, and quickly carry out the primary assessment. Begin an IV of normal saline. Transport the patient rapidly, without lights or sirens. If the blood pressure is dangerously high (diastolic > 110), medical direction may request the administration of hydralazine (Apresoline) or similar antihypertensives that are safe for use in pregnancy. If the transport time is long, the administration of magnesium sulphate may also be ordered.
- *Eclampsia.* If the patient has already suffered a seizure or a seizure appears to be imminent, then, in addition to the above measures, administer oxygen, and manage the airway appropriately. If you are still unable to control the seizures, you may consider diazepam (Valium) or other sedative. Also, monitor your patient closely for signs of abruptio placentae (vaginal bleeding or abdominal rigidity) or developing pulmonary edema. Transport immediately to a hospital with surgical obstetric and neonatal care availability.

> *Preeclampsia and eclampsia are life threatening. Keep the patient calm. Dim the lights. Place patient in left lateral recumbent position, and transport quickly without lights or sirens. Administer magnesium sulphate to control seizures if they occur. Medical direction may request administration of antihypertensive or sedative drugs.*

Supine-Hypotensive Syndrome

Supine-hypotensive syndrome usually occurs in the third trimester of pregnancy. Also known as vena caval syndrome, supine hypotensive syndrome occurs when the gravid uterus compresses the inferior vena cava when the mother lies in the supine position (Figure 40-7).

Assessment Supine-hypotensive syndrome usually occurs in a patient late in her pregnancy who has been supine for a period of time. The patient may complain of dizziness, which results from the decrease in venous return to the right atrium and consequent lowering of the patient's blood pressure. Question the patient about prior episodes of a similar nature and about any recent hemorrhage or fluid loss. Direct the secondary assessment at determining whether the patient is volume depleted.

Management If there are no indications of volume depletion, such as decreased skin turgor or thirst, place the patient in the left lateral recumbent position, or elevate her right hip. Monitor the FHTs and maternal vital signs frequently. If there is clinical evidence of volume depletion, administer oxygen, and start an IV of normal saline. Check for orthostatic changes (a decrease in blood pressure and increase in heart rate when rising from the supine position), and place electrodes for cardiac monitoring. Transport the patient promptly in the left lateral recumbent position.

> *Treat supine hypotensive syndrome by placing the patient in the left lateral recumbent position or elevating her right hip. Monitor fetal heart tones and maternal vital signs. If volume depletion is evident, initiate an IV of normal saline.*

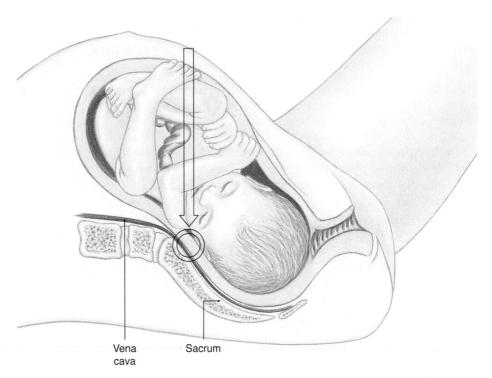

Vena
cava

Sacrum

FIGURE 40-7 The supine-hypotensive syndrome results from compression of the inferior vena cava by the gravid uterus.

Gestational Diabetes

Diabetes mellitus occurs in approximately 4 percent of all pregnancies. Hormonal influences cause an increase in insulin production as well as an increased tissue response to insulin during the first 20 weeks of gestation. However, during the last 20 weeks, placental hormones cause an increased resistance to insulin and a decreased glucose tolerance. This causes catabolism (the "breaking down" phase of metabolism) between meals and during the night. At these times, ketones may be present in the urine because fats are metabolized more rapidly. Further, maternal glucose stores are used up, as they are the sole source of glucose to meet the energy needs of the growing fetus. This is known as the *diabetogenic* (diabetes-causing) *effect of pregnancy*. Gestational diabetes usually subsides after pregnancy.

Routine prenatal care includes screening to detect diabetes throughout the pregnancy. Women who are considered to be at high risk for developing gestational diabetes are given a glucose tolerance test at their first prenatal visit. High risk is associated with maternal age (over 35), obesity, hypertension, family history of diabetes, and history of prior stillbirth.

Management of gestational diabetes requires meticulous prenatal care. The mother will be instructed on diabetic management and the importance of balancing diet and exercise as well as on how to monitor her glucose levels and administer insulin. Fetal development will be monitored on an ongoing basis throughout the pregnancy.

Consider hypoglycemia when encountering a pregnant patient with altered mental status.

Assessment When you encounter a pregnant patient with an altered mental status, consider hypoglycemia as a likely cause. Remember that the clinical signs and symptoms of hypoglycemia are many and varied. An abnormal mental status is the most important. Physical signs may include diaphoresis and tachycardia. If the blood sugar falls to a critically low level, she may sustain a hypoglycemic seizure or become comatose, which poses a potential life threat to the mother and fetus. Obtaining an accurate history of associated signs and symptoms, such as nausea, vomiting, abdominal pain, increased urination, or a recent infection, will allow you to ascertain whether diabetic ketoacidosis might be the cause of your patient's altered mental status. Determine the blood glucose level in addition to obtaining baseline vital signs and FHTs.

Management If the blood glucose level is noted to be less than 4 mmol/L start an IV of normal saline. Next, administer 25 g of 50-percent dextrose intravenously. If the patient is conscious and able to swallow, complete glucose administration with orange juice, sugared soft drinks, or commercially available glucose pastes.

If the blood glucose level is in excess of 11.1 mmol/L, establish IV access to administer one litre of 0.9-percent sodium chloride per protocol.

If blood glucose is below 4 mmol/L, start an IV of normal saline, and administer 25 g of 50-percent dextrose.

BRAXTON-HICKS CONTRACTIONS

It is occasionally difficult to determine the onset of labour. As early as the 13th week of gestation, the uterus contracts intermittently, thus conditioning itself for the birth process. It is also believed that these contractions enhance placental circulation. These painless, irregular contractions are known as Braxton-Hicks contractions. As the EDC approaches, these contractions become more frequent. Ultimately, the contractions become stronger and more regular, signalling the onset of labour. Labour consists of uterine contractions that cause the dilation and **effacement** (thinning and shortening) of the cervix. The contractions of labour are firm, fairly regular, and quite painful. Prior to the onset of labour, Braxton-Hicks contractions, occasionally called *false labour,* increase in intensity and frequency but do not cause cervical changes.

It is virtually impossible to distinguish false labour from true labour in the field. Distinguishing the two requires repeated vaginal examinations, over time, to determine whether the cervix is effacing and dilating. *Remember: Internal vaginal exams should not be performed in the field.* Therefore, all patients with uterine contractions should be transported to the hospital for additional evaluation.

Braxton-Hicks contractions do not require treatment by the paramedic aside from reassurance of the patient and, if necessary, transport for evaluation by a physician.

✱ **effacement** the thinning and shortening of the cervix during labour.

PRETERM LABOUR

As you have already learned, normal gestation is 40 weeks, and in terms of fetal development, the fetus is not considered to be full term until the 38th week. True labour that begins before the 38th week of gestation is called *preterm labour* and frequently requires medical intervention. A variety of maternal, fetal, or placental factors may cause this potentially life-threatening situation for the mother and fetus.

- Maternal Factors
  - Cardiovascular disease
  - Renal disease
  - Pregnancy-induced hypertension (PIH)
  - Diabetes
  - Abdominal surgery during gestation
  - Uterine and cervical abnormalities
  - Maternal infection

- Trauma, particularly blows to the abdomen
- Contributory factors: history of preterm birth, smoking, and cocaine use
- Placental Factors
  - Placenta previa
  - Abruptio placentae
- Fetal Factors
  - Multiple gestation
  - Excessive amniotic fluid
  - Fetal infection

In many cases, physicians attempt to stop preterm labour to give the fetus additional time to develop in the uterus. Prematurity is the primary neonatal health problem in the nation and occurs in 7–10 percent of all live births. All of the preterm infant's organ systems are immature to some degree, but lung development is of greatest concern. Although technological advances in the care of preterm infants have improved the prognosis dramatically, the consequences of a preterm birth can last a lifetime.

Assessment With a patient having uterine contractions, first determine the approximate gestational age of the fetus. If it is fewer than 38 weeks, then suspect preterm labour. If gestational age is greater than 38 weeks, treat the patient as a term patient, as described later in this chapter.

After determining gestational age, obtain a brief obstetrical history. Then, question the mother about the urge to push or the need to move her bowels or urinate. Also, ask if her membranes have ruptured. Any sensation of fluid leakage or "gushing" from the vagina should be interpreted as ruptured membranes until proven otherwise. Next, palpate the contractions by placing your hand on the patient's abdomen. Note the intensity and length of the contractions, as well as the interval between contractions.

Commonly reported signs and symptoms of preterm labour include contractions that occur every 10 minutes or less, low abdominal cramping that is similar to menstrual cramps, or a sensation of pelvic pressure. Other complaints, such as low backache, changes in vaginal discharge, and abdominal cramping with or without diarrhea, may also be reported. Rupture of the membranes is confirmatory for preterm labour.

Management Preterm labour, especially if quite early in the pregnancy, should be stopped if possible. The process of stopping labour, or **tocolysis,** is frequently practised in obstetrics. However, it is infrequently done in the field.

There are three general approaches to tocolysis. The first is to sedate the patient, often with narcotics or barbiturates, thus allowing her to rest. Often, after a period of rest, the contractions stop on their own. The second approach is to administer a fluid bolus intravenously. The administration of approximately one litre of fluid intravenously increases the intravascular fluid volume, thus inhibiting antidiuretic hormone (ADH) secretion from the posterior pituitary. Since oxytocin and ADH are secreted from the same area of the pituitary gland, the inhibition of ADH secretion also inhibits oxytocin release, often causing cessation of uterine contractions. Ultimately, if the above methods fail, a beta agonist, such as terbutaline or ritodrine, or magnesium sulphate may be administered to stop labour by inhibiting uterine smooth muscle contraction. Current research in tocolysis includes the administration of calcium channel blockers, such as nifedipine, and prostaglandin inhibitors, such as indomethacin. You may also find that a patient in preterm labour has been given corticosteroids to accelerate fetal lung maturity.

As a rule, tocolysis in the field is limited to sedation and hydration, especially if transport time is long. Critical care paramedics may, however, transport

The patient with suspected preterm labour should be transported immediately.

✳ **tocolysis** the process of stopping labour.

a patient from one medical facility to another, with beta agonist administration underway. You should therefore be familiar with its use. Commonly associated side effects include being jittery, tachycardia usually described by the patient as palpitations, and occasionally abdominal pain. You will, of course, want to transport your patient to the nearest facility that has neonatal intensive care capabilities. Careful and frequent monitoring of maternal vital signs and FHTs is imperative during tocolysis.

THE PUERPERIUM

The **puerperium** is the time period surrounding delivery. Childbirth generally occurs in a hospital or similar facility with appropriate equipment. Occasionally, prehospital personnel may be called upon to attend a delivery in the field. Therefore, you should be familiar with the birth process and some of the complications that may be associated with it.

LABOUR

Childbirth, or the delivery of the fetus, is the culmination of pregnancy. The process by which delivery occurs is called **labour,** the physiological and mechanical process in which the baby, placenta, and amniotic sac are expelled through the birth canal. The duration of labour is widely variable.

Prior to the onset of true labour, the head of the fetus descends into the bony pelvic area. The frequency and intensity of the Braxton-Hicks contractions increase in preparation for true labour. Increased vaginal secretions and softening of the cervix occur. Bloody show—pink-tinged secretions—is generally considered a sign of imminent labour as the mucous plug is expelled from the cervix. Labour then usually begins within 24 to 48 hours. Many people also consider the rupture of the membranes (ROM) as a sign of impending labour. If labour does not begin spontaneously within 12 to 24 hours after ROM, labour will likely require induction because of the risk of infection.

Pressure exerted by the fetus on the cervix causes changes that lead to the subsequent expulsion of the fetus. Muscular uterine contractions increase in frequency, strength, and duration. You can assess the frequency and duration of contractions by placing one hand on the fundus of the uterus. Time the contractions from the beginning of one contraction until the beginning of the next. It is important to note whether the uterus relaxes completely between contractions. It is also advisable to monitor FHTs during and between contractions. Occasional fetal bradycardia occurs during contractions, but the heart rate should increase to a normal rate (120–160) after contraction ends. Failure of the heart rate to return to normal between contractions is a sign of fetal distress.

Labour is generally divided into three stages:

- *Stage One (Dilation Stage).*   The first stage of labour begins with the onset of true labour contractions and ends with the complete dilation and effacement of the cervix. Early in pregnancy the cervix is quite thick and long, but after complete *effacement,* it is short and paper-thin. Effacement usually begins several days before active labour ensues. *Dilation* is the progressive stretching of the cervical opening. The cervix dilates from its closed position to 10 cm, which is considered complete dilation. This stage lasts approximately 8–10 hours for the woman in her first labour (the nullipara) and about 5–7 hours in the woman who has given birth previously (the multipara). Early in this stage the contractions are usually mild, lasting

Content Review
STAGES OF LABOUR
Stage one: dilation
Stage two: expulsion
Stage three: placental

for 15–20 seconds with a frequency of 10–20 minutes. As labour progresses, the contractions increase in intensity and occur approximately every 2–3 minutes with duration of 60 seconds each.

- *Stage Two (Expulsion Stage).* The second stage of labour begins with the complete dilation of the cervix and ends with the delivery of the fetus. In the nullipara, this stage lasts 50–60 minutes, while it takes about half that amount of time for the multipara. The contractions are very strong, occurring every 2 minutes and lasting for 60–75 seconds. Often, the patient feels pain in her lower back as the fetus descends into the pelvis. The urge to push or "bear down" usually begins in the second stage. The membranes usually rupture at this time, if they have not ruptured previously. Crowning during contractions is evident as the delivery of the fetus nears. Crowning occurs when the head (or other presenting part of the fetus) is visible at the vaginal opening during a contraction and is the definitive sign that birth is imminent. The most common presentation is for the infant to be delivered headfirst, face down (vertex position).

- *Stage Three (Placental Stage).* The third and final stage of labour begins immediately after the birth of the infant and ends with the delivery of the placenta. The placenta generally delivers within 5–20 minutes. There is no need to delay transport to wait for its delivery. Classic signs of placental separation include a gush of blood from the vagina; a change in size, shape, or consistency of the uterus; lengthening of the umbilical cord protruding from the vagina; and the mother reporting that she has the urge to push.

MANAGEMENT OF A PATIENT IN LABOUR

Transport the patient in labour unless delivery is imminent. Maternal urge to push or the presence of crowning indicates imminent delivery. Delivery at the scene or in the ambulance will be necessary.

Probably one of the most important decisions you must make with a patient in labour is whether to attempt to deliver the infant at the scene or to transport the patient to the hospital. It is generally preferable to transport the mother unless delivery is imminent. There are several factors to take into consideration when making this decision. They include the patient's number of previous pregnancies, the length of labour during the previous pregnancies, the frequency of contractions, the maternal urge to push, and the presence of crowning. Some women have rapid labours and may be completely dilated in a short period of time. Also, as mentioned above, multiparas generally have shorter labours than nulliparas. The maternal urge to push or the presence of crowning indicates that delivery is imminent. In such cases, the infant should be delivered at the scene or in the ambulance.

Traditionally, a woman who had previously delivered by a cesarean section was advised to have all subsequent deliveries by cesarean section. However, current thinking encourages women to attempt *vaginal birth after cesarean* (VBAC). If your patient has had prenatal care during the current pregnancy, she has probably already discussed this with her health-care provider. The only absolute contraindication for VBAC is a classic vertical uterine incision. However, nowadays most cesarean sections are done using a low transverse uterine incision. (Note that a horizontal skin incision does not mean that the uterine incision is also horizontal.) A patient who is opting for VBAC requires no more special care than any other patient does.

However, certain factors should prompt immediate transport, despite the imminent delivery. These include prolonged rupture of membranes (> 24 hours), since prolonged time between rupture and delivery often leads to fetal infection;

abnormal presentation, such as breech or transverse; a prolapsed cord; or fetal distress, as evidenced by fetal bradycardia or meconium staining (the presence of meconium—the first fetal stools—in the amniotic fluid). The presence of multiple fetuses may also contribute to your decision to transport. You will read more about these conditions later in this chapter.

FIELD DELIVERY

If delivery is imminent, you can assist the mother to deliver the baby in the field (Procedure 40-1 and Figures 40-8 through 40-16). Equipment and facilities must be quickly prepared. Set up a delivery area. This should be out of public view, such as in a bedroom or the back of the ambulance. Administer oxygen to the mother via a nasal cannula or nonrebreather mask. If time permits, establish intravenous access, and administer normal saline at a keep-open rate. Place the patient on her back with knees and hips flexed and buttocks slightly elevated. It should be noted that this position is easier on you than on the mother. She may prefer to squat or lie in a semi-Fowler's position with her knees and hips flexed. Either of these positions enables gravity to facilitate the delivery. If time permits, drape the mother with towelling from the OB kit. Place one towel under the buttocks, another below the vaginal opening, and another across the lower abdomen.

Until delivery, the fetal heart rate should be monitored frequently. A drop in the fetal heart rate to fewer than 90 beats per minute (bpm) indicates fetal distress and should prompt immediate transport of the mother in the left lateral recumbent position. Coach the mother to breathe deeply between contractions and to push with contractions. If the baby does not deliver after 20 minutes of contractions every 2–3 minutes, *transport immediately*.

Prepare the OB equipment, and don sterile gloves, gown, and goggles. If time permits, wash your hands and forearms prior to gloving. As the head crowns, control it with gentle pressure. Providing support to the head and perineum decreases the likelihood of vaginal and perineal tearing and decreases the potential for rapid expulsion of the baby's skull through the birth canal which may cause intracranial injury. Support the head as it emerges from the vagina and begins to turn. If it is still enclosed in the amniotic sac, tear the sac open to permit release of the amniotic fluid and to enable the baby to breathe.

Gently slide your finger along the head and neck to ensure that the umbilical cord is not wrapped around the baby's neck. If it is, try to gently slip it over the baby's shoulder and head. If this cannot be done and it is wrapped so tightly as to inhibit delivery, carefully place two umbilical cord clamps approximately 5 cm apart and cut the cord between the clamps. As soon as the infant's head is clear of the vagina, instruct the mother to stop pushing. While supporting the head, suction the baby's mouth and then the nose using a bulb syringe or DeLee suction. If meconium-stained fluid is seen, suction the baby's mouth, nares, and pharynx with mechanical suction to prevent aspiration. Then, tell the mother to resume pushing, while you support the infant's head as it rotates.

Gently guide the baby's head downward to allow delivery of the upper shoulder. *Do not pull!* Gently guide the baby's body upward to allow delivery of the lower shoulder. Once the head and shoulders have been delivered, the rest of the body will follow rapidly. Be prepared to support the infant's body as it emerges. Remember to keep the baby at the level of the vagina to prevent over- or under-transfusion of blood from the cord. Never "milk" the cord. Clamp and cut the cord as shown in Figure 40-17: Supporting the baby's body, place the first umbilical clamp approximately 10 cm from the baby. Place the second clamp approximately 5 cm above the first. Then, carefully cut the umbilical cord between the clamps. Wipe the baby's face clean of blood and mucus and repeat suctioning of

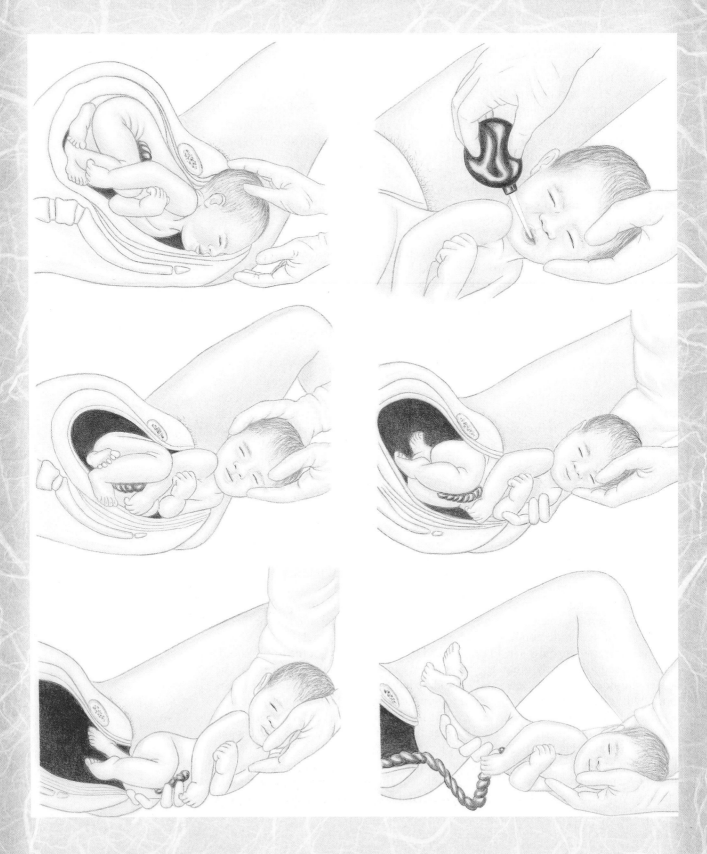

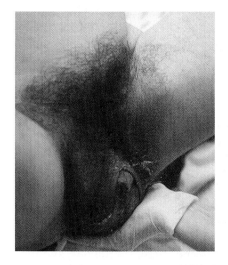

FIGURE 40-8   Crowning.

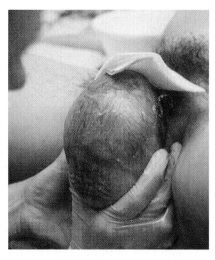

FIGURE 40-9   Delivery of the head.

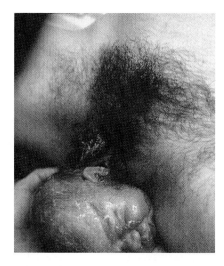

FIGURE 40-10   External rotation of the head.

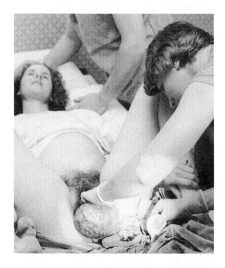

FIGURE 40-11   As soon as possible, suction the mouth, then the nose.

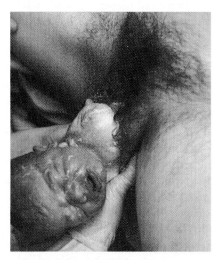

FIGURE 40-12   Delivery of the anterior shoulder.

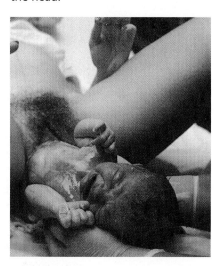

FIGURE 40-13   Complete delivery of the infant.

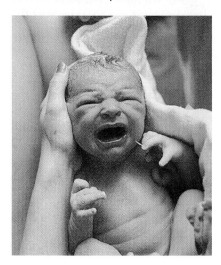

FIGURE 40-14   Dry the infant.

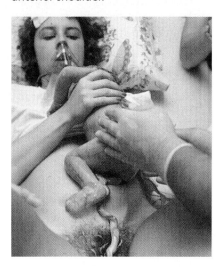

FIGURE 40-15   Place the infant on the mother's abdomen.

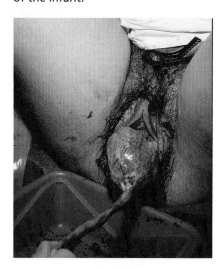

FIGURE 40-16   Deliver the placenta. and save it for transport with the mother and infant.

FIGURE 40-17   Clamp and cut the cord.

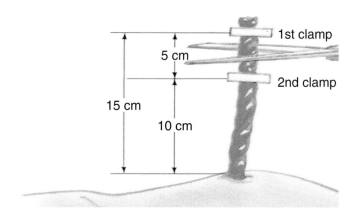

the mouth and nose until the airway is clear. Dry the infant thoroughly, and then cover with warm, dry blankets or towels, and position him on his side. Record the time of birth.

Usual maternal blood loss with delivery is about 500 mL. Following delivery, if the uterus is contracting normally, the fundus should be at the level of the umbilicus and be the size and consistency of a grapefruit. After birth, the mother's vagina should continue to ooze blood. Do not pull on the umbilical cord. Eventually, the cord will appear to lengthen, which indicates separation of the placenta. The placenta should be delivered and transported with the mother to the hospital. If it does deliver, place it in a plastic biohazard bag, and bring it to the hospital for evaluation. Retained placenta may cause maternal hemorrhage or become a source of infection. However, there is no need to delay transport for delivery of the placenta. At this time, massage the uterine fundus by placing one hand immediately above the symphysis pubis and the other on the uterine fundus. Cup the uterus between both hands and support it. Massage until the uterus assumes a woody hardness. Avoid overmassaging. Putting the baby to the mother's breast also stimulates uterine contractions, which will further decrease bleeding.

Following delivery, inspect the mother's perineum for tears. If any tears are present, apply direct pressure. Continuously monitor vital signs. If there is continued hemorrhage, report it to medical direction. In some systems, paramedics may administer oxytocin (Pitocin) to facilitate uterine contractions in the control of postpartum hemorrhage. Oxytocin should only be administered *after* the delivery of the placenta has been confirmed. Following stabilization, transport the mother and infant to the hospital.

NEONATAL CARE

* **neonate** newborn infant

Care of the **neonate** will be discussed in detail in Chapter 41. Initial care of the neonate has been described in the preceding section. Several additional important considerations regarding routine care of the neonate, APGAR scoring, and neonatal resuscitation are briefly discussed in the following sections.

Routine Care of the Neonate

Newborns are slippery; use both of your hands to support the head and torso. Position yourself so that you can work close to the surface where you have placed the infant.

Maintain warmth! Cold infants rapidly become distressed infants. Quickly dry the infant with towels, discarding each as it becomes wet. Then, cover the infant with a dry receiving blanket, or use a commercial warming blanket made of a material such as Thinsulate™.

Support the infant's head and torso, using both hands. Maintain warmth, repeat suctioning of the mouth and nose as needed, and assess using APGAR scoring.

Repeat suctioning of the mouth and nose as needed until the infant's airway is clear. Generally, suctioning and drying the baby will stimulate respirations, crying, and activity. This should cause the infant to "pink up." Do not be alarmed if the extremities remain dusky. This is known as *acrocyanosis* and is very common in the first hours of life. If the infant doesn't respond well, you may try flicking your finger against the soles of the feet or rubbing gently in a circular motion in the middle of the back (Figure 40-18).

Assess the neonate as soon as possible after birth. The normal neonatal respiratory rate should average 30–60 breaths per minute, while the heart rate should be about 100–180 beats per minute. If resuscitation is not indicated, assign APGAR scores. Do not however, delay resuscitative efforts and transport in order to complete APGAR scoring.

APGAR Scoring

Named for Dr. Virginia Apgar, who developed the assessment tool, the APGAR scoring system is a means of evaluating the status of a newborn's vital functions at 1 minute and 5 minutes after delivery. There are five parameters, and each is given a score from a low value of 0 to a normal value of 2. APGAR is also an acronym for the names of the five parameters, which are *a*ppearance (skin colour), *p*ulse rate, *g*rimace (irritability), *a*ctivity (muscle tone), and *r*espiratory effort (Table 40-2).

The majority of infants are healthy and active and have total scores of 7–10, requiring only routine care. Infants scoring 4–6 are moderately depressed and require oxygen and stimulation to breathe. Infants scoring 0–3 are severely depressed and require immediate ventilatory and circulatory assistance. By repeating the score at 1 and 5 minutes, it is possible to determine whether intervention has caused a change in infant status.

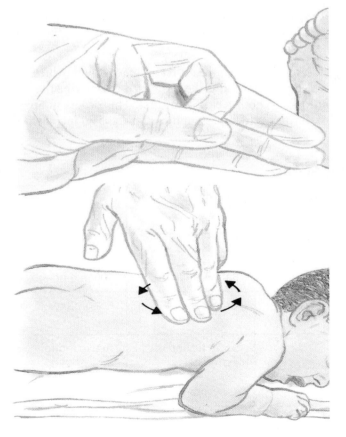

FIGURE 40-18 Stimulate the infant as required.

Neonatal Resuscitation

If the infant's respirations are fewer than 30 per minute and tactile stimulation does not increase the rate to a normal range, immediately assist ventilations using a pediatric bag-valve-mask with high-flow oxygen. If the heart rate is less than 80 and does not respond to ventilations, initiate chest compressions. Transport to a facility with neonatal intensive care capabilities.

It is estimated that approximately 6 percent of all neonates born in a hospital require resuscitation. It is likely that this percentage is higher for out-of-hospital deliveries, although the exact numbers are not available. Factors that contribute to the need for resuscitation include prematurity, pregnancy and delivery complications, maternal health problems, or inadequate prenatal care.

If tactile stimulation does not increase the neonate's respiratory rate, immediately assess heart rate. Reassess after 15 to 30 seconds.

Assess the heart rate using a stethoscope to auscultate the apical pulse, by feeling the pulse at the base of the umbilical cord, or by palpating the brachial or femoral artery. The heart rate should normally be 100–180 beats per minute with a range of 140–160 beats per minute being optimal. If the pulse is 100 or greater with spontaneous respirations, continue assessment. If less than 100, continue positive pressure ventilations. If less than 60 and not responding to ventilations, initiate chest compressions. Continue to reassess respiratory status and heart rate frequently.

Make every effort to expedite transport to a facility capable of providing neonatal intensive care while you continue resuscitative efforts. If you have a long transport time, it may be necessary to initiate vascular access in order to administer medications or fluid resuscitation. The most logical (and easiest) access is the umbilical vein. If this is not feasible, consider peripheral veins or an intraosseous access. While many medications (epinephrine, atropine, lidocaine, and naloxone) can be administered via the endotracheal route, this route is not suitable for fluid resuscitation. During transport, continue to maintain warmth while supporting ventilations, oxygenation, and circulation. Refer to Chapter 41 for more information on neonatal resuscitation.

ABNORMAL DELIVERY SITUATIONS

Breech Presentation

Most infants present headfirst and face down, which is called the vertex position. Breech presentation is the term used to describe the situation in which either the buttocks or both feet present first. This occurs in approximately 4 percent of all live births. In such presentations, there is an increased risk for delivery trauma to

Content Review

ABNORMAL DELIVERIES
Breech presentation
Prolapsed cord
Limb presentation
Occiput posterior

Table 40-2 THE APGAR SCORE

Element	0	1	2	Score
Appearance (skin colour)	Body and extremities blue, pale	Body pink, extremities blue	Completely pink	
Pulse rate	Absent	Below 100/min	100/min or above	
Grimace (Irritability)	No response	Grimace	Cough, sneeze, cry	
Activity (Muscle tone)	Limp	Some flexion of extremities	Active motion	
Respiratory effort	Absent	Slow and irregular	Strong cry	
			TOTAL SCORE =	

the mother, as well as an increased potential for cord prolapse, cord compression, or anoxic insult for the infant. Although the cause is unknown, breech presentations are most commonly associated with preterm birth, placenta previa, multiple gestation, and uterine and fetal anomalies.

Management Because cesarean section is often required, delivery of the breech presentation is best accomplished at the hospital. However, if field delivery is unavoidable, the following manoeuvres are recommended. First, position the mother with her buttocks at the edge of a firm bed. Ask her to hold her legs in a flexed position. She will often require assistance in doing this. As the infant delivers, do not pull on the infant's legs. Simply support them. Allow the entire body to be delivered with contractions, while you merely continue to support the infant's body (Figure 40-19).

As the head passes the pubis, apply gentle upward traction until the mouth appears over the perineum. If the head does not deliver, and the baby begins to breathe spontaneously with his face pressed against the vaginal wall, place a gloved hand in the vagina with the palm toward the infant's face. Form a "V" with the index and middle fingers on either side of the infant's nose, and push the vaginal wall away from the infant's face to allow unrestricted respiration (Figure 40-20). If necessary, continue this during transport.

Prolapsed Cord

A *prolapsed cord* occurs when the umbilical cord precedes the fetal presenting part. This causes the cord to be compressed between the fetus and the bony pelvis, shutting off fetal circulation (Figure 40-21). This occurs once in every 250 deliveries. Predisposing factors include prematurity, multiple births, and premature rupture of the membranes before the head is fully engaged. It is a serious emergency, and fetal death will occur quickly without prompt intervention.

Management If the umbilical cord is seen in the vagina, gently check the cord for pulsations, but take great care to ensure that you do not compress the cord. Place the mother in the Trendelenburg or knee-chest position (Figure 40-22). Administer high-flow oxygen to the mother, and transport her immediately, with the fingers continuing to hold the presenting part off the umbilical cord. If assistance is available, apply a dressing moistened with sterile saline to the exposed cord. *Do not attempt delivery! Do not pull on the cord! Do not attempt to push the cord back into the vagina!*

If there is no cord pulsation, insert a gloved hand to raise the presenting part of the fetus off the cord.

Limb Presentation

Sometimes, if the baby is in a transverse lie across the uterus, an arm or leg is the presenting part protruding from the vagina. This is seen in less than 1 percent of births and is more commonly associated with preterm birth and multiple gestation.

Management When examination of the perineum reveals a single arm or leg protruding from the birth canal, a cesarean section becomes necessary. Under no circumstance should you attempt a field delivery. Do not touch the extremity, as doing so may stimulate the infant to gasp, risking inhalation and aspiration of amniotic fluid. *Do not pull on the extremity or attempt to push it back into vagina!*

Assist the mother into a knee-chest position as is also done when there is a prolapsed cord, and administer oxygen via a nonrebreather mask. Provide reas-

If the infant starts to breathe with his face pressed against the vaginal wall, form a "V" with the index and middle fingers on either side of the infant's nose and push the vaginal wall away from the infant's face. If necessary, continue during transport.

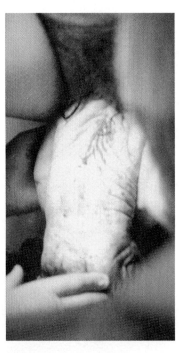

FIGURE 40-19 Breech delivery.

If the umbilical cord is seen in the vagina, insert two gloved fingers to raise the fetus off the cord. Place the mother in Trendelenburg or knee-chest position, administer oxygen, and transport immediately. Do not attempt delivery.

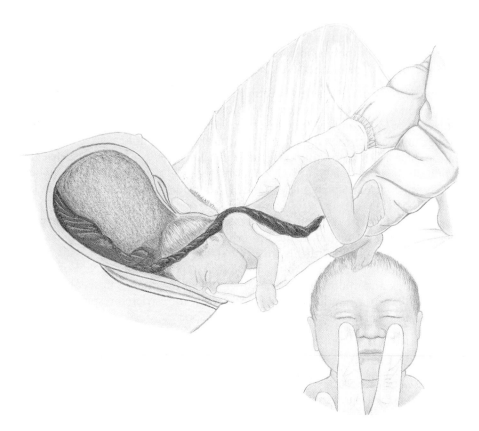

FIGURE 40-20   Placement of the fingers to maintain the airway in a breech birth.

With limb presentation, place the mother in knee-chest position, administer oxygen, and transport immediately. Do not attempt delivery.

Whenever an abnormal presentation or position of the fetus makes normal delivery impossible, reassure the mother, administer oxygen, and transport immediately. Do not attempt field delivery in these circumstances.

surance to the mother. Transport her (still in knee-chest position) immediately for emergency cesarean section.

Other Abnormal Presentations

Other abnormal presentations can complicate delivery. One of the most common is the *occiput posterior position*. Normally, as the infant descends into the pelvis, its face is turned posteriorly. This is important, as the extension of the head assists delivery. However, if the infant descends facing forward, or in the occiput posterior position, his passage through the pelvis is delayed. This presentation occurs most frequently in primigravidas. In multigravidas, it usually resolves spontaneously.

The presenting part may also be the face or brow, rather than the crown of the head. Occasionally, during these presentations, the face or brow can be seen high in the pelvis during a contraction. Usually, vaginal delivery is impossible in these cases.

As described earlier for a limb presentation, the fetus can lie transversely in the uterus. In such a case, the fetus cannot enter the pelvis for delivery. If the membranes rupture, the umbilical cord can prolapse, or an arm or leg can enter the vagina. Vaginal delivery is then impossible.

Management   Early recognition of an abnormal presentation is important. If one is suspected, the mother should be reassured, placed on oxygen, and transported immediately, since forceps or cesarean delivery is often required.

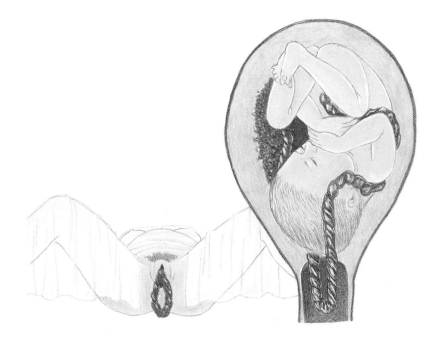

- Elevate hips, administer oxygen, and keep warm.
- Keep baby's head away from cord.
- Do not attempt to push cord back.
- Wrap cord in sterile moist towel.
- Transport mother to hospital, continuing pressure on baby's head.

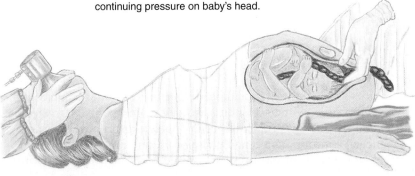

FIGURE 40-21   Prolapsed cord.

OTHER DELIVERY COMPLICATIONS

Although most deliveries proceed without incident, complications can arise. Therefore, you should be prepared to deal with them.

Multiple Births

Multiple births are fairly rare, with twins occurring approximately once in every 90 deliveries, about 40 percent of those being preterm. Usually, the mother knows or at least suspects the presence of more than one fetus. Multiple births should also be suspected if the mother's abdomen remains large after delivery of one baby and labour continues.

Content Review

OTHER DELIVERY COMPLICATIONS
Multiple births
Cephalopelvic disproportion
Precipitous delivery
Shoulder dystocia
Meconium staining

FIGURE 40-22 Patient positioning for prolapsed cord.

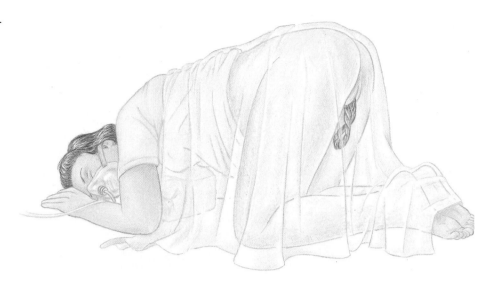

Management Manage this situation with the normal delivery guidelines, recognizing that you will need additional personnel and equipment to manage a multiple birth. In twin births, labour often begins earlier than expected, and the infants are generally smaller than babies in single births. Usually, one twin presents vertex and the other breech. There may be one shared placenta or two placentas. After delivery of the first baby, clamp and cut the cord. Then, deliver the second baby. Because prematurity is common in multiple births, low birth weight is common and prevention of hypothermia is even more crucial.

Cephalopelvic Disproportion

Cephalopelvic disproportion occurs when the infant's head is too big to pass through the maternal pelvis easily. This may be caused by an oversized fetus. Large fetuses are associated with diabetes, multiparity, or postmaturity. Fetal abnormalities, such as hydrocephalus, conjoined twins, or fetal tumours, may make vaginal delivery impossible. Women of short stature or women with contracted pelvises are at increased risk for this problem. If cephalopelvic disproportion is not recognized and managed appropriately, fetal demise or uterine rupture may occur.

Cephalopelvic disproportion tends to develop most frequently in the primigravida. There may be strong contractions for an extended period of time. On secondary assessment, the fetus may feel large. Also, labour generally does not progress. The fetus may be in distress, as evidenced by fetal bradycardia or meconium staining.

Management The usual management of cephalopelvic disproportion is cesarean section. Administer oxygen to the mother, and establish intravenous access. Transport should be immediate and rapid.

Precipitous Delivery

A *precipitous delivery* is a delivery that occurs after less than three hours of labour. This type of delivery occurs most frequently in the grand multipara and is associated with a higher-than-normal incidence of fetal trauma, tearing of the umbilical cord, or maternal lacerations.

Management The best way to handle precipitous delivery is to be prepared. Do not turn your attention from the mother. Be ready for a rapid delivery, and attempt to control the infant's head. Once delivered, the baby may have some difficulty with temperature regulation and must be kept warm.

Shoulder Dystocia

A *shoulder dystocia* occurs when the infant's shoulders are larger than its head. This occurs most frequently with diabetic and obese mothers and in postterm pregnancies. In shoulder dystocia, labour progresses normally, and the head is delivered routinely. However, immediately after the head is delivered, it retracts back into the perineum because the shoulders are trapped between the symphysis pubis and the sacrum ("turtle sign").

Management If a shoulder dystocia occurs, *do not pull on the infant's head*. Administer oxygen to the mother and have her drop her buttocks off the end of the bed. Then flex her thighs upward to facilitate delivery and apply firm pressure with an open hand immediately above the symphysis pubis. If delivery does not occur, transport the patient immediately.

Meconium Staining

Meconium staining occurs when the fetus passes feces into the amniotic fluid. About 10–30 percent of all deliveries have meconium-stained fluid. It is always indicative of a fetal hypoxic incident. Hypoxia causes an increase in fetal peristalsis along with relaxation of the anal sphincter, causing meconium to pass into the amniotic fluid. In addition to the stress that caused the incident, there is a risk of aspiration of the meconium-stained fluid.

Meconium staining is often associated with prolonged labour but may be seen in term, postterm, and low-birth-weight infants. The incident may occur a few days prior to delivery or during labour. Some meconium staining is virtually always associated with breech deliveries. This is due to vagal stimulation, which occurs as a result of the pressure of the contracting uterus on the fetus's head.

Evidence of meconium staining is readily observable. Normally, the amniotic fluid is clear or possibly light straw-coloured. When meconium is present, the colour varies from a light yellowish-green to light green or in the worst case, dark green, which is sometimes described as "pea soup." As a rule, the thicker and darker the colour, the higher is the risk of fetal morbidity.

Management As noted earlier, once the head of the newborn is out of the birth canal, you should suction the infant's mouth and nose, on the perineum. If the meconium is thin and light coloured, no further treatment is required, and you should continue with the delivery and routine care. However, if the meconium is thick, a thorough suction of the infant's mouth and nose must be performed with the bulb or DeLee suction. As an ACP or CCP, visualize the glottis, and suction the hypopharynx and trachea using an endotracheal tube until you have cleared all of the meconium from the newborn's airway. Failure to do so will cause the meconium to be pushed farther into the airway and down into the lungs during the delivery process.

> *If meconium is thick, visualize the infant's glottis, and suction the hypopharynx and trachea using an endotracheal tube until all meconium has been cleared from the airway (if you are an ACP/CCP).*

MATERNAL COMPLICATIONS OF LABOUR AND DELIVERY

Several maternal problems can arise during and after delivery. These include postpartum hemorrhage, uterine rupture, uterine inversion, and pulmonary embolism.

> **Content Review**
>
> **MATERNAL COMPLICATIONS**
> Postpartum hemorrhage
> Uterine rupture
> Uterine inversion
> Pulmonary embolism

Postpartum Hemorrhage

Postpartum hemorrhage is the loss of more than 500 mL of blood immediately following delivery. It occurs in approximately 5 percent of deliveries. The most common cause of postpartum hemorrhage is *uterine atony,* or lack of uterine muscle tone. This tends to occur most frequently in the multigravida and is most common following multiple births or births of large infants. Uterine atony also occurs after precipitous deliveries and prolonged labours. In addition to uterine atony, postpartum hemorrhage can be caused by placenta previa, abruptio placentae, retained placental parts, clotting disorders in the mother, or vaginal and cervical tears. Occasionally, the uterus fails to return to its normal size during the postpartum period, and postpartum hemorrhage occurs long after the birth, potentially as much as two weeks postpartum.

Assessment of the patient with postpartum hemorrhage should focus on the history and the predisposing factors described above. You must rely heavily on the clinical appearance of the patient and her vital signs. Often, the uterus will feel boggy and soft on secondary assessment. Vaginal bleeding is usually obvious as a steady, free flow of blood. Counting the number of sanitary pads used is a good way to monitor the bleeding. When postpartum bleeding takes place in the hospital setting, the pads are often weighed, since 500 mL of blood weighs approximately 2.2 kg. You should also examine the perineum for evidence of traumatic injury, which may be the source of the bleeding.

Management When dealing with a patient with postpartum hemorrhage, complete the primary assessment immediately. Administer oxygen, and begin fundal massage. Establish at least one, preferably two, large-bore IVs of normal saline. Never attempt to force delivery of the placenta or pack the vagina with dressings.

> *When there is a loss of more than 500 mL of blood immediately following delivery, administer oxygen, and begin fundal massage. Establish two large-bore IVs of normal saline. Treat for shock as necessary.*
>
>

Uterine Rupture

Uterine rupture is the actual tearing, or rupture, of the uterus. It usually occurs with the onset of labour. However, it can also occur before labour as a result of blunt abdominal trauma. During labour, it often results from prolonged uterine contractions or a surgically scarred uterus, such as occurs from previous cesarean sections, especially in those with the classic vertical incision. It can also occur following a prolonged or obstructed labour, as in the case of cephalopelvic disproportion or in conjunction with abnormal presentations. Although it is a rare occurrence, it carries with it extremely high maternal and fetal mortality rates.

The patient with uterine rupture will complain of excruciating abdominal pain and will often be in shock. Uterine rupture is virtually always associated with the cessation of labour contractions. If the rupture is complete, the pain usually subsides. On secondary assessment, there is often profound shock without evidence of external hemorrhage, although it is sometimes associated with vaginal bleeding. Fetal heart tones (FHTs) are absent. The abdomen is often tender and rigid and may exhibit rebound tenderness. It is often possible to palpate the uterus as a separate hard mass found next to the fetus.

Management Management is the same as for any patient in shock. Administer oxygen at high concentration. Next, establish two large-bore IVs with normal saline, and begin fluid resuscitation. Monitor vital signs and FHTs continuously. Transport the patient rapidly. If the fetus is still viable, the definitive treatment is cesarean section with subsequent repair or removal of the uterus.

Uterine Inversion

Uterine inversion is a rare emergency occurring only once in every 2500 live births. It occurs when the uterus turns inside out after delivery and extends through the cervix. When uterine inversion occurs, the supporting ligaments and blood vessels supplying blood to the uterus are torn, usually causing profound shock. The average blood loss associated with uterine inversion ranges from 800 to 1800 mL. Uterine inversion usually results from pulling on the umbilical cord while awaiting delivery of the placenta or from attempts to express the placenta when the uterus is relaxed.

Management If uterine inversion occurs, you must act quickly. First, place the patient in the supine position, and begin oxygen administration. *Do not* attempt to detach the placenta or pull on the cord. Initiate two large-bore IVs of normal saline, and begin fluid resuscitation. Make one attempt to replace the uterus using the following technique. With the palm of the hand, push the fundus of the inverted uterus toward the vagina. If this single attempt is unsuccessful, cover the uterus with towels moistened with saline, and transport the patient immediately.

In the rare occurrence of uterine inversion, begin fluid resuscitation and then make one attempt to replace the uterus. If this fails, cover the uterus with towels moistened with saline, and transport immediately.

Pulmonary Embolism

Pulmonary embolism is the presence of a blood clot in the pulmonary vascular system (see Chapter 27). It can occur after pregnancy, usually as a result of venous thromboembolism. It is one of the most common causes of maternal death and appears to occur more frequently following cesarean section than vaginal delivery. Pulmonary embolism may occur at any time during pregnancy. There is usually a sudden onset of severe dyspnea accompanied by sharp chest pain. Some patients also report a sense of impending doom. On secondary assessment, the patient may show tachycardia, tachypnea, jugular vein distention, and, in severe cases, hypotension.

Management Management of pulmonary embolism consists of administration of high-flow oxygen and ventilatory support as needed. Also, establish an IV of normal saline at a keep-open rate. Initiate cardiac monitoring, and carefully monitor the patient's vital signs and oxygen saturation while transporting her rapidly.

Pulmonary embolism usually presents with sudden severe dyspnea and sharp chest pain. Administer high-flow oxygen, and support ventilations as needed. Establish an IV of normal saline. Transport immediately, monitoring the heart, vital signs, and oxygen saturation.

ʃUMMARY

Childbirth is a normal process, and obstetrical emergencies are fairly uncommon. However, all pregnant patients are at risk for developing complications, and it is impossible to predict which ones will actually occur. It is therefore important to recognize these complications and act accordingly. Keep in mind that you are caring for two patients, and as long as you remember the priorities of patient care, the situation should normally go smoothly. Relax and enjoy the opportunity to help bring a new life into the world.

DIVISION 5
SPECIAL CONSIDERATIONS

Chapter 41 Neonatology   906

Chapter 42 Pediatrics   937

Chapter 43 Geriatric Emergencies   1021

Chapter 44 Abuse and Assault   1074

Chapter 45 The Challenged Patient   1088

Chapter 46 Acute Interventions for the Chronic-Care Patient   1106

CHAPTER 41

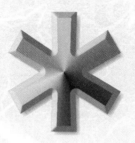

Neonatology

Objectives

After reading this chapter, you should be able to:

1. Define newborn and neonate. (p. 907)
2. Identify important antepartum factors that can affect childbirth. (p. 908)
3. Identify important intrapartum factors that can determine high-risk newborn patients. (p. 908)
4. Identify the factors that lead to premature birth and low-birth-weight newborns. (pp. 924, 926, 929–930)
5. Distinguish between primary and secondary apnea. (p. 909)
6. Discuss pulmonary perfusion and asphyxia. (p. 909)
7. Identify the primary signs employed for evaluating a newborn during resuscitation. (p. 918)
8. Identify the appropriate use of the APGAR scale. (pp. 911–912)
9. Calculate the APGAR score given various newborn situations. (p. 912; see also Chapter 40)
10. Formulate an appropriate treatment plan for providing initial care to a newborn. (p. 912)

Continued

Objectives Continued

11. Describe the indications, equipment needed, application, and evaluation of the following management techniques for the newborn in distress:
    a. Blow-by oxygen (p. 921)
    b. Ventilatory assistance (p. 921)
    c. Endotracheal intubation (pp. 916, 918, 919)
    d. Orogastric tube (p. 922)
    e. Chest compressions (pp. 922–923)
    f. Vascular access (pp. 923–924)
12. Discuss the routes of medication administration for a newborn. (pp. 923–924)
13. Discuss the signs of hypovolemia in a newborn. (p. 931)
14. Discuss the initial steps in resuscitation of a newborn. (pp. 915–924)
15. Discuss the effects of maternal narcotic usage on the newborn. (pp. 924, 926)
16. Determine the appropriate treatment for the newborn with narcotic depression. (p. 924)
17. Discuss appropriate transport guidelines for a newborn. (p. 926)
18. Determine appropriate receiving facilities for low- and high-risk newborns. (p. 926)
19. Describe the epidemiology, including the incidence, morbidity/mortality, risk factors and prevention strategies, pathophysiology, assessment findings, and management for the following neonatal problems:
    a. Meconium aspiration (pp. 912, 916, 926–927)
    b. Apnea (p. 928)
    c. Diaphragmatic hernia (pp. 928–929)
    d. Bradycardia (p. 929)
    e. Prematurity (pp. 929–930)
    f. Respiratory distress/cyanosis (p. 930)
    g. Seizures (pp. 931–932)
    h. Fever (p. 932)
    i. Hypothermia (pp. 932–933)
    j. Hypoglycemia (pp. 933–934)
    k. Vomiting (p. 934)
    l. Diarrhea (pp. 934–935)
    m. Common birth injuries (pp. 935–936)
    n. Cardiac arrest (p. 936)
    o. Postarrest management (p. 936)
20. Given several neonatal emergencies, provide the appropriate procedures for assessment, management, and transport. (pp. 907–936)

INTRODUCTION

Babies pass through stages of physical and emotional development. This chapter concerns itself with babies one month old and under. Babies less than one month old are called **neonates.** Recently born neonates—those in the first few hours of their lives—may also be called **newborns** or *newly born infants* (Figure 41-1).

After an unscheduled delivery in the field, you have two patients to manage—the mother and the baby. You can review the information on care of the mother in Chapter 40. The present chapter describes the initial care of newborns, focusing on the special needs of distressed and premature newborns.

* **neonate** an infant from the time of birth to one month of age.

* **newborn** a baby in the first few hours of its life; also called a *newly born infant.*

After an unscheduled delivery in the field, you have two patients to manage—the mother and the baby.

FIGURE 41-1 Term newborn.

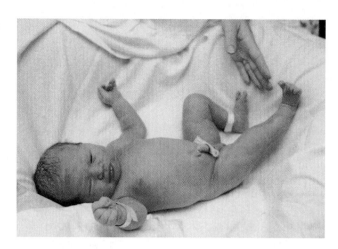

GENERAL PATHOPHYSIOLOGY, ASSESSMENT, AND MANAGEMENT

For newborns that require additional care, your quick actions can make the difference between life and death.

✱ **antepartum** before the onset of labour.

✱ **intrapartum** occurring during childbirth.

Your success in treating at-risk newborns increases with training, ongoing practice, and proper stocking of equipment on board the ambulance.

The care of newborns follows the same priorities as for all patients. You should complete the primary assessment first. Correct any problems detected during the primary assessment before proceeding to the next step. The vast majority of newborns require no resuscitation beyond suctioning the airway, mild stimulation, and maintenance of body temperature. However, for newborns who require additional care, your quick actions can make the difference between life and death.

EPIDEMIOLOGY

Approximately 6 percent of field deliveries require life support. The incidence of complications increases as the birth weight decreases. About 80 percent of newborns weighing less than 1500 g at birth require resuscitation. Determine at-risk newborns by considering the **antepartum** and **intrapartum** factors that may indicate complications at the time of delivery (Table 41-1).

Your success in resuscitating these at-risk infants increases with training, ongoing practice, and proper stocking of equipment on board the ambulance. Make sure your ambulance carries a basic OB kit and resuscitation equipment for newborns of various sizes. (See the list under "Resuscitation," later in this chapter.)

Table 41-1	RISK FACTORS INDICATING POSSIBLE COMPLICATIONS IN NEWBORNS	
Antepartum Factors		**Intrapartum Factors**
Multiple gestation		Premature labour
Inadequate prenatal care		Meconium-stained amniotic fluid
Mother's age (< 16 or > 35)		Rupture of membranes more than 24 hours prior to delivery
History of perinatal morbidity or mortality		
Postterm gestation		Use of narcotics within four hours of delivery
Drugs/medications		Abnormal presentation
Toxemia, hypertension, diabetes		Prolonged labour or precipitous delivery
		Prolapsed cord or bleeding

Plan transport in advance. Know the type of facilities available in your locality and local protocols governing use of these facilities. A nearby neonatal intensive care unit (NICU) makes the best choice for at-risk newborns. However, if you must transport to a distant NICU, determine whether it might be in the best interests of the infant to transport her to the nearest facility for stabilization. Follow local protocols and consult medical direction as needed.

PATHOPHYSIOLOGY

Upon birth, dramatic changes occur within the newborn to prepare it for **extrauterine** life. The respiratory system, which is essentially nonfunctional when the fetus is in the uterus, must suddenly initiate and maintain respirations. While in the uterus, fetal lung fluid fills the fetal lungs. The capillaries and arterioles of the lungs are closed. Most blood pumped by the heart bypasses the nonfunctional respiratory system by flowing through the **ductus arteriosus.**

Approximately one-third of fetal lung fluid is removed through compression of the chest during vaginal delivery. Under normal conditions, the newborn takes her first breath within the first few seconds after delivery. The timing of the first breath is unrelated to the cutting of the umbilical cord. Factors that stimulate the baby's first breath include

- Mild acidosis
- Initiation of stretch reflexes in the lungs
- Hypoxia
- Hypothermia

With the first breaths, the lungs rapidly fill with air, which displaces the remaining fetal fluid. The pulmonary arterioles and capillaries open, decreasing pulmonary vascular resistance. At this point, the resistance to blood flow in the lungs is now less than the resistance of the ductus arteriosus. Because of this pressure difference, blood flow is diverted from the ductus arteriosus to the lungs, where it picks up oxygen for transport to the peripheral tissues (Figure 41-2).

Soon, there is no need for the ductus arteriosus, and it eventually closes. However, if hypoxia or severe acidosis occurs, the pulmonary vascular bed may constrict again and the ductus may reopen. This will retrigger fetal circulation with its attendant shunting and ongoing hypoxia. (This condition is called **persistent fetal circulation.**) To help the newborn make her transition to extrauterine life, it is very important for the paramedic to facilitate her first few breaths and to prevent ongoing hypoxia and acidosis.

Remain alert at all times to signs of respiratory distress. Infants are susceptible to hypoxemia, which can lead to permanent brain damage. After initial hypoxia, the infant rapidly gasps for breath. If the asphyxia continues, respiratory movements cease altogether, the heart rate begins to fall, and neuromuscular tone gradually diminishes. The infant then enters a period of apnea known as *primary apnea.* In most cases, simple stimulation and exposure to oxygen will reverse bradycardia and assist in the development of pulmonary perfusion.

With ongoing asphyxia, however, the infant will enter a period known as *secondary apnea.* During secondary apnea, the infant takes several last deep gasping respirations. The heart rate, blood pressure, and oxygen saturation in the blood continue to fall. The infant becomes unresponsive to stimulation and will not spontaneously resume respiration on her own. Death will occur unless you promptly initiate resuscitation. For this reason, always assume that apnea in the newborn is secondary apnea, and rapidly treat it with ventilatory assistance with oxygen and, when appropriate, chest compressions.

✱ extrauterine outside the uterus.

Upon birth, dramatic changes take place within the newborn to prepare it for extrauterine life.

✱ ductus arteriosus channel between the main pulmonary artery and the aorta of the fetus.

The time of a newborn's first breath is unrelated to the cutting of the umbilical cord.

✱ persistent fetal circulation condition in which blood continues to bypass the fetal respiratory system, resulting in ongoing hypoxia.

Always assume that apnea in the newborn is secondary apnea, and rapidly treat it with ventilatory assistance.

FIGURE 41-2 Hemodynamic changes in the newborn at birth.

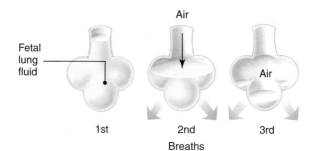

Air

Fetal lung fluid

Air

1st 2nd 3rd

Breaths

Following birth, the lungs expand as they are filled with air. The fetal lung fluid gradually leaves the alveoli.

Arterioles dilate, and blood flow increases.

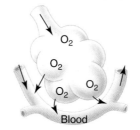

O_2

O_2

O_2

O_2

O_2

Blood

At the same time as the lungs are expanding and the fetal lung fluid is clearing, the arterioles in the lung begin to open, allowing a considerable increase in the amount of blood flowing through the lungs.

Pulmonary blood flow increases.

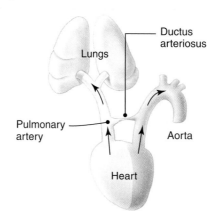

Ductus arteriosus

Lungs

Pulmonary artery

Aorta

Heart

Blood previously diverted through the ductus arteriosus flows through the lungs, where it picks up oxygen to transport to tissues throughout the body. Soon, there is no need for the ductus, and it eventually closes.

Congenital Anomalies

Approximately 2 percent of infants are born with some sort of congenital problem. Congenital problems typically arise from a problem in fetal development. Most fetal development occurs during the first trimester of pregnancy. It is during this time that the developing fetus is most sensitive to environmental factors and substances that can affect normal development.

There are many types of congenital anomalies. These may affect a single organ or structure or may affect many organs or structures. There are several recognized patterns, called *syndromes,* that can occur. It is not within the scope of this text to discuss all the various congenital anomalies. However, there are a few congenital anomalies that can make resuscitation more difficult. For example, some children may be born with a defect in the diaphragm that allows some of the abdominal contents to enter the chest. This abnormality is referred to as a **diaphragmatic hernia.** If you suspect a diaphragmatic hernia, do not treat the infant with bag-valve-mask ventilation. This procedure will distend the stomach, which protrudes into the chest cavity, thus decreasing ventilatory capacity. Instead, immediately intubate the infant. (Diaphragmatic hernias will be discussed in more detail later in this chapter.)

Newborns may have congenital anomalies that make resuscitation more difficult.

✱ **diaphragmatic hernia** protrusion of abdominal contents into the thoracic cavity through an opening in the diaphragm.

Some infants are born with a defect in their spinal cords. In some cases, the spinal cord and associated structures may be exposed. This abnormality is called a **meningomyelocele**. Infants born with a meningomyelocele should not be placed on their backs. Instead, place them on their stomachs or sides and conduct resuscitation in this position, if possible. Cover the spinal defect with sterile gauze pads soaked in warm sterile saline and inserted in a plastic covering.

A newborn may exhibit a defect in the area of the umbilicus. In some cases, the abdominal contents will fill this defect, resulting in an **omphalocele**. If you encounter a newborn with an omphalocele, cover the defect with an occlusive plastic covering to decrease water and heat loss.

Since newborns are obligate nose breathers, **choanal atresia** can cause upper airway obstruction and respiratory distress. Choanal atresia is the most common birth defect involving the nose and is due to the presence of a bony or membranous septum between the nasal cavity and the pharynx. Suspect this condition if you are unable to pass a catheter through either nare into the oropharynx. An oral airway will usually bypass the obstruction.

A fairly common congenital anomaly is cleft lip or cleft palate. During fetal development, the lip and palate come together in the middle forming the oral cavity. Failure of the palate to completely close during fetal development can result in a defect known as **cleft palate**. Cleft palate may also be associated with failure of the upper lip to close. This condition, referred to as **cleft lip**, can make it difficult to obtain an adequate seal for effective mask ventilation. If a child with a cleft lip or cleft palate will require more than brief mechanical ventilation, you should place an endotracheal tube.

Pierre Robin syndrome is a congenital condition characterized by a small jaw and large tongue in conjunction with a cleft palate. In this condition, the tongue is likely to obstruct the upper airway. A nasal or oral airway usually bypasses the obstruction. If the obstruction cannot be bypassed with a simple airway, then intubation will be necessary, although it can be very difficult to carry out on newborns with this condition.

* **meningomyelocele** herniation of the spinal cord and membranes through a defect in the spinal column.

* **omphalocele** congenital hernia of the umbilicus.

* **choanal atresia** congenital closure of the passage between the nose and pharynx by a bony or membranous structure.

* **cleft palate** congenital fissure in the roof of the mouth, forming a passageway between oral and nasal cavities.

* **cleft lip** congenital vertical fissure in the upper lip.

* **Pierre Robin syndrome** unusually small jaw, combined with a cleft palate, downward displacement of the tongue, and an absent gag reflex.

ASSESSMENT

Assess the newborn immediately after birth. (Ideally, if two paramedics are available, one paramedic attends the mother, while the other attends the newborn.) Make a mental note of the time of birth, and then quickly obtain vital signs. Remember that newborns are slippery and you will need to use both hands to support the head and torso. Position yourself so that you can work close to the surface where you have placed the infant.

The newborn's respiratory rate should average 40–60 breaths per minute. If respirations are not adequate or if the newborn is gasping, immediately start positive-pressure ventilation.

Expect a normal heart rate of 150–180 beats per minute at birth, slowing to 120–140 beats per minute thereafter. A pulse rate of less than 100 beats per minute indicates distress and requires emergency intervention.

Evaluate the skin colour as well. Some cyanosis of the extremities is common immediately after birth. However, cyanosis of the central part of the body is abnormal, as is persistent peripheral cyanosis. In such cases, administer 100 percent oxygen until the cause is determined or the condition is corrected.

> **Content Review**
> ### APGAR
> - Appearance
> - Pulse rate
> - Grimace
> - Activity
> - Respiratory effort

* **APGAR score** a numerical system of rating the condition of a newborn. It evaluates the newborn's heart rate, respiratory rate, muscle tone, reflex irritability, and colour.

If a newborn is not breathing, DO NOT withhold resuscitation in order to determine the APGAR score.

THE APGAR SCALE

As discussed in Chapter 40, as soon as possible, assign the newborn an **APGAR score** (See Table 40-2 in Chapter 40.) Ideally, try to do this at 1 and 5 minutes after birth. However, if the newborn is not breathing, DO NOT withhold resuscitation in order to determine the APGAR score. The APGAR scoring system helps distinguish between newborns who need only routine care and those who need greater assistance. The system also predicts long-term survival. A score of 0, 1, or 2 is given for each of the parameters. The minimum total score is 0 and the maximum is 10. A score of 7–10 indicates an active and vigorous newborn who requires only routine care. A score of 4–6 indicates a moderately distressed newborn who requires oxygenation and stimulation. Severely distressed newborns, those with APGAR scores of less than 4, require immediate resuscitation.

TREATMENT

Treatment starts prior to delivery. Begin care by preparing the environment and assembling the equipment needed for delivery and immediate care of the newborn. The initial care of a newborn follows the same priorities as for all patients. Complete the primary assessment first. Correct any problems detected during the primary assessment before proceeding to the next step. The vast majority of term newborns—approximately 80 percent—require no resuscitation beyond suctioning of the airway, mild stimulation, and maintenance of body temperature by drying and warming with blankets.

Establishing the Airway

Airway management is one of the most critical steps in caring for the newborn. During delivery, fluid is forced out of the baby's lungs, into the oropharynx, and out through the nose and mouth. Fluid drainage occurs independently of gravity. As soon as you deliver the newborn's head, suction the mouth and then the nose, using a bulb suction. Always suction the mouth first so that there is nothing for the infant to aspirate if she gasps when the nose is suctioned.

Immediately following delivery, maintain the newborn at the same level as the mother's vagina, with the head approximately 15 degrees below the torso. This facilitates the drainage of secretions and helps prevent aspiration. If there appears to be a large amount of secretions, attach a **DeLee suction trap** to a suction source. As previously explained, suction the mouth first and then the nose (Figure 41-3a). Repeat these steps until the airway is clear. If you detect **meconium**, prepare intubation equipment and a meconium aspirator (Figure 41-3b). (Meconium staining will be discussed in more detail in several later sections of this chapter.)

Drying and suctioning produce enough stimulation to initiate respirations in most newborns. If the newborn does not immediately cry, stimulate her by flicking the soles of her feet or gently rubbing her back (Figure 41-4). DO NOT spank or vigorously rub a newborn baby.

Prevention of Heat Loss

Heat loss can be a life-threatening condition in newborns. Cold infants quickly become distressed infants. Heat loss occurs through evaporation, convection, conduction, and radiation. Most heat loss in newborns results from evaporation. The newborn comes into the world wet, and the amniotic fluid quickly evaporates. Immediately after birth, the newborn's core temperature can drop 1°C or more from its birth temperature of 38°C.

Loss of heat can also occur through convection, depending on the temperature of the room and the movement of the air around the newborn. The newborn can lose additional heat through contact with surrounding surfaces (convection) or by radiating heat to colder objects nearby.

FIGURE 41-3a   Suctioning of the mouth using flexible suction catheter.

When head is delivered

As soon as the baby's head is delivered (prior to delivery of the shoulders) *the mouth, oropharynx, and hypopharynx should be thoroughly suctioned*, using a 10-Fr. DeLee suction catheter or other flexible suction catheter. Any catheter used should be no smaller than a 10-Fr.

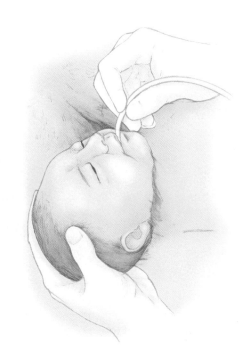

FIGURE 41-3b   Intubation for removal of residual meconium.

Following delivery

After delivery of the infant, if a great deal of meconium is present, the trachea should be intubated and any residual meconium removed from the lower airway.

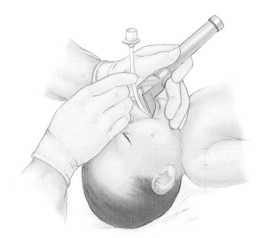

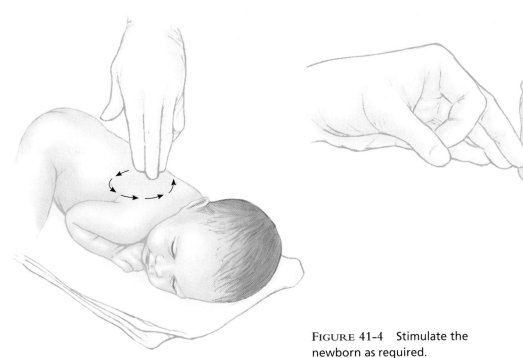

FIGURE 41-4   Stimulate the newborn as required.

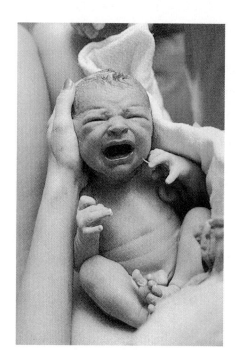

FIGURE 41-5 Dry the infant to prevent loss of evaporative heat.

To prevent heat loss, take these steps.

- Dry the newborn immediately to prevent evaporative cooling (Figure 41-5).
- Maintain the ambient temperature—the temperature in the delivery room or ambulance—at a *minimum* of 23–24°C.
- Close all windows and doors.
- Discard the towel used to dry the newborn and swaddle the infant in a warm, dry receiving blanket or other suitable material. Cover the head.
- In colder areas, place well-insulated water bottles or rubber gloves filled with warm water (40°C) around the newborn to help maintain a warm body temperature. To avoid burns, do not place these items against the skin. Be sure the newborn is wrapped in a blanket and place the water bottle or rubber glove against the blanket.

> *Do not "milk" or strip the umbilical cord.*
>
>

✱ **polycythemia** an excess of red blood cells. In a newborn, the condition may reflect hypovolemia or prolonged intrauterine hypoxia.

✱ **hyperbilirubinemia** an excessive amount of bilirubin—the orange-coloured pigment associated with bile—in the blood. In newborns, the condition appears as jaundice. Precipitating factors include maternal Rh or ABO incompatibility, neonatal septicemia, anoxia, hypoglycemia, and congenital liver or gastrointestinal defects.

Cutting the Umbilical Cord

After you have stabilized the newborn's airway and minimized heat loss, clamp and cut the umbilical cord. You can prevent over- and undertransfusion of blood by maintaining the baby at the same level as the vagina, as previously described. Do not "milk" or strip the umbilical cord, since this increases blood viscosity, or **polycythemia.** Polycythemia can cause cardiopulmonary problems. It can also contribute to excessive red blood cell destruction, which may, in turn, lead to **hyperbilirubinemia**—an increased level of bilirubin in the blood that causes jaundice.

Apply the umbilical clamps within 30–45 seconds after birth. Place the first clamp approximately 10 cm from the newborn. Place the second clamp about 5 cm farther away than the first. Then, cut the cord between the two clamps (see Figure 40-17 in Chapter 40). After the cord is cut, inspect it periodically to make sure there is no additional bleeding.

THE DISTRESSED NEWBORN

The distressed newborn can be either full term or premature. (See "Premature Infants" later in this chapter.) The presence of fetal meconium at birth indicates that fetal distress has occurred at some point during pregnancy. If the newborn is simply meconium stained, then distress may have occurred at a remote time. If you see *particulate* meconium, however, distress may have occurred recently and the newborn should be managed accordingly.

Aspiration of meconium can cause significant respiratory problems and should be prevented. Whenever you spot meconium during delivery, do not induce respiratory effort until you have removed the meconium from the trachea by suctioning under direct visualization with the laryngoscope. (There will be more about this topic under "Meconium-Stained Amniotic Fluid" later.) Be sure to report the presence of meconium to the medical direction physician.

The most common problems experienced by newborns during the first minutes of life involve the airway. For this reason, resuscitation usually consists of ventilation and oxygenation. Except in special situations, the use of IV fluids, drugs, or cardiac equipment is usually not indicated. (See "Inverted Pyramid for Resuscitation" on the next page.) The most important procedures include suctioning, drying, and stimulating the distressed newborn.

Of the vital signs, fetal heart rate is the most important indicator of neonatal distress. The newborn has a relatively fixed stroke volume. Thus, cardiac output depends more on heart rate. Bradycardia, as caused by hypoxia, results in decreased cardiac output and, ultimately, poor perfusion. A pulse rate of less than 60 beats per minute in a distressed newborn should be treated with chest compressions. In distressed newborns, monitor the heart rate manually. Do not depend on external electronic monitors.

> *Of the vital signs, fetal heart rate is the most important indicator of neonatal distress.*
>

RESUSCITATION

The vast majority of newborns do not require resuscitation beyond stimulation, maintenance of the airway, and maintenance of body temperature. Unfortunately, it is difficult to predict which newborns ultimately will require resuscitation. Each EMS unit, therefore, should contain a neonatal resuscitation kit containing the following items:

- Neonatal bag-valve-mask unit
- Bulb syringe
- DeLee suction trap
- Meconium aspirator
- Laryngoscope with size 0 and 1 blades
- Uncuffed endotracheal tubes (2.5, 3.0, 3.5, 4.0) with appropriate suction catheters
- Endotracheal tube stylet
- Tape or device to secure endotracheal tube
- Umbilical catheter and 10-mL syringe
- Three-way stopcock
- 20-mL syringe and 8-French feeding tube for gastric suction
- Glucometer
- Assorted syringes and needles
- Towels (sterile)

- Medications:
  - Epinephrine 1:10 000 and 1:1000
  - Neonatal naloxone (Narcan)
  - Volume expander (Ringer's Lactate solution or saline)
  - Sodium bicarbonate (10 mEq in 10 mL)

INVERTED PYRAMID FOR RESUSCITATION

Resuscitation of the newborn follows an inverted pyramid (Figure 41-6). As this pyramid indicates, most distressed newborns respond to relatively simple manoeuvres. Few require cardiopulmonary resuscitation (CPR) or advanced life support measures.

The following are steps for the initial care of the newborn. Also, see the resuscitation steps illustrated in Procedure 41–1 and Figure 41-7.

Step 1: Drying, Warming, Positioning, Suctioning, and Tactile Stimulation

Resuscitation begins with drying, warming, positioning, suctioning, and stimulating the newborn. Immediately on delivery, minimize heat loss by drying the newborn. Next, place the newborn in a warm, dry blanket. Make sure the environment is warm and free of drafts.

After you have dried the newborn, place the infant on her back with her head slightly below her body and her neck slightly extended (Figure 41-8). This facilitates drainage of secretions and fluids from the lungs. Place a small blanket, folded to a 2-cm thickness, under the newborn's shoulders to help maintain this position.

Next, suction the newborn again, using a bulb syringe or DeLee suction trap. Deep suctioning can cause a **vagal response**, resulting in bradycardia. Because of this, suctioning should last no longer than 10 seconds. If meconium is present, avoid stimulating the infant, and visualize the airway with a laryngoscope. Suction the meconium, preferably with a DeLee suction trap. If there is a great deal of meconium, place an appropriately sized endotracheal tube (Table 41-2) and suction the meconium directly through the tube. Remove the tube and discard. Do not use the same tube for mechanical ventilation. (See Procedure 41-2.) Following adequate tracheal suctioning, stimulate the newborn by flicking the soles of her feet or rubbing her back.

✱ **vagal response** stimulation of the vagus nerve causing a parasympathetic response.

Suctioning of a newborn should last no longer than 10 seconds.

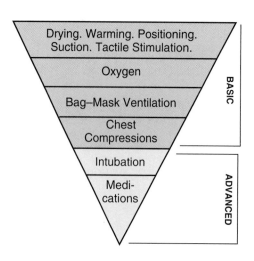

FIGURE 41-6 The inverted pyramid of neonatal resuscitation showing approximate relative frequencies of neonatal care and resuscitative efforts. Note that a majority of infants respond to the simple measures noted at the top, wide part of the pyramid.

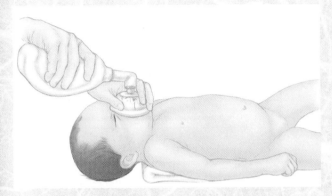

41-1a   Ventilate with 100-percent oxygen for 15–30 seconds.

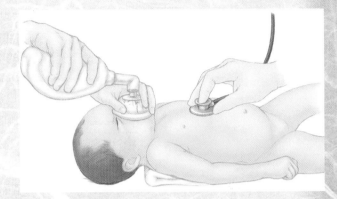

41-1b   Evaluate heart rate.

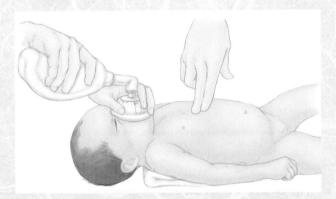

41-1c   Initiate chest compressions if heart rate less than 60.

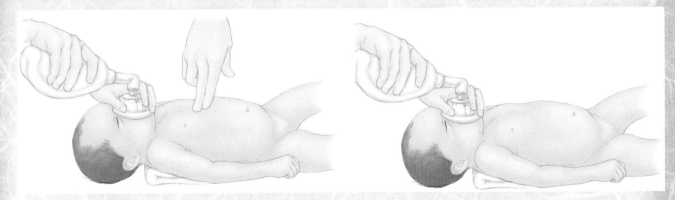

41-1d   Evaluate heart rate: Below 60—Continue chest compressions; 60 or above—Discontinue chest compressions.

NORMAL NEWBORN ASSESSMENT AND SUPPORT

Temperature: Dry, warm
Airway: Position, suction
Breathing: Gentle stimulation to cry
Circulation: Pulse rate, colour

ASSISTANCE SOME NEWBORNS MAY REQUIRE
(Note: Moving down the list, progressively
fewer patients will require the listed interventions.)

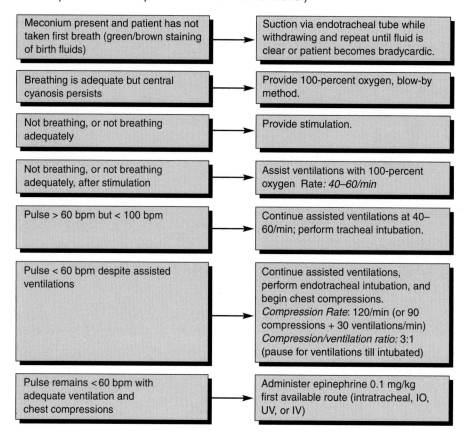

Meconium present and patient has not taken first breath (green/brown staining of birth fluids)	Suction via endotracheal tube while withdrawing and repeat until fluid is clear or patient becomes bradycardic.
Breathing is adequate but central cyanosis persists	Provide 100-percent oxygen, blow-by method.
Not breathing, or not breathing adequately	Provide stimulation.
Not breathing, or not breathing adequately, after stimulation	Assist ventilations with 100-percent oxygen Rate: *40–60/min*
Pulse > 60 bpm but < 100 bpm	Continue assisted ventilations at 40–60/min; perform tracheal intubation.
Pulse < 60 bpm despite assisted ventilations	Continue assisted ventilations, perform endotracheal intubation, and begin chest compressions. *Compression Rate:* 120/min (or 90 compressions + 30 ventilations/min) *Compression/ventilation ratio:* 3:1 (pause for ventilations till intubated)
Pulse remains <60 bpm with adequate ventilation and chest compressions	Administer epinephrine 0.1 mg/kg first available route (intratracheal, IO, UV, or IV)

FIGURE 41-7   Resuscitation of the newborn. (Adapted from David S. Markenson, *Pediatric Prehospital Care,* Prentice Hall, 2002.)

After carrying out the preceding procedures, assess the newborn as noted below.

Newborn Assessment Parameters

• *Respiratory effort.* The rate and depth of the newborn's breathing should increase immediately with tactile stimulation. If the respiratory response is adequate, evaluate the heart rate next. If the respiratory rate is inadequate, begin positive-pressure ventilation (see Step 3).

• *Heart rate.* As noted earlier, heart rate is critical in the newborn. Check the heart rate by listening to the apical area of the heart with a stethoscope, feeling the pulse by lightly grasping the umbilical cord, or feeling either the brachial or femoral pulse. If the heart rate is greater than 100 and spontaneous respirations are present, continue the assessment. If the heart rate is less than 100, immediately begin positive-pressure ventilation (see Step 3).

CORRECT

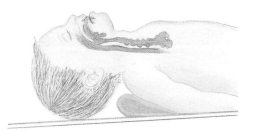

Neck slightly extended

Care should be taken to prevent hyperextension or underextension of the neck, since either may decrease air entry.

INCORRECT

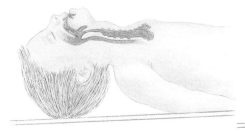 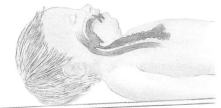

Neck hyperextended   Neck underextended

FIGURE 41-8 Positioning the newborn to open the airway.

- *Colour.* A newborn may be cyanotic despite a heart rate greater than 100 and spontaneous respirations. If you note central cyanosis, or cyanosis of the chest and abdomen, in a newborn with adequate ventilation and a pulse rate greater than 100, administer supplemental oxygen (see Step 2). Newborns with peripheral cyanosis do not usually need supplemental oxygen UNLESS the cyanosis is prolonged.
- *APGAR score.* Unless resuscitation is required, obtain 1- and 5-minute APGAR scores.

Content Review

NORMAL NEWBORN VITAL SIGNS
- Respirations 30–60
- Heart rate 100–180
- Blood pressure 60–90 systolic
- Temperature 36.7°–37.8°C

Table 41-2 GUIDELINES FOR TRACHEAL TUBE SIZES AND DEPTH OF INSERTION IN THE NEWBORN

Tube Size, mm ID	Depth of Insertion from Upper Lip, cm	Weight, g	Gestation, wk
2.5	6.5–7	< 1000	< 28
3.0	7–8	1000–2000	28–34
3.5	8–9	2000–3000	34–38
3.5–4.0	> 9	> 3000	> 38

American Heart Association: *2000 Handbook of Cardiovascular Care for Healthcare Providers* © 2000, American Heart Association.

Procedure 41-2   Endotracheal Intubation and Tracheal Suctioning in the Newborn

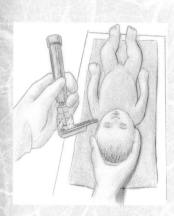
41-2a   Position the infant.

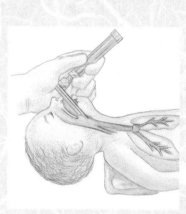
41-2b   Insert the laryngoscope.

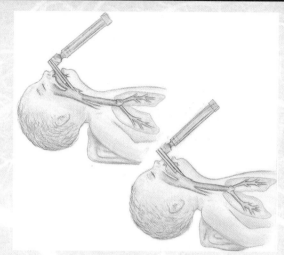
41-2c   Elevate the epiglottis by lifting.

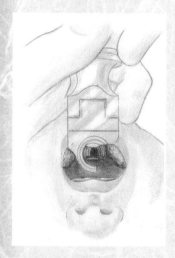
41-2d   Visualize the cords.

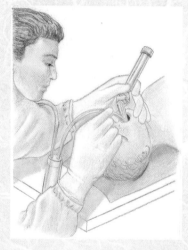
41-2e   Suction any meconium present.

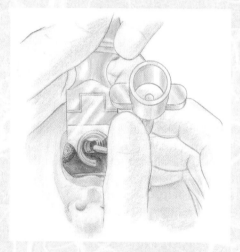
41-2f   Insert a fresh tube for ventilation.

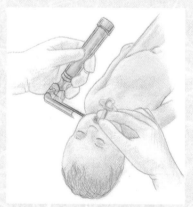
41-2g   Remove the laryngoscope.

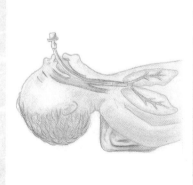
41-2h   Check proper tube placement.

Step 2: Supplemental Oxygen

If central cyanosis is present or the adequacy of ventilation is uncertain, administer supplemental oxygen by blowing oxygen across the newborn's face (Figure 41-9). If possible, the oxygen should be warmed and humidified. Continue oxygen administration until the newborn's colour has improved. Although oxygen toxicity is a concern, this condition usually results from prolonged usage over several days. Administration of blow-by oxygen in the prehospital setting will not cause problems. NEVER DEPRIVE A NEWBORN OF OXYGEN IN THE PREHOSPITAL SETTING FOR FEAR OF OXYGEN TOXICITY.

Never deprive a newborn of oxygen in the prehospital setting for fear of oxygen toxicity.

Step 3: Ventilation

Begin positive-pressure ventilation if *any* of the following conditions is present:

- Heart rate less than 100 beats per minute
- Apnea
- Persistence of central cyanosis after administration of supplemental oxygen

A ventilatory rate of 40–60 breaths per minute is usually adequate. A bag-valve-mask unit is the device of choice. A self-inflating bag of an appropriate size (450 mL is optimal) should be used. Many self-inflating bags have a pressure-limiting pop-off valve that is preset at 30–45 cm H_2O. However, since the initial pressures required to ventilate a newborn may be as high as 60 cm/H_2O, you may have to depress the pop-off valve to deactivate it and ensure adequate ventilation. If prolonged ventilation is required, it may be necessary to disable the pop-off valve.

Face masks in various sizes must be available. The most effective ones are designed to fit the contours of the newborn's face and have a low dead space volume (less than 5 mL). When a mask is correctly sized and positioned, it covers the newborn's nose and mouth but not the eyes.

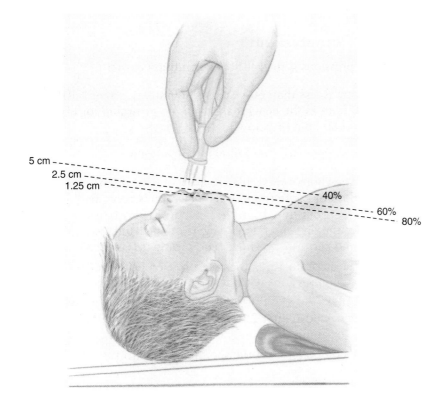

FIGURE 41-9 Guidelines for estimating oxygen concentration. Based on oxygen flow rate of five litres per minute.

Endotracheal intubation of a newborn should be carried out in the following situations:

- The bag-valve-mask unit does not work.
- Tracheal suctioning is required (such as in cases of thick meconium).
- Prolonged ventilation will be required.
- A diaphragmatic hernia is suspected.
- Inadequate respiratory effort is found.

Because of the narrowness of the neonatal airway at the level of the cricoid cartilage, always use an *uncuffed* endotracheal tube. (Review Table 41-2.) After inserting it, ensure proper placement by noting symmetrical chest wall motion and equal breath sounds. (Review Procedure 41-2.)

✱ glottic function opening and closing of the glottic space.

✱ PEEP positive end-expiratory pressure.

Intubation has several effects in the newborn. First, it bypasses **glottic function**. Second, it eliminates **PEEP**—the physiological positive end-expiratory pressure created during normal coughing and crying. To maintain adequate functional residual capacity, a PEEP of 2–4 cm/H_2O should be provided when mechanical ventilation is initiated by adding a magnetic-disk PEEP valve to the bag-valve outlet.

✱ nasogastric tube/orogastric tube a tube that runs through the nose or mouth and esophagus into the stomach; used for administering liquid nutrients or medications or for removing air or liquids from the stomach.

Gastric distention, caused by a leak around an uncuffed endotracheal tube, may compromise ventilation of a newborn. This can be minimized by using a properly sized endotracheal tube. If there is significant gastric distension, a **nasogastric tube** or **orogastric tube** should be inserted (through the nose or mouth, then through the esophagus into the stomach) as soon as the airway is controlled. It is recommended that the endotracheal tube be in place before the gastric tube is placed to avoid wrongly placing the gastric tube into the trachea.

Make sure the newborn is well oxygenated before attempting to insert a gastric tube. To determine the depth of insertion, measure a nasogastric tube from the tip of the nose, around the ear, to below the xiphoid process. Measure an orogastric tube from the lips to below the xiphoid process. Lubricate the end of the tube, and pass it gently along the nasal floor or the mouth and into the esophagus. Confirm that the tube is in the stomach by injecting 10 mL of air into the tube and auscultating a bubbling sound, or sound of rushing air, over the epigastrium.

Step 4: Chest Compressions

Initiate chest compressions if the following condition exists:

- The heart rate is less than 60 beats per minute. (Current NRP guidelines use 60 bpm as the benchmark, with no provision for 80 bpm or above and 80 bpm or below.)

Perform chest compressions by following these steps:

- Encircle the newborn's chest, placing both of your thumbs on the lower one-third of the sternum. If the newborn is very small, you may need to overlap your thumbs. If the newborn is very large, you may need to place the ring and middle fingers of one hand just below the nipple line and perform two-finger compressions (Figure 41-10).
- Compress the sternum 1.5–2.0 cm at a rate of 120 times per minute. Accompany compressions with positive-pressure ventilation. Maintain a ratio of 3 compressions to 1 ventilation.
- Reassess the newborn after 20 cycles of compressions and ventilations, or at approximately one-minute intervals.
- Discontinue compressions if the spontaneous heart rate exceeds 60.

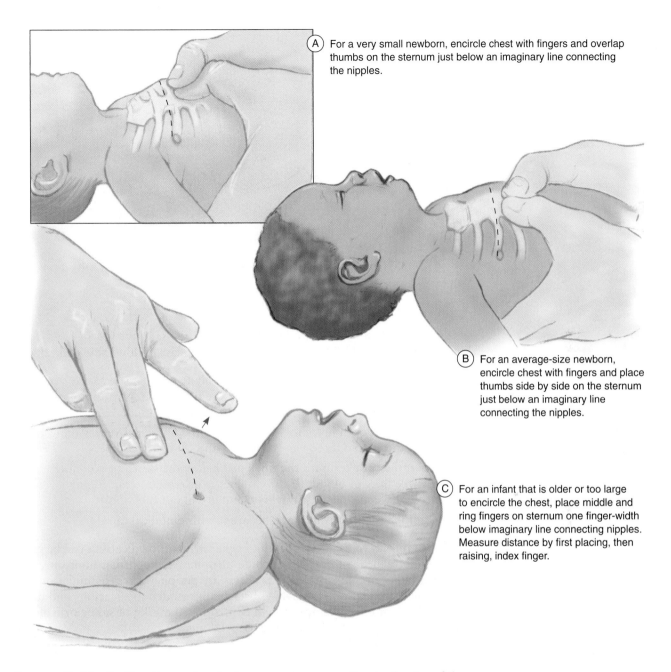

A For a very small newborn, encircle chest with fingers and overlap thumbs on the sternum just below an imaginary line connecting the nipples.

B For an average-size newborn, encircle chest with fingers and place thumbs side by side on the sternum just below an imaginary line connecting the nipples.

C For an infant that is older or too large to encircle the chest, place middle and ring fingers on sternum one finger-width below imaginary line connecting nipples. Measure distance by first placing, then raising, index finger.

FIGURE 41-10   Position fingers for chest compressions according to the size of the infant.

Step 5: Medications and Fluids

Most cardiopulmonary arrests in newborns result from hypoxia. Because of this, initial therapy consists of ventilation and oxygenation. However, when these measures fail, fluid and medications should be administered. They may also be necessary in cases of persistent bradycardia, hypovolemia, respiratory depression secondary to narcotics, and metabolic acidosis.

Vascular access for the administration of fluids and drugs can most readily be managed by using the umbilical vein. The umbilical cord contains three

Vascular access for the administration of fluids and drugs can most readily be managed by using the umbilical vein.

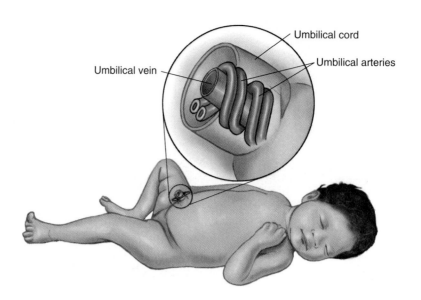

FIGURE 41-11 The umbilical cord contains two arteries and one vein. The umbilical vein can be accessed for vascular administration of fluids and drugs. The vein is larger than the arteries and has a thinner wall.

Umbilical vein

Umbilical cord

Umbilical arteries

vessels—two arteries and one vein. The vein is larger than the arteries and has a thinner wall (Figure 41-11). To establish venous access, follow these procedures:

- Trim the umbilical cord with a scalpel blade to 1 cm above the abdomen. Be sure to save enough of the umbilical cord stump in case neonatal personnel have to place additional lines.
- Insert a 5-French umbilical catheter into the umbilical vein. Connect the catheter to a three-way stopcock, and fill it with saline.
- Insert the catheter until the tip is just below the skin and you note the free flow of blood. (If the catheter is inserted too far, it may become wedged against the liver, and it will not function.)
- After the catheter is in place, secure it with umbilical tape.

If an umbilical vein catheter cannot be placed, some medications can be given via the endotracheal tube. They include atropine, epinephrine, lidocaine, and naloxone. Other options for vascular access are peripheral vein cannulation and intraosseous cannulation. Table 41-3 lists recommended medications and doses for the newborn. Fluid therapy should consist of 10 mL/kg of saline or Ringer's Lactate solution given by syringe as a slow IV push.

MATERNAL NARCOTIC USE

Maternal abuse of narcotics—either illegal or prescribed—can complicate field deliveries. Maternal narcotic use has been shown to produce low-birth-weight infants. Such infants may demonstrate withdrawal symptoms—tremors, startles, and decreased alertness. They also face a serious risk of respiratory depression at birth.

Naloxone (Narcan), which is extremely safe even at high doses, is the treatment of choice for respiratory depression secondary to maternal narcotic use *within four hours of delivery*. Ventilatory support must be provided prior to administration of naloxone. Because the duration of the narcotics may exceed that of the naloxone, repeat administration as necessary.

Keep in mind, however, that the naloxone may induce a withdrawal reaction in an infant born to *a narcotic-addicted* mother. Medical direction may advise that naloxone NOT be administered if the mother is an addict and may recommend that prolonged ventilatory support be provided instead.

Keep in mind that naloxone may induce a withdrawal reaction with an infant born to a narcotic-addicted mother.

Table 41-3   NEONATAL RESUSCITATION DRUGS

Medication	Concentration to Administer	Preparation	Dosage/Route*	Total Dose/Infant		Rate/Precautions
Epinephrine	1:10 000	1 mL	0.1–0.3 mL/kg I.V. or I.T.	*weight . . . total mLs* 1 kg 0.1–0.3 mL 2 kg 0.2–0.6 mL 3 kg 0.3–0.9 mL 4 kg 0.4–1.2 mL		Give rapidly.
Volume Expanders	Whole Blood 5% Albumin Normal Saline Ringer's Lactate	40 mL	10 mL/kg I.V.	*weight . . . total mLs* 1 kg 10 mL 2 kg 20 mL 3 kg 30 mL 4 kg 40 mL		Give over 5–10 min.
Sodium Bicarbonate	0.5 mEq/mL	20 mL or two 10-mL prefilled syringes	2 mEq/kg I.V.	*weight . . . total dose . . . mLs* 1 kg 2 mEq 4 mL 2 kg 4 mEq 8 mL 3 kg 6 mEq 12 mL 4 kg 8 mEq 16 mL		Give slowly, over at least 2 min. Give only if infant is being effectively ventilated.
Narcan Neonatal	1.0 mg/mL or 0.4 mg/mL (dilute 1.0 mg in 9 mL of Saline)	2 mL	0.1 mg/kg I.V., I.M., S.Q., I.T.	*weight . . . total mLs* 1 kg 1.0 mL 2 kg 2.0 mL 3 kg 3.0 mL 4 kg 4.0 mL		Give rapidly.
Dopamine	$6 \times \dfrac{\text{weight} \times \text{desired dose}}{(\text{kg})\ (\mu g/kg/min)}{\text{desired fluid (mL/hr)}} = \dfrac{\text{mg of dopamine}}{\text{per 100 mL of solution}}$		Begin at 5 μg/kg/min (may increase to 20 μg/kg/min if necessary) I.V.	*weight . . . total μg/min* 1 kg 5–20 μg/min 2 kg 10–40 μg/min 3 kg 15–60 μg/min 4 kg 20–80 μg/min		Give as continuous infusion using an infusion pump. Monitor HR and BP closely. Seek consultation.

Adapted from *Textbook of Neonatal Resuscitation* © 2001, American Heart Association.

* I.M. = Intramuscular
  I.T. = Intratracheal
  I.V. = Intravenous
  S.Q. = Subcutaneous

HR = Heart rate
BP = Blood pressure

The dosage of naloxone is 0.1 mg/kg. The initial dose may be repeated every 2–3 minutes as needed. Naloxone may be given by intravenous, intraosseous, endotracheal, subcutaneous, or intramuscular routes.

As with other newborns, continue all resuscitative measures until the newborn is resuscitated or until the emergency staff assumes care.

NEONATAL TRANSPORT

Healthy newborns should be allowed to begin the bonding process with the mother as soon as possible (Figure 41-12). Distressed newborns, however, must be positioned on their sides to prevent aspiration and be rapidly transported.

In addition to field deliveries, paramedics are frequently called upon to transport a high-risk newborn from a facility where stabilization has occurred to a neonatal intensive care unit (NICU). The trip may be across the street or across the province. Usually, a pediatric nurse, respiratory therapist, and, often, a physician accompany the newborn. During transport, a paramedic crew will help maintain a newborn's body temperature, control oxygen administration, and maintain ventilatory support. Often, a transport **isolette** with its own heat, light, and oxygen source is available. In such cases, intravenous medications are usually infused through the umbilical vein. The umbilical artery is catheterized as well.

If a self-contained isolette is not available for transport, it is important to keep the ambulance warm. Wrap the newborn in several blankets, keep the infant's head covered, and place hot-water bottles containing water heated to no more than 40°C near, but not touching, the newborn. Do not use chemical packs to keep the newborn warm. These can generate excessive heat and may burn the infant.

SPECIFIC NEONATAL SITUATIONS

Rapid assessment and treatment of a distressed newborn is the key to the infant's survival. The following information will help you to formulate treatment plans for specific emergencies involving newborns. Remember that, unless otherwise directed, it will be necessary to transport these infants to a facility that is able to handle high-risk neonates. Whenever possible, keep the parents advised of what is happening and the reason for any treatments being given to the infant. However, do not discuss "chances of survival" with the family or caregivers.

MECONIUM-STAINED AMNIOTIC FLUID

Meconium-stained amniotic fluid occurs in approximately 10–15 percent of deliveries, mostly in postterm or in small-for-gestational-age (SGA) newborns. The mortality rate for meconium-stained infants is considerably higher than the mor-

✳ **isolette** also known as an *incubator*; a clear plastic enclosed bassinet used to keep prematurely born infants warm. The temperature of an isolette can be adjusted regardless of the room temperature. Some isolettes also provide humidity control.

Do not discuss "chances of survival" with a newborn's family or caregivers.

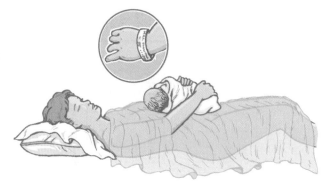

FIGURE 41-12 A healthy newborn can be placed on the mother's abdomen. Write the mother's last name and time of delivery on a tape, and place it around the infant's wrist. (Do not allow adhesive to contact the infant's skin.)

tality rate for nonstained infants, and meconium aspiration accounts for a significant proportion of neonatal deaths.

Fetal distress and hypoxia can cause the passage of meconium into the amniotic fluid. Meconium is a dark green substance found in the digestive tract of full-term newborns. It arises from secretions of the various digestive glands and amniotic fluid. Either in utero, or more often with the first breath, thick meconium is aspirated into the lungs, resulting in small-airway obstruction and aspiration pneumonia. This may produce respiratory distress within the first hours, or even minutes, of life as evidenced by tachypnea, retraction, grunting, and cyanosis in severely affected newborns.

The partial obstruction of some airways may lead to pneumothorax. A pneumothorax may occur in an infant, cause no distress, and require no active treatment. If, however, the infant has significant respiratory distress, then the pneumothorax must be evacuated. If tension pneumothorax has occurred, needle decompression may be required.

An infant born through thin meconium may not require treatment, but depressed infants born through thick, particulate (pea-soup) meconium-stained fluid should be intubated immediately, prior to the first ventilation (Figure 41-13). Aspiration of meconium by a newborn can result in either partial or complete airway obstruction. Complete airway obstruction causes atelectasis (collapsed or airless lungs). In addition, some aspects of fetal blood flow resume a right-to-left shunt of blood across the foramen ovale (the opening between the atria of the fetal heart). This results from increased pulmonary pressures. Incomplete obstruction can act as a ball-valve in the smaller airways, thus preventing exhalation. Also, the newborn is at increased risk of developing a pneumothorax.

Before stimulating the infant to breathe, apply suction with a meconium aspirator attached to an endotracheal tube. Connect to suction at 100 cm/H_2O or less to remove meconium from the airway. Withdraw the endotracheal tube as suction is applied.

Repeat intubation and suction until the meconium clears, usually not more than two times. Once the airway is clear and the infant is able to breathe on her own, ventilate with 100-percent oxygen. If the infant is found to be hypotensive, consider a fluid challenge. Remember to warm the infant to prevent hypothermia. The parents will probably question the treatment being performed on the infant. Explain what you are doing and why, without discussing chances of survival. Stress the need for rapid transport to a facility able to handle high-risk infants.

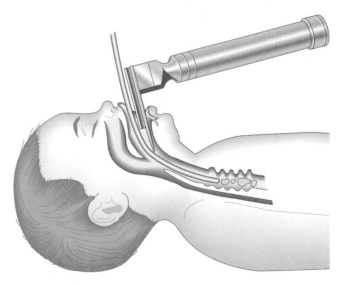

FIGURE 41-13 Intubate the infant born through particulate, thick meconium immediately—prior to the first ventilation.

CAUSES OF APNEA IN NEWBORNS

- Hypoxia
- Hypothermia
- Narcotics
- Respiratory muscle weakness
- Septicemia
- Metabolic disorder
- Central nervous system disorder

DO NOT utilize narcotic antagonists if the mother is a drug abuser.

✱ **herniation** protrusion or projection of an organ or part of an organ through the wall of the cavity that normally contains it.

APNEA

Apnea is a common finding in preterm infants, infants weighing under 1500 g, infants exposed to drugs, or infants born after prolonged or difficult labour and delivery. Typically, the infant fails to breathe spontaneously after stimulation, or the infant experiences respiratory pauses of greater than 20 seconds.

While apnea is usually due to hypoxia or hypothermia, there may be other causative factors. These include

- Narcotic or central nervous depressants
- Weakness of the respiratory muscles
- Septicemia
- Metabolic disorders
- Central nervous system disorders

Begin management of apnea with tactile stimulation. Flick the soles of the infant's feet or gently rub her back. If necessary, ventilate using a bag-valve mask with the pop-off valve disabled. If the infant still does not breathe on her own, or if she has a heart rate of less than 60 with adequate ventilation and chest compressions, perform tracheal intubation with direct visualization. Gain circulatory access, and monitor the heart rate continuously. If the apnea is due to narcotics taken within the previous four hours, consider naloxone. As noted earlier, however, the use of narcotic antagonists is generally contraindicated if the mother is a drug abuser.

Early and aggressive treatment of apnea usually results in a good outcome. Throughout treatment, keep the infant warm to prevent hypothermia. Also explain the procedures to parents and the need for rapid transport.

DIAPHRAGMATIC HERNIA

Diaphragmatic hernias rarely occur. They are seen in approximately 1 out of every 2200 live births. When they do appear, the **herniation** takes place most often in the posterolateral segments of the diaphragm, and most commonly (90 percent) on the left side. The defect is caused by the failure of the pleuroperitoneal canal (foramen of Bochdalek) to close completely. The survival rate for infants who require mechanical ventilation in the first 18 to 24 hours is approximately 50 percent. However, if there is no respiratory distress in the first 24 hours of life, the survival rate approaches 100 percent.

Protrusion of abdominal viscera through the hernia into the thoracic cavity occurs in varying degrees. In severe cases, the stomach, a large part of the intestines, and the spleen, liver, and kidneys displace the lungs and heart to the opposite side. The lung on the affected side is compressed, causing diminished total lung volume. In at least one-third of patients, pulmonary hypertension is present. With a patent ductus arteriosus, there may be severe right-to-left shunting, further aggravating tissue hypoxia.

Assessment findings may include

- Little to severe distress present from birth
- Dyspnea and cyanosis unresponsive to ventilations
- Small, flat (scaphoid) abdomen
- Bowel sounds in the chest
- Heart sounds displaced to the right

As soon as you suspect a diaphragmatic hernia, position the infant with her head and thorax higher than the abdomen and feet (Figure 41-14). This will help facilitate the downward displacement of the abdominal organs. Place a naso-

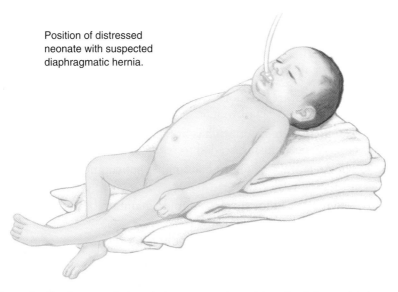

Position of distressed neonate with suspected diaphragmatic hernia.

FIGURE 41-14   If a diaphragmatic hernia is suspected, position the infant with her head and thorax higher than the abdomen and feet to facilitate downward displacement of abdominal organs.

gastric or orogastric tube, and apply low, intermittent suctioning. This will decrease the entrapment of air and fluid within the herniated viscera and will lessen the degree of ventilatory compromise. DO NOT use bag-valve-mask ventilation, which can worsen this condition by causing gastric distention. If necessary, cautiously administer positive-pressure ventilation through an endotracheal tube.

This condition usually requires surgical repair. Explain the possible need for surgery to parents, assuring them that their newborn child will be transported quickly to the facility best able to handle this procedure.

If you suspect a diaphragmatic hernia, DO NOT use bag-valve-mask ventilation, which can worsen the condition by causing gastric distention.

BRADYCARDIA

Bradycardia in the newborn is most commonly caused by hypoxia. However, it may also be due to several other factors, including increased intracranial pressure, hypothyroidism, or acidosis.

In cases of hypoxia, the infant experiences minimal risk if the hypoxia is corrected quickly. In providing treatment, follow the procedures in the inverted pyramid, as discussed earlier. Check for secretions in the airway, check tongue and soft tissue positioning, and check for possible foreign body obstruction. Resist the inclination to treat the bradycardia with pharmacological measures alone. While epinephrine may be necessary, in all likelihood, you will be able to correct the problem with suctioning, positioning, administration of oxygen (blow-by or bag-valve mask), or tracheal intubation. Throughout treatment, keep the newborn warm, and transport to the nearest facility.

Resist the temptation to treat bradycardia in a newborn with pharmacological measures alone.

PREMATURE INFANTS

A premature newborn is an infant born prior to 37 weeks of gestation or with weight ranging from 0.6 to 2.2 kg. Healthy premature infants weighing more than 1700 g have a survivability and outcome approximately that of full-term infants. The mortality rate decreases weekly as the gestational age surpasses the age of fetal viability. With the technology currently available, fetal viability is considered to be 23–24 weeks of gestation.

Premature newborns are at greater risk of respiratory depression, head or brain injury caused by hypoxemia, changes in blood pressure, intraventricular hemorrhage, and fluctuations in serum osmolarity. They are also more susceptible to hypothermia than are full-term newborns. Reasons premature newborns lose heat more readily include the following:

- The premature newborn has a relatively large body surface area and comparatively small weight.
- The premature newborn has not sufficiently developed the various control mechanisms needed to regulate body temperature.
- The premature newborn has smaller subcutaneous stores of insulating fat.
- Newborns cannot shiver and must maintain body temperature through other mechanisms.

The degree of immaturity determines the physical characteristics of a premature newborn (Figure 41-15). Premature newborns often appear to have a larger head relative to body size. They may have large trunks and short extremities, transparent skin, and few wrinkles.

Prematurity should not be a factor in short-term treatment. Resuscitation should be attempted if there is any sign of life.

Prematurity should not be a factor in short-term treatment. Resuscitation should be attempted if there is any sign of life, and the measures of resuscitation should be the same as those for newborns of normal weight and maturity. Maintain a patent airway, and avoid potential aspiration of gastric contents. Medical direction may advise administration of epinephrine. Throughout treatment, maintain the newborn's body temperature, and transport to a facility with special services for low-birth-weight newborns.

RESPIRATORY DISTRESS/CYANOSIS

Prematurity is the single most common factor causing respiratory distress and cyanosis in the newborn. The problem occurs most frequently in infants less than 1200 g and 30 weeks of gestation. Premature infants have an immature central respiratory control centre and are easily affected by environmental or metabolic changes. Multiple gestations or prenatal maternal complications may also increase the risk of respiratory distress and cyanosis.

The severely ill newborn with respiratory distress and cyanosis presents a difficult diagnostic challenge. There may be many contributing factors, including lung or heart disease, central nervous system disorders, meconium aspira-

FIGURE 41-15 The premature newborn.

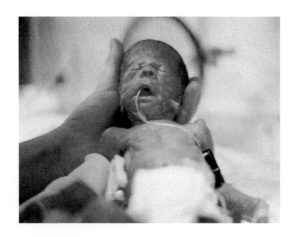

tion, metabolic problems, obstruction of the nasal passages, shock and sepsis, diaphragmatic hernia, and more. Assessment findings include

- Tachypnea
- Paradoxical breathing
- Intercostal retractions
- Nasal flaring
- Expiratory grunt

Follow the inverted pyramid of treatment, paying particular attention to airway and ventilation. Suction as needed, and provide a high concentration of oxygen. Ventilate as needed with a BVM. If prolonged ventilation will be required, consider placing an endotracheal tube. Perform chest compressions if indicated. Sodium bicarbonate may be helpful for prolonged resuscitation. Consider dextrose ($D_{10}W$ or $D_{25}W$) solution if the newborn is hypoglycemic. Maintain body temperature, and transport. Be sure to keep the parents informed and provide needed psychological support.

HYPOVOLEMIA

Hypovolemia is the leading cause of shock in newborns. It may result from dehydration, hemorrhage, or third-spacing of fluids. Dehydration is by far the most common cause. Signs of hypovolemia include

- Pale colour
- Cool skin
- Diminished peripheral pulses
- Delayed capillary refill, despite normal ambient temperature
- Mental status changes
- Diminished urination (oliguria)

When you observe these signs, administer a fluid bolus, and assess the infant's response. If signs of shock continue, administer a second bolus. Additional boluses should be infused as indicated by repeated assessments. A hypovolemic infant may often need 40 to 60 mL/kg of fluid during the first hour of resuscitation.

Fluid bolus resuscitation consists of 20 mL/kg of an isotonic crystalloid solution, such as Ringer's Lactate or normal saline. Administer the bolus over 5–10 minutes as soon as intravascular or intraosseous access is obtained. Do not use solutions containing dextrose, as they can produce hypokalemia or worsen ischemic brain injury.

In treating hypovolemia in a newborn, do not use solutions containing dextrose, as they can produce hypokalemia or worsen ischemic brain injury.

SEIZURES

Although seizures occur in a very small percentage of all newborns, they usually indicate a serious underlying abnormality and represent a medical emergency. Prolonged and frequent multiple seizures may result in metabolic changes and cardiopulmonary difficulties.

Neonatal seizures differ from seizures in a child or an adult because generalized tonic-clonic convulsions normally do not occur during the first month of life. Seizures in neonates include

- *Subtle seizures.* These seizures consist of chewing motions, excessive salivation, blinking, sucking, swimming movements of the arms, pedalling movements of the legs, apnea, and changes in colour.
- *Tonic seizures.* These seizures are characterized by rigid posturing of the extremities and trunk. They are sometimes associated with fixed

deviation of the eyes. They occur more commonly in premature infants, especially those with an intraventricular hemorrhage.

- *Focal clonic seizures.* These seizures consist of rhythmic twitching of muscle groups, particularly in the extremities and face. They may occur in both full-term and premature infants.
- *Multifocal seizures.* These seizures are similar to focal clonic seizures, except that multiple muscle groups are involved. Clonic activity randomly migrates. These seizures occur primarily in full-term newborns.
- *Myoclonic seizures.* These seizures involve brief focal or generalized jerks of the extremities or parts of the body that tend to involve distal muscle groups. They may occur singly or in a series of repetitive jerks.

Causes of neonatal seizures include sepsis, fever, hypoglycemia, hypoxic-ischemic encephalopathy, metabolic disturbances, meningitis, developmental abnormalities, or drug withdrawal. Assessment findings include a decreased level of consciousness and seizure activities, such as those described above. Treatment focuses on airway management and oxygen saturation. With medical direction, consider administration of an anticonvulsant. You might also administer a benzodiazepine (usually lorazepam) for status epilepticus or dextrose ($D_{10}W$ or $D_{25}W$) for hypoglycemia. As with all distressed newborns, maintain body temperature and transport rapidly.

FEVER

Average normal temperature in a newborn is 37.5°C. A rectal temperature of 38.0°C or higher is considered fever. Neonates do not develop fever as readily as older children do. Thus, any fever in a neonate requires extensive evaluation because it may be caused by life-threatening conditions, such as pneumonia, sepsis, or meningitis. Fever may be the only sign of meningitis in a neonate. Because of their immature development, they do not develop the classic symptoms, such as a stiff neck. Thus, any neonate with a fever should be considered to have meningitis until proven otherwise.

In assessing a neonate with fever, remember that infants have a limited ability to control their body temperature. As a result, fever can be a serious problem. Assessment findings will probably include the following:

- Mental status changes (irritability/somnolence)
- Decreased feeding
- Skin warm to the touch
- Rashes or *petechia* (small, purplish, hemorrhagic spots on the skin)

Term infants may produce beads of sweat on their brow but not on the rest of their body. Premature infants will have no visible sweat at all.

Treatment of a neonate with fever will, for the most part, be limited to ensuring a patent airway and adequate ventilation. Do not use cold packs, which may drop the temperature too quickly and may also cause seizures. If the newborn becomes bradycardic, provide chest compressions. In the prehospital setting, administration of an antipyretic agent to a neonate is of questionable benefit and should be avoided. Select the appropriate treatment facility, and explain the need for transport to the parents or caregivers.

HYPOTHERMIA

As previously noted, hypothermia presents a common and life-threatening condition for newborns. Adults sometimes fail to realize that a newborn may die because of exposure to temperatures that adults find comfortable. The increased

Any neonate with a fever should be considered to have meningitis until proven otherwise.

In assessing a neonate with fever, remember that infants have a limited ability to control their body temperature. As a result, fever can be a serious condition.

surface-to-volume relationship in newborns makes them extremely sensitive to environmental temperatures, especially right after delivery when they are wet. As a result, it is important to control the four methods of heat loss—evaporation, conduction, convection, and radiation.

In treating hypothermia—a body temperature below 35°C—keep in mind that it can also be an indicator of sepsis in the newborn. Regardless of the cause, the increased metabolic demands created by hypothermia can produce a variety of related conditions, including metabolic acidosis, pulmonary hypertension, and hypoxemia.

In assessing hypothermic newborns, remember that they do not shiver. Instead, expect these findings:

- Pale colour
- Skin cool to the touch, particularly in the extremities
- **Acrocyanosis**
- Respiratory distress
- Possible apnea
- Bradycardia
- Central cyanosis
- Initial irritability
- Lethargy in later stages

✱ **acrocyanosis** cyanosis of the extremities.

Management focuses on ensuring adequate ventilations and oxygenation. Chest compressions may be performed, if necessary. With medical direction, you might administer warm fluids through an IV fluid heater. Do not microwave fluids, as there can be a great variation in fluid temperature. Dextrose ($D_{10}W$ or $D_{25}W$) may also be given if the newborn is hypoglycemic. Above all, the newborn must be kept warm. Set the ambulance temperature at 24–26°C. Also, remember to warm your hands before touching the newborn. Select the appropriate receiving facility, and transport rapidly.

Remember to warm your hands before touching a neonate.

HYPOGLYCEMIA

Newborns are the only age group that can develop severe hypoglycemia and not have diabetes mellitus. Hypoglycemia may be due to inadequate glucose intake or increased glucose utilization. Stress and other factors can also cause the blood sugar to fall, sometimes to a critical level.

Hypoglycemia is more common in premature or small-for-gestational-age (SGA) infants, the smaller twin, and newborns of a diabetic mother, as these infants often have decreased glycogen stores. Hypoglycemia can also develop due to increased glucose utilization. Causes include respiratory illnesses, hypothermia, toxemia, central nervous system (CNS) hemorrhage, asphyxia, meningitis, and sepsis. In an older infant, hypoglycemia may be due to an inadequate glucose intake or increased utilization of glucose. Infants receiving glucose infusions can develop hypoglycemia if the infusion is suddenly stopped.

Infants with hypoglycemia may be asymptomatic, or they may exhibit such symptoms as apnea, colour changes, respiratory distress, lethargy, seizures, acidosis, and poor myocardial contractility.

Persistent hypoglycemia can have catastrophic effects on the brain. The normal newborn's glycogen stores are sufficient to meet glucose requirements for only 8–12 hours. This time frame is diminished in infants with decreased glycogen stores or the presence of other problems where glucose utilization increases. As a result, you should determine the blood glucose on all sick infants. A blood glucose screening test level of less than 2.5 mmol/L indicates hypoglycemia.

Because hypoglycemia can have a catastrophic effect on a neonate's brain, you should determine the blood glucose on all sick infants.

In response to hypoglycemia, the newborn's body will release counter-regulatory hormones, such as glucagon, epinephrine, cortisol, and growth hormone. These hormones help raise the blood glucose level by mobilizing glucose stores. In fact, this hormone response may cause transient symptoms of hyperglycemia that may last for several hours. However, when the infant's glucose stores are depleted, the glucose level will again fall.

In assessing hypoglycemic newborns, expect these findings:

- Twitching or seizures
- Limpness
- Lethargy
- Eye-rolling
- High-pitched cry
- Apnea
- Irregular respirations
- Possible cyanosis

Treatment begins with management of the airway and ventilations. Ensure adequate oxygenation. Perform chest compressions if indicated. With medical direction, administer dextrose ($D_{10}W$ or $D_{25}W$). Maintain a normal body temperature in the newborn, and transport to the appropriate facility.

VOMITING

Vomiting in a neonate may result from a variety of causes and rarely presents as an isolated symptom. Vomiting (a forceful ejection of stomach contents) is uncommon during the first weeks of life and may be confused with regurgitation (a simple backflow of stomach contents into the mouth, or "spitting up"). Vomiting in the neonate usually occurs because of an anatomical abnormality, such as a tracheoesophageal fistula or upper gastrointestinal obstruction. More often, it may be a symptom of some disease, such as increased intracranial pressure (ICP) or an infection. Vomitus containing dark blood often signals a life-threatening illness. Keep in mind, however, that vomiting of mucus—which may occasionally be blood streaked—in the first few hours after birth is not uncommon.

Assessment findings may include a distended stomach, signs of infection, increased ICP, or drug withdrawal. Because vomitus can be aspirated, management considerations focus on ensuring a patent airway. If you detect respiratory difficulties or obstruction of the airway, suction or clear vomitus from the airway, and ensure adequate oxygenation. Fluid administration may be needed to prevent dehydration. Also remember that as with older patients, vagal stimulation may cause bradycardia in the neonate.

After you have protected the airway, place the infant on her side, and transport to an appropriate facility. As with all other situations involving distressed neonates, advise parents or caregivers of steps taken and why.

DIARRHEA

Diarrhea in a neonate can cause severe dehydration and electrolyte imbalances. Although diarrhea may be harder to assess in neonates than in other patients, consider five to six stools per day as normal, especially in breast-fed infants.

Causes of diarrhea in a neonate include

- Bacterial or viral infection
- Gastroenteritis

- Lactose intolerance
- **Photothcrapy**
- **Neonatal abstinence syndrome (NAS)**
- **Thyrotoxicosis**
- Cystic fibrosis

In treating neonates with diarrhea, remember to take appropriate body substance isolation (BSI) precautions, just as you would do in any situation involving body fluids. Expect to find loose stools, decreased urinary output, and other signs of dehydration, such as prolonged capillary refill time, cool extremities, and listlessness or lethargy. It is often difficult for the parents to estimate the frequency of stools. In such cases, it might be better to inquire about the number of diapers used.

Management consists of maintenance of airway and ventilations, adequate oxygenation, and chest compressions if indicated. With medical direction, you might also consider fluid therapy. Explain all treatments to parents or caregivers, and transport the neonate to a facility able to handle high-risk infants.

COMMON BIRTH INJURIES

A **birth injury** occurs in an estimated 2–7 of every 1000 live births in Canada. About 3 of every 100 000 infants die of birth trauma. Risk factors for birth injury include

- Prematurity
- Postmaturity
- Cephalopelvic disproportion
- Prolonged labour
- Breech presentation
- Explosive delivery
- Diabetic mother

Birth injuries take various forms. Cranial injuries may include moulding of the head and overriding of the parietal bones, erythema (reddening of the skin), abrasions, ecchymosis (black-and-blue discoloration) and subcutaneous fat necrosis, subconjunctival and retinal hemorrhage, subperiosteal hemorrhage, and fracture of the skull. Intracranial hemorrhage may result from trauma or asphyxia. Often, the infant will develop a large scalp hematoma during the birth process. This injury, called *caput succedaneum,* will usually resolve over a week's time. There may be damage to the spine and spinal cord from strong traction exerted when the spine is hyperextended or when there is a lateral pull. Other birth injuries include peripheral nerve injury, injury to the liver, rupture of the spleen, adrenal hemorrhage, fractures of the clavicle or extremities, and, of course, hypoxia-ischemia.

Assessment findings may include

- Diffuse, sometimes ecchymotic, edematous swelling of soft tissues around the scalp
- Paralysis below the level of the spinal cord injury
- Paralysis of the upper arm with or without paralysis of the forearm
- Diaphragmatic paralysis
- Movement on only one side of the face when crying
- Inability to move the arm freely on the side of the fractured clavicle

✱ **phototherapy** exposure to sunlight or artificial light for therapeutic purposes. In newborns, light is used to treat hyperbilirubinemia or jaundice.

✱ **neonatal abstinence syndrome (NAS)** a generalized disorder presenting a clinical picture of CNS hyperirritability, gastrointestinal dysfunction, respiratory distress, and vague autonomic symptoms. It may be due to intrauterine exposure to heroin, methadone, or other less potent opiates. Nonopiate CNS depressants may also cause NAS.

✱ **thyrotoxicosis** toxic condition characterized by tachycardia, nervous symptoms, and rapid metabolism due to hyperactivity of the thyroid gland.

In treating a neonate with diarrhea, remember to take appropriate BSI precautions.

✱ **birth injury** avoidable and unavoidable mechanical and anoxic trauma incurred by the newborn during labour and delivery.

- Lack of spontaneous movement of the affected extremity
- Hypoxia
- Shock

Management of a newborn, especially one with birth injuries, usually centres on protection of the airway, provision of adequate ventilation and oxygen, and, if needed, chest compressions. With medical direction, you may administer medications or take other nonpharmacological steps to support the specific injury. Newborns with birth injuries usually require treatment at specialized facilities. As in the management of other neonatal emergencies, provide professional and compassionate communication to parents or caregivers.

CARDIAC RESUSCITATION, POST RESUSCITATION, AND STABILIZATION

The incidence of neonatal cardiac arrest is related primarily to hypoxia. As previously explained, the outcome will be poor unless you immediately initiate appropriate interventions. As you might expect, cases involving cardiac arrest have an increased chance of brain and organ damage. Risk factors for cardiac arrest in newborns include

- Bradycardia
- Intrauterine asphyxia
- Prematurity
- Drugs administered to or taken by the mother
- Congenital neuromuscular diseases
- Congenital malformations
- Intrapartum hypoxemia

Cardiac arrest can be caused by primary or secondary apnea, bradycardia, persistent fetal circulation, or pulmonary hypertension. Assessment findings may include peripheral cyanosis, inadequate respiratory effort, and ineffective or absent heart rate.

In managing neonatal cardiac arrest, follow the inverted pyramid for resuscitation. Administer drugs or fluids according to medical direction. Maintain normal body temperature while transporting the distressed newborn to the appropriate facility. This situation will require delicate handling of the parents or caregivers. Explain what is being done for the infant, without discussing the possibilities of survival.

SUMMARY

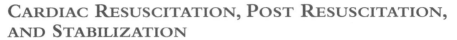

After a woman gives birth, you are caring for two patients—the mother and her newborn child. The newborn has several special needs, the most important of which are protection of the airway and support of ventilations. The newborn must be kept warm at all times. If assessment reveals a distressed newborn, you should initiate ventilatory support, stimulation, and, if required, CPR. If possible, newborns should be transported to a facility with an NICU. Maintain communications with family members or caregivers, explaining all procedures performed on the newborn.

CHAPTER 42

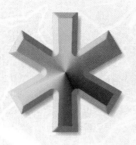

Pediatrics

Objectives

After reading this chapter, you should be able to:

1. Discuss the paramedic's role in the reduction of infant and childhood morbidity and mortality from acute illness and injury. (pp. 939–940)

2. Identify methods/mechanisms that prevent injuries to infants and children. (pp. 939–940)

3. Identify the common family responses to acute illness and injury of an infant or child. (pp. 941–942)

4. Describe techniques for successful inter-action with families of acutely ill or injured infants and children. (pp. 941–942)

5. Identify key anatomical, physiological, growth, and developmental characteristics of infants and children and their implications. (pp. 942–945)

6. Outline differences in adult and childhood anatomy, physiology, and "normal" age-group-related vital signs. (pp. 945–949, 953)

7. Describe techniques for successful assessment and treatment of infants and children. (pp. 950–959)

8. Discuss the appropriate equipment used to obtain pediatric vital signs. (pp. 957–959)

9. Determine appropriate airway adjuncts, ventilation devices, and endotracheal intubation equipment; their proper

Continued

Objectives Continued

use; and complications of use for infants and children. (pp. 961–964)

10. List the indications and methods of gastric decompression for infants and children. (pp. 969–970, 971)

11. Define pediatric respiratory distress, failure, and arrest. (pp. 977–978)

12. Differentiate between upper-airway obstruction and lower-airway disease. (pp. 979–986)

13. Describe the general approach to the treatment of children with respiratory distress, failure, or arrest from upper-airway obstruction or lower-airway disease. (pp. 979–986)

14. Discuss the common causes and relative severity of hypoperfusion in infants and children. (pp. 986–987)

15. Identify the major classifications of pediatric cardiac rhythms. (pp. 991–994)

16. Discuss the primary etiologies of cardiopulmonary arrest in infants and children. (pp. 977–978, 986)

17. Discuss age-appropriate sites, equipment, techniques, and complications of vascular access for infants and children. (pp. 970, 972–973)

18. Describe the primary etiologies of altered level of consciousness in infants and children. (pp. 976–1003, 1008, 1019)

19. Identify common lethal mechanisms of injury in infants and children. (pp. 1003–1005)

20. Discuss anatomical features of children that predispose them to or protect them from certain injuries. (pp. 1009–1011)

21. Describe aspects of infant and child airway management that are affected by potential cervical spine injury. (pp. 975, 1006)

22. Identify infant and child trauma patients who require spinal immobilization. (pp. 1006–1007)

23. Discuss fluid management and shock treatment for infant and child trauma patients. (pp. 987–990, 1007)

24. Determine when pain management and sedation are appropriate for infants and children. (p. 1008)

25. Define child abuse, child neglect, and sudden infant death syndrome (SIDS). (pp. 1012–1016, 1011)

26. Discuss the parent/caregiver responses to the death of an infant or child. (p. 1012)

27. Define children with special health-care needs and technology-assisted children. (pp. 1016–1020)

28. Discuss basic cardiac life support (CPR) guidelines for infants and children. (pp. 959–964)

29. Integrate advanced life support skills with basic cardiac life support for infants and children. (pp. 964–975, 991–994)

30. Discuss the indications, dosage, route of administration, and special considerations for medication administration in infants and children. (pp. 973–975)

31. Discuss appropriate transport guidelines for low- and high-risk infants and children. (pp. 955, 975–976)

32. Describe the epidemiology, including the incidence, morbidity/mortality, risk factors, prevention strategies, pathophysiology, assessment, and treatment of infants and children with
   a. Respiratory distress/failure (pp. 977–978)
   b. Hypoperfusion (pp. 986–990)
   c. Cardiac dysrhythmias (pp. 991–994)
   d. Neurological emergencies (pp. 994, 996–997)
   e. Trauma (pp. 1003–1011)
   f. Abuse and neglect (pp. 1012–1016)
   g. Special health-care needs, including technology-assisted children (pp. 1016–1020)
   h. SIDS (pp. 1011–1012)

33. Given several preprogrammed simulated pediatric patients, provide the appropriate assessment, treatment, and transport. (pp. 939–1020)

INTRODUCTION

The ill or injured child presents special concerns for prehospital personnel. The leading causes of death are age specific. They include motor-vehicle collisions, burns, drownings, suicides, and homicides. These alarming facts become even more troublesome when experts theorize that many of them could have been prevented by early intervention. Tragedies involving children—neonates to adolescents—account for some of the most stressful incidents that you will encounter in EMS practice.

Treatment of pediatric patients presents a number of challenges for the paramedic. Children, especially young ones, often cannot describe what is bothering them or what has happened to them. In addition to the child patient, you must deal with the parents or caregivers. Finally, a child's size often makes routine procedures more difficult. Keep in mind that children are not simply small adults. They have special considerations and needs. This chapter will present the topic of pediatric emergencies as it applies to advanced prehospital care.

ROLE OF PARAMEDICS IN PEDIATRIC CARE

When considering the reduction of pediatric morbidity and mortality, your role as a paramedic centres on two key concepts. First, you must realize that pediatric injuries have become a major health concern. Second, you should remember that children are at a higher risk of injury than are adults and that they are more likely to be adversely affected by the injuries that they suffer.

Numerous factors account for the high pediatric injury rates. Some factors, such as geography and weather, cannot be altered. However, other factors, particularly dangers within the home and community, can be eliminated or minimized. As health-care professionals, we must all get involved in identifying and implementing methods and mechanisms that prevent injuries to infants and children. Those of us who deliver prehospital care must do more than simply enter the picture after an injury has taken place.

In addition to pediatric injuries, paramedics are often responsible for treating the ill child. There are many aspects of disease and disease processes that are unique to children. It is important that the paramedic be familiar with these, as early intervention is often the key to reduced morbidity and mortality.

CONTINUING EDUCATION AND TRAINING

Your role in improving the health care offered to pediatric patients begins with your own training. Because you will encounter pediatric patients less frequently than adult patients, you have a professional responsibility to maintain and improve on your pediatric knowledge, particularly your clinical skills. Continuing education programs include

- Pediatric Advanced Life Support (PALS)
- Pediatric Basic Trauma Life Support (PBTLS)
- Advanced Pediatric Life Support (APLS)

In addition to these programs, you can also attend regional conferences and seminars designed to increase your knowledge of pediatric care. These are often conducted by regional children's hospitals. You can further enhance your clinical skills by spending time in pediatric emergency departments, pediatric hospitals, or pediatric departments in local hospitals.

For self-study, you can choose among many excellent pediatric textbooks currently available or read articles on pediatric care in the various EMS journals. Many good pediatric educational sites are available on the Internet.

As prehospital care providers, we see the consequences of pediatric trauma all too often. You can help reduce the rate of injury by taking advantage of opportunities to share "teaching points" in your daily life, both personally and professionally. Take part in, or offer to organize, school or community programs in injury prevention or health care. Engage student interest in the EMS profession by volunteering to speak at "career days," emphasizing those aspects of your job that relate to young people. Use nonurgent ambulance calls as an opportunity to educate family members or caregivers on the importance of "childproofing" a home or neighbourhood or inspecting childcare seats in vehicles. Work with appropriate agencies in initiating or conducting safety inspections, block watches, and more.

There has been an increased effort to identify the severity and nature of prehospital pediatric emergencies. Many regions now have both pediatric and trauma registries. These, in addition to standard epidemiological research conducted by local health departments, are dependent on quality prehospital documentation. If your area is participating in a registry program or research study, be sure to obtain and record all required data. Information gained from these registries will help identify the need for more or specialized resources.

GENERAL APPROACH TO PEDIATRIC EMERGENCIES

The approach to the pediatric patient varies with the age of the patient and with the problem being treated. Foremost in approaching any pediatric emergency is consideration of the patient's emotional and physiological development. Care also involves the family members or caregivers responsible for the child. They will demand information, express fears, and, ultimately, give or refuse consent for treatment and/or transport.

COMMUNICATION AND PSYCHOLOGICAL SUPPORT

Treatment of an infant, child, or teenager begins with communication and psychological support.

Treatment of an infant, child, or teenager begins with communication and psychological support. Interaction with pediatric patients and related adults continues throughout assessment and management. When obtaining the medical history of the pediatric patient, you should gather information as quickly and as accurately as possible. The parents and caregivers are often the primary source of information, especially in the case of infants. However, as children become older, they can also be a good source of information. Older children, for example, can often give accurate descriptions of symptoms or other details. Treat pediatric patients with respect, allowing them to express opinions and ask questions. Your listening skills will play an important role in alleviating the fears of child patients. You can communicate a calm and caring attitude even to infants, who respond to touch and voice just like any other human being does.

Responding to Patient Needs

As previously mentioned, a child's response to an emergency will vary, depending on the age and emotional maturity of the child. The child's most common response to illness or injury is fear. Common fears of children include

- Fear of being separated from the parents or caregivers
- Fear of being removed from a family place, such as the home, and never returning

- Fear of being hurt
- Fear of being mutilated or disfigured
- Fear of the unknown

These fears may be intensified if the child detects fear or anxiety from the parents or caregivers. The general chaos and panic that often surround pediatric emergency situations may further distress the child.

Remember that children have the right to know what is being done to them. You should be as honest as possible with them. If a procedure, such as an IV needle stick, will hurt, tell them so. Tell them immediately before performing a procedure. Do not say that a procedure will be painful and then take five minutes to prepare the equipment, allowing time for the child's anticipation of pain to build.

Always use language that is appropriate for the age of the child. Medical and anatomical terms that we routinely use may be completely foreign to children. Telling a child that you are going to "apply a cervical collar" means nothing. Instead, tell the child: "I'm going to put this collar around your neck to keep it from moving." "Try to hold your head still." "Tell me if the collar is too tight." This will involve children in their own care and reduce their feelings of helplessness.

> *Remember that children have the right to know what is being done to them. Be as honest as possible.*
>

Responding to Parents or Caregivers

As you might expect, the reaction of parents or caregivers to a pediatric emergency will vary. Initial reactions might include shock, grief, denial, anger, guilt, fear, or complete loss of control. Their behaviour may change during the course of the emergency. Communication is the key. Preferably only one paramedic will speak with adults at the scene. This will avoid any chance of conflicting information and allow a second paramedic to focus on the child. If parents or caregivers sense your confidence and professionalism, they will regain control and trust your suggestions for care. As with the child, most parents and caregivers feel overwhelmed by fear. They often express their fears in such questions as the following:

"Is my child going to die?"
"Did my child suffer brain damage?"
"Is my child going to be all right?"
"What are you doing to my child?"
"Will my child be able to walk?"

It may be difficult to answer these questions in the prehospital setting. However, the following actions may help allay parents' fears:

- Tell them your name and qualifications.
- Acknowledge their fears and concerns.
- Reassure them that it is all right to feel the way they do.
- Redirect their energies toward helping you care for the child.
- Remain calm and appear in control of the emergency.
- Keep the parents or caregivers informed as to what you are doing.
- Don't "talk down" to them.
- Assure them that everything possible is being done for their child.

If conditions permit, you should allow one of the parents or caregivers to remain with the child at all times. Some family members may be extremely emotional in emergency situations. The child will react more positively to a family member who appears calm and reassuring. If a parent or caregiver is "out of control," have another person take him away from the immediate area to settle down. Maintain a reasonable level of suspicion if a child shows a pattern of injuries, some old and some new. In such cases, the parent or caregiver may try to cover up what may be an abusive situation. They may also try to block any examination and treatment. (There will be more on potential abuse or neglect later in this chapter.)

GROWTH AND DEVELOPMENT

Children progress through developmental stages on their way to adulthood. You should tailor your approach to the developmental level of your pediatric patient.

Newborns (First Hours after Birth)

Although the terms "newborn" and "neonate" are often used interchangeably, "newborn" refers to a baby in the first hours of extrauterine life. The term "neonate" describes infants from birth to one month of age. The method most frequently used to assess newborns is the *APGAR scoring system*, which was described in Chapter 40. Resuscitation of the newborn generally follows the inverted pyramid described in Chapter 41 and the guidelines established in the Neonatal Advanced Life Support (NALS) curriculum.

Neonates (Ages Birth–1 Month)

The neonate, as noted above (and described in Chapter 41), is an infant up to one month of age. This is a major stage of development. Soon after birth, the neonate typically loses up to 10 percent of his birth weight as he adjusts to extrauterine life. This lost weight, however, is ordinarily recovered within 10 days. Gestational age affects early growth. Children born at term (40 weeks) should follow accepted developmental guidelines. Infants born prematurely will not be as developed, either neurologically or physically, as their term counterparts.

The neonatal stage of development centres on reflexes. The neonate's personality also begins to form. The infant is close to the mother and may stare at faces and smile. The mother, and occasionally the father, can comfort and quiet the child. Obviously, the history must be obtained from the parents or caregivers. However, it is also important to observe the child. Common illnesses in this age group include jaundice, vomiting, and respiratory distress. Serious illnesses, such as meningitis, are difficult to distinguish from minor illnesses in neonates. Often, fever is the only sign, although the majority of neonates with fever have minor illnesses (96–97 percent). The few that are seriously ill can be easily missed. For this reason, any fever in a neonate requires extensive evaluation.

The approach to this age group should include several factors. First, the child should always be kept warm. Observe skin colour, tone, and respiratory activity. The absence of tears when crying may indicate dehydration. The lungs should be auscultated early during the assessment, while the infant is quiet. You might find it helpful to have the child suck on a pacifier during the assessment. Allowing the infant to remain in a parent's or caregiver's lap may help keep the child calm.

Infants (Ages 1–5 Months)

Infants should have doubled their birth weight by 5–6 months of age. They should be able to follow the movements of others with their eyes. Muscle control develops in a cephalocaudal progression. This means, literally, that development of muscular control begins at the head (cephalo) and moves toward the tail (caudal). Muscular control also spreads from the trunk toward the extremities during this period. The infant's personality at this stage still centres closely on the parents or caregivers. The history must be obtained from these individuals, with close attention to possible illnesses and accidents, including sudden infant death syndrome (SIDS), vomiting, dehydration, meningitis, child abuse, and household accidents.

Concentrate on keeping these patients warm and comfortable. Allow the infant to remain in the parent's or caregiver's lap. A pacifier or bottle can be used to help keep the baby quiet during the assessment.

Infants (Ages 6–12 Months)

Infants in this age group may stand or even walk with assistance. They are quite active and enjoy exploring the world with their mouths. In this stage of development, the risk of **foreign body airway obstruction (FBAO)** becomes a serious concern.

Infants six months and older have more fully formed personalities and express themselves more readily. They have considerable anxiety toward strangers. They do not like lying on their backs. Children in this age group tend to cling to the mother, though the father "will do" in many cases. Common illnesses and accidents include febrile seizures, vomiting, diarrhea, dehydration, bronchiolitis, car accidents, croup, child abuse, poisonings, falls, airway obstructions, and meningitis.

These children should be assessed while sitting in the lap of the parent or caregiver (Figure 42–1). The assessment should progress in a toe-to-head order, since starting at the face may upset the child. If time and conditions permit, allow the child to become familiar with you before beginning the assessment.

✱ **foreign body airway obstruction (FBAO)** blockage or obstruction of the airway by an object that impairs respiration; in the case of pediatric patients, tongues, abundant secretions, and deciduous (baby) teeth are most likely to block airways.

Examine infants and toddlers in a toe-to-head order.

Toddlers (Ages 1–3 Years)

Great strides occur in gross motor development during this stage. Children tend to run underneath or stand on almost everything. They seem to always be on the move. As they grow older, toddlers become braver and more curious or stubborn. They begin to stray away from the parents or caregivers more frequently. Yet these remain the only people who can comfort them quickly, and most children will cling to a parent or caregiver if frightened.

At ages 1–3 years, language development begins. Often, children can understand better than they can speak. Therefore, the majority of the medical history will still come from the parents or caregivers. Remember, however, that you can ask toddlers simple and specific questions.

Accidents of all types are the leading cause of injury deaths in pediatric patients ages 1–15 years. Common accidents in this age group include motor-vehicle collisions, homicides, burn injuries, drownings, and pedestrian accidents. Common illnesses and injuries in the toddler age group include vomiting, diarrhea, febrile seizures, poisonings, falls, child abuse, croup, and meningitis. Keep in mind that FBAO is still a high risk for toddlers.

Be cautious when treating toddlers. Approach toddlers slowly, and try to gain their confidence. Conduct the assessment in a toe-to-head order. The child may be difficult to examine and may resist being touched. Speak softly, and use only simple words. Avoid asking questions to which the child can say "no." If the situation permits, allow toddlers to hold transitional objects, such as a favourite blanket or toy. Be sure to tell the child if something will hurt. If at all possible, avoid procedures on the dominant arm/hand, which the child will try to pull away.

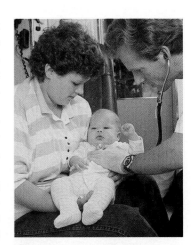

FIGURE 42-1 Infants and young children should be allowed to remain in their parent's arms.

Preschoolers (Ages 3–5 Years)

Children in this age group show a tremendous increase in fine and gross motor development. Language skills increase greatly. Children in this age group know how to talk. However, if frightened, they often refuse to speak, especially to strangers. They often have vivid imaginations and may see monsters as part of their world. Preschoolers may have tempers and will express them. During this stage of development, children fear mutilation and may feel threatened by treatment. Avoid frightening or misleading comments.

Preschoolers often run to a particular parent or caregiver, depending on the occasion. They stick up for the people they love and are openly affectionate. They still seek support and comfort from within the home.

When evaluating children in this age group, question the child first, keeping in mind that imagination may interfere with the facts. The child often has a distorted sense of time, and therefore you must rely on the parents or caregivers to fill in the gaps. Common illnesses and accidents in this age group include croup, asthma, poisonings, auto accidents, burns, child abuse, ingestion of foreign bodies, drownings, epiglottitis, febrile seizures, and meningitis.

Treatment of preschoolers requires tact. Avoid baby talk. If time and situation permit, give the child health-care choices. Often, the use of a doll or stuffed animal will ease the assessment. Allow the child to hold a piece of equipment, such as a stethoscope, and to use it. Let the child sit on your lap. Start the assessment with the chest, and evaluate the head last. Avoid misleading comments. Do not trick or lie to the child, and always explain what you are going to do.

Do not trick or lie to the child, and always explain what you are going to do.

School-Aged Children (Ages 6–12 Years)

Children in this age group are active and carefree. Growth spurts sometimes lead to clumsiness. The personality continues to develop. School-aged children are protective and proud of their parents or caregivers and seek their attention. They value peers but also need home support.

When examining school-aged children, give them the responsibility of providing the history. However, remember that children may be reluctant to provide information if they sustained an injury while doing something forbidden. The parents or caregivers can fill in the pertinent details. When assessing children in this age group, it is important to respect their modesty. Be honest and tell the child what is wrong. A small toy may help to calm the child (Figure 42-2). Common illnesses and injuries for this age group include drownings, auto collisions, bicycle accidents, falls, fractures, sports injuries, child abuse, and burns.

Adolescents (Ages 13–18 Years)

Adolescence covers the period from the end of childhood to the start of adulthood (age 18). It begins with puberty, roughly age 13 for male children and age 11 for female children. (For this reason, adolescence is often defined as including ages 11 to 18, rather than 13 to 18.) Puberty is highly child specific and can begin at various ages. A female child, for example, may experience her first menstrual period as early as age 7 or 8.

Adolescents vary significantly in their development. Those over age 15 are physically nearer to adults in terms of their vital signs but emotionally may still be children. Regardless of physical maturity, remember that teenagers as a group are "body conscious." They worry about their physical image more than any other pediatric age group. You should tactfully address their stated concerns about body integrity or disfigurement. The slightest possibility of a lasting scar may be a tremendous issue to the adolescent patient.

Although patients in this age are not yet legally adults, most consider themselves to be grown up. They take offence at the use of the word "child." They have a strong desire to be liked by their peers and to be included. Relationships with parents and caregivers may at times be strained as the adolescent demands greater independence. They value the opinions of other adolescents, especially members of the opposite sex. Generally, these patients make good historians. Do

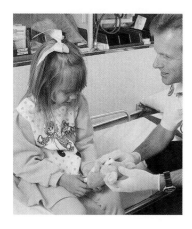

FIGURE 42-2 A small toy may calm a child in the 6–10-year age range.

not be surprised, however, if their perception of events differs from that of their parents or caregivers.

Common illnesses and injuries in this age group include mononucleosis, asthma, auto collisions, sports injuries, drug and alcohol problems, suicide gestures, sexual abuse. Remember that pregnancy is also possible in female adolescents. When assessing teenagers, remember that vital signs will approach those of adults. In gathering a history, be factual, and address the patient's questions. It may be wise to interview the patient away from the parents or caregivers. Listen to what the teenager is saying, as well as what he is *not* saying. If you suspect substance abuse or endangerment of the patient or others, approach the subject with tact and compassion. If you must perform a detailed secondary assessment, respect the teenager's sense of privacy. If the patient is shy or has a poor body image, have a paramedic of the same sex as the teenager conduct the assessment, if possible. Regardless of the situation, provide psychological support and reassurance.

It may be wise to interview the adolescent patient away from the parents or caregivers.

ANATOMY AND PHYSIOLOGY

The differences between the anatomy and physiology of infants and children and that of adults form the basis for the differences in the emergency medical care offered to the two groups (Table 42-1). As previously mentioned, children are not

Table 42-1 ANATOMICAL AND PHYSIOLOGICAL CHARACTERISTICS OF INFANTS AND CHILDREN

Differences in Infants and Children as Compared with Adults	Potential Effects That May Impact Assessment and Care
Tongue proportionately larger	More likely to block airway
Smaller airway structures	More easily blocked
Abundant secretions	Can block the airway
Deciduous (baby) teeth	Easily dislodged; can block the airway
Flat nose and face	Difficult to obtain good face mask seal
Head heavier relative to body and less developed neck structures and muscles	Head may be propelled more forcefully than body producing a higher incidence of head injury in trauma
Fontanelle and open sutures (soft spots) palpable on top of young infant's head	Bulging fontanelle can be a sign of increased intracranial pressure (but may be normal if infant is crying); shrunken fontanelle may indicate dehydration
Thinner, softer brain tissue	Susceptible to serious brain injury
Head larger in proportion to body	Tips forward when supine; possible flexion of neck, which makes neutral alignment of airway difficult
Shorter, narrower, more elastic (flexible) trachea	Can close off trachea with hyperextension of neck
Short neck	Difficult to stabilize or immobilize
Abdominal breathers	Difficult to evaluate breathing
Faster respiratory rate	Muscles easily fatigue, causing respiratory distress
Newborns breathe primarily through the nose (obligate nose breathers)	May not automatically open mouth to breathe if nose is blocked; airway more easily blocked
Larger body surface relative to body mass	Prone to hypothermia
Softer bones	More flexible, less easily fractured; traumatic forces may be transmitted to internal organs, causing injury without fracturing the ribs; lungs easily damaged with trauma
Spleen and liver more exposed	Organ injury likely with significant force to abdomen

simply small adults. They possess bodies well suited to growth. As a rule, they have healthier organs, a greater ability to compensate for most illnesses, and softer, more flexible tissues. Because you will probably have infrequent contact with pediatric patients, you need to regularly review the physical characteristics that distinguish them from the adult patients whom you encounter more often.

Head

The pediatric patient's head is proportionally larger than an adult's, and the occipital region is significantly larger. In comparison with their head size, most pediatric patients have small faces and flat noses, which makes it difficult to obtain a good face mask seal.

With infants, pay special attention to the fontanelles—areas of the skull that have not yet fused. The fontanelles allow for compression of the head during childbirth and for rapid growth of the brain during early life. The posterior fontanelle generally closes by four months of age. The anterior fontanelle diminishes after six months of age and usually closes between 9 and 18 months.

During assessment, always inspect the anterior fontanelle. Normally, it should be level with the surface of the skull or slightly sunken. It also may pulsate. With increased intracranial pressure, as with meningitis or head trauma, the fontanelle may become tight and bulging, and pulsations may diminish or disappear. In the presence of dehydration, the anterior fontanelle often falls below the level of the skull and appears sunken.

The heavy head relative to body size places an infant or a child at risk of blunt head trauma. In accidents, the head may be propelled more forcefully than the body, resulting in a higher incidence of brain injury. Head size also affects the airway positioning techniques you should use in treating pediatric patients. In general, follow these guidelines:

- In treating seriously injured patients less than three years of age, place a thin layer of padding under the back to obtain a neutral position. This will prevent the head from tipping forward when supine, causing flexion of the neck (Figure 42-3).

> *In assessing infants, pay special attention to the fontanelles, especially the anterior fontanelle.*
>

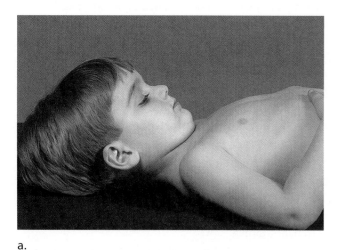
a.

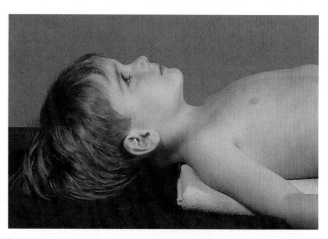
b.

FIGURE 42-3   a. In the supine position, an infant's or child's larger head tips forward, causing airway obstruction. b. Placing padding under the patient's back and shoulders will bring the airway to a neutral or slightly extended position.

- In treating medically ill children over three years of age, place a folded sheet or towel under the occiput to obtain a sniffing position (neck flexed slightly forward, head extended slightly backward to align pharynx and trachea).

Airway

In managing the airway of an infant or child, keep in mind these anatomical and physiological considerations:

- Pediatric patients have narrower airways at all levels and these are more easily blocked by secretions or obstructions.
- Infants are obligate nose breathers. If their noses are blocked by secretions, for example, they may not automatically "know" to open their mouths to breathe.
- The tongue takes up more space proportionately in a child's mouth and can more easily obstruct breathing in an unconscious patient.
- The trachea is softer and more flexible in a child and can collapse if the neck and head are hyperextended.
- A child's larynx is higher (C-3 to C-4) and extends into the pharynx.
- In young children, the cricoid ring is the narrowest part of the airway.
- Infants have an omega-shaped (horseshoe-shaped) epiglottis that extends at a 45-degree angle into the airway. Because epiglottic folds in pediatric patients have softer cartilage than in adults, they can be more floppy, especially in infants.

Take these anatomical and physiological differences into account by following these general procedures: Always keep the nares clear in infants less than six months of age. Do not overextend the neck, which may collapse the trachea. Open the airway gently to avoid soft-tissue injury. Because any device placed in the infant's or child's airway further narrows the passage's diameter and may result in localized swelling, consider use of an oral or a nasal airway only after other manual manoeuvres have failed to keep the airway open. (There will be more information on pediatric airway management later in this chapter.)

Consider use of an oral or nasal airway in a pediatric patient only after other manual manoeuvres have failed to keep the airway open.

Chest and Lungs

In evaluating the chest and lungs of an infant or child, remember that tissues and muscles are more immature than in adults. Chest muscles tire easily, and lung tissues are more fragile. The soft, pliable ribs offer less protection to organs. Expect the ribs to be positioned horizontally and the mediastinum to be more mobile.

Take into account the following anatomical and physiological considerations when assessing the chest and lungs of a pediatric patient:

- Infants and children are diaphragmatic breathers.
- Pediatric patients, especially young infants, are prone to gastric distention.
- Although rib fractures occur less frequently in children, they are not uncommon in cases of child abuse.
- Because of the softness of a child's ribs, greater energy can be transmitted to underlying organs following trauma. As a result, significant internal injury can be present without external signs.

- Pulmonary contusions are more common in pediatric patients who have been subjected to major trauma.
- An infant's or child's lungs are more prone to pneumothorax following barotrauma.
- The mediastinum of a child or an infant will shift more with tension pneumothorax than in an adult.
- Thin chest walls in infants and children allow for easily transmitted breath sounds. This may result in perception of breath sounds from elsewhere in the chest, which may cause you to miss a pneumothorax or misplaced intubation.

Abdomen

Note that the liver and spleen, both very vascular organs, are proportionately larger in the pediatric patient than in the adult patient. Abdominal organs lie closer together. Because of the immature abdominal muscles in an infant or child, expect to find more frequent damage to the liver and spleen and more multiple organ injuries than in an adult.

Extremities

Until pediatric patients reach adolescence, they have softer and more porous bones than adults. Therefore, you should treat "sprains" and "strains" as fractures and immobilize them accordingly.

During early stages of development, injuries to the **growth plate** may also disrupt bone growth. Keep this in mind when inserting an intraosseous needle, which could mistakenly pierce the plate. (Intraosseous infusion is discussed later in this chapter.)

Skin and Body Surface Area

There are three distinguishing features of the pediatric patient's skin and body surface area (BSA). First, the skin of an infant or child is thinner than that of an adult. Second, infants and children generally have less subcutaneous fat. Finally, they have a larger BSA-to-weight ratio.

As a result of these features, children risk greater injury from extremes in temperature or thermal exposure. They lose fluids and heat more quickly than adults do and have a greater likelihood of dehydration and hypothermia. They also burn more easily and deeply than adults, explaining why burns account for one of the leading causes of death among pediatric trauma patients.

Respiratory System

Although infants and children have a tidal volume proportionately similar to that of adolescents and adults, they require double the metabolic oxygen. They also have proportionately smaller oxygen reserves. The combination of increased oxygen requirements and decreased oxygen reserves makes infants and children especially susceptible to hypoxia.

Cardiovascular System

Cardiac output is rate dependent in infants and small children. They possess vigorous, but limited, cardiovascular reserves. Although infants and children have a circulating blood volume proportionately larger than adults, their absolute

* **growth plate** the area just below the head of a long bone in which growth in bone length occurs; the epiphyseal plate.

During the early stages of development, injuries to the growth plate by an intraosseous needle may disrupt bone growth.

Infants and children increase their cardiac output by increasing their heart rate. They have a very limited capacity to increase their stroke volume.

blood volume is smaller. As a result, they can maintain blood pressure longer than an adult can but still be at risk of shock (hypoperfusion). In assessing a pediatric patient for shock, keep in mind the following points:

- A smaller absolute volume of fluid/blood loss is needed to cause shock in infants and children.
- A larger proportional volume of fluid/blood loss is needed to cause shock in these same patients.
- As with all categories of patients, hypotension is a late sign of shock. In pediatric patients, it is an ominous sign of imminent cardiopulmonary arrest.
- A child may be in shock despite a normal blood pressure.
- Shock assessment in children and infants is based on clinical signs of tissue perfusion. (See the later discussion of circulation assessment.)
- Suspect shock if tachycardia is present.
- Monitor the pediatric patient carefully for the development of hypotension.

Once again, remember that children are not small adults. Bleeding that would not be dangerous in an adult may be a serious and life-threatening condition in an infant or child. Shock can develop in the small child who has a laceration to the scalp (with its many blood vessels) or in the three-year-old who loses as little as a cup of blood. (Management of shock in pediatric patients will be discussed in detail later in the chapter.)

Bleeding that would not be dangerous in an adult may be life threatening in an infant or a child.

Nervous System

The nervous system develops continuously throughout childhood. Even so, the neural tissue remains more fragile than in adults. The skull and spinal column, which are softer and more pliable than in adults, offer less protection of the brain and spinal cord. Therefore, greater force can be transmitted to a child's neural tissue with more devastating consequences. These injuries can occur without injury to the skull or to the spinal column. (Treatment of head and neck trauma will be discussed later in the chapter.)

Metabolic Differences

You may have noticed the repeated emphasis on the need to keep neonatal and pediatric patients warm during treatment and transport. The emphasis on warming techniques is based on the following metabolic considerations:

- Infants and children have a limited store of glycogen and glucose.
- Pediatric patients are prone to hypothermia because of their greater BSA-to-weight ratio.
- Significant volume loss can result from vomiting and diarrhea.
- Newborns and neonates lack the ability to shiver.

To prevent heat loss, always cover the patient's head and maintain adequate temperature controls in the ambulance. Ensure that the ambulance is always stocked with an adequate supply of blankets and, if you live in a cold area, hot water bottles.

GENERAL APPROACH
TO PEDIATRIC ASSESSMENT

Priorities in the management of the pediatric patient, as with all patients, are established on a threat-to-life basis. If life-threatening problems are not present, you will complete each of the general steps discussed in the following sections.

BASIC CONSIDERATIONS

Many of the components of the primary patient assessment can be done during a visual assessment of the scene. (This is sometimes called the "assessment from across the room," during which you quickly note signs of an ill child, such as lethargy.) Whenever possible, involve the parent or caregiver in efforts to calm or comfort the child. Depending on the situation, you may decide to allow the parent or caregiver to remain with the child during treatment and transport. As previously mentioned, the developmental stage of the patient and the coping skills of the parents or guardians will be key factors in making this decision.

When interacting with parents or other responsible adults, keep in mind the communication techniques suggested earlier. Pay attention to the way in which parents or caregivers interact with the child. Are the interactions appropriate to the emergency? Are family members concerned? Are they angry? Are they overly emotional or entirely indifferent?

From the time of dispatch, you will continually acquire information relative to the patient's condition. As with all patients, personal safety must be your first priority. In treating pediatric patients, follow the same guidelines in approaching the scene as you would with any other patient. Observe for potentially hazardous situations, and make sure you take appropriate BSI precautions. Remember that infants and young children are at especially high risk of an infectious process.

Remember to take appropriate BSI precautions when treating infants and children.

SCENE ASSESSMENT

On arrival, conduct a quick scene assessment. Dispatch information received en route, as well as your own observations, can provide critical indicators of scene safety. Be aware of the increased anxiety and stress in any situation involving an infant or a child. Try to set aside thoughts of your own children, if you have children, and adopt the professional, systematic approach to assessment necessary for scene safety and effective patient management. If you find yourself getting angry or upset, temporarily turn over care to another paramedic until you compose yourself.

As you survey the scene, look for clues to the mechanism of injury (MOI) or the nature of the illness (NOI). These clues will help guide your assessment and determine appropriate interventions. Note the presence of dangerous substances—for example, medicine bottles, household chemicals, or poisonous plants—that the child may have ingested. Spot hazards in the environment, such as unprotected stairwells, kerosene heaters, and so on. Identify possible causes of trauma, especially in motor-vehicle collisions. Remain alert for evidence of child abuse, particularly in cases in which the injury and history do not match. As already mentioned, pay attention to the way parents or caregivers respond to the child and the way the child responds to them.

Keep the child in mind while conducting your scene assessment. Pace your approach to give the child time to adjust to your presence. Speak in a soft voice, using simple words. As soon as you reach the child, position yourself at eye level with the patient, and make every effort to win his trust. If the child bonds more readily with one member of the team than another, allow that person to remain with the child and, if possible, to conduct most of the secondary assessment.

PRIMARY ASSESSMENT

The patient's condition determines the course of your primary assessment. An active and alert child will allow for a more comfortable approach, with more time spent on communication with the child and appropriate adults. A critically ill or injured child, however, may require quick intervention and rapid transport. Your choice of action depends on your general impression of the patient.

General Impression

The major points in forming your general impression are outlined in an assessment tool called the *pediatric assessment triangle.* Many experts recommend this assessment tool as a way of quickly evaluating the level of severity and the need for immediate intervention. It is a rapid "eyes-open, hands-on" approach that allows you to detect a life-threatening situation without the use of a stethoscope, blood pressure cuff, pulse oximeter, or other medical device. The triangle's three components are:

- *Appearance*—focuses on the child's mental status and muscle tone
- *Breathing*—directs attention to respiratory rate and respiratory effort
- *Circulation*—uses skin signs and colour as well as capillary refill as indicators of the patient's circulatory status

Vital Functions

After quickly applying the pediatric assessment triangle to form a general impression, you will evaluate vital functions—mental status (level of consciousness) and the ABCs—as they apply to infants and children. Although assessment steps are basically the same as for adults, certain modifications must be made to collect accurate data.

Level of Consciousness Employ the AVPU method (*a*lert, responds to *v*erbal stimuli, responds to *p*ainful stimuli, *u*nresponsive) to evaluate the pediatric patient's level of consciousness. Adjust the techniques for the child's age. With an infant, you may need to shout to elicit a response (perhaps crying) to verbal stimulus. An infant should withdraw from a noxious stimulus. *Never shake an infant or a child.*

Airway Assess the airway using the techniques shown in Figures 42-4 to 42-7. If at any point the patient shows little or no movement of air, intervene immediately. Keep this fact in mind: *Airway and respiratory problems are the most common cause of cardiac arrest in infants and young children.*
    As you inspect the airway, ask yourself the following questions:

- Is the airway patent?
- Is the airway maintainable with head positioning, suctioning, or airway adjuncts?
- Is the airway *not* maintainable? If so, what action is required? (Airway management techniques are discussed later in this chapter.)

Breathing In assessing the breathing of a pediatric patient, recall the CPR certification courses in which you learned to "Look, Listen, and Feel." *Look* at the patient's chest and abdomen for movement. *Listen* for breath sounds—both normal and abnormal. *Feel* for air movement at the patient's mouth.
    Keep in mind that pediatric patients have small chests. For this reason, place the stethoscope near each of the armpits in order to minimize transmitted breath

Never shake an infant or a child.

Airway and respiratory problems are the most common cause of cardiac arrest in infants and young children.

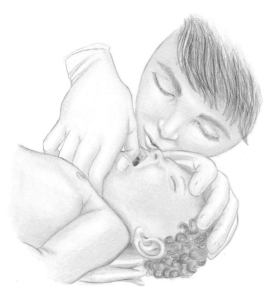

FIGURE 42-4   Opening the airway in a child.

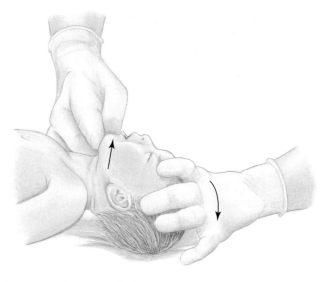

FIGURE 42-5   Head-tilt/chin-lift method.

sounds. When considering the respiratory rate, remember that pain or fear can increase a child's respiratory efforts. Tachypnea, an abnormally rapid rate of breathing, may indicate fear, pain, inadequate oxygenation, or, in the case of neonates, exposure to cold.

If you suspect trauma, check the infant or child for life-threatening chest injuries. Keep in mind that even a minor injury to the chest can interfere with a child's breathing efforts. A chest injury can also interfere with your effort to provide adequate oxygenation or ventilation.

Your goal is to identify any evidence of compromised breathing. Evaluation of breathing includes assessment of the following conditions:

- *Respiratory Rate.* Tachypnea is often the first manifestation of respiratory distress in infants. Regardless of the cause, an infant breathing at a rapid rate will eventually tire. Keep in mind that a decreasing respiratory rate may be a result of tiring and is not necessarily a sign of improvement. A slow respiratory rate in an acutely ill infant or child is an ominous sign. (Normal respiratory rates are listed in Table 42-2.) In short, be alert for a respiratory rate that is *either* abnormally fast *or* abnormally slow.

FIGURE 42-6   Jaw-thrust method.

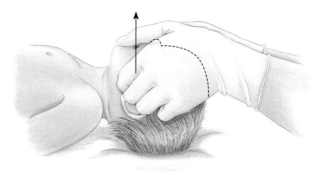

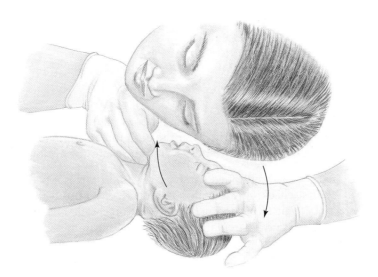

FIGURE 42-7 Assessing breathing.

Table 42-2 NORMAL VITAL SIGNS: INFANTS AND CHILDREN*

Normal Pulse Rates (Beats per Minute, at Rest)

Newborn	100 to 180
Infant (0–5 Months)	100 to 160
Infant (6–12 Months)	100 to 160
Toddler (1–3 Years)	80 to 110
Preschooler (3–5 Years)	70 to 110
School Age (6–10 Years)	65 to 110
Early Adolescence (11–14 Years)	60 to 90

Normal Respiration Rates (Breaths per Minute, at Rest)

Newborn	30 to 60
Infant (0–5 Months)	30 to 60
Infant (6–12 Months)	30 to 60
Toddler (1–3 Years)	24 to 40
Preschooler (3–5 years)	22 to 34
School Age (6–10 Years)	18 to 30
Early Adolescence (11–14 Years)	12 to 26

Normal Blood Pressure Ranges (mmHg, at Rest)

	Systolic Approx. 90 plus 2 × age	Diastolic Approx. 2/3 systolic
Preschooler (3–5 Years)	average 98 (78 to 116)	average 65
School age (6–10 Years)	average 105 (80 to 122)	average 69
Early Adolescence (11–14 Years)	average 114 (88 to 140)	average 76

*Adolescents ages 15 to 18 approach the vital signs of adults.

Note: A high pulse in an infant or child is not as great a concern as a low pulse. A low pulse may indicate imminent cardiac arrest. Blood pressure is usually not taken in a child under three years of age. In cases of blood loss or shock, a child's blood pressure will remain within normal limits until near the end, then fall swiftly.

- *Respiratory Effort.* The quality of air entry can be assessed by observing for chest rise, breath sounds, stridor, or wheezing. An increased respiratory effort in the infant or child is also evidenced by nasal flaring and the use of accessory respiratory muscles. (Signs of respiratory effort are listed in Table 42-3.)
- *Colour.* Cyanosis is a fairly late sign of respiratory failure and is most frequently seen in the mucous membranes of the mouth and the nail beds. Cyanosis of the extremities alone is more likely due to circulatory failure (shock) than to respiratory failure.

Circulation As mentioned earlier, you should assess a pediatric patient's circulation by first checking the child's colour. Keep in mind that the pediatric patient tends to become hypothermic; therefore, you should check the capillary refill time in an area of central circulation, such as the sternum or forehead. (Note that capillary refill time, as discussed later in this chapter, is considered reliable as a sign of perfusion primarily in children less than six years of age.) In general, evaluate the following conditions when assessing circulation during the primary assessment:

- *Heart Rate.* As previously mentioned, infants develop sinus tachycardia in response to stress. Thus, any tachycardia in an infant or a child requires further evaluation to determine the cause. Bradycardia in a distressed infant or child may indicate hypoxia and is an ominous sign of cardiac arrest. (Normal heart rates are listed in Table 42-2.)
- *Peripheral Circulation.* The presence of peripheral pulses is a good indicator of the adequacy of end-organ perfusion. Loss of central pulses is an ominous sign.
- *End-Organ Perfusion.* End-organ perfusion is most evident in the skin, kidneys, and brain. Decreased perfusion of the skin is an early sign of shock. A capillary refill time of greater than two seconds is indicative of low cardiac output. Impairment of brain perfusion is usually evidenced by a change in mental status. The child may become confused or lethargic. Seizures may occur. Failure of the child to recognize the parents' faces is often an ominous sign. Urine output directly relates to kidney perfusion. Normal urine output is 1–2 mL/kg/hr. Urine flow of less than 1 mL/kg/hr is an indicator of poor renal perfusion.

Table 42-3 SIGNS OF INCREASED RESPIRATORY EFFORT

Retraction	Visible sinking of the skin and soft tissues of the chest around and below the ribs and above the collarbone
Nasal flaring	Widening of the nostrils; seen primarily on inspiration
Head bobbing	Observed when the head lifts and tilts back as the child inhales and then moves forward as the child exhales
Grunting	Sound heard when an infant attempts to keep the alveoli open by building back pressure during expiration
Wheezing	Passage of air over mucous secretions in bronchi; heard more commonly on expiration; a low- or high-pitched sound
Gurgling	Coarse, abnormal bubbling sound heard in the airway during inspiration or expiration; may indicate an open chest wound
Stridor	Abnormal, musical, high-pitched sound, more commonly heard on inspiration

Remember that evaluation of mental status and ABCs during the primary assessment is rapid and not detailed—aimed at discovering and correcting immediate life threats. More thorough measurements will be performed during the focused history and secondary assessment.

Anticipating Cardiopulmonary Arrest

Your primary assessment—and the repeated assessments that follow—help you recognize and prevent cardiopulmonary arrest. At each stage of evaluating vital functions, ask yourself this question: *"Does this child have pulmonary or circulatory failure that may lead to cardiopulmonary arrest?"* Early recognition of the physiologically unstable child is one of the main goals of pediatric advanced life support (PALS). Conditions that place a pediatric patient at risk of cardiopulmonary arrest include

- Respiratory rate greater than 60
- Heart rate greater than 180 or less than 80 (under five years)
- Heart rate greater than 180 or less than 60 (over five years)
- Respiratory distress
- Trauma
- Burns
- Cyanosis
- Altered level of consciousness
- Seizures
- Fever with petechiae (small purple spots resulting from skin hemorrhages)

Evaluate the patient for these conditions throughout assessment and transport. Cardiopulmonary arrest in infants and children is usually not a sudden event. Instead, it is the end result of progressive deterioration in respiratory and cardiac function. Therefore, you need to determine whether the patient's condition is deteriorating or improving. Any decompensation or change in the patient's status will prompt you to perform basic or advanced life support measures as appropriate.

Transport Priority

On the basis of your primary assessment, you will assign the patient one of the following transport priorities:

- *Urgent*—Proceed with the rapid trauma assessment, if trauma is suspected, then transport immediately with further assessment and treatment performed en route.
- *Nonurgent*—Complete the focused history and secondary assessment at the scene, and then transport.

Transitional Phase

The way in which the pediatric patient is transferred to EMS care depends entirely on the seriousness of the patient's condition. A transitional phase is intended for the conscious, nonacutely ill child. This phase of assessment allows the infant or child to become familiar with you and the equipment that you will be using. When

> *At each stage of evaluating vital functions, ask yourself "Does this child have pulmonary or circulatory failure that may lead to cardiopulmonary arrest?"*

dealing with the unconscious or acutely ill patient, however, you will skip this phase and proceed directly to the treatment and transport phases of assessment. In essence, you assign the patient an "urgent" status or higher priority.

FOCUSED HISTORY AND SECONDARY ASSESSMENT

After you have prioritized patient care at the end of the primary assessment, you will obtain a history and perform a secondary assessment. If the patient has a medical illness, the history will precede the secondary assessment. If the patient is suffering from trauma, the secondary assessment will take precedence. If partners are working together, the history and secondary assessment may be performed simultaneously.

History

Whenever a patient is identified as a priority patient, then the focused history taking will occur en route to the hospital, after essential treatments or interventions for life-threatening conditions have been performed.

To obtain the history of a pediatric patient, you will probably need to involve a family member or caregiver. Remember, however, that school-aged children and adolescents like to take part in their own care. As previously mentioned, you can elicit valuable information from even very young patients. As a general precaution, question older adolescent patients in private, especially about such issues as sexual activity, pregnancy, or illicit drug and alcohol use. If you question adolescents about these subjects in the presence of an adult, they will probably be more reticent for fear of later repercussions.

As with any patient, you will use the history to uncover additional pertinent injuries or medical conditions. The history should centre on the chief complaint and past medical history.

To evaluate the nature of the chief complaint, determine each of the following:

- Nature of the illness/injury
- Length of time the patient has been sick/injured
- Presence of fever
- Effects of the illness/injury on patient behaviour
- Bowel/urine habits
- Presence of vomiting/diarrhea
- Frequency of urination

The past medical history identifies chronic illnesses, use of medications, and allergies. Be sure to inquire whether the infant or child is currently under a doctor's care. If so, obtain the name of the physician and present it at the receiving hospital. In the case of trauma patients, reconsider the mechanism of injury and the results of your on-scene secondary assessment (which, as noted earlier, will precede the history in the case of trauma).

Secondary Assessment

Focused Assessment Carry out the secondary assessment after all life-threatening conditions have been identified and addressed. If there is a significant mechanism of injury or if the patient is unresponsive, perform a complete rapid trauma assessment or rapid medical assessment. Use the toe-to-head approach with the younger child (or begin with the chest and examine the head last) and the head-to-

toe approach in the older child. If the injury is minor or if the patient is responsive, perform a secondary assessment that is focused on the affected areas and systems.

Perform the secondary assessment as described in Chapter 6. Depending on the particular situation, some or all of the following techniques may be appropriate to include in the assessment:

- *Pupils.* Inspect the patient's pupils for uniformity and reaction to light.
- *Capillary Refill.* As noted earlier, this technique is valuable for pediatric patients less than six years of age. Blanch the nail bed, base of the thumb, or sole of one of the feet. Remember that normal capillary refill is two seconds or less. Recall that this technique is less reliable in cold environments.
- *Hydration.* Note skin turgor, presence of tears and saliva and, with infants, the condition of the fontanelles.
- *Pulse Oximetry.* Use this mechanical device on moderately injured or ill infants and children. Readings will give you immediate information regarding peripheral oxygen saturation and allow you to follow trends in the patient's pulse rate and oxygenation status. Keep in mind, however, that hypothermia or shock can affect readings.

Glasgow Coma Scale In cases of trauma, you may need to apply the Glasgow Coma Scale (GCS)—a scoring system for monitoring the neurological status of patients with possible head injuries. The GCS assigns scores based on verbal responses, motor functions, and eye movements.

In using the GCS with pediatric patients, you will have to make certain modifications. The younger the patient, the more adjustments you will need to make. Verbal responses, for example, will not be possible for neonates and infants. However, motor function may be assessed in very young children by observing voluntary movement. Infants under four months of age should have a grasp reflex when an object is placed on the palmar surface of their hand. The grasp should be immediate. Children over three years of age will follow directions, when encouraged. Sensory function can be observed by the withdrawal reaction from "tickling" the patient. (See Table 42-4 for a modified GCS for infants.)

After you score the GCS for the patient, prioritize the patient according to severity. Guidelines are

- *Mild*—GCS 13 to 15
- *Moderate*—GCS 9 to 12
- *Severe*—GCS less than or equal to 8

Vital Signs Remember that poorly taken vital signs are of less value than not taking them at all. The following guidelines will help you obtain accurate pediatric readings. (Review Table 42-2 for normal pediatric vital signs.)

- Take vital signs with the patient in as close to a resting state as possible. If necessary, allow the child to calm down before attempting to take the vital signs. Vital signs in the field should include pulse, respiration, blood pressure, and temperature.
- Obtain blood pressure with an appropriate-sized cuff. The cuff should be two-thirds the width of the upper arm. Note that the pulse pressure (the difference between the systolic and diastolic blood pressure) narrows as shock develops. *Note that hypotension is a late and often sudden sign of cardiovascular decompensation.*

In using the Glasgow Coma Scale with pediatric patients, you will have to make certain modifications. The younger the patient, the more adjustments you will need to make.

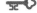

Remember that poorly taken vital signs are of less value than not taking them at all.

Table 42-4	GLASGOW COMA SCALE MODIFICATIONS FOR INFANTS		
Category	**Response**		**Score**
Verbal	Happy, coos, babbles, or cries spontaneously		5
	Irritable crying, but consolable		4
	Cries to pain, weak cry		3
	Moans to pain		2
	None		1
Motor	Spontaneous movement		6
	Withdraws to touch		5
	Withdraws to pain		4
	Abnormal flexion		3
	Abnormal extension		2
	None		1
Eye Opening (same as adult)	Spontaneous		4
	To speech		3
	To pain		2
	None		1

Source: Adapted from James, H.E., (1986): "Neurological evaluation and support in the child with acute brain insult," *Pediatric Annals*, 15(1): 17.

Even mild hypotension should be taken seriously in infants and young children.

Even mild hypotension should be taken seriously and treated quickly and vigorously, since cardiopulmonary arrest is probably imminent.

- Feel for peripheral, brachial, or femoral pulses. There is often a significant variation in pulse rate in children due to varied respirations. Therefore, it is important to monitor the pulse for at least 30 seconds, a full minute if possible.

- It is generally not possible to weigh the child. However, if medications are required, make a good estimate of the child's weight. Often, the parents or caregivers can provide a fairly reliable weight from a recent visit to the doctor.

- Observe respiratory rate before beginning the assessment. After the assessment is started, the child will often begin to cry. It will then be impossible to determine the respiratory rate. For an estimate of the upper limit of respiratory rate, subtract the child's age from 40. It is also important to identify the respiratory pattern, as well as retractions, nasal flaring, or paradoxical chest movement.

- Measure temperature early in the encounter, and repeat toward the end. IV fluid administration and exposure to the environment can cause a drop in core temperature.

- Continue to observe the child for level of consciousness. There may be a wide variety in levels of consciousness and activity during treatment.

Noninvasive Monitoring Modern noninvasive monitoring devices all have their application in pediatric emergency care (Figure 42-8). These may include the pulse oximeter, automated blood pressure devices, self-registering thermometers, and electrocardiograms (ECGs). To promote the goal of early recognition of cardiopulmonary arrest, every seriously ill or injured child should receive continuous pulse oximetry. This will provide you with essential information regarding the patient's heart rate and peripheral O_2 saturation. It will also help you to monitor the effects of any medications administered. ECG and automated blood pressure/pulse monitor should also be considered. However, these devices may frighten the child. Before

Every seriously ill or injured child should receive continuous ECG monitoring.

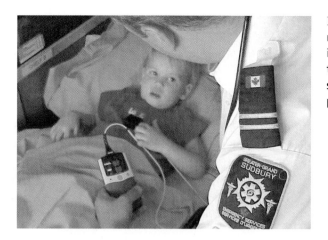

FIGURE 42-8 If available, noninvasive monitoring, including pulse oximetry and temperature measurement, should be used in prehospital pediatric care.

applying any monitoring device, explain what you are going to do. Demonstrate the display or lights. If the monitoring device makes noise, allow the child to hear the noise before you apply it. Reassure the child that the device will not hurt him.

ONGOING ASSESSMENT

Because a pediatric patient's condition can rapidly improve or deteriorate, it is necessary to repeat relevant portions of the assessment. (For this reason, ongoing assessment is sometimes called "reassessment.") You should continually monitor the patient's respiratory effort, skin colour, mental status, temperature, and pulse oximetry. Retake vital signs, and compare them with baseline vitals. In general, reassess stable patients every 15 minutes, critical patients every 5 minutes.

GENERAL MANAGEMENT OF PEDIATRIC PATIENTS

The same ABCs that guide the management of adult patients apply to pediatric patients: Your top priorities in treating an infant or a child are airway, breathing, and circulation. However, because of the special anatomical and physiological considerations that influence the management of pediatric patients, you need to practise these skills on an ongoing and regular basis.

BASIC AIRWAY MANAGEMENT

In treating the pediatric patient, basic life support (BLS) should be applied according to current standards and protocols. BLS should include maintenance of the airway, artificial ventilation, and, if required, chest compressions. (See Table 42-5.) As with all patients, your priority is to ensure an open airway. The following modifications of BLS airway skills will ensure that you take into account the clinical implications of the pediatric airway.

Manual Positioning

Allow the pediatric patient to assume a position of comfort, if possible. When placing the patient in a supine position, avoid hyperextension of the neck. As previously mentioned, infants and small children risk collapsed tracheas from hyperextension of the neck. For trauma patients less than three years old, place support under the torso. For supine medical patients three years old and older, provide occipital elevation.

Table 42-5	SUMMARY OF BLS MANOEUVRES IN INFANTS AND CHILDREN	
Target of Manoeuvre	**Infant (< 1 year)**	**Child (1 to 8 years)**
Airway		
Open airway	Head tilt/chin lift (unless trauma present)	Head tilt/chin lift (unless trauma present)
	Jaw thrust	Jaw thrust
Clear foreign body obstruction	Back blows/chest thrusts	Heimlich manoeuvre
Breathing		
Initial	2 breaths at 1 to 1.5 seconds/breath	2 breaths at 1 to 1.5 seconds/breath
Subsequent	20 breaths/minute	20 breaths/minute
Circulation		
Pulse check	Brachial/femoral	Carotid
Compression area	Lower third of sternum	Lower third of sternum
Compression width	2 or 3 fingers	Heel of 1 hand
Depth	Approximately 1–3 cm (Newborn 1–2 cm)	Approximately 3–4 cm
Rate	At least 100/minute (Newborn 120/minute)	100/minute
Compression–ventilation ratio	5:1 (Newborn 3:1)	5:1

Foreign Body Airway Obstruction (FBAO)

Before administering treatment, determine if an airway obstruction is partial or complete. Infants or children with a partial airway obstruction will have a cough, hoarse voice or cry, stridor, or some other evidence that at least some air is passing through the airway. Avoid any manoeuvres that will turn a partial obstruction into a complete obstruction. Instead, place the patient in a position of comfort and transport immediately.

In the case of complete airway obstruction, take one of the following age-specific manoeuvres:

- *Children.* For children older than one year of age, perform a series of abdominal thrusts if conscious and chest thrusts if unconscious.
- *Infants.* For infants less than one year old, deliver a series of five back blows followed by five chest thrusts. Inspect the infant's mouth upon completion of each series.

Never use blind finger sweeps in a pediatric patient.

As you recall from the basic cardiopulmonary resuscitation (CPR) courses, never check a pediatric patient's mouth with blind finger sweeps.

Suctioning

Apply suctioning whenever you detect heavy secretions in the nose or mouth of a pediatric patient, especially if the patient has a diminished level of consciousness. You can use a bulb syringe, flexible suction catheter, or rigid-tip suction catheter, depending on the patient's age or size (Figure 42-9). Make sure that flexible catheters are the correct size (Table 42-6).

Although pediatric suctioning techniques vary very little from adult suctioning techniques, keep the following modifications in mind:

- Decrease suction pressure to less than 100 mmHg in infants.

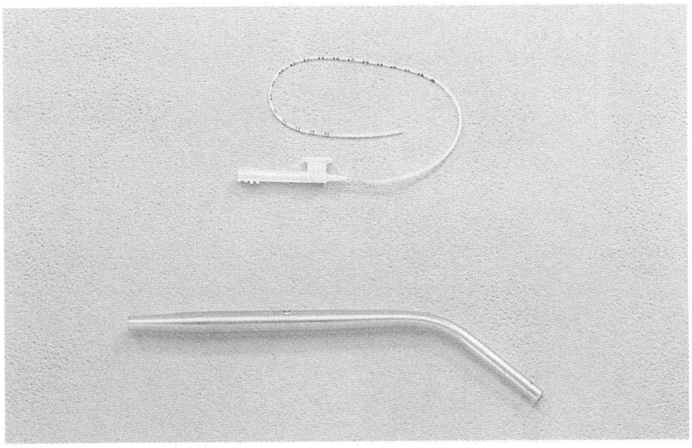

FIGURE 42-9 Pediatric-size suction catheters. Top: soft suction catheter. Bottom: rigid or hard suction catheter.

- Avoid excessive suctioning time (suction less than 10 seconds) in order to decrease the possibility of hypoxia.
- Avoid stimulation of the vagus nerve, which may produce bradycardia. As a general rule, suction no deeper than you can see and for no more than 15 seconds per attempt.
- Frequently check the patient's pulse. If bradycardia occurs, stop suctioning immediately, and oxygenate.

Oxygenation

Adequate oxygenation is the hallmark of pediatric patient management. Methods of oxygen delivery include "blow-by" techniques (especially for neonates) and via pediatric-sized nonrebreather masks. Although nonrebreather masks provide the highest concentration of supplemental oxygen, children may resist their use. Try to overcome their fear by demonstrating the use of the mask on yourself (Figure 42-10). Better yet, enlist the support of a parent or caregiver, and ask them to demonstrate the mask. As an alternative, you might place the mask over the face of a stuffed animal.

If the child refuses to accept the nonrebreather mask, resort to high-flow, blow-by oxygen. Some units place oxygen tubing through the bottom of a colourful paper cup, and use it to deliver the blow-by supplemental oxygen. Children often find a familiar object less frightening than complicated medical equipment.

Adequate oxygenation is the hallmark of pediatric patient management.

Airway Adjuncts

As a general rule, use airway adjuncts in pediatric patients only if prolonged artificial ventilations are required. There are two reasons for this. First, infants and children often improve quickly through the administration of 100-percent

Use airway adjuncts in pediatric patients only if prolonged artificial ventilations are required.

Table 42-6	SUCTION CATHETER SIZES FOR INFANTS AND CHILDREN	
Age	**Suction Catheter Size (French)**	
Up to 1 Year	8	
2 to 6 Years	10	
7 to 15 Years	12	
16 Years	12 to 14	

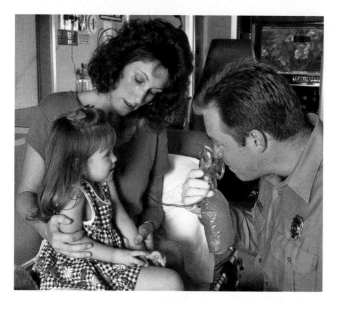

FIGURE 42-10 To overcome the child's fear of the non-rebreather mask, try it on yourself, or have the parent try it on before attempting to place it on the child.

oxygen. Second, airway adjuncts may create greater complications in children than in adults. Pediatric patients risk soft-tissue damage, vomiting, and stimulation of the vagus nerve.

Oropharyngeal Airways Oropharyngeal airways should be used only in pediatric patients who do not have a gag reflex. (Patients with a gag reflex risk vomiting and bradycardia.) Size the airway by measuring from the corner of the mouth to the front of the earlobe. Remember: Oropharyngeal airways that are too small can obstruct breathing; ones that are too large can both block the airway and cause trauma. (For general sizing suggestions, see Table 42-7.)

In placing an oropharyngeal airway, use a tongue blade to depress the tongue and jaw (Figure 42-11). If you detect a gag reflex, continue to maintain an open airway with a manual manoeuvre (jaw-thrust or head tilt/chin lift), and consider the use of a nasal airway. Remember that with a pediatric patient, the oral airway is inserted with the tip pointing toward the tongue and pharynx.

FIGURE 42-11 Inserting an oropharyngeal airway in a child with the use of a tongue blade.

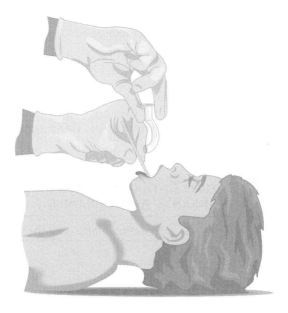

Table 42-7 — EQUIPMENT GUIDELINES ACCORDING TO AGE AND WEIGHT

Equipment	Age (50th Percentile Weight)					
	Preemie (1–2.5 kg)	Neonate (2.5–4.0 kg)	6 Months (7.0 kg)	1–2 Years (10–12 kg)	5 Years (16–18 kg)	5–10 Years (24–30 kg)
Airway *Oral*	infant 50 mm	infant (small) 50 mm	small 55 mm	small 60 mm	medium 70 mm	medium large 80 mm
Breathing *Self-inflating bag*	infant	infant	child	child	child	child/adult
O₂ ventilation mask	premature	newborn	infant/child	child	child	small adult
Endotracheal tube	2.5–3.0 (uncuffed)	3.0–3.5 (uncuffed)	3.5–4.0 (uncuffed)	4.0–4.5 (uncuffed)	5.0–5.5 (uncuffed)	5.5–6.5 (uncuffed)
Laryngoscope blade	0 (straight)	1 (straight)	1 (straight)	1–2 (straight)	2 (straight or curved)	2–3 (straight or curved)
Suction/stylet (F)	6–8/6	8/6	8–10/6	10/6	14/14	14/14
Circulation *BP cuff*	newborn	newborn	infant	child	child	child/adult
Venous access *Angiocath*	22–24	22–24	22–24	20–22	18–20	16–20
Butterfly needle	25	23–25	23–25	23	20–23	18–21
Intracath	—	—	19	19	16	14
Arm board	15 cm	15 cm	15–20 cm	20 cm	20–45 cm	45 cm
Orogastric tube (F)	5	5–8	8	10	10–12	14–18
Chest tube (F)	10–14	12–18	14–20	14–24	20–32	28–38

Reproduced with permission of the American Heart Association.

Nasopharyngeal Airways Use nasopharyngeal airways for those children who possess a gag reflex and who require prolonged artificial ventilations. DO NOT use them on any child with midface or head trauma. You might mistakenly pass the airway through a fracture into the sinuses or the brain.

Size a nasal airway in the same fashion as for adult patients. (Use the outside diameter of the patient's little finger as a measure.) Although nasopharyngeal airways come in a variety of sizes, they are not readily available for infants less than one year old. Equipment required for insertion of a nasal airway includes

- Appropriately sized soft, flexible latex tubing
- Water-based lubricant

When inserting the nasal airway, follow the same basic method as you would in an adult patient. It is important to remember that younger children often have enlarged adenoids (lymphatic tissues in the nasopharynx), which can be easily lacerated when inserting a nasopharyngeal airway. Because of this, always use care when inserting a nasopharyngeal airway in a younger child. If resistance is met, do not force the airway as significant bleeding can result.

> *Do not use nasal airways on a child with midface or head trauma.*
>

Ventilation

Adequate tidal volume and ventilatory rate provide more than just a high oxygen saturation for your patient. Ventilation is a two-way physiological street: Maintenance of appropriate oxygen levels results in appropriate carbon dioxide levels as well. However, you will achieve neither of these clinically important events without tailoring the ventilatory device and technique to your pediatric patient. Important points to remember include the following:

- Avoid excessive bag pressure and volume. Ventilate at an age-appropriate rate, using only enough ventilation to make the chest rise.
- Use a properly sized mask to ensure a good fit. In general, the mask should fit on the bridge of the nose and the cleft of the chin (Figure 42-12).
- Obtain a chest rise with each breath.
- Allow adequate time for exhalation.
- Assess bag-valve-mask (BVM) ventilation. (Provide 100-percent oxygen by using a reservoir attached to the BVM.)
- Remember that flow-restricted, oxygen-powered ventilation devices are contraindicated in pediatric resuscitation.
- Do not use BVMs with pop-off valves unless they can be readily occluded if necessary. (Ventilatory pressures required during pediatric CPR may exceed the limit of the pop-off valve.)
- Apply cricoid pressure through application of the Sellick manoeuvre to minimize gastric inflation and passive regurgitation (Figure 42-13).
- Ensure correct positioning to avoid hyperextension of the neck.

ADVANCED AIRWAY AND VENTILATORY MANAGEMENT

As the advanced or critical care paramedic, you will be expected to master the advanced life support (ALS) procedures that make you a leader in the EMS system. Your clinical skills will help save the lives of pediatric patients whose respiratory systems have failed so severely that basis life support (BLS) measures are insufficient. When signs of impending cardiopulmonary arrest have been identified (as discussed earlier), you may be called upon to implement the following pediatric advanced life support (PALS) techniques, either in your own unit or in a transfer of care from a primary care paramedic (PCP) unit. The success of these techniques requires knowledge of the procedures that set pediatric skills apart from the advanced life support skills used on adults. (Review the advanced airway skills for adults discussed in Chapter 27, Part 2.)

Foreign-Body Airway Obstruction

One advantage of being able to perform endotracheal intubation is that it gives you another treatment modality for children with foreign-body airway obstructions. If a child's airway cannot be cleared by basic airway procedures, visualize the airway with the laryngoscope. Often, the obstructing foreign body can be seen. Once visualized, grasp the foreign body with the Magill forceps, and remove it. If you cannot remove the foreign body with Magill forceps, try to intubate around the obstruction. This often requires using an endotracheal tube smaller than you

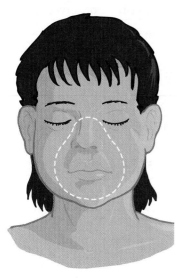

FIGURE 42-12   While placing a mask on a child, ensure that it fits on the bridge of the nose and the cleft of the chin.

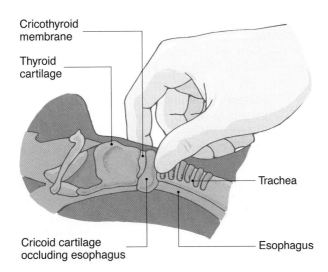

FIGURE 42-13 In the Sellick manoeuvre, pressure is placed on the cricoid cartilage, compressing the esophagus. This reduces regurgitation and helps bring the vocal cords into view, which is useful if intubation is to be performed.

Cricothyroid membrane

Thyroid cartilage

Trachea

Cricoid cartilage occluding esophagus

Esophagus

would normally choose. However, this will provide an adequate airway until the foreign body can be removed at the hospital.

Needle Cricothyrostomy

Needle cricothyrostomy in children is the same as for adult patients (as discussed in Chapter 27). It is important to remember that the anatomical landmarks are smaller and more difficult to identify. For years, it was taught that needle cricothyrostomy was contraindicated in children less than one year of age. However, current thinking is that the possible benefit (life) exceeds the risks (bleeding, local tissue damage). Remember, the only indication for cricothyrostomy is failure to obtain an airway by any other method and is not usually practised in Canadian prehospital care.

Endotracheal Intubation

Endotracheal intubation allows direct visualization of the lower airway through the trachea, bypassing the entire upper airway. It is the most effective method of controlling a patient's airway, whether it be an adult or a child. However, endotracheal intubation is not without complications. It is an invasive technique with little room for error. A tube that is wrongly sized or placed, especially in an apneic patient, can quickly lead to hypoxia and death.

Anatomical and Physiological Concerns Although endotracheal intubation of a child and an adult follow the same basic procedures, the special features of the pediatric airway complicate placement of any orotracheal tube. In fact, variations in the airway size of children discourage the use of certain airways, including esophageal-tracheal combitubes (ETC). In using an endotracheal tube, keep in mind these points:

- In infants and small children, it is often more difficult to create a single clear visual plane from the mouth, through the pharynx, and into the glottis. A straight-blade laryngoscope is preferred, since it provides greater displacement of the tongue and better visualization of the relatively cephalad and anterior glottis. For bigger children, a curved blade may sometimes be used. (Review Table 42-7.)
- Variations in the sizes of pediatric airways, coupled with the fact that the narrowest portion of the airway is at the level of the cricoid

Remember: An endotracheal tube that is wrongly sized or placed, especially in the apneic patient, can quickly lead to hypoxia and death.

A properly sized laryngeal mask airway (LMA) can be used in the pediatric patient. However, you should remember that LMAs do not protect the airway from aspiration.

ring, makes proper sizing of the endotracheal tube crucial. To determine correct size, apply any of the following methods:
- Use a resuscitation tape, such as the Broselow™ tape, to estimate tube size based on height.
- Estimate the correct tube size by using the diameter of the patient's little finger or the diameter of the nasal opening.
- Calculate the correct tube size by using this simple numerical formula:
  (Patient's age in years + 16) ÷ 4 = Tube size
  or Age ÷ 4 + 4 = Tube size

- The depth of insertion can be estimated on the basis of age (Table 42-8). However, the best method of determining depth is direct visualization. Due to the distance between the mouth and the trachea, a stylet is rarely needed to position the tube properly. When a stylet is used, select a malleable yet rigid style.

- Because the pediatric airway narrows at the level of the cricoid cartilage, uncuffed tubes should be used in children younger than eight years old. The tubes should display a vocal cord marker to ensure correct placement.

- Infants and small children may have greater vagal response than adults. Therefore, laryngoscopy and passage of an endotracheal tube are likely to cause a vagal response, dramatically slowing the child's heart rate and decreasing the cardiac output and blood pressure. As a result, pediatric intubations must be carried out swiftly, accurately, and with continuous monitoring.

Pediatric intubation must be carried out swiftly, accurately, and with continuous monitoring.

Indications The indications for endotracheal intubation in a pediatric patient are the same as those for an adult. They include

- Need for prolonged artificial ventilations
- Inadequate ventilatory support with a bag-valve mask
- Cardiac or respiratory arrest
- Control of an airway in a patient without a cough or gag reflex
- Necessary for providing a route for drug administration
- Need to gain access to the airway for suctioning

Additionally, if local protocols allow it, endotracheal intubation may be used in a child who is suffering from an increasingly compromised airway.

Techniques for Pediatric Intubation To perform endotracheal intubation on a pediatric patient, follow the basic steps in Procedure 42-1. Detailed steps include

1. While maintaining ventilatory support, hyperoxygenate the patient with 100-percent oxygen. If time allows, hyperoxygenate for a full two minutes.

Table 42-8 INFANT/CHILD ENDOTRACHEAL TUBES

Age of Patient	Measurement of the Endotracheal Tube at the Teeth
6 Months to 1 Year	12 cm—teeth to mid-trachea
2 Years	14 cm—teeth to mid-trachea
4 to 6 Years	16 cm—teeth to mid-trachea
6 to 10 Years	18 cm—teeth to mid-trachea
10 to 12 Years	20 cm—teeth to mid-trachea

2. Assemble and check your equipment. As stated earlier, a straight-blade laryngoscope is preferred. Assorted sizes of endotracheal tubes, both cuffed and uncuffed, should be stocked in the pediatric kit aboard your ambulance.

3. Place the patient's head and neck into an appropriate position. With a pediatric patient, the head should be maintained in a sniffing position.

4. Hold the laryngoscope in your left hand.

5. Insert your laryngoscope blade into the right side of the patient's mouth. With a sweeping action, displace the tongue to the left.

6. Move the blade slightly toward the midline, and then advance it until the distal end is positioned at the base of the tongue (Figure 42-14).

7. Look for the tip of the epiglottis, and place the laryngoscope blade into its proper position. Keep in mind that a child—particularly an infant—has a shorter airway and a higher glottis than an adult does. Because of this, you will see the cords much sooner than you may expect.

8. With your left wrist straight, use your shoulder and arm to lift the mandible and tongue at a 45-degree angle to the floor until the glottis is exposed. Use the little finger of your left hand to apply gentle downward pressure to the cricoid cartilage. This will permit easier visualization of the cords.

9. Grasp the endotracheal tube in your right hand. To pass the tube into your patient's mouth, it may be helpful to hold it so that its curve is in a horizontal plane (bevel sideways). Insert the tube through the right corner of the child's mouth.

10. Under direct observation, insert the endotracheal tube into the glottic opening, and pass it through until its distal cuff disappears past the vocal cords—approximately 5 to 10 cm. As the tube is

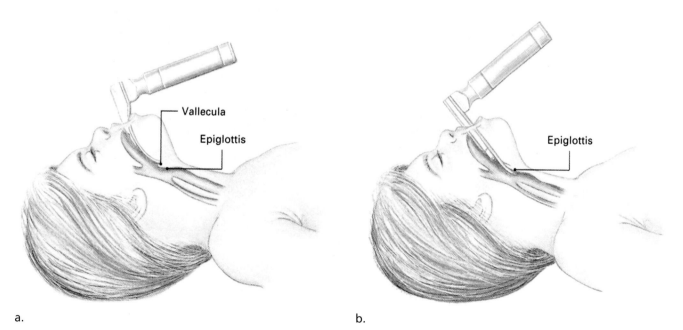

a. b.

FIGURE 42-14 Placement of the laryngoscope: a. MacIntosh (curved) blade;
b. Miller (straight) blade.

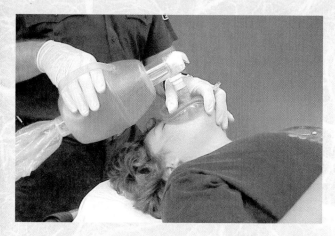

42-1a   Hyperoxygenate the child.

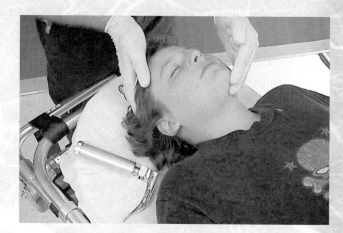

42-1b   Position the head.

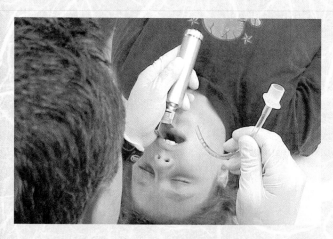

42-1c   Insert the laryngoscope, and visualize the airway.

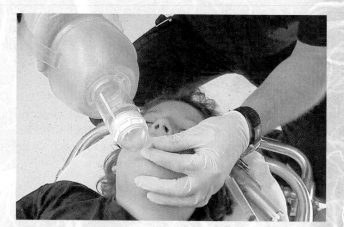

42-1d   Insert the tube, and oxygenate the child.

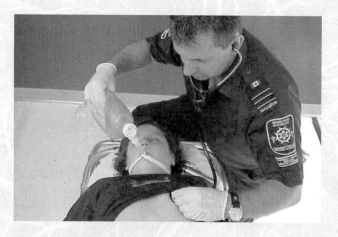

42-1e   Confirm tube placement.

advanced, it should be rotated into the proper plane. In some cases, it will be difficult to advance the endotracheal tube at the level of the cricoid. DO NOT force the tube through this region, as it may cause laryngeal edema.

11. Hold the tube in place with your left hand. Attach an infant- or child-sized bag-valve device to the 15/22-mm adapter, and deliver several breaths.

12. Check for proper tube placement. Watch for chest rise and fall with each ventilation and listen for equal, bilateral breath sounds. There should also be an absence of sounds over the epigastrium with ventilations. Confirm placement with an $ETCO_2$ detector.

13. If the tube has a distal cuff, inflate it with the recommended amount of air.

14. Recheck for proper placement of the tube, and hyperoxygenate the patient with 100-percent oxygen.

15. Secure the endotracheal tube with umbilical tape while maintaining ventilatory support.

16. Continue supporting the tube manually while maintaining ventilations. Check periodically to ensure proper tube position. As with adults, allow no more than 30 seconds to pass without ventilating your patient.

Nasogastric Intubation

If gastric distention is present in a pediatric patient, you may consider placing a nasogastric tube (NG tube) if within your scope of practice (CCP). In infants and children, gastric distention may result from overly aggressive artificial ventilations or from air swallowing. Placement of an NG tube will allow you to decompress the stomach and proximal bowel of air. An NG tube can also be used to empty the stomach of blood or other substances. Indications for use of a nasogastric intubation include

- Inability to achieve adequate tidal volumes during ventilation due to gastric distention
- Presence of gastric distention in an unresponsive patient

As with nasopharyngeal airways, an NG tube is contraindicated in pediatric patients who have sustained head or facial trauma. Because the NG tube might migrate into the cranial sinuses, consider the use of an orogastric tube instead. Other contraindications include possible soft-tissue damage in the nose and inducement of vomiting.

Equipment for placing an NG tube includes

- Age-appropriate NG tubes
- 20-mL syringe
- Water-soluble lubricant
- Emesis basin
- Tape
- Suctioning equipment
- Stethoscope

In sizing the NG tube, keep in mind the following recommended guidelines:

- Newborn/infant: #8 French
- Toddler/preschooler: #10 French
- School-aged children: #12 French
- Adolescents: #14–16 French

In determining the correct length, measure the tube from the top of the patient's nose, over the ear, to the tip of the xiphoid process. The steps for inserting the tube can be followed in Procedure 42-2. Keep in mind as you examine these steps that many experts believe that an NG tube should only be inserted when an endotracheal tube is in place. This precaution will prevent misplacement of the tube into the trachea instead of the esophagus. Consult protocols in your area on the use of NG tubes.

NG tube insertion is safest when the airway is protected with an ET tube.

Rapid Sequence Intubation

Advanced airway management by a CCP may sometimes be indicated in pediatric patients with a significant level of consciousness and the presence of a gag reflex. Examples may include a combative child with head trauma or an adolescent with a drug overdose. In such cases, clenched teeth and resistance may make intubation difficult or impossible. As a result, medical direction may authorize the use of "paralytics" to induce a state of neuromuscular compliance. All skeletal muscles, including the muscles of respiration, respond to these drugs, known as neuromuscular blocking agents. Following their administration, the patient will require mechanical ventilation.

An example of a commonly used neuromuscular blocker is succinylcholine (Anectine). Typically, it is administered at 1–2 mg/kg IV push. It acts in 60–90 seconds and lasts approximately 3–5 minutes. Remember that succinylcholine has no effect on consciousness or pain. Thus, a sedative agent must be used in all children, except those who are unconscious. Commonly used drugs include midazolam (Versed), diazepam (Valium), thiopental, and fentanyl. A bite block should be placed to prevent the patient from biting the endotracheal tube. Medical direction may authorize sedation to minimize the emotional trauma to the patient or such drugs as pancuronium or vecuronium if paralysis for a longer period is required.

CIRCULATION

As mentioned earlier, the respiratory and cardiovascular systems are interdependent. In pediatrics, you are encouraged to look at the total child. You should assess the child by assessing the various body systems. For example, instead of simply checking a pulse, you should look for end-organ changes that indicate the effectiveness of respiratory and cardiovascular functions. These include such factors as mental status, skin colour, skin temperature, urine output, and others. There are two problems that lead to cardiopulmonary arrest in children: shock and respiratory failure. Both must be identified and corrected early. The following section will address assessment of the cardiovascular system. Particular emphasis is placed on venous access and fluid resuscitation, as these are essential skills for prehospital advanced life support (ALS) personnel who treat pediatric patients.

There are two problems that lead to cardiopulmonary arrest in children: shock and respiratory failure.

In obtaining venous access, the external jugular vein should only be used in life-threatening situations.

Vascular Access

Intravenous techniques for children are basically the same as for adults. (See Chapter 15.) However, additional veins may be accessed in the infant. These include veins of the neck and scalp, as well as of the arms, hands, and feet. The external jugular vein, however, should only be used in life-threatening situations.

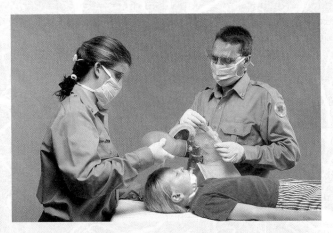

42-2a Oxygenate, and continue to ventilate if possible.

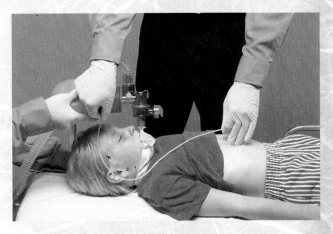

42-2b Measure the NG tube from the tip of the nose, over the ear, to the tip of the xiphoid process.

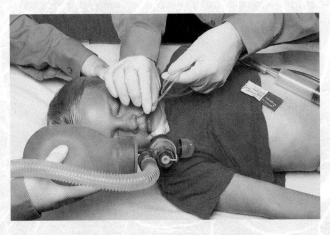

42-2c Lubricate the end of the tube. Then, pass it gently downward along the nasal floor to the stomach.

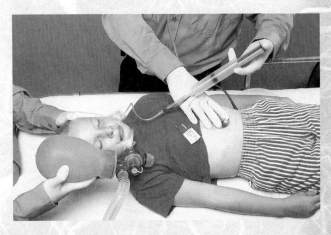

42-2d Ausculate over the epigastrium to confirm correct placement. Listen for bubbling while injecting 10–20 mL of air into the tube.

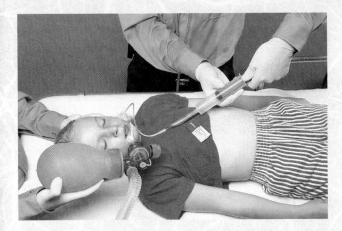

42-2e Use suction to aspirate stomach contents.

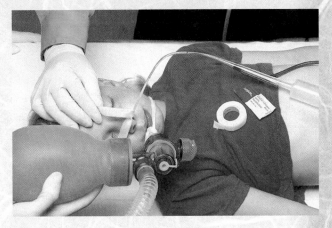

42-2f Secure the tube in place.

Intraosseous Infusion

The use of intraosseous (IO) infusion has become popular in the pediatric patient (see Figure 42-15a). This is especially true when large volumes of fluid must be administered, as occurs in hypovolemic shock, and when other means of venous access are unavailable. Certain drugs can be administered intraosseously, including epinephrine, atropine, dopamine, lidocaine, sodium bicarbonate, and dobutamine. Indications for intraosseous infusion include

- Children less than seven years old
- Existence of shock or cardiac arrest
- An unresponsive patient
- Unsuccessful attempts at peripheral IV insertion

The primary contraindications for IO infusion include

- Presence of a fracture in the bone chosen for infusion
- Fracture of the pelvis or extremity fracture in the bone proximal to the chosen site

In performing IO perfusion, you can use a standard 16- or 18-gauge needle (either hypodermic or spinal). However, an intraosseous needle is preferred and significantly better (Figure 42-15b). The anterior surface of the leg below the

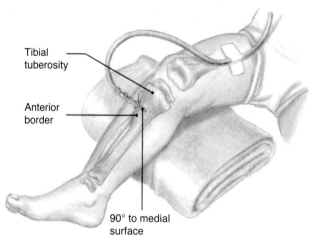

a.

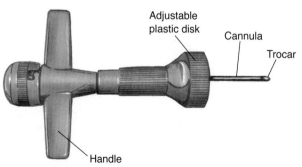

b.

FIGURE 42-15   a. Intraosseous administration in the pediatric patient. b. An intraosseous needle.

knee should be prepped with antiseptic solution, such as povidone iodine. The needle is then inserted, in a twisting fashion, 1–3 cm below the tuberosity. Insertion should be slightly inferior in direction (to avoid the growth plate) and perpendicular to the skin (Figure 42-16). Placement of the needle into the marrow cavity can be determined by noting a lack of resistance as the needle passes through the bony cortex. Other indications include the needle standing upright without support, the ability to aspirate bone marrow into a syringe, or free flow of the infusion without infiltration into the subcutaneous tissues. (See also the discussion of intraosseous infusion in Chapter 15.)

Fluid Therapy

The accurate dosing of fluids in children is crucial. Too much fluid can result in heart failure and pulmonary edema. Too little fluid can be ineffective. The initial dosage of fluid in hypovolemic shock should be 20 mL/kg of an isotonic solution, such as Ringer's Lactate or normal saline, as soon as IV access is obtained. After the infusion, the child should be reassessed. A child with hypovolemic shock may require 40–60 mL/kg, while a child with septic shock may require at least 60–80 mL/kg. Fluid therapy should be guided by the child's clinical response.

Intravenous infusions in children should be closely monitored with frequent patient reassessment. Minidrip administration sets, flow limiters (e.g., buretrol), or infusion pumps should be routinely used in pediatric cases.

Medications

Cardiopulmonary arrest in infants and children is almost always due to a primary respiratory problem, such as drowning, choking, or smoke inhalation. The major aim in pediatric resuscitation is airway management and ventilation, as well as replacement of intravascular volume if indicated. In certain cases, medications may be required. The objectives of medication therapy in pediatric patients include

- Correction of hypoxemia
- Increased perfusion pressure during chest compressions
- Stimulation of spontaneous or more forceful cardiac contractions
- Acceleration of the heart rate
- Correction of metabolic acidosis
- Suppression of ventricular ectopy
- Maintenance of renal perfusion

The accurate dosing of fluids in children is crucial. Too much fluid can result in heart failure and pulmonary edema. Too little fluid can be ineffective.

Do not allow a full litre bag of fluid to be directly connected to a small child or infant without having a flow limiter attached, such as buretrol.

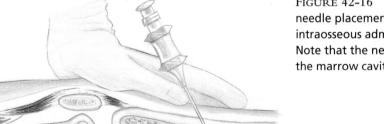

FIGURE 42-16 Correct needle placement for intraosseous administration. Note that the needle tip is in the marrow cavity.

The dosages of medications must be modified for the pediatric patient. Tables 42-9 and 42-10 illustrate recommended pediatric drug dosage in advanced cardiac life support.

ELECTRICAL THERAPY

You are less likely to use electrical therapy on pediatric patients than on adult patients. This is because ventricular fibrillation is much less common in children than in adults. However, you should review and keep the following principles in mind for times when these emergencies arise:

- Administer an initial dosage of two joules per kilogram of body weight.
- If this is unsuccessful, increase the dosage to four joules per kilogram.
- If this is unsuccessful, focus your attention on correcting hypoxia and acidosis.
- Transport to a pediatric critical care unit, if possible.

Table 42-9 DRUGS USED IN PEDIATRIC ADVANCED LIFE SUPPORT*

Drug	Dose	Remarks
Adenosine	0.1 to 0.2 mg/kg Maximum strength dose 12 mg	Rapid IV bolus
Amiodarone	5 mg/kg IV/IO	Rapid IV bolus
Atropine sulphate	0.02 mg/kg per dose	Minimum dose 0.1 mg Maximum single dose: 0.5 mg in child; 1.0 mg in adolescent
Calcium chloride 10 percent	20 mg/kg/dose	Give slowly
Dopamine hydrochloride	2–10 µg/kg/min.	Adrenergic action dominates at ≥ 15–20 µg/kg per minute
Epinephrine *for bradycardia*	IV/IO 0.01 mg/kg (1:10 000) ET: 0.1 mg/kg (1:1000)	Be aware of effective dose of preservatives administered (if preservatives are present in epinephrine preparation) when high doses are used
for asystolic or pulseless arrest	*First dose:* IV/IO: 0.01 mg/kg (1: 10 000) ET: 0.1 mg/kg (1:1000) *Subsequent doses:* IV/IO/ET: 0.1 mg/kg (1:1000)	Be aware of effective dose of preservatives administered (if preservatives are present in epinephrine preparation) when high doses are used
Epinephrine infusion	Initial at 0.1 µg/kg/min Higher infusion dose used if asystole present	Titrate to desired effect (0.1–1.0 µg/kg/min.)
Lidocaine	1 mg/kg per dose	Rapid bolus
Lidocaine infusion	20–50 µg/kg/min	
Sodium bicarbonate	1 mEq/kg/dose or 0.3 × kg × base deficit	Infuse slowly and only if ventilation is adequate

*IV indicates intravenous route; IO, intraosseous route; ET, endotracheal route.

Table 42-10 **PREPARATION OF INFUSIONS**

Drug	Preparation*	Dose
Epinephrine	0.6 × body weight (kg) equals milligrams added to diluent[†] to make 100 mL	Then 1 mL/h delivers 0.1 µg/kg/min; titrate to effect
Dopamine/ dobutamine	0.6 × body weight (kg) equals milligrams added to diluent[†] to make 100 mL	Then 1 mL/h delivers 0.3 µg/kg/min; titrate to effect
Lidocaine	120 mg of 40 mg/mL solution added to 97 mL of 5 percent dextrose in water, yielding 1200 µg/mL solution	Then 1 mL/kg/h delivers 20 µg/kg/min

*Standard concentration may be used to provide more dilute or more concentrated drug solution, but then individual dose must be calculated for each patient and each infusion rate:

$$\text{Infusion Rate (mL/h)} = \frac{\text{Weight (kg)} \times \text{Dose (µg/kg/min)} \times 60 \text{ min/h}}{\text{Concentration (µg/mL)}}$$

[†]Diluent may be 5 percent dextrose in water, 5 percent dextrose in half-normal, normal saline, or Ringer's Lactate.

CERVICAL SPINE IMMOBILIZATION

Spinal injuries in children are not as common as in adults. However, because of a child's disproportionately larger and heavier head, the cervical spine (C-spine) is vulnerable to injury. Any time an infant or child sustains a significant head injury, assume that a neck injury may also be present. Children can suffer a spinal cord injury with no noticeable damage to the vertebral column as seen on C-spine x-rays. Thus, negative C-spine x-rays do not necessarily mean that a spinal cord injury does not exist. Because of this, children should remain immobilized until a spinal cord injury has been excluded by hospital personnel. As previously noted, even a child secured in a car safety seat can suffer neck injuries if the head is propelled forward during an accident or sudden stop.

Any time an infant or a child sustains a head injury, assume that a neck injury may also be present.

Always make sure that you use the appropriate-sized pediatric immobilization equipment. These supplies may include rigid cervical collars, towel or blanket rolls, foam head blocks, commercial pediatric immobilization devices, vest-type devices, and long boards with the appropriate padding. For pediatric patients found in car seats, you can also use the seat for immobilization. The Kendrick Extrication Device (KED) can be quickly modified to immobilize a pediatric patient. Because of the significant variations in the size of children, you must be creative in devising a plan for pediatric immobilization.

In securing the pediatric patient to the backboard, use appropriate amounts of padding to secure infants, toddlers, and preschoolers in a supine, neutral position. Never use sandbags when immobilizing a pediatric patient's head. If you must tip the board to manage vomiting, the weight of the sand bag may worsen the head injury.

Any time you immobilize a pediatric patient, remember that many children, especially those under age 5, will protest or fight restraint. Try to minimize the emotional stress by having a parent or caretaker stand near or touch the child. Often, the child will quit struggling when secured totally in an immobilization device. Ideally, a rescuer or family member should remain with the child at all times to reassure and calm the child if possible.

In managing a pediatric patient, never delay transport to perform a procedure that can be done en route to the hospital.

TRANSPORT GUIDELINES

In managing a pediatric patient, never delay transport to perform a procedure that can be done en route to the hospital. After deciding on necessary interventions—

first BLS, then ALS—determine the appropriate receiving facility. In reaching your decision, consider three factors:

- Time of transport
- Specialized facilities
- Specialized personnel

If you live in an area with specialized prehospital crews, such as critical care crews and neonatal nurses, their availability should weigh in your decision as well. Consider whether the patient would benefit by transfer to one of these crews. If so, request support. If not, determine the closest definitive care facility for the infant or child placed in your care. If time allows, continue to reduce the fear involved in transition of care from the family to the hospital. If you have won the trust of the child, and conditions permit, you might allow the patient to sit on your lap en route to the hospital (Figure 42-17). Think of what you would do or say to calm your own child or the child of a close relative or friend.

SPECIFIC MEDICAL EMERGENCIES

As you already realize from your earlier training and experience, a variety of pediatric medical problems can activate the EMS system. Although the majority of childhood medical emergencies involve the respiratory system, other body systems can be involved as well. To help you recognize and treat pediatric medical emergencies, the following sections cover some of the specific conditions you may encounter.

INFECTIONS

Infectious diseases account for the majority of pediatric illnesses.

Childhood is a time of frequent illnesses because of the relative immaturity of the pediatric immune system. Infectious diseases may be caused by the infection or infestation of the body by an infectious agent, such as a virus, bacterium, fungus, or parasite. Most infections are minor and self-limiting. There are, however, several infections that can be life threatening. These include meningitis, pneumonia, and septicemia—a systemic infection (usually bacterial) in the bloodstream.

The impact of an infection on physiological processes depends on the type of infectious agent and the extent of the infection. Signs and symptoms also vary, depending on the type of infection and the time since exposure. Any of the following conditions may indicate the presence of an infection: fever, chills, tachycardia,

FIGURE 42-17 Emotional support of the infant or child continues during transport.

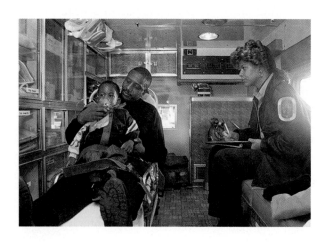

cough, sore throat, nasal congestion, malaise, tachypnea, cool or clammy skin, petechiae, respiratory distress, poor appetite, vomiting, diarrhea, dehydration, hypoperfusion (especially with septicemia), purpura (purple blotches resulting from hemorrhages into the skin that do not disappear under pressure), seizures, severe headache, irritability, stiff neck, or bulging fontanelle (infants).

The management of infections depends on the body system or systems affected. Treatment of some of the most common and serious infections will be found in the sections that follow. As a general rule, you should adhere to these guidelines when treating an infectious illness:

- Take all body substance isolation (BSI) precautions because of the unknown cause of the infection.
- Become familiar with the common pediatric infections encountered in your area.
- If possible, try to determine which, if any, pediatric infections you have not been exposed to or vaccinated against. For example, if you did not have chicken pox (varicella) or measles (rubeola) as a child, and were not vaccinated against them, then you should consider receiving vaccination against these illnesses. If you encounter a child suspected of having an infectious disease to which you may be susceptible, consider allowing another rescuer to be the primary person to care for the child.

RESPIRATORY EMERGENCIES

Respiratory emergencies constitute the most common reason EMS is summoned to care for a pediatric patient. Respiratory illnesses can cause respiratory compromise due to their effect on the alveolar/capillary interface. Some illnesses are quite minor, causing only mild symptoms, while others can be rapidly fatal. Your approach to the child with a respiratory emergency will depend on the severity of respiratory compromise. If the child is alert and talking, then you can take a more relaxed approach. However, if the child appears ill and is exhibiting marked respiratory difficulty, then you must immediately intervene to prevent respiratory arrest and possible cardiopulmonary arrest.

Severity of Respiratory Compromise

The severity of respiratory compromise can be quickly classified into the following categories:

- Respiratory distress
- Respiratory failure
- Respiratory arrest

Respiratory emergencies in pediatric patients may quickly progress from respiratory distress to respiratory failure to respiratory arrest. You must learn to recognize the phase your patient is in and take the appropriate interventions. Prompt recognition and treatment can literally mean the difference between life and death for an infant or child suffering from respiratory compromise.

Respiratory Distress The mildest form of respiratory impairment is classified as respiratory distress. The most noticeable finding is an increased work of breathing. One of the earliest indicators of respiratory distress is an increase in respiratory rate. Unfortunately, respiratory rate is one of the vital signs that is most often "estimated." As mentioned previously, it is essential to obtain an accurate

Prompt recognition of a respiratory emergency in an infant or child can literally mean the difference between life and death.

respiratory rate in children. Ideally, the respiratory rate should be measured for an entire minute. If time does not allow it, or if the child is deteriorating, then the respiratory rate should be measured for at least 30 seconds and multiplied by two to obtain the respiratory rate.

In addition to an increased work of breathing, the child in respiratory distress will initially have a slight decrease in the arterial carbon dioxide tension as the respiratory rate increases. However, as respiratory distress increases, the carbon dioxide tension will gradually increase.

The signs and symptoms of respiratory distress include

- Normal mental status deteriorating to irritability or anxiety
- Tachypnea
- Retractions
- Nasal flaring (in infants)
- Good muscle tone
- Tachycardia
- Head bobbing
- Grunting
- Cyanosis that improves with supplemental oxygen

If not corrected immediately, respiratory distress will lead to respiratory failure.

Respiratory Failure Respiratory failure occurs when the respiratory system is not able to meet the demands of the body for oxygen intake and for carbon dioxide removal. It is characterized by inadequate ventilation and oxygenation. During respiratory failure, the carbon dioxide level begins to rise as the body is not able to remove carbon dioxide. This ultimately leads to respiratory acidosis.

The signs and symptoms of respiratory failure include

- Irritability or anxiety deteriorating to lethargy
- Marked tachypnea later deteriorating to bradypnea
- Marked retractions later deteriorating to agonal respirations
- Poor muscle tone
- Marked tachycardia later deteriorating to bradycardia
- Central cyanosis

Respiratory failure is a very ominous sign. If immediate intervention is not provided, the child will deteriorate to full respiratory arrest.

Respiratory Arrest The end result of respiratory impairment, if untreated, is respiratory arrest. The cessation of breathing typically follows a period of bradypnea and agonal respirations.

Signs and symptoms of respiratory arrest include

- Unresponsiveness deteriorating to coma
- Bradypnea deteriorating to apnea
- Absent chest wall motion
- Bradycardia deteriorating to asystole
- Profound cyanosis

Respiratory arrest will quickly deteriorate to full cardiopulmonary arrest if appropriate interventions are not made. The child's chances of survival markedly decrease when cardiopulmonary arrest occurs.

Management of Respiratory Compromise

The management of respiratory compromise should be based on the severity of the problem. The goals of management include increasing ventilation and increasing oxygenation. You should try to identify the signs and symptoms of respiratory distress early so that you can intervene before the child deteriorates.

Your initial attention should be directed at the airway. Is it patent? Is it maintainable with simple positioning? Is endotracheal intubation required?

After assessing the airway, ensure continued maintenance of the airway by positioning, placement of an airway adjunct (oropharyngeal or nasopharyngeal airway), or endotracheal intubation.

For children in respiratory distress or early respiratory failure, administer oxygen at high flow. Some children will tolerate a nonrebreather mask. Others may not and may require that someone (perhaps a parent) hold blow-by oxygen for them to breathe. If the child fails to improve with supplemental oxygen administration, the patient should be treated more aggressively. Often, it is necessary to separate the parents from the child so that you can provide the necessary care without interruption or distraction.

Pediatric patients with late respiratory failure or respiratory arrest require aggressive treatment. This includes

- Establishment of an airway
- High-flow supplemental oxygen administration
- Mechanical ventilation with a bag-valve-mask device attached to a reservoir delivering 100-percent oxygen
- Endotracheal intubation if mechanical ventilation does not rapidly improve the patient's condition
- Consideration of gastric decompression with an orogastric or nasogastric tube if abdominal distension is impeding ventilation
- Consideration of needle decompression of the chest if a tension pneumothorax is thought to be present

In addition to the above, you should obtain venous access. The child should be promptly transported to a facility staffed and equipped to handle critically ill children. While en route, continue to reassess the child. Signs of improvement include an improvement in skin colour and temperature. As end-organ perfusion improves, the child will exhibit an increase in pulse rate, an increase in oxygen saturation, and an improvement in mental status. Provide emotional and psychological support to the parents, and keep them abreast of the results of your care.

SPECIFIC RESPIRATORY EMERGENCIES

Respiratory problems typically arise from obstruction of a part of the respiratory tract or impairment of the mechanics of respiration. In the following discussion we will present the common pediatric respiratory emergencies based on the part of the airway they most affect.

Upper-Airway Obstruction

Obstruction of the upper airway can be caused by many factors. As previously mentioned, upper-airway obstruction may be partial or complete. It can be caused by inflamed or swollen tissues caused by infection or by an aspirated foreign body. Appropriate care depends on prompt and immediate identification of the disorder and its severity. Whenever you find an infant, a toddler, or a young

Whenever you find an infant, a toddler, or a young child in respiratory or cardiac arrest, assume complete upper airway obstruction until proven otherwise.

child in respiratory or cardiac arrest, assume complete upper airway obstruction until proven otherwise.

Croup Croup, medically referred to as *laryngotracheobronchitis*, is a viral infection of the upper airway. It most commonly occurs in children six months to four years of age and is prevalent in the fall and winter. Croup causes an inflammation of the upper respiratory tract involving the subglottic region. The infection leads to edema beneath the glottis and larynx, thus narrowing the lumen of the airway. Severe cases of croup can lead to complete airway obstruction. Another form of croup called *spasmodic croup* occurs mostly in the middle of the night without any prior upper respiratory infection.

Assessment The history for croup is fairly classic. Often, the child will have a mild cold or other infection and be doing fairly well until evening. After dark, however, a harsh, barking or brassy cough develops. The attack may subside in a few hours but can persist for several nights.

The secondary assessment will often reveal inspiratory stridor. There may be associated nasal flaring, tracheal tugging, or retraction. You *should never* examine the oropharynx. Often, in the prehospital setting, it is difficult to distinguish croup from **epiglottitis**. (See Table 42-11 and Figure 42-18.) If epiglottitis is present, examination of the oropharynx may result in laryngospasm and complete airway obstruction. If the attack of croup is severe and progressive, the child may develop restlessness, tachycardia, and cyanosis. Although croup can result in complete airway obstruction and respiratory arrest, this is a rare event.

Management Management of croup consists of appropriate airway maintenance. Place the child in a position of comfort and administer cool mist oxygen at 4–6 L/min. Oxygen can be delivered by face mask or blow-by method. If the attack is severe, paramedics may administer nebulized epinephrine or salbutamol (Ventolin).

In preparing the patient for transport, remember that the journey from the house to the ambulance will often allow the child to breathe in cool air. Because cool air causes a decrease in subglottic edema, the child may be clinically improved by the time you reach the ambulance. If appropriate, keep the parent or caregiver with the infant or child. Do not agitate the patient, which could worsen the croup, by administering nonessential measures such as IVs or blood pressure readings.

Epiglottitis Epiglottitis is an acute infection and inflammation of the epiglottis and is potentially life threatening. (Recall that the epiglottis is a flap of cartilage that protects the airway during swallowing.) Epiglottitis, unlike croup, is caused by a bacterial infection, usually *Hemophilus influenza* type B. Due to the availability of influenza vaccination, epiglottitis has become an uncommon occurrence. When it does occur, it tends to strike preschool and school-age children ages 3–7 years.

* **croup** laryngotracheobronchitis; a common viral infection of young children, resulting in edema of the subglottic tissues; characterized by barking cough and inspiratory stridor.

* **epiglottitis** bacterial infection of the epiglottis, usually occurring in children older than age four; a serious medical emergency.

Table 42-11	Symptoms of Croup and Epiglottitis	
Croup	**Epiglottitis**
Slow onset	Rapid onset
Generally wants to sit up	Prefers to sit up
Barking cough	No barking cough
No drooling	Drooling; painful to swallow
Fever approx. 37.7–38.3°C	Fever approx. 38.8–40°C
	Occasional stridor

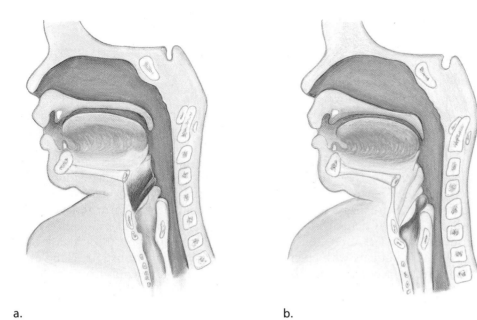

a.   b.

FIGURE 42-18   a. Epiglottitis is characterized by inflammation of the epiglottis and supraglottic tissues. b. Croup is characterized by subglottic edema.

Assessment   Epiglottitis presents similarly to croup. Often, the child will go to bed feeling relatively well, usually with what parents or caregivers consider to be a mild infection of the respiratory tract. Later, the child awakens with a high temperature and a brassy cough. The progression of symptoms can be dramatic. There is often pain on swallowing, sore throat, high fever, shallow breathing, dyspnea, inspiratory stridor, and drooling (Figure 42-19).

On secondary assessment, the child will appear acutely ill and agitated. *Never attempt to visualize the airway.* If the child is crying, the tip of the epiglottis can be seen posterior to the base of the tongue. In epiglottitis, the epiglottis is cherry red and swollen. As airway obstruction develops, the child will exhibit retractions, nasal flaring, and pulmonary hyperexpansion. As the epiglottis swells, the child may not be able to swallow his saliva and will begin to drool. Often, he will want to remain seated. Patients often assume the "tripod position" to help maximize the airway. If they lean backward or lie flat, the epiglottis can fall back and completely obstruct the airway.

Never attempt to visualize the airway in patients with epiglottitis.

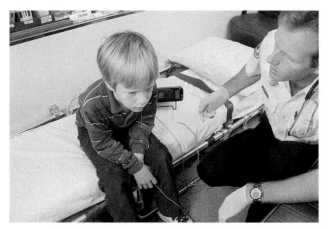

FIGURE 42-19   Posturing of the child with epiglottitis. Often, there will be excessive drooling.

Management Management of epiglottitis consists of appropriate airway maintenance and oxygen administration via a face mask (Figure 42-20) or by the blow-by technique. Ideally, the oxygen should be humidified to minimize drying of the epiglottis and airway. To reduce the child's anxiety, you might ask the parent or caregiver to administer the oxygen. If the airway becomes obstructed, two-rescuer ventilation with a bag-valve mask (BVM) is almost always effective. Make sure that all intubation equipment is available, including an appropriate-sized endotracheal tube. Remember, however, that intubation is contraindicated unless complete obstruction has occurred.

Also, do not intubate in a situation involving short transport times. If endotracheal intubation is required, it may be necessary to use a smaller endotracheal tube because of narrowing of the glottic opening. If you perform chest compression on glottic visualization during intubation, a bubble may form at the tracheal opening. This may help to establish upper airway landmarks that are distorted by the disease. As a last resort, consider needle cricothyrostomy per medical direction.

Pediatric patients with epiglottitis require immediate transport. Handle the child gently, since stress could lead to total airway obstruction from spasms of the larynx and swelling tissues. Avoid IV sticks, do not take a blood pressure reading, and do not attempt to look into the mouth. During transport, allow the child to sit on the lap of the parent or caregiver if appropriate. Constantly monitor the child, and notify the hospital of any changes in status. Remember, if the patient is maintaining his airway, *do not put anything in the child's mouth,* including a thermometer. At all times, consider epiglottitis a critical condition.

Bacterial Tracheitis Bacterial tracheitis is a bacterial infection of the airway, in the subglottic region. Although the condition is very uncommon, it is most likely to appear following episodes of viral croup. It afflicts mainly infants and toddlers 1–5 years of age.

Assessment In assessing this condition, parents or caregivers will typically report that the child has experienced an episode of croup in the preceding few days. They will also indicate the presence of high-grade fever accompanied by coughing up of pus and/or mucus. The patient may exhibit a hoarse voice and, if able to talk, may complain of a sore throat. A secondary assessment may reveal inspiratory or expiratory stridor.

Management As with all respiratory emergencies, the child must be carefully monitored, since respiratory failure or arrest may be an end result. Carefully manage airway and breathing, providing oxygenation via a face mask or by blow-by technique. Keep in mind that ventilations may require high pressure in order to adequately ventilate the patient. This may require depressing the pop-

Do not put anything in the mouth of an epiglottitis patient, including a thermometer.

At all times, consider epiglottitis a critical condition.

✱ **bacterial tracheitis** bacterial infection of the airway, in the subglottic region; in children, most likely to appear after episodes of croup.

FIGURE 42-20 The child with epiglottitis should be administered humidified oxygen and transported in a comfortable position.

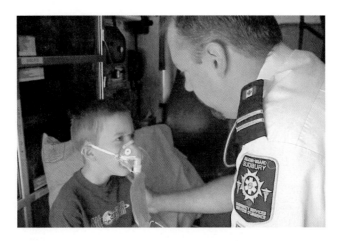

off valve of the pediatric bag-valve-mask device, if the valve is present. Consider intubation only in cases of complete airway obstruction. Transport guidelines are similar to those for cases of epiglottitis.

Foreign Body Aspiration Children—especially toddlers and preschoolers ages 1–4—like to put objects into their mouths. As a result, these children are at increased risk of aspirating foreign bodies, especially when they run or fall. In fact, foreign body aspiration is the number one cause of in-home accidental deaths in children under six years of age. In addition, many children choke on, or aspirate, food given to them by their parents or other well-meaning adults. Young children have not yet developed coordinated chewing motions in their mouth and pharynx and cannot adequately chew food. Common foods associated with aspiration and airway obstruction in children include hard candy, nuts, seeds, hot dogs, sausages, and grapes. Nonfood items include coins, balloons, and other small objects.

Assessment The child with a suspected aspirated foreign body may present in one of two ways. If the obstruction is complete, the child will have minimal or no air movement. If the obstruction is partial, the child may exhibit inspiratory stridor, a muffled or hoarse voice, drooling, pain in the throat, retractions, and cyanosis.

Management Whenever you suspect that a child has aspirated a foreign body, immediately assess the patient's respiratory efforts. If the obstruction is partial, make the child as comfortable as possible, and administer humidified oxygen. If the child is old enough, place him in a sitting position. Do not attempt to look in the mouth. Intubation equipment should be readily available, since complete airway obstruction can occur. Transport the child to a hospital, where the foreign body can be removed by hospital personnel in a controlled environment.

If the obstruction is complete, clear the airway with accepted BLS techniques. Sweep visible obstructions with your gloved finger. Do not perform blind finger sweeps, as this can push a foreign body deeper into the airway. Following BLS foreign body removal procedures, attempt ventilation with a BVM. An ACP/CCP should visualize the airway with a laryngoscope. If the foreign body is seen and readily accessible, try to remove it with Magill forceps. Intubate if possible. Transport following appropriate guidelines, avoiding any agitation of the child.

Lower-Airway Distress

As already discussed, suspect lower-airway distress when the following conditions exist: absence of stridor, presence of wheezing during exhalation, and increased work of breathing. Common causes of lower-airway distress include respiratory diseases, such as asthma, bronchiolitis, and pneumonia. Although infrequent, you may also encounter cases of foreign body lower-airway aspiration, especially in toddlers and preschoolers.

Asthma Asthma is a chronic inflammatory disorder of the lower respiratory tract. It occurs before age 10 in approximately 50 percent of the cases and before age 30 in another 33 percent of cases. The disease tends to run in families. It is also commonly associated with atopic conditions, such as eczema and allergies. Although deaths from other respiratory conditions have been steadily declining, asthmatic deaths have risen significantly in recent decades. Hospitalization of children for treatment of asthma has increased by more than 200 percent over the past 20 years. Because children can readily succumb to asthma, prompt prehospital recognition and treatment are essential. In Canada, approximately 20 children and 500 adults die each year from asthma.

Pathophysiology Asthma is a chronic inflammatory disorder of the airways, characterized by bronchospasm and excessive mucus production. In susceptible

> ### Content Review
> **COMMON CAUSES OF UPPER-AIRWAY OBSTRUCTIONS**
> - Croup
> - Epiglottitis
> - Bacterial tracheitis
> - Foreign body aspiration

✱ **asthma** a condition marked by recurrent attacks of dyspnea with wheezing due to spasmodic constriction of the bronchi, often as a response to allergens or by mucous plugs in the arterial walls.

children, this inflammation causes widespread, but variable, airflow obstruction. In addition to airflow obstruction, the airways become hyperresponsive.

Asthma may be induced by one of many different factors, commonly called "triggers." The triggers vary from one child to the next. Common triggers include environmental allergens, cold air, exercise, foods, irritants, emotional stress, and certain medications.

Within minutes of exposure to the trigger, a two-phase reaction occurs. The first phase of the reaction is characterized by the release of chemical mediators, such as histamine. These cause bronchoconstriction and bronchial edema that effectively decreases expiratory airflow, causing the classic "asthmatic attack." If treated early, asthma may respond to inhaled bronchodilators. If the attack is not aborted, or does not resolve spontaneously, a second phase may occur. The second phase is characterized by inflammation of the bronchioles as cells of the immune system invade the respiratory tract. This causes additional edema and further decreases expiratory airflow. The second phase is typically unresponsive to inhaled bronchodilators. Instead, anti-inflammatory agents, such as corticosteroids, are often required.

As the attack continues and the swelling of the mucous membranes lining the bronchioles worsens, there may be plugging of the bronchi by thick mucus. This further obstructs airflow. As a result, there is an increase in sputum production. In addition, the lungs become progressively hyperinflated, since airflow is more restricted in exhalation. This effectively reduces vital capacity and results in decreased gas exchange by the alveoli, resulting in hypoxemia. If allowed to progress untreated, hypoxemia will worsen, and unconsciousness and death may ensue.

Assessment Asthma can often be differentiated from other pediatric respiratory illnesses by the history. In many cases, there is a prior history of asthma or reactive airway disease. The child's medications may also be an indicator. Children with asthma often have an inhaler or take a theophylline or oral beta agonist preparation.

On secondary assessment, the child is usually sitting up, leaning forward, and tachypneic. Often, there is an associated unproductive cough. Accessory respiratory muscle usage is usually evident. Wheezing may be heard. However, in a severe attack, the patient may not wheeze at all. This is an ominous finding. Some children will not wheeze but will cough—often continuously. Generally, there is associated tachycardia, and this should be monitored, since virtually all medications used to treat asthma increase the heart rate.

Management The primary therapeutic goals in treating the asthmatic are to correct hypoxia, reverse bronchospasm, and decrease inflammation. First, it is imperative that you establish an airway. Next, administer supplemental, humidified oxygen as necessary. Initial pharmacological therapy is the administration of an inhaled beta agonist (Figure 42-21). All paramedic units should have the capability of administering nebulized bronchodilator medications, such as salbutamol. Alternatively, a metered-dose inhaler (MDI) may be used.

Status Asthmaticus Status asthmaticus is defined as a severe, prolonged asthma attack that cannot be broken by aggressive pharmacological management. This is a serious medical emergency, and prompt recognition, treatment, and transport are required. Often, the child suffering status asthmaticus will have a greatly distended chest from continued air trapping. Breath sounds, and often wheezing, may be absent. The patient is usually exhausted, severely acidotic, and often dehydrated. The management of status asthmaticus is basically the same as for asthma. However, you should recognize that respiratory arrest is imminent and remain prepared for endotracheal intubation. Transport should be immediate, with aggressive treatment continued en route. Subcutaneouse epinephrine may be given to a child in a pre–respiratory arrest state.

If an asthmatic attack is allowed to progress untreated, hypoxemia will worsen, and unconsciousness and death may result.

In severe asthmatic attacks, the patient may not wheeze at all. This is an ominous finding.

Subcutaneous epinephrine or terbutaline may be used when inhaled medications are poorly tolerated or are unavailable.
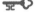

Status asthmaticus requires immediate transport with aggressive treatment administered en route.

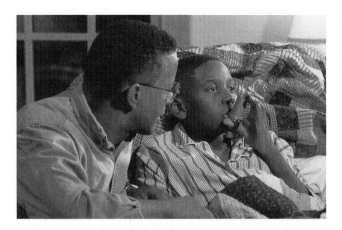

FIGURE 42-21 The young asthma patient may be making use of a prescribed inhaler to relieve symptoms. (© The Stock Market Photo Agency.)

Brochiolitis **Brochiolitis** is a respiratory infection of the medium-sized airways—the bronchioles—that occurs in early childhood. It should not be confused with bronchitis, which is an infection of the larger bronchi. Bronchiolitis is caused by a viral infection, most commonly *respiratory syncytial virus (RSV)*, that affects the lining of the bronchioles.

* **bronchiolitis** viral infection of the medium-sized airways, occurring most frequently during the first year of life.

Bronchiolitis is characterized by prominent expiratory wheezing and clinically resembles asthma. It most commonly occurs in winter in children less than two years of age. Bronchiolitis often spreads quickly through daycare and preschool facilities. Most children will develop life-long immunity to RSV following infection. The exception is the very young infant who has an immature immune system.

Assessment A history is necessary to distinguish bronchiolitis from asthma. Often, with bronchiolitis, there is a family history of asthma or allergies, although neither is yet present in the child. In addition, there is often a low-grade fever. A major distinguishing factor is age. Asthma rarely occurs before the age of one year, whereas bronchiolitis is more frequent in this age group.

Your secondary assessment should be systematic. Pay particular attention to the presence of crackles or wheezes. Also, note any evidence of infection or respiratory distress.

Management Prehospital management of suspected bronchiolitis is much the same as with asthma. Place the child in a semi-sitting position, if he is old enough, and administer humidified oxygen via a mask or by blow-by method. Ventilations should be supported as necessary. Equipment for intubation should be readily available. If respiratory distress is present, consider administration of a bronchodilator, such as salbutamol (Ventolin) by small-volume nebulizer. The cardiac rhythm should be constantly monitored. Pulse oximetry, if available, should be used continuously.

Pneumonia Pneumonia is an infection of the lower airway and lungs. It may be caused by a bacterium or a virus. Pneumonia can occur at any age, but in pediatric patients, it most commonly appears in infants, toddlers, and preschoolers aged 1–5 years. Most cases of pneumonia in children are viral and self-limiting. As children get older, they can contract bacterial pneumonias as do adults. A pneumonia vaccine is available. However, its use is reserved for patients with an immune system problem or who are asplenic.

Assessment Persons with pneumonia often have a history of a respiratory infection, such as a severe cold or bronchitis. Signs and symptoms include a low-grade fever, decreased breath sounds, crackles, rhonchi, and pain in the chest area. Conduct a systematic assessment of a patient with suspected pneumonia, paying particular attention to evidence of respiratory distress.

Management   Prehospital management of pneumonia is supportive. Place the patient in a position of comfort. Ensure a patent airway, and administer supplemental oxygen via a nonrebreather device. If respiratory failure is present, support ventilations with a bag-valve-mask device. If prolonged ventilation will be required, perform endotracheal intubation (if ACP or CCP). Transport the patient in a position of comfort. Provide emotional and psychological support to the parents.

Lower-Airway Foreign-Body Obstruction   The same pediatric patients who are at risk for upper-airway obstruction are also at risk for lower-airway obstruction. A foreign body can enter the lower airway if it is too small to lodge in the upper airway. The object is often food (nuts, seeds, candy), small toys, or parts of toys. The child will take a deep breath or will fall and accidentally aspirate the foreign body. The foreign body will fall into the lower airway until it reaches the airway that is smaller than the foreign body. Depending on positioning, the foreign body can act as a one-way valve either trapping air in distal lung tissues or preventing aeration of distal lung tissues, causing a ventilation–perfusion mismatch.

Assessment   There will often be a history that the child had a foreign body in the mouth and then it was gone. The parents may be unsure whether the child swallowed it, aspirated it, or simply lost the object. If the aspirated object was fairly large, then respiratory distress may be present. There is often considerable, often intractable, coughing. The child will be anxious and may have diminished breath sounds in the part of the chest affected by the foreign body. There may be crackles or rhonchi, usually unilateral. In some cases, there may be unilateral wheezing where some air is getting past the object. Unilateral wheezing should be considered to be due to an aspirated foreign body until proven otherwise.

Management   The management of an aspirated foreign body is supportive. Place the child in a position of comfort, and avoid agitation. Provide supplemental oxygen. Transport the child to a facility that has the capability of performing pediatric fibreoptic bronchoscopy. The bronchoscope can be used to visualize the airway and remove any foreign objects detected.

SHOCK (HYPOPERFUSION)

The second major cause of pediatric cardiopulmonary arrest—after respiratory impairment—is shock. Shock can most simply be defined as inadequate perfusion of the tissues with oxygen and other essential nutrients and inadequate removal of metabolic waste products. This ultimately results in tissue hypoxia and metabolic acidosis. Ultimately, if untreated, cellular death will occur.

When compared with the incidence of shock in adults, shock is an unusual occurrence in children because their blood vessels constrict highly efficiently. However, when blood pressure does drop, it drops so far and so fast that the child may quickly develop cardiopulmonary arrest. A number of factors place infants and young children at risk of shock. As mentioned in Chapter 41, newborns and neonates can develop shock as a result of loss of body heat. Other causes include dehydration (from vomiting and/or diarrhea), infection (particularly septicemia), trauma (especially from abdominal injuries), and blood loss. Less common causes of shock in infants and children include allergic reactions, poisoning, and cardiac events (rare).

The definitive care of shock takes place in the emergency department of a hospital. Because shock is a life-threatening condition in pediatric patients, it is important to recognize early signs and symptoms—or even the possibility of shock in a situation where signs and symptoms have not yet developed. In a situation in which you suspect a possibility of shock, provide oxygen to boost tissue perfusion, and transport the patient as quickly as possible. Also, keep him in

Content Review

COMMON CAUSES OF LOWER-AIRWAY DISTRESS

- Asthma
- Bronchiolitis
- Pneumonia
- Lower-airway foreign-body obstruction

Content Review

PREDISPOSING FACTORS OF PEDIATRIC SHOCK

- Hypothermia
- Dehydration (vomiting, diarrhea)
- Infection
- Trauma
- Blood loss
- Allergic reactions
- Poisoning
- Cardiac events (rare)

The definitive care of shock takes place in the emergency department of a hospital. However, early detection of shock by EMS personnel makes sure the patient gets to the hospital.

a supine position, and take steps to protect the child from hypothermia and agitation that might worsen the condition.

Severity of Shock

Shock is classified by degrees of severity as compensated, decompensated, and irreversible. The child responds to decreased perfusion by increasing heart rate and by increasing peripheral vascular resistance. The child has very little capacity to increase stroke volume. The key to early identification of shock is detecting the subtle signs that result from the body's various compensatory mechanisms.

Compensated Shock Early shock is known as *compensated shock* because the body is able to compensate for decreased tissue perfusion through various physiological mechanisms. In compensated shock, the patient exhibits a normal blood pressure. The signs and symptoms of compensated shock include

- Irritability or anxiety
- Tachycardia
- Tachypnea
- Weak peripheral pulses, full central pulses
- Delayed capillary refill (more than two seconds in children less than six years of age)
- Cool, pale extremities
- Systolic blood pressure within normal limits
- Decreased urinary output

A slight increase in the heart rate is one of the earliest signs of shock.

Compensated shock is generally reversible if appropriate treatment measures are instituted. Again, the key to a good outcome is prompt detection of the early signs and symptoms and initiation of therapy based on this. Management is directed at correcting the underlying problem. High-flow oxygen should be administered and venous access obtained. If the patient is hypovolemic, then fluid replacement should be initiated. If the cause is cardiogenic, then medications should be administered to support cardiac output and increase peripheral vascular resistance. Sometimes, definitive care of shock is surgical. However, in these cases, fluid therapy and oxygen administration will help buy time until the patient can be taken to surgery.

Decompensated Shock *Decompensated shock* develops when the body can no longer compensate for decreased tissue perfusion. The hallmark of decompensated shock is a fall in blood pressure (an ominous sign in children). This results in hypoperfusion and inadequate end-organ perfusion. It is important to remember that a child's compensatory mechanisms are quite efficient. Thus, when a child develops decompensated shock, there has been a significant loss of fluid or a significant impairment of cardiac output. The signs and symptoms of decompensated shock (Figure 42-22) include

The hallmark of decompensated shock is a fall in blood pressure (an ominous sign in children).

- Lethargy or coma
- Marked tachycardia or bradycardia
- Absent peripheral pulses, weak central pulses
- Markedly delayed capillary refill
- Cool, pale, dusky, mottled extremities
- Hypotension
- Markedly decreased urinary output
- Absence of tears

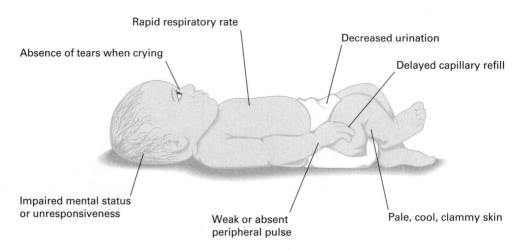

Rapid respiratory rate

Absence of tears when crying

Decreased urination

Delayed capillary refill

Impaired mental status
or unresponsiveness

Weak or absent
peripheral pulse

Pale, cool, clammy skin

FIGURE 42-22   Signs and symptoms of shock (hypoperfusion) in a child.

*The child in decompensated
shock is critically ill, and death
will ensue rapidly without
aggressive intervention.*

Decompensated shock can become irreversible if aggressive treatment measures are not undertaken. In some cases, it may be irreversible despite providing aggressive treatment measures. Management is directed at treatment of the underlying cause. You should have a low threshold for initiating mechanical ventilation with a bag-valve-mask device and 100-percent oxygen. Consider intubating the patient if mechanical ventilation will be prolonged.

Irreversible Shock *Irreversible shock* occurs when treatment measures are inadequate or too late to prevent significant tissue damage and death. Sometimes, blood pressure and pulse can be restored. However, the patient later succumbs due to organ failure. The best treatment for irreversible shock is prevention.

Categories of Shock

There are a number of ways of categorizing shock. Shock can be categorized as *cardiogenic* (caused by impaired pumping power of the heart), *hypovolemic* (caused by decreased blood or water volume), *obstructive* (caused by an obstruction that interferes with return of blood to the heart, such as a pulmonary embolism, cardiac tamponade, or tension pneumothorax), and *distributive* (caused by abnormal distribution and return of blood resulting from vasodilation, vasopermeability, or both, as in septic, anaphylactic, or neurogenic shock).

Often, shock is classified into two general categories—cardiogenic and noncardiogenic. As noted above, **cardiogenic shock** results from an inability of the heart to maintain an adequate cardiac output to the circulatory system and tissues. Cardiogenic shock in a pediatric patient is ominous and often fatal. **Noncardiogenic shock** includes types of shock that result from causes other than inadequate cardiac output. Causes may include hemorrhage, abdominal trauma, systemic bacterial infection, spinal cord injury, and others.

Noncardiogenic Shock

Noncardiogenic shock is more frequently encountered than is cardiogenic shock in prehospital pediatric care. (Recall that children have a much lower incidence

* **cardiogenic shock** the inability of the heart to meet the metabolic needs of the body, resulting in inadequate tissue perfusion.

* **noncardiogenic shock** types of shock that result from causes other than inadequate cardiac output.

of cardiac problems than have adults.) The forms that you will most commonly assess and manage are hypovolemic and distributive shock. (See also the discussion of metabolic problems in children later in the chapter.)

Hypovolemic Shock Hypovolemic shock results from loss of intravascular fluids. In pediatric patients, the most common causes include severe dehydration from vomiting and/or diarrhea and blood loss, usually as a result of trauma. Trauma may include blood loss into a body cavity (particularly the abdomen) or frank external hemorrhage. Children are also at risk of fluid loss as a result of burns, but this is not evident in the Canadian statistics. The statistics available conclude that burns are the number one cause of death among children in Canada.

Treatment of hypovolemic shock involves administration of supplemental oxygen and establishment of intravenous access. This should be followed by a 20 mL/kg bolus of Ringer's Lactate or normal saline. Following the bolus, the child should be reassessed. If signs and symptoms of compensated shock still exist, then administer a second bolus. Some children may require 80–100 mL/kg of fluid, depending on the volume of fluid lost.

Distributive Shock Distributive shock presents with a marked decrease in peripheral vascular resistance, usually due to a loss of vasomotor tone. In pediatric patients, causes include septicemia from bacterial infection, anaphylactic reaction, and damage to the brain and/or spinal cord. Cardiac output and fluid volume are adequate.

Septic Shock This condition is caused by sepsis, an infection of the bloodstream by some pathogen, usually bacterial. Sepsis commonly occurs as a complication of an infection at some other site, such as pneumonia, an ear infection, or a urinary tract infection. Meningitis is frequently associated with sepsis. The etiology can be varied, as can be the signs and symptoms.

The septic child is critically ill. Septic shock may develop when the pathogen causing the infection releases deadly toxins. These toxins cause peripheral vasodilation, leading to a drop in blood pressure and decreased tissue perfusion. Sepsis can be rapidly fatal if not promptly identified and treated.

Signs of sepsis include

- Ill appearance
- Irritability or altered mental status
- Fever
- Vomiting and diarrhea
- Cyanosis, pallor, or mottled skin
- Nonspecific respiratory distress
- Poor feeding

Signs and symptoms of septic shock include

- Very ill appearance
- Altered mental status
- Tachycardia
- Capillary refill time greater than two seconds
- Hyperventilation, leading to respiratory failure
- Cool and clammy skin
- Inability of child to recognize parents

* **hypovolemic shock** decreased amount of intravascular fluid in the body; often due to trauma that causes blood loss into a body cavity or frank external hemorrhage; in children, can be the result of vomiting and diarrhea.

* **distributive shock** marked decrease in peripheral vascular resistance with resultant hypotension; examples include septic shock, neurogenic shock, and anaphylactic shock.

Sepsis can be rapidly fatal if not promptly identified and treated. Your goal in treating sepsis is to prevent the development of septic shock.

Septic shock kills!

The child in septic shock may require pressor therapy (dopamine or epinephrine).

Your goal in treating sepsis is to prevent the development of septic shock. Supplemental oxygen should be administered and intravenous access obtained. Administer a 20 mL/kg bolus of Ringer's Lactate or normal saline. Consider initiating pressor therapy with dopamine. Begin at 2 μg/kg/min. and gradually increase the dose until the blood pressure improves or there is evidence of improved end-organ perfusion. Definitive treatment includes antibiotics and other therapy. Transport should be rapid, with care provided en route.

Anaphylactic Shock   Anaphylactic shock results from exposure to an antigen to which the patient has been previously exposed. Milder cases may simply result in an allergic reaction. More severe reactions can impair tissue perfusion. This primarily occurs as a result of the release of histamine and other similar chemicals. Histamine causes peripheral vasodilation and leakage of fluid from the intravascular space into the interstitial space. Anaphylactic shock can be differentiated from a severe allergic reaction by the presence of signs and symptoms of impaired end-organ perfusion. These include

- Tachycardia
- Tachypnea
- Wheezing
- Urticaria (hives)
- Anxiety
- Edema
- Hypotension

Allergic reactions can usually be managed with subcutaneous epinephrine 1:1000, while severe allergic reactions require intravenous epinephrine 1:10 000.

Treatment of a severe allergic reaction includes administration of subcutaneous epinephrine 1:1000. Treatment of anaphylactic shock includes supplemental oxygen administration and intravenous access. Patients not exhibiting hypotension may be given an initial dose of epinephrine subcutaneously. Salbuterol may also be given if wheezes are present from anaphylaxis.

Neurogenic Shock   Neurogenic shock is due to sudden peripheral vasodilation resulting from interruption of nervous control of the peripheral vascular system. The most common cause is injury to the spinal cord. Cardiac output and intravascular fluid volume are usually adequate.

Treatment is directed at increasing peripheral vascular resistance. This is primarily through administration of a pressor agent, such as dopamine. Care should also include stabilization of the injury and administration of supplemental oxygen.

Cardiogenic Shock

Cardiogenic shock results from inadequate cardiac output. In children, cardiogenic shock usually results from a secondary cause, such as near-drowning or a toxin ingestion. Children, unlike adults, rarely have primary cardiac disease. The exceptions are congenital heart disease and cardiomyopathy.

Congenital heart disease is an abnormality or defect in the heart that is present at birth. Many congenital cardiac problems are detected at birth. However, some may not be detected until later in life. Cardiomyopathy causes a decrease in cardiac output due to impairment of cardiac muscle contraction. Dysrhythmias, although rare in children, can cause a decrease in cardiac output. Rapid dysrhythmias may impair ventricular filling and thus cause a decrease in cardiac output. Likewise, slow dysrhythmias may cause decreased cardiac output simply due to their slow rate.

In the following sections, we will discuss in more detail congenital heart disease, cardiomyopathy, and dysrhythmias which, as noted, are primary causes of pediatric cardiogenic shock. Remember, however, cardiogenic shock in children most often results from secondary causes.

✱ **congenital** present at birth.

Congenital Heart Disease

Congenital heart disease is the primary cause of heart disease in children. As noted above, although most congenital heart problems are detected at birth, some problems may not be discovered until later in childhood. A common symptom of congenital heart disease is cyanosis. This occurs when blood going to the lungs for oxygenation mixes with blood bound for other parts of the body. This may result from holes in the internal walls of the heart or from abnormalities of the great vessels.

The child with congenital heart disease may develop respiratory distress, congestive heart failure, or a "cyanotic spell." *Cyanotic spells* occur when oxygen demand exceeds that provided by the blood. They begin as irritability, inconsolable crying, or altered mental status, and progressive cyanosis in conjunction with severe dyspnea. In severe and prolonged cases, seizures, coma, or cardiac arrest may result. Noncyanotic problems associated with congenital heart disease include respiratory distress, tachycardia, decreased end-organ perfusion, drowsiness, fatigue, and pallor.

Tetralogy of Fallot, a type of congenital heart disease with a right-to-left shunt, is often characterized by cyanotic episodes ("tet" spells) which are relieved by squatting.

Treatment includes the standard primary assessment. Administer oxygen at a high concentration. If necessary, provide ventilatory support. If the patient is having a cyanotic spell, place the child in the knee-chest position facing downward. This will help increase the cardiac return. Apply the electrocardiography (ECG) monitor, and start an intravenous line at a keep-open rate. Transport immediately.

Cardiomyopathy

Cardiomyopathy is a disease or dysfunction of the cardiac muscle. Although fairly rare, cardiomyopathy can result from congenital heart disease or infection. A frequent cause of infectious cardiomyopathy is Coxsackie virus. Cardiomyopathy causes mechanical pump failure, which is usually biventricular. It often develops slowly and is not detectable until heart failure develops.

The signs and symptoms of cardiomyopathy include early fatigue, crackles, jugular venous distension, engorgement of the liver, and peripheral edema. Later, as the disease progresses, the signs and symptoms of shock can develop.

The prehospital treatment of cardiomyopathy is supportive. Supplemental oxygen should be administered via a nonrebreather mask. Fluids should be restricted. If possible, IV access should be obtained. Severe cases resulting in the development of severe dyspnea should be treated with furosemide and pressor agents (dobutamine, dopamine). The child should be transported to a facility capable of managing critically ill children. Most cases of cardiomyopathy are managed with medication. Definitive care in severe cases may include cardiac transplantation.

Dysrhythmias

Dysrhythmias in children are uncommon. When dysrhythmias occur, bradydysrhythmias are the most common. Supraventricular tachydysrhythmias are uncommon, and ventricular tachydysrhythmias are extremely rare. Dysrhythmias can cause pump failure ultimately leading to cardiogenic shock. Children have a very limited capacity to increase stroke volume. The primary mechanism through which they increase cardiac output is through changes in the heart rate. The treatment of dysrhythmias is specific for the dysrhythmia in question.

Tachydysrhythmias Tachydysrhythmias are dysrhythmias in which the rate is greater than the estimated maximum normal heart rate for the child. These can result from primary cardiac disease or from secondary causes. Tachydysrhythmias from any cause are relatively uncommon in children.

Supraventricular Tachycardia   True supraventricular tachycardia is a narrow complex tachycardia with a heart rate of 220 per minute or greater. Supraventricular tachycardia is typically due to a problem in the cardiac conductive system. Rarely, it can be due to a secondary cause, such as drug ingestion. It is occasionally seen in infants with no prior history. The cause is uncertain but may be due to immaturity of the cardiac conductive system. Rapid heart rates often do not allow time for adequate cardiac filling, eventually causing congestive heart failure and cardiogenic shock.

The signs and symptoms of supraventricular tachycardia include irritability, poor feeding, jugular vein distension, hepatomegaly (enlarged liver), and hypotension. The ECG will show a narrow complex (supraventricular) tachycardia with a rate greater than 220 per minute. Children can often tolerate the rapid rate well.

Prehospital treatment of supraventricular tachycardia depends on the clinical findings. Children who are tolerating the heart rate (normal blood pressure) and are stable should receive supplemental oxygen and be transported. Adenosine should be considered if the child is stable. If the child is exhibiting signs of decompensation (hypotension, mental status change, poor skin colour), then synchronized cardioversion should be attempted at an initial dose of 0.5 to 1.0 joules/kg of body weight. This can be increased to 2 joules/kg if the initial shock is unsuccessful. The child should be transported to the appropriate facility.

Ventricular Tachycardia with a Pulse   Ventricular tachycardia and ventricular fibrillation are exceedingly rare in children. They are occasionally seen following drowning or following a prolonged resuscitation attempt. Unlike adults, whose ventricular tachydysrhythmias result from primary heart disease, ventricular tachydysrhythmias in children are almost always due to a secondary cause. The exception is congenital structural heart disease.

The signs and symptoms of ventricular tachycardia with a pulse include poor feeding, irritability, and a rapid, wide-complex tachycardia. Children are unable to tolerate this dysrhythmia very long. They soon develop signs of shock.

The prehospital management of ventricular tachycardia with a pulse include supplemental oxygen and intravenous access. Ventricular tachycardia due to structural heart disease often does not respond to antidysrhythmic drugs. If the patient is unstable or deteriorating, administer synchronized cardioversion at 0.5–1.0 joules/kg. This can be increased to 2 joules/kg if needed. Transport emergently, and provide care en route.

Bradydysrhythmias   Bradydysrhythmias are the most common type of pediatric dysrhythmia. They most frequently result from hypoxia. Although rare, they can also result from vagal stimulation from such causes as marked gastric distension.

The signs and symptoms of bradycardia include a slow, narrow-complex rhythm. The child may be lethargic or exhibiting early signs of congestive heart failure.

Stable children with bradydysrhythmias should receive supportive care. Unstable children should be ventilated with a bag-valve-mask unit and 100-percent oxygen. If the heart rate does not readily increase, consider endotracheal intubation. Perform chest compressions if oxygenation and ventilation do not increase the heart rate. Consider administering epinephrine or atropine down the endotracheal tube until intravenous access can be obtained. Transport emergently with care provided en route. (See the algorithm for treatment of pediatric bradycardia, Figure 42-23.)

Absent Rhythm   The absence of a cardiac rhythm is an ominous finding. Most cases are asystole. However, some cases may be a very fine ventricular fibrillation. If necessary, turn up the gain on the ECG to distinguish between the two.

Wide-complex tachycardia should be treated with amiodarone, procainamide, or lidocaine if stable. If unstable, go directly to synchronized cardioversion.

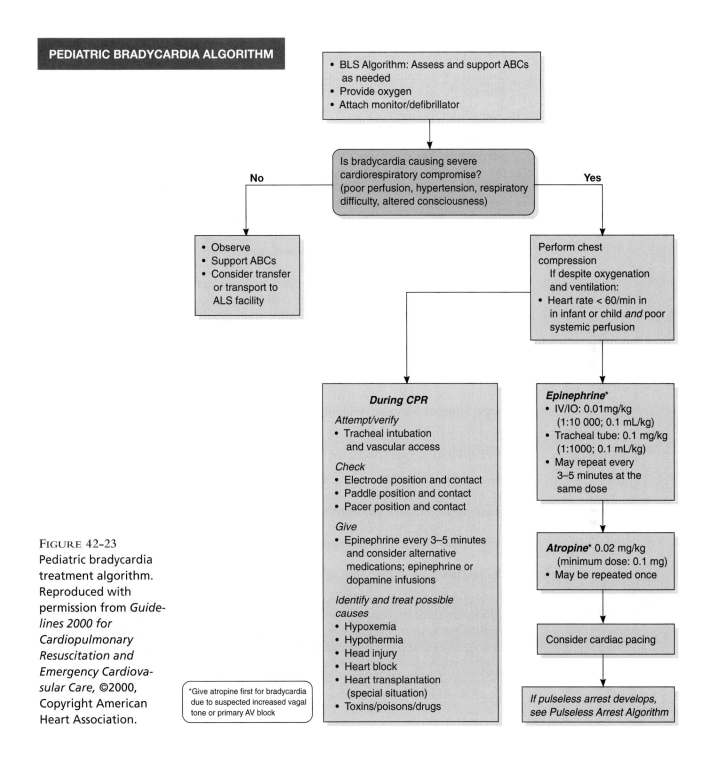

PEDIATRIC BRADYCARDIA ALGORITHM

- BLS Algorithm: Assess and support ABCs as needed
- Provide oxygen
- Attach monitor/defibrillator

Is bradycardia causing severe cardiorespiratory compromise? (poor perfusion, hypertension, respiratory difficulty, altered consciousness)

No

- Observe
- Support ABCs
- Consider transfer or transport to ALS facility

Yes

Perform chest compression
If despite oxygenation and ventilation:
- Heart rate < 60/min in in infant or child *and* poor systemic perfusion

During CPR

Attempt/verify
- Tracheal intubation and vascular access

Check
- Electrode position and contact
- Paddle position and contact
- Pacer position and contact

Give
- Epinephrine every 3–5 minutes and consider alternative medications; epinephrine or dopamine infusions

Identify and treat possible causes
- Hypoxemia
- Hypothermia
- Head injury
- Heart block
- Heart transplantation (special situation)
- Toxins/poisons/drugs

*Give atropine first for bradycardia due to suspected increased vagal tone or primary AV block

Epinephrine*
- IV/IO: 0.01mg/kg (1:10 000; 0.1 mL/kg)
- Tracheal tube: 0.1 mg/kg (1:1000; 0.1 mL/kg)
- May repeat every 3–5 minutes at the same dose

Atropine* 0.02 mg/kg (minimum dose: 0.1 mg)
- May be repeated once

Consider cardiac pacing

If pulseless arrest develops, see Pulseless Arrest Algorithm

FIGURE 42-23
Pediatric bradycardia treatment algorithm. Reproduced with permission from *Guidelines 2000 for Cardiopulmonary Resuscitation and Emergency Cardiovasular Care,* ©2000, Copyright American Heart Association.

Asystole   Asystole is the absence of a rhythm and may be the initial rhythm seen in cardiopulmonary arrest. (Remember, children rarely develop ventricular fibrillation, which is often the precursor to arrest in adults.) Bradycardias can degenerate to asystole if appropriate intervention is not provided. The mortality rate associated with asystole in children is very high.

The child with asystole is pulseless and apneic. The cardiac rhythm is a straight line that should be confirmed in two leads. Treatment is often futile. However, cardiopulmonary resuscitation (CPR) should be initiated. The patient should be intubated and ventilated with 100-percent oxygen. Chest compressions should be continued. Emergency resuscitative drugs (epinephrine) should be administered through the endotracheal tube until intravenous access can be obtained. (See the algorithm for pediatric asystole and cardiac arrest, Figure 42-24.)

Ventricular Fibrillation/Pulseless Ventricular Tachycardia   Ventricular fibrillation and pulseless ventricular tachycardia are functionally the same rhythm. They are exceedingly rare in children. Causes include electrocution and drug overdoses. The mortality rate is very high.

The child with ventricular fibrillation/pulseless ventricular tachycardia will be pulseless and apneic. The ECG will exhibit a wide-complex tachycardia or fibrillation. In unmonitored patients, provide CPR. If the patient was monitored at the time of the arrest, then defibrillate three times (2 joules/kg, then 4 joules/kg, then repeat at 4 joules/kg). Ventilate the patient with 100-percent oxygen, and intubate. Continue chest compressions. Resuscitative medications (epinephrine or lidocaine) can be administered through the endotracheal tube until intravenous access can be obtained. Transport as soon as possible.

Pulseless Electrical Activity   Pulseless electrical activity (PEA) is the presence of a cardiac rhythm without an associated pulse. This is due to noncardiogenic causes, such as hypoxia, pericardial tamponade, tension pneumothorax, trauma, acidosis, hypothermia, hypoglycemia, and others.

The patient with PEA is pulseless and apneic. Resuscitation should be directed toward correcting the underlying cause. The patient should receive CPR, be intubated and ventilated, and given the standard resuscitative medications (epinephrine). Transport should be prompt, with care provided en route.

NEUROLOGICAL EMERGENCIES

Neurological emergencies in childhood are fairly uncommon. However, seizures can and do occur in children. In fact, they are a frequent reason for summoning EMS. In addition to seizures, meningitis tends to show up more often in children than in adults. Although your chances of encountering either of these two conditions are small, both are life threatening and should be promptly identified and treated.

Seizures

Seizures result from an abnormal discharge of neurons in the brain. Many people suffer seizures, and it is a common reason that EMS is summoned. People with chronic seizure disorders can often control their seizures with medications. A seizure can be an exceptionally scary event for the parents and the child. This is especially true if the child has never had a seizure before.

Although the etiology for seizures is often unknown, several risk factors have been identified. They include

- Fever
- Hypoxia
- Infections
- Idiopathic epilepsy (epilepsy of unknown origin)
- Electrolyte disturbances
- Head trauma
- Hypoglycemia
- Toxic ingestions or exposure
- Tumour
- Central nervous system (CNS) malformations

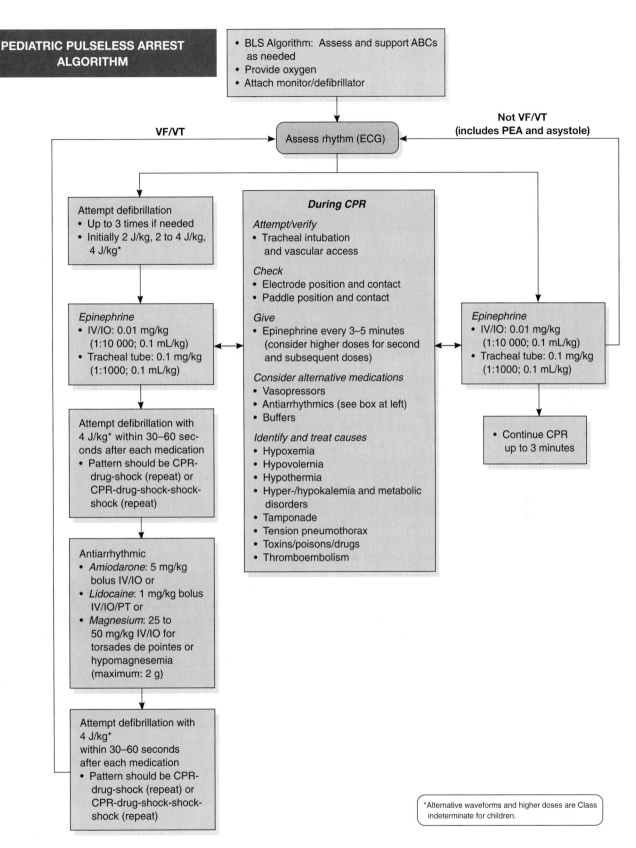

PEDIATRIC PULSELESS ARREST ALGORITHM

- BLS Algorithm: Assess and support ABCs as needed
- Provide oxygen
- Attach monitor/defibrillator

Assess rhythm (ECG)

VF/VT

Not VF/VT (includes PEA and asystole)

Attempt defibrillation
- Up to 3 times if needed
- Initially 2 J/kg, 2 to 4 J/kg, 4 J/kg*

Epinephrine
- IV/IO: 0.01 mg/kg (1:10 000; 0.1 mL/kg)
- Tracheal tube: 0.1 mg/kg (1:1000; 0.1 mL/kg)

Attempt defibrillation with 4 J/kg* within 30–60 seconds after each medication
- Pattern should be CPR-drug-shock (repeat) or CPR-drug-shock-shock-shock (repeat)

Antiarrhythmic
- *Amiodarone*: 5 mg/kg bolus IV/IO or
- *Lidocaine*: 1 mg/kg bolus IV/IO/PT or
- *Magnesium*: 25 to 50 mg/kg IV/IO for torsades de pointes or hypomagnesemia (maximum: 2 g)

Attempt defibrillation with 4 J/kg* within 30–60 seconds after each medication
- Pattern should be CPR-drug-shock (repeat) or CPR-drug-shock-shock-shock (repeat)

During CPR

Attempt/verify
- Tracheal intubation and vascular access

Check
- Electrode position and contact
- Paddle position and contact

Give
- Epinephrine every 3–5 minutes (consider higher doses for second and subsequent doses)

Consider alternative medications
- Vasopressors
- Antiarrhythmics (see box at left)
- Buffers

Identify and treat causes
- Hypoxemia
- Hypovolemia
- Hypothermia
- Hyper-/hypokalemia and metabolic disorders
- Tamponade
- Tension pneumothorax
- Toxins/poisons/drugs
- Thromboembolism

Epinephrine
- IV/IO: 0.01 mg/kg (1:10 000; 0.1 mL/kg)
- Tracheal tube: 0.1 mg/kg (1:1000; 0.1 mL/kg)

- Continue CPR up to 3 minutes

*Alternative waveforms and higher doses are Class indeterminate for children.

FIGURE 42-24   Pediatric pulseless arrest treatment algorithm. Reproduced with permission from *Guidelines 2000 for Cardiopulmonary Resuscitation and Emergency Cardiovasular Care,* ©2000, Copyright American Heart Association.

Seizures in pediatric patients may be either partial or generalized. (Recall that generalized seizures normally do not occur during the first month of life.) Simple partial seizures, sometimes called focal motor seizures, involve sudden jerking of a particular part of the body, such as an arm or a leg. Other characteristics include lip smacking, eye blinking, staring, confusion, and lethargy. There is usually no loss of consciousness. Generalized seizures involve sudden jerking of both sides of the body, followed by tenseness and relaxation of the body. In a generalized seizure, patients typically experience a loss of consciousness.

Keep in mind that children can have **status epilepticus**—a series of one or more generalized seizures without any intervening periods of consciousness. Status epilepticus is a serious medical emergency because it involves a prolonged period of apnea, which, in turn, can cause hypoxia of vital brain tissues. (For more on seizures and status epilepticus, see Chapter 29.)

Most of the pediatric seizures that you will probably encounter are febrile seizures. **Febrile seizures** are those seizures that occur as a result of a sudden increase in body temperature. They occur most commonly between the ages of six months and six years. Febrile seizures seem related to the rate at which the body temperature increases, not to the degree of fever. Often, the parents or caregivers will report the recent onset of fever or cold symptoms. The diagnosis of febrile seizure should not be made in the field. All pediatric patients suffering a seizure must be transported to the hospital so that other etiologies can be excluded.

Assessment The history is a major factor in determining seizure type. Febrile seizure should be suspected if the temperature is above 39.2°C. The history of a previous seizure may suggest idiopathic epilepsy or another CNS problem. However, there is also a tendency for recurrence of febrile seizures in children.

When dealing with a seizing child, determine whether there is a history of seizures or seizures with fever. Has the child had a recent illness? Also, determine how many seizures occurred during the incident. If the child is not seizing on your arrival, elicit a description of the seizure activity. Note the condition and position of the child when found. Question parents, caregivers, or bystanders about the possibility of head injury. A history of irritability or lethargy prior to the seizure may indicate CNS infection. If possible, find out whether the child suffers from diabetes or has recently complained of a headache or a stiff neck. Note any current medications, as well as possible ingestions.

The secondary assessment should be systematic. Pay particular attention to the adequacy of respirations, the level of consciousness, neurological evaluation, and signs of injury. Also, inspect the child for signs of dehydration. Dehydration may be evidenced by the absence of tears or, in an infant, by the presence of a sunken fontanelle.

Management Management of pediatric seizures is essentially the same as for seizing adults. Place the patient on the floor or on the bed. Be sure to lay him on his side, away from the furniture. Do not restrain him, but take steps to protect him from injury. Maintain the airway, but do not force anything, such as a bite stick, between the teeth. Administer supplemental oxygen. Then, take and record all vital signs. If the patient is febrile, remove excess layers of clothing while avoiding extreme cooling. If status epilepticus is present, institute the following steps:

- Start an IV of normal saline or Ringer's Lactate and perform a glucometer evaluation.
- Administer diazepam as follows:
  - *Children 1 month to 5 years:* 0.2–0.5 mg slowly IV push every 2–5 minutes up to a maximum of 2.5 mg.
  - *Children 5 years and older:* 5 mg IV push every 2–5 minutes to a maximum of 2 doses.

- Contact medical direction for additional dosing. Diazepam can be administered rectally if an IV cannot be established, usually twice the IV dose.

As mentioned previously, all pediatric patients should be transported. Reassure and support the parents or caregivers, since this is a very stressful and frightening situation for them.

Meningitis

Meningitis is an infection of the meninges, the lining of the brain and spinal cord. Meningitis can result from both bacteria and viruses. Viral meningitis is frequently called *aseptic meningitis,* since an organism cannot be routinely cultured from the cerebrospinal fluid (CSF). Aseptic meningitis is generally less severe than bacterial meningitis and self-limiting. Bacterial meningitis most commonly results from *Streptococcus pneumoniae, Haemophilus influenzae,* and *Neisseria meningitides.* These infections can be rapidly fatal if they are not promptly recognized and treated appropriately.

Assessment Meningitis is more common in children than in adults. Findings in the history that may suggest meningitis include a child who has been ill for one day to several days, recent ear or respiratory tract infection, high fever, lethargy or irritability, a severe headache, or a stiff neck. Infants generally do not develop a stiff neck. They will generally become lethargic and will not feed well. Some babies may simply develop a fever.

On secondary assessment, the child with meningitis will appear very ill. With an infant, the fontanelle may be bulging or full unless accompanied by dehydration. Extreme discomfort with movement, due to irritability of the meninges, may be present.

Be alert for rapid cardiopulmonary collapse in the child with fulminant meningitis, or severe meningitis with a rapid onset.

Management Prehospital care of the pediatric patient with meningitis is supportive. Rapidly complete the primary assessment, and transport the child to the emergency department. If shock is present, treat the child with intravenous fluids (20 mL/kg) and oxygen.

GASTROINTESTINAL EMERGENCIES

Childhood gastrointestinal (GI) problems almost always present with nausea and vomiting as a chief complaint. As a child gets older, other GI system emergencies, such as appendicitis, become more common.

Nausea and Vomiting

Nausea and vomiting are not diseases themselves but are symptoms of other disease processes. Virtually any medical problem can cause these conditions in an infant or child. The most common causes include fever, ear infections, and respiratory infections. In addition, many viruses and certain bacteria can infect the GI system. These infections—collectively known as *gastroenteritis*—readily cause vomiting, diarrhea, or both.

The biggest risks associated with nausea and vomiting in children are dehydration and electrolyte abnormalities. Infants and toddlers can quickly become dehydrated from bouts of vomiting. If diarrhea or fever is also present, fluid loss is further accelerated, worsening the situation. Dehydration in infants and toddlers is more difficult to detect than in older children. (See Table 42-12 for a description of the signs and symptoms of dehydration.)

Vomiting and diarrhea carry the potential for dehydration and electrolyte abnormalities— serious conditions in the pediatric patient.

Table 42-12 SIGNS AND SYMPTOMS OF DEHYDRATION

Signs/Symptoms	Mild	Moderate	Severe
Vital Signs			
Pulse	normal	increased	markedly increased
Respirations	normal	increased	tachypneic
Blood pressure	normal	normal	hypotensive
Capillary refill	normal	2–3 seconds	> 2 seconds
Mental Status	alert	irritable	lethargic
Skin	normal	dry and ashen	dry, cool, mottled
Mucous Membranes	dry	very dry	very dry/no tears

Treatment of pediatric nausea and vomiting is primarily supportive. If the child is dehydrated and unable to keep oral fluids down, intravenous fluid therapy may be indicated. Severe dehydration, as evidenced by prolonged capillary refill time, should be treated with 20 mL/kg boluses of Ringer's Lactate solution or 0.9-percent sodium chloride solution (normal saline).

Diarrhea

Diarrhea is a common occurrence in childhood. Often, what parents call diarrhea is actually loose bowel movements. Generally, 10 or more stools per day is considered diarrhea. As with nausea and vomiting, the main concern associated with diarrhea is dehydration. Often, diarrhea is due to viral infections of the GI system or secondary to infections elsewhere in the body. However, certain bacterial infections can cause significant, even life-threatening, diarrhea.

Treatment of the child suffering from diarrhea is primarily supportive. If dehydration is evident, administer fluids. Severe dehydration should be treated with 20 mL/kg boluses of intravenous fluids (Ringer's Lactate or normal saline).

METABOLIC EMERGENCIES

Metabolic problems are uncommon in children. However, diabetes can occur in very young children. It is rarely diagnosed until the child comes to the hospital in diabetic ketoacidosis. Diabetic children can have great swings in their blood glucose levels due to diet, growth, and physical activity. Because of this, hypoglycemia and hyperglycemia are possible. It is important to remember that very young children, unlike adults, can develop hypoglycemia without having diabetes. This can occur with severe illnesses, such as meningitis and pneumonia. The following section will present the prehospital treatment of pediatric hypoglycemia and hyperglycemia.

Hypoglycemia

Hypoglycemia is an abnormally low concentration of sugar (glucose) in the blood. It is a true medical emergency that must be treated immediately. Without treatment, a low blood sugar may progress to unconsciousness and convulsions.

In the prehospital setting, hypoglycemia in pediatric patients usually occurs in newborn infants and children with Type I diabetes. Diabetic children increase their risk of hypoglycemia through overly strenuous exercise, too much insulin, and dehydration from illness. Nondiabetic children can develop hypoglycemia from physical activity, diet changes, illness, and growth.

✱ hypoglycemia abnormally low concentration of glucose in the blood.

Hypoglycemia is a true medical emergency that must be treated immediately.

In known diabetics or hypoglycemics, preventive steps include

- Taking extra snacks for extra activity
- Eating immediately after taking insulin if the blood sugar is less than 5.5 mmol/L
- Eating regular meals
- Regularly monitoring blood sugar
- Eating an extra snack of carbohydrate and protein if the blood sugar is less than 6.6 mmol/L at bedtime
- Replacing carbohydrates in the meal plan with such things as regular soda pop or regular Popsicles on days when the child is sick

Assessment Suspect hypoglycemia when the patient exhibits such signs and symptoms as weakness, dizziness, tachypnea, tachycardia, pallor, sweating, tremors, vomiting, or altered mental status. Measure blood glucose with a glucometer, and elicit a history of conditions known to cause hypoglycemia in infants and children. Treatment should be initiated whenever you have a high index of suspicion and/or blood sugar level below 4.0 mmol/L.

Management As with all patients, continually monitor the ABCs. Be sure to find out if parents or caregivers have given the patient any glucose tablets, gels, foods (cake icing, honey, maple syrup, sugar, raisins), or drinks (juice, regular soda pop, milk) to correct the situation. If so, find out what was given, how much was given, and when it was given. Administer a blood glucose test.

In the conscious, alert patient, administer oral fluids with sugar or oral glucose. (Amounts are age and/or weight specific.) If there is no response or if the patient exhibits an altered level of consciousness or an unconscious state, treat according to local protocol and paramedic scope of practice. For infants less than one year old, administer 0.5 mg Glucagon subcutaneously or 2 mg/kg of $D_{25}W$. Twenty-five percent dextrose can be prepared by diluting 50 percent dextrose solution (1:1) with sterile water or saline. It is easier to dose infants with this concentration, and it does not cause as much discomfort as intravenous administration. Typical doses for children greater than one year old are weight specific. Glucagon is administered in 1-mg doses for children weighing over 20 kg and $D_{50}W$ is administered as a 1 mL/kg bolus.

In treating diabetic pediatric patients, remember that most children have been educated about their condition and can participate, in varying degrees, in their care. Most understand how glucometers work, for example, and can hand you a test strip (Figure 42-25). Also, they may be sensitive about their condition. So, avoid labelling any tests as "good" or "bad."

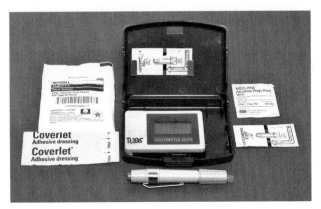

FIGURE 42-25 Many diabetic children have home glucometers to test their blood glucose levels. Older children know what the readings mean and will be curious about any glucose testing device that you may use.

Hyperglycemia

Hyperglycemia is an abnormally high concentration of blood sugar. For patients with Type I diabetes, hyperglycemia may lead to dehydration and **diabetic ketoacidosis,** a very serious medical emergency. Left untreated, the condition will deteriorate to coma. Hyperglycemia and diabetic ketoacidosis are the most common findings in new-onset diabetics.

In the prehospital setting, pediatric hyperglycemia is commonly associated with Type I diabetes. Causes include

- Eating too much food relative to injected insulin
- Missing an insulin injection
- Defective insulin pump, blockage of tubing, or disconnection of insulin pump infusion set
- Illness or stress

Hyperglycemia can occur with other severe illnesses and not necessarily mean that the child is developing diabetes mellitus.

Assessment In cases of hyperglycemia, glucose is spilled into the urine, taking water with it through osmotic diuresis. This can result in a signficant fluid loss with resultant dehydration.

Keep in mind that acidosis results from the accumulation of ketones, a by-product of fat metabolism. A continual increase in the ketones eventually leads to metabolic acidosis, which produces the fruity breath odour commonly associated with hyperglycemia. For other signs and symptoms, see Table 42-13.

As with hypoglycemia, elicit a history to determine causes linked with hyperglycemia. If possible, confirm your suspicions with blood glucose test. A blood sugar reading of greater than 11.1 mmol/L typically indicates hyperglycemia.

Management Carefully monitor the ABCs and vital signs. Confirm the presence of hyperglycemia with a blood glucose test. If intravenous access is possible, consider initiating an IV of either normal saline or Ringer's Lactate. Administer an IV bolus of 20 mL/kg, and repeat the bolus if the patient's vital signs do not change. Monitor the patient's mental status, and be prepared to intubate if the respirations continue to decrease.

Table 42-13 SIGNS AND SYMPTOMS OF HYPERGLYCEMIA

Early	Late	Ketoacidosis
Increased thirst	Weakness	Continued decreased level level of consciousness progressing to coma
Increased urination	Abdominal pain	
Weight loss	Generalized aches	Kussmaul respirations (deep and slow)
	Loss of appetite	Signs of dehydration
	Nausea	
	Vomiting	
	Signs of dehydration, except increased urinary output	
	Fruity breath odour	
	Tachypnea	
	Hyperventilation	
	Tachycardia	

Remember this is a potentially life-threatening situation. Consult with medical direction on all actions taken, and transport immediately.

POISONING AND TOXIC EXPOSURE

Accidental poisoning or toxic exposure is a common reason for summoning the EMS. Pediatric patients account for the majority of poisonings treated by the EMS. Most poisonings result from accidental ingestion of a toxic substance, usually by a young child. Toddlers and preschoolers like to taste things, especially colourful objects and substances that look like food or beverages. They also mimic their parents or caregivers, swallowing pills or drinking alcohol "just like Mommy and Daddy." Teenagers on antidepressants are also at risk of misusing or abusing their prescriptions, especially if given a one- or two-month supply of a medication.

Poisonings are the leading cause of preventable death in children under age five. Because of their immature respiratory and cardiovascular systems, even a single pill can poison or, in some cases, kill a child. Iron-containing supplements are the leading cause of poisonings, especially in toddlers and preschoolers.

The most dangerous rooms in a house in terms of poisons are the kitchen, where household cleaners are stored, and the bathroom, where many people keep their over-the-counter and prescription medications. Garages and utility rooms also contain toxic substances, attracting children when these substances are stored in everyday containers, such as coffee cans, soda bottles, or plastic cups. Living rooms may have poisonous plants and liquor bottles.

The best way to prevent pediatric poisonings is by helping the families in your communities learn how to "poison proof" their homes. Poisoning prevention should be a major goal of EMS prevention and community education programs.

Assessment Common substances involved in pediatric poisonings include

- Alcohol, barbiturates, sedatives
- Amphetamines, cocaine, hallucinogens
- Anticholinergic agents (jimson weed, belladonna products)
- Aspirin, acetaminophen
- Lead
- Vitamins and iron-containing supplements
- Corrosives
- Digitalis and beta-blockers
- Hydrocarbons
- Narcotics
- Organic solvents (inhaled)
- Organophosphates (insecticides)

Poisoning can cause many different signs and symptoms (Figure 42-26). Narcotics and some of the hydrocarbons can cause respiratory system depression. Digitalis, beta-blockers, and many of the antihypertensive agents can cause circulatory depression or collapse. The CNS can be impaired by a great many agents, including alcohol, barbiturates, narcotics, cocaine, and others. Thinking and behaviour can be affected by virtually any substance. Common agents include the anticholinergics, alcohol, narcotics, hydrocarbons, and many others. Aspirin, corrosives, and hydrocarbons can irritate or destroy the GI system. Acetaminophen can cause liver necrosis and liver failure.

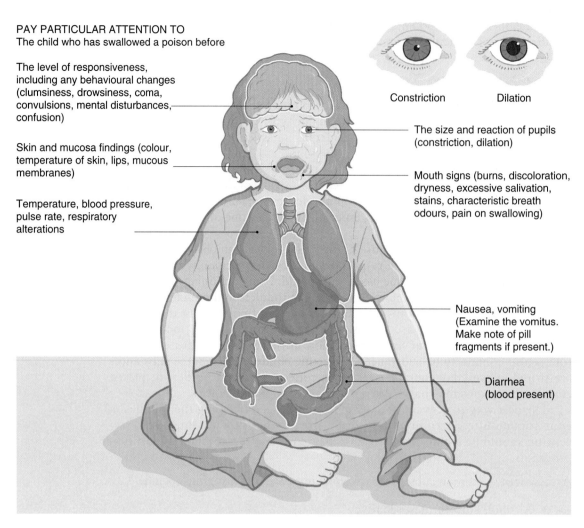

PAY PARTICULAR ATTENTION TO
The child who has swallowed a poison before

The level of responsiveness, including any behavioural changes (clumsiness, drowsiness, coma, convulsions, mental disturbances, confusion)

Skin and mucosa findings (colour, temperature of skin, lips, mucous membranes)

Temperature, blood pressure, pulse rate, respiratory alterations

Constriction   Dilation

The size and reaction of pupils (constriction, dilation)

Mouth signs (burns, discoloration, dryness, excessive salivation, stains, characteristic breath odours, pain on swallowing)

Nausea, vomiting (Examine the vomitus. Make note of pill fragments if present.)

Diarrhea (blood present)

FIGURE 42-26   Possible indicators of ingested poisoning in children.

Management Although scenarios vary, take these general steps in managing a pediatric poisoning patient:

Responsive patient

- Administer oxygen.
- Obtain IV access.
- Transport. (Be sure to take all pills, substances, and containers to the hospital.)
- Monitor the patient continuously in case the child suddenly becomes unresponsive.

Unresponsive patient

- Ensure a patent airway. Apply suctioning if necessary, and utilize airway adjuncts.
- Administer oxygen.

- Be prepared to provide artificial ventilations if respiratory failure or cardiac arrest is present.
- Contact medical direction and/or the poison control centre.
- Transport.
- Monitor the patient continuously, and rule out trauma as a cause of altered mental status.

For more on poisonings and toxic exposure, see Chapter 34.

TRAUMA EMERGENCIES

Trauma is the number one cause of death in infants and children. Most pediatric injuries result from blunt trauma. As previously mentioned, children have thinner body walls that allow forces to be more readily transmitted to body contents, increasing the possibility of injury to internal tissues and organs. If you serve in an urban area, you can expect to see a higher incidence of penetrating trauma, mostly intentional and mostly from gunfire or knife wounds. There is also a significant incidence of penetrating trauma outside the cities, mostly unintentional from hunting accidents and agricultural accidents.

MECHANISMS OF INJURY

Children tend to be more susceptible to certain types of injuries than are grownups. The following categories describe the most common mechanisms of injury among infants and children.

Falls

Falls are the single most common cause of injury in children (Figure 42-27). Fortunately, serious injury or death from accidental falls, unless from a significant height, is relatively uncommon. Falls from bicycles account for a significant number of injuries. The incidence of head injuries is declining, primarily because of bicycle safety helmets.

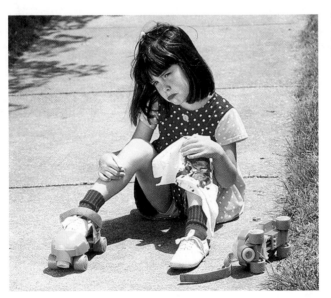

FIGURE 42-27 Falls are the most common cause of injury in young children.

Motor-Vehicle Collisions

Motor-vehicle collisions are the leading cause of traumatic death in children aged 1–14 years. In addition, motor-vehicle collisions are the leading cause of permanent brain injury and the new onset of epilepsy. Improperly seated children are at increased risk of sustaining injury or death from automobile airbags when they deploy (Figure 42-28). This is an area where EMS prevention strategies can make a difference. Public education programs on drunk driving, safe driving, airbags, and proper use of children's car seats can be a major focus of EMS personnel.

Car-versus-Pedestrian Injuries

Car-versus-child-pedestrian injuries are more common in cities, where children play close to the street. Car–pedestrian injuries are a particularly lethal form of trauma in children, as their short stature tends to push them down under the car. There are two phases of injury in car-versus-pedestrian accidents. The first group of injuries occur when the auto impacts the child. Because of the energy present, the child may be propelled away from the car or pushed down underneath the car. It is at this point that the second group of injuries occur as the child contacts the ground or other objects. Head and spinal injuries often occur with the secondary impact. The best treatment for car-versus-child-pedestrian accidents is prevention. This, too, can be a major area of emphasis for prehospital prevention programs.

Drownings and Near-Drownings

Drowning accounts for 11 percent of deaths due to unintentional injury among children and youth, ranking second after motor-vehicle collisions. The term *drowning* is used to describe deaths that occur within 24 hours of the accident. *Near-drowning* refers to incidents in which the child did not die or where the death occurred more than 24 hours after the injury. Many children who do not die from drowning suffer severe and irreversible brain injuries as a result of anoxia. Approximately 20–25 percent of near-drowning survivors exhibit severe

FIGURE 42-28 A deploying airbag can propel a child safety seat back into the vehicle's seat, seriously injuring the child secured in it.

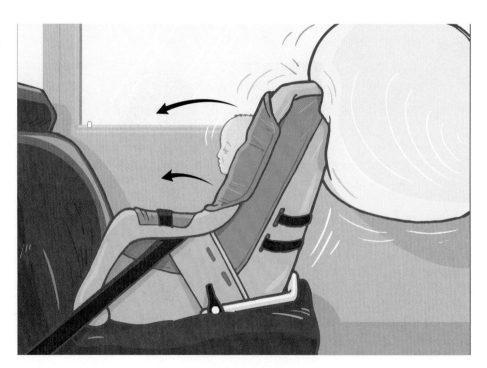

neurological deficits. The outcomes are better when the water is cold, as the body's protective mechanisms protect against brain injury.

Again, as with the other injury processes, the best treatment is prevention. EMS systems, in conjunction with local building inspectors, can inspect pools for safety. A pool should be fenced off with a gate that closes automatically. Essential rescue equipment (pole, life saver) should be immediately available, and the local emergency number must be posted. The best time for drowning-prevention education is late spring and early summer. Encourage parents to enroll their children in water safety classes as soon as possible.

Penetrating Injuries

Until 20 years ago, penetrating injuries in children were fairly uncommon. Since then, an increase in violent crime (although violent crime rates have both risen and fallen within that period) has resulted in an increasing number of children sustaining penetrating trauma. Stab wounds and firearm injuries account for approximately 10–15 percent of all pediatric trauma admissions. The risk of death increases with age. Children are usually innocent victims of crimes involving adults. However, children are sometimes the intended targets of gunfire and stabbings, as in the school shootings that have occurred recently.

It is important to remember that visual inspection of external injuries does not provide adequate evaluation of internal injuries. This is especially true with high-energy, high-velocity weapons that can cause massive internal injury with only minimal external trauma.

Paramedics can play a major role in preventing pediatric shooting accidents. During public education and community service programs, it is prudent to talk about gun safety, including such measures as using trigger locks or locking weapons in places where children cannot reach them. You might emphasize the fact that children have an uncanny ability to find and gain access to weapons that adults think they have hidden and secured. As with many other pediatric emergencies, the best treatment is prevention.

Burns

Burn injuries are the leading cause of accidental death in the home among children under 14 years of age. Children can sustain both burn injuries and smoke inhalation in house fires. Unsupervised children with matches or cigarette lighters are responsible for many fires that result in pediatric injury.

Fire prevention programs are a major area of emphasis for fire departments. The importance of smoke detectors cannot be overemphasized. People should be encouraged to change the batteries in their smoke detectors when the clock is moved backward or forward for daylight savings time. Many fire departments replace smoke detector batteries as a part of their fire prevention program. Part of the fire prevention program should be specifically directed at children. It is especially important to teach children how to exit their houses in case of a fire.

Physical Abuse

Unfortunately, children are at risk for physical abuse by adults and older children. Factors leading to child abuse are known to include social phenomena, such as poverty, domestic disturbances, younger-aged parents, substance abuse, and community violence. Paramedics are often the first members of the healthcare team to come into contact with the abused child. It is very important to not accuse the parents or to confront a suspected abuser. Instead, document all pertinent findings, treatments, and interventions, and report these to the proper authorities. (Child abuse is discussed in more detail later in this chapter.)

SPECIAL CONSIDERATIONS

As mentioned previously, children are not small adults. You should keep this in mind and modify treatment accordingly. Specific items to consider are discussed below.

Airway Control

Special considerations are related to characteristics of the child's airway. These include the following:

- Maintain in-line stabilization in neutral position instead of the sniffing position to prevent possible pinching of the trachea (Figure 42-29).
- Administer 100-percent oxygen to all trauma patients.
- Maintain a patent airway with suctioning and the jaw-thrust manoeuvre.
- Be prepared to assist ineffective respirations. Remember that airway pressures can be high in children and it may be necessary to depress the pop-off valve to ventilate the child adequately.
- Intubate the child when the airway cannot be simultaneously maintained with cervical spine stabilization (Figure 42-30).
- A gastric tube should be placed following intubation to decompress the stomach.
- Needle cricothyrostomy is rarely indicated for traumatic upper airway obstruction.

Immobilization

Use appropriate-sized pediatric immobilization equipment, including

- Rigid cervical collar
- Towel or blanket roll
- Child safety seat
- Pediatric immobilization device
- Vest-type device (KED, Kendrick Extrication Device)
- Short wooden backboard

FIGURE 42-29   In the pediatric trauma victim, use the combination of jaw-thrust/spine stabilization manoeuvre to open the airway.

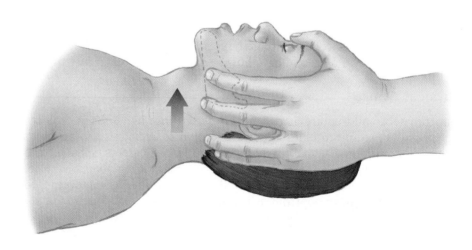

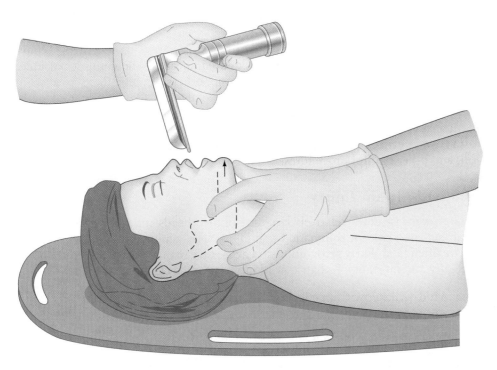

FIGURE 42-30   Simultaneous cervical spine immobilization and intubation in a pediatric patient.

- Straps and cravats
- Tape
- Padding

Keep infants, toddlers, and preschoolers supine with the cervical spine in a neutral in-line position by placing padding from the shoulders to the hips. (Review the discussion of pediatric immobilization earlier in this chapter.)

Fluid Management

Management of the airway and breathing takes priority over management of circulation, as circulatory compromise is less common in children than in adults. When obtaining vascular access, remember the following:

- If possible, insert a large-bore intravenous catheter into a peripheral vein.
- Do not delay transport to gain venous access.
- Intraosseous access in children less than six years of age is an alternative when a peripheral IV cannot be obtained.
- Administer an initial fluid bolus of 20 mL/kg of Ringer's Lactate solution or normal saline.
- Reassess the vital signs, and administer another 20 mL/kg bolus if there is no improvement.
- If improvement does not occur after the second bolus, there is likely to be a significant blood loss that may require surgical intervention. Rapid transport is essential.

Pediatric Analgesia and Sedation

An often overlooked aspect of prehospital pediatric care is pain control. Many pediatric injuries are painful, and analgesics are indicated. These injuries include burns, long-bone fractures, dislocations, and others. Unless there is a contraindication, pediatric patients should receive analgesics. Commonly used analgesics include morphine and fentanyl. Also, certain cases of pediatric emergencies may benefit from sedation. These include such problems as penetrating eye injuries, prolonged rescue from entrapment in machinery, cardioversion, and other painful procedures.

Traumatic Brain Injury

Children, because of the relatively large size of their heads and weak neck muscles, are at increased risk for traumatic brain injury. These injuries can be devastating and are often fatal. Early recognition and aggressive management can reduce both morbidity and mortality. Pediatric head injuries can be classified as follows:

- Mild—Glasgow Coma Scale (GCS) score is 13–15
- Moderate—GCS score is 9–12
- Severe—GCS score is less than or equal to 8

Traumatic head injuries can cause intracranial bleeding or swelling. This ultimately results in an increase in intracranial pressure. The signs of increased intracranial pressure can be subtle. They include

- Elevated blood pressure
- Bradycardia
- Rapid, deep respirations progressing to slow, deep respirations
- Bulging fontanelle in infants

Increased intracranial pressure will eventually lead to herniation of a portion of the brain through the foramen magnum. This is an ominous development that is often associated with irreversible injury. Signs and symptoms of herniation include

- Asymmetrical pupils
- Decorticate posturing
- Decerebrate posturing

Specific management of traumatic head injuries in children is similar to that for adults. As a rule, follow these steps:

- Administer high-concentration oxygen for mild to moderate head injuries.
- Intubate children with a GCS score less than or equal to 8 (severe head injury) and ventilate at a normal rate with 100-percent oxygen.
- Consider using intravenous or tracheal lidocaine prior to intubation to blunt the rise in intracranial pressure that often occurs in association with this procedure.

Consider hyperoxygenation if there is deterioration in the child's condition as evidenced by asymmetric pupils, active seizures, or neurological posturing. Children with traumatic head injuries do best at facilities that treat a great number of children and that have pediatric neurosurgeons on staff. Consider diverting to a pediatric trauma facility if a moderate or severe traumatic head injury is present.

SPECIFIC INJURIES

As previously mentioned, more pediatric patients die of trauma than of any other cause. Statistics reveal that nearly 50 percent of these deaths occur within the first hour of injury. The quick arrival of EMS at the scene can literally mean the difference between life and death for a child. Although management of trauma is basically the same for children as for adults, anatomical and physiological differences cause different patterns of injury in pediatric patients.

Head, Face, and Neck

The majority of children who sustain multiple trauma will suffer associated head and/or neck injuries. As previously mentioned, the larger relative mass of the head and lack of neck muscle strength provide for increased momentum in acceleration-deceleration injuries and a greater stress on the cervical spine. The fulcrum of cervical mobility in the younger child is at the C2–C3 level. As a result, nearly 60–70 percent of pediatric fractures occur in C1–C2.

Injuries to the head are the most common cause of death in pediatric trauma victims. School-age children tend to sustain head injuries from bicycle accidents, falls from trees, or auto–pedestrian accidents. Older children most commonly suffer head injuries from sporting events. Heads injuries in all age groups may result from abuse.

In treating head injuries, remember that diffuse injuries are common in children, while focal injuries are rare. Because the skull is softer and more compliant in children than in adults, brain injuries occur more readily in infants and young children. Because of open fontanelles and sutures, infants up to an average age of 16 months may be more tolerant to an increase in intracranial pressure and can have delayed signs. (Keep this fact in mind when taking the history of children in the one-month to two-year age range.)

Children also frequently injure their faces. The most common facial injuries are lacerations secondary to falls. Young children are uncoordinated when they first start walking. A fall onto a sharp object, such as the corner of a coffee table, can result in a laceration. Older children sustain dental injuries in falls from bicycles, skateboard accidents, fights, and sports activities.

Spinal injuries in children are not as common as in adults. However, as discussed earlier, a child's proportionately larger and heavier head makes the cervical spine vulnerable to injury. Any time a child sustains a severe head injury, always assume that a neck injury may also be present.

Chest and Abdomen

Most injuries to the chest and abdomen result from blunt trauma. As noted earlier, infants and young children lack the rigid rib cages of adults. Therefore, they suffer fewer rib fractures and more intrathoracic injuries. Likewise, their relatively undeveloped abdominal musculature affords minimal protection to the viscera.

Because of the high mortality associated with blunt trauma, children with significant blunt abdominal or chest trauma should be transported immediately to a pediatric trauma centre with appropriate care provided en route.

Injuries to the Chest Chest injuries are the second most common cause of pediatric trauma deaths. Because of the compliance of the chest wall, severe intrathoracic injury can be present without signs of external injury. Pneumothorax and hemothorax can occur in the pediatric patient, especially if the mechanism of injury was a motor vehicle collision. Tension pneumothorax can also occur in children. The condition is poorly tolerated by pediatric patients and a needle

Children tend to develop pulmonary contusions, sometimes massive, following blunt trauma to the chest.

thoracostomy may be life saving. Tension pneumothorax presents with the following signs and symptoms:

- Diminished breath sounds over the affected lung
- Shift of the trachea to the opposite side
- A progressive decrease in ventilatory compliance

Keep in mind that children with cardiac tamponade may have no physical signs of tamponade other then hypotension. Also, remember that flail chest is an uncommon injury in children. When noted without a significant mechanism of injury, suspect child abuse.

Injuries to the Abdomen Significant blunt trauma to the abdomen can result in injury to the spleen or liver. In fact, the spleen is the most commonly injured organ in children. Signs and symptoms of a splenic injury include tenderness in the left upper quadrant of the abdomen, abrasions on the abdomen, and hematoma of the abdominal wall. Symptoms of liver injury include right upper quadrant abdominal pain and/or right lower chest pain. Both splenic and hepatic injuries can cause life-threatening internal hemorrhage.

In treating blunt abdominal trauma, keep in mind the small size of the pediatric abdomen. Be certain to palpate only one quadrant at a time. In cases of both chest and abdominal trauma, treat for shock with positioning, fluids, and maintenance of body temperature.

Extremities

Extremity injuries in children are typically limited to fractures and lacerations. Children rarely sustain amputations and other serious extremity injuries. An exception includes farm children who are vulnerable to becoming entangled in agricultural equipment.

The most common injuries are fractures, usually resulting from falls. Because children have more flexible bones than adults do, they tend to have incomplete fractures, such as **bend fractures, buckle fractures,** and **greenstick fractures.** In younger children, the bone growth plates have not yet closed. Some types of growth plate fractures can lead to permanent disability if not managed correctly.

Whenever indicated, perform splinting in order to decrease pain and prevent further injury and/or blood loss.

Burns

Burns are the second leading cause of death in children. They are the leading cause of accidental death in the home for children under 14. Burns may be chemical, thermal, or electrical. The most common type of burn injury encountered by EMS personnel is scalding. Children can scald themselves by pulling hot liquids off tables or stoves. In cases of abuse, they can be scalded by immersion in hot water.

Estimation of the burn surface area (BSA) is slightly different for children from that for adults (Figure 42-31). In adults, the "rule of nines" assigns 9 percent of the BSA to each of 11 body regions: the entire head and neck; the anterior chest; the anterior abdomen; the posterior chest; the lower back (posterior abdomen); the anterior surface of each lower extremity; the posterior surface of each lower extremity; and the entirety of each upper extremity. The remaining 1 percent is assigned to the genitalia.

In a child, the head accounts for a larger percentage of BSA, while the legs make up a smaller percentage. So, for children, the rule of nines is modified to take away 8 percent from the lower extremities (2 percent from the front and 2 percent from the back of each leg) plus the 1 percent assigned to the adult geni-

* **bend fractures** fractures characterized by angulation and deformity in the bone without an obvious break.

* **buckle fractures** fractures characterized by a raised or bulging projection at the fracture site.

* **greenstick fractures** fractures characterized by an incomplete break in the bone.

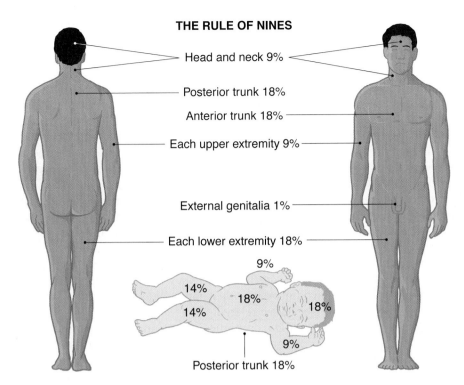

THE RULE OF NINES

Head and neck 9%

Posterior trunk 18%

Anterior trunk 18%

Each upper extremity 9%

External genitalia 1%

Each lower extremity 18%

9%

14%

18%

14%

18%

9%

Posterior trunk 18%

FIGURE 42-31   The rule of nines helps estimate the extent of a burn in adults and children. Note the modifications for the child.

talia. This 9 percent that is taken from the lower part of the body is reassigned to the head. So, whereas the adult's entire head and neck are counted as 9 percent, in the child, the anterior head and neck count as 9 percent and the posterior head and neck count as another 9 percent.

You can also use the child's palm as a guide (the "rule of palm"). The palm equals about 1 percent of the BSA. You can calculate a burn area by estimating how many palm areas it equals. Usually, the rule of nines works best for more extensive burns. The rule of palm works best for less extensive ones.

Management considerations for pediatric burn patients include the following:

- Provide prompt management of the airway, as swelling can develop rapidly.
- If intubation is required, you may need to use an endotracheal tube up to two sizes smaller than normal.
- Children with thermal burns are very susceptible to hypothermia. Be sure to maintain body heat.
- When treating serious electrical burn patients, suspect musculoskeletal injuries, and perform spinal immobilization.

SUDDEN INFANT DEATH SYNDROME (SIDS)

Sudden infant death syndrome (SIDS) is defined as the sudden death of an infant during the first year of life from an illness of unknown etiology. The incidence of SIDS in Canada is approximately 1 death per 2000 births. SIDS is the leading cause of death between two weeks and one year of age. It is responsible for a

✳ **sudden infant death syndrome (SIDS)** illness of unknown etiology that occurs during the first year of life, with the peak at ages 2–4 months.

significant number of deaths between 1 and 6 months, with peak incidence occurring at 2–4 months. SIDS is the leading cause of death in Canada for infants between the ages of one month and one year, claiming three babies every week.

SIDS occurs most frequently in the fall and winter months. It tends to be more common in males than in females. It is more prevalent in premature and low-birth-weight infants, in infants of young mothers, and in infants whose mothers did not receive prenatal care. Infants of mothers who used cocaine, methadone, or heroin during pregnancy are at greater risk. Occasionally, a mild upper respiratory infection will be reported prior to the death. SIDS is not caused by external suffocation from blankets or pillows. Neither is it related to allergies to cow's milk or regurgitation and aspiration of stomach contents. It is not thought to be hereditary.

Current theories vary about the etiology of SIDS. Some authorities feel it may result from an immature respiratory centre in the brain that leads the child to simply stop breathing. Others think there may be an airway obstruction in the posterior pharynx as a result of pharyngeal relaxation during sleep, a hyper-mobile mandible, or an enlarged tongue. Studies strongly link SIDS to a prone sleeping position. Soft bedding, waterbed mattresses, adults smoking in the home, and/or an overheated environment are other potential associations. A small percentage of SIDS cases may be abuse related.

Although research into SIDS continues, the Canadian Pediatric Society (www.cps.ca) suggests that infants be placed in the supine position unless medical conditions prevent this. In addition, the academy urges parents or caregivers to avoid smoking before and after pregnancy, placing infants in overheated environments, overwrapping them with too many clothes or blankets, and filling the crib with soft bedding.

Assessment Autopsies of infants dying due to SIDS show similar physical findings. Externally, there is a normal state of nutrition and hydration. The skin may be mottled. There are often frothy, occasionally blood-tinged, fluids in and around the mouth and nostrils. Vomitus may be present. Occasionally, the infant may be in an unusual position as a result of muscle spasm or high activity at the time of death. Other common findings noted at autopsy include intrathoracic petechiae (small hemorrhages) in 90 percent of cases. There is often associated pulmonary congestion and edema. Sometimes, stomach contents are found in the trachea. Microscopic examination of the trachea often reveals the presence of inflammatory changes.

Management The immediate needs of the family with a SIDS baby are many. Unless the infant is obviously dead, undertake active and aggressive care of the infant to assure the family that everything possible is being done. Other personnel should be assigned to assist the parents and to explain the procedures. At all points, use the baby's name.

After arrival at the hospital, direct management at the parents or caregivers, since nothing can be done for the child. Allow the family to see the dead child. Expect a normal grief reaction. Initially, there may be shock, disbelief, and denial. Other times, the parents or caregivers may express anger, rage, hostility, blame, or guilt. Often, there is a feeling of inadequacy as well as helplessness, confusion, and fear. The grief process is likely to last for years. SIDS has major long-term effects on family relations. It may also affect you, the on-scene paramedic. If so, do not be reluctant to request a Critical Incident Stress Debriefing.

Active and aggressive care of the infant should continue until delivery to the emergency room unless the infant is obviously dead.

At all points in a SIDS case, use the baby's name when speaking with parents or caregivers.

CHILD ABUSE AND NEGLECT

A tragic fact is that some people cause physical and psychological harm to children, either through intentional abuse or through intentional or unintentional neglect. In fact, child abuse is the second leading cause of death in infants less than six months of age. In Canada, in 1998, there were 135 573 child maltreatment investigations, and abuse was confirmed in 45 percent of the cases.

There are several characteristics common to abused children. Often, the child is seen as "special" and different from others. Premature infants and twins stand a higher risk of abuse than other children. Many abused children are less than five years of age. Children with physical or mental disabilities as well as those with other special needs are also at greater risk. So are uncommunicative (autistic) children. Boys are more often abused than girls. A child who is not what the parents wanted (e.g., the "wrong" gender) is at increased risk of abuse, too.

PERPETRATORS OF ABUSE OR NEGLECT

Abuse or neglect may be instigated by a parent, a legal guardian, or a foster parent. It can be carried out by a person, an institution, or an agency or program entrusted with custody. Abuse or neglect can also result from the actions of a caregiver, such as a babysitter or a "nanny."

The person who abuses or neglects a child can come from any geographic, religious, ethnic, racial, occupational, educational, or socioeconomic background. Despite their diversity, people who abuse children tend to share certain traits. The abuser is usually a parent or a full-time caregiver. When the mother spends the majority of the time with the child, she is the parent most frequently identified as the abuser. Most abusers were abused themselves as children.

Three conditions can alert you to the potential for abuse:

- A parent or adult who seems capable of abuse—especially one who exhibits evasive or hostile behaviour
- A child in one of the high-risk categories
- The presence of a crisis, particularly financial stress, marital or relationship stress, or physical illness in a parent or child

TYPES OF ABUSE

Child abuse can take several forms. These forms include

- Psychological abuse
- Physical abuse
- Sexual abuse
- Neglect (either physical or emotional)

Abused children suffer every imaginable kind of maltreatment. They are battered with fists, belts, broom handles, hair brushes, baseball bats, electric cords, and any other objects that can be used as weapons (Figure 42-32). They are locked in closets, denied food, or deprived of access to a toilet. They are intentionally burned or scalded with anything from hot water to cigarette butts to open flames (Figure 42-33). They are severely shaken, thrown into cribs, pushed down stairs, or shoved into walls. Some are shot, stabbed, or suffocated.

Sexual abuse ranges from adults exposing themselves to children to overt sexual acts to sexual torture. Sexual abuse can occur at any age, and the victims may be male or female. Generally, the sexual abuser is someone the child knows and, perhaps, trusts. Stepchildren or adopted children face a greater risk for sexual abuse than do biological children. Cases in which sexual abuse causes physical harm may get reported. Other cases, especially those with emotional or minor physical injury, may go undetected.

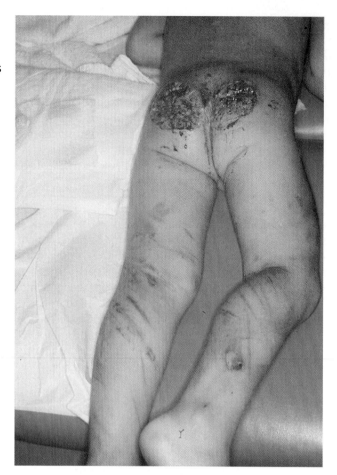

FIGURE 42-32   An abused child. Note the marks on the legs associated with beatings with an electric wire. The burns on the buttocks are from submersion in hot water. (Courtesy of Scott and White Hospital and Clinic.)

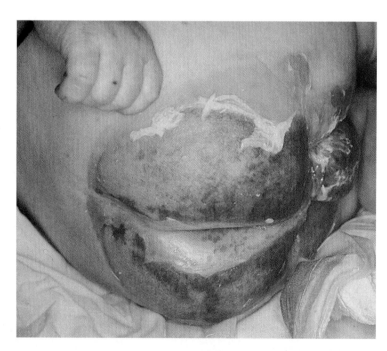

FIGURE 42-33   Burn injury from placing a child's buttocks in hot water as a punishment. (Courtesy of Scott and White Hospital and Clinic.)

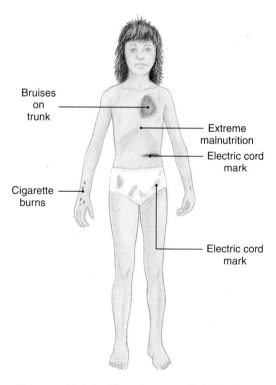

Bruises on trunk

Extreme malnutrition

Electric cord mark

Cigarette burns

Electric cord mark

FIGURE 42-34   The stigmata of child abuse.

ASSESSMENT OF THE POTENTIALLY ABUSED OR NEGLECTED CHILD

Signs of abuse or neglect can be startling (Figure 42-34, previous page). As a guide, the following findings should trigger a high index of suspicion:

- Any obvious or suspected fractures in a child under two years of age
- Multiple injuries in various stages of healing, especially burns and bruises (Figure 42-35)
- More injuries than usually seen in children of the same age or size
- Injuries scattered on many areas of the body
- Bruises or burns in patterns that suggest intentional infliction
- Increased intracranial pressure in an infant
- Suspected intra-abdominal trauma in a young child
- Any injury that does not fit with the description of the cause given

Information in the medical history may also raise the index of suspicion. Examples include

- A history that does not match the nature or severity of the injury
- Vague parental accounts or accounts that change during the interview
- Accusations that the child injured himself intentionally
- A delay in seeking help
- A child dressed inappropriately for the situation
- Revealing comments by bystanders, especially siblings

Suspect child neglect if you spot any of the following conditions:

- Extreme malnutrition
- Multiple insect bites
- Longstanding skin infections
- Extreme lack of cleanliness
- Verbal or social skills far below those you would expect for a child of similar age and background
- Lack of appropriate medical care (Figure 42-36)

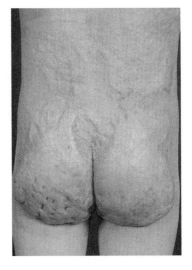

FIGURE 42-35 The effects of child abuse, both physical and mental, can last a lifetime. (Courtesy of Scott and White Hospital and Clinic.)

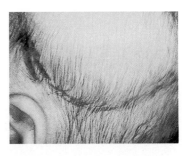

FIGURE 42-36 Child neglect from a lack of appropriate medical care.

MANAGEMENT OF THE POTENTIALLY ABUSED OR NEGLECTED CHILD

In cases of child abuse or neglect, the goals of management include appropriate treatment of injuries, protection of the child from further abuse, and notification of proper authorities. You should obtain as much information as possible, in a nonjudgmental manner. Document all findings or statements in the patient report. Do not "cross-examine" the parents—this job belongs to the police or other authorities. Try to be supportive toward the parents, especially if it helps you transport the child to the hospital. Remember: Never leave transport to the alleged abuser.

On arrival at the emergency department, report your suspicions to the appropriate personnel. Complete the patient report and all available documentation at this time, since delay may inhibit accurate recall of data.

Never leave transport of an abused child to an alleged abuser.

In Canada paramedics are required by law to report suspected child abuse or neglect to the appropriate authorities.

Child abuse and neglect are particularly stressful aspects of emergency medical services. You must recognize and deal with your feelings, perhaps taking them up at a Critical Incident Stress Debriefing.

RESOURCES FOR ABUSE AND NEGLECT

You can contact your local child protection agency for additional information on child abuse. Consider taking a course in the recognition of child abuse and neglect. These are often offered by children's hospitals. The Internet has several sites that provide up-to-date information on child abuse.

INFANTS AND CHILDREN WITH SPECIAL NEEDS

For most of human history, infants and children with devastating congenital conditions or diseases either died or remained confined to a hospital. In recent decades, however, medical technology has lowered infant mortality rates and allowed a greater number of children with special needs to live at home. (See more about home care in Chapter 46.) Some of these infants and children include

- Premature babies
- Infants and children with lung disease, heart disease, or neurological disorders
- Infants and children with chronic diseases, such as cystic fibrosis, asthma, childhood cancers, cerebral palsy, and others
- Infants and children with altered functions from birth (Examples include cerebral palsy, spina bifida, and other congenital birth defects.)

In caring for these children, family members receive education relative to the special equipment required by the infant or child. Even so, they may feel a great deal of apprehension when care moves from the hospital to the home. As a result, they may summon the EMS at the first indication of trouble. This is especially true in the initial weeks following discharge.

COMMON HOME CARE DEVICES

Devices you might commonly find in the home include tracheostomy tubes, apnea monitors, home artificial ventilators, central intravenous lines, gastric feeding tubes, gastrostomy tubes, and shunts. In treating children with special needs, remember that the parents and caregivers are often highly knowledgeable about their children and the devices that sustain their lives. Listen to them. They know their children better than anybody else.

Tracheostomy Tubes

* **tracheostomy** a surgical incision in the neck held open by a metal or plastic tube.

Patients who are on prolonged home ventilators or who have chronic respiratory problems may have surgically placed tubes in the inferior trachea (Figure 42-37). A **tracheostomy** (trach) tube may be utilized as a temporary or a permanent device. Although there are various types of tubes, you might expect some common complications. They include

- Obstruction, usually by a mucus plug

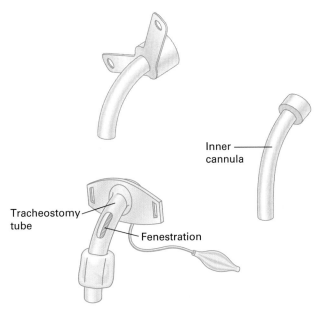

Inner cannula

Tracheostomy tube

Fenestration

- Site bleeding, either from the tube or around the tube
- An air leakage
- A dislodged tube
- Infection—a condition that will worsen an already impaired breathing function

Management steps for a patient with a tracheostomy include

- Maintaining an open airway
- Suctioning the tube as needed
- Allowing the patient to remain in a position of comfort if possible
- Administering oxygen in cases of respiratory distress
- Assisting ventilations in cases of respiratory failure/arrest by
  - Intubating orally in the absence of an upper-airway obstruction
  - Intubating via the **stoma** if there is an upper-airway obstruction
- Transporting the patient to the hospital

✳ stoma a permanent surgical opening in the neck through which the patient breathes.

Apnea Monitors

Apnea monitors are used to alert parents or caregivers to the cessation of breathing in an infant, especially a premature infant. Some types of monitors signal changes in heart rate, such as bradycardia or tachycardia. They operate via pads attached to the baby's chest and connected to the monitor by wires. If the device does not detect a breath within a specific time frame or if the infant's heart rate is too slow or too fast, an alarm will sound.

When an apnea monitor is placed in a home, the parents are typically instructed on what to do if the alarm sounds (stimulate the child, provide artificial respirations, and so on). If these fail, the EMS may be summoned. Also, nervous parents who have just brought home a baby on an apnea monitor may panic the first couple of times the alarm sounds and call 911. Be patient and kind while instructing them on what to do when the alarm sounds.

Most parents who have infants on apnea monitors have received training in pediatric CPR.

Home Artificial Ventilators

Various configurations exist for home ventilators. Demand ventilators sense the rate and quality of a patient's respiration as well as several other parameters, including pulse oximetry. They typically respond to preset limits. Other devices provide a constant PEEP (positive end-expiratory pressure) and a set oxygen concentration for the patient.

Two complications commonly result in EMS calls: (1) a device's mechanical failure, and (2) shortages of energy during an electrical failure. Treatment typically includes

- Maintaining an open airway
- Administering artificial ventilations via an appropriate-sized BVM with oxygen
- Transporting the patient to hospital care while the home ventilator is being repaired

Central Intravenous Lines

Children who require long-term IV therapy will often have central lines placed into the superior vena cava near the heart. In cases where IV therapy is necessary for only several weeks, PIC (percutaneous intravenous catheter) lines may be placed in the arm and threaded into the superior vena cava. Otherwise, the lines are placed through subclavian venipuncture. **Central IV lines** are commonly used to administer intravenous nutrition, antibiotics, or chemotherapy for cancer.

Possible complications for central IV lines include

* **central IV line** intravenous line placed into the superior vena cava for the administration of long-term fluid therapy.

- Cracked line
- Infection, either at the site or at more distal aspects of the line
- Loss of patency—for example, clotting
- Hemorrhage, which can be considerable
- Air embolism

Emergency medical care steps include control of any bleeding through direct pressure. If a large amount of air is in the line, try to withdraw it with a syringe. If this fails, clamp the line, and transport the patient. In cases of a cracked line, place a clamp between the crack and the patient. If the patient exhibits an altered mental status following the cracked line, position the child on the left side with head down. Transport the child to the hospital as quickly as possible.

Gastric Feeding Tubes and Gastrostomy Tubes

Children who are unable to swallow or eat receive nutrition through a gastric feeding tube or a gastrostomy tube. (A gastric feeding tube is placed through the nostrils into the stomach. A gastrostomy tube is placed through the abdominal wall directly into the stomach.) These special devices are commonly used in disorders of the digestive system or in situations in which the developmental ability of the patient hinders feeding. Food consists of nutritious liquids.

Possible emergency complications include

- Bleeding at the site
- Dislodged tube

- Respiratory distress, particularly if a tube feeding backs up into the esophagus and is aspirated into the trachea and lungs

- In the case of diabetics, altered mental status due to missed feedings

Emergency medical care involves supporting the ABCs, including possible suctioning and administration of supplemental oxygen. Patients should be transported to a definitive care facility, either in a sitting position or lying on the right side with the head elevated. The goal is to reduce the risk of aspiration, a serious condition.

Shunts

A **shunt** is a surgical connection that runs from the brain to the abdomen. It removes excess cerebrospinal fluid from the brain through drainage. A subcutaneous reservoir is usually palpable on one side of the patient's head. A pathological rise in intracranial pressure, secondary to a blocked shunt, is a primary complication. Shunt failure may also result when the shunt's connections separate, usually because of a child's growth.

Cases of shunt failure present as altered mental status. The patient may exhibit drowsiness, respiratory distress, or the classic signs of pupil dysfunction or posturing. Be aware that an altered mental status may be caused by infection—a distinction to be made in a hospital setting.

Care steps involve maintenance of an open airway, administration of ventilations as needed, and immediate transport. Shunt failures require correction in the operating room, where the cerebrospinal fluid can be drained or, in rare cases, an infection identified and treated.

✱ shunt surgical connection that runs from the brain to the abdomen for the purpose of draining excess cerebrospinal fluid, thus preventing increased intracranial pressure.

GENERAL ASSESSMENT AND MANAGEMENT PRACTICES

Remember that pediatric patients with special needs require the same assessment as other patients. Always evaluate the airway, breathing, and circulation. (Recall that in the primary assessment, "disability" refers to patient's neurological status—not to the child's special need.) If you discover life-threatening conditions in the primary assessment, begin appropriate interventions. Keep in mind that the child's special need is often an ongoing process. In most cases, you should concentrate on the acute problem.

During the assessment, ask pertinent questions of the patient, parent, or caregiver, such as: "What unusual situation caused you to call for an ambulance?" As already mentioned, the parent or caregiver is usually very knowledgeable about the patient's condition.

In most cases, the secondary assessment is essentially the same as with other patients. It is important to explain everything that is being done, even if the patient does not seem to understand. Do not be distracted by the special equipment. Be aware of the help that the patient, parent, or caregiver may be able to provide in handling home care devices.

In managing patients with special needs, try to keep several thoughts in mind.

- Avoid using the term "disability" (in reference to the child's special need). Instead, think of the patient's many abilities.

- Never assume that the patient cannot understand what you are saying.

Remember that pediatric patients with special needs require the same assessment as other patients.

In most cases, concentrate on the acute problem, rather than the ongoing special need.

- Involve the parents, caregivers, and the patient, if appropriate, in treatment. They manage the illness or congenital condition on a daily basis.
- Treat the patient with a special need with the same respect as you would any other patient.

SUMMARY

Pediatric emergencies can be stressful for both you and the adults responsible for the child's well-being. Most pediatric emergencies result from trauma, respiratory distress, ingestion of poisons, or febrile seizure activity. In addition, you must always be on the lookout for signs and symptoms of child abuse or neglect. The approach and management of pediatric emergencies must be modified for the age and size of the child. Certain skills generally considered routine, such as IV administration, become difficult in the pediatric patient because of size and other factors. It is important to remember that children are not "small adults." They have special considerations—both physical and emotional—that must be managed accordingly.

CHAPTER 43

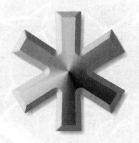

Geriatric Emergencies

Objectives

_____

After reading this chapter, you should be able to:

1. Discuss the demographics demonstrating the increasing size of the elderly population in Canada. (pp. 1023–1025)
2. Assess the various living environments of elderly patients. (p. 1024)
3. Discuss society's view of aging and the social, financial, and ethical issues facing the elderly. (p. 1024)
4. Discuss common emotional and psychological reactions to aging, including causes and manifestations. (pp. 1023–1029)

5. Apply the pathophysiology of multisystem failure to the assessment and management of medical conditions in the elderly patient. (p. 1026)
6. Compare the pharmacokinetics of an elderly patient with those of a young patient, including drug distribution, metabolism, and excretion. (pp. 1026–1027)
7. Discuss the impact of polypharmacy, dosing errors, increased drug sensitivity, and medication noncompliance on the assessment and management of the elderly patient (pp. 1026–1027)

Continued

8. Discuss the use and effects of drugs commonly prescribed to the elderly patient (pp. 1026–1027, 1064–1066)
9. Discuss the problem of mobility in the elderly and develop strategies to prevent falls. (pp. 1027–1028)
10. Discuss age-related changes in sensations in the elderly and describe the implications of these changes for communication and patient assessment. (pp. 1028, 1031–1033)
11. Discuss the problems with continence and elimination in the elderly patient and develop communication strategies to provide psychological support. (pp. 1028–1029)
12. Discuss factors that may complicate the assessment of the elderly patient. (pp. 1026, 1030–1034)
13. Discuss the principles that should be employed when assessing and communicating with the elderly. (pp. 1028, 1030–1034)
14. Compare the assessment of a young patient with that of an elderly patient. (pp. 1030–1031, 1035–1041)
15. Discuss the common complaints of elderly patients. (pp. 1026, 1041–1068)
16. Discuss the normal and abnormal changes of age in relation to the:
    a. Pulmonary system (pp. 1035–1037)
    b. Cardiovascular system (pp. 1037–1038)
    c. Nervous system (p. 1038)
    d. Endocrine system (pp. 1038, 1039)
    e. Gastrointestinal (GI) system (p. 1039)
    f. Thermoregulatory system (p. 1039)
    g. Integumentary system (pp. 1040, 1057)
    h. Musculoskeletal system (pp. 1040, 1058)
17. Describe the incidence, morbidity/mortality, risk factors, prevention strategies, pathophysiology, assessment, need for intervention and transport, and management for elderly medical patients with
    a. Pneumonia, chronic obstructive disease, and pulmonary embolism (pp. 1042–1045)
    b. Myocardial infarction, heart failure, dysrhythmias, aneurysm, and hypertension (pp. 1045–1049)
    c. Cerebral vascular disease, delirium, dementia, Alzheimer's disease, and Parkinson's disease (pp. 1049–1054)
    d. Diabetes and thyroid diseases (pp. 1054–1055)
    e. GI problems, GI hemorrhage, and bowel obstruction (pp. 1055–1057)
    f. Skin diseases and pressure ulcers (p. 1057–1058)
    g. Osteoarthritis and osteoporosis (pp. 1058)
    h. Hypothermia and hyperthermia (pp. 1061–1062)
    i. Toxicological problems, including drug toxicity, substance abuse, alcohol abuse, and drug abuse (pp. 1062–1066)
    j. Psychological disorders, including depression and suicide (pp. 1066–1068)
18. Describe the incidence, morbidity/mortality, risk factors, prevention strategies, pathophysiology, assessment, need for intervention and transport, and management of the elderly trauma patient with
    a. Orthopedic injuries (pp. 1071–1072)
    b. Burns (pp. 1072–1073)
    c. Head injuries (p. 1073)
19. Given several preprogrammed simulated geriatric patients with various complaints, provide the appropriate assessment, management, and transport. (pp. 1023–1073)

INTRODUCTION

Aging—the gradual decline of biological functions—varies widely from one individual to another. Most people reach their biological peak in the years before age 30. For practical purposes, however, the aging process does not affect their daily lives until later years. Many of the decrements commonly ascribed to aging are caused by other factors, such as lifestyle, diet, behaviour, or environment. The aging process becomes even more complicated if we remember that age-related changes in organ functions also occur at different rates. For example, a person's kidneys may decline rapidly with age, while the heart remains strong, and vice versa.

As people age, they actually become less alike, both physiologically and psychologically. Although some functional losses in old age are due to normal age-related changes, many others result from abnormal changes, particularly disease. In assessing and treating older patients, it is important to distinguish, when possible, normal age-related changes from abnormal changes. The purpose of this chapter is to present some of the most common physiological changes associated with aging and the implications of these changes to the quality of EMS care provided to the **elderly**—one of the fastest-growing segments of our population.

Many of the decrements commonly ascribed to aging are caused by other factors, such as lifestyle, diet, behaviour, or environment.

* **elderly** a person age 65 or older.

EPIDEMIOLOGY AND DEMOGRAPHICS

The twentieth century—with its tremendous medical and technological advances—witnessed both a reduction in infant mortality rates and an increase in life expectancies. The cumulative effect was a population boom worldwide, with the greatest gains seen among people aged 65 or older. During the 1900s, the population of Canada increased threefold, while the number of elderly increased tenfold. The growing number of elderly patients presents a challenge to all health-care services, including EMS, not only in terms of resources, but also in the enormous impact that aging has on our society.

POPULATION CHARACTERISTICS

In 1996, persons aged 65+ made up 12 percent of the population. This was up from 8 percent in 1971 and 5 percent in 1921. By 2020, most experts estimate that this group will approach or surpass 20 percent. People are living longer, not only in Canada but also around the world. Never before in history have people lived so long. A Canadian born in 1960, for example, can expect to live 20 years longer than a Canadian born in 1900. Meanwhile, birth rates have declined so that a growing proportion of the population is over 65. At age 65, a woman can expect to live another 19 years and a man another 15 years.

- The mean survival rate of older persons is increasing.
- The birth rate is declining.
- There has been an absence of major wars and other catastrophes.
- Health care and standards of living have improved significantly since World War II.

The number of Canadians aged 65 or over is expected to triple to 7.8 million (20 percent of the population) by the year 2031. In other words, 1 in 5 Canadians will be aged 65 or older. The rapid growth of the senior population is also expected to continue well into the future. Whether longer life spans mean longer years of active living or longer years of disease or disability is unknown.

* **gerontology** scientific study of the effects of aging and of age-related diseases on humans.

* **geriatrics** the study and treatment of diseases of the aged.

* **ageism** discrimination against aged or elderly people.

Emotional, physical, and/or financial difficulties can create a context in which illnesses can occur. Successful medical treatment of elderly patients involves an understanding of the broader social context in which they live.

Gerontology—the study of the effects of aging on humans—is a relatively new science. Gerontologists still do not fully understand the underlying causes of aging. However, most believe that some form of cellular damage or loss, particularly of nerve cells (neurons), is involved. The result is a general decline in the body's efficiency, such as a reduction in the size and function of most internal organs.

To treat age-related changes, physicians and other health-care workers have increasingly specialized in the care of the elderly. This aspect of medicine, known as **geriatrics,** is essential in caring for our aging population.

The demographic changes will also affect your EMS career. Today, nearly 56 percent of all EMS calls involve the elderly. The percentage is expected to grow. Therefore, you will need to be familiar with the fundamental principles of geriatrics, especially those related to advanced prehospital care. You will also need to be aware of the social issues that can affect the health and mental well-being of the elderly patients that you will be treating.

SOCIETAL ISSUES

For a typical working person, the postretirement years can be up to one-third of an average life span. The years include a series of transitions, such as reduced income, relocation, and loss of friends, family members, spouse, or partner.

After years of working and/or raising a family, an elderly person must not only find new roles to fulfill, but in many cases, must also overcome the societal label of "old person." A lot of elderly people disprove **ageism**—and all the stereotypes it engenders—by living happy, productive, and active lives (Figure 43-1). Others, however, feel a sense of social isolation or uselessness. Physical and financial difficulties reinforce these feelings and create an emotional context in which illnesses can occur. Therefore, successful medical treatment of elderly patients involves an understanding of the broader social situation in which they live.

The elderly live in either independent or dependent living environments. Many continue to live alone or with their partner well into their 80s or 90s. The "oldest" old are the most likely to live alone, and, in fact, nearly half of those aged 85 and over live by themselves. The great majority of these people—an estimated 78 percent—are women. This is because men tend to die before their wives, and widowed men tend to remarry more often than widowed women.

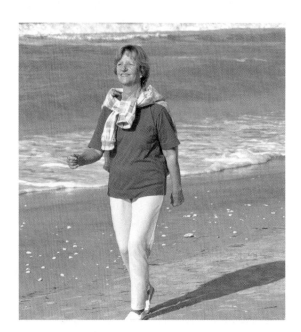

FIGURE 43-1 Many older adults live active lives, participating in sports and exercises popular among people of all ages.
(© The Stock Market Photo Agency.)

Prevention and Self-Help

In treating the elderly, remember that the best intervention is prevention (Table 43-1). The goal of any health-care service, including EMS, should be to help keep people from becoming sick or injured in the first place. As previously mentioned, disease and disability in later life are often linked to earlier unhealthy or unsafe behaviour. As a paramedic, you can reduce morbidity among the elderly by taking part in community education programs and by cooperating with agencies or organizations that support the elderly. Some possible resources are described in the following sections.

In treating the elderly, remember that the best intervention is prevention.

GENERAL PATHOPHYSIOLOGY, ASSESSMENT, AND MANAGEMENT

In treating elderly patients, it is important to recall several facts. First, medical disorders in the elderly often present as **functional impairment** and should be treated as an early warning of a possibly undetected medical problem. Second, signs and symptoms do not necessarily point to the underlying cause of the problem or illness. For example, while confusion often indicates a brain disease in younger patients, this may not be the case in an elderly patient. The confused patient may be suffering from a wide range of disorders, including drug toxicity, malnutrition, or accidental hypothermia.

* **functional impairment** decreased ability to meet daily needs on an independent basis.

Table 43-1	PREVENTION STRATEGIES FOR THE OLDER PERSON	
Issues	**Strategies**	
Lifestyle		
Exercise:	Weight-bearing and cardiovascular exercise (walking) for 20–30 minutes at least three times a week	
Nutrition:	Varies, but generally low fat, adequate fibre (complex carbohydrates), reduced sugar (simple carbohydrates), moderate protein; adequate calcium, especially for women*	
Alcohol/tobacco:	Moderate alcohol, if any; abstinence from tobacco	
Sleep:	Generally 7–8 hours a night	
Accidents	Maintain good physical condition; add safety features to home (handrails, nonskid surfaces, lights, etc.); modify potentially dangerous driving practices (driving at night with impaired night vision, travelling in hazardous weather, etc.)	
Medical Health		
Disease/Illness:	Routine screening for hearing, vision, blood pressure, hemoglobin, cholesterol, etc.; regular physical examinations; immunizations (tetanus booster, influenza vaccine, once-in-a-lifetime pneumococcal vaccine)	
Pharmacological:	Regular review of prescription and over-the-counter medications, focusing on potential interactions and side effects	
Dental:	Regular dental checkups and good oral hygiene (important for nutrition and general well-being)	
Mental/emotional:	Observe for evidence of depression, disrupted sleep patterns, psychosocial stress; ensure effective support networks and availability of psychotherapy; compliance with prescribed antidepressants	

*Vitamin supplements may be required but should be taken only in correct dosages and after other medications are reviewed. Excessive doses of vitamin A or D, for example, can be toxic.

A thorough evaluation must always be done to detect possible causes of an impairment. If identified early, an environmental- or disease-generated impairment can often be reversed. Your success depends on knowledge of age-related changes and the implications of these changes for patient assessment and management.

PATHOPHYSIOLOGY OF THE ELDERLY PATIENT

As mentioned, patients become less alike as they enter their elderly years, Even so, certain generalizations can be made about age-related changes and the disease process in the elderly.

Multiple-System Failure

The elderly often suffer from more than one illness or disease at a time.

✱ **old-old** an elderly person aged 80 or older.

✱ **comorbidity** having more than one disease at a time.

✱ **dysphagia** inability to swallow or difficulty swallowing.

Content Review

COMMON COMPLAINTS IN THE ELDERLY

- Fatigue/weakness
- Dizziness/vertigo/syncope
- Falls
- Headaches
- Insomnia
- Dysphagia
- Loss of appetite
- Inability to void
- Constipation/diarrhea

The existence of multiple chronic diseases in the elderly often leads to the use of multiple medications. Keep this in mind throughout the assessment.

✱ **polypharmacy** multiple drug therapy in which there is a concurrent use of a number of drugs.

There is no escaping the fact that the body becomes less efficient with age, increasing the likelihood of malfunction. The body is susceptible to all the disorders of young people, but its maintenance, defence, and repair processes are weaker. As a result, the elderly often suffer from more than one illness or disease at a time. On average, six medical disorders may coexist in an elderly person and perhaps even more in the **old-old**. Neither the patient nor the patient's doctor may be aware of all of these problems. Furthermore, disease in one organ system may result in the deterioration of other systems, compounding existing acute and/or chronic conditions.

Because of concomitant diseases (**comorbidity**) in the elderly, complaints may not be specific to any one disorder. Common complaints of the elderly include fatigue and weakness, dizziness/vertigo/syncope, falls, headaches, insomnia, **dysphagia**, loss of appetite, inability to void, and constipation/diarrhea.

Elderly patients often accept medical problems as a part of aging and neglect to monitor changes in their condition. In some cases, such as a silent myocardial infarction, pain may be diminished or absent. In others, an important complaint, such as constipation, may seem trivial.

Although many medical problems in the young and middle-aged populations present with a standard set of signs and symptoms, the changes involved in aging lead to different presentations. In pneumonia, for example, the classic symptom of fever is often absent in the elderly. Chest pain and a cough are also less common. Finally, many cases of pneumonia among the elderly are due to aspiration, not infection. The presentation of pneumonia and other diseases commonly found in the elderly will be covered later in the chapter.

Pharmacology in the Elderly

The existence of multiple chronic diseases in the elderly leads to the use of multiple medications. Persons aged 65 and older use approximately one-third of all prescription drugs in Canada, taking an average of 4.5 medications per day. This does not include over-the-counter medications, vitamin supplements, or herbal remedies.

If medications are not correctly monitored, **polypharmacy** can lead to a number of problems among the elderly. In general, a person's sensitivity to drugs increases with age. When compared with younger patients, the elderly experience more adverse drug reactions, more drug–drug interactions, and more drug–disease interactions. Because of age-related pharmacokinetic changes, such as a loss of body fluid and atrophy of organs, drugs concentrate more readily in the plasma and tissues of elderly patients. As a result, drug dosages often must be adjusted to prevent toxicity. (The problem of toxicity will be discussed in more detail later in the chapter.)

In taking a medical history of an elderly patient, remember to ask questions to determine if a patient is taking a prescribed medication as directed. Noncompliance with drug therapy, usually underadherence, is common among the elderly. Up to 40 percent do not take medications as prescribed. Factors that can decrease compliance in the elderly include

- Limited income
- Memory loss due to decreased or diseased neural activity
- Limited mobility
- Sensory impairment (cannot hear/read/understand directions)
- Multiple or complicated drug therapies
- Fear of toxicity
- Difficult-to-open childproof containers (especially with arthritic patients)
- Duration of drug therapy (The longer the therapy, the less likely it is that a patient will stick with it.)

Factors that can increase compliance among the elderly include

- Good patient–physician communication
- Belief that a disease or illness is serious
- Drug calendars or reminder cards
- Compliance counselling
- Blister-pack packaging or other easy-to-open packaging
- Multicompartment pill boxes
- Transport or home delivery services by a pharmacy
- Clear, simple directions written in large type
- Ability to read

In taking a medical history of an elderly patient, remember to ask if the patient is taking a prescribed medication as directed.

Problems with Mobility and Falls

Regular exercise and a good diet are two of the most effective preventive measures for ensuring mobility among the elderly. However, not all elderly take these measures. They may suffer from a severe medical problem, such as crippling arthritis. They may fear for their personal safety, either from accidental injury or from intentional injury, such as in a robbery. Certain medications also may increase their lethargy. Whatever the cause, a lack of mobility can have detrimental physical and emotional effects. Some of these include

- Poor nutrition
- Difficulty with elimination
- Poor skin integrity
- A greater predisposition for falls
- Loss of independence and/or confidence
- Depression from "feeling old"
- Isolation and lack of a social network

Fall-related injuries represent the leading cause of accidental death among the elderly. Intrinsic factors include a history of repeated falls, dizziness, a sense of weakness, impaired vision, an altered gait, central nervous system (CNS) problems, decreased mental status, or use of certain medications. Extrinsic factors include environment-related hazards, such as slippery floors, a lack of handrails, or loose throw rugs.

In assessing an elderly patient who has fallen, remember that a fall often has multiple causes.
⚷

In assessing an elderly patient who has fallen, remember that a fall often has multiple causes. An overmedicated patient, for example, trips over a throw rug. A fall may also be a presenting sign of an acute illness, such as a myocardial infarction, or a sign that a chronic illness has worsened. Bear in mind the possibility of physical abuse, especially if the injury does not match the story.

Communication Difficulties

Most elderly patients suffer from some form of age-related sensory changes. Normal physiological changes may include impaired vision or blindness, impaired or loss of hearing, an altered sense of taste or smell, and/or a lower sensitivity to pain (touch). Any of these conditions can affect your ability to communicate with the patient. For communication strategies, see Table 43-2. (A discussion on the implications of sensory impairment on patient assessment appears later in the chapter.)

Problems with Continence and Elimination

The elderly often find it embarrassing to talk about problems with continence and elimination. They may feel stigmatized, isolated, and/or helpless. When confronted with these problems, DO NOT make a big deal out of them. Respect the patient's dignity, and assure the person that, in many cases, the problem is treatable.

✱ **incontinence** inability to retain urine or feces because of loss of sphincter control or cerebral or spinal lesions.

Incontinence The problem of **incontinence** can affect nearly any age group but is most commonly associated with the elderly. Incontinence may be either urinary or fecal. An estimated 15 percent of the elderly who live at home experience some form of urinary incontinence. Nearly 30 percent of the hospitalized elderly and 50 percent of those living in nursing homes suffer from the same condition. Although fecal, or bowel, incontinence is less common, it seriously impairs activity and may lead to dependent care. About 16–60 percent of the institutionalized elderly have some kind of fecal incontinence.

Incontinence can lead to a variety of conditions, such as rashes, skin infections, skin breakdown (ulcers), urinary tract infections, sepsis, and falls or fractures. As mentioned, the condition takes a high emotional toll on both the patient and the caregiver. Management of incontinence costs billions of dollars each year.

Table 43-2 AGE-RELATED SENSORY CHANGES AND IMPLICATIONS FOR COMMUNICATION

Sensory Change	Result	Communication Strategy
Clouding and thickening of lens in eye	Cataracts; poor vision, especially peripheral vision	Position yourself in front of the patient where you can be seen; put your hand on the arm of the blind patient to let the patient know where you are; locate a patient's glasses if necessary.
Shrinkage of structure in ear	Decreased hearing, especially ability to hear high-frequency sounds; diminished sense of balance	Speak clearly; check hearing aids as necessary; write notes if necessary; help the patient to use the stethoscope, while you speak into it like a microphone.
Deterioration of teeth and gums	Patient needs dentures, but since they may inflict pain on sensitive gums, patient does not always wear them	If the patient's speech is unintelligible, ask the patient to put in dentures if possible.
Lowered sensitivity to pain and altered sense of taste and smell	Patient underestimates the severity of the problem or is unable to provide a complete pertinent history	Probe for significant symptoms, asking questions aimed at functional impairment.

In general, effective continence requires several physical conditions. These include

- An anatomically correct GI/GU tract
- Competent sphincter mechanism
- Adequate cognition and mobility

Although incontinence is not necessarily caused by aging, several factors predispose older patients to this condition. As mentioned, the elderly tend to have several medical disorders, each of which may require drug therapy. These disorders and/or the drugs used to treat them may compromise the integrity of either the urinary or the bowel tract. In addition, bladder capacity, urinary flow rate, and the ability to postpone voiding appear to decline with age. Certain diseases, such as diabetes and autonomic neuropathy, may also cause sphincter dysfunction. Diarrhea or lack of physical sensation may produce bowel incontinence as well.

Management of incontinence depends on the cause, which cannot be easily diagnosed in the field. Some cases of incontinence can be managed surgically. In most cases, however, patients use some type of absorptive devices, such as leak-proof underwear or pads. Indwelling catheters are less common and may cause infections when used, particularly if not properly managed. Of critical importance is respect for the patient's modesty and dignity.

In treating incontinence, remember to respect the patient's modesty and dignity.

Elimination Difficulty with elimination can be a sign of a serious underlying condition (Table 43-3). It can also lead to other complications. Straining to eliminate may have serious effects on the cerebral, coronary, and peripheral arterial circulations. In elderly people with cerebrovascular disease or impaired baroreceptor reflexes, efforts to force a bowel movement can lead to a **transient ischemic attack (TIA)** or syncope. In the case of prolonged constipation, the elderly may experience colonic ulceration, intestinal obstruction, and urinary retention.

In assessing a patient with difficulty eliminating, remember to inquire about her medications. Any of the following drugs can cause constipation:

Difficulty with elimination can be a sign of a serious underlying condition.

✱ **transient ischemic attacks (TIA)** reversible interruptions of blood flow to the brain; often seen as a precursor to a stroke.

- Opioids
- Anticholinergics (e.g., antidepressants, antihistamines, muscle relaxants, antiparkinsonian drugs)
- Cation-containing agents (e.g., antacids, calcium supplements, iron supplements)
- Neurally active agents (e.g., opiates, anticonvulsants)
- Diuretics

Table 43-3 POSSIBLE CAUSES OF ELIMINATION PROBLEMS

Difficulty in Urination	Difficulty with Bowel Movements
Enlargement of the prostate in men	Diverticular disease
Urinary tract infection	Constipation*
Acute or chronic renal failure	Colorectal cancer

*Constipation may be related to dietary, medical, or surgical conditions. It could also be the result of a malignancy, intestinal obstruction, or hypothyroidism. Treat constipation as a serious medical problem.

Assessment Considerations

Because of the increased risk of tuberculosis in the patients who are in nursing homes, consider using a HEPA or N-95 respirator.

As with all patients, be sure to take appropriate body substance isolation (BSI) precautions when assessing an elderly patient. Because of the increased risk of tuberculosis in patients who are in nursing homes, consider wearing a HEPA or N-95 respirator. Remain alert to the environment, particularly the temperature of the surroundings and evidence of prescription medications.

In general, assessment of the elderly patient follows the same basic approach used with any patient. However, you need to keep in mind several factors that will improve the quality of your evaluation and make subsequent treatment more successful.

General Health Assessment

Content Review

FACTORS IN FORMING A GENERAL ASSESSMENT
- Living situation
- Level of activity
- Network of social support
- Level of independence
- Medication history
- Sleep patterns

As already mentioned, you need to set a context for illness when assessing an elderly patient. When performing a general health assessment, take into account the patient's living situation, level of activity, network of social support, level of independence, medication history (both prescription and nonprescription), and sleep patterns.

Pay particularly close attention to the patient's nutrition. Elderly patients often have a decreased sense of smell and taste, which decreases their pleasure in eating. They also may be less aware of internal cues of hunger and thirst. Although caloric requirements generally decrease with age, an elderly patient may still suffer from malnutrition. Conditions that may complicate or discourage eating among the elderly include

- Breathing or respiratory problems
- Abdominal pain
- Nausea/vomiting, sometimes a drug-induced condition, as with antibiotics or aspirin
- Poor dental care
- Medical problems, such as hyperthyroidism, hypercalcemia, and chronic infections (e.g., cancer or tuberculosis)
- Medications (e.g., digoxin, vitamin A, fluoxetine)
- Alcohol or drug abuse
- Psychological disorders, including depression and **anorexia nervosa**
- Poverty
- Problems with shopping or cooking

* anorexia nervosa eating disorder marked by excessive fasting.

Content Review

BYPRODUCTS OF MALNUTRITION
- Vitamin deficiencies
- Dehydration
- Hypoglycemia

As with any person, nutrition greatly affects a patient's overall health. Because of reasons cited above, patients may suffer from a number of byproducts of malnutrition, including vitamin deficiencies, dehydration, and hypoglycemia. Also, remember that when a malnourished elderly person is fed, the food may produce yet other side effects, including electrolyte abnormalities, hyperglycemia, aspiration pneumonia, and a significant drop in blood pressure.

Pathophysiology and Assessment

Try to distinguish the patient's chief complaint from the primary problems.

Assessment of the elderly reflects the pathophysiology of this age group. As already mentioned, the chief complaint of the elderly may seem trivial or vague at first. Also, the patient may fail to report important symptoms. Therefore, you should try to distinguish the patient's chief complaint from the patient's primary problem. A patient may report nausea, which is the chief complaint.

The primary problem, however, may be the rectal bleeding that the patient neglected to mention.

The presence of multiple diseases also complicates the assessment process. The presence of chronic problems may make it more difficult to assess an acute problem. It is easy to confuse symptoms from a chronic illness with those of an acute condition. When confronted with an elderly patient who has chest pain, for example, it is difficult to determine whether the presence of frequent premature ventricular contractions is acute or chronic. Lacking access to the patient's medical record, you should treat the patient on a "threat-to-life" basis.

Other complications stem from age-related changes in an elderly patient's response to illness and injury. Pain may be diminished, causing both you and the patient to underestimate the severity of the primary problem. In addition, the temperature-regulating mechanism may be altered or depressed. This can result in the absence of fever, or a minimal fever, even in the face of a severe infection. Alterations in the temperature-regulating mechanism, coupled with changes in the sweat glands, also make the elderly more prone to environmental thermal problems.

Because of the complexity of factors that can affect assessment, you must probe for significant symptoms, and ultimately, the primary problem. Patience, respect, and kindness will elicit the answers needed for a pertinent medical history.

Age-related alterations in the temperature-regulating mechanism, coupled with changes in the sweat glands, make the elderly more prone to environmental thermal problems.

History

You should be prepared to spend more time obtaining histories from elderly patients. You may need to split the interview into sessions. For example, you might need to allow patients time to rest, if they become fatigued during the interview, or you might take a break to talk with caregivers.

When gathering the history, keep in mind the complications that arise from multiple diseases and multiple medications. Medications can be an especially important indicator of the patient's diseases. Therefore, you should find the patient's medications and take them to the hospital with the patient. Try to determine which of the medications, including over-the-counter medications, are currently being taken. In cases of multiple medications, there is an increased incidence of medication errors, drug interactions, and noncompliance.

Be prepared to spend more time obtaining a history from an elderly patient.

Communication Challenges As previously mentioned, communications may be more difficult when dealing with the aged. **Cataracts** (Figure 43-2) and **glaucoma** can diminish sight. Blindness, often resulting from diabetes and stroke, is more common in the elderly. The level of anxiety increases when a patient is unable to see her surroundings clearly. As a result, you should talk calmly to the visually impaired patient. Yelling does not help. Instead, position yourself so the patient can see or touch you.

Age also affects hearing. Overall hearing decreases, and patients may suffer from auditory disorders, such as **tinnitus** or **Meniere's disease.** Diminished hearing or deafness can make it virtually impossible to obtain a history. In such cases, try to determine the history from a friend or family member. DO NOT shout at the patient. This will not help if the patient is deaf, and it may distort sounds and make it difficult for the patient who still has some hearing to understand you. Write notes if necessary. If the patient can lip-read, speak slowly and directly toward the patient. Whenever possible, verify the history with a reliable source. Also, because loss of hearing may result from other causes (such as a build up of earwax), confirm whether deafness is a preexisting condition.

Patients may also have trouble with speech. They may have difficulty finding the words. They will often speak slowly and exhibit changes in voice quality, which may be a normal age-related change. If a patient has forgotten to put in dentures, politely ask the person to do so.

* **cataracts** medical condition in which the lens of the eye loses its clearness.

* **glaucoma** medical condition where the pressure within the eye increases.

* **tinnitus** subjective ringing or tingling sound in the ear.

* **Meniere's disease** a disease of the inner ear characterized by vertigo, nerve deafness, and a roar or buzzing in the ear.

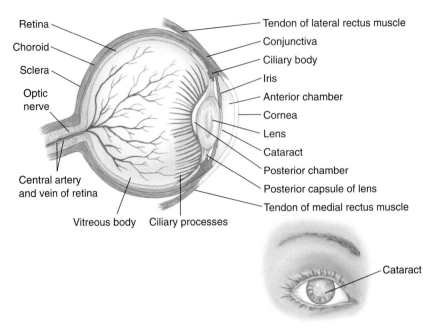

Retina
Choroid
Sclera
Optic nerve

Central artery and vein of retina

Vitreous body   Ciliary processes

Tendon of lateral rectus muscle
Conjunctiva
Ciliary body
Iris
Anterior chamber
Cornea
Lens
Cataract
Posterior chamber
Posterior capsule of lens
Tendon of medial rectus muscle

Cataract

FIGURE 43-2   Cataracts, which cloud the lens, can diminish eyesight in the elderly.

To improve your skill at communicating with the elderly, keep these techniques in mind:

- Always introduce yourself.
- Speak slowly, distinctly, and respectfully.
- Speak to the patient first, rather than to family members, caregivers, or bystanders.
- Speak face to face, at eye level, with eye contact (Figure 43-3).
- Locate the patient's hearing aid or eyeglasses if needed (Figure 43-4).
- Help the patient to put on the stethoscope, while you speak into it like a microphone.
- Turn on the room lights.
- Use verbal and nonverbal signs of concern and empathy.

FIGURE 43-3   If possible, talk *to* the elderly patient, rather than talking about the patient to others.

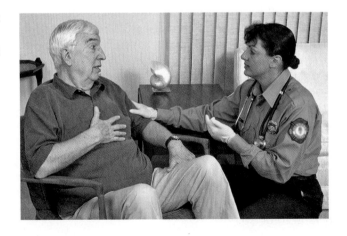

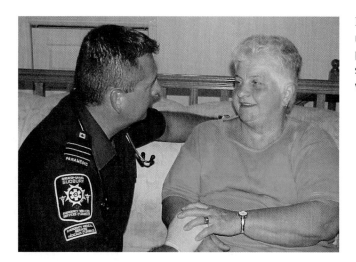

FIGURE 43-4 The paramedic must move closer to the patient and talk clearly and slightly louder to a patient who is hearing impaired.

- Remain polite at all times.
- Preserve the patient's dignity.
- Always explain what you are doing and why.
- Use your power of observation to recognize anxiety—tempo of speech, eye contact, tone of voice—during the telling of the history.

Altered Mental Status and Confusion Remember that age sometimes diminishes mental status. The patient can be confused and unable to remember details. In addition, the noise of radios, electrocardiograph (ECG) equipment, and strange voices may add to the confusion. Both senility and organic brain syndrome may manifest themselves similarly. Common symptoms include

- Delirium
- Confusion
- Distractibility
- Restlessness
- Excitability
- Hostility

When confronted with a confused patient, try to determine whether the patient's mental status represents a significant change from normal. DO NOT assume that a confused, disoriented patient is "just senile," thus failing to assess for a serious underlying problem (Figure 43-5). Alcoholism, for example, is more common in the elderly than was once recognized. It can further complicate taking the history.

Another complication results from depression, which can be mistaken for many other disorders. It can often mimic senility and organic brain syndrome. Depression may also inhibit patient cooperation. The depressed patient may be malnourished, dehydrated, overdosed, contemplating suicide, or simply imagining physical ailments for attention. If you suspect depression, question the patient regarding drug ingestion or suicidal ideation. It is important to remember that suicide is now the fourth leading cause of death among the elderly in the United States.

Concluding the History After obtaining the history, and if time allows, try to verify the patient's history with a credible source. This will often be less offensive to the patient if done away from her presence. While at the scene, it is important

DO NOT assume that a confused, disoriented patient is "just senile," thus failing to assess for a serious underlying problem.

Treat depression as a warning sign of substance abuse and/or suicide ideation—both more common among the elderly than previously understood.

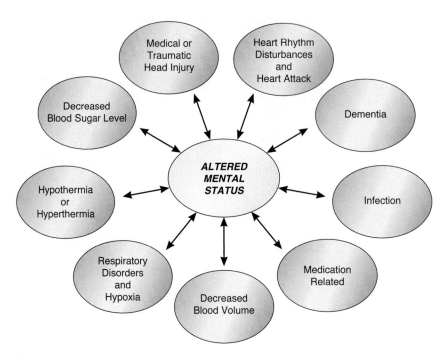

FIGURE 43-5   DO NOT assume that an altered mental status is a normal age-related change. A number of serious underlying problems may be responsible for changes in consciousness.

to observe the surroundings for indications of the patient's self-sufficiency. Look for evidence of drug or alcohol ingestion or for Medic-Alert or Vial-of-Life items. It is also important to spot signs of abuse or neglect, particularly in dependent living arrangements.

Secondary Assessment

Certain considerations must be kept in mind when assessing the elderly patient. Remember that some patients are often easily fatigued and cannot tolerate a long assessment. Also, because of the problems with temperature regulation, the patient may be wearing several layers of clothing, which can make assessment difficult. Be sure to explain all actions clearly before initiating the assessment, especially to patients with impaired vision. Be aware that the patient may minimize or deny symptoms because of a fear of being institutionalized or losing self-sufficiency.

Try to distinguish signs of chronic disease from an acute problem. Peripheral pulses may be difficult to evaluate because of peripheral vascular disease and arthritis. The elderly may also have nonpathological crackles (rales) on lung auscultation. In addition, the elderly often exhibit an increase in mouth breathing and a loss of skin elasticity, which may be easily confused with dehydration. Dependent edema may be caused by inactivity, not congestive heart failure. Only experience and practice will enable you to distinguish acute from chronic physical findings.

Only experience and repeated practice will enable you to distinguish acute from chronic physical findings in the elderly patient.

MANAGEMENT CONSIDERATIONS

As you have read, people become less alike as they age. Therefore, each elderly patient presents a unique challenge in terms of assessment and management. You will need to tailor your management plan to fit a patient's illness, injury, and overall general health. Because of the potential for rapid deterioration among the elderly, you must quickly spot conditions requiring rapid transport. As with any other patient, your first concern is ensuring the ABCs (airway, breathing, circulation). Remain alert at all times for changes in an elderly patient's neurological status, vital signs, and general cardiac status. (Management of specific disorders is covered in other sections of this chapter.)

In general, remember that transport to a hospital is often more stressful to the elderly than to any other age group, except for the very young. Avoid lights and sirens in all but the most serious cases, such as when you suspect a pulmonary embolism or bowel infarction. A calm, smooth transport helps reduce patient anxiety—and the resulting strain on an elderly patient's heart.

Provide emotional support at every phase of the call. Nearly any serious illness or injury in the elderly can provoke a sense of impending doom. Death is a very real possibility to this age group. To help reduce patient fears, keep these guidelines in mind:

- Encourage patients to express their feelings.
- DO NOT trivialize their fears.
- Acknowledge nonverbal messages.
- Avoid questions that are judgmental.
- Confirm what the patient says.
- Recall all you have learned about communicating with the elderly, thus avoiding communication breakdowns.
- Assure patients that you understand that they are adults on an equal footing with their care providers, including you.

SYSTEM PATHOPHYSIOLOGY IN THE ELDERLY

Although aging begins at the cellular level, it eventually affects virtually every system in the body. Age-related changes in the structure and function of organs increase the probability of disease, modify the threshold at which signs and symptoms appear, and affect assessment and treatment of the elderly patient (Table 43-4). You should be familiar with normal systemic changes related to aging so that you can more easily identify the abnormal changes that may point to a serious underlying problem.

RESPIRATORY SYSTEM

The effects of aging on the respiratory system begin as early as age 30. Age-related changes in the respiratory system include

- Decreased chest wall compliance
- Loss of lung elasticity
- Increased air trapping due to collapse of the smaller airways
- Reduced strength and endurance of the respiratory muscles

Functionally, by the time we reach age 65, vital capacity may be reduced by as much as 50 percent. In addition, the maximum breathing capacity may decrease by as much as 60 percent, while the maximum oxygen uptake may decrease by as much as 70 percent. These changes ultimately result in decreased ventilation and progressive hypoxemia. Any presence of underlying pulmonary diseases, such as emphysema and chronic bronchitis, further reduces respiratory function.

Table 43-4	COMMON AGE-RELATED SYSTEMIC CHANGES

Body System	Changes with Age	Clinical Importance
Respiratory	Loss of strength and coordination in respiratory muscles Cough and gag reflex reduced	Increased likelihood of respiratory failure
Cardiovascular	Loss of elasticity and hardening of arteries Changes in heart rate, rhythm, efficiency	Hypertension common Greater likelihood of strokes, heart attacks Great likelihood of bleeding from minor trauma
Neurological	Brain tissue shrinks Loss of memory Clinical depression common Altered mental status common Impaired balance	Delay in appearance of symptoms with head injury Difficulty in patient assessment Increased likelihood of falls
Endocrinological	Lowered estrogen production (women) Decline in insulin sensitivity Increase in insulin resistance	Increased likelihood of fractures (bone loss) and heart disease Diabetes mellitus common with greater possibility of hyperglycemia
Gastrointestinal	Diminished digestive functions	Constipation common Greater likelihood of malnutrition
Thermoregulatory	Reduced sweating Decreased shivering	Environmental emergencies more common
Integumentary (Skin)	Thins and becomes more fragile	More subject to tears and sores Bruising more common Heals more slowly
Musculoskeletal	Loss of bone strength (osteoporosis) Loss of joint flexibility and strength (osteoarthritis)	Greater likelihood of fractures Slower healing Increased likelihood of falls
Renal	Loss of kidney size and function	Increased problems with drug toxicity
Genitourinary	Loss of bladder function	Increased urination/incontinence Increased urinary tract infection
Immunological	Diminished immune response	More susceptible to infections Impaired immune response to vaccines
Hematological	Decrease in blood volume and/or red blood cells	Slower recuperation from illness/injury Greater risk of trauma-related complications

In addition, there is a decrease in an effective cough reflex and the activity of the cilia—the small hair-like fibres that trap particles and infectious agents. The decline of these two defence mechanisms leave the lungs more susceptible to recurring infection.

Other factors that may affect pulmonary function in the elderly include

* **kyphosis** exaggeration of the normal posterior curvature of the spine.

- **Kyphosis**
- Chronic exposure to pollutants
- Long-term cigarette smoking

The management of respiratory distress in elderly patients is essentially the same as for all age groups. Position the patient for adequate breathing, usually in the upright or sitting position. Teach breathing techniques that assist in exhalation, such as "pursed-lip breathing." (Tell patients to pretend they are blowing out a candle with each exhalation.) Use bronchodilators as needed, and provide high-concentration supplemental oxygen.

At all points, remain attentive for possible complications, such as **anoxic hypoxemia**. Monitor ventilations closely, as an elderly patient can become easily fatigued from any increase in the work of breathing. Remember that many elderly patients with respiratory disease have underlying cardiac disease. With this in mind, such drugs as the beta agonists should be used with extreme caution. Monitor cardiovascular status, and administer IV fluids judiciously. DO NOT OVERLOAD FLUIDS. When infusing fluids, frequently reassess lung sounds to check for the pressure of pulmonary edema.

✳ anoxic hypoxemia an oxygen deficiency due to disordered pulmonary mechanisms of oxygenation.

In treating respiratory disorders in the elderly patient, DO NOT OVERLOAD FLUIDS.

CARDIOVASCULAR SYSTEM

A number of variables unrelated to aging influence cardiovascular function. They include diet, smoking and alcohol use, education, socioeconomic status, and even personality traits. Of particular importance is the level of physical activity. Even though maximum exercise capacity and maximum oxygen consumption decline with age, a well-trained elderly person can match—or even exceed—the aerobic capacity of an unfit younger person.

This said, the cardiovascular system still experiences, in varying degrees, age-related deterioration. The wall of the left ventricle may thicken and enlarge (**hypertrophy**), often by as much as 25 percent. This is even more pronounced if there is associated hypertension. In addition, **fibrosis** develops in the heart and peripheral vascular system, resulting in hypertension, arteriosclerosis, and decreased cardiac function.

✳ hypertrophy an increase in the size or bulk of an organ.

✳ fibrosis the formation of fibre-like connective tissue, also called scar tissue, in an organ.

The aorta also becomes stiff and lengthens. This results from deposits of calcium and changes in the connective tissue. These changes predispose the aorta to partial tearing, resulting in dissection (thoracic) or aneurysm (abdominal).

As a person ages, the pattern of ventricular filling changes. Less blood enters the left ventricle during early diastole when the mitral valve is open. Therefore, filling and stretch (preload) depend on atrial contraction. Loss of the atrial kick (as will occur with atrial fibrillation) is not well tolerated in the elderly.

Over time, the conductive system of the heart degenerates, often causing dysrhythmias and varying degrees of heart block. Ultimately, the stroke volume declines and the heart rate slows, leading to decreased cardiac output. Because of this, the heart's ability to respond to stress diminishes. In such situations, expect exercise intolerance—an inability of the heart to meet an exercising muscle's need for oxygen.

To adequately manage complaints related to the cardiovascular system, ask the patient to stop all activity. This reduces the myocardial oxygen demand. DO NOT walk a patient with a cardiovascular complaint to the ambulance. Take the following basic steps according to local protocols.

DO NOT walk a patient with a cardiovascular disorder to the ambulance.

- Provide high-concentration supplemental oxygen.
- Start an IV for medication administration. Medications will vary with the complaint but may include
  - Antianginal agents
  - Aspirin
  - Diuretics
  - Antidysrhythmics

- Inquire about age-related dosages.
- Monitor vital signs and rhythm.
- Acquire a 12-lead ECG if obtainable.
- Remain calm, professional, and empathetic. A heart attack is one of the most fearful situations for the elderly.

NERVOUS SYSTEM

Unlike cells in other organ systems, cells in the central nervous system (CNS) cannot regenerate. The brain can lose as much as 45 percent of its cells in certain areas of the cortex. Overall, there is an average 10-percent reduction in brain weight from age 20 to age 90. Keep in mind that reductions in brain weight and ventricular size are not well correlated with intelligence, and elderly people may still be capable of highly creative and productive thinking. Once again, DO NOT assume that an elderly person possesses less cognitive skill than a younger person. Slight changes that may be expected include

- Difficulty with recent memory
- Psychomotor slowing
- Forgetfulness
- Decreased reaction times

Although brain size may not have clinical implications in terms of intelligence, it does have implications for trauma. A reduction in brain size leaves room for increased bleeding following a blow to the head, making the elderly more prone to subdural hematomas. In cases of altered mental status, maintain a suspicion of trauma, especially when an accident has been reported.

In assessing an elderly patient with altered mental status, presume the patient to have been mentally sharp unless proven otherwise.

Whenever you assess an elderly patient for mental status, determine a baseline. Presume your patient to have been mentally sharp unless proven otherwise. (Talk with partners, caregivers, family members, and so on.) Focus on the patient's perceptions, thinking processes, and communication. In questioning an elderly patient, provide an environment with minimal distractions. As already mentioned, ask clear questions in an unhurried manner.

In forming a patient plan, observe for weakness, chronic fatigue, changes in sleep patterns, and syncope or near-syncope. If you suspect a stroke, think "brain attack," and assign the patient a priority status. (Additional material on strokes will appear later in the chapter.) Consider blood pressure control per local protocol—but remember that perfusion of the brain tissue depends on an adequate blood pressure. DO NOT plan to reduce the blood pressure to an average of 120/80 as cerebral blood flow may be diminished. Consider the causes of changes in mental status, keeping in mind the possibility of trauma. Apply oxygen, and monitor ventilations. Depending on the situation, you may be called on to administer dextrose, thiamine, and naloxone.

ENDOCRINE SYSTEM

Early diagnosis of disorders in the endocrine system offers some of the greatest opportunities to prevent disabilities through appropriate hormonal therapy and/or lifestyle changes. Diabetes mellitus, for example, is extremely common among the elderly. However, normalization of glucose levels—through diet, exercise, and/or drug therapy—can reduce some of the devastating vascular and neurological complications.

In women, menopause—a normal age-related hormonal deficiency—can be similarly treated in a variety of ways, including hormone replacement therapy (HRT). By taking preventive measures, women can reduce and/or delay the incidence of heart disease, bone loss, and possibly Alzheimer's disease.

Thyroid disorders are "clinical masqueraders," especially in the elderly. Common signs and symptoms may be absent or diminished. When signs and symptoms are present, they may be attributed to aging or tied to other diseases, such as cardiovascular, gastrointestinal, or neuromuscular disorders. However, it has been shown that thyroid disorders, especially hypothyroidism and thyroid nodules, increase with age. (For more on thyroid disorders, see "Metabolic and Endocrine Disorders" later in the chapter.)

With the exception of glucose disorders, most endocrine disorders cannot be easily determined in the field. Many endocrine emergencies will present as altered mental status, especially with insulin-related diseases. Monitor for cardiovascular effects of endocrine changes, such as aortic aneurysm in a patient with **Marfan's syndrome**—a disorder resulting in abnormal growth of distal tissues and a dilatation of the root of the aorta. Also, remain alert to blood pressure swings in thyroid disorders, such as hyperthyroidism and hypothyroidism.

GASTROINTESTINAL SYSTEM

Age affects the gastrointestinal (GI) system in various ways. The volume of saliva may decrease by as much as 33 percent, leading to complaints of dry mouth, nutritional deficiencies, and a predisposition to choking. Gastric secretions may decrease to as little as 20 percent of the quantity present in younger people. Esophageal and intestinal motility also decrease, making swallowing more difficult and delaying digestive processes. The production of hydrochloric acid also declines, further disrupting digestion and, in some adults, contributing to nutritional anemia. Gums atrophy, and the number of taste buds decrease, reducing even further the desire to eat.

Other conditions may also develop. **Hiatal hernias** are not age related per se but can have serious consequences for the elderly. They may incarcerate, strangulate, or, in the most severe cases, result in massive GI hemorrhage. A diminished liver function, which is associated with aging, can delay or impede detoxification. A common drug toxicity problem for EMS personnel is the use of lidocaine for ventricular arrythmias. (See "Toxicological Emergencies" later in the chapter.) A diminished liver function can also reduce the production of clotting proteins, which, in turn, leads to bleeding abnormalities.

Complications in the GI system can be life threatening. Use shock protocols as necessary, and remember that not all fluid loss occurs outside the body.

THERMOREGULATORY SYSTEM

The elderly and infants are highly susceptible to variations in environmental temperatures. This occurs in the elderly because of altered or impaired thermoregulatory mechanisms. Aging seems to reduce the effectiveness of sweating in cooling the body. Older persons tend to sweat at higher core temperatures and have less sweat output per gland than younger people. As people age, they also experience deterioration of the autonomic nervous system, including a decrease in shivering and lower resting peripheral blood flow. In addition, the elderly may have a diminished perception of the cold. Drugs and disease can further affect an elderly patient's response to temperature extremes, resulting in hyperthermia or accidental hypothermia.

Many endocrine emergencies encountered in the field present as altered mental status, especially with insulin-related disorders.

* **Marfan's syndrome** hereditary condition of connective tissue, bones, muscles, ligaments, and skeletal structures characterized by irregular and unsteady gait, tall lean body type with long extremities, flat feet, stooped shoulders. The aorta is usually dilated and may become weakened enough to allow an aneurysm to develop.

* **hiatal hernia** protrusion of the stomach upward into the mediastinal cavity through the esophageal hiatus of the diaphragm.

A diminished liver function, which is associated with aging, can delay or impede detoxification. A common drug toxicity problem for EMS personnel is the use of lidocaine for ventricular arrythmias.

Environment-related emergencies are common causes of EMS calls, especially among the elderly living alone or in poverty. For more on these emergencies, see the discussion of heatstroke, hypothermia, and hyperthermia later in the chapter.

INTEGUMENTARY SYSTEM

As people age, the skin loses collagen, a connective tissue that gives elasticity and support to the skin. Without this support, the skin is subject to a greater number of injuries from bumping or tearing. The lack of support also makes it more difficult to start an IV, as the veins "roll away." Furthermore, the assessment of tenting skin becomes an inaccurate indicator of fluid status in the elderly. Without elasticity, the skin often will remain tented regardless of water balance.

As the skin thins, cells reproduce more slowly. Injury to skin is often more severe than in younger patients, and healing time is increased. As a rule, the elderly are at a higher risk of secondary infection, skin tumours, drug-induced eruptions, and fungal or viral infections. Decades of exposure to the sun also makes the elderly vulnerable to melanoma and other sun-related carcinomas (for example, basal cell carcinoma, squamous cell carcinoma).

MUSCULOSKELETAL SYSTEM

* **osteoporosis** softening of bone tissue due to the loss of essential minerals, principally calcium.

An aging person may lose as much as 5–8 cm of height from narrowing of the intervertebral discs and **osteoporosis**. Osteoporosis is the loss of mineral from the bone, resulting in softening of the bones. This is especially evident in the vertebral bodies, thus causing a change in posture. The posture of the aged individual often reveals an increase in the curvature of the thoracic spine, commonly called kyphosis, and slight flexion of the knee and hip joints. The demineralization of bone makes the patient much more susceptible to hip and other fractures. Some fractures may even occur from simple actions, such as sneezing.

In addition to skeletal changes, a decrease in skeletal muscle weight commonly occurs with age—especially with sedentary individuals. To compensate, elderly women develop a narrow, short gait, while older men develop a wide gait. These changes make the elderly more susceptible to falls and, consequently, a possible loss of independence.

Many extremity injuries should be splinted as found because of changes in the bone and joint structure in the elderly.

Because of the changes in the musculoskeletal system, simple trauma in the elderly can lead to complex injuries. In treating musculoskeletal disorders, supply supplemental oxygen, initiate an IV line, and consider pain control. Many extremity injuries should be splinted as found because of changes in the bone and joint structure of the elderly. To determine the cause of any injury, be sure to look beyond the obvious. Keep in mind the possibility of underlying medical conditions, drug complications, abuse or neglect, and ingestion of alcohol or drugs.

RENAL SYSTEM

* **nephrons** the functional units of the kidneys.

Aging affects the renal system through a reduction in the number of functioning **nephrons**, which may be decreased by 30–40 percent. Renal blood flow may also be reduced by up to 45 percent, increasing the waste products in the blood and upsetting the fluid and electrolyte balance. Because the kidneys are responsible for the production of erythropoietin (which stimulates the production of red blood cells in the bone marrow) and renin (which stimulates vasoconstriction), a decrease in renal function may result in anemia or hypertension in the older patient.

Prehospital treatment of complaints involving the renal and urinary systems is directed toward adequate oxygenation, fluid status, monitoring output, and pain control. Pay attention to the airway as nausea and vomiting are complications of pain secondary to renal obstruction. Also, monitor vital signs to detect changes in blood pressure and pulse.

GENITOURINARY SYSTEM

As people age, they experience a progressive loss of bladder sensation and tone. The bladder does not empty completely, and consequently the patient may sense a frequent need to urinate. This urge increases the risk of falls, especially during the middle of the night when lighting is dim or the patient is sleepy. Furthermore, the failure of complete emptying increases the likelihood of urinary tract infection and perhaps sepsis. In the male, the prostate often becomes enlarged (benign prostatic hypertrophy), causing difficulty in urination or urinary retention. As already mentioned, the elderly also commonly develop, in varying degrees, problems with incontinence.

Treatment for a complaint in the genitourinary system is described in the preceding section on the renal system and in the earlier discussion of incontinence.

IMMUNE SYSTEM

As a person ages, the function of T cells declines, making them less able to notify the immune system of invasion by antigens. A diminished immune response, sometimes called **immune senescence**, increases the susceptibility of the elderly to infections. It also increases the duration and severity of an infection.

✳ **immune senescence** diminished vigour of the immune response to the challenge and rechallenge by pathogens.

Unless contraindicated, the elderly should receive the vaccinations suggested by Health Canada. However, keep in mind that aging impairs the immune response to vaccines. The best prevention is adequate nutrition, infection control measures (for example, washing hands), and exercise. Recognition and treatment of such diseases as diabetes mellitus, congestive heart failure, thyroid disease, and occult malignancy also reduce the risk and severity of infections. As a paramedic, you should treat alterations in immune status as life threats and seek to prevent exposure of patients to infectious agents. DO NOT transmit any infection—even a mild cold—to an elderly patient.

HEMATOLOGICAL SYSTEM

DO NOT transmit an illness—even a mild cold—to an elderly patient.

The hematological system is affected by a failure of the renal system to stimulate the production of red blood cells (RBCs). Nutritional abnormalities may also produce abnormal RBCs. Since there is less body water present in the elderly, blood volume similarly decreases. This makes it difficult for an elderly patient to recuperate from an illness or injury. Intervention must be started early in order to make a lasting difference.

In addition to providing supplemental oxygen, you should prepare for increases in bleeding time. Monitor the elderly patient closely as deterioration is difficult to stop.

COMMON MEDICAL PROBLEMS IN THE ELDERLY

In general, the elderly suffer from the same kinds of medical emergencies as younger patients. However, illnesses may be more severe, complications more likely, and classic signs and symptoms absent or altered. In addition, the elderly are more likely to react adversely to stress and deteriorate much more quickly than young or middle-aged adults. The following are some of the medical disorders that you may encounter.

PULMONARY/RESPIRATORY DISORDERS

Respiratory emergencies are some of the most common reasons elderly persons summon EMS or seek emergency care. Most elderly patients with a respiratory disorder present with a chief complaint of dyspnea. However, coughing, congestion, and wheezing are also common chief complaints.

Many factors can trigger respiratory distress among the elderly (Figure 43-6). Descriptions of the most common ones follow.

Pneumonia

Pneumonia is an infection of the lung. It is usually caused by a bacterium or virus. However, aspiration pneumonia may also develop as a result of difficulty swallowing.

Pneumonia is a serious disease for the elderly. It is the fourth leading cause of death in people aged 65 and older. Its incidence increases with age at a rate of 10 percent for each decade beyond age 20. It is found in up to 60 percent of the autopsies performed on the elderly. Reasons the elderly develop pneumonia more frequently than younger patients include

- Decreased immune response
- Reduced pulmonary function
- Increased colonization of the pharynx by gram-negative bacteria
- Abnormal or ineffective cough reflex
- Decreased effectiveness of mucociliary cells of the upper respiratory system

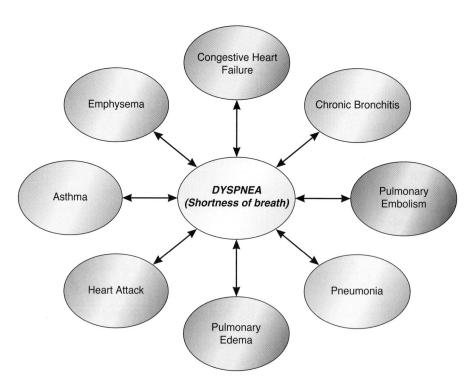

FIGURE 43-6 Dyspnea can be caused by a number of respiratory and cardiac problems in the elderly.

The elderly who are at greatest risk for contracting pneumonia include frail adults and those with chronic, multiple diseases or compromised immunity. Institutionalized patients—either in hospitals or nursing homes—are especially vulnerable because of increased exposure to microorganisms and limited mobility. A patient in an institutional setting is up to 50 times more likely to contract pneumonia than is an elderly patient receiving home care.

Common signs and symptoms of pneumonia include increasing dyspnea, congestion, fever, chills, tachypnea, sputum production, and altered mental status. Occasionally, abdominal pain may be the only symptom. Because of thermoregulatory changes, a fever may be absent in an elderly patient.

Prevention strategies include prophylactic treatment with antibiotics. Efforts should also be taken to reduce exposure to hospital infections and to promote patient mobility.

In treating an elderly patient with pneumonia, manage all life threats. Maintain adequate oxygenation. Transport the patient to the hospital for diagnosis, keeping in mind that patients with respiratory disease often have other underlying problems.

Chronic Obstructive Pulmonary Disease

Chronic obstructive pulmonary disease (COPD) is really a collection of diseases, characterized by chronic airflow obstruction with reversible and/or irreversible components. Although each COPD has its own distinct features, elderly patients commonly have two or more types at the same time. COPD usually refers to some combination of emphysema, chronic bronchitis, and, to a lesser degree, asthma. Pneumonia, as well as other respiratory disorders, can further complicate chronic obstructive pulmonary disease in the elderly.

In Canada, chronic obstructive pulmonary disease is among the leading causes of death. Its prevalence has been increasing over the past 20 years. Several factors combine to produce the damage of COPD. They include

- Genetic disposition
- Exposure to environmental pollutants
- Existence of a childhood respiratory disease
- Cigarette smoking, a contributing factor in up to 80 percent of all cases of COPD

The physiology of COPD varies but may include inflammation of the air passages with increased mucus production or actual destruction of the alveoli. The outcome is decreased airflow in the alveoli, resulting in reduced oxygen exchange. Usual signs and symptoms include

- Cough
- Increased sputum production
- Dyspnea
- Accessory muscle use
- Pursed-lip breathing
- Tripod positioning
- Exercise intolerance
- Wheezing
- Pleuritic chest pain
- Tachypnea

COPD is progressive and debilitating (Figure 43-7). The patient can often keep the signs and symptoms under control until the body is stressed. When the condition becomes disabling, it is called exacerbation of COPD. This condition can lead rapidly to death as hypoxia and hypercapnia alter acid-base balance and deprive the tissues of the oxygen needed for efficient energy production.

The most effective prevention involves elimination of tobacco products and reduced exposure to cigarette smoke (in nonsmokers). Recent legislation has sought to keep public places smoke free and to discourage cigarette smoking in the young. Once the disease has been diagnosed, patients are taught to identify stresses that exacerbate the condition. Appropriate self-care includes exercise, avoidance of infections, appropriate use of drugs, and, when necessary, calling EMS.

When dealing with an elderly patient with COPD, treatment is essentially the same as for all age groups. Supply supplemental oxygen and possibly drug therapy, usually for reducing dyspnea.

Pulmonary Embolism

Pulmonary embolism (PE) should always be considered as a possible cause of respiratory distress in the elderly. Although statistics for the elderly are unavailable, nearly 11 percent of PE deaths take place in the first hour and 38 percent in the second hour.

Blood clots are the most frequent cause of pulmonary embolism. However, the condition may also be caused by fat, air, bone marrow, tumour cells, or foreign bodies. Risk factors for developing pulmonary embolism include

- Deep venous thrombosis
- Prolonged immobility, common among the elderly
- Malignancy (tumours)
- Paralysis
- Fractures of the pelvis, hip, or leg
- Obesity
- Trauma to the leg vessels
- Major surgery
- Presence of a venous catheter
- Use of estrogen (in women)
- Atrial fibrillation

Pulmonary emboli usually originate in the deep veins of the thigh and calf. The condition should be suspected in any patient with the acute onset of dyspnea. Often, it is accompanied by pleuritic chest pain and right heart failure. If the pulmonary embolus is massive, you can expect severe dyspnea, cardiac dysrhythmias, and, ultimately, cardiovascular collapse.

Definitive diagnosis of a pulmonary embolism takes place in a hospital setting. The goals of field treatment are to manage and minimize complications of the condition. General treatment considerations include delivery of high-flow oxygen via a mask, maintaining oxygen levels above an SaO_2 of 90 percent. Establishment of an IV for possible administration of medications is appropriate, but vigorous fluid therapy should be avoided, if possible. Prehospital pharmacological therapy for pulmonary embolism is limited.

The risk of death from pulmonary embolism is greatest in the first few hours. Therefore, rapid transport is essential. Position the patient in an upright position, and avoid lifting the patient by the legs or knees, which may dislodge thrombi in

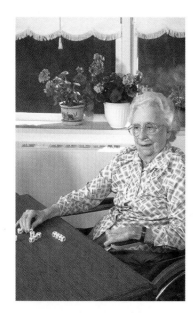

FIGURE 43-7 The COPD patient may use a nasal cannula with a home oxygen unit.

The risk of death from pulmonary embolism is greatest in the first few hours. Therefore, rapid transport is essential.

the lower extremities. During transport, continue to monitor changes in skin colour, pulse oximetry, and changes in breathing rate and rhythm. Your field assessment and interventions can save the patient's life and guide the hospital physician in a direction that will result in an accurate diagnosis and rapid treatment.

Pulmonary Edema

Pulmonary edema is an effusion or escape of serous fluids into the alveoli and interstitial tissues of the lungs. Acute pulmonary edema can develop rapidly in the elderly. Although most commonly associated with acute myocardial infarction, it can also occur due to other factors, including pulmonary infections, inhaled toxins, narcotic overdose, pulmonary embolism, and decreased atmospheric pressure.

Pulmonary edema causes severe dyspnea associated with congestion. Other signs and symptoms include rapid laboured breathing, cough with blood-stained sputum, cyanosis, and cold extremities. Secondary assessment usually reveals the presence of moist crackles and accessory muscle use. Severe cases will exhibit rhonchi.

Treatment is directed toward altering the cause of the condition. The existence of pulmonary edema can be life threatening and is often the symptom of a fatal cardiovascular disease.

The existence of pulmonary edema can be life-threatening and is often the symptom of a fatal cardiovascular disease.

Lung Cancer

North America has the highest incidence of lung cancer in the world. The incidence increases with age, with about 65 percent of all lung cancer deaths occurring among people aged 65 and older. The leading cause of lung cancer is cigarette smoking.

Often, progressive dyspnea will be the first presentation of a cancerous lesion. Hemoptysis (bloody sputum), chronic cough, and weight loss are also common symptoms.

Treatment of lung cancer occurs in a hospital setting. However, you may be called to assist in the follow-up home care or, in terminal stages, a hospice. (See Chapter 46 for more information on this subject.)

CARDIOVASCULAR DISORDERS

The leading cause of death in the elderly is cardiovascular disease. Assessment and treatment of cardiovascular disease in the elderly patient is often complicated by non-age-related factors and disease processes in other organ systems. In conducting your history, determine the patient's level of cardiovascular fitness, changes in exercise tolerance, recent diet history, use of medications, and use of cigarettes and/or alcohol. Ask questions about breathing difficulty, especially at night, and evidence of palpitations, flutter, or skipped beats.

In performing the secondary assessment, look for hypertension and orthostatic hypotension (a decrease in blood pressure and an increase in heart rate when rising from a seated or supine position). Watch for dehydration or dependent edema. When taking an elderly patient's blood pressure, consider checking both arms. Routinely determine pulses in all the extremities. In auscultating the patient, remember that a bruit or noise in the neck, abdomen, or groin indicates a high probability of carotid, aortorenal, or peripheral vascular disease. Keep in mind, too, that heart sounds are generally softer in the elderly, probably because of a thickening of lung tissue between the heart and chest wall.

In evaluating the problem, recall the cardiovascular disorders commonly found in elderly patients. They include angina pectoris, myocardial infarction, congestive heart failure, dysrhythmias, aortic dissection, aneurysm, hypertension, and syncope.

In auscultating a patient, remember that a bruit in the neck, abdomen, or groin indicates a high probability of carotid, aortorenal, or peripheral vascular disease.

Keep in mind that heart sounds are generally softer in the elderly, probably because of a thickening of lung tissues between the heart and chest wall.

Angina Pectoris

The likelihood of developing angina increases dramatically with age. This is especially true of women, who are estrogen protected until after menopause. Angina is usually triggered by physical activity, especially after a meal, and by exposure to very cold weather. Attacks vary in frequency, from several a day to occasional episodes separated by weeks or months.

Angina pectoris literally means "pain in the chest." However, the pain of angina is actually felt in only about 10–20 percent of elderly patients. The changes in sensory nerves, combined with the myocardial changes of aging, make dyspnea a more likely symptom of angina than is pain.

Angina develops when narrowing of coronary vessels due to plaque or vasospasm lead to an inability to meet the oxygen demands of the heart muscle. The heart muscle usually responds by sending out pain signals, which represent a buildup of lactic acid. In an elderly patient, exercise intolerance is a key symptom of angina. In obtaining a history, you should ask the patient about sudden changes in routine. In addition, inquire about any increased stresses on the heart, such as anemia, infection, dysrhythmias, and thyroid changes.

General prevention strategies in the elderly are similar to those in young patients. Blood pressure control, combined with diet, exercise, and smoking cessation reduces the risk in all groups.

In an elderly patient, exercise intolerance is a key symptom of angina.

Myocardial Infarction

A myocardial infarction (MI) involves actual death of muscle tissue due to a partial or complete occlusion of one or more of the coronary arteries. The greatest number of patients hospitalized for acute myocardial infarction are older than 65. The elderly patient with myocardial infarction is less likely to present with classic symptoms, such as chest pain, than a younger counterpart. Atypical presentations that may be seen in the elderly include

The elderly patient with myocardial infarction is less likely to present with classic symptoms than is a younger counterpart.

- Absence of pain
- Exercise intolerance
- Confusion/dizziness
- Syncope
- Dyspnea—common in patients over age 85
- Neck, dental, and/or epigastric pain
- Fatigue/weakness

The mortality rate associated with myocardial infarction and/or resulting complications doubles after age 70. Unlike younger patients, the elderly are more likely to suffer a **silent myocardial infarction.** They also tend to have larger myocardial infarctions. The majority of deaths that occur in the first few hours following a myocardial infarction are due to dysrhythmias.

A myocardial infarction is most commonly triggered by some form of physical exertion or a preexisting heart disease. Because of the high mortality associated with myocardial infarctions in the elderly, early detection and emergency management are critical.

 silent myocardial infarction a myocardial infarction that occurs without exhibiting obvious signs and symptoms.

Heart Failure

Heart failure takes place when cardiac output cannot meet the body's metabolic demands. The incidence rises exponentially after age 60. The condition is widespread among the elderly and is the most common diagnosis in hospitalized patients over age 65. The causes of heart failure fall in one of four categories: impairment to flow, inadequate cardiac filling, volume overload, and myocardial failure.

Typical age-related factors, such as prolonged myocardial contractions, make the elderly vulnerable to heart failure. Other factors that place them at risk include

- Noncompliance with drug therapy
- Anemia
- Ischemia
- Thermoregulatory disorders (hypothermia/hyperthermia)
- Hypoxia
- Infection
- Use of nonsteroidal anti-inflammatory drugs

Signs and symptoms of heart failure vary. In most patients, regardless of age, some form of edema exists. However, edema in the elderly can indicate a range of problems, including musculoskeletal injury. Assessment findings specific to the elderly include

- Fatigue (left failure)
- **Two pillow orthopnea**
- Dyspnea on exertion
- Dry, hacking cough progressing to productive cough
- Dependent edema (right failure)
- **Nocturia**
- Anorexia, **hepatomegaly,** ascites

Nonpharmacological management of heart failure includes modifications in diet (e.g., less fat and cholesterol), exercise, and reduction in weight, if necessary. Pharmacological management may include treatment with diuretics, vasodilators, antihypertensive agents, or inotropic agents. Check to see if the patient is already on any of these medications and if the patient is compliant with scheduled doses.

Dysrhythmias

Many cardiac dysrhythmias develop with age. Atrial fibrillation is the most common dysrhythmia encountered.

Dysrhythmias occur primarily as a result of degeneration of the patient's conductive system. Anything that decreases myocardial blood flow can produce a dysrhythmia. They may also be caused by electrolyte abnormalities.

To complicate matters further, the elderly do not tolerate extremes in heart rate as well as a younger person would. For example, a heart rate of 140 in an older patient may cause syncope, while a younger patient can often tolerate a heart rate greater than 180. In addition, dysrhythmias can lead to falls due to cerebral hypoperfusion. They can also result in congestive heart failure (CHF) or a transient ischemic attack (TIA).

Treatment considerations depend on the type of dysrhythmia. Patients may already have a pacemaker in place. In such cases, keep in mind that pacemakers have a low but significant rate of complications, such as a failed battery, fibrosis around the catheter site, lead fracture, or electrode dislodgment. In a number of situations, drug therapy may be indicated. Whenever you discover a dysrhythmia,

* **two-pillow orthopnea** the number of pillows—in this case, two—needed to ease the difficulty of breathing while lying down; a significant factor in assessing the level of respiratory distress.

* **nocturia** excessive urination during the night.

* **hepatomegaly** enlarged liver.

Content Review

POSSIBLE PACEMAKER COMPLICATIONS

- Failed battery
- Fibrosis around the catheter site
- Lead fracture
- Electrode dislodgment

Remember that an abnormal or disordered heart rhythm may be the only clinical finding in an elderly patient suffering acute myocardial infarction.

remember that an abnormal or disordered heart rhythm may be the only clinical finding in an elderly patient suffering acute myocardial infarction.

Aortic Dissection/Aneurysms

✱ **aortic dissection** a degeneration of the wall of the aorta.

✱ **aneurysm** abnormal dilation of a blood vessel, usually an artery, due to a congenital defect or a weakness in the wall of the vessel.

Aortic dissection is a degeneration of the wall of the aorta, either in the thoracic or in the abdominal cavity. It can result in an **aneurysm** or in a rupture of the vessel.

Approximately 80 percent of thoracic aneurysms are due to atherosclerosis combined with hypertension. The remaining cases occur secondary to other factors, including Marfan's syndrome or blunt trauma to the chest. Patients with dissections will often present with tearing chest pain radiating through to the back or, if rupture occurs, cardiac arrest.

The distal portion of the aorta is the most common site for abdominal aneurysms. Approximately 1 in 250 people over age 50 die from a ruptured abdominal aneurysm. The aneurysm may appear as a pulsatile mass in a patient with a normal girth, but lack of an identifiable mass does not eliminate this condition. Patients may present with tearing abdominal pain or unexplained low back pain. Pulses in the legs are diminished or absent and the lower extremities feel cold to the touch. There may be sensory abnormalities, such as numbness, tingling, or pain in the legs. The patient may fall when attempting to stand.

Most abdominal aortic aneurysms occur below the renal arteries.

Treatment of an aneurysm depends on its size, location, and the severity of the condition. In the case of thoracic aortic dissection, continuous IV infusion and/or administration of drug therapy to lower the arterial pressure and to diminish the velocity of left ventricle contraction may be indicated. Rapid transport is essential, especially for the older patient who most commonly requires care and observation in an intensive care unit.

Hypertension

Hypertension appears to be a product of the industrialized society. In the developed nations, such as Canada, the systolic and diastolic pressures have a tendency to rise until age 60. Systolic pressure may continue to rise after that time, but diastolic pressure stabilizes. Since this rise in blood pressure is not seen in the less developed nations, experts believe that hypertension is not a normal age-related change.

Today, more than 50 percent of Canadians over age 65 have clinically diagnosed hypertension—defined as blood pressure greater than 140/90 mmHg. Prolonged elevated blood pressure will eventually damage the heart, brain, or kidneys. As a result of hypertension, elderly patients are at greater risk for heart failure, stroke, blindness, renal failure, coronary heart disease, and peripheral vascular disease. In men with blood pressure greater than 160/95 mmHg, the risk of mortality nearly doubles.

Hypertension increases with atherosclerosis, which is more common with the elderly than other age groups. Other contributing factors include obesity and diabetes. The condition can be prevented or controlled through diet (sodium reduction), exercise, cessation of smoking, and compliance with medications.

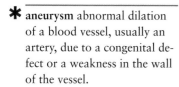

Content Review

HYPERTENSION PREVENTION STRATEGIES

- Modified diet (low sodium)
- Exercise
- Cessation of smoking
- Compliance with medications

✱ **epistaxis** nosebleed.

Hypertension is often a silent disease that produces no clinically obvious signs or symptoms. It may be associated with nonspecific complaints, such as headache, tinnitus, **epistaxis**, slow tremors, or nausea and vomiting. An acute onset of high blood pressure without any kidney involvement is often a telltale indicator of thyroid disease.

Management of hypertension depends on its severity and the existence of other conditions. For example, hypertension is often treated with beta-blockers—medications that are contraindicated in patients with chronic obstructive lung disease, asthma, or heart block greater than first degree. Diuretics, another common drug used in treating hypertension, should be prescribed with care for patients on digitalis. Keep in mind that centrally acting agents are more likely to produce negative side effects in the elderly. Unlike younger patients, the elderly may experience depression, forgetfulness, sleep problems, or vivid dreams and/or hallucinations.

Syncope

Syncope is a common presenting complaint among the elderly. The condition results when blood flow to the brain is temporarily interrupted or decreased. It is most often caused by problems with either the nervous system or the cardiovascular system. In general, syncope has a higher incidence of death in elderly patients than in younger individuals. The following are some of the common presentations that you may encounter:

- *Vasodepressor Syncope.* Vasodepressor syncope is the common faint. It may occur following emotional distress, pain, prolonged bed rest, mild blood loss, prolonged standing in warm, crowded rooms, anemia, or fever.

- *Orthostatic Syncope.* Orthostatic syncope occurs when a person rises from a seated or supine position. There are several possible causes. First, there may be a disproportion between blood volume and vascular capacity. That is, there is a pooling of blood in the legs, reducing blood flow to the brain. Causes of this include hypovolemia, venous **varicosities,** prolonged bed rest, and **autonomic dysfunction.** Many drugs, especially blood pressure medicines, can cause drug-induced orthostatic syncope due to the effects of the medications on the capacitance vessels.

- *Vasovagal Syncope.* Vasovagal syncope occurs as a result of a **valsalva manoeuvre,** which happens during defecation, coughing, or similar manoeuvres. This effectively slows the heart rate and cardiac output, thus decreasing blood flow to the brain.

- *Cardiac Syncope.* Cardiac syncope results from transient reduction in cerebral blood flow due to a sudden decrease in cardiac output. It can result from several mechanisms. Syncope can be the primary symptom of silent myocardial infarction. In addition, many dysrhythmias can cause syncope. Dysrhythmias that have been shown to cause syncope include bradycardias, **Stokes-Adams syndrome,** heart block, tachydysrhythmia, and **sick sinus syndrome.**

- *Seizures.* Syncope may result from a seizure disorder, or syncope (prolonged) may cause seizure activity. Syncope due to seizures tends to occur without warning. It is associated with muscular jerking or convulsions, incontinence, and tongue biting. Postictal confusion may follow.

- *Transient Ischemic Attacks.* Transient ischemic attacks occur more frequently in the elderly. They may cause syncope.

NEUROLOGICAL DISORDERS

Elderly patients are at risk for several neurological emergencies. Often, the exact cause is not initially known and may require probing at the hospital.

Many of the patients with neurological disorders whom you will encounter in the field will exhibit an alteration in mental status. You may discover a range

* **varicosities** an abnormal dilation of a vein or group of veins.

* **autonomic dysfunction** an abnormality of the involuntary aspect of the nervous system.

* **valsalva manoeuvre** forced exhalation against a closed glottis, such as with coughing. This manoeuvre stimulates the parasympathetic nervous system via the vagus nerve, which, in turn, slows the heart rate.

* **Stokes-Adams syndrome** a series of symptoms resulting from heart block, most commonly syncope. The symptoms result from decreased blood flow to the brain caused by the sudden decrease in cardiac output.

* **sick sinus syndrome** a group of disorders characterized by dysfunction of the sinoatrial node in the heart.

of underlying causes from stroke to degenerative brain disease. Some of the most common causes of altered mental status include

- Cerebrovascular disease (stroke or transient ischemic attack)
- Myocardial infarction
- Seizures
- Medication-related problems (drug interactions, drug underdose, and drug overdose)
- Infection
- Fluid and electrolyte abnormalities (dehydration)
- Lack of nutrients (hypoglycemia)
- Temperature changes (hypothermia, hyperthermia)
- Structural changes (dementia, subdural hematoma)

As mentioned, it is often impossible in the field to distinguish the cause of an altered mental status. Even so, you should carry out a thorough assessment. Administer supplemental oxygen. As soon as practical, obtain a blood glucose level to exclude hypoglycemia as a possible cause. Overall, the approach to the elderly patient with altered mental status is the same as with any other patient presenting with similar symptoms.

Cerebrovascular Disease (Stroke/Brain Attack)

Stroke is the fourth leading cause of death in Canada. Each year, about 16 000 Canadians die from stroke. More women than men die from stroke. There are between 40 000 and 50 000 strokes in Canada each year, with about 300 000 Canadians living with the effects of stroke. Of every 100 people who are hospitalized for stroke

- 20 die before leaving the hospital
- 50 return home
- 10 go to an inpatient rehabilitation program
- 15 require long-term care

Strokes cost the Canadian economy $2.7 billion a year. Incidence of stroke and the likelihood of dying from a stroke increase with age. Occlusive stroke is statistically more common in the elderly and relatively uncommon in younger individuals. Older patients are at higher risk of stroke because of atherosclerosis, hypertension, immobility, limb paralysis, congestive heart failure, and atrial fibrillation. Transient ischemic attacks (TIAs) are also more common in older patients. More than one-third of patients suffering TIAs will develop a major, permanent stroke. As previously mentioned, TIAs are a frequent cause of syncope in the elderly.

Strokes usually fall in one of two major categories. **Brain ischemia**—injury to brain tissue caused by an inadequate supply of oxygen and nutrients—accounts for about 80 percent of all strokes. Brain hemorrhage, the second major category, may be either **subarachnoid hemorrhage** or **intracerebral hemorrhage**. These different patterns of bleeding have different presentations, causes, and treatments. However, together they account for a high percentage of all stroke deaths.

Because of the various kinds of strokes, signs and symptoms can present in many ways—altered mental status, coma, paralysis, slurred speech, a change in mood, and seizures. Stroke should be highly suspect in any elderly patient with a sudden change in mental status.

Whenever you suspect a stroke, it is essential that you complete the Glasgow Coma Scale rating for later comparison in the emergency department. Thrombolytic agents administered to a patient suffering an occlusive (ischemic) stroke

---

As soon as practical, obtain a blood glucose level to exclude hypoglycemia as a possible cause of altered mental status in an elderly patient.

✽ **stroke** injury to or death of brain tissue resulting from interruption of cerebral blood flow and oxygenation.

✽ **brain ischemia** injury to brain tissues caused by an inadequate supply of oxygen and nutrients.

✽ **subarachnoid hemorrhage** bleeding that occurs between the arachnoid and dura mater of the brain.

✽ **intracerebral hemorrhage** bleeding directly into the brain.

can decrease the severity of damage if administered within six hours of onset. Rapid transport is essential for avoiding brain damage or limiting its extent. In the case of stroke, "time is brain tissue."

By far the most preferred treatment is prevention of strokes in the first place. Strategies include

- Control of hypertension
- Treatment of cardiac disorders, including dysrhythmias and coronary artery disease
- Treatment of blood disorders, such as anemia and **polycythemia**
- Cessation of smoking
- Cessation of recreational drug use
- Moderate use of alcohol
- Regular exercise
- Good eating habits

Seizures

Seizures may be easily mistaken for stroke in the elderly. Also, a first-time seizure may occur due to damage from a previous stroke. Not all seizures experienced by the elderly are of the major motor type. Some are more subtle. Many causes of seizure activity in the elderly have been identified. Common causes include

- Seizure disorder (epilepsy)
- Syncope
- Recent or past head trauma
- Mass lesion (tumour or bleed)
- Alcohol withdrawal
- Hypoglycemia
- Stroke

Often, the cause of the seizure cannot be determined in the field. As a result, treat the condition as a life-threatening emergency, and transport as quickly as possible to eliminate the possibility of stroke. If the patient has fallen during a seizure, check for evidence of trauma, and treat accordingly.

Dizziness/Vertigo

Dizziness is a frightening experience and a frequent complaint of the elderly. The complaint of dizziness may actually mean that the patient has suffered syncope, presyncope, lightheadedness, or true **vertigo.** Vertigo is a specific sensation of motion perceived by the patient as spinning or whirling. Many patients will report that they feel as though they are spinning. Vertigo is often accompanied with sweating, pallor, nausea, and vomiting. Meniere's disease can cause severe, **intractable** vertigo. It is often, however, associated with a constant "roaring" sound in the ears, as well as ear "pressure."

Vertigo results from so many factors that it is often hard, even for the physician, to determine the actual cause. Any factor that impairs visual input, inner-ear function, peripheral sensory input, or the central nervous system can cause dizziness. In addition, alcohol and many prescription drugs can cause dizziness. So can hypoglycemia in its early stages. It is virtually impossible to distinguish dizziness, syncope, and presyncope in the prehospital setting.

Whenever you suspect stroke, it is essential that you complete the Glasgow Coma Scale rating for later comparison in the emergency department.

* **polycythemia** an excess of red blood cells.

Treat seizures in the elderly as a life-threatening condition, and transport as quickly as possible to eliminate the possibility of stroke.

* **vertigo** the sensation of faintness or dizziness; may cause a loss of balance.

* **intractable** resistant to cure, relief, or control.

Delirium, Dementia, Alzheimer's Disease

Approximately 12 percent of all Canadians over age 65 have some degree of dementia or delirium. **Dementia** is a chronic global cognitive impairment, often progressive or irreversible. The best-known form of dementia is **Alzheimer's disease. Delirium** is a global mental impairment of sudden onset and self-limited duration. (For differences between dementia and delirium, see Table 43-5.) About 420 000 Canadians over age 65 have Alzheimer's disease or other dementia (287 660 women and 132 560 men). One in 13 of all Canadians aged 65 and over has Alzheimer's disease or other dementia.

Delirium Many conditions can cause delirium. The cause may be either organic brain disease or disorders that occur elsewhere in the body. Delirium in the elderly is a serious condition. According to some estimates, about 18 percent of hospitalized elderly patients with delirium die. Possible etiologies or causes include

- Subdural hematoma
- Tumours and other mass lesions
- Drug-induced changes or alcohol intoxication
- CNS infections
- Electrolyte abnormalities
- Cardiac failure
- Fever
- Metabolic disorders, including hypoglycemia
- Chronic endocrine abnormalities, including hypothyroidism and hyperthyroidism
- Postconcussion syndrome

The presentation of delirium varies greatly and can change rapidly during assessment. Common signs and symptoms include the acute onset of anxiety, an inability to focus, disordered thinking, irritability, inappropriate behaviour, fearfulness, excessive energy, or psychotic behaviour, such as hallucinations or paranoia. Aphasic or speaking errors and/or prominent slurring may be present. Normal patterns of eating and sleeping are almost always disrupted.

In distinguishing between delirium, and dementia, err on the side of delirium. The condition is often caused by life-threatening, but reversible, conditions. Causes of delirium such as infections, drug toxicity, and electrolyte imbalances, generally have a good prognosis if identified quickly and managed promptly.

Table 43-5	DISTINGUISHING DEMENTIA AND DELIRIUM*	
Dementia		**Delirium**
Chronic, slowly progressive development		Rapid in onset, fluctuating course
Irreversible disorder		May be reversed, especially if treated early
Greatly impairs memory		Greatly impairs attention
Global cognitive deficits		Focal cognitive deficits
Most commonly caused by Alzheimer's disease		Most commonly caused by systemic disease, drug toxicity, or metabolic changes
Does not require immediate treatment		Requires immediate treatment

*These are general characteristics that apply to most, but not all, cases. For example, some forms of dementia, such as those caused by hypothyroidism, may be reversed.

Dementia Dementia is more prevalent than delirium in the elderly. Over 50 percent of all nursing home patients have some form of dementia. It is usually due to an underlying neurological disease. This mental deterioration is often called "organic brain syndrome," **"senile dementia,"** or "senility." It is important to find out whether an alteration in mental status is acute or chronic. Causes of dementia include

- Small strokes
- Atherosclerosis
- Age-related neurological changes
- Neurological diseases
- Certain hereditary diseases (e.g., Huntington's disease)
- Alzheimer's disease

⁕ **senile dementia** general term used to describe an abnormal decline in mental functioning seen in the elderly; also called "organic brain syndrome" or "multi-infarct dementia."

Signs and symptoms of dementia include progressive disorientation, shortened attention span, **aphasia** or nonsense talking, and hallucinations. Dementia often hampers treatment through the patient's inability to communicate and exhausts caregivers. In moderate to severe cases, you will need to rely on the caregiver for information. (Remain alert to signs of abuse or neglect, which occurs in a disproportionate number of elderly suffering from dementia.)

⁕ **aphasia** absence or impairment of the ability to communicate through speaking, writing, or signing as a result of brain dysfunction.

Alzheimer's Disease Alzheimer's disease is a particular type of dementia. It is a chronic degenerative disorder that attacks the brain and results in impaired memory, thinking, and behaviour. It accounts for more than half of all forms of dementia in the elderly.

Alzheimer's disease generally occurs in stages, each with different signs and symptoms. These stages include:

- *Early Stage.* Characterized by loss of recent memory, inability to learn new material, mood swings, and personality changes. Patients may believe someone is plotting against them when they lose items or forget things. Aggression or hostility is common. Poor judgment is evident.
- *Intermediate Stage.* Characterized by a complete inability to learn new material; wandering, particularly at night; increased falls; loss of ability for self-care, including bathing and use of the toilet.
- *Terminal Stage.* Characterized by an inability to walk and regression to infant stage, including the loss of bowel and bladder functions. Eventually, the patient loses the ability to eat and swallow.

Families caring for an Alzheimer's patient at home also present signs of stress. Remember to treat both the Alzheimer patient and the family and/or caregivers with respect and compassion. Evaluate the needs of the family, and make an appropriate report at your facility. There are support groups available to assist families.

Remember to treat both the Alzheimer patient and family and/or caregivers with respect and compassion.

Parkinson's Disease

Parkinson's disease is a degenerative disorder characterized by changes in muscle response, including tremors, loss of facial expression, and gait disturbances. It mainly appears in people over age 50 and peaks at age 70. The disease affects about 100 000 Canadians. It is the fourth most common neurodegenerative disease among the elderly.

The cause of primary Parkinson's disease remains unknown. However, it affects the basal ganglia in the brain, an area that deciphers messages going to

⁕ **Parkinson's disease** chronic, degenerative nervous disease characterized by tremors, muscular weakness and rigidity, and a loss of postural reflexes.

muscles. Secondary Parkinson's disease is distinguished from primary Parkinson's disease by having a known cause. Some of the most common causes include:

- Viral encephalitis
- Atherosclerosis of cerebral vessels
- Reaction to certain drugs or toxins, such as antipsychotics or carbon monoxide
- Metabolic disorders, such as anoxia
- Tumours
- Head trauma
- Degenerative disorders, such as **Shy-Drager syndrome**

It is impossible in a field setting to distinguish primary and secondary Parkinson's disease. The most common initial sign of a Parkinson's disorder is a resting tremor combined with a **pill-rolling motion**. As the disease progresses, muscles become more rigid and movements become slower and/or more jerky. In some cases, patients may find their movements halted while carrying out some routine task. Their feet may feel "frozen to the ground." Gaits becomes shuffled with short steps and unexpected bursts of speed, often to avoid falling. Kyphotic deformity is a hallmark of the disease.

Patients with Parkinson's disease commonly develop mask-like faces devoid of all expression. They speak in slow, monotone voices. Difficulties in communication, coupled with a loss of mobility, often lead to anxiety and depression.

There is no known cure for Parkinson's disease, with the exception of drug-induced secondary Parkinson's disorders. Exercise may help maintain physical activity or teach the patient adaptive strategies. In calls involving a Parkinson's patient, observe for conditions that may have involved the EMS system, such as a fall or the inability to move. Manage treatable conditions, and transport the patient as needed.

METABOLIC AND ENDOCRINE DISORDERS

As previously mentioned, the endocrine system undergoes a number of age-related changes, which affect hormone levels. The most common endocrine disorders include diabetes mellitus and problems related to the thyroid gland. Of the two, you will more often treat diabetic-related emergencies, particularly hypoglycemia.

Diabetes Mellitus

An estimated 20 percent of older adults have diabetes mellitus, primarily Type II diabetes. Almost 40 percent have some type of glucose intolerance. Reasons that the elderly develop these disorders include

- Poor diet
- Decreased physical activity
- Loss of lean body mass
- Impaired insulin production
- Resistance by body cells to the actions of insulin

Diagnosis of Type II diabetes usually occurs during screening in routine checkups. In some cases, urine tests may register negative because of an increased renal glucose threshold in the elderly. The condition may present, in its early stages, with such vague constitutional symptoms as fatigue or weakness. Allowed to progress, diabetes can result in neuropathy and visual impairment.

✳ Shy-Drager syndrome chronic orthostatic hypotension caused by a primary autonomic nervous system deficiency.

✳ pill-rolling motion an involuntary tremor, usually in one hand or sometimes in both, in which fingers move as if they were rolling a pill back and forth.

These manifestations often lead to more aggressive blood testing, which in most cases will reveal elevated glucose levels.

The treatment of diabetes involves diet, exercise, the use of sulphonylurea agents, and/or insulin. Many diabetics use self-monitoring devices to test glucose levels. Unfortunately, the cost of these devices and the accompanying test strips sometimes discourages the elderly from using them. Elderly patients on insulin also risk hypoglycemia, especially if they accidentally take too much insulin or do not eat enough food following injection. The lack of good nutrition can be particularly troublesome to elderly diabetics. They often find it difficult to prepare meals, fail to enjoy food because of altered taste perceptions, have trouble chewing food, or are unable to purchase adequate and/or the right type of food because of limited income.

Management of diabetic and hypoglycemic emergencies for the elderly are generally the same as for any other patient. DO NOT rule out alcohol as a complicating factor, especially in cases of hypoglycemia. In addition, remember that diabetes places the elderly at increased risk of other complications, including atherosclerosis, delayed healing, **retinopathy,** blindness, altered renal function, and severe peripheral vascular disease, leading to foot ulcers and even amputations.

> *DO NOT rule out alcohol as a complicating factor in cases of hypoglycemia.*

> ***** **retinopathy** any disorder of the retina.

Thyroid Disorders

With normal aging the thyroid gland undergoes moderate atrophy and changes in hormone production. An estimated 2–5 percent of people over age 65 experience hypothyroidism, a condition resulting from inadequate levels of thyroid hormones. It affects women in greater numbers than men, and the prevalence rises with age.

Less than 33 percent of the elderly present with typical signs and symptoms of hypothyroidism. When they do, their complaints are often attributed to aging. Common nonspecific complaints in the elderly include mental confusion, anorexia, falls, incontinence, and decreased mobility. Some patients also experience an increase in muscle or joint pain. Treatment involves thyroid hormone replacement.

Hyperthyroidism is less common among the elderly but may result from medication errors, such as an overdose of thyroid hormone replacement. The typical symptom of heat intolerance is often present. Otherwise, hyperthyroidism presents atypically in the elderly. Common nonspecific features or complaints include atrial fibrillation, failure to thrive (weight loss and apathy combined), abdominal distress, diarrhea, exhaustion, and depression.

The diagnosis and treatment of thyroid disorders do not take place in the field. Elderly patients with known thyroid problems should be encouraged to go to the hospital for medical evaluation.

GASTROINTESTINAL DISORDERS

Gastrointestinal (GI) emergencies are common among the elderly. The most frequent emergency is GI bleeding. However, older people will also describe a variety of other GI complaints—nausea, poor appetite, diarrhea, and constipation, to name a few. Remember, that like other presenting complaints, these conditions may be symptomatic of more serious diseases. Bowel problems, for example, may point to cancer of the colon or other abdominal organs.

Regardless of the complaint, remember that prompt management of a GI emergency is essential for young and old alike. For the elderly, there is a significant risk of hemorrhage and shock. There is a tendency to take GI patients less seriously than those suffering moderate or severe external hemorrhage. This is a serious mistake. Patients with GI complaints should be aggressively managed, especially the

> *Patients with gastrointestinal complaints should be aggressively managed, especially the elderly.*

elderly. Keep in mind that older patients are far more intolerant of hypotension and anoxia than are younger patients. Treatment should include

- Airway management
- Support of breathing and circulation
- High-flow oxygen therapy
- IV fluid replacement with a crystalloid solution
- Rapid transport

Some of the most critical GI problems that you may encounter in the field will involve internal hemorrhage and bowel obstruction. You may also be called on to treat **mesenteric infarct**—a serious and life-threatening condition in an elderly patient. The following will help you to recognize each of these gastrointestinal disorders.

GI Hemorrhage

Gastrointestinal bleeding falls into two general categories: upper GI bleed and lower GI bleed.

Upper GI Bleed This form of gastrointestinal bleeding includes

- *Peptic Ulcer Disease.* Injury to the mucous lining of the upper part of the gastrointestinal tract due to stomach acids, digestive enzymes, and other agents, such as anti-inflammatory drugs.
- *Gastritis.* An inflammation of the lining of the stomach.
- *Esophageal Varices.* An abnormal dilation of veins in the lower esophagus; a common complication of cirrhosis of the liver.
- *Mallory-Weiss Tear.* A tear in the lower esophagus that is often caused by severe and prolonged retching.

Lower GI Bleed Conditions categorized as lower GI bleeding include

- *Diverticulosis.* The presence of small pouches on the colon that tend to develop with age; causes 70 percent of life-threatening lower GI bleeds.
- *Tumours.* Tumours of the colon can cause bleeding when the tumour erodes into blood vessels within the intestine or surrounding organs.
- *Ischemic Colitis.* An inflammation of the colon due to impaired or decreased blood supply.
- *Arteriovenous Malformations.* An abnormal link between an artery and a vein.

Signs of significant GI blood loss include the presence of "coffee ground" emesis; black tar-like stools (**melena**); obvious blood in the emesis or stool; orthostatic hypotension; pulse greater than 100 (unless on beta-blockers); and confusion. Gastrointestinal bleeding in the elderly may result in such complications as a recent increase in angina symptoms, congestive heart failure, weakness, or dyspnea.

Bowel Obstruction

Bowel obstruction in the elderly typically involves the small bowel. Causes include tumours, prior abdominal surgery, use of certain medications, and occasionally the presence of vertebral compression fractures. The patient will typically complain of diffuse abdominal pain, bloating, nausea, and vomiting. The abdomen may feel distended when palpated. Bowel sounds may be hypoactive or absent. If the obstruction has been present for a prolonged period of time, the patient may have fever, weakness, shock, and various electrolyte disturbances.

Mesenteric Infarct

Vessels arising from the superior or inferior mesenteric arteries generally serve the bowel. An infarct occurs when a portion of the bowel does not receive enough blood to survive. Certain age-related changes make the elderly more vulnerable to this condition. First, as a person ages, changes in the heart (such as atrial fibrillation) or the vessels (atherosclerosis) predispose the patient to a clot lodging in one of the branches serving the bowel. Second, changes in the bowel itself can promote swelling that effectively cuts off blood flow.

The primary symptom of a bowel infarct is pain out of proportion to the secondary assessment. Signs include

- Bloody diarrhea, but usually not a massive hemorrhage
- Some tachycardia, although there may be a vagal effect masking the sign
- Abdominal distention

The patient is at great risk for shock as the dead bowel attracts interstitial and intravascular fluids, thus removing them from use. Necrotic products are released to the peritoneal cavity, leading to a massive infection. The prognosis is poor due, in part, to decreased physiological reserves on the part of the older patient.

SKIN DISORDERS

Younger and older adults experience common skin disorders at about the same rates. However, age-related changes in the immune system make the elderly more prone to certain chronic skin diseases and infections. They are also more likely to develop **pressure ulcers** (bedsores) than any other age group.

Skin Diseases

Elderly patients commonly complain about **pruritus** or itching. This condition can be caused by dermatitis (eczema) or environmental conditions, especially during winter, that is, from hot dry air in the home and cold dry air outside. Keep in mind that generalized itching can also be a sign of systemic diseases, particularly liver and renal disorders. When itching is strong and unrelenting, suspect an underlying disease, and encourage the patient to seek medical evaluation.

Slower healing and compromised tissue perfusion in the elderly makes them more susceptible to bacterial infection of wounds, appearing as cellutitis, impetigo, and, in the case of immunocompromised adults, staphylococcal scalded skin. The elderly also experience a higher incidence of fungal infections, partly because of decreases in the cutaneous immunological response. In addition, they suffer higher rates of **herpes zoster** (shingles), which peaks between ages 50 and 70. Although these skin disorders occur in the young, their duration and severity increases markedly with age.

In treating skin disorders, remember that many conditions may be drug induced. Beta-blockers, for example, can worsen psoriasis, which occurs in about 3 percent of elderly patients. Question patients about their medications, keeping in mind that certain prescription drugs, for example, penicillins and

Content Review

SIGNS AND SYMPTOMS OF BOWEL OBSTRUCTION

- Diffuse abdominal pain
- Bloating
- Nausea
- Vomiting
- Distended abdomen
- Hypoactive/absent bowel sounds

✳ **pressure ulcer** ischemic damage and subsequent necrosis affecting the skin, subcutaneous tissue, and often the muscle; result of intense pressure over a short time or low pressure over a long time; also known as pressure sore or bedsore.

✳ **pruritus** itching; often occurs as a symptom of some systemic change or illness.

Keep in mind that generalized itching can also be a sign of systemic diseases, particularly liver and renal disorders.

✳ **herpes zoster** an acute eruption caused by a reactivation of latent varicella virus (chicken pox) in the dorsal root ganglia; also known as shingles.

sulphonamides, and some over-the-counter drugs can cause skin eruptions. Also ask about topical home remedies, such as alcohol or soaps, that may cause or worsen the disorder. Find out if the patient is compliant with prescribed topical treatments. Finally, remember that some drugs and topical medications commonly used to treat skin disorders in the young can worsen or cause other problems for the elderly. Antihistamines and corticosteroids are two to three times more likely to provoke adverse reactions in the elderly than in younger adults.

Pressure Ulcers (Decubitus Ulcers)

Most pressure ulcers occur in people over age 70. As many as 20 percent of patients enter the hospital with a pressure ulcer or develop one while hospitalized. The highest incidence occurs in nursing homes, where up to 25 percent of patients may develop this condition.

Pressure ulcers typically develop from the waist down, usually over bony prominences, in bedridden patients. However, they can occur anywhere on the body and with the patient in any position. Pressure ulcers usually result from tissue hypoxia and affect the skin, subcutaneous tissues, and muscle. Factors that can increase the risk of this condition include

* External compression of tissues (i.e., pressure)
* Altered sensory perception
* **Maceration,** caused by excessive moisture
* Decreased activity
* Decreased mobility
* Poor nutrition
* Friction or shear

To reduce the development of pressures ulcers or to alleviate them, you may take these steps.

* Assist the patient in changing position frequently, especially during extended transport, to reduce the length of time pressure is placed on any one point.
* Use a pull sheet to move the patient, reducing the likelihood of friction.
* Reduce the possibility of shearing by padding areas of skin prior to movement.
* Unless a life-threatening condition is present, take time to clean and dry areas of excessive moisture, such as due to urinary or fecal incontinence and excessive perspiration.
* Clean ulcers with normal saline solution, and cover with hydrocolloid or hydrogel dressings, if available. With severe ulcers, pack with loosely woven gauze moistened with normal saline.

* **maceration** process of softening a solid by soaking in a liquid.

MUSCULOSKELETAL DISORDERS

The skeleton, as you know, is a metabolically active organ. Its metabolic processes are influenced by a number of factors, including age, diet, exercise, and hormone levels. The musculoskeletal system is also subject to disease. In fact, musculoskeletal diseases are the leading cause of functional impairment in the elderly. Although usually not fatal, musculoskeletal disorders often produce chronic disability, which, in turn, creates a context for illness. Two of the most widespread musculoskeletal disorders include **osteoarthritis** and **osteoporosis.**

* **osteoarthritis** a degenerative joint disease, characterized by a loss of articular cartilage and hypertrophy of bone.

* **osteoporosis** softening of bone tissue due to the loss of essential minerals, principally calcium.

Osteoarthritis

Osteoarthritis is the leading cause of disability among people age 65 and older. Many experts think the condition may not be one disease but several with similar presentations. While wear-and-tear as well as age-related changes, such as loss of muscle mass, predisposes the elderly to osteoarthritis, other factors may play a role as well. Presumed contributing causes include

- Obesity
- Primary disorders of the joint, such as inflammatory arthritis
- Trauma
- Congenital abnormalities, such as hip dysplasia

Osteoarthritis in the elderly presents initially as joint pain, worsened by exercise and improved by rest. As the disease progresses, pain may be accompanied by diminished mobility, joint deformity, and crepitus or grating sensations. Late signs include tenderness on palpation or during passive motion.

The most effective treatment involves management before the disability develops or worsens. Prevention strategies include stretching exercises and activities that strengthen stress-absorbing ligaments (Figure 43-8). Immobilization, even for short periods, can exacerbate the condition. Drug therapy is usually aimed at lessening pain and/or inflammation. Surgery—that is, total joint replacement—is usually the last resort after more conservative methods have failed.

Wear-and-tear is the most common factor leading to osteoarthritis.

Osteoporosis

Osteoporosis affects an estimated 1.4 million Canadians and is largely responsible for fractures of the hip, wrist, and vertebral bones following a fall or other injury. Risk factors include

- *Age.* Peak bone mass for men and women occurs in their third and fourth decades of life and declines at varying rates thereafter. Decreased bone density generally becomes a treatment consideration at about age 50.
- *Gender.* The decline of estrogen production places women at a higher risk of developing osteoporosis than are men. Women are more than twice as likely to have brittle bones, especially if they experience early menopause (before age 45) and do not take estrogen replacement therapy. One in four women over the age of 50 has osteoporosis.

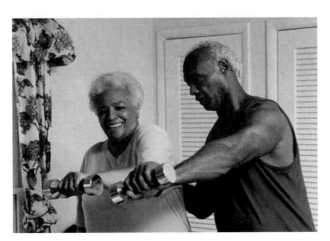

FIGURE 43-8 Regular stretching and weight-bearing exercises help prevent the development of osteoarthritis. (© The Stock Market Photo Agency.)

- *Race.* Whites and Asians are more likely to develop osteoporosis than are African Americans and Hispanics, who have higher bone mass at skeletal peak.
- *Body Weight.* Thin people, or people with low body weight, are at greater risk of osteoporosis than obese people. Increased skeletal weight is thought to promote bone density. However, weight-bearing exercise can confer the same benefit.
- *Family History.* Genetic factors—that is, peak bone mass attainment—and a family history of fractures may predispose a person to osteoporosis.
- *Miscellaneous.* Late menarche, nulliparity, and use of caffeine, alcohol, and cigarettes are all thought to be important determinants of bone mass.

Unless a bone density test is conducted, persons with osteoporosis are usually asymptotic until a fracture occurs. The precipitating event can be as slight as turning over in bed, lifting a package, or even sneezing forcefully. Management includes prevention of fractures through exercise and drug therapy, such as the administration of calcium, vitamin D, estrogen, and other medications or minerals. Once the condition occurs, pain management also becomes a consideration.

RENAL DISORDERS

* **glomerulonephritis** a form of nephritis, or inflammation of the kidneys; primarily involves the glomeruli, one of the capillary networks that are part of the renal corpuscles in the nephrons.

The most common renal diseases in the elderly include renal failure, **glomerulonephritis,** and renal blood clots. These problems may be traced to two age-related factors: (1) loss in kidney size, and (2) changes in the walls of the renal arteries and in the arterioles serving the glomeruli. In general, the kidney loses approximately one-third of its weight between the ages of 30 and 80. Most of this loss occurs in the tissues that filter blood. When filtering tissue is gone, blood is shunted from the precapillary side directly to venules on the postcapillary side, thus bypassing any tissue still capable of filtering. The result is a reduction in kidney efficiency. This condition is complicated by changes in renal arteries, which promote the development of renal emboli and thrombi.

With renal changes, elderly patients are more likely to accumulate toxins and medications within the bloodstream. Occasionally, this will be obvious to the patient as she experiences a substantial decrease in urine output. More often, however, the elderly are prone to a type of renal failure in which urine output remains normal to high while the kidney remains ineffective in clearing wastes.

Processes that precipitate acute renal failure include hypotension, heart failure, major surgery, sepsis, angiographic procedures (the dye is nephrotoxic), and use of nephrotoxic antibiotics, that is, gentamicin, tobramycin. Ongoing hypertension also figures in the development of chronic renal failure.

URINARY DISORDERS

* **urosepsis** septicemia originating from the urinary tract.

Urinary tract infections (UTIs) affect as much as 10 percent of the elderly population each year. Younger women generally suffer more UTIs than do young men, but the distribution is almost even in the elderly. Most of these infections result from bacteria and easily lead to **urosepsis** due to reduced immune system function among the elderly.

A number of factors contribute to the high rate of UTIs among the elderly. They include

- Bladder outlet obstruction from benign prostatic hyperplasia (in men)
- Atrophic vaginitis (in women)

- Stroke
- Immobilization
- Use of indwelling bladder catheters
- Diabetes
- Upper urinary tract stone
- Dementia, with resulting poor hygiene

Signs or symptoms of a UTI range from cloudy, foul-smelling urine to the typical complaints of bladder pain and frequent urination. Urosepsis presents as an acute process, including fever, chills, abdominal discomfort, and other signs of septic shock. The septicemia generally begins within 24–72 hours after catheterization or cystoscopy.

Treatment of urosepsis commonly includes placement of a large-bore IV catheter for administration of fluids and parenteral antibiotics. Diagnosis of urosepsis is based on history and other physical findings. Prompt transport is critical. The prognosis for elderly patients with urosepsis is poor, with a mortality rate of approximately 30 percent. Maintenance of fluid balance as well as adequate blood pressure is essential.

ENVIRONMENT-RELATED EMERGENCIES

As previously mentioned, environmental extremes represent a great health risk for the elderly. Nearly 50 percent of all **heatstroke** deaths occur among people over age 50. The elderly are just as susceptible to low temperatures. As you may already know from your paramedic experience, thermoregulatory emergencies represent some of the most common EMS calls involving the elderly.

Hypothermia

A number of factors predispose the elderly to hypothermia. These include

- Accidental exposure to cold
- Central nervous system (CNS) disorders, including head trauma, stroke, tumours, or subdural hematomas
- Endocrine disorders, including hypoglycemia and diabetes (Patients with diabetes are six times as likely to develop hypothermia as other patients.)
- Drugs that interfere with heat production, including alcohol, antidepressants, and tranquilizers
- Malnutrition or starvation
- Chronic illness
- Forced inactivity as a result of arthritis, dementia, falls, paralysis, or Parkinson's disease
- Low or fixed income, which discourages the use of home heating
- Inflammatory dermatitis
- A-V shunts, which increase heat loss

Signs and symptoms of hypothermia can be slow to develop. Many times, elderly patients with hypothermia lose their sensitivity to cold and fail to complain. As a result, hypothermia may be missed. Nonspecific complaints may suggest a metabolic disorder or stroke. Hypothermic patients may exhibit slow speech,

Prompt transport is critical for elderly patients with suspected urosepsis, as the condition has a mortality rate of approximately 30 percent.

* heatstroke life-threatening condition caused by a disturbance in temperature regulation; in the elderly, characterized by extreme fever and, in extreme cases, delirium or coma.

confusion, and sleepiness. In the early stages, patients will exhibit hypertension and an increased heart rate. As hypothermia progresses, however, blood pressure drops, and the heart rate slows, sometimes to a barely detectable level.

Remember that the elderly hypothermic patient often does not shiver.

Remember that the elderly patient with hypothermia often does not shiver. Check the abdomen and back to see if the skin is cool to the touch. Expect subcutaneous tissues to be firm. If your unit has a low-temperature thermometer, check the patient's core temperature.

As with other medical disorders, prevention is the preferred treatment. However, once elderly patients develop hypothermia, they become progressively impaired. Treat even mild cases of hypothermia, or suspected hypothermia, as a medical emergency. Focus on the rewarming techniques used with other patients and rapid transport. Maintain ongoing assessment to ensure that the hypothermia does not complicate existing medical problems or untreated disorders. Death most commonly results from cardiac arrest or ventricular fibrillation.

Treat even a mild case of hypothermia, or suspected hypothermia, as a medical emergency.

Hyperthermia (Heatstroke)

Age-related changes in sweat glands and increased incidence of heart disease place the elderly at risk of heat stress. They may develop heat cramps, heat exhaustion, or heatstroke. While the first two disorders rarely result in death, heatstroke is a serious medical emergency. Risk factors for severe hyperthermia include

Heatstroke in the elderly is a serious medical emergency.

- Altered sensory output, which would normally warn a person of overheating
- Inadequate liquid intake
- Decreased functioning of the thermoregulatory centre
- Commonly prescribed medications that inhibit sweating, such as antihistamines and tricyclic antidepressants
- Low or fixed income, which may result in a lack of air conditioning or adequate ventilation
- Alcoholism
- Concomitant medical disorders
- Use of diuretics, which increase fluid loss

Like hypothermia, early heatstroke may present with nonspecific signs and symptoms, such as nausea, lightheadedness, dizziness, or headache. High temperature is the most reliable indicator, but consider even a slight temperature elevation as symptomatic if coupled with an absence of sweating and a neurological impairment. Severe hypotension also exists in many critical patients.

Prevention strategies include adequate fluid intake, reduced activity, shelter in an air-conditioned environment, and use of light clothing. If hyperthermia develops, however, rapid treatment and transport are necessary.

TOXICOLOGICAL EMERGENCIES

As previously mentioned, aging alters pharmacokinetics and pharmacodynamics in the elderly. Functional changes in the kidneys, liver, and gastrointestinal system slow the absorption and elimination of many medications. In addition, the various compensatory mechanisms that help buffer against medication side effects are less effective in the elderly than these mechanisms are in younger patients.

Approximately 30 percent of all hospital admissions are related to drug-related illnesses. About 50 percent of all drug-related deaths occur in people over age 60. Accidental overdoses may occur more frequently in the aged due to confusion, vision impairment, self-medication, forgetfulness, and concurrent drug use. Intentional drug overdose also occurs in attempts at self-destruction. Another complicating factor is the abuse of alcohol among the elderly.

It is essential for the paramedic to be familiar with the range of side effects that can be caused by the polypharmacy (use of multiple medications) in geriatric patients. In assessing the geriatric patient, always take these steps:

- Obtain a full list of medications currently taken by the patient, including prescribed medications, over-the-counter medications, and herbal and other dietary supplements.
- Elicit any medications that are newly prescribed. (Some side effects appear within a few days of taking a new medication.)
- Obtain a good past medical history. Find out if your patient has a history of renal or hepatic depression.
- Know your medications, their routes of elimination, and their potential side effects.
- If possible, always take all medications to the hospital along with the patient.

A knowledge of pharmacology is important in all patients. However, it is critical in recognizing potential toxicological emergencies in the geriatric patient. Some of the drugs or substances that have been identified as commonly causing toxicity in the elderly are described in the following sections.

Lidocaine

Lidocaine is used for the treatment of ventricular dysrhythmias. It is also a commonly used local anesthetic. The drug is primarily metabolized by the liver and excreted through the kidneys. In older patients, hepatic impairment can cause elevated lidocaine levels and possible toxicity. It is recommended that the lidocaine dose be reduced by 50 percent in patients greater than 70 years of age.

Beta-Blockers

Beta-blockers are used as antihypertensives and antidysrhythmics and for glaucoma. In the elderly, beta-blockers can cause depression, lethargy, and orthostatic hypotension. It is important to remember that patients taking beta-blockers may not be able to increase their heart rate, which can mask the early signs of shock.

Antihypertensives/Diuretics

Diuretics can cause electrolyte abnormalities. In the elderly, decreased drug clearance can result in hypotension or dehydration. Other types of antihypertensives may affect the elderly differently. Because of this, it is sometimes necessary to reduce the dose or change to a less toxic agent.

Angiotensin-Converting Enzyme (ACE) Inhibitors

ACE inhibitors are popular antihypertensive agents because they have a good safety profile and are well tolerated by most patients. ACE inhibitors are also used to decrease afterload in congestive heart failure (CHF) and pulmonary edema. In the elderly, ACE inhibitors can cause plasma volume reduction and hypotension. Also, they have been associated with dizziness, lightheadedness, skin rashes, and cough.

Digitalis (Digoxin, Lanoxin)

Most patients who take digitalis on a regular basis are elderly. The drug is extremely effective at controlling the heart rate in tachydysrhythmias and at increasing cardiac output in CHF. Digitalis toxicity is the most common adverse drug effect that is seen in the elderly. It can cause visual disturbances, nausea, anorexia, abdominal discomfort, headache, and vomiting. Virtually any dysrhythmia can be seen in digitalis toxicity.

Antipsychotics/Antidepressants

Psychoactive medications affect mood, behaviour, and other aspects of mental functioning. They are used in the elderly for depression and psychosis. The elderly are more vulnerable to the side effects of these medications and should be closely monitored. Be particularly alert for extrapyramidal system reactions with the antipsychotic medications.

Antiparkinsonion Agents

Drugs used in the treatment of Parkinson's disease can affect other body systems. Common complications include dyskinesia and psychological disturbances (such as hallucinations and nightmares).

Antiseizure Medications

Medications that prevent seizures can cause sedation in the elderly. They can also cause GI distress, headache, lack of coordination, and skin rashes. The doses of these drugs often must be reduced in the elderly.

Analgesics and Anti-inflammatory Agents

Pain medications, especially the narcotics, can cause sedation, mood changes, nausea, vomiting, and constipation. The anti-inflammatory agents can cause GI distress, including gastritis and peptic ulcers. Elderly patients taking these classes of medications should be closely monitored.

Corticosteroids

Corticosteroids are necessary for the treatment of several diseases seen in the aged, including chronic obstructive pulmonary disease, rheumatoid arthritis, and other inflammatory conditions. These drugs can cause ulcers, hypertension, glaucoma, and increased risk of infection. These side effects are more prevalent in the elderly.

For additional information on pharmacology, pharmacokinetics, and pharmacodynamics, review Chapter 14, Pharmacology. For more information on specific drugs, consult the Brady publication *Drug Guide for Paramedics*.

SUBSTANCE ABUSE

✱ **substance abuse** misuse of chemically active agents, such as alcohol, psychoactive chemicals, and therapeutic agents; typically results in clinically significant impairment or distress.

Substance abuse is a widespread problem in Canada. It affects nearly all age groups, including the elderly.

In general, the factors that contribute to substance abuse among the elderly are different from those of younger people. They include

- Age-related changes
- Loss of employment

- Loss of spouse or partner
- Multiple prescriptions
- Malnutrition
- Loneliness
- Moving from a long-loved house to an apartment

Like other age groups, the elderly may intentionally abuse substances, to escape pain or life itself. Other times, particularly in the case of prescription drugs, the abuse is accidental. Substance abuse in the elderly may involve drugs, alcohol, or both drugs and alcohol.

Drug Abuse

As previously mentioned, compared with younger adults, people aged 65 and older have more illnesses, consume more drugs, and are more sensitive to adverse drug reactions. The sheer number of medications taken by the elderly make them vulnerable to drug abuse. People aged 65 and older fill an average of 13 prescriptions per year. The elderly also use a disproportionate percentage of over-the-counter drugs.

Polypharmacy, coupled with impaired vision and/or memory, increase the likelihood of complications. The elderly might experience drug–drug interactions, drug–disease interactions, and drug–food interactions.

The elderly who become physically and/or psychologically dependent on drugs (or alcohol) are more likely to hide their dependence and less likely to seek help than other age groups. Common signs and symptoms of drug abuse include

- Memory changes
- Drowsiness
- Decreased vision/hearing
- Orthostatic hypotension
- Poor dexterity
- Mood changes
- Falling
- Restlessness
- Weight loss

In cases of suspected drug abuse, carefully document your findings. Collect medications for identification at the hospital, where the patient can be evaluated and, if necessary, referred for substance abuse treatment.

Alcohol Abuse

In a national survey, nearly 50 percent of the elderly reported abstinence from alcohol. However, the same survey found that 15 percent of the men and 12 percent of the women interviewed regularly drank in excess of the one-drink-a-day limit. Those percentages are expected to rise with the aging of the baby-boom generation, which has generally used alcohol more frequently than their predecessors.

The use or abuse of alcohol places the elderly at high risk of toxicity. Physiological changes, such as organ dysfunction, makes older adults more susceptible to the effects of alcohol. Consumption of even moderate amounts of alcohol can interfere with drug therapy, often leading to dangerous consequences. Severe stress and a history of heavy and/or regular drinking predisposes a person to alcohol dependence or abuse in later life.

Unless a patient is openly intoxicated, discovery of alcohol abuse is only possible from a thorough history. Signs and symptoms of alcohol abuse in the elderly may be very subtle or confused with other conditions. Remember that even small amounts of alcohol can cause intoxication in an older person. If possible, question family, friends, or caregivers about the patient's drinking patterns. Pertinent findings include

- Mood swings, denial, and hostility (especially when questioned about drinking)
- Confusion
- History of falls
- Anorexia
- Insomnia
- Visible anxiety
- Nausea

Treatment follows many of the same steps as for any other patient with a pattern of abusive drinking. DO NOT judge the patient. Evaluate the need for fluid therapy, and keep in mind the possibility of withdrawal. Transport the patient to the hospital for evaluation and referral for treatment. Ideally, these patients will seek support from community organizations, such as Alcoholics Anonymous (AA). Many communities have AA groups specifically for senior citizens.

BEHAVIOURAL/PSYCHOLOGICAL DISORDERS

When behavioural or psychological problems develop later in life, they are often dismissed as normal age-related changes. This attitude denies an elderly person the opportunity to correct a treatable condition and/or overlooks an underlying physical disorder. Studies have shown that the elderly retain their basic personalities and their adaptive cognitive abilities. In other words, intellectual decline and/or regressive behaviour are not normal age-related changes. Unless an organic brain disorder is involved, alterations in behaviour should be considered symptomatic of a possible psychological problem.

It is important to keep in mind the emotionally stressful situations facing many elderly people—isolation, loneliness, loss of self-dependence, loss of strength, fear of the future, and more. The elderly also face a higher incidence of secondary depression as a result of neuroleptic medications, such as Haldol and Thorazine. Some of the common classifications of psychological disorders related to age include

- Organic brain syndrome
- Affective disorders (depression)
- Personality disorders (dependent personality)
- Dissociative disorders (paranoid schizophrenia)

As with other people, the emotional well-being of the elderly affects their overall physical health. Therefore, it is important that you note evidence of altered behaviour in any elderly patient whom you assess. Common signs and symptoms of a psychological disorder include lapses in memory, cognitive difficulty, changes in sleep patterns, fear of death, changes in sexual interest, thoughts of suicide, or withdrawal from society.

In general, management of psychological disorders in the elderly is the same as for other age groups. Two of the most common emotional disturbances that you may encounter in the elderly are depression and suicide.

Depression

Up to 15 percent of the noninstitutionalized elderly experience depression. Within institutions, that figure rises to about 30 percent. The incidence of depression among the elderly is expected to rise as the baby boomers—with their larger numbers and more prevalent depression at an earlier age—enter their 60s.

Some of the general signs and symptoms noted previously may indicate depression. Ask the patient about feelings of sadness or despair. Determine if she has suffered episodes of crying. Inquire about past psychological treatment and current stressful events, particularly the death of a loved one. Keep in mind that sensory changes—especially deafness and blindness—may make the patient vulnerable to depression. Serious acute diseases can have the same effect. If the patient recognizes the depression, ask about the duration and any prior bouts. Find out if the patient has been given any medications to treat the depression. If so, check compliance.

Some depressed patients may exhibit **hypochondriasis** (hypochondria). If this condition is a side effect of the depression, the patient will still show some degree of emotional pain and/or **dysphoria**. Although you may not be able to identify hypochondria in the field, remember that the condition is an illness and requires treatment by trained medical personnel.

In general, depressed patients should receive supportive care. Encourage them to talk, delicately raising questions about suicidal thoughts. The seriously depressed patient should be transported to the hospital. Treatment of depression usually entails psychotherapy and/or antidepressants.

Suicide

Depression is the leading cause for suicide among the elderly. As a group, the elderly are less likely to seek help than are the young. They are also less likely to express their anger or sorrow, turning their feelings inward instead. Other stressors that put the elderly at risk of suicide include

- Chronic illness
- Physical impairment
- Unrelieved pain
- Living in a youth-oriented society
- Family issues
- Financial problems
- Isolation and loneliness
- Substance abuse
- Low serotonin levels (Serotonin declines with age.)
- Bereavement
- Family history of suicide

Suicidal behaviour is related to stress. As a paramedic, you should try to evaluate the stress from an elderly patient's point of view, keeping the preceding factors in mind. In cases of a seriously depressed patient, elicit behaviour patterns from family, friends, or caregivers. Warning signs may include

- Loss of interest in activities that were once enjoyable
- Curtailing social interaction, grooming, and self-care
- Breaking from medical or exercise regimens

* **hypochondriasis** an abnormal concern with one's health, with the false belief of suffering from some disease, despite medical assurances to the contrary; commonly known as hypochondria.

* **dysphoria** an exaggerated feeling of depression or unrest, characterized by a mood of general dissatisfaction, restlessness, discomfort, and unhappiness.

Remember that hypochondriasis is an illness, too.

- Grieving a personal loss ("I don't want to live without him/her.")
- Feeling useless ("Nobody would miss me.")
- Putting affairs in order, giving away things, finalizing a will
- Stock-piling medications or obtaining other lethal means of self-destruction, including firearms

Be particularly alert to suicide among the acutely ill. With more patients being returned home to care for themselves, there is a higher incidence of suicide among the terminally ill, especially cancer victims. A lack of postacute hospital care can be interpreted as a lack of caring in general.

Prevention of suicide among the elderly involves intervention by all levels of society, from family to EMS to hospital workers. It is important to dispel the common myths about aging and age-related diseases. Recognition of warning signs and involvement of appropriate individuals and agencies are critical.

Your first priorities in the management of a suicidal elderly patient are to protect yourself and then to protect the patient from self-harm. To do this, you must gain access to the patient. This may require breaking into a house or room, particularly if the patient is unconscious or can be readily seen. Remember to summon law enforcement personnel as necessary. DO NOT RULE OUT FIREARMS USE AMONG THE ELDERLY.

If you reach the patient, emergency care has the highest priority following crew safety. Conduct a brief interview with the patient, if possible, to determine the need for further action. DO NOT leave the suicidal patient alone. Administer medications with caution, keeping in mind polypharmacy and drug interactions in the elderly. ALL SUICIDAL ELDERLY PATIENTS SHOULD BE TRANSPORTED TO THE HOSPITAL.

Do not rule out firearms use among the elderly.

All suicidal elderly patients should be transported to the hospital.

TRAUMA IN THE ELDERLY PATIENT

Trauma is the leading cause of death among the elderly. Older patients who sustain moderate to severe injuries are more likely to die than their younger counterparts. Postinjury disability is also more common in the elderly than in the young.

CONTRIBUTING FACTORS

A number of factors contribute to the high incidence and severity of trauma among the elderly. Slower reflexes, arthritis, and diminished eyesight and hearing predispose the elderly to accidents, especially falls. Because of their physical state and vulnerability, the elderly are also at high risk from trauma caused by criminal assault. Purse snatching, armed robbery, and assault occur all too frequently in the elderly population, especially among those living in urban areas.

Age-related factors that place the elderly at risk of severe injury and complications include

- Osteoporosis and muscle weakness—increased likelihood of fractures
- Reduced cardiac reserve—decreased ability to compensate for blood loss
- Decreased respiratory function—increased likelihood of **acute respiratory distress syndrome (ARDS)**
- Impaired renal function—decreased ability to adapt to fluid shifts
- Decreased elasticity in the peripheral blood vessels—greater susceptibility to tearing

 acute respiratory distress syndrome (ARDS) respiratory insufficiency marked by progressive hypoxemia, due to severe inflammatory damage.

GENERAL ASSESSMENT

As with any other trauma patient, determine the mechanism of injury. Leading causes of trauma in the elderly include falls, motor vehicle crashes, burns, assault or abuse, and underlying medical problems, such as syncope.

In assessing elderly trauma patients, remember that blood pressure readings may be deceptive. Older patients typically have a higher blood pressure than younger patients. Although a blood pressure of 110/70 may be normal for a 30-year-old, it could represent a low blood pressure, and possibly shock, for an older patient. Elderly trauma patients also may not exhibit an elevated pulse—a common early sign of hypoperfusion. This may be because of chronic heart disease or the use of medications to treat hypertension or a myocardial infarction. Fractures may also be obscured or concealed because of a diminished sense of pain among the elderly. One of the best indicators of shock in the elderly is an altered mental status or changes in consciousness during assessment. Elderly trauma patients who exhibit confusion or agitation are candidates for rapid transport.

In assessing elderly trauma patients, remember that blood pressure and pulse readings can be deceptive in hypoperfusion.

Observing for Abuse/Neglect

Make sure you observe the scene for signs of abuse and neglect. Abuse of the elderly is as big a problem in North American society as child abuse and neglect. **Geriatric abuse** is defined as a syndrome in which an elderly person has received serious physical or psychological injury from family members or other caregivers. Abuse of the elderly knows no socioeconomic bounds. It often occurs when an older person is no longer able to be totally independent, and the family has difficulty upholding their commitment to care for the patient. It can also occur in nursing homes and other health-care facilities. The profile for the potential geriatric abuser may often show a great deal of life stress. In many cases, there is sleep deprivation, marital discord, financial problems, and work-related problems. As the abuser's life gets in further disarray, and as the patient further deteriorates, abuse may be the outcome.

Signs and symptoms of geriatric abuse and neglect are often obvious (Figure 43-9). Unexplained trauma is usually the primary presentation. The average

✱ **geriatric abuse** a syndrome in which an elderly person is physically or psychologically injured by another person.

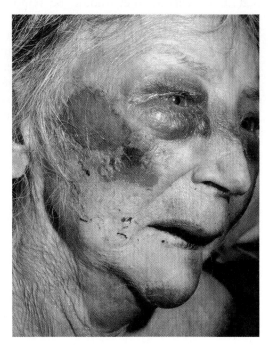

FIGURE 43-9 When you encounter evidence of serious head injury, maintain suspicion of geriatric abuse until proven otherwise.

abused patient is older than 80 and has multiple medical problems, such as cancer, congestive heart failure, heart disease, and incontinence. Senile dementia is often present. In these cases, it can be hard to determine whether the dementia is chronic or acute, especially if there is an increased likelihood of head trauma from abuse.

Whenever you suspect geriatric abuse, obtain a complete patient and family history. Pay particular attention to inconsistencies. *DO NOT confront the family.* Instead, report your suspicions to the emergency department and the appropriate governmental authority. Many provinces and territories have very strong laws protecting the elderly from abuse or neglect. In fact, many provinces and territories consider it a criminal offence *not* to report suspected geriatric abuse.

Many provinces and territories have laws that require prehospital personnel to report suspected cases of geriatric abuse and/or neglect.

GENERAL MANAGEMENT

The priorities of care for the elderly trauma patient are similar to those for any trauma patient. However, you must keep in mind age-related systemic changes and the presence of chronic diseases. This is especially true of the cardiovascular, respiratory, and renal systems.

Cardiovascular Considerations

Recent or past myocardial infarctions may contribute to the risk of dysrhythmia or congestive heart failure in the trauma patient. In addition, there may be a decreased response of the heart, in adjusting heart rate and stroke volume, to hypovolemia. An elderly trauma patient may require higher than usual arterial pressures for perfusion of vital organs, due to increased peripheral vascular resistance and hypertension. Care must be taken in intravenous fluid administration because of decreased myocardial reserves. Hypotension, hypovolemia, and hypervolemia are poorly tolerated in the elderly patient.

Respiratory Considerations

In managing the airway and ventilation in an elderly trauma patient, you must consider the physical changes that may affect treatment. Check for dentures and determine whether they should be removed. Keep in mind that age-related changes can decrease chest wall movement and vital capacity. Age also reduces the tolerance of all organs for anoxia. Remember, too, that chronic obstructive pulmonary disease (COPD) is widespread among the elderly.

Make necessary adjustments in treatment to provide adequate oxygenation and appropriate CO_2 removal. It is important to remember that use of 50-percent nitrous oxide (Nitronox) for elderly patients may result in more respiratory depression than would occur in younger patients. Positive pressure ventilation (PPV) should also be used cautiously. There is an increased danger of resultant alkalosis and rupture of emphysematous bullae, making the elderly more vulnerable to pneumothorax.

Renal Considerations

The decreased ability of the kidneys to maintain normal acid/base balance and to compensate for fluid changes can further complicate the management of the elderly trauma patient. Any preexisting renal disease can decrease the kidney's ability to compensate. The decrease in renal function, along with a decreased cardiac reserve, places the elderly injured patient at risk for fluid overload and pulmonary edema. Remember, too, that renal changes allow toxins and medications to accumulate more readily in the elderly.

Transport Considerations

You may have to modify the positioning, immobilization, and packaging of the elderly trauma patient before transport. Be attentive to physical deformities, such as arthritis, spinal abnormalities, or frozen limbs, that may cause pain or special care (Figure 43-10a–c). Recall the frailty of an elderly person's skin and avoid creating skin tears or pressure sores. Keep in mind that trauma places an elderly person at increased risk of hypothermia. Ensure that the patient is kept warm at all times.

Keep in mind that trauma places an elderly person at increased risk of hypothermia. Ensure that the patient is kept warm at all times.

SPECIFIC INJURIES

The elderly can be subject to a variety of injuries, just like any other age group. The three most common categories of injuries among the elderly include orthopedic injuries, burns, and injuries of the head and spine.

Orthopedic Injuries

As previously mentioned, the elderly suffer the greatest mortality and greatest incidence of disability from falls. Approximately 33 percent of falls in the elderly result in at least one fractured bone. The most common fall-related fracture is a fracture of the hip or pelvis (Figure 43-11). Osteoporosis and general frailty

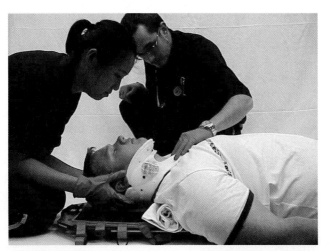

FIGURE 43-10a In an elderly patient with curvature of the spine, place padding behind the neck when immobilizing a patient to a long spine board.

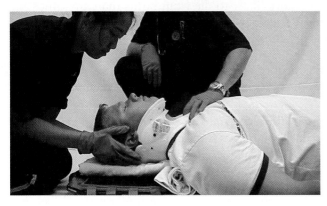

FIGURE 43-10b Additional padding, such as rolled blankets or towels behind the head, may be needed to keep the head in a neutral, in-line position.

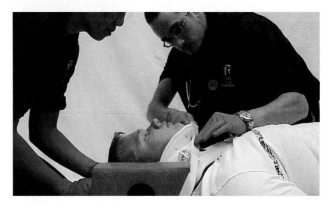

FIGURE 43-10c Secure the patient's head with a head immobilizer device. To prevent spinal damage, maintain manual stabilization until the head is secured.

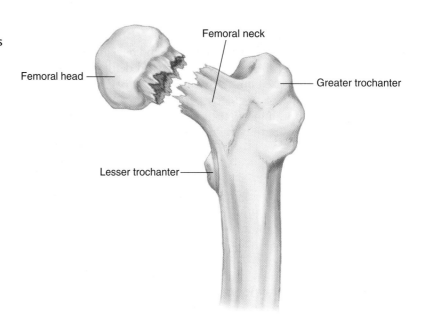

FIGURE 43-11 Subcapital femoral neck fracture. Patients with a displaced femoral neck fracture present with groin pain and a shortened externally rotated leg.

Femoral neck

Femoral head

Greater trochanter

Lesser trochanter

contribute to this. The older patient who has fallen should be assumed to have a hip fracture until proven otherwise. Signs and symptoms of a hip fracture include tenderness over the affected joint and shortening and external rotation of the leg. The patient is unable to bear weight on the affected leg. Those patients who live alone may not be able to get to a phone to summon help. Because of this, they may remain on the floor for a prolonged period of time. This can lead to hypothermia, hyperthermia, and/or dehydration.

Falls also result in a variety of other stress fractures in the elderly, including fractures of the proximal humerus, distal radius, proximal tibia, and thoracic and lumbar bodies. Falls may also lead to soft-tissue injuries and hot water burns, if the incident occurred in a hot tub or shower.

In treating orthopedic injuries, remember to ask questions aimed at detecting an underlying medical condition. Ask if the patient recalls "blacking out." Remain alert for evidence of potential cardiac emergencies. Package and transport the patient according to the general guidelines mentioned earlier.

Burns

People aged 60 and older are more likely to die from burns than any other age group, except neonates and infants. Several factors help explain the high mortality rate among elderly burn victims. They include

- Reaction time slows as people age, so the elderly often stay in contact with thermal sources longer than their younger counterparts would.

- Preexisting diseases place the elderly at risk of medical complications, particularly pulmonary and cardiac problems.

- Age-related skin changes (thinning) result in deeper burns and slower healing time.

- Immunological and metabolic changes increase the risk of infection.

- Reductions in physiological function and the reduced reserve of several organ systems make the elderly more vulnerable to major systemic stress.

Management of elderly burn patients follows the same general procedures as for other patients. However, remember that the elderly are at increased risk of shock. Administration of fluids are important to prevent renal tubular damage. Assess hydration in the initial hours after a burn injury by blood pressure, pulse, and urine output (at least 1–2 mL/kg/h).

In the case of the elderly, complications from a burn may manifest themselves in the days and weeks following the incident. For serious burns to heal, the body may use up to 20 000 calories a day. Elderly patients with altered metabolisms and such complications as diabetes may not be able to meet this demand, increasing the chances for infection and systemic failure. Part of your job may be to prepare the family for such a delayed response and to provide necessary psychological support.

Head and Spinal Injuries

As a group, the elderly experience more head injuries, even from relatively minor trauma, than their younger counterparts. A major factor is the difference in proportion between the brain and the skull. As mentioned earlier, the brain decreases in size and weight with age. The skull, however, remains constant in size, allowing the brain more room to move, thus increasing the likelihood of brain injury. Because of this, signs of brain injury may develop more slowly in the elderly, sometimes over days and weeks. In fact, the patient may often have forgotten the offending injury.

The cervical spine is also more susceptible to injury due to osteoporosis and spondylosis. **Spondylosis** is a degeneration of the vertebral body. The elderly often have a significant degree of this disease. In addition, arthritic changes can gradually compress the nerve rootlets or spinal cord. Thus, injury to the spine in the elderly makes the patient much more susceptible to spinal cord injury. In fact, sudden neck movement, even without fracture, may cause spinal cord injury. This can occur with less than normal pain, due to the absence of fracture. Therefore, it is important to provide older patients with suspected spinal injuries, especially those involved in motor-vehicle collisions, with immediate manual cervical spinal stabilization at the time of primary assessment.

✷ **spondylosis** a degeneration of the vertebral body.

$\int$ UMMARY

Emergency medical services in the twenty-first century means treating a growing elderly population. The "Greying of Canada" has resulted in a greater number of people aged 65 and older, many of whom will be in home settings. When treating elderly patients, keep in mind the anatomical, physiological, and emotional changes that occur with age. However, never jump to conclusions based solely on age. Weigh normal age-related changes against abnormal changes—that is, those resulting from a medical condition or trauma. Recall that elderly patients are much more susceptible to medication side effects and toxicity than are younger patients. They also are more susceptible to trauma and environment-related stressors. Abuse of the elderly does occur, and you should bear this in mind whenever injuries do not match the history. Any suspected abuse or neglect of an elderly patient should be reported to the emergency department and/or the appropriate governmental authorities.

CHAPTER 44

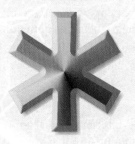

Abuse and Assault

Objectives

After reading this chapter, you should be able to:

1. Discuss the incidence of abuse and assault. (p. 1075)
2. Describe the categories of abuse. (pp. 1075–1085)
3. Discuss examples of spouse, elder, child, and sexual abuses. (pp. 1075–1085)
4. Describe the characteristics associated with the profile of a typical spouse, elder, or child abuser and the typical assailant in sexual abuse. (pp. 1077, 1079, 1080–1081)
5. Identify the profile of the "at-risk" spouse, elder, and child.

(pp. 1077, 1079, 1081, 1084–1085)
6. Discuss the assessment and management of the abused patient. (pp. 1077–1078, 1079–1081, 1084–1086)
7. Discuss the legal aspects associated with abuse situations. (pp. 1078, 1084, 1086–1087)
8. Identify community resources that are able to assist victims of abuse and assault. (pp. 1078, 1086)
9. Discuss the documentation necessary when caring for abused and assaulted patients. (pp. 1078, 1084, 1086)

INTRODUCTION

Because of underreporting, it is difficult to provide accurate statistics on the incidence of abuse and assault in Canada today. That makes available figures even more overwhelming in their seriousness. To grasp the magnitude of the problem, consider these facts.

- Fifty-one percent of all Canadian women have experienced at least one incident of sexual abuse or violence. Close to 60 percent of these women have survived more than one incident of violence.
- Elder abuse occurs at an incidence of between 700 000 and 1.1 million annually.
- Twenty-five percent of all female postsecondary students in 1993 had been physically and/or sexually assaulted by a male date or boyfriend.
- It is hard to find reliable Canadian statistics on child abuse. Health Canada is sponsoring the National Incidence Study on Child Abuse and Neglect. This study will look at the nature and extent of child abuse and neglect.

Abuse and assaults transcend gender, race, age, and socioeconomic status. The effects are serious and long-lasting. Victims may die as a result of their injuries or have long-term health-care problems. No victim ever forgets his pain. Even after the physical wounds have healed, the emotional injuries never completely fade.

Canada has some of the most thorough and advanced laws in the world to protect women and children. Yet violence against them continues to be a major problem. It is estimated by the Canadian Health Network that fewer than 1 in 10 child abuse cases is ever reported to authorities.

Unfortunately, the pattern of abuse and assault forms a cycle that is difficult to break. Parents who harm each other are more likely to abuse their children. Children who suffer abuse have a greater likelihood of becoming abusers themselves. At some point in their lives, they may abuse their dates, their partners, their children, their elders, or others.

The EMS system is involved with many cases of abuse. Although law enforcement is not always present, you have a responsibility to identify victims of abuse and initiate some kind of action. In many areas, laws require health-care personnel to report actual or suspected incidences of abuse. Early detection is critical to breaking the cycle of abuse through social services support and alterations in behaviour.

> *Abuse and assaults transcend gender, race, age, and socio-economic status.*

> *Early detection is critical to breaking the cycle of abuse through social services support and alterations in behaviour.*

PARTNER ABUSE

The potential for **partner abuse** has existed for as long as couples have interacted. It results when a man or woman subjects a domestic partner to some form of physical or psychological violence. The victim may be a husband or wife, someone who shares a residence, or simply a boyfriend or girlfriend.

The most widespread and best-known form of abuse involves the abuse of women by men. However, battery is not limited to women. Men can be—and are—abused by women. They suffer the same feelings of guilt, humiliation, and a loss of control. A battered man feels trapped just like a battered woman but is often even less likely to report the abuse, either out of a sense of shame or a lack of resources for support, or both.

✳ **partner abuse** physical or emotional violence from a man or woman toward a domestic partner.

Battery also affects same-sex couples. Abusive relationships between men or between women follow the same patterns and the same conditioning as those seen in heterosexual relationships. What can be said of women battered by men can generally be said of most battery situations, regardless of the sex of the victim or the abuser.

REASONS FOR NOT REPORTING ABUSE

Victims of partner abuse hesitate or fail to report the problem for a number of reasons. Fear presents one of the biggest obstacles to taking action. Most battered partners fear reprisals, either to themselves or to their children. They also feel humiliated by their powerlessness or inability to stop the violence, especially if the battered partner is a male.

Reporting abuse is usually the last resort. Many partners hope the abusive behaviour will simply just end. This hope is fuelled when the abuser promises to change—a common reaction after a violent episode. The abused partner may also be in denial—claiming that the situation is less serious than it is or rationalizing that the violence is somehow justified. Some abused women, for example, believe they are the cause of the abusive behaviour or that the abuse is part of the marriage and should be endured to preserve the family.

Finally, many victims of abuse lack the knowledge or financial means to seek help. They may not know where to turn or whom to trust. They may also lack the money to seek counselling, intervention, or a safe place to live. A partner who lacks job training and/or who must support dependent children may find the prospect of starting life anew more frightening than the abuse. Unfortunately, an abusive situation rarely ceases without some kind of separation or intervention. Escalation of violence is common, with injuries becoming more severe. Over time, abuse becomes more frequent, often occurring without provocation, and more inclusive. If children were not initially involved, they may become victims as the episodes escalate.

IDENTIFICATION OF PARTNER ABUSE

Partner abuse can fall into several categories. The most obvious form is physical abuse, which involves the application of force in ways too numerous to list here. In addition to direct personal injury, physical abuse may exacerbate existing medical conditions, such as hypertension, diabetes, or asthma. These conditions can also be affected by verbal abuse, which consists of words chosen to control or harm a person. Verbal abuse may leave no physical mark, but it damages a person's self-esteem and can lead to depression, substance abuse, or other self-destructive behaviour.

Sexual abuse, which is a form of physical abuse, can also occur between partners. It involves forced sexual contact and includes marital or date rape. (For more on sexual abuse and assault, see material later in the chapter.)

In identifying an abusive family situation, keep in mind the following 10 generic risk factors. These factors, based on research on battered women, include

In addition to direct personal injury, physical abuse may exacerbate existing medical conditions, such as hypertension, diabetes, or asthma.

1. Male is unemployed.
2. Male uses illegal drugs at least once a year.
3. Partners have different religious backgrounds.
4. Family income is below the poverty level.
5. Partners are unmarried.
6. Either partner is violent toward children at home.
7. Male did not graduate from high school.
8. Male is unemployed or has a blue-collar job.

9. Male is between 18 and 30 years old.

10. Male saw his father hit his mother.

CHARACTERISTICS OF PARTNER ABUSERS

As already indicated, partner abuse occurs in all demographic groups. However, abuse is more common in lower socioeconomic levels in which wage earners have trouble paying bills, holding down jobs, or keeping pace with technological changes that make their job skills outdated or obsolete.

A history of family violence makes a person more likely to repeat the pattern as an adult. Typically, the abuser does not like being out of control but at the same time feels powerless to change. The situation is made worse if both parties do not know how to back down from a conflict. Lacking any alternative, one or both of the partners may turn to physical and/or verbal violence. In some cases, abusers will think they are demonstrating discipline rather than violent behaviour.

Abusers usually exhibit overly aggressive personalities—an outgrowth of low self-esteem. They often feel insecure and jealous, flying into sudden and unpredictable rages. Use of alcohol or drugs increases the likelihood that the abuser will lose control and may not even clearly remember his actions.

In the aftermath of an abusive incident, the abuser often feels a sense of remorse and shame. The person may seek to relieve his guilt by promising to change or even seeking help. For a time, the abuser may appear charming or loving, convincing an abused partner to think that perhaps the pattern has finally been broken. All too often, however, the cycle of violence repeats itself in just a few days, weeks, or months.

CHARACTERISTICS OF ABUSED PARTNERS

It may be difficult to identify the abused partner. As mentioned, the primary risk factor for abuse is a history of violence between parents, a factor that will not be immediately known to you or other EMS providers. However, studies have revealed that abused partners share certain common characteristics. They include:

- *Pregnancy:* Forty-five percent of women suffer some form of battery during pregnancy.
- *Substance abuse:* Abused partners often seek the numbing effect of alcohol and/or drugs.
- *Emotional disorders:* Abused partners frequently exhibit depression, evasiveness, anxiety, or suicidal behaviour.

As mentioned earlier, the victim may seek to protect his attacker, either by delaying care and/or by providing alternative explanations for injuries. Remain alert to subtle signs that the patient is being less than honest. Many victims, for example, avoid eye contact, exhibit nervous behaviour, and/or watch the abuser, if present. The victim may also provide verbal clues, saying such things as "we've been having some problems lately" or "I always seem to be causing some kind of trouble."

APPROACHING THE BATTERED PATIENT

In assessing the battered patient, direct questioning usually works best. Convey an awareness that the person's partner may have caused the harm or created conditions that led to the injury and/or the emotional trauma. Once the subject of abuse has been introduced, exhibit a willingness to discuss it. Remember to avoid

In assessing the battered patient, direct questioning usually works best.

judgmental questions, such as "Why don't you leave?" and judgmental statements, such as "How awful!"

Throughout the assessment, listen carefully to the patient. Indicate your attention by saying, "I hear what you are telling me." Often, victims of abuse feel a sense of relief when someone else knows about the situation. This can be the first step toward seeking help.

When speaking with abused patients, encourage them to regain control over their lives. Do this by helping them identify what they want for themselves and, in many cases, for their children. Also, be prepared to share your knowledge of community resources, such as shelters and counselling services, that may offer help. Find out about the support services, both for the victim and the abuser, that are available in your area.

> *Do not leave the scene of suspected abuse without advising the patient to take all necessary precautions.*

Finally, do not leave the scene without advising the patient to take all necessary precautions. Rehearse the quickest way to leave the home. Find out where the patient will go and/or who the patient will call. If the patient drives, suggest carrying the keys to the vehicle at all times. Remind the patient that beating another person is a crime and that, depending on the type of injury, assault is either a misdemeanour or a felony.

Keep in mind that in cases of partner abuse, the abuser may be reported and taken into custody by the police. However, the person may soon be released on his own recognizance, sometimes within a matter of hours. The patient may already know this and therefore be reluctant to take any action. If the patient does not know this, it is your duty to inform her of this possibility and to tell the person about available protection programs.

ELDER ABUSE

As noted in Chapter 43, elder abuse is a widespread medical and social problem caused by many factors. They include

- Increased life expectancies
- Increased dependency on others, as a result of longevity
- Decreased productivity in later years
- Physical and mental impairments, especially among the "old-old"
- Limited resources for long-term care of the elderly
- Economic factors, such as strained family finances
- Stress on middle-aged caregivers responsible for two generations—their children and parents

The problem of elder abuse is expected to grow along with the size of the elderly population, which will increase dramatically within the next 20–30 years as baby boomers turn 65 and older. It is your responsibility to be aware of this situation and to remain alert to signs of elder abuse.

IDENTIFICATION OF ELDER ABUSE

* **domestic elder abuse** physical or emotional violence or neglect when an elder is being cared for in a home-based setting.

* **institutional elder abuse** physical or emotional violence or neglect when an elder is being cared for by a person paid to provide care.

There are basically two types of elder abuse—domestic and institutional. **Domestic elder abuse** takes place when an elder is being cared for in a home-based setting, usually by relatives. **Institutional elder abuse** occurs when an elder is being cared for by a person with a legal or contractual responsibility to provide care, such as paid caregivers, nursing home staff, or other professionals. Both types of abuse can be either acts of commission (acts of physical, sexual, or emotional violence) or acts of omission (neglect).

In some cases, signs of elder abuse are subtle, such as theft of the victim's belongings or loss of freedom. Other signs, such as wounds, untreated decubitus ulcers, or poor hygiene, are more obvious. For additional information on the signs of elder abuse, see Chapter 43.

THEORIES ABOUT DOMESTIC ELDER ABUSE

There are four main theories about the causes of domestic elder abuse. (1) Commonly, caregivers feel stressed and overburdened. They are ill-equipped to provide care or simply lack the knowledge to do the job correctly. (2) Another cause of elder abuse is their physical and/or mental impairment. Elders in poor health are more likely to be abused than elders in good health. This situation results, in part, from their inability to report the abuse. (3) Yet another cause of elder abuse is family history, or the cycle of violence mentioned earlier. (4) Finally, elder abuse increases proportionately with the personal problems of the caregivers. Abusers of the elderly tend to have more difficulties, either financial or emotional, than nonabusers.

CHARACTERISTICS OF ABUSED ELDERS

Like partner abuse, elder abuse cuts across all demographic groups. As a result, it is difficult to outline an accurate profile of the abused elder. The most common cases involve elderly women abused by their sons. However, this pattern is skewed by the fact that women live longer than men. Elder abuse most frequently occurs among people who are dependent on others for their care, especially among those elders who have mental or physical disabilities. In such cases, elders may be repeatedly abused by relatives who believe the elder will not or cannot ask for help.

In cases of neglect, abused elders most commonly live alone. They may be mentally competent but fear asking for help because relatives have complained about providing care or have threatened to place them in a nursing home. Like abused partners, they may be reluctant to give information about their abusers for fear of retaliation.

CHARACTERISTICS OF ELDER ABUSERS

It is also difficult to profile the people who are most likely to abuse elders. According to the National Aging Resource Center on Elder Abuse, the percentages in Table 44-1 reflect the reported perpetrators of elder abuse in domestic settings. As you can see, the most typical abusers are adult children, who are either overstressed by care of the elder or who were abused themselves. The Canadian data on elder abuse are very similar.

As with partner abusers, there are several characteristics commonly found in abusers of the elderly. Often, the perpetrators exhibit alcoholic behaviour, drug addiction, or some mental impairment. The abuser may also be dependent on the income or assistance of the elder—a situation that can cause resentment, anger, and, in some cases, violence.

For more on the management of elder abuse, see Chapter 43.

CHILD ABUSE

As pointed out in Chapters 41 and 42, child abuse is one of the most difficult circumstances that you will face as a paramedic. **Child abuse** may range from physical or emotional impairment to neglect of a child's most basic needs (Figure 44-1). It can occur from infancy to age 18 and can be inflicted by any number of

✳ **child abuse** physical or emotional violence or neglect toward a person from infancy to 18 years of age.

Table 44-1	PERPETRATORS OF DOMESTIC ELDER ABUSE
Group	Percentage
Adult children	32.5
Grandchildren	4.2
Spouse	14.4
Sibling	2.5
Other relatives	12.5
Friend/neighbour	7.5
All others	18.2
Unknown	8.2

Child abuse can occur from infancy to age 18 and can be inflicted by any number of caregivers.

caregivers—parents, foster parents, stepparents, babysitters, siblings, stepsiblings, or other relatives or friends charged with a child's care.

Although you may be familiar with some of the following information from your training or from earlier chapters in this book, it bears repeating. The damage done to a child can last a lifetime and, as stressed, perpetuate a cycle of violence in generations to come.

CHARACTERISTICS OF CHILD ABUSERS

As with other types of abusers, you cannot relate child abuse to social class, income, or education. However, certain patterns do emerge, most notably a history of abuse within the abusers' own families. Most child abusers were physically or emotionally

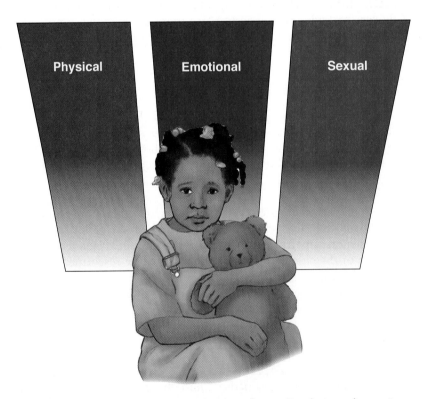

FIGURE 44-1   Child abuse comes in many forms. Be alert, and report any concerns you may have regarding abuse or neglect.

abused as children. They often would prefer to use other forms of discipline, but under stress they regress to the earliest and most familiar patterns. Once resorting to physical discipline, the punishments become more severe and more frequent.

In cases of reported physical abuse, perpetrators tend to be men. However, the statistics for men and women even out when neglect is taken into account. As indicated earlier, potential child abusers can include a wide variety of caregivers. In most cases, however, one or both parents are the most likely abusers. Frequent behavioural traits include

- Use or abuse of drugs and/or alcohol
- Immaturity and preoccupation with self
- Obvious lack of feeling for the child, rarely looking at or touching the child
- Seemingly unconcerned about the child's injury, treatment, or prognosis
- Openly critical of the child, with little indication of guilt or remorse for involvement in the child's condition
- Little identification with the child's pain, whether it be physical or emotional

Any one of these signs should raise suspicion in your mind of possible child abuse. The infant or child will provide other clues, even before you begin your secondary assessment.

CHARACTERISTICS OF ABUSED CHILDREN

A child's behaviour is one of the most important indicators of abuse. Some behaviour is age-related. For example, abused children under age six usually appear excessively passive, while abused children over age six seem aggressive. Other behavioural clues include

A child's behaviour is one of the most important indicators of abuse.

- Crying, often hopelessly, during treatment or not crying at all
- Avoiding the parents or showing little concern for their absence
- Unusually wary or fearful of physical contact
- Apprehensive and/or constantly on the alert for danger
- Prone to sudden behavioural changes
- Absence of nearly all emotions
- Neediness, constantly requesting favours, food, or things

In general, use your instincts and knowledge of age-appropriate behaviour (see Chapters 41 and 42) to form your first impression of the child. If the child's behaviour is atypical, maintain an index of suspicion throughout your assessment.

Use your instincts and knowledge of age-appropriate behaviour to form your first impression of a child whom you suspect may have been abused.

IDENTIFICATION OF THE ABUSED CHILD

As you know, children very commonly get injured, and not all injured children are abused. If a child volunteers the story of his injury without hesitation and if it matches the story told by the parents and the symptoms of injury, child abuse is very unlikely. However, in cases in which the behaviour of a caregiver and/or child has raised an index of suspicion, you may face a challenge in distinguishing between an intentional injury and an authentic accident. Conditions commonly mistaken for abuse are car seat burns, staphylococcal scalded skin syndrome, chicken pox (cigarette burns), and hematological disorders that can

Content Review

COMMON CONDITIONS MISTAKEN FOR ABUSE
- Car seat burns
- Staphylococcal scalded skin syndrome
- Chicken pox (cigarette burns)
- Hematological disorders that cause easy bruising

cause bruising. In assessing a child, look for common patterns of physical abuse, evidence of emotional abuse, and/or environmental clues of neglect.

Secondary Assessment

In most cases, signs of physical mistreatment of a child should be the easiest type of abuse for you to recognize. Soft-tissue injuries are the most common indicators, especially multiple bruises in different planes of the body, in different stages of healing, and with distinctive shapes (Table 44-2 and Figure 44-2). Other common warning signs include defensive wounds on the hands and forearms and symmetrical injuries, such as bites or burns. Any of these conditions carry a high index of suspicion of abuse.

Burns and Scalds Abusive burns often have distinctive patterns that indicate the implement or source used to injure the child. The burns tend to be in certain common locations—the soles of the feet, palms of the hands, back, or buttocks. They may or may not be found in conjunction with other injuries.

Because children have thinner skin than adults (other than elders), they also tend to scald more easily. The temperature of hot water in most residences is about 60°C, which can scald an adult in only about five seconds. (Bath water for children should be kept below 49°C.) When children accidentally get into water that is too hot, you can expect to see "splash" burns—marks created by spattering water as children try to get out. Intentional scalding, however, is characterized by the conspicuous lack of splash burns. Such "dipping injuries" are a common form of child abuse.

Fractures Fractures constitute the second most common form of child abuse. Sites of fractures include the skull, nose, facial structures, and upper extremities. Twisting and jerking fractures result from grabbing a child by an extremity, while neck injuries occur from shaking a child. Because children have soft, pliable ribs, they rarely experience accidental fractures to this region. As a result, you should maintain a high index of suspicion of abuse whenever you encounter a child with fractured ribs.

Head Injuries Over time, injuries from abuse tend to progress from the extremities and trunk to the head. Head injuries commonly found in abused children include scalp wounds, skull fractures, subdural or subgaleal hematomas, and repeated contusions.

Injuries to the head claim the largest number of lives among abused children. They also account for most of the long-term disabilities associated with child abuse.

Shaken Baby Syndrome Shaken baby syndrome frequently occurs when a parent or caregiver becomes frustrated with a crying infant and all other attempts to

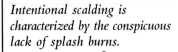

Soft-tissue injuries are common indicators of abuse, especially multiple bruises in different places on the body, in different stages of healing, and/or with distinctive shapes.

Intentional scalding is characterized by the conspicuous lack of splash burns.

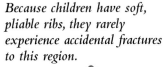

Because children have soft, pliable ribs, they rarely experience accidental fractures to this region.

Table 44-2	COLOUR OF BRUISES AND THEIR AGE*
Age	**Skin Appearance**
0 to 2 days	tender and swollen, red
0 to 5 days	blue, purple
5 to 7 days	green
7 to 10 days	yellow
10 or more days	brown
2 or more weeks	cleared

*Adapted from Richardson, A.C., "Cutaneous Manifestations of Abuse" in Reece, R.M. *Child Abuse: Medical Diagnosis and Management.*

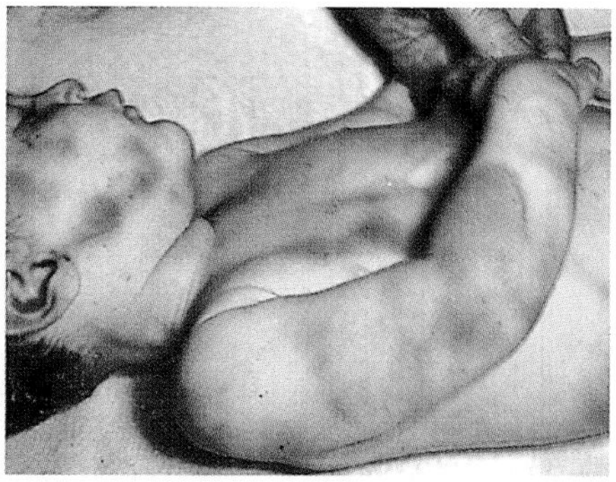

FIGURE 44-2   Severe multiple bruises can lead to death.

quiet the baby have failed. It happens when a person picks up the infant and shakes the baby vigorously. The movement can cause permanent brain damage, such as subdural hematomas or diffuse swelling. It may also result in injuries to the neck and spine or retinal hemorrhages, which, in turn, can lead to blindness. If the infant is shaken hard enough or repeatedly, he may die from the injuries.

Abdominal Injuries Although abdominal injuries represent a small proportion of the injuries suffered by abused children, they are usually very serious. Blunt force can result in trauma to the liver, spleen, or mesentery. You should look for pain, swelling, and vomiting, as well as hemodynamic compromise from these injuries.

Signs of Neglect

Some forms of child abuse are less obvious than physical injuries. Abuse may result from neglect. Caregivers simply do not provide children with adequate food, clothing, shelter, or medical care.

As a paramedic, you may be in a unique position to observe and report neglect. Unlike many other health-care or public-safety workers, EMS personnel get an opportunity to see the child's home environment for themselves. Unhealthy or unclean conditions are clear evidence of a caregiver's inability to provide for a child's safety or well-being.

In examining a child, keep in mind the following common signs of neglect:

- Malnutrition (Neglected children are often underweight, sometimes by up to 30 percent.)
- Severe diaper rash
- Diarrhea and/or dehydration
- Hair loss
- Untreated medical conditions
- Inappropriate, dirty, or torn clothing
- Tired and listless attitudes
- Near constant demands for physical contact or attention

Signs of Emotional Abuse

Emotional abuse is often the hardest form of abuse to identify. It may take any one of the following six forms:

1. Parents or caregivers simply ignore the child, showing indifference to the child's needs and failing to provide any stimulation.

2. Parents or caregivers reject, humiliate, or criticize the child.

3. The child may be isolated and deprived of normal human contact or nurturing.

4. A child may be terrorized or bullied through verbal assaults and threats, creating feelings of fear and anxiety.

5. A parent or caregiver may encourage destructive or antisocial behaviour.

6. The child may be overpressured by unrealistic expectations of success.

RECORDING AND REPORTING CHILD ABUSE

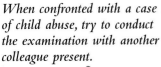

As with all other forms of abuse, you have a responsibility to report suspected cases of child abuse.

As with all other forms of abuse, you have a responsibility to report suspected cases of child abuse. In some instances, you might have a chance to provide early intervention. An abusive adult may actively seek help or may send out signals for help. For example, a potential abuser may make several calls within a 24-hour period. The person may also summon help for inconsequential symptoms or demonstrate an inability to handle an impending crisis. These are warning signs and should be duly noted.

When confronted with a case of child abuse, try to conduct the examination with another colleague present.

When confronted with an actual case of child abuse, try to conduct the examination with another colleague present. You must keep your personal reactions to yourself and record only your objective observations. Assumptions must not be included in your report. The final document should be objective, legible, and written with the knowledge that it may be used in a future court or child custody case. At all times, put the child's interest first, treating him with utmost kindness and gentleness. (For more on your EMS and legal responsibilities, see material later in the chapter.)

SEXUAL ASSAULT

Sexual assault is any unwanted sexual act committed by one person on another. This can mean anything from unwanted touching of a sexual nature to rape. There are many types of sexual assault that appear in the Criminal Code. They include descriptions of a variety of acts (for example, the use of a weapon causing bodily harm and making threats) as well as the types of relationships in which sexual contact is or may be a criminal offence (for example, where one person is in a position of authority over the other or where one person is dependent on the other). The penalties for committing these different types of sexual offences vary depending on the severity of the offence.

✱ **sexual assault** unwanted oral, genital, rectal, or manual sexual contact.

The courts generally interpret **sexual assault** as unwanted sexual contact, whether it be genital, oral, rectal, or manual. **Rape** is usually defined as penile penetration of the genitalia or rectum (however slight) without consent of the victim. Both forms of sexual violence are prosecuted as crimes, with rape constituting a felony offence. As a result, your actions at the scene and the report that you file will, in all likelihood, affect the outcome of a trial.

✱ **rape** usually defined as penile penetration of the genitalia or rectum (however slight) without the consent of the victim.

CHARACTERISTICS OF VICTIMS OF SEXUAL ASSAULT/RAPE

It is difficult to profile a victim of sexual assault or rape because of the variety of victims. However, statistics reveal certain patterns. The group most likely to be victimized is made up of adolescent females younger than age 18. Nearly two-thirds of all rapes and sexual assaults take place between the hours of 6 P.M. and 6 A.M. at the victim's home or at the home of a friend, relative, or acquaintance.

Particularly alarming is the number of children who suffer some form of sexual abuse. A Canadian study shows that 1 in 2 girls and 1 in 3 boys will have unwanted sexual experience by age 18. Of girls under the age of sixteen, 54 percent have experienced some form of unwanted sexual attention. Twenty-four percent have experienced rape or coercive sex, and 17 percent have experienced incest. In 2000, 77 percent of female victims of sexual assault were assaulted by someone they knew, such as a friend, a casual acquaintance, a family member, a partner, or ex-partner. Eighty-five percent of women with disabilities will be assaulted in their lifetime. The disturbing fact is that only 6 percent of assaults are reported to authorities.

Typically, contact involves a male assailant and a female victim, but not always. The contact can range from exposure to fondling to penetration. Although sexual abuse can occur in families of all descriptions, children raised in families where there is domestic violence are eight times more likely to be sexually molested within that family.

Sexual assault and rape carry serious consequences for the victim. Victims may be physically injured during the assault or even killed. They commonly suffer internal injuries, particularly if multiple assailants are involved in the attack. Rape can result in infections, sexually transmitted diseases, and unwanted pregnancies. The psychological damage is deep and long-lasting. Shame, anger, and a lack of trust may persist for years—or even a lifetime.

Children, in particular, find it difficult to speak about molestation. It is likely that they know the person and fear reprisal or, in some instances, even seek to protect the individual. In many cases, the assailants physically explore the child without intercourse or force the child to touch or fondle them. Victims, especially very young children, may be confused about the situation or, lacking physical evidence of abuse, fear that nobody will believe them. Symptoms of sexual abuse, regardless of its form, may include

- Nightmares
- Restlessness
- Withdrawal tendencies
- Hostility
- Phobias related to the offender
- Regressive behaviour, such as bed wetting
- Truancy
- Promiscuity, in older children and teens
- Drug and alcohol abuse

CHARACTERISTICS OF SEXUAL ASSAILANTS

Like the victims of sexual assaults, the assailants can come from almost any background. However, the violent victimizers of children are substantially more likely than the victimizers of adults to have been physically or sexually abused as children. Many assailants, particularly adolescents and abusive adults, think domination is part of any relationship. Such thinking can lead to date rape or marital rape. In a significant percentage of all cases, the assailants are under the influence of alcohol or drugs. Nearly 30 percent of all rapists use weapons, which underscores the fact that sexual assaults are violent crimes.

In cases of date rape, the assailant may have drugged the unsuspecting victim with flunitrazepam (Rohypnol), known by the street names of "roofie," "roche," "rib," or "rope." The victim may exhibit extreme intoxication without a corresponding strong smell of alcohol or may have drug-induced amnesia (a common effect), making questioning difficult or impossible. More often than not, the alleged assailant in such cases lives on a college or university campus, the location of most EMS calls involving what is known as the "date rape drug."

EMS RESPONSIBILITIES

In calls involving abuse or assault, your primary responsibility is safety—both your own and that of the patient.

Your response to a call involving a sexual assault is in many ways similar to your response to any abusive situation. In both instances, your primary responsibility is safety—both your own and that of the patient. You should never enter a scene if your safety is compromised, and you should leave the scene as soon as you feel unsafe.

You can expect victims of assault or abuse to feel unsafe as a result of the violence they have suffered. One of your primary responsibilities is to provide a safe environment for an already traumatized patient. Sometimes, you can provide safety merely by your official presence. Other times, you may have to move the patient to the ambulance where you can lock the doors or move to a different location entirely. In still other instances, you may have to summon additional personnel. (For more on crime scene management, see Chapter 3.)

In many cases, a same-sex paramedic—you or a colleague—should maintain contact with the victim of an alleged sexual assault.

You are also responsible for providing proper psychosocial care for the victims of abuse and assault. Privacy is a major consideration. In many cases, a same-sex paramedic—you or a colleague—should maintain contact with the victim. Although you may need to expose the victim during assessment, you should cover the patient and remove him from public view as soon as possible.

When talking with a victim of sexual assault, use open-ended questions to help the patient regain a sense of self-control.

When talking with the patient, use open-ended questions to reestablish a sense of control. You might say, for example, "Would you like to sit on a seat or ride on the stretcher?" Or you might ask, "Is there someone you would like us to call?" As mentioned in earlier sections, remain nonjudgmental throughout care, avoiding subjective comments both of the patient and of the assailant. In a reassuring voice, encourage the patient to report the rape, explaining the importance of preserving evidence.

Medical treatment of victims of abuse and assault is essentially the same as with other patients. However, you should always remember the source of the patient's injuries and provide appropriate emotional support. Keep in mind that the patient has been harmed by another human being, in many cases a person that he knows intimately.

LEGAL CONSIDERATIONS

As noted throughout this chapter, abuse and assault constitute crimes. Although the nature and extent of the crime often are determined by local laws, you have a responsibility to report suspected cases to the appropriate law enforcement officials. Because the assailants may be detained only a short time, you also have an obligation to find out about the victim and witness protection programs available in your area.

Specialized resources include both private and provincially, territorially, or federally funded programs. Make a point of learning about hospital units for the victims of sexual assault, public and private shelters for battered persons, and government agencies responsible for youths and their families.

As you have read, your actions can affect the prosecution of a crime. Clothing should only be removed from a patient when necessary for assessment and treatment. All items should then be turned over to the proper authorities.

In the case of rape, patients should not urinate, defecate, douche, bathe, eat, drink, or smoke. Some jurisdictions have specific rules for evidence protection, such as using paper bags to collect evidence or placing bags over the patient's hands to preserve trace evidence. Remember that any evidence that you collect must remain in your custody until you can give it directly to a law enforcement official to preserve the **chain of evidence.**

As indicated, it is important that you carefully and objectively document all your findings. You may have to defend your words in a court of law. Regardless of the emotions evoked by the call, you must remain professional at all times.

Finally, you should study the local laws and protocols regarding cases of abuse and assault. All provinces and territories require health-care workers to report suspected cases of child abuse. Some provinces and territories require EMS personnel to report even a suspicion of abuse or assault. Regardless of where you live, take time to learn the rules and regulations that affect your practice, both for your sake and for the sake of your patients.

 chain of evidence legally retaining items of evidence and accounting for their whereabouts at all times to prevent loss or tampering.

Your actions in the case of alleged sexual assaults can affect the prosecution of a crime. Protect the evidence.

Regardless of the emotions evoked by a call involving abuse or assault, you must remain professional at all times.

$\int$UMMARY

The incidence of abuse is widespread today, and you will encounter many cases during your paramedic career. You should learn the hallmarks of partner abuse, elder abuse, child abuse, and sexual assaults. You should also learn to recognize significant physical and emotional assessment findings as well as characteristics of the victims and assailants. Proper treatment of victims of abuse and assault includes knowing the legal requirements of your area, protecting evidence, and properly documenting your findings and actions.

CHAPTER 45

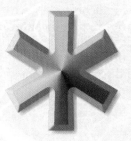

The Challenged Patient

Objectives

After reading this chapter, you should be able to:

1. Describe the various etiologies and types of hearing impairments. (pp. 1090–1091)
2. Recognize the patient with a hearing impairment. (p. 1091)
3. Anticipate accommodations that may be needed in order to properly manage the patient with a hearing impairment. (pp. 1091–1092)
4. Describe the various etiologies and types of, recognize patients with, and anticipate accommodations that may be needed in order to properly

manage each of the following conditions:

a. Visual impairments (pp. 1092–1093)
b. Speech impairments (pp. 1093–1094)
c. Obesity (pp. 1094–1095)
d. Paraplegia/quadriplegia (pp. 1096)
e. Mental illness (p. 1096)
f. Developmental disability (pp. 1096–1098)
g. Down syndrome (pp. 1097–1098)
h. Emotional impairment/mental challenges (p. 1096)

Continued

5. Describe, identify possible presenting signs of, and anticipate accommodations for the following diseases/illnesses:
   a. Arthritis (p. 1099)
   b. Cancer (pp. 1099–1100)
   c. Cerebral palsy (pp. 1100–1101)
   d. Cystic fibrosis (pp. 1101–1102)
   e. Multiple sclerosis (p. 1102)
   f. Muscular dystrophy (p. 1102)
   g. Myasthenia gravis (p. 1104)
   h. Poliomyelitis (pp. 1102–1103)
   i. Spina bifida (pp. 1103–1104)
   j. Patients with a previous head injury (p. 1103)
6. Define, recognize, and anticipate accommodations needed to properly manage patients who
   a. are culturally diverse (pp. 1104–1105)
   b. are terminally ill (p. 1105)
   c. have a communicable disease (p. 1105)
7. Given several patients with disabilities, provide the appropriate assessment, management, and transport. (pp. 1089–1105)

INTRODUCTION

Throughout your EMS career, you can expect to encounter a number of patients who live with a variety of impairments or disabilities. Many will have met these challenges so successfully that you may not notice the problem right away. For example, people with hearing impairments might lip read so well that you may not initially realize they cannot hear. People with more obvious disabilities, such as paralysis, may have accepted their impairments and built active and rewarding lives. A patient with a history of polio, for example, may have lived with the problem so long that she neglects to tell you about it right away. Instead the patient talks about a more immediate problem—the reason for summoning EMS.

The one thing that challenged patients share is their variety. They might have any number of physical, mental, or emotional impairments. They might have contracted a pathological illness that necessitates a special living or working arrangement. They might be suffering from a terminal illness or a communicable disease. They may come from a cultural or financial situation that dictates medical practices contrary to those of the EMS community. The key to treating these patients is to understand and recognize the special condition or situation and to make any accommodations that may be needed for proper patient care.

PHYSICAL DISABILITIES

A number of physical disabilities—conditions that limit the use of one or more parts of the body—can affect patient assessment and/or treatment. These impairments may be the result of accidents, birth injuries, chronic illnesses, aging,

✱ **deafness** the inability to hear.

✱ **conductive deafness** deafness caused when there is a blocking of the transmission of the sound waves through the external ear canal to the middle or inner ear.

✱ **sensorineural deafness** deafness caused by the inability of nerve impulses to reach the auditory centre of the brain because of nerve damage either to the inner ear or to the brain.

✱ **otitis media** middle ear infection.

✱ **cerumen** earwax.

and more. Impairments can limit the ability of a patient to hear, see, speak, or move. Patients will react to their impairments in different ways—from acceptance, to denial, to anger, to shame. It is important that you quickly recognize the impairment and exhibit knowledge and sensitivity to assure the patient that you understand her special needs.

HEARING IMPAIRMENTS

Hearing impairments involve a decrease or loss in the ability to distinguish or hear sounds, particularly those involving speech. An inability to hear is commonly described as **deafness.** A person may be completely deaf or partially deaf. Deafness may be in one ear or both ears. The condition may be present at birth or may occur later in life as a result of an accident, illness, or aging.

Types of Hearing Impairments

There are basically two types of deafness—**conductive deafness** and **sensorineural deafness.** Many forms of conductive deafness may be treated and cured, especially if caught early. Sensorineural deafness, conversely, is often incurable.

Conductive Deafness Conductive deafness results from any condition that prevents sound waves from being transmitted from the external ear to the middle or inner ear. The condition can be either temporary or permanent.

If an infant or child does not respond to verbal stimulation or questions, rule out the possibility of conductive deafness when performing your assessment of disability. Congenital malformation of the ear is a possible but rare cause of conductive deafness in the neonate. A more common cause of conductive deafness in children is **otitis media,** an infection of the middle ear. This condition often arises from various childhood illnesses, particularly those involving the upper respiratory tract. To prevent hearing loss, children under age six who experience recurrent otitis media may need to take daily prophylactic antibiotics or have tympanostomy (myringotomy) tubes placed.

In addition to infection, a number of other conditions can result in a temporary loss of hearing. Anyone can experience conductive deafness during an airline flight, where changes in air pressure can affect hearing. A deep-water dive can have a similar effect. Impacted **cerumen,** or earwax, is yet another common and easily treatable cause of conductive deafness.

Other causes might be the temporary blockage of the ear canal by various irritants, such as dust, hair spray, insects, or water ("swimmer's ear"). Patient attempts to clean the canal with cotton applicators may disrupt the ear's natural cleaning process and push the debris deeper into the ear, which sets the stage for bacterial infections and conductive deafness.

Obstructions can also be caused by hematomas, which may result from blunt trauma to the ear. Force to the mandible, such as a fractured jaw, can also produce a temporary loss of hearing and may, in fact, result in fragments of bone displaced to the ear canal. Although these conditions cannot be treated in the field, they should be taken into account when a trauma patient appears not to respond to, or "hear," your questions.

Sensorineural Deafness Sensorineural deafness arises from the inability of nerve impulses to reach the auditory centre of the brain because of damage either to the inner ear or to the brain itself. It is usually a permanent condition.

In the case of infants and children, sensorineural deafness often results from congenital defects or birth injuries. Preterm infants are particularly at risk for sensorineural deafness, especially those with severe asphyxia or recurrent apnea in the neonatal period. Ototoxic drugs, such as furosemide (Lasix) and gentamicin, can also cause sensorineural deafness if administered to infants in neonatal intensive care units. Finally, many children who develop this type of hearing loss have mothers who contracted rubella (German measles) or cytomegalovirus (CMV), during the first three months of pregnancy.

Diseases, such as bacterial meningitis, or viral illnesses, such as **labrynthitis** (inner ear infection), can lead to sensorineural deafness at any age. Taking high does of ototoxic drugs, such as aspirin, can also cause sensorineural deafness in both children and adults. A common symptom of aspirin toxicity is "ringing in the ears" (tinnitus). Other causes of sensorineural deafness include tumours of the brain or middle ear, concussion, severe blows to the ear, and repeated loud noises, such as those from chainsaws, heavy machinery, gun fire, rock music, or sudden blasts of sound.

Conditions associated with aging can also lead to permanent hearing loss. **Presbycusis** is a progressive sensorineural hearing loss that begins after age 20 but is usually significant only in people over age 65. More common in men than women, this type of hearing loss affects high-frequency sounds first, then low-frequency sounds. Eventually, human voices becomes harder to detect, especially if background noise is present. Elderly people with this condition will often tell others not to "mumble" or will ask them to speak louder.

✱ labrynthitis inner ear infection that causes vertigo, nausea, and an unsteady gait.

✱ presbycusis progressive hearing loss that occurs with aging.

Recognition of Deafness

As mentioned, it is important to detect deafness early in your assessment. A partially deaf person may ask questions repeatedly, misunderstand answers to questions, or respond inappropriately. Such reactions can easily be mistaken for head injury, leading to misdirected treatment.

The most obvious sign of deafness is a hearing aid. Unfortunately, hearing aids do not work for all types of deafness. Also, many people do not wear hearing aids, even when they have been prescribed. In addition, deaf people may have poor diction due to partial hearing loss or hearing loss later in life. They might use their hands to gesture or use sign language. As noted, deaf people may ask you to speak louder, or they may speak excessively loudly themselves. Finally, deaf people will commonly want to face you so that they can read your lips. Be sure that you are fully facing deaf patients before you speak to them.

A partially deaf person may ask questions repeatedly, misunderstand answers to questions, or respond inappropriately. Such reactions can easily be mistaken for head injury, leading to misdirected treatment.

Accommodations for Deaf Patients

When managing a patient with a hearing impairment, you can do several things to ease communication. Begin by identifying yourself and making sure the patient knows that you are speaking to her. Get the patient's attention by moving so you can be seen or by gently touching the person if appropriate. By addressing deaf patients face to face, you give them the opportunity to read your lips and interpret your expression.

When talking with a deaf patient, speak slowly in a normal voice. Never yell or use exaggerated gestures. These techniques often distort your facial and body language, making you seem angry or threatening. Keep in mind that nearly 80 percent of hearing loss is related to high-pitched sounds. Therefore, you could use a low-pitched voice to speak directly into the patient's ear. Whatever you do, make sure that background noise is reduced as much as possible, turning off the TV, radio, or other sources of sound.

If you are called to a deaf patient's home during the night, you may need to help find or adjust a hearing aid. If you cannot locate the device, you might make use of an "amplified" listener—for example, an ear microphone.

Do not forget one of the simplest and most effective means of communication—use of writing. As long as you do not need to move quickly, you can write

By addressing deaf patients face to face, you give them the opportunity to read your lips and interpret your expression.

out notes for the patient to read and wait for the person to respond in the same way. You can also draw pictures to illustrate basic needs or procedures. This approach can ease a patient's anxiety, reducing the fear of miscommunication or lack of control over her treatment.

Finally, many people with hearing impairments know sign language, usually American Sign Language (ASL). If this is the case, try to utilize an interpreter, often a family member or even a neighbour. Make sure that you document the name of the person who did the interpreting and the information received. Also, notify the receiving hospital of the need to have an interpreter on hand if the person is unable to accompany you.

VISUAL IMPAIRMENTS

When caring for the patient with a visual impairment, it is important to note if the impairment is a permanent disability or if it is a new symptom as a result of the illness or injury for which you were called. It is necessary to understand the causes of blindness before this determination can be made.

Etiologies

Visual impairments can result from a number of causes. Possible etiologies include injury, disease, congenital conditions, infection (such as cytomegalovirus [CMV]), and degeneration of the retina, optic nerve, or nerve pathways. A description of each of the etiologies follows.

Injury A previous injury to the eye can cause a permanent vision loss. An injury to the orbit usually includes injury to the tissue around the orbit as well as to the eye itself. This can cause muscle and nerve damage that may lead to permanent loss of eyesight. Penetrating injuries can result in **enucleation,** which is removal of the eyeball. Chemical and thermal burns to the eye can result in damage to the cornea and can also lead to permanent vision loss if not treated quickly. A temporary loss of vision can result from an injury, such as the chemical burn that may occur with the deployment of an airbag, or from a corneal abrasion. Once treated, these injuries rarely lead to permanent loss of vision.

Disease Visual impairments may also be caused by a disease of the eye, or as a secondary result of the primary disease process. **Glaucoma,** for example, is a group of eye diseases that result in increased intraocular pressure on the optic nerve. If not treated, glaucoma leads to loss of peripheral vision and blindness.

The are two different types of glaucoma, primary and secondary. The cause of primary glaucoma remains unknown. However, secondary glaucoma results from other eye diseases. The incidence of glaucoma is higher in blacks than in whites. A black person between the ages of 45 and 65 is 15 times more likely to have glaucoma than a white person in the same age group.

Diabetic retinopathy is another disease-related visual impairment. It results from diabetes mellitus, which causes disorders in the blood vessels that lead to the retina. Small hemorrhages in these blood vessels leads to a slow loss of vision and possible blindness.

Congenital and Degenerative Disorders A congenital disorder that causes visual disturbances is cerebral palsy. Premature birth can lead to blindness in the neonate. Degeneration of the eyeball, optic nerve, or nerve pathways is most commonly caused by aging and can slowly lead to loss of vision. Cytomegalovirus (CMV), an opportunistic infection often seen in AIDS patients, can lead to blindness by causing retinitis—an inflammation of the retina.

Content Review

CAUSES OF VISUAL IMPAIRMENTS
- Injury
- Disease
- Congenital conditions
- Infection
- Degeneration of the retina, optic nerve, or nerve pathways

✱ enucleation removal of the eyeball after trauma or illness.

✱ glaucoma group of eye diseases that results in increased intraocular pressure on the optic nerve; if left untreated, it can lead to blindness.

✱ diabetic retinopathy slow loss of vision as a result of damage caused by diabetes.

Recognizing and Accommodating Visual Impairments

Many visually impaired people live independent, active lives (Figure 45-1). Depending on the degree of impairment and a person's adjustment to the loss of vision, you may or may not recognize the condition right away. In cases of obvious blindness, identify yourself as you approach the patient so that the person knows you are there. Also, describe everything you are doing while you do it.

Many blind people have aids to assist them in their activities of daily living. The most obvious is a seeing eye dog. When approaching a person with a seeing eye dog, DO NOT pet the dog or disturb it while the dog is in its harness. For the dog, the harness means that it is working. Ask permission from the patient to touch the dog. Never grab the leash, the harness, or the patient's arm without asking permission. Doing this may place the dog or the owner—or you—in danger.

Accommodation must be made for transporting the guide dog with the patient. Circumstances and local protocols will dictate whether you transport the dog in the ambulance with the patient or have the dog transported in another vehicle.

If your patient does not have a guide dog, inquire about other aids that the person may want brought to the hospital. If the patient is ambulatory, have the person take your arm for guidance, rather than taking the patient's arm.

SPEECH IMPAIRMENTS

When performing an assessment, you may come across a patient who is awake, alert, and oriented but cannot communicate with you due to a speech impairment. Possible miscommunication can hinder both the care you provide and the information that you provide to the receiving facility.

Types of Speech Impairments

You may encounter four types of speech impairments—language disorders, articulation disorders, voice production disorders, and fluency disorders. A discussion of each disorder follows.

Language Disorders A language disorder is an impaired ability to understand the spoken or written word. In children, language disorders result from a number of causes, such as congenital learning disorders, cerebral palsy, or hearing impairments. A child who receives inadequate language stimulation in the first year of life may also experience delayed speaking ability.

In an adult patient, language disorders may result from a variety of illnesses or injuries. The person may have suffered a stroke, aneurysm, head injury, brain tumour, hearing loss, or some kind of emotional trauma. The loss of ability to communicate in speech, writing, or signs is known as **aphasia**. Aphasia can manifest itself in the following ways:

- **Sensory aphasia**—a person can no longer understand the spoken word. Patients with sensory aphasia will not respond to your questions because they cannot understand what you are saying.

- **Motor aphasia**—a person can no longer use the symbols of speech. Patients with motor aphasia, also known as expressive aphasia, will understand what you say but cannot clearly articulate a response. They may respond to your questions slowly, use the wrong words, or act out answers. It is important to allow such patients to express their responses in whatever way they can.

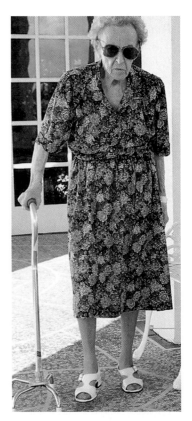

FIGURE 45-1 Individuals who are visually impaired can still maintain active, independent lives.

Content Review

TYPES OF SPEECH IMPAIRMENTS
- Language disorders
- Articulation disorders
- Voice production disorders
- Fluency disorders

✳ **aphasia** occurs when the individual suffers a brain injury due to stroke or head injury and no longer has the ability to speak or read.

✳ **sensory aphasia** occurs when the patient cannot understand the spoken word.

✳ **motor aphasia** occurs when the patient cannot speak but can understand what is said.

✱ **global aphasia** a combination of motor and sensory aphasia.

• **Global aphasia**—occurs when a person has both sensory and motor aphasia. These patients can neither understand nor respond to your questions. A brain tumour in Broca's region can cause this condition.

Articulation Disorders Articulation disorders, also known as dysarthria, affect the way a person's speech is heard by others. These disorders occur when sounds are produced or put together incorrectly or in a way that makes it difficult to understand the spoken word. Articulation disorders may start at an early age, when the child learns to say words incorrectly or when a hearing impairment is involved. This type of disorder can also occur in both children and adults when neural damage causes a disturbance in the nerve pathways leading from the brain to the larynx, mouth, or lips.

When speaking with someone who has an articulation disorder, you will notice that they pronounce their words incorrectly or that their speech is slurred. They may leave certain sounds out of a word because they are too difficult for them to pronounce. Again, it is important for you to listen carefully and let the person complete a response.

Voice Production Disorders When a patient has a voice production disorder, the quality of the person's voice is affected. This can be caused by trauma due to overuse of the vocal cords or infection. Cancer of the larynx can also cause a speech failure by impeding air from passing through the vocal cords. A patient with a production disorder will exhibit hoarseness, harshness, an inappropriate pitch, or abnormal nasal resonance.

Fluency Disorders Fluency disorders present as stuttering. Although the cause of stuttering is not fully understood, the condition is found more often in men than in women. Stuttering occurs when sounds or syllables are repeated and the patient cannot put words together fluidly. When speaking with patients who stutter, do not interrupt or finish their answers out of frustration. Let patients complete what they have to say, and do not correct how they say it.

Accommodations for Speech Impairments

When speaking to a patient with a speech impairment, never assume that the person lacks intelligence. It will be difficult, if not impossible, to complete a thorough interview if you have insulted the patient. Do not to rush the patient or predict an answer. Try to form questions that require short, direct answers. Prepare to spend extra time during your interview.

When asking questions, look directly at the patient. If you cannot understand what the person has said, politely ask her to repeat it. Never pretend to understand when you do not. You might miss valuable information about the patient's chief complaint—the reason for the call. If all else fails, give the patient an opportunity to write the responses to your questions.

OBESITY

According to Statistics Canada, 48 percent of Canadians have a body-mass index (BMI) of 25 or more, meaning that they are overweight. Fifteen percent of Canadians are obese. In 1996, 57 percent of Canadian men were deemed overweight. This is up from 48 percent in 1981. Among women, 35 percent were overweight in 1996, up from 30 percent in 1981.

Obesity among Canadian children has increased dramatically in the last 15 years, doubling among boys and tripling among girls. In 1996, 33 percent of Canadian boys (aged 7–13) were likely to be overweight when they became adults (age 18). This is up from 11 percent in 1981. For girls, in 1996, 27 percent were likely to be overweight by the time they were adults, compared with 13 percent in 1981.

The estimated total cost of obesity in Canada in 1997 was 1.8 billion dollars. This was about 2.4 percent of the total health budget. The three contributors to obesity were hypertension, Type 2 diabetes mellitus, and coronary artery disease.

An obese patient can make a difficult job even more difficult for an EMS provider. Besides the obvious difficulty of lifting and moving the obese patient, excess weight can exacerbate the complaint for which you were called. Obesity can also lead to a number of serious medical conditions, including hypertension, heart disease, stroke, diabetes, and joint and muscle problems.

Etiologies

People require a certain amount of body fat in order to metabolize vitamins and minerals. Obesity occurs when a person has an abnormal amount of body fat and a weight 20 to 30 percent heavier than is normal for people of the same age, sex, and height.

Obesity occurs for a number of reasons. In many cases, it happens when a person's caloric intake is higher than the amount of calories required to meet her energy needs. In such cases, diet, exercise, and lifestyle choices play a role in the person's condition. Genetic factors may also predispose a patient toward obesity. In rare cases, an obese patient may have a low basal metabolic rate, which causes the body to burn calories at a slower rate. In such cases, the condition may be produced by an illness, particularly hypothyroidism.

Accommodations for Obese Patients

Regardless of the cause of your patient's obesity, your primary responsibility is to provide thorough and professional medical care. Conduct an extensive medical history, keeping in mind the chronic medical conditions commonly associated with obesity.

Obese patients often mistakenly blame signs and symptoms of an untreated illness on their weight. For example, they may quickly dismiss shortness of breath by saying, "When you're as heavy as I am, you can't expect to walk up a flight of stairs without some extra breathing." Do not accept such an answer. The shortness of breath may be caused by congestive heart failure. Obtain a complete history of the symptoms and the activities the person was engaged in when the symptoms appeared. While the patient usually experiences shortness of breath when climbing stairs, this time the condition may have started while sitting down or may have been more severe than usual.

When doing your patient assessment, you may also have to make accommodations for the person's weight. For example, if the patient's adipose tissue presents an obstruction, you may need to place ECG monitoring electrodes on the arms and thighs instead of on the chest. You may also need to auscultate lung sounds anteriorly on a patient who is too obese to lean forward. In assessing an obese patient, flexibility is the key. Keep in mind that no two patients and no two environments will be exactly alike.

Positioning an obese patient for transport may prove especially difficult, as many EMS transport devices are not designed or rated for high weights. Always be sure you have enough lifting assistance for the circumstances. Never compromise your health or safety during the transport process. Another EMS crew or the fire department may be necessary to move your patient safely. Finally, remember to let the emergency department know that extra lifting assistance and special stretchers will be needed on your arrival.

If the adipose tissue on an obese patient presents an obstruction, you may need to place ECG monitoring electrodes on the arms and thighs instead of on the chest.

When transporting an extremely obese patient, summon adequate assistance. Try not to draw excess attention to the patient in order to avoid causing further embarrassment.

Be prepared to be extremely innovative when determining how to transport a morbidly obese patient who will not fit the ambulance stretcher.

PARALYSIS

Always expect the unexpected in EMS. During your career, you may respond to a call and find that your patient is paralyzed from a previous traumatic or medical event. You will have to treat the chief complaint while taking into account the accommodations that must be made with a patient who cannot move some or all of her extremities.

A paralyzed patient may be paraplegic or quadriplegic. A paraplegic patient has been paralyzed from the waist down, while a quadriplegic patient has paralysis of all four extremities. In addition, spinal cord injuries in the area of C3 to C5 and above may also paralyze the patient's respiratory muscles and compromise the ability to breathe.

If your patient depends on a home ventilator, it is important to maintain a patent airway and to keep the ventilator functioning. Also, a paralyzed patient may have been breathing through a tracheostomy for some time. Therefore, you should keep suction nearby in case the person experiences an airway obstruction. You may also need to use a bag-valve mask while transporting the patient to the ambulance if the ventilator does not transport easily. If your ambulance is equipped, use the ventilator with an onboard power supply to save the ventilator's batteries. This is an already anxious time for your patient, and so you may need to spend some extra time reassuring the person before making any changes in the life-support system.

If the patient has suffered a recent spinal cord injury, halo traction may still be intact. Be sure to stabilize the traction before transport. The patient can probably tell you how to assist with the halo traction; if not, a call to the patient's physician may be necessary.

While performing your physical assessment, you may come across a **colostomy.** This device is necessary when the patient does not have normal bowel function due to paralysis of the muscles needed for proper elimination. Be sure to take any other assisting devices, such as canes or wheelchairs, so that the patient can get around once out of your care. (For more on acute interventions for patients with physical disabilities and other chronic-care patients, see Chapter 46.)

If a patient still has halo traction intact, be sure to stabilize the traction before transport.

* colostomy a surgical diversion of the large intestine through an opening in the skin where the fecal matter is collected in a pouch; may be temporary or permanent.

MENTAL CHALLENGES AND EMOTIONAL IMPAIRMENTS

Mental and emotional illnesses present a special challenge to the EMS provider. They may range from the psychoses caused by complex biochemical brain diseases, such as bipolar disorder (manic depression), to the personality disorders related to personality development, to traumatic experiences. Emotional impairments can include such conditions as hysteria, compulsive behaviour, and anxiety. For a detailed discussion on the etiologies, assessment, management, and treatment of these patients, see Chapter 38.

DEVELOPMENTAL DISABILITIES

People with developmental disabilities are those individuals with impaired or insufficient development of the brain who are unable to learn at the usual rate. In recent years, a large number of people with developmental disabilities have been mainstreamed into the day-to-day activities of life. They hold jobs and live in residential settings, either on their own, with their families, or in group homes.

Developmental disabilities can result from a variety of reasons. They can be genetic, such as in Down syndrome, or they can be the result of brain injury caused by some hypoxic or traumatic event. Such injuries can take place before birth, during birth, or anytime thereafter.

ACCOMMODATIONS FOR DEVELOPMENTAL DISABILITIES

Unless a patient has Down syndrome, it may be difficult to recognize someone with a developmental disability unless the person lives in a group home or other special residential setting. The disability may only become obvious when you start your interview, and even then the person may be able to provide adequate information (Figure 45-2). Remember that a person with a developmental disability can recognize body language, tone, and disrespect just like anyone else. Treat them as you would any other patient, listening to their answers, particularly if you suspect physical or emotional abuse. As mentioned in previous chapters, this group has a higher than average chance of being abused, particularly by someone they know.

If a patient has a severe cognitive disability, you may need to rely on others to obtain the chief complaint and history. In this case, plan to spend a little extra time on your secondary assessment because the patient may not be able to tell you what is wrong. Also, many children or young people with developmental disabilities have been taught to be wary of strangers who may seek to touch them. You will have to establish a basis of trust with the patient, perhaps by making it clear that you are a member of the medical community or by asking for the support of a person the patient does trust. Also, some people with developmental disabilities may have been judged "stupid" or "bad" for behaviour that had resulted in an accident and they may try to cover up the events that led up to the call.

At all times, keep in mind that a person with a developmental disability may not understand what is happening. The ambulance, special equipment, and even your uniform may confuse or scare them. In cases of severe disabilities, it will be important to keep the primary caregiver with you at all times, even in the back of the ambulance. Talk to patients who have disabilities in terms they will understand, and demonstrate what you are doing, as much as possible, on yourself or your partner.

Remember that a person with a developmental disability can recognize body language, tone, and disrespect just like anyone else. Treat them as you would any other patient.

DOWN SYNDROME

Until the mid-1900s, people with Down syndrome lived largely out of public view and tended to die at an early age. Today, however, people with Down syndrome

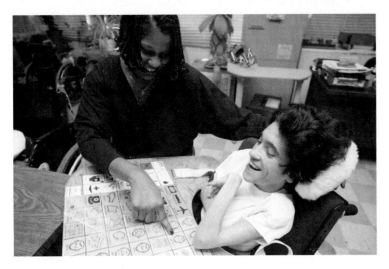

FIGURE 45-2 People with developmental disabilities may have trouble communicating but can often still understand what you say.

people attend special schools, hold paid jobs, and, because of improved medical care, can live long lives.

Down syndrome is named after J. Langdon Down, the British physician who studied and identified the condition. It results from an extra chromosome, usually on chromosome 21 or 22. Instead of 46 chromosomes, a person with Down syndrome has 47.

Although the cause is unknown, the chromosomal abnormality increases with the age of the mother, especially after age 40. It also occurs at a higher rate in parents with a chromosomal abnormality, such as the translocation of chromosome 21 to chromosome 14. In such cases, the parent, usually the mother, is phenotypically normal but has 45 chromosomes. Theoretically, the chance is one in three that the mother will have a Down syndrome child.

Typically, Down syndrome presents with easily recognized physical features. They include

- Eyes sloped up at the outer corners
- Folds of skin on either side of the nose that cover the inner corner of the eye
- Small face and features
- Large and protruding tongue
- Flattening of the back of the head
- Short and broad hands

Patients with Down syndrome are often loving and trusting. Be sure to treat them with respect and patience.

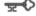

In addition to mild to moderate developmental disability, patients with Down syndrome may have other physical ailments, such as heart defects, intestinal defects, and chronic lung problems. People with Down syndrome are also at risk of developing cataracts, blindness, and Alzheimer's disease at an early age.

When assessing the patient with Down syndrome, consider the level of her developmental delay and follow the general guidelines mentioned earlier. Transport to the hospital should be uneventful, especially if the caregiver accompanies you.

FETAL ALCOHOL SPECTRUM DISORDER

Fetal alcohol spectrum disorder (FASD) is sometimes confused with Down syndrome because of similar facial characteristics. Unlike Down syndrome, FASD is a preventable disorder, caused by excessive alcohol consumption during pregnancy. Children who suffer FASD have characteristic features, including

- Small head with multiple facial abnormalities
- Small eyes with short slits
- Wide, flat nose bridge
- Lack of a groove between the nose and lip
- Small jaw

FASD patients often exhibit delayed physical growth, mental disabilities, and hyperactivity. Again, follow the preceding general guidelines when treating children with FASD.

PATHOLOGICAL CHALLENGES

As you will learn in Chapter 46, "Acute Interventions for the Chronic-Care Patient," you will encounter a number of patients with chronic conditions. It is important for you to be aware of most common of these conditions, since chronic-care patients require higher-than-average interventions and transport.

Arthritis

The three most common types of arthritis include

- Juvenile rheumatoid arthritis (JRA)—a connective tissue disorder that strikes before age 16
- Rheumatoid arthritis—an autoimmune disorder
- Osteoarthritis—a degenerative joint disease, the most common arthritis seen in elderly patients

All forms of arthritis cause painful swelling and irritation of the joints, making everyday tasks sometimes impossible. Patients with arthritis commonly have joint stiffness and limited range of motion. Sometimes the smaller joints of the hands and feet become deformed (Figure 45-3). In addition, children with JRA may suffer complications involving the spleen or liver.

Treatment for arthritis includes aspirin, nonsteroidal anti-inflammatory drugs (NSAIDS), and/or corticosteroids. It is important for you to recognize the side effects of these medications because you may have been called on to treat a medication side effect, rather than the disease. NSAIDS can cause stomach upset and vomiting, with or without bloody emesis. Corticosteroids, such as prednisone, can cause hyperglycemia, bloody emesis, and decreased immunity. You should also take note of all the patient's medications so that you do not administer a medication that can interact with the ones already taken by the patient.

When transporting patients with arthritis, keep in mind their high level of discomfort. Use pillows to elevate affected extremities. The most comfortable patient position might not be the best position to start an IV, but try to make the patient as comfortable as possible. Special padding techniques may be required.

Most cases of arthritis encountered in emergency medicine are due to osteoarthritis.

When transporting patients with arthritis, keep in mind their high level of discomfort.

Cancer

Many volumes of books have been written on the subject of cancer. It is impossible to list all that a health-care provider needs to know about cancer in a small part of a single chapter. In fact, "cancer" is really many different diseases, each with its own characteristics. However, there are some basic points that a paramedic should keep in mind when treating a patient with cancer.

Cancer is caused by the abnormal growth of cells in normal tissue. The primary site of origin of the cancer cells determines the type of cancer that the patient has. If the cancer starts in epithelial tissue, it is called a carcinoma. If the cancer forms in connective tissue, it is called a sarcoma. It may be difficult for you to recognize a cancer patient because the disease often has few obvious signs and symptoms. Rather, the treatments for the disease take on telltale signs, such as anorexia leading to weight loss or alopecia (hair loss). Tattoos may be left on the skin by radiation oncologists to mark positioning of radiation therapy equipment. In addition, physical changes, such as loss of a breast (mastectomy), may be obvious.

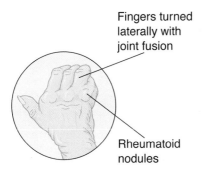

Fingers turned laterally with joint fusion

Rheumatoid nodules

FIGURE 45-3 Rheumatoid arthritis causes joints to become painful and deformed.

neutropenic a condition that results from an abnormally low neutrophil count in the blood (less than 2000/mm^3).

If a person has recently undergone chemotherapy, assume that the patient is neutropenic. For this reason, keep a mask on the patient during transport and during transfer at the emergency department.

Management of the patient with cancer can present a special challenge to the paramedic. Many patients undergoing chemotherapy treatments become **neutropenic.** This is a condition in which chemotherapy creates a dangerously low level of neutrophils—the white blood cells responsible for the destruction of bacteria and other infectious organisms. Frequently during chemotherapy, the neutrophils are destroyed along with the cancer cells, severely increasing the patient's risk for infection.

If patients have recently undergone chemotherapy, assume that they are neutropenic. Decrease their exposure to infection as much as possible. Remember that once infected, a neutropenic patient can quickly go into septic shock, sometimes in a matter of hours. For this reason, keep a mask on a patient both during transport and during transfer at the emergency department (Figure 45-4).

In treating patients with cancer, also keep in mind that their veins may have become scarred and difficult to access due to frequent IV starts, blood draws, and chemotherapy transfusions. Patients with cancer may also have an implanted infusion port, found just below the skin, with the catheter inserted into the subclavian vein or brachial artery. This port is accessed for infusion of chemotherapy drugs or IV fluids using sterile technique.

You need special training to use these ports and should not attempt to access them unless you have such training. Local protocols usually dictate whether an EMS provider may access one of these devices. The patient may request that you do not start a peripheral IV if their port can be accessed at the hospital. In such cases, you need to consider if your IV is a life-saving necessity that cannot wait or if the patient can indeed wait for access at the emergency department.

Patients with cancer may also have a peripheral access device, such as a Groshong catheter or Hickman catheter, which has access ports that extend outside the skin. In this situation, it may simply be a matter of flushing the line and then hooking up your IV fluids to this external catheter. Whatever you decide to do, involve the patient in the decision-making process whenever possible. Patients with cancer lose much control over their lives during treatment, and so it is important for them to maintain as much control over their EMS care as possible.

CEREBRAL PALSY

Cerebral palsy is a group of a disorders caused by damage to the cerebrum in utero or by trauma during birth. Prenatal exposure of the mother to German measles (rubella) can cause cerebral palsy, along with any event that leads to hypoxia in the fetus. Premature birth or brain damage from a difficult delivery

FIGURE 45-4 Make every effort to protect patients with cancer from infection. Both you and the patient should wear masks during transport and during transfer at the hospital.

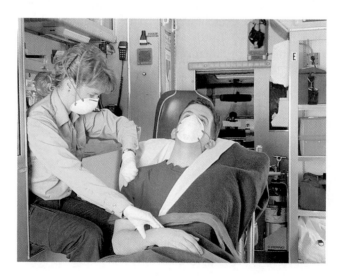

can also lead to cerebral palsy. Other causes include encephalitis, meningitis, or head injury from a fall or the abuse of an infant.

Patients with cerebral palsy have difficulty controlling motor functions, causing spasticity of the muscles. This condition may affect a single limb or the entire body. About two-thirds of cerebral palsy patients have a below normal intellectual capacity, and about half experience seizures. Conversely, a full third of cerebral palsy patients have normal intelligence, and a few are highly gifted.

There are three main types of cerebral palsy—spastic paralysis, athetosis, and ataxia. Spastic paralysis, which is the most common form of cerebral palsy, forces the muscles into a state of permanent stiffness and contracture. When both legs are affected, the knees turn inward, causing the characteristic "scissor gait." Athetosis causes an involuntary writhing movement, usually affecting arms, feet, hands, and legs. If the patient's face is affected, the person may demonstrate drooling or grimacing. Ataxic cerebral palsy is the rarest form of the disease and causes problems with coordination of gait and balance.

In treating patients with cerebral palsy, keep this fact in mind: Many people with atheotoid and diplegic cerebral palsy are highly intelligent. Do not automatically assume that a person with cerebral palsy cannot communicate with you. Also, as you might expect, many cerebral palsy patients rely on special devices to help them with their mobility. Diplegic patients, for example, may be dependent on wheelchairs.

When transporting cerebral palsy patients, make accommodations to prevent further injury. If they experience severe contractions, the patients may not rest comfortably on a stretcher. Use pillows and extra blankets to pad extremities that are not in proper alignment. Have suction available if a patient drools. If a patient has difficulty communicating, make sure that the caregiver helps in your assessment. Be alert for cerebral palsy patients who use sign language. If you do not know sign language, find someone who does, and alert the emergency department.

CYSTIC FIBROSIS (MUCOVISCIDOSIS)

Cystic fibrosis (CF) is an inherited disorder that involves the exocrine (mucus-producing) glands, primarily in the lungs and the digestive system. Thick mucus forms in the lungs, causing bronchial obstruction and atelectasis, or collapse of the alveoli. In addition, the thick mucus causes blockages in the small ducts of the pancreas, **mucoviscidosis**, leading to a decrease in the pancreatic enzymes needed for digestion. This results in malnutrition, even in patients on healthy diets.

Obtaining a complete medical history is important to the recognition of a patient with CF. A unique characteristic of CF is the high concentration of chloride in the sweat, leading to the use of a diagnostic test known as the "sweat test." A patient with CF may also complain of frequent lung infections, clay-coloured stools, or clubbing of the fingers or toes.

Recent medical advances have extended the lives of patients with CF so that some live well into their thirties. However, because of the poor prognosis, most of the patients with CF whom you see will be children and adolescents. In treating these patients, remember that they have been chronically ill for their entire lives. The last thing they want is another trip to the hospital. For this reason, transport can be difficult for both the patient and the family members. To allay their fears, keep in mind the developmental stage of your patient. A child with cystic fibrosis is still a child. So, recall everything you have learned about the treatment of pediatric patients.

Because of the high probability of respiratory distress in a patient with CF, some form of oxygen therapy may be necessary. You may need to have a family member or caregiver hold blow-by oxygen, rather than use a mask, if that is all the patient will tolerate. Suctioning may be necessary to help the patient clear the thick

Content Review

MAIN TYPES OF CEREBRAL PALSY
- Spastic paralysis
- Athetosis
- Ataxia

Many people with atheotoid and diplegic cerebral palsy are highly intelligent. Do not automatically assume that they cannot communicate with you.

✱ **mucoviscidosis** cystic fibrosis of the pancreas resulting in abnormally viscous mucoid secretion from the pancreas.

In treating patients with cystic fibrosis, remember that they have been chronically ill for their entire lives. The last thing they want is another trip to the hospital.

secretions from the airway. Patients with CF patients may be taking antibiotics to prevent infection and using inhalers or Mucomyst to thin their secretions. Make sure that you take along all medications so that the hospital staff can continue with the patient's regimen.

MULTIPLE SCLEROSIS

Multiple sclerosis (MS) is a disorder of the central nervous system that usually strikes between the ages of 20 and 40, affecting women more than men. The exact cause of MS is unknown, but it is considered to be an autoimmune disorder. Characteristically, repeated inflammation of the myelin sheath surrounding the nerves leads to scar tissue, which, in turn, blocks nerve impulses to the affected area.

The onset of MS is slow. It starts with a slight change in the strength of a muscle and a numbness or tingling in the affected muscle. For example, a patient may start to drop things, blaming it on clumsiness. Doctors encourage patients with MS to lead as normal a life as possible, but the patients become increasingly tired. Their gait may become unsteady, and their speech may slur. Patients with MS may also develop eye problems, such as double vision due to weakness of the eye muscles or eye pain due to neuritis of the optic nerve.

The initial signs of MS are usually temporary. However, they return and become more frequent and long lasting. As the symptoms progress, they become more permanent, leading to a weak extremity or paralysis. Over time, some patients may become bedridden and lose control of bladder function. Eventually, a patient with MS may develop a lung or urinary infection, which may lead to death. As with other chronically ill patients, people with MS may experience mood swings and seek medical attention for those feelings.

Transport of a patient with MS to the hospital may require supportive care, such as oxygen therapy. Make sure the patient is comfortable, and help position the person as necessary. Do not expect patients with MS to walk to the ambulance. Even if normally ambulatory, they may be in a more weakened state than usual. Again, be sure to bring along assistive devices, such as a wheelchair or cane so that the patient can maintain as much independence as possible (Figure 45-5).

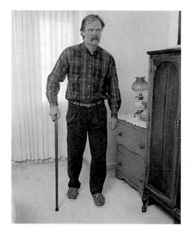

FIGURE 45-5 Patients with multiple sclerosis and muscular dystrophy may use canes to aid in ambulation. Be sure to take such devices with you on the ambulance.

MUSCULAR DYSTROPHY

Muscular dystrophy (MD) is a group of hereditary disorders characterized by progressive weakness and wasting of muscle tissue. It is a genetic disorder, leading to gradual degeneration of muscle fibres. The most common form of MD is Duchenne muscular dystrophy, which typically affects boys between the ages of 3 and 6. It leads to progressive muscle weakness in the legs and pelvis and to paralysis by age 12. Ultimately, the disease affects the respiratory muscles and heart, causing death at an early age. The other various MD disorders are classified by the age of the patient at onset of symptoms and by the muscles affected.

Since MD is a hereditary disease, you should obtain a complete family history. You should also note the particular muscle groups that the patient cannot move. Again, since patients with MD are primarily children, use age-appropriate language. Respiratory support, such as oxygen, may be needed, especially in the later stages of the disease.

POLIOMYELITIS

Poliomyelitis is a communicable disease that affects the grey matter of the brain and the spinal cord. Although it is highly contagious, immunization has made outbreaks of polio extremely rare in the developed nations. It is expected that polio will be completely eradicated soon all over the world. However, it is important to know about the disease since many people born before development of the polio vaccination in the 1950s were affected by the disease.

Typically, the polio virus enters the body through the gastrointestinal tract. It circulates through the digestive tract and then enters the bloodstream. Once there, it is carried to the central nervous system, where the virus enters the nerve cells and alters them. In cases of paralytic poliomyelitis, patients experience asymmetrical muscle weakness that leads to permanent paralysis.

Although most patients recover from the disease itself, they are left with permanent paralysis of the affected muscles. You may recognize a polio survivor by the use of assistive devices for ambulation or by the reduced size of the affected limb due to muscle atrophy. Some patients may have experienced paralysis of the respiratory muscles, requiring assisted ventilation. Patients on long-term ventilators will typically have tracheostomies.

Along with polio, you should know about a related disorder called postpolio syndrome. Postpolio syndrome affects those patients who suffered severely from polio more than 30 years ago. Although the cause of postpolio syndrome remains unknown, researchers think the condition results from the stress of long-term weakness in the affected nerves. Patients with this condition quickly tire, especially after exercise, and develop an intolerance for cold in their extremities.

Many patients with polio or postpolio syndrome try to maintain their independence. They may insist on walking to the ambulance but should not be encouraged to do so. The idea of hospitalization will frustrate them, since many polio survivors have memories of spending months or even years in hospitals as children. Unlike other chronically ill patients, most do not require frequent trips to the hospital. Therefore, this may be their first time in an ambulance. Try to alleviate their anxiety as much as possible.

PREVIOUS HEAD INJURIES

A patient with a previous head injury may not be easily recognizable. You may not notice anything different about the patient until the person starts to speak. A patient with a head injury may display symptoms similar to that of a stroke, without the hemiparesis, or paralysis to one side of the body. The presenting symptoms will be related to the area of the brain that has been injured. The patient may have aphasia, slurred speech, and loss of vision or hearing or may develop a learning disability. Such patients may also exhibit short-term memory loss and may not even have any recollection of their original injury.

Obtaining a medical history from these patients is very important, especially if you are responding to a traumatic event. Note any new symptoms the patient may be having or the recurrence of old ones. Conduct the secondary assessment slowly. If the patient cannot speak, look for obvious physical signs of trauma or for facial expressions of pain. Transport considerations will depend on the condition for which you were called. However, information about the previous head injury should be an important part of the patient's transfer procedures.

SPINA BIFIDA

Spina bifida is a congenital abnormality that falls under the category of neural tube defects. It presents when there is a defect in the closure of the backbone and the spinal canal. In spina bifida occulta, the patient exhibits few outward signs of the deformity. In spina bifida cystica, the failure of the closure allows the spinal cord and covering membranes to protrude from the back, causing an obvious deformity.

Symptoms depend on which part of the spinal cord is protruding through the back. The patient may have paralysis of both lower extremities and lack of bowel or bladder control. A large percentage of children born with spina bifida have hydrocephalus, which results from the accumulation of fluid in the brain. Permanent disabilities caused by spina bifida are difficult to assess before the defect is surgically corrected. If the patient has hydrocephalus, a shunt will need to be inserted to drain off the excess fluid.

When treating patients with spina bifida, keep several things in mind. Recent research has shown that between 18 percent and 73 percent of children and adolescents with spina bifida have latex allergies. For safety, assume that all patients with spina bifida have this problem. In transporting a spina bifida patient, be sure to take along any devices that aid the patient.

For safety, assume that all patients with spina bifida have a latex allergy.

MYASTHENIA GRAVIS

Myasthenia gravis is an autoimmune disease characterized by chronic weakness of voluntary muscles and progressive fatigue. The condition results from a problem with the neurotransmitters, which causes a blocking of nerve signals to the muscles. It occurs most frequently in women between the ages of 20 and 50.

A patient with myasthenia gravis may complain of a complete lack of energy, especially in the evening. The disease commonly involves muscles in the face. You may note eyelid drooping or difficulty in chewing or swallowing. The patient may also complain of double vision. In severe cases, a patient may experience paralysis of the respiratory muscles, leading to respiratory arrest. These patients may need assisted ventilations en route to the emergency facility.

As a health-care provider, you are ethically required to take care of all patients in the same manner, regardless of their race, religion, gender, ethnic background, and living situation.

OTHER CHALLENGES

In addition to the challenges described in the preceding sections, you can expect to meet a whole range of special situations that will affect the quality of the patient service that you provide. The following are some of the special situations or conditions that you will encounter, if you have not already done so.

CULTURALLY DIVERSE PATIENTS

Many ethnic groups believe in and practise various forms of folk medicine. You should respect these beliefs but remember that some folk remedies may interact with scientific medical therapies. If you work in an area predominantly populated by a specific ethnic group, learn more about the group's folk medicine beliefs and practices.

As a health-care provider, you are ethically required to take care of all patients in the same manner, regardless of their race, religion, gender, ethnic background, or living situation. What may make it difficult for you to treat culturally different patients may not be the differences per se but your inability to understand them. Do not consider this a reason for refusing treatment. Rather, consider it a learning experience that will prepare you for a similar situation on another run. With North American society becoming more diverse, tolerance of cultural differences will become an important part of your career (Figure 45-6).

FIGURE 45-6 North American society is becoming diverse.

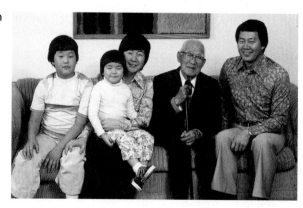

From time to time, you may encounter a patient who will make a decision about medical care you do not agree with. For example, Christian Scientists do not believe in human intervention in sickness through the use of drugs or other therapies. You cannot force these patients to accept care. You should, however, obtain a signed document indicating informed refusal of care.

Accommodation of a culturally diverse population will require patience and, in some cases, ingenuity. If your patient does not speak English, communication may be a problem. You may need to rely on a family member to act as an interpreter or on a translator device, such as telephone language line for non-English-speaking people. Notify the receiving facility of the need for an interpreter.

TERMINALLY ILL PATIENTS

Caring for a terminally ill patient can be an emotional challenge. Many times, the patient may choose to die at home, but at the last minute the family may override those wishes by calling for an ambulance. In other cases, the patient may call for an ambulance so that a newly developed condition can be treated or a medication adjusted. See Chapter 46 for a fuller discussion.

PATIENTS WITH COMMUNICABLE DISEASES

When treating people with communicable diseases, you should withhold all personal judgment. Although you will have to take body substance isolation (BSI) precautions just as you would with any patient, keep in mind the heightened sensitivity of a person with a communicable disease. Most of these patients are familiar with the health-care setting and understand why you must take certain protective measures. However, you should still explain that you take these measures with other patients that have a similar disease. Also, you do not need to take additional precautions that are not required by departmental policy. The patient will generally spot these extra measures and feel guilt, shame, or anger. For more information on the etiologies and treatment of communicable diseases, see Chapter 37.

SUMMARY

It is important to be aware of the pathophysiology of diseases that you may encounter throughout your career. You should also know the characteristics of impairments that are commonly found in the medical setting. They may be the primary reason that your patient seeks help, or they may not be the reason your patient called at all. Whatever the circumstances, it is important to learn the various etiologies of these impairments and illnesses in order to treat your patient with the knowledge and respect that every patient deserves every day.

CHAPTER 46

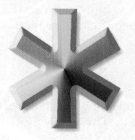

Acute Interventions for the Chronic-Care Patient

Objectives

After reading this chapter, you should be able to:

1. Compare and contrast the primary objectives of the paramedic and the home care provider. (pp. 1108, 1112–1113)
2. Identify the importance of home health care medicine as it relates to emergency medical services. (pp. 1107–1108)
3. Differentiate between the role of the paramedic and the role of the home care provider. (pp. 1108, 1112–1113)
4. Compare and contrast the primary objectives of acute care, home care, and hospice care. (pp. 1108, 1112–1113, 1138)
5. Discuss aspects of home care that enhance the quality of patient care

and aspects that have the potential to become detrimental. (pp. 1107–1123)
6. List pathologies and complications in home care patients that commonly result in ALS intervention. (pp. 1108–1113)
7. Compare the mortality and quality of care for a given patient in the hospital versus the home care setting. (pp. 1107–1108)
8. Discuss the significance of palliative care programs as related to a patient in a home health care or hospice setting. (pp. 1112–1113, 1138)
9. Define hospice care, comfort care, and DNR/DNAR as they relate to local

Continued

practice, law, and policy. (pp. 1112–1113, 1118, 1138–1140)

10. List and describe the characteristics of typical home care devices related to airway maintenance, artificial and alveolar ventilation, vascular access, drug administration, and the GI/GU tract. (pp. 1111–1112, 1119, 1123–1135)

11. Discuss the complications of assessing each of the devices described above. (pp. 1123–1135)

12. Describe indications, contraindications, and techniques for urinary catheter insertion in the male and female patient in an out-of-hospital setting. (p. 1132)

13. Identify failure of GI/GU, ventilatory, vascular access, and drain devices found in the home care setting. (pp. 1123–1135)

14. Discuss the relationship between local home care treatment

protocols/SOPs and local EMS Protocols/SOPs. (p. 1113)

15. Discuss differences in the ability of individuals to accept and cope with their own impending death. (p. 1140)

16. List the stages of the grief process and relate them to an individual in hospice care. (p. 1140)

17. Discuss the rights of the terminally ill patient. (pp. 1138–1140)

18. Summarize the types of home health care available in your area and the services provided. (pp. 1107–1112)

19. Given a series of home care scenarios, determine which patients should receive follow-up home care and which should be transported to an emergency care facility. (pp. 1113–1118)

20. Given a series of scenarios, demonstrate interaction and support with the family members/support persons for a patient who has died. (pp. 1138–1140)

INTRODUCTION

One of the major trends in modern health care involves the shifting of patients out of the hospital and back into their homes as soon as possible. The result has been a huge increase in home health-care needs and services.

EPIDEMIOLOGY OF HOME CARE

A number of factors have promoted the growth of home care, including improved medical technology and studies showing improved recovery rates and lower costs with home care. The shift to home care has important implications for EMS providers. As patients assume greater responsibility for their own treatment and recovery, the likelihood of advanced life support (ALS) intervention for the chronic-care patient increases. Calls may come from the patient, the patient's family, or a home health-care provider.

In home care settings, sometimes you can expect to encounter a dizzying array of devices, machines, and equipment designed to provide anything from supportive to life-sustaining care. As a paramedic, you should become familiar with the basic functions of the common home care devices and, just as importantly, recognize the underlying need for them. The failure or malfunction of this type of equipment has the potential to become a life-threatening or life-altering event. New technologies and machines are being developed constantly. It is your responsibility to stay informed of these changes and the assessment complications that may be involved with the use of each device.

The primary driving force in home health care is cost containment.

As a paramedic, you should become familiar with the basic functions of many of the common home care devices and, just as importantly, recognize the underlying need for them.

ALS Response to Home Care Patients

A number of situations may involve you in the treatment of a home care patient—equipment failure, unexpected complications, absence of a caregiver, need for transport, inability of the patient or caregiver to operate a device, and more. As already mentioned, you might also be called on to provide emotional support or intervention. Taking responsibility for an illness or an ill family member can be a stressful and overwhelming experience. Some people may be ill-equipped to deal with complicated directions, mechanical problems, or the stress of long-term care. Do not minimize their frustrations or allow them to interfere with your care.

Your primary role as a paramedic is to identify and treat any life-threatening problems. An important source of information is the home care provider—whether it be a nurse, nurse's aid, family member, or friend. Remember that this person usually knows the patient better than anyone else does. The provider will often spot subtle changes in the patient's condition that may seem insignificant to the outsider. Listen carefully to what this person says (Figure 46-1).

Home care providers are often health-care professionals; be sensitive in questioning their training or background. You must obtain certain information to care for your patient, and the home care provider may be the only source you have for such critical items as the patient's baseline mental status. If you meet resistance, due to either from the home care provider's lack of training or a misunderstanding of your needs, try rephrasing your question or using less technical language. You may also find evidence of neglect or improper patient care by the home care provider. Correct any immediate life-threats that you find, and document your findings in your patient report. You should also report the situation to your supervisors for corrective action. However, do not confront the home care worker yourself.

At all times, keep in mind the presence of the patient. Involve him in the questioning process. If the caregiver mentions a change or reaction, you might say: "Did you notice this change, too?" "How do you think you reacted?"

Typical Responses

Many of the medical problems that you will encounter in a home care setting are the same as the ones that you will encounter elsewhere in the field. However, you must always keep in mind that the home care patient is in a more fragile state to begin with. A member of the medical community has already decided that the person needs extra help. A home care patient is more likely to decompensate and go into crisis more quickly than the general population. As a result, you need to monitor the home care patient carefully and be ready to intervene at all times. Some of the typical responses involve airway complications, respiratory failure, cardiac decompensation, alterations in peripheral circulation, altered mental status, gastrointestinal/genitourinary (GI/GU) crises, infections and/or septic complications, and equipment malfunction. (For more specific information on examples, see later sections of the chapter.)

Airway Complications The airway is always your paramount concern, and the home care patient is no exception. In the absence of documentation proving the patient's request to withhold intubation and mechanical ventilation, you should protect the airway at all costs. However, even if the patient has a valid do not resuscitate (DNR) order, remember that in certain situations, you still can use basic airway techniques and suctioning to protect the airway.

Airway compromise can be the result of many different etiologies. Problems that you might encounter include inadequate pulmonary toilet, inadequate alveolar ventilation, and inadequate alveolar oxygenation. (For more on airway problems, see material later in the chapter.)

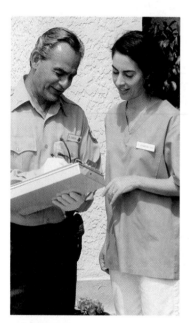

FIGURE 46-1 The home health-care provider usually knows the patient better than anyone else and will often spot subtle changes in the patient's condition.

A home care patient is more likely to decompensate and go into crisis more quickly than the general population.

Respiratory Failure As you will read later in the chapter, any number of respiratory problems can be treated in a home care setting. Some of the most common conditions that will lead to respiratory failure or acute crisis include

- Emphysema
- Bronchitis
- Asthma
- Cystic fibrosis
- Congestive heart failure
- Pulmonary embolus
- Sleep apnea
- **Guillain-Barré syndrome**
- **Myasthenia gravis**

Cardiac Decompensation Regardless of the setting, cardiac decompensation is a true medical emergency that can lead to life-threatening shock. This condition requires aggressive identification and treatment. Home care patients who have borderline cardiac output may be placed at risk if their cardiac demand increases from stress or illness and their system cannot compensate. Some other common causes of cardiac decompensation include

- Congestive heart failure
- Acute myocardial infarction (MI) (Home care patients are at higher risk.)
- Cardiac **hypertrophy**
- Calcification or degeneration of the heart's conductive system
- Heart transplantation
- Sepsis

Alterations in Peripheral Circulation You already know that the heart circulates blood throughout the body. However, remember that bodily movement also aids in circulation. If a home care patient has limited mobility, expect the entire circulatory system to be less effective and weaker. As muscle tone declines, so does the flow of blood. When circulation slows, movement becomes more difficult, thus creating a vicious cycle that leads to poorer circulation overall.

Keep in mind that alterations in peripheral circulation can complicate or worsen the course of treatment for a home care patient. Slowed circulation may result in delayed healing, increased risk of infections, or even **gangrene**. The number of Canadians aged 12 and over with diabetes is estimated at 1.2–1.4 million (4.9–5.8 percent of the population > 12 years), including undiagnosed cases of diabetes. These patients commonly develop poor circulation, especially to the extremities. They are at high risk of unhealed wounds or ulcers, particularly on the feet.

Altered Mental Status A common ALS response to a home care patient involves some kind of subtle or obvious change in mental status. In the home care patient, always suspect an exacerbation of his condition as well as other causes. Never forget that these patients are at higher risk than the general population of developing new medical problems. Some common causes of altered mental status include

- Hypoxia (from any number of respiratory or airway problems)
- Hypotension (from any number of cardiac problems or shock)

✱ **Guillain–Barré syndrome** acute viral infection that triggers the production of autoantibodies, which damage the myelin sheath covering the peripheral nerves; causes rapid, progressive loss of motor function, ranging from muscle weakness to full-body paralysis.

✱ **myasthenia gravis** disease characterized by episodic muscle weakness triggered by an autoimmune attack of the acetylcholine receptors.

Regardless of the setting, cardiac decompensation is a true medical emergency that can lead to life-threatening shock.

✱ **hypertrophy** an increase in the size or bulk of an organ or structure; caused by growth rather than by a tumour.

If a patient has limited mobility, expect the entire circulatory system to be less effective and weaker.

✱ **gangrene** death of tissue or bone, usually from an insufficient blood supply.

- Sepsis
- Altered electrolytes or blood chemistries (common in dialysis patients)
- Hypoglycemia (diabetes)
- Alzheimer's disease
- Cancerous tumour or brain lesions
- Overdose
- Stroke (brain attack)

GI/GU Crises EMS personnel find themselves involved in a number of calls involving home care patients with GI/GU problems. The problem often revolves around a misplaced or removed catheter, such as a Foley or a percutaneous endoscopic gastrostomy (PEG) tube. This may not seem like an emergency to you, but the inability to eat or urinate for a period of time can easily compromise an already weakened patient. In addition, home interventions, such as peritoneal dialysis, can alter fluid balances or electrolytes, creating a subtle but life-threatening problem.

Infections and Septic Complications You should always maintain a high index of suspicion for infection in a home care patient with a decreased immune response, either from poor general health or from a specific disease. Be particularly alert to infections in patients with indwelling devices, such as gastrostomy tubes, peripherally-inserted central catheter (PICC) lines, Foley catheters, or colostomies. Also remember that patients with limited lung function or tracheostomies cannot clear their airway easily, putting them at a higher risk of lung infections.

Patients who have decreased **sensorium** from a variety of conditions may have wounds and ulcers that they are unaware of, especially if they have been bedridden or inactive for long periods of time. Surgically implanted drains or wound closures may become infected without the patient realizing it. A bedbound patient may also develop decubitus wounds, or bedsores (Figure 46-2). If these problems are not identified or treated, they can progress from a generalized infection to gangrene and sepsis.

In identifying infections, look for the following general signs:

- Redness and/or swelling, especially at the insertion site of an indwelling device
- Purulent discharge at the insertion site
- Warm skin at the insertion site
- Fever

Infection at the cellular level is called **cellulitis** and is not life threatening. When an infection spreads systemically, however, it can lead to sepsis—a serious medical emergency. This may cause a patient's immune system to fail, resulting in septic shock. Signs and symptoms of sepsis include

- Redness at an insertion site
- Fever
- Altered mental status
- Poor skin colour or **turgor**
- Signs of shock
- Vomiting
- Diarrhea

You should always maintain a high index of suspicion for infection in a home care patient with a decreased immune response.

✱ **sensorium** sensory apparatus of the body as a whole; also that portion of the brain that functions as a centre of sensations.

✱ **cellulitis** inflammation of cellular or connective tissue.

✱ **turgor** ability of the skin to return to normal appearance after being subjected to pressure.

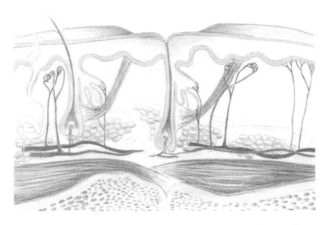

FIGURE 46-2a **Stage 1** Inflammation or redness of the skin that does not return to normal after 15 minutes of removal of pressure. Edema is present. It involves the epidermis. Skin may or may not be broken.

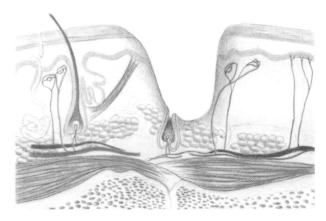

FIGURE 46-2b **Stage 2** Skin blister or shallow skin ulcer. Involves the epidermis. Looks like a shallow crater. Area is red and warm and may or may not have drainage.

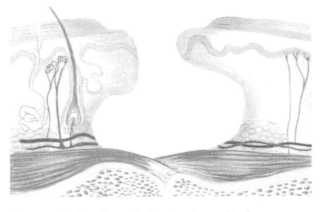

FIGURE 46-2c **Stage 3** Full thickness skin loss exposing subcutaneous tissue may extend into the next layer. Edema, inflammation, and necrosis are present. Drainage is present and may or may not have an odour.

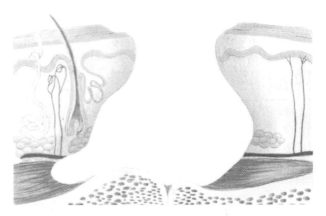

FIGURE 46-2d **Stage 4** Full thickness ulcer. Muscle and/or bone can be seen. Infection and necrosis are present. Drainage is present and may or may not have an odour.

FIGURE 46-2   Pressure sores are classified by the depth of tissue destruction.

Keep in mind that home care patients may already be receiving treatment for a generalized infection that has, in fact, worsened or spread. Inquire if a pattern of deterioration has been seen by the caregiver or home care provider. In cases of septic shock, ALS treatment is mainly supportive. Provide fluid for hypotension and necessary airway and oxygen support.

Equipment Malfunction Home care equipment has the normal limitations of any machine. The power may go out and stop the machine from functioning. The machine may break down and/or need maintenance. Some machines, if inoperative, can create a life threat to a patient. Common examples include home ventilators, oxygen delivery systems, apnea monitors, and home dialysis machines.

In cases of equipment malfunction, you may be called on to take the place of a device (such as a ventilator) or to treat problems that have arisen as a result of the malfunction. Even the malfunction of a glucometer for a diabetic can be a difficult situation for some patients to handle, especially if they suspect hypoglycemia. Your job is to assess the problem and take the appropriate actions.

Other Medical Disorders and Home Care Patients As already mentioned, you can expect to find a wide variety of problems treated in the home care setting. They can range from an infant on an apnea monitor to progressive dementia in a family member to psychosocial support of the family of a home care patient.

Some other conditions that may be treated at home include

- Brain or spinal trauma
- Arthritis
- Psychological disorders
- Cancer
- Hepatitis
- Acquired immune deficiency syndrome (AIDS)
- Transplantations (including patients awaiting transplantations)

Commonly Found Medical Devices

As previously mentioned, home care patients use a vast number of devices. They range from the simplicity of a nasal cannula to the complexity of a home ventilator. If you encounter an unfamiliar device—which may happen at some time in your career—do not panic. Find out what it is used for, and you will then have an idea on how to proceed. Do not think that you will look foolish if you ask questions. You will not. You will be foolish, and endanger the patient, if you pretend to understand a device, but do not. Some commonly used devices include

You will be foolish, and endanger the patient, if you pretend to understand a device, but don't.

- Glucometers
- IV infusions and indwelling IV sites
- Nebulized and aerosolized medication administrators
- Shunts, fistulas, and venous grafts
- Oxygen concentrators, oxygen tanks, and liquid oxygen systems
- Oxygen masks and nebulizers
- Tracheostomies and home ventilators
- G-tubes, colostomies, and urostomies
- Surgical drains
- Apnea monitors, cardiac monitors, and pulse oximeters
- Wheelchairs, canes, and walkers

Spend some time at the hospital talking with health-care personnel about new devices being introduced for the home care setting. Study or make copies of the brochures that come with these devices. You might also talk with manufacturers or vendors, the people who commonly deliver equipment to home care patients.

Intervention by a Home Health-Care Practitioner or Physician

Most calls involving home care patients will require acute intervention in such problems as inadequate respiratory support, acute respiratory events, acute cardiac events, acute sepsis, or GI/GU crises. Keep in mind, however, that you may not be the first person to provide intervention. If home care patients have a good relationship with their home health-care practitioner or physician, they may contact this person first. In fact, they may be required to do so in order to receive reimbursement for medical services.

Remain especially alert to home care patients receiving medications for pain management. They are at risk for pharmacological side effects and possible overdose. The patient may also be taking nonprescription drugs that could interact with prescribed medications. Substance abuse, especially in critically ill patients, is also a possibility.

Hospice patients have unique psychological needs due to the terminal nature of their illness. Although they and their families will have been counselled about the disease process, emotional support is still part of your job. If a call involves a hospice patient, the situation will almost always require intervention by specially trained health-care professionals. Find out the names of these people as quickly as possible, and determine the advisability of consultation versus rapid transport. (For more on hospice care, see the closing sections of this chapter.)

Injury Control and Prevention

As always, the most effective intervention is prevention. Before the patient comes home, steps should be taken to prepare the home. For example, purchasing a shower chair, raised toilet seat, and grab bars for the bathroom, rearranging furniture for free movement, having a bedpan or commode chair within patient reach, removing hazards to mobility, such as throw rugs and electrical cords, providing a cordless phone. You should also keep in mind the matrix, or strategy, for injury prevention developed by William Haddon in 1972. Its 10 steps are

1. Prevent the creation of hazard to begin with.
2. Reduce the amount of the hazard brought into existence.
3. Prevent the release of the hazard that already exists.
4. Modify the rate of distribution of the hazard from the source.
5. Separate the hazard and that which is to be protected in both time and space.
6. Separate the hazard and that which is to be protected by a barrier.
7. Modify the basic qualities of the hazard.
8. Make that which is to be protected more resistant to the hazard.
9. Counter the damage already done by the hazard.
10. Stabilize, repair, and rehabilitate the object of the damage.

These 10 steps can be used to protect paramedics from the hazards they encounter in the workplace or to protect patients from injuries at home. The steps can be seen in such simple areas as body substance isolation (BSI) precautions (barrier protection), the use of side rails to prevent falls, or the use of home rehabilitation to stabilize or repair a patient's injuries.

GENERAL SYSTEM PATHOPHYSIOLOGY, ASSESSMENT, AND MANAGEMENT

Assessment and management of home care patients can be challenging. You can gain confidence by becoming familiar with the pathophysiology of the diseases most commonly found in home care settings. You must also keep in mind the emotional needs of both the home care patient and the caregivers or family members affected by the patient's condition. Some caregivers love what they do and treat caring for the patient' as part of their daily lives. Other families feel constant, unremitting stress and possibly resentment toward the patient's condition.

Getting a feel for the emotional context of a patient's care should be a part of any call. However, in the case of home care patients, you must exhibit extra sensitivity. The way in which you interact with the patient and family can greatly affect the ease and efficiency with which you assess the patient and gather information. Developing a consistent, comprehensive approach to patient assessment and treatment can be your best strategy for dealing with these sometimes complex responses. The one thing home care calls have in common is their diversity. Be prepared to draw on all your EMS skills and to think quickly as you figure out the most effective management plan.

The one thing home care calls have in common is their diversity.

ASSESSMENT

Assessment of the home care patient follows the same basic steps as any other patient—scene assessment, primary assessment, focused history and secondary assessment, ongoing assessment, and continued management. However, you will need to modify your mind set for the home care patient—that is, observe for conditions that you might not ordinarily look for in the general population. This section highlights some of the points you should keep in mind or emphasize when assessing the home care patient. (For more on assessment, see the Patient Assessment division, Chapters 4 through 15. For information on assessment-based management, see Chapter 11.)

Scene Assessment

As with any call, your assessment of the scene begins before you get out of your vehicle. In the case of home care patients, note any special equipment you may observe on entering the home. This will alert you to any possible chronic problems that the patient might have. As you approach the scene, keep the following questions in mind:

- Is there a wheelchair ramp next to the front steps?
- Is there oxygen equipment in view?
- Is there a trail of oxygen tubing that leads into the patient's bedroom?
- Are there infection control supplies on the counter?
- Is there a sharps container present? (This means there are sharps, too!)
- Is the patient in a hospital bed?

Introduce yourself to any other medical personnel on the scene—nurse, aide, hospice worker, and so on. By creating personal interaction, you will help form a health-care team that can pool resources and share information. It is a serious mistake to arrive on the scene with a "takeover" mentality that all but eliminates the home care provider from the assessment process.

It is a serious mistake to arrive on the scene with a "takeover" mentality that all but eliminates the home care provider from the assessment process.

Scene Safety After you have identified the scene as a home care situation, remain alert for special hazards that might be present. As mentioned earlier, emotions often run high in a home care situation. Evaluate whether any of the people present have a threatening attitude that could be directed toward you. If at any time you do not feel comfortable, withdraw from the scene and seek assistance, either from the police or additional personnel. Ask someone to put any pets in another room and have all sources of sound (TV, radio, and so on) turned off so that you can work in a quiet, focused environment. As in any patient's home, look for weapons that the patient might use for self-defence—firearms, knives, or chemical sprays.

Other special hazards that you may face in a home care situation include infectious wastes, medical supplies, such as needles, and potentially dangerous equipment. You would hope that all home care providers are meticulous with the safe disposal of sharps. However, do not take it for granted. You would cease to be useful as a paramedic if you contracted hepatitis or AIDS from a needle stick injury. Look around carefully.

In responding to any home care situation, keep in mind the following guidelines:

- Any patient with limited movement may be soiled with feces, urine, or **emesis.**
- Any bed-bound patient may have weeping wounds, bleeding, or decubitus ulcers (bedsores).
- Sharps may be present.
- Collection bags for urine or feces sometimes leak.
- Tracheostomy patients clear mucus by coughing, which can spray.
- Any electrical equipment has the potential for causing electric shock.
- A hospital bed, wheelchair, or walker could be contaminated by bodily fluid.
- Contaminated medical devices, such as nebulizers, may be left around unprotected.
- Oxygen in the presence of an open flame has the potential for causing a fire or explosion.
- Equipment may be in the way and cause you to fall—or it may be unstable and fall on you.
- Medical wastes may not be properly contained or discarded.

Do not minimize the impact of any of these hazards. You can always be contaminated by any patient, but treatment of the home care patient has the potential for a broader range of exposures. Be sure to remove any medical waste you generate to ensure that the patient does not return to an unsafe environment. If at all possible, you should also remove any medical waste that is already there for the same reason. Always use BSI precautions, and be careful!

Patient Milieu Another important part of the scene assessment involves an evaluation of the patient's environment. Is the house clean or filthy? Is there nutritious food available? Are the sanitary facilities clean? Is the house heated and/or air conditioned? Is there adequate electricity? Is there insect or vermin infestation? The answers to such questions obviously have an impact on the patient's health and his ability to recover.

Also, note the condition of the patient's specific medical devices. For example, is the nasal cannula clean? Is the wheelchair in good working order? Is the ventilator well situated for safety and effectiveness? Again, these observations provide important clues to the quality of the home care received by the patient and the ability or willingness of the patient to comply with a prescribed treatment regimen.

Remember that you not only have a responsibility to treat the patient but also to act as an advocate. If a patient is living in a hazardous or unhealthy environment, you have an obligation to notify the proper agency to ensure that the person receives the necessary help. Often, hospital social services will be of assistance. The patient's home care agency or the police might also intervene, depending on the situation.

Remain alert to signs of abuse and/or neglect. In many provinces and territories, you are required by law to report signs of child or elder abuse. (See

✱ emesis vomitus.

Be sure to remove any medical wastes that you generate to ensure that the patient does not return to an unsafe environment.

If the patient is living in a hazardous or unhealthy environment, you have an obligation to notify the proper agency to ensure that the person receives the necessary help.

Chapters 42, 43, and 44.) Know the laws in your province or territory. Home care patients, whether old or young, may be helpless to improve their situations. It is the responsibility of all health-care workers to look out for their safety and well-being.

Primary Assessment, Focused History, Secondary Assessment

At this point in your assessment, you may already have a good base of information without actually having seen the patient! As you approach the patient, begin your primary assessment by observing general appearance, skin colour and quality, quality of respiration, and level of distress. Also, note any medical equipment that the patient may be currently using.

As you continue to assess the patient for the ABCs (airway, breathing, circulation), try to ascertain from the primary care provider (if present) a baseline presentation for the patient. Were you called because his condition has gotten worse? Or are you here for a new problem? For some home care patients, respiratory distress may be a chronic condition. For example, a patient with chronic obstructive pulmonary disease (COPD) might always have difficulty breathing. Your first impulse may be to reach for your airway supplies only to find that this is the patient's norm and that you were called to treat an unrelated problem. You must be flexible in your judgments and listen carefully to the report provided by the caregiver or family member who summoned EMS.

As with any patient, treat it as you see it! Once you have established the patient's baseline, assess for changes from the norm. Airway and breathing are always your first concern, followed by circulation. If there are any serious threats to the ABCs, you must treat them. If you are unable to stabilize the patient, complete your rapid assessment, and transport immediately. In such cases, your detailed and ongoing assessments will be performed en route to the hospital, if possible.

With noncritical patients, you might take the opportunity to compare current vital signs to the bedside records, if they are kept. The focus of your assessment should be on the chief complaint and how it might relate to the patient's chronic condition. Be meticulous in your assessment, especially with the home care patient. As stated earlier, home care patients are more susceptible to complications than most other patients and can deteriorate rapidly—that is, a noncritical patient can quickly become a critical patient.

In examining a home care patient, be sure to inspect, palpate, and auscultate all potential problem areas. In bed-bound patients, look for decubiti (pressure sores or bed sores) on parts of the body subjected to constant pressure or friction. As mentioned, decubiti pose a significant danger to the patient through infection or sepsis and may require surgical débridement.

Mental Status If your patient has a preexisting altered mental status, such as dementia or Alzheimer's disease, you must have a good understanding of his usual mentation before transport. This information is vital to the physician evaluating and treating the patient at the receiving facility. As stressed in Chapter 43, depression can mimic senility and senility can mimic organic brain syndrome. Dementia can also be a sign or symptom of a number of other serious medical problems, such as hypoglycemia and AIDS.

In general, assessment of mental status follows the same general procedure as with other patients. However, you must tailor your questions to the home care setting (Figure 46-3). For example, a person who does not work may be oriented but not know the date or even the day of the week. Also, keep in mind the high level of stress in many home care situations and the effect this may have on patient confusion.

To avoid the possibility of insulting the patient with what may appear to be simplistic questions, preface your assessment by saying, "Since I don't know your

Try to ascertain from the primary health-care provider (if present) a baseline presentation for the patient.

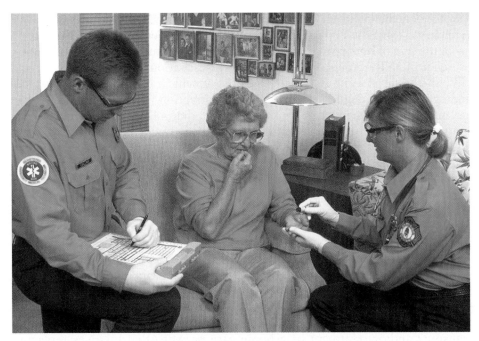

FIGURE 46-3 When assessing a chronic-care patient, tailor your questions to the home care setting. Remember that the stress in many home care settings, or fear of removal from the home, can increase patient confusion.

condition very well, I need to ask you some very basic questions." If patients understand that you are following a systematic assessment procedure, they usually cooperate in what, for them, is often a tedious process.

If a patient cannot or will not answer questions, rely on the explanations by family members or health-care providers as to whether the patient's current mental status is a departure from the norm. For example, belligerent behaviour might be normal in a home care patient. If this is the case, find out what is different this time from other times. Perhaps, as pointed out earlier, nothing may be different—the family member or caregiver may have just reached the breaking point and is in need of outside assistance.

Remember that home care patients, especially older or terminal patients, are fearful of being removed from the home environment. This can trigger depression, which, in turn, worsens a preexisting altered mental status. The key in such cases is tactful questioning combined with your own powers of observation. Pay particular attention to body language and interactions among household members. Note any evidence that the altered mental condition may have been triggered or worsened by a treatable cause, and present this information as part of your focused history.

Other Considerations In preparing your history, take into account any long-term medical problems—that is, the conditions that necessitated home care—and the specific events that led to the current crisis. Use the home health history and written orders from the physician, if available. As mentioned, talk to the health-care provider and to the patient. What changes, if any, have taken place in the patient's life in the recent past? Has patient treatment and/or compliance changed? Are medical devices operating correctly?

Keep in mind that eating habits, fluid intake, and minor illnesses or injuries can have a dramatic effect on a seriously ill home-bound patient. Have a high index of suspicion for any new conditions that the patient may be developing. For example, evidence of dementia in an AIDS patient is a serious sign. Correlate this with your secondary assessment, and use this information in developing your care plan.

In the case of home care patients, you may more commonly encounter do not resuscitate (DNR) orders, do not attempt resuscitation (DNAR) orders, living wills, and so on. Ascertain whether these documents are in existence before beginning any life-saving treatments. If that information is unavailable, act in the best interests of the patient. Also, keep in mind, that a DNR or DNAR does not mean that you have to withhold *all* treatment. For example, if a congestive heart failure patient with crackles and shortness of breath has a DNR, you may still be able to start a line, give nitroglycerine, administer an IV diuretic, and/or transport the patient to the hospital. However, you must read the specific instructions contained within the advance directives and consult with medical control.

Advance directives are designed to prevent useless treatment and invasion of the body when natural death occurs. However, many people who have advance directives can be treated in crisis situations and recover. You must use your judgment on a case-by-case basis to determine what qualifies as a resuscitative or life-sustaining measure. (Additional material on advance directives appears later in the chapter.)

TRANSPORT AND MANAGEMENT TREATMENT PLAN

Transport and/or treatment of a home care patient often involves replacing home health treatment modalities with ALS modalities. Airway and ventilatory support should be straightforward, as EMS providers are usually equipped and trained in the use of most necessary supplies. Some home care interventions, such as Foley catheters, can simply be brought along with the patient. Other interventions, such as percutaneous endoscopic gastrostomy (PEG) tubes, must be flushed and capped, which you may not be trained or equipped to do. In this case, the home care provider should assist you.

In some instances, you may be forced to take the support mechanism in your ambulance if you cannot find a suitable replacement. Certain infusion pumps or other devices may be essential to the patient's well-being, and you must bring them along. You should critically assess the risks of discontinuing the home care intervention versus transporting the mechanism. Seek advice from medical direction if you are unfamiliar with the intervention and if the home health provider is unable to help.

You should critically assess the risks of discontinuing the home health care intervention versus transporting the mechanism.

When taking a home care patient to a receiving facility, be sure to notify family members and caregivers, if they are not present. Before leaving the scene, secure the home, making sure that doors and windows are locked. In all likelihood, you will need to notify the patient's physician and/or the appropriate health-care agency, if you have not already done so.

Document your findings and all care steps carefully. Your call report will become part of the home care patient's record and may, in fact, suggest modifications in the treatment plan. If the patient is not already using a home care agency, provide names of services in your community, or refer the person to the proper social service agency. You might also mention nonmedical attendant care, such as housekeeping services and Meals-on-Wheels. As mentioned earlier, if you suspect the need for intervention in patient care, report your suspicions to the appropriate agency.

Content Review

COMMON ACUTE HOME CARE SITUATIONS
- Respiratory disorders
- Cardiac problems
- Use of VADs
- GI/GU disorders
- Acute infections

SPECIFIC ACUTE HOME HEALTH SITUATIONS

Although you will undoubtedly intervene in a wide variety of home care situations during your EMS career, you can expect to encounter certain conditions more commonly than others. The chronic-care patients that will most likely require acute ALS intervention include those with respiratory disorders, cardiac problems, vascular access devices (VADs), GI/GU disorders, and acute infections. You may also be called upon to intervene in the home care of mothers and their newborn infants and to provide assistance in hospice settings. A discussion of each of these situations will help you to prepare for your increasing involvement in the home health-care system of the present time.

RESPIRATORY DISORDERS

Respiratory disorders account for more than 60 000 of the hospital patients discharged for home care each year. Nearly 37 percent of patients with simple pneumonia and pleurisy and more than 50 percent of patients with chronic obstructive pulmonary disease (COPD) often receive home care within one day of their discharge from the hospital.

Some of the most common home care devices used to treat respiratory disorders include oxygen equipment, portable suctioning machines, aerosol equipment and nebulizers, incentive spirometers, various home ventilators, and tracheostomy tubes and collars. In order to provide intervention with these devices, you need to review pertinent respiratory anatomy and physiology as they relates to home oxygen and respiratory therapy. (See Chapter 27, "Pulmonology.") You also need to review the pathophysiology of the disorders that most frequently require home respiratory support.

Select respiratory disorders and the medical therapy used to treat them are discussed in the following sections. As you read this material, keep in mind earlier comments on the increased risk of airway infections and respiratory compromise in the home care patient.

Chronic Diseases Requiring Home Respiratory Support

Many home care patients have a lung capacity that is only minimally able to meet their normal requirements. Sometimes, even simple activities, such as climbing stairs, can severely stress their systems. Unlike patients with normal lung capacities, they simply do not have the ability for any increased workload. Even walking from one room to another may require the use of oxygen equipment. The following is a review of some of the conditions you may find in the respiratory-compromised patient.

COPD As you know, COPD is a triad of diseases—emphysema, chronic bronchitis, and asthma. Some patients may have one, two, or all three disorders. All three are outflow obstructive diseases, impeding the exhalation of air from the lungs. This causes an increase in carbon dioxide and a decrease in oxygenation.

COPD patients work harder to breathe than do healthy people. When that work becomes too much, they tire quickly. If the home equipment fails for any reason, they often panic, worsening their problem. As with any COPD patient, direct your treatment toward increasing oxygen flow. Be prepared to assist their breathing as soon as patients can no longer move enough oxygen to sustain themselves. In some cases, this may mean fixing or replacing home respiratory equipment and/or transport to the hospital (Figure 46-4).

In treating the COPD patient, keep in mind the following disease-specific information.

Bronchitis and Emphysema These two diseases go hand-in-hand. Most often, they result from smoking but can have other causes as well. Bronchitis involves the chronic overproduction of mucus, which narrows bronchial passages and restricts airflow. Emphysema typically leads to stiffening and enlargement of the alveoli. This loss of elasticity and compliance requires higher pressures in the lungs to facilitate

COMMON HOME RESPIRATORY EQUIPMENT
- Oxygen equipment
- Portable suctioning machines
- Aerosol equipment and nebulizers
- Incentive spirometers
- Home ventilators
- Tracheostomy tubes and collars

Many home care patients have a lung capacity that is only minimally able to meet their normal requirements.

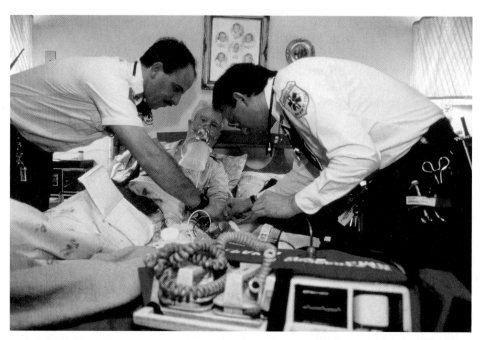

FIGURE 46-4   If the patient's home equipment fails, transport the patient to the hospital until arrangements can be made by family to have equipment replaced.

gas exchanges at the alveolar level. Usually, these patients are thin (because breathing takes up a large portion of their daily caloric intake) and barrel chested (due to the retention of air in the lungs as a result of outflow obstruction).

In cases of acute exacerbation, these patients have a difficult time compensating. They may exhibit wheezing, with diminished lung sounds, use of accessory muscles, retractions, tripod positioning, and the inability to speak in full sentences. Home treatments that you may see include oxygen, nebulized or aerosol medications, and possibly a ventilator utilizing **PEEP, CPAP,** or **BiPAP.** PEEP is provided through an endotracheal tube, while CPAP and BiPAP are provided through a tightly fitted mask.

When providing intervention, do not forget that home care patients usually have a high-dosing regimen, which may make them less immediately responsive to medications. Always provide these patients with high-flow oxygen. Medications that may be helpful include

- Nebulized beta-2 specific agonist bronchodilators, such as salbutamol
- IV or oral corticosteroids, such as methylprednisolone (Solu-Medrol)
- Nebulized anticholinergics (ipratropium)

Asthma   Asthma, sometimes referred to as reactive airway disease, can be seen in patients of any age. A crisis often occurs when some reactant causes an acute constriction of the bronchial passages. Home care asthma patients can usually handle these episodes on their own. If the episode becomes severe, however, you may be called by a caregiver or parent. (Asthma in children can be especially stressful for the family; be sure to review its treatment in Chapter 42.)

With asthmatic patients, look for wheezing with diminished lung sounds, use of accessory muscles, and the inability to speak in full sentences. Head bobbing in children is an ominous sign of impending respiratory failure.

* PEEP positive end expiratory pressure.

* CPAP continuous positive airway pressure.

* BiPAP bilevel positive airway pressure.

When providing intervention, do not forget that home care patients usually have a high dosing regimen, which may make them less responsive to their medications.

Home treatments you may see include oxygen, oral medications, and a variety of nebulizers and/or inhalers. In providing support, always administer high-flow oxygen. Medications that may be helpful include the same ones used to treat bronchitis and emphysema. You may also consider IV or SQ epinephrine. However, use this medication with caution when treating elderly or very weak patients.

Long-term care of asthma involves the avoidance or elimination of reactants that can trigger the problem. Try to gather as much information as possible about the cause of the attack so that the physician and patient can take action to avoid future episodes.

Congestive Heart Failure (CHF) CHF often presents as a respiratory problem. For more information on this condition, see "Cardiac Problems" in Chapter 28, "Cardiology."

Cystic Fibrosis (CF) Cystic fibrosis is a genetic disorder usually identified during childhood, sometimes in the late teenage years. It is characterized by chronic and copious overproduction of mucus, inflammation of the small airways and hyperinflation of the alveoli, chronic infections, and erosion of the pulmonary blood vessels secondary to infection. CF is an **exocrine** disease that causes other systemic problems, such as GI disturbances, pancreatic disorders, and glucose intolerance.

> ✱ **exocrine** disorder involving external secretions.

> *In the later stages, most patients with CF will be colonized with respiratory system pathogens such as Pseudomonas aeruginosa.*
>

Treatment of CF typically involves frequent postural drainage of mucus and chest percussion. Some patients may use mechanical vibrators to facilitate the percussions. They usually take medications aimed at mucus reduction and control of bacterial infection.

CF can be regarded as a terminal disease. Few patients live to the age of 40. Take this fact into account when treating the patient. At all times, remain sensitive to the emotional state of both the patient and any members of the family who may be present.

You may be summoned to help a patient with CF for a variety of reasons. The vigorous coughing associated with the disease can result in **hemoptysis** and pneumothorax. Severe or fatal pulmonary hemorrhage can occur at any time. Patients can also suffer **cor pulmonale,** or right ventricular hypertrophy secondary to pulmonary hypertension.

> ✱ **hemoptysis** expectoration of blood arising from the oral cavity, larynx, trachea, bronchi, or lungs; characterized by sudden coughing with production of salty sputum with frothy bright red blood.

> ✱ **cor pulmonale** congestive heart failure secondary to pulmonary hypertension.

In treating a CF patient, ascertain the stage of the disease and inquire about any standing medical orders. Also, find out if the patient or family has initiated any advance directives. Your treatment will flow from this information and your own assessment. There is no specific in-field treatment for acute problems stemming from CF. As a general rule, you will provide respiratory support, ventilation, and intubation, if indicated. Be sure to counsel the family or summon the proper counsellor to do so, especially if the patient is in the terminal stage of the disease.

> *In treating a patient with CF, ascertain the stage of the disease and inquire about any standing orders.*
>

Bronchopulmonary Dysplasia (BPD) This disease primarily affects infants of low birth weight. It is characterized by an ongoing need for mechanical ventilation in newborns who have been treated for respiratory distress from any cause. These infants may simply fail to wean from mandatory ventilation or from oxygen. They are also at increased risk of lower respiratory tract infections, especially viral infections, and may require immediate hospitalization if signs of respiratory infection or increased distress develop.

> ✱ **Intermittent Mandatory Ventilation (IMV)** respirator setting where a patient-triggered breath does not result in assistance by the machine.

Home care providers will have been advised to wean infants to lower **Intermittent Mandatory Ventilation (IMV)** settings. However, if the process occurs too quickly, the infant may be at risk of becoming hypoxemic. Arterial oxygenation should be maintained at or above 88 to 90 percent saturation and should be monitored continuously with a pulse oximeter.

Keep in mind that pulmonary congestion and edema may develop in BPD infants if excessive fluids have been administered. Question caregivers about fluid

> *Keep in mind that pulmonary congestion and edema may develop in infants with BPD if excessive fluids have been administered.*
>

intake, which may need to be restricted to about 120 mL/kg per day. Inquire, too, about the use of diuretic therapy, which is sometimes prescribed to these patients.

Even after an infant is weaned from a ventilator, supplemental oxygen may still be required for weeks or even months. In such cases, it is usually delivered via a nasal cannula.

Remember that BPD is a serious condition in infants. Reduced lung compliance and increased airway resistance may persist for several years. The best treatment is adequate ventilatory support and prompt transport to the nearest neonatal unit.

Neuromuscular Degenerative Diseases As a group, these diseases affect respiratory action through degeneration of the muscles used for breathing. Patients who suffer from neuromuscular degeneration may at some point require respiratory support. Other problems, particularly an inability to ambulate, will have a huge impact on the patient's life.

Many patients with neuromuscular degenerative diseases will be cared for by family members. However, if the condition worsens, professional home care providers may be involved and ALS may be summoned. In cases of respiratory compromise, there is little that you can do other than provide airway and respiratory support and transport. Expect to see all manner of respiratory home care devices, including oxygen and ventilators.

In treating and transporting these patients, keep in mind the following information on the leading neuromuscular degenerative diseases.

Muscular Dystrophy This genetically inherited disorder causes a defect in the intracellular metabolism of muscle cells. The condition leads to degeneration and atrophy of muscles, which are eventually replaced by fatty and connective tissue. There is no cure as yet, and treatment is multidisciplinary because of the many muscle systems involved. These patients have difficulty moving and may need assistance with daily tasks. ALS involvement would almost certainly be for respiratory failure or accidental injuries, usually related to falls.

Poliomyelitis Poliomyelitis is an infectious disease rarely seen today because of effective vaccines. When it does occur, the disease causes destruction of motor neurons, leading to muscular atrophy, muscle weakness, and paralysis. Patients have difficulty ambulating. However, unless the respiratory muscles are involved, there may be no systemic effects. Children who contract the disease may suffer permanent disability or deformity. But once the disease is resolved, further degeneration will cease.

It has been shown that after polio patients recover normal functioning they sometimes experience a **demylenation** of affected neurons and a return of the disability. This condition is known as postpolio syndrome. Its pathophysiology is unknown.

Guillain–Barré Syndrome This syndrome is thought to be an autoimmune response to a viral (rarely bacterial) infection. It is usually preceded by a febrile episode with a respiratory and/or GI infection. The disease is characterized by muscle weakness leading to paralysis caused by nerve demylenation. It usually starts in the distal extremities and progresses proximally.

Progression of this disorder may take several days. Once it reaches the patient's trunk, respiratory involvement becomes an obvious concern. One way to differentiate Guillain–Barré syndrome from a spinal injury is the increased motor involvement. In other words, motor deficits are greater than sensory deficits. As a rule, there is no cognitive or CNS involvement with the disease. With supportive ventilatory care, the patient can be expected to recover.

Myasthenia Gravis Myasthenia gravis is a rare disease that affects the neuronal junction. Due to the breakdown in acetylcholine receptors, nerve impulses are dampened. This disease is characterized by muscle weakness and can be more apparent in muscles proximal to the body than distally.

There is no cure for this disorder, and treatment is aimed at relieving symptoms. If the disease progresses to the diaphragm or intercostal muscles, respira-

✱ **demylenation** destruction or removal of the myelin sheath of nerve tissue; found in Guillain–Barré syndrome.

tory compromise can result. Sometimes, patients may have an acute exacerbation of the disease brought on by infection or stress. In such cases, intubation or artificial ventilation may be required. These episodes are most commonly preceded by difficulty swallowing or breathing.

Sleep Apnea Sleep apnea is a complex condition not yet fully understood by experts. It is characterized by long pauses in the respiratory cycle that can be caused by a relaxation of the pharynx or lack of respiratory drive. It can result in hypertension, cardiac arrhythmias, and chronic fatigue.

As a general rule, the muscles of the airway become more relaxed as the mind falls deeper and deeper into sleep. This is what leads to snoring and, in some cases, blockage of the airway. With sleep apnea, decreased oxygen levels cause a partial awakening of the patient. Breathing then resumes and the patient returns to sleep, often with no memory of the incident. Repeated over and over, such interruptions destroy normal sleep patterns and the patient spends much of the sleeping period in a hypoxic state.

People with sleep apnea often suffer alterations in their blood pressure and stroke volume. They lose the normal effect of declining blood pressure as they sleep, and their pulse oximetry may fall to 80 percent or less. In patients who have ingested alcohol, the reading can fall to 50 percent.

Treatment of sleep apnea may include surgical alteration of the airway, medications, prescribed loss of weight, avoidance of any CNS depressant or alcohol, or use of a CPAP ventilator.

Patients Awaiting Lung Transplantations Patients receive lung transplantations for a variety of cardiopulmonary diseases. Single-lung transplantations are performed for pulmonary fibrosis, COPD, or reversible hypertension or cardiac disease. Double-lung transplantations are performed for cystic fibrosis, COPD, or **bronchiectasis.** Patients may also receive heart-lung transplants for primary pulmonary hypertension or various congenital diseases. Remember that patients awaiting organ transplants are in the end-stages of their diseases and traditional therapies are unlikely to be effective.

✱ **bronchiectasis** chronic dilation of a bronchus or bronchi, with a secondary infection typically involving the lower portion of the lung.

Medical Therapy Found in the Home Setting

The treatment of chronic respiratory disorders in the home setting requires a wide range of devices. The following are some of the most common types of medical therapy that you can expect to encounter.

Home Oxygen Therapy Oxygen therapy has many advantages for the home care patient. First, it is relatively simple to manage. Second, most patients tolerate it easily. Third, oxygen therapy can add much to the quality of a patient's life. Studies have shown that long-term oxygen use raises the life expectancy of COPD patients considerably. It also prevents hypoxic states that may result in permanent cognitive damage or degeneration.

A medical equipment supplier usually delivers, sets up, and educates patients on the home oxygen delivery systems that they will use. In most cases, the systems include:

- A source of oxygen—for example, concentrator, cylinder, or liquid oxygen reservoir
- Regulator-flow meter
- Nasal cannula, face mask, tracheostomy collar, oxygen tubing (large-bore for face tents or tracheostomy collars)
- Humidifier
- Sterile water for respiratory therapy (Make sure it is sterile!)

Very few problems arise from the systems themselves. When they do occur, patients or home care providers can usually correct the situation on their own. However, you may be called upon to provide oxygen while a home system is repaired or to transport the patient to the hospital until the system is replaced. You may also be summoned if a condition unexpectedly worsens and the home oxygen system proves insufficient.

When you arrive at the scene, review the physician's prescription for the type of therapy and the source of the oxygen supply. As already noted, the three sources include

- *Oxygen concentrators.* These systems supply the lowest concentrations of home oxygen. They extract oxygen from room air and add to the flow received by the patient. Home concentrators usually provide no more than six litres of oxygen per minute.
- *Oxygen cylinders.* Cylinders or tanks are used by patients who may require more than six litres/minute or for some reason cannot have a concentrator. Cylinders involve the same technology that you use on your own portable oxygen systems.
- *Liquid oxygen.* Patients who require constant oxygen may have a liquid oxygen system. This allows much more oxygen to be stored in the home. Patients will use this system as a reservoir to fill portable tanks that they make take outside the home.

Although these systems are relatively safe, any high-pressure tank or liquid system has the potential for explosion. In a polite manner, ensure that the patient and home care provider adhere to these safety tips:

- Alert the local fire department to the presence of oxygen in the home.
- Keep a fire extinguisher on hand.
- If a fire does start, turn the oxygen off immediately, and leave the house.
- Do not smoke—and do not allow others to smoke—near the oxygen system. (No open flames or smoking within 25 cm of oxygen.)
- Do not use electrical equipment near oxygen administration.
- Store the oxygen tank in an approved, upright position.
- Keep a tank or reservoir away from direct sunlight or heat.
- Ground all oxygen cylinders.

In terms of the oxygen therapy itself, keep these guidelines in mind:

- Ensure the ability of the patient/home care provider to administer oxygen.
- Make sure the patient knows what to do in case of a power failure.
- Evaluate sterile conditions, especially disinfection of reusable equipment.
- As with any patient with chronic respiratory problems, remain alert to signs and symptoms of hypoxemia.

Artificial Airways/Tracheostomies Patients who have long-term upper airway problems often have a tracheostomy. A **tracheostomy** is a small surgical opening that a surgeon makes from the anterior neck into the trachea. The tracheostomy may be temporary or permanent. The technique is used on any patient who requires artificial ventilation for a long period of time. (Endotracheal or nasal in-

✱ **tracheostomy** small surgical opening that a surgeon makes from the anterior neck into the trachea.

tubation can only be used on a short-term basis. Pressure on the tracheal tissues, from the inflated cuff, can cause necrosis.) Tracheostomies may also be used on patients who have had damage to their larynx, epiglottis, or upper airway structures from surgery or trauma. They may also be performed on patients who have cancer of the larynx or neck.

The tracheostomy consists of the surgical opening (stoma), an outer cannula, and an inner cannula. The outer cannula keeps the stoma open and is held in place with twill tape or Velcro around the neck. The inner cannula is similar to a mini ET tube and slides down into the trachea a few inches. Due to the small size of the airway, the inner cannula usually has a low-pressure cuff at the end to hold it in place and provide a good seal. In the case of infants, there is no inner cannula because of the small size of their airways. Also, the airways of infants are more pliable than those of older patients and more susceptible to blockage.

Tracheostomy patients who have had a laryngectomy may have some ability for speech, and some may have an air connection to the oropharynx or nasopharynx. Keep this in mind if you need to ventilate a person with a tracheostomy. It may be necessary to block off the nose and mouth to prevent air from escaping upwardly instead of being pushed into the lungs.

Those patients who are unable to speak will use an artificial larynx. This device looks like a small flashlight. It creates an electronic vibration, which the patient manipulates by pressing the device up against the neck and by changing the shape of his mouth (much as you do when you speak). If the patient does not have an artificial larynx, you will need to resort to writing or signing for communication. Remember that an inability to communicate can create a lot of stress and frustration for the patient. Try to be part of the solution, not part of the problem.

Routine care of the tracheostomy includes

- Keeping the stoma clean and dry
- Periodically changing the outer cannula
- Changing and cleaning the inner cannula every few weeks to every few months, depending on the patient
- Routinely changing the ventilator hose connections for ventilator patients
- Suctioning frequently, due to increased secretions

It is important to remember that a tracheostomy eliminates a large part of the normal air-filtering process. The trapping of bacteria in the nasopharynx and oropharynx no longer occurs. Neither does the humidification and heating of air by the nasal passages. This means that bacteria have a more direct route to the lungs, and the air received in the lungs is drier and cooler than normal. Therefore, people with a tracheostomy have a higher incidence of lung infections, mucus production, and irritation. Since they have less control over their airway, it is also more difficult for them to clear blocked airways.

If a patient is not currently using a tracheostomy, it may be closed with a trach-button. This device simply plugs up the opening until it is needed again.

Common Complications The most common problems faced by tracheostomy patients include blockage of the airway by mucus and a dislodged cannula. The patient can usually clear the obstructing mucus by coughing. (Be careful—the mucus can fly out of the stoma to quite a distance.) Sometimes, suctioning, either by the patient or by the caregiver, will suffice. Cannulas can become dislodged by patient movement, or, in the case of children, by their growth. In assessing a child with a cannula problem, find out when it was last changed. Maybe the child is ready for the next size. Children can also have their stoma blocked by foreign objects that enter by accident or are put there by another child. Other complications include

Use sterile technique when changing or adjusting tracheostomy tubes to avoid colonizing the site with flora from your own skin.

In assessing a child with a cannula problem, find out when it was last changed. Maybe the child is ready for the next size.

infection of the stoma, drying of the tracheal mucus leading to crusting or bleeding, and tracheal erosion from an overinflated cuff (causing necrosis).

Management If EMS has been called, it means that neither the patient nor the caregiver has been able to solve the problem. If the tracheostomy patient is on a ventilator, you must rapidly determine if the problem is with the ventilator or with the airway itself. If the problem is simply a loose fitting or disconnected tube, fix it. If the problem is not immediately apparent, do not waste time trying to troubleshoot the machine. Your bag-valve device will connect directly to where the ventilator tubing connects. Remove the tubing, connect the bag-valve device to the trach connector, and ventilate (Figure 46-5).

If the problem is with the patient's airway, you will need to clear it. If the patient is hypoxic, always hyperoxygenate before suctioning. Be sure to evaluate any postural or positional considerations. If the patient is slumped over, straighten him up. Remember to ensure that ventilations are directed downward into the lungs, not upward into the mouth. (Ask the home care provider if there is a connection from the trachea to the upper airway.)

If you are unable to ventilate, clearing the airway is your first priority. Visualize as much of the airway as possible, and check for obstructions. If none is visible, introduce a suction catheter, and suction while withdrawing—no more than 10–15 seconds for an adult, 5 seconds for a child. Again, always hyperoxygenate before and after suctioning.

If it appears that the inner cannula is blocked or dislodged, you may remove it. If cuffed, you must first deflate the cuff. Connect a 10 mL syringe to the cuff valve and withdraw the air. If a syringe is unavailable, you can cut off the valve, and the air will escape. You can then remove the inner cannula, hyperoxygenate, and continue to suction as needed.

If necessary, you may intubate the stoma. The inner cannula must always be removed first. Use an appropriate-sized tube to pass through the outer cannula, and advance so that the ET cuff (if a cuffed tube is used) is 1–2 cm inside the trachea. Inflate the cuff, and verify placement by auscultating the epigastrum and both lungs. Attach an end tidal CO_2 device to the end of the tube. Pulse oximetry should also be used to monitor patient oxygenation.

Once the airway is secure, you may proceed with the rest of your assessment. It is inappropriate to proceed until you have protected the airway.

Home Ventilation Although you will see positive-pressure ventilators with most home care patients, you may also encounter negative-pressure ventilators. Both devices are used to ventilate patients for a wide variety of diseases and conditions.

If the problem is not immediately apparent, do not waste time troubleshooting the machine.

The tracheostomy stoma will close fairly quickly if a tube is not promptly replaced.

FIGURE 46-5 Artificial ventilation can be accomplished in the patient with a tracheostomy tube by attaching the bag-valve device directly to the tube.

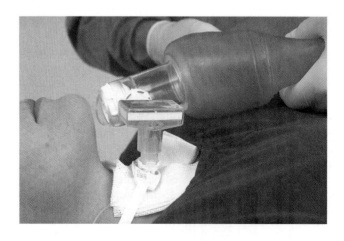

Some of the most common reasons patients may be on a ventilator include

- Decreased respiratory drive
  – spinal cord injury
- Ventilatory muscle weakness
  – muscular dystrophy
  – poliomyelitis
  – myasthenia gravis
  – Guillian–Barré syndrome
- Obstructive pulmonary disorders
  – COPD
  – sleep apnea
  – cystic fibrosis
  – bronchopulmonary dysplasia
- Other disorders
  – pediatric sleep apnea
  – chest wall deformities

Ventilators provide ventilation in several different ways. They also have a number of operating controls and options, depending on the manufacturer. Volume-cycled ventilation, for example, has long been the standard type of ventilatory support for all forms of severe respiratory failure. All modern ventilators can provide this feature as well as several other modes that vary in ventilatory waveform, method of terminating the machine-aided cycle, and so on.

Positive-Pressure Ventilators According to current practice, positive-pressure ventilation (PPV) is the recommended form of support for acute respiratory disorders. A positive-pressure ventilator pushes air into the lungs, either through a face mask, nasal mask, or tracheostomy. Features of this type of ventilator include variations in tidal volume, respiratory rate, flow rate, and pressure. Optional connectors will be available for oxygen and a humidifier.

There are too many types of positive-pressure ventilators to list here. However, any home care provider should be familiar with a patient's particular machine—including the small ventilators that attach to a mobile patient's wheelchair.

Negative-Pressure Ventilators Ventilators that apply negative pressure to the chest—tank, cuirass, or poncho-wrap—require a rigid structure to support the vacuum department. When they expand, they pull on the chest, causing it to expand and allowing air to flow into the lungs. This mimics the normal breathing process.

The iron lung is one of the best known examples of negative-pressure ventilators. However, some home care patients may also be fitted with a poncho-wrap—a suit that is sealed at all openings. Patients most commonly use this device at night.

PEEP, CPAP, and BiPAP These three ventilator options add pressure at various times in the respiratory cycle. They may be used by full-time or part-time ventilator patients. Keep in mind that there is a danger of pneumothorax because of the increased pulmonary pressure. Take this into account during your assessment of PEEP.

PEEP PEEP, or positive end-expiratory pressure, is used to keep alveoli from collapsing. It works by providing a little back pressure at the end of expiration. This option can be used for newborns—usually premature—who have insufficient surfactant to keep the alveoli inflated or in adults who have surfactant washout from acute pulmonary edema, **ARDS,** or drowning.

PEEP also has a use in treating COPD. However, due to stiffening and degeneration of the alveoli in emphysema, patients require higher diffusion pressures for gas exchange. If you ever see COPD patients pursing their lips as they exhale, they are providing their own PEEP. By blowing against a slight resistance, they will keep

According to current practice, positive-pressure ventilation (PPV) is the recommended form of support for acute respiratory disorders.

✱ ARDS acute respiratory distress syndrome.

their alveoli open. A COPD patient who is getting worse may deteriorate to the point where he needs occasional assistance from a ventilator with PEEP.

CPAP CPAP, or continuous positive airway pressure, is used to keep pharyngeal structures from collapsing at the end of a breath. This option is often prescribed for sleep apnea patients who need help in keeping their airways open. Most of these patients will use nasal CPAP—a mask that encompasses the nose (Figure 46-6). In these cases, patients must learn to keep their mouths closed for the mask to work correctly. Otherwise the pressure will be lost. The idea behind mask CPAP or nasal CPAP is the same as PEEP, except that CPAP is provided by mask, while PEEP is provided by endotracheal tube.

BiPAP BiPAP, or bilevel positive airway pressure, provides two levels of pressure—one on inspiration and one on exhalation. This option is used for patients who require more or higher levels of pressure than CPAP. Although the settings on the patient's home ventilator may be useful to the emergency department or to follow up patient care, they are not essential to your assessment. Try to gather this information at the scene, but do not let it delay your management of any serious airway or breathing problems.

As you may already have inferred, a home care patient with a chronic respiratory problem might eventually progress from home oxygen, to occasional ventilator support (PEEP, CPAP, BiPAP), to full ventilator dependency. Knowing each stage of the illness and how it relates to the various ventilatory options will give you a more complete understanding of the patient's clinical progress.

General Assessment Considerations Assessment of the respiratory patient should focus on the patient's entire respiratory apparatus. Any deficit found in the system must be rapidly identified and managed.

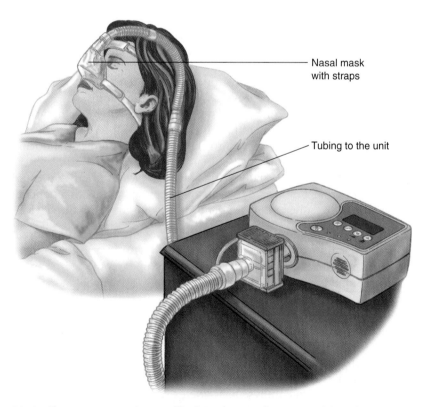

Nasal mask
with straps

Tubing to the unit

FIGURE 46-6   Sleep apnea patients will often use continuous positive airway pressure—CPAP—to keep their airways open.

As you approach the patient, look at the effort required to breathe. Observe for head bobbing, retractions, respiratory rate, tripod posturing, pursed lips, cyanosis, and depth of respiration. Listen for sounds of wheezing or rales. Note any devices or medications that the patient is currently using.

Immediately assess the patient's mental status by talking to him as you approach. Patients will indicate understanding with their eyes even if they are unable to speak due to dyspnea. Note the number of words that they can speak without stopping for a breath. Rapidly confirm the patient's baseline respiratory effort and mental status from the home care worker, if present.

Next, auscultate the lungs to identify the type of problem that the patient may be having and to determine tidal volume. Look at the patient's chest to spot any irregularities, retractions, or abdominal breathing. You can use pulse oximetry as an adjunct to your assessment, but do not rely on it alone. If the patient has poor peripheral circulation, it may not give an accurate reading.

Finally, complete your assessment by considering the full range of problems that might have caused the patient's current complaint. Whenever assessing a home care patient, you must remain vigilant for complications other than the chronic medical condition being treated at home. An asthma patient, for example, might be having a myocardial infarction (MI).

General Management Considerations As always, your first considerations when intervening in the care of a chronically ill patient centre on the ABCs. In the absence of documentation or a valid prehospital DNR, you must maintain a patent airway or improve on the airway that is already in place. This may be as simple as suctioning secretions from an airway device, such as a tracheostomy tube. You should also assess the placement of airway devices that you did not insert. It is easy for a device to become dislodged, obstructing the airway or failing to ensure patency. You may be forced to remove home airway devices and replace them with your own interventions, such as endotracheal tubes.

Ventilatory problems are traditionally easy to fix in the prehospital environment. If a home ventilator fails, you should begin manual positive pressure ventilation immediately. The failure may be easy to remedy, such as in the case of unplugged power cords or a temporary loss of electricity. If you are familiar with the ventilator, you can adjust the settings to restore or improve ventilations. However, if you are unfamiliar with the ventilator, play it safe and support ventilations with your own equipment.

As with ventilation, oxygenation problems are also generally easy for EMS providers to fix. First, assess the patency of the patient's home oxygen delivery system. The power may be off, the tubing damaged, or the oxygen supply depleted.

Whatever interventions you choose, you will have to make arrangements for the devices to be transported to the hospital along with the patient. Flexibility is the key to transporting home care patients. You should reassure the patient that you will properly care for their needs, as they will be physically as well as psychologically dependent on their home care systems.

If you are having problems ventilating patients with their home health equipment, remove it and use equipment from the EMS unit.

If a home ventilator fails, you should begin manual positive-pressure ventilation immediately.

VASCULAR ACCESS DEVICES

Vascular access devices (VADs) are used to provide any parenteral treatment on a long-term basis. The type of device and treatment depends on the disease process involved. Patients may have chemotherapy, hemodialysis, peritoneal dialysis, total parenteral nutrition (TPN) feedings, or antibiotic therapy provided through a VAD.

Types of VADs

Some of the most common VADs that you can expect to find in the home are described in the following sections. Consult your local protocols and procedures for accessing VADs.

Hickman, Broviac, and Groshong Catheters These catheters may be single, double, or triple lumen and can be inserted into any central vein in the trunk of the body. The subclavian vein is the most common anatomical insertion site, as it is usually easy to locate and secure.

Although these catheters have slight differences, each has an external port that looks like a typical intravenous port. The external hub of the catheter is sutured to the skin and has a cuff that promotes fibrous in-growth. This growth helps anchor the catheter to the body and prevents infection from travelling down the catheter. The highest risk of infection or accidental removal of the catheter is during the first two weeks after insertion. Care of these devices consists of keeping the site clean and dry and the administration of anticoagulant therapy to prevent clot formations.

VADs will often be routed through a subcutaneous tunnel to protect the site of venous puncture.

Peripherally Inserted Central Catheters Peripherally inserted central catheters, or PICC lines, are inserted into a peripheral vein, such as the median cubital vein in the antecubital fossa. These veins are easily accessible and allow a physician to thread a catheter from the insertion site into central venous circulation. PICC lines are inserted under fluoroscopy by radiology, rather than in an operating room. As a result, the procedure has a relatively low complication rate.

Surgically Implanted Medication Delivery Systems Surgically implanted devices, such as the Port-A-Cath or Medi-Port, are similar to Hickman-style catheters. However, the infusion port is implanted completely below the skin. These devices are disc-shaped and have a diaphragm that requires a specially shaped needle, such as the Huber needle, to access. They are typically found in the upper chest and can be felt through the skin.

Never access a surgically implanted port unless local protocols allow you to do so and only if you have the training and equipment to complete the procedure.

Never access a surgically implanted port unless local protocols allow you to do so. If such protocols exist, only properly trained personnel with proper equipment should complete the procedure. A regular intravenous catheter or needle will permanently damage an implanted port. Surgically implanted medication delivery devices should only be accessed using sterile technique.

Dialysis Shunts Dialysis shunts are used for patients undergoing hemodialysis to filter their blood. An arteriovenous (A-V) shunt is a loop connecting an artery and a vein, usually in the distal arm, where the dialysis apparatus draws out and returns blood (Figure 46-7). A fistula connects an artery and a vein, creating an artificially large blood vessel for access. It is also usually found in the upper extremity.

Avoid obtaining vascular access and blood pressure in the extremity where a shunt is located.

Both shunts and fistulas are created surgically and are very delicate. As a result, you should avoid vascular access and application of blood pressure cuffs in the extremity where they are located. You will be able to see the shunt in the extremity, and you should be able to auscultate a bruit over the area. Failure to auscultate a bruit over the shunt area may indicate an obstruction, either a thrombus that has formed or an embolus that has lodged there.

Anticoagulant Therapy

It is prudent to have an orientation session on VADs used by the home health agencies in your area.

Patients with vascular access devices will be on some type of anticoagulant therapy. The most commonly found anticoagulants will be those used to flush the device to prevent clot formation. Some patients may be on systemic anticoagulants as well. Because VADs are artificial, the body's natural clotting mechanism must be suppressed in order to ensure that the devices function properly. As a result, these pa-

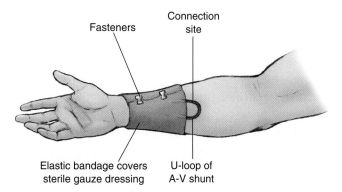

Fasteners

Connection site

FIGURE 46-7 An A-V shunt is a loop connecting an artery and a vein, usually in the distal arm, where the dialysis apparatus draws and returns blood. It is used in home care patients requiring dialysis.

Elastic bandage covers sterile gauze dressing

U-loop of A-V shunt

tients will be much more prone to bleeding disorders. The most common manifestations of hemorrhage are gastrointestinal bleeding, strokes, and extremity bruising.

VAD Complications

In treating patients with VADs, keep in mind possible complications. The most common complications result from various types of obstructions. A thrombus may form at the catheter site, or an embolus may lodge there after formation elsewhere in the body. Inactivity increases the risk for clot formation. Other obstructive problems include catheter kinking or catheter tip embolus.

With central venous access devices, you should always be aware of the potential for an air embolus. The devices provide a clear pathway for air to enter central circulation. Signs and symptoms of an air embolus include

- Headache
- Shortness of breath with clear lungs
- Hypoxia
- Chest pain
- Other indications of myocardial ischemia
- Altered mental status

Of course, any device implanted in the body has a risk of infection or hemorrhage. Look for redness, swelling, tenderness, localized heat, or discharge for a potentially infected catheter site. Because these catheters provide a channel into the central circulation, patients may quickly become septic, especially if they are weakened or immunosuppressed.

CARDIAC CONDITIONS

Many chronic-care patients receive treatment for a wide variety of cardiac conditions. You may be called to intervene in the following situations:

- Post MI recovery
- Post cardiac surgery
- Heart transplantation
- Congestive heart failure
- Hypertension
- Implanted pacemaker
- Atherosclerosis
- Congenital malformation (pediatric)

Home care for the cardiac patient can consist of oxygen, monitoring devices, and regular visits by a home health-care provider. You can expect to find a variety of medications associated with the specific cardiac problem, bedside cardiac monitors (for adults and children), diagnostic devices, such as a halter monitor, and possibly a defibrillator. For a review of the assessment, treatment, and management of cardiac problems, see Chapter 28.

GI/GU CRISIS

Patients with various long-term devices to support gastrointestinal (GI) or genitourinary (GU) functions may need ALS intervention. Your response may be directly related to a problem with the GI or GU device, or you may simply need to be aware of the device and provide support during transport.

Urinary Tract Devices

There are various medical devices designed to support patients with urinary tract dysfunction. External devices, such as Texas catheters (also called condom catheters), attach to the male external genitalia to collect urine (Figure 46-8). Because these devices are not inserted into the urethra, they reduce the risk of infection. However, they do not collect urine in a sterile manner, nor are they adequate for long-term use.

Internal catheters, such as Foley or indwelling catheters, are the most commonly used devices in the treatment for urinary tract dysfunction. They are long catheters with a balloon tip that is inserted through the urethra into the urinary bladder. The balloon is then inflated with saline to keep the device in place (Figure 46-9). Internal catheters are well tolerated for long-term use and are frequently found in hospitals, skilled nursing facilities, or home care situations.

Suprapubic catheters are similar in purpose to internal catheters. However, they are inserted directly through the abdominal wall into the urinary bladder. Suprapubic catheters may be used instead of indwelling catheters in the event of surgery or other problems with the genitalia or bladder.

Urostomies are a surgical diversion of the urinary tract to a stoma, or hole, in the abdominal wall. A collection device will be attached to the stoma outside the body to collect urine. Urostomies are used when the bladder is unable to effectively collect urine.

Urinary Device Complications

Most complications related to urinary tract support devices result from infection or device malfunctions. Infection is a very common problem with urinary tract devices because the area is rich with pathogens and because the catheter provides a pathway directly into the body. Remain alert to foul-smelling urine or altered urine colour, such as "tea" coloured, cloudy, or blood-tinged urine. Also, look for signs and symptoms of systemic infection, or urosepsis, as urinary infections can quickly spread in the immunocompromised patient. Suprapubic catheters or urostomies may also have infections at the abdominal wall site. You should note redness, swelling, heat, discharge, or loss of skin integrity.

Device malfunctions typically include accidental displacement of the device, obstruction, balloon ruptures in devices that use a balloon as an anchor, or leaking collection devices. Changes in the patient's anatomy, such as a shortened urinary tract or tissue necrosis can also cause malfunctions. Ensure that the collection device is empty, and record the amount of urine output. Look for kinks or other obstructions in the device, and make sure that the collection bag is placed below the patient.

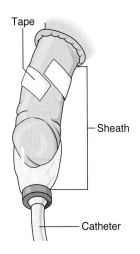

FIGURE 46-8 An external urinary tract device.

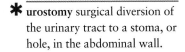

✳ **urostomy** surgical diversion of the urinary tract to a stoma, or hole, in the abdominal wall.

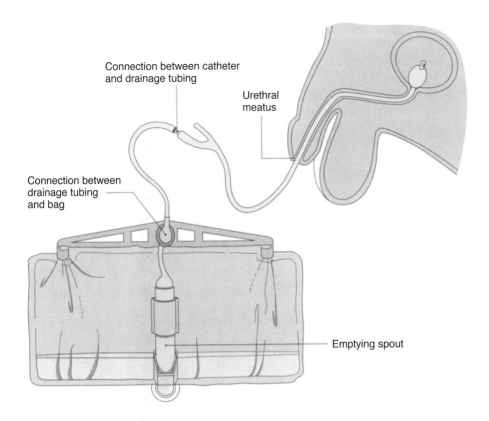

FIGURE 46-9   An internal urinary catheter with balloon. Note sites where bacteria can enter.

Connection between catheter and drainage tubing

Urethral meatus

Connection between drainage tubing and bag

Emptying spout

Gastrointestinal Tract Devices

You can expect to encounter a wide variety of devices to support the GI tract. Nasogastric (NG) tubes are commonly seen by EMS personnel, as they are often used to decompress gastric contents in the prehospital environment (Figure 46-10). NG tubes may also be used to lavage the GI system in various situations, such as GI bleeding or substance ingestion. NG tubes are not usually long-term devices, as they cause discomfort and may lead to tissue necrosis in the nasal passages if left in for an extended period.

Feeding tubes are more substantial than NG tubes and come to rest in either the duodenum or jejunum. Often, they are weighted to help them pass through the pyloric sphincter and have a steel filament to facilitate insertion. Feeding tubes are used for supplemental nutrition when a person cannot swallow due to dysphagia, paralysis, or unconsciousness.

For longer-term supplemental nutrition, a gastric tube may be inserted through the abdominal wall into the small intestine (Figure 46-11). Indications for a gastrostomy tube include Alzheimer's disease, neurological deficits from strokes or head trauma, or mental retardation. Gastrostomy tubes come in many forms, such as percutaneous endoscopic gastrostomy (PEG) tubes, surgical gastrostomy tubes, and jejunal tubes, to name a few. These tubes have different means of insertion (surgical versus endoscopic), location (stomach versus duodenum), and function (feeding versus aspiration prevention).

A **colostomy** is used to bypass part of the large intestine and allow feces to be collected outside the body in a collection bag, on either a temporary or permanent basis. Indications for a colostomy include cancer of the bowel or

✱ **colostomy** opening of a portion of the colon through the abdominal wall, allowing feces to be collected outside the body.

FIGURE 46-10 A nasogastric feeding tube.

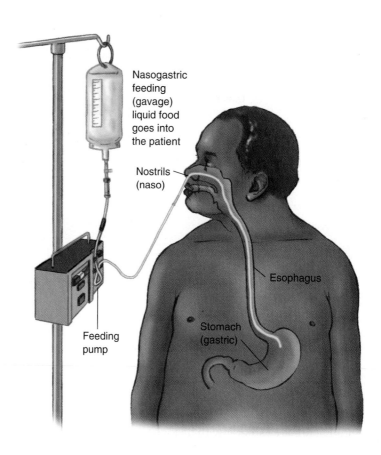

Nasogastric feeding (gavage) liquid food goes into the patient

Nostrils (naso)

Esophagus

Stomach (gastric)

Feeding pump

rectum, diverticulitis, Crohn's disease, or trauma. A surgical connection of the bowel to an ostomy created in the skin results in diversion of feces into the collection bag (Figure 46-12).

Gastrointestinal Tract Device Complications

Complications from GI tract devices include tube misplacement, obstruction, or infection. Because misplaced tubes can obstruct the airway or GI system, you should always ensure device patency if you have doubts about placement of the tube. First, have the patient speak to you. If he cannot speak, the tube may be in the airway and need to be removed. Second, to ensure patency of an NG tube, use a 60-mL syringe to insert air into the stomach. Use your stethoscope to listen over the epigastrum for air movement within the stomach. A low-pitched, rumbling should be heard. You may also note stomach contents spontaneously moving up the tube, or they may be aspirated with a 60 mL syringe. In such cases, patients may be repositioned to return patency, or the device may be reinserted.

Tubes are also prone to obstructions. Colostomies may become clogged or otherwise obstructed. Feeding tubes can become clogged due to the thick consistency of supplemental feedings or pill fragments. As a result, the tubes may require irrigation with water. In addition, the thick consistency of food may cause bowel obstructions or constipation.

As might be expected, ostomies can become infected (or lose skin integrity from pressure). Look for signs and symptoms of skin or systemic infection. In addition, remember that digestive enzymes may leak from various ostomies and begin to digest the skin and abdominal contents.

A displaced gastrostomy or jeuojenostomy tube must be replaced as soon as possible after dislodgement.

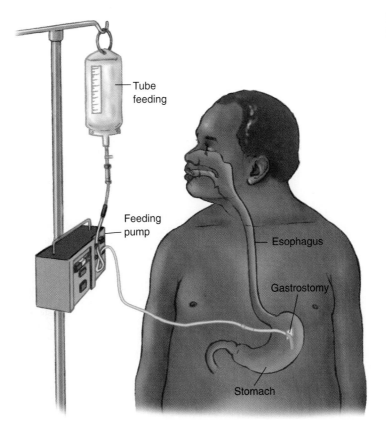

FIGURE 46-11   A gastrostomy feeding tube.

- Tube feeding
- Feeding pump
- Esophagus
- Gastrostomy
- Stomach

Psychosocial Implications

Many patients with GI or GU support devices lead active and otherwise normal lives. These patients may be understandably self-conscious about their conditions and many experience embarrassment, avoidance, anger, or discomfort when questioned. You should be sensitive to the patient's emotions during your patient assessment and treatment.

ACUTE INFECTIONS

After physicians or hospital personnel treat open wounds, they typically release patients to home care. These wounds may be surgical wounds or loss of skin integrity for other reasons. In such instances, you may see dressings covering wounds to protect against infection, absorb drainage, or immobilize the wound area. Gauze packing may also be inserted in infected spaces to absorb drainage.

Drains may sometimes be inserted in a wound site to remove blood, serum bile, or pus from the area. Drains are typically soft rubber tubes that have one end in the wound and the other end attached to a bag or suction device. Common drains include the Penrose drain, which is a simple rubber tube, and the Jackson-Pratt drain, which includes a suction bulb.

Wounds are typically closed with sutures, wires, staples, or cyanoacrylate adhesives. The type of closure used depends on the wound and the preferences of the physician closing it. Sutures are the most common means used to secure a wound, but staples and adhesives are becoming more widespread due to their ease of use. Wires are typically used to secure musculoskeletal structures, such as the ribs or the sternum after a sternotomy.

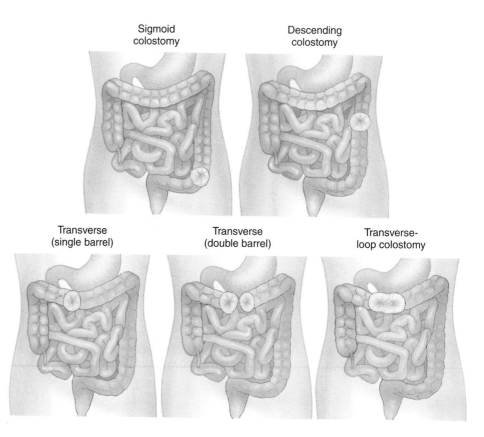

Sigmoid colostomy

Descending colostomy

Transverse (single barrel)

Transverse (double barrel)

Transverse-loop colostomy

FIGURE 46-12   Examples of colostomy stoma locations.

In assessing wounds, always be aware of the potential for improper wound healing. As already mentioned, home care patients are at increased risk of infection. The immunological response and rate of wound healing expected in the general population is compromised in the home care patient by poor peripheral perfusion, a sedentary existence, the presence of percutaneous and implanted medical devices, the existences of chronic diseases, and more.

An infected superficial wound may quickly lead to major infections or sepsis in the immunocompromised or weakened patient. Keep in mind that the chronically ill or homebound patient, particularly the elderly, often has a decreased ability to perceive pain or to perform self-care. Pay particular attention to signs of infection in wounds found in home care patients. If you inspect a wound, be sure to use sterile technique and redress the wound. For more on the treatment of bedsores and shear, see Chapter 43.

Pay particular attention to signs of infection in wounds found in home care patients.

MATERNAL AND NEWBORN CARE

Today, many women who deliver their babies in a hospital are being discharged in 24 hours or less. This trend, fuelled by rising health-care costs, greatly shortens the transition time from hospital to home. Some parents may not yet be emotionally prepared to care for a new baby, especially first-time parents. Rapid discharge may also leave a mother or newborn with an unrecognized problem or complication stemming from delivery. As a result, you might be summoned to the home for ALS care and called on to utilize the neonatology and pediatrics skills that you learned in Chapters 40, 41, and 42.

Common Maternal Complications

For the mother, postpartum bleeding and embolus (especially after a cesarean section) are the most common complications. Management of an embolus would be the same as with any patient with a similar complaint. Postpartum bleeding can be a serious condition. Management steps include

- Massage of uterus, if it has not already contracted
- Administration of fluids to correct hypotension
- Administration of certain medications, such as Pitocin (if ordered)
- Rapid transport to the hospital, if necessary

Mothers may also experience **postpartum depression.** In such cases, women may have difficulty caring for both themselves and their neonate/infant. In extreme cases, babies have been neglected or even harmed.

When entering the home, be sensitive to the needs of the parents. First-time mothers and/or fathers may be inexperienced in childrearing and may call EMS for what more experienced parents might regard as normal. It is important that you always take any parent's concerns seriously and, if no medical support is needed, provide emotional reassurance. If you suspect neglect or abuse of the neonate, take actions recommended in Chapters 41, 42, and 44.

✱ **postpartum depression** the "let down" feeling experienced during the period following birth occurring in 70–80 percent of mothers.

Common Infant/Child Complications

As pointed out in Chapter 41, newborns must rapidly adapt to a new environment and may well not have reached a state where they can thrive on their own. Newborns must be positioned properly to breathe, their noses must be clear (newborns are nose breathers), and they must be kept warm because of their immature thermoregulation. Newborns also have immature immune systems and can rapidly develop life-threatening infections or septicemia.

Infants with recognized problems may already be receiving home care. They may have cardiac or respiratory abnormalities or other congenital defects. Premature or low-birth-weight babies—as well as babies with any number of respiratory disorders—are at risk for sleep apnea. Such babies may wear apnea monitors around their chest so that an alarm sounds at any pause in their breathing pattern. Some infants may also be on pulse oximetry. If you are summoned because of an alarm and find a normal breathing pattern, still encourage the parents or caregivers to have the baby examined as soon as possible.

As noted, neonates may also be discharged from the hospital with an undetected cardiac or respiratory condition. Signs and symptoms of cardiac or respiratory insufficiency include:

- Cyanosis
- Bradycardia (< 100 bpm)
- Crackles
- Respiratory distress

In such cases, resuscitation should be initiated immediately. Management should be toward respiratory support with bag-valve-mask ventilation or intubation, as necessary. If any neonate has a heart rate < 60 bpm despite 30 seconds or more of oxygenation, start cardiopulmonary resuscitation (CPR). Preserve warmth, and obtain a record from the parents of feeding intake since birth. If the infant has not been feeding or has been vomiting and has diarrhea, he may be dehydrated. In this case, a fluid bolus of 20 mL/kg is indicated. If a peripheral IV cannot be obtained in two attempts or two minutes, obtain access via the intraosseus route. If blood sugar is below 4 mmol/L administer $D_{25}W$ (some experts suggest $D_{10}W$) at a dosage of 0.5 mg/kg or 2 mL/kg.

In a newborn with infection or septicemia, look for fever, tachycardia, and irritability. If septicemia progresses to septic shock, you should initiate resuscitation as previously described.

Children who have serious, long-term health problems are usually cared for by their parents at home—with or without the help of a home care professional. Commonly found medical therapies for children who are home care patients include

- Mechanical ventilators
- IV medications or nutrition
- Oxygen therapy
- Tracheostomies
- Feeding tubes
- Pulse oximeters
- Apnea monitors

Parents of children with special needs are often highly educated regarding their child's problem. Always listen to them even when their attitude may appear condescending.

Education of the parents or caregivers by doctors and nurses forms a critical component in their ability to deal with a crisis. Some people adapt well to the task and can deal with their child's chronic problems in a professional manner. Others, however, may become panicked or, either through misunderstanding or denial, have little comprehension of the situation. As with any difficult call, maintain a professional demeanour at all times.

When dealing with children, remember to keep the parents or caregivers informed of your assessment and treatment plans. Children quickly pick up on a person's emotions. Therefore, it is your job to act in a supportive and controlled manner. Calming a child could make a huge difference in the long-term effects of the current episode.

HOSPICE AND COMFORT CARE

The goal of hospice care is to provide palliative or comfort care rather than curative care.

Currently, hospices provide support for terminally ill patients and their families. The goal of hospices is to provide palliative or comfort care, rather than curative care. This is a very different role from that of most other branches of the health-care profession, including EMS. For an ALS team, care is usually geared toward aggressive and life-saving treatment. A hospice team, conversely, seeks to relieve symptoms, manage pain, and give patients control over the end of their lives. It is important to remember that these patients have, for the most part, exhausted or declined curative resources.

ALS Intervention

Involvement in a hospice situation can be a difficult and stressful call. In most cases, family members, caregivers, and health-care workers have been instructed to call a hospice, rather than EMS. However, you may be summoned for intervention, particularly in situations involving transport. You should always keep in mind that the hospice patient is at the end stage of a disease and has already expressed wishes to withhold resuscitation. However, even a valid DNR order should not prevent you from performing palliative and/or comfort care.

Common diseases that you can expect to see in a hospice include

- Congestive heart failure (CHF)
- Cystic fibrosis

- Chronic obstructive pulmonary disease (COPD)
- AIDS (Figure 46-13)
- Alzheimer's disease
- Cancer

In some instances, particularly with cancer, you may also be confronted with patients on high dosages of pain medications. In cases of cancer, for example, morphine is the drug of choice. It is important for you to know that patients, who often take doses of up to 1500 mg a day, will have few side effects other than constipation. They will have grown used to the drug, and normal side effects will not be seen. Other drugs that may be administered include Percocet, Oxycontin, or a Duragesic patch. Some patients may also have a portable pump that provides a continuous infusion of medication through a PICC line. The pumps can be small and hidden by clothing.

In a hospice, you need to establish communication with the home health-care worker as quickly as possible. Your inclination may be to intubate, start a line, or administer medications. However, as noted, palliative care supersedes curative care. A hospice worker, when faced with the end stage of a disease, may do nothing in accordance with the patient's wishes. Therefore, it is vital that you gain a clear understanding of these wishes, whether through a family member or a written document. If you are called to the house, it is your responsibility to respect the wishes of the patient and the ideals of hospice care.

In a hospice situation, family members might panic at the though of a patient's imminent death, and appropriate care might involve support for the family, rather than resuscitation of the patient. Local protocols may also vary in respect to DNRs, DNARs, living wills, and durable power of attorney documents. Be sure that you are familiar with these legal statements and their implications for care of the terminally ill. (See Chapter 2, "Medical-Legal Aspects of Prehospital Care.")

Terminally ill patients may take up to 1500 mg of morphine a day with few side effects other than constipation.

If you are called to the house of a terminally ill patient, it is your responsibility to respect the wishes of the patient and the ideals of hospice care.

Caring for a hospice patient can be a challenge for paramedics as they must act within the scope of the patient's wishes.

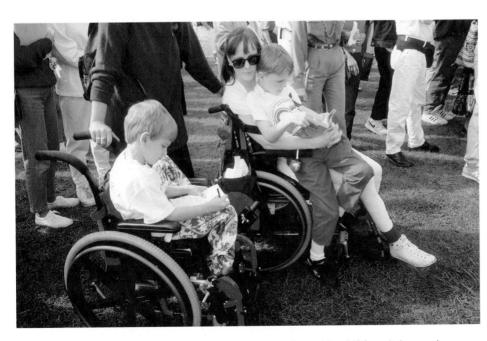

FIGURE 46-13   The incidence of HIV infection and AIDS in children is increasing worldwide. These children may be among the patients that you may encounter in a hospice setting.

Terminally ill patients who are not involved in a hospice present a potentially grey area. Remember that while hospice care prepares families for the impending death of their loved ones, families without hospice care may be ill-prepared for the end stages of life. Do not assume that all terminal patients are under hospice care. A simple question to determine the presence of hospice care may alter your course of treatment and approach to the family.

Regardless of whether a patient is in hospice care or not, keep in mind the stages of the grief process—denial, anger, depression, bargaining, and acceptance. Remember that both the patient and the family will go through these stages, and, in the case of the terminally ill, the patient may have reached acceptance well ahead of others around him.

SUMMARY

The shift toward home health care is one of the most important current trends and will have a great impact on the ALS profession. You can expect in your career to provide acute intervention for a growing number of chronic-care patients of all ages and in all stages of diseases. These calls will challenge you to use all of your assessment skills in developing an effective management plan, which in many cases will be based on input from an extended team of home health-care workers.

Appendix A

PCP AND ACP COMPETENCIES

The following table correlates the Paramedic Association of Canada's *National Occupational Competency Profiles for Paramedic Practitioners* with text content. Please refer to the legend below to understand the degree of competency required as a primary care paramedic (PCP) or an advanced care paramedic (ACP).

N   The competency is not applicable to the practitioner.

X   The practitioner should have a basic awareness of the subject matter of the competency.

A   The practitioner must have demonstrated an academic understanding of the competency.

S   The practitioner must have demonstrated the competency in a simulated setting (including practical scenarios, skill stations). In Competency Areas 4 and 5, skills must be demonstrated on a human subject where legally and ethically acceptable.

C   The practitioner must have demonstrated the competency in a clinical setting with a patient.

P   The practitioner must have demonstrated the competency in a field preceptorship with a patient.

AREA 1 PROFESSIONAL RESPONSIBILITIES

Specific Competency	PCP	ACP	Reference Chapter(s)
General Competency 1.1 Function as a professional			
Maintain patient dignity	P	P	**1, 41, 43, 45, 46**
Reflect professionalism through use of appropriate language	P	P	**1, 4, 5**
Dress appropriately and maintain personal hygiene	P	P	**1, 4, 5**
Maintain appropriate personal interaction with patients	A	A	**1, 4**
Maintain patient confidentiality	P	P	**2**
Participate in quality assurance and enhancement programs	A	A	**1, 16**
Utilize community support agencies as appropriate	A	A	**1**
Promote awareness of emergency medical system and profession	P	P	**1**
Participate in professional association	A	A	**1**
Behave ethically	P	P	**1, 2**
Function as patient advocate	P	P	**1, 2**
General Competency 1.2 Participate in continuing education			
Develop personal plan for continuing professional development	A	A	**1**
Self-evaluate and set goals for improvement, as related to professional practice	A	A	**1**
Interpret evidence in medical literature and assess relevance to practice	A	A	**1, Appendix B**

General Competency 1.3 Possess an understanding of the medicolegal aspects of the profession

	PCP	ACP	
Comply with scope of practice	P	P	1, 2, 10, 11
Recognize "patient rights" and the implications on the role of the provider	A	A	1, 2
Include all pertinent and required information on ambulance call report forms	P	P	1, 2, 6, 9

General Competency 1.4 Recognize and comply with relevant provincial and federal legislation

Function within relevant legislation, policies, and procedures	A	A	1, 2, 3, 8

General Competency 1.5 Function effectively in a team environment

Work collaboratively with a partner	P	P	1, 11
Accept and deliver constructive feedback	P	P	1
Work collaboratively with other emergency response agencies	P	P	1, 3, 16
Work collaboratively with other members of the health care team	P	P	1, 3, 16

General Competency 1.6 Make decisions effectively

Exhibit reasonable and prudent judgement	P	P	10, 11
Practise effective problem-solving	P	P	10, 11
Delegate tasks appropriately	P	P	11

AREA 2 COMMUNICATION

Specific Competency	PCP	ACP	Reference Chapter(s)

General Competency 2.1 Practise effective oral communication skills

Deliver an organized, accurate, and relevant report utilizing telecommunication devices	P	P	8
Deliver an organized, accurate, and relevant verbal report	P	P	8, 11
Deliver an organized, accurate, and relevant patient history	P	P	8, 11
Provide information to patient about their situation and how they will be treated	P	P	4, 42
Interact effectively with the patient, relatives, and bystanders who are in stressful situations	P	P	5, 38, 41, 42, 43
Speak in language appropriate to the listener	P	P	4, 5, 42
Use appropriate terminology	P	P	5, 8, 9

General Competency 2.2 Practise effective written communication skills

Record organized, accurate, and relevant patient information	P	P	2, 9
Prepare professional correspondence	P	P	8, 9

General Competency 2.3 Practise effective non-verbal communication skills

Exhibit effective non-verbal behaviour	S	S	4
Practise active listening techniques	P	P	4, 5, 6
Establish trust and rapport with patients and colleagues	P	P	4, 5, 6
Recognize and react appropriately to non-verbal behaviours	P	P	3, 4, 38

General Competency 2.4 Practise effective interpersonal relations

Treat others with respect	P	P	1, 4, 5, 38, 42, 43
Exhibit empathy and compassion while providing care	P	P	1, 4, 5, 22, 43
Recognize and react appropriately to individuals and groups manifesting coping mechanisms	P	P	1, 42
Act in a confident manner	P	P	1, 4, 5, 10

	PCP	ACP	Reference Chapter(s)
Act assertively as required	P	P	1, 4
Manage and provide support to patients, bystanders, and relatives manifesting emotional reactions	P	P	1, 5, 42
Exhibit diplomacy, tact, and discretion	P	P	1, 5
Exhibit conflict resolution skills	S	S	1, 4

AREA 3 HEALTH AND SAFETY

Specific Competency	PCP	ACP	Reference Chapter(s)

General Competency 3.1 Maintain good physical and mental health

	PCP	ACP	Reference Chapter(s)
Maintain balance in personal lifestyle	A	A	1
Develop and maintain an appropriate support system	A	A	1
Manage personal stress	A	A	1
Practise effective strategies to improve physical and mental health related to shift work	A	A	1
Exhibit physical strength and fitness consistent with the requirements of professional practice	A	A	1

General Competency 3.2 Practise safe lifting and moving techniques

	PCP	ACP	Reference Chapter(s)
Practise safe biomechanics	P	P	1
Transfer patient from various positions using applicable equipment and/or techniques	P	P	24, 1
Transfer patient using emergency evacuation techniques	S	S	3, 24, 1
Secure patient to applicable equipment	P	P	3, 24, 1
Lift patient and stretcher in and out of ambulance with partner	P	P	1

General Competency 3.3 Create and maintain a safe work environment

	PCP	ACP	Reference Chapter(s)
Assess scene for safety	P	P	1, 3, 7
Address potential occupational hazards	P	P	1, 3, 7
Conduct basic extrication	S	S	3
Exhibit defusing and self-protection behaviours appropriate for use with patients and bystanders	S	S	1, 4, 5, 23, 38
Conduct procedures and operations consistent with Workplace Hazardous Materials Information System (WHMIS) and hazardous materials management requirements	A	A	3
Practise infection control techniques	P	P	1, 7, 19, 37
Clean and disinfect equipment	P	P	1, 7, 37
Clean and disinfect an emergency vehicle	P	P	1, 3, 37

AREA 4 ASSESSMENT AND DIAGNOSTICS

Specific Competency	PCP	ACP	Reference Chapter(s)

General Competency 4.1 Conduct triage

	PCP	ACP	Reference Chapter(s)
Rapidly assess a scene based on the principles of a triage system	S	S	3
Assume different roles in a mass casualty incident	A	A	3
Manage a mass casualty incident	A	A	3

General Competency 4.2 Obtain patient history

	PCP	ACP	Reference Chapter(s)
Obtain a list of patient's allergies	P	P	5, 7
Obtain a list of patient's medications	P	P	5, 7
Obtain chief complaint and/or incident history from patient, family members, and/or bystanders	P	P	5, 7

Obtain information regarding patient's past medical history	P	P	5, 7
Obtain information about patient's last oral intake	P	P	5, 7
Obtain information regarding incident through accurate and complete scene assessment	P	P	5

General Competency 4.3 Conduct complete physical assessment demonstrating appropriate use of inspection, palpation, percussion, and auscultation, and interpret findings

Conduct primary patient assessment and interpret findings	P	P	7, 10, 11
Conduct secondary patient assessment and interpret findings	P	P	5, 6, 7, 10, 11
Conduct cardiovascular system assessment and interpret findings	P	P	5, 6, 7, 12, 13, 28, 41, 42, 43
Conduct neurological system assessment and interpret findings	P	P	5, 6, 7, 13, 23, 24, 29, 37, 42, 43, 45, 46
Conduct respiratory system assessment and interpret findings	P	P	5, 6, 7, 12, 25, 27, 27a, 42, 43
Conduct obstetrical assessment and interpret findings	S	C	5, 26, 40, 41
Conduct gastrointestinal system assessment and interpret findings	S	P	5, 6, 7, 26, 32, 43
Conduct genitourinary system assessment and interpret findings	S	P	5, 6, 7, 13, 26, 33, 39, 43
Conduct integumentary system assessment and interpret findings	S	S	5, 6, 7, 20, 21, 31, 37, 42, 43
Conduct musculoskeletal assessment and interpret findings	P	P	5, 6, 7, 20, 22, 24, 42, 43
Conduct assessment of the immune system and interpret findings	P	P	13, 31, 43
Conduct assessment of the endocrine system and interpret findings	P	P	5, 13, 30, 43
Conduct assessment of the ears, eyes, nose, and throat and interpret findings	S	S	5, 6, 23, 42
Conduct multisystem assessment and interpret findings	P	P	7, 13, 19, 20, 31, 34, 35, 36, 37, 44
Conduct neonatal assessment and interpret findings	S	C	41
Conduct psychiatric assessment and interpret findings	S	S	5, 38, 43

General Competency 4.4 Assess vital signs

Assess pulse	P	P	6, 7, 41, 42
Assess respiration	P	P	6, 7, 41, 42
Conduct non-invasive temperature monitoring	C	C	6, 42
Measure blood pressure by auscultation	P	P	6, 42
Measure blood pressure by palpation	P	P	6
Measure blood pressure with non-invasive blood pressure monitor	C	C	6, 42
Assess skin condition	P	P	6, 7, 41, 42
Assess pupils	P	P	6, 7, 41, 42
Assess level of mentation	P	P	4, 6, 7, 23, 29, 41, 42

General Competency 4.5 Utilize diagnostic tests

Conduct oximetry testing and interpret findings	C	C	6, 27, 27a, 29
Conduct end-tidal carbon dioxide monitoring and interpret findings	N	C	6, 27, 27a, 29
Conduct glucometric testing and interpret findings	P	P	6
Conduct peripheral venipuncture	N	X	15
Obtain arterial blood samples via radial artery puncture	N	X	Glossary
Conduct invasive core temperature monitoring and interpret findings	N	X	Glossary
Conduct pulmonary artery catheter monitoring and interpret findings	N	X	Glossary
Conduct central venous pressure monitoring and interpret findings	N	X	Glossary
Conduct arterial line monitoring and interpret findings	N	X	Glossary
Interpret laboratory and radiological data	X	A	Glossary
Conduct 3-lead electrocardiogram (ECG) and interpret findings	S	P	6, 7, 28
Obtain 12-lead electrocardiogram and interpret findings	X	A	6, 7, 28

AREA 5 THERAPEUTICS

Specific Competency	PCP	ACP	Reference Chapter(s)
General Competency 5.1 Maintain patency of upper airway and trachea			
Use manual manoeuvres and positioning to maintain airway patency	C	C	27a, 42
Suction oropharynx	S	C	23, 27a, 42
Suction beyond oropharynx	A	C	27a
Utilize oropharyngeal airway	S	C	23, 27a, 41, 42
Utilize nasopharyngeal airway	S	S	23, 27a, 42
Utilize airway devices not requiring visualization of vocal cords and not introduced endotracheally	A	S	27a
Utilize airway devices not requiring visualization of vocal cords and introduced endotracheally	A	S	10, 20, 27a
Utilize airway devices requiring visualization of vocal cords and introduced endotracheally	A	C	27a, 41, 42
Remove airway foreign bodies (AFB)	S	S	7, 27, 42
Remove foreign body by direct techniques	X	S	7, 27, 27a, 42
Conduct percutaneous cricothyroidotomy	X	S	20, 23, 27a, 42
Conduct surgical cricothyroidotomy	N	A	20, 23, 27a, 42
General Competency 5.2 Prepare oxygen delivery devices			
Recognize indications for oxygen administration	A	A	27a, 42
Take appropriate safety precautions	A	A	46
Ensure adequacy of oxygen supply	A	A	27a
Recognize different types of oxygen delivery systems	A	A	27a, 46
General Competency 5.3 Deliver oxygen and administer manual ventilation			
Administer oxygen using nasal cannula	C	C	27a, 42
Administer oxygen using low concentration mask	C	C	27a
Administer oxygen using controlled concentration mask	X	X	27a
Administer oxygen using high concentration mask	C	C	27a, 42
Administer oxygen using pocket mask	S	S	27a
Provide oxgenation and ventilation using bag-valve-mask	C	C	27, 27a, 7, 42, 46
Recognize indications for mechanical ventilation	A	A	27, 27a
Prepare mechanical ventilation equipment	A	A	27a, 46
Provide mechanical ventilation	N	C	27a, 46
General Competency 5.5 Implement measures to maintain hemodynamic stability			
Conduct cardiopulmonary resuscitation (CPR)	S	S	28, 41, 42
Control external hemorrhage through the use of direct pressure and patient positioning	S	S	19, 23
Maintain peripheral intravenous (IV) access devices and infusions of crystalloid solutions without additives	C	P	15, 19, 42
Conduct peripheral intravenous cannulation	A	P	15
Conduct intraosseous needle insertion	X	S	15, 42
Utilize direct pressure infusion devices and intravenous infusions	A	S	19
Administer volume expanders (colloid and non-crystalloid)	X	S	13, 15, 19
Administer blood and/or blood products	X	A	13, 15, 35
Conduct automated external defibrillation	S	S	28
Conduct manual defibrillation	X	S	28
Conduct cardioversion	X	S	28
Conduct transcutaneous pacing	X	S	28
Maintain transvenous pacing	N	A	Glossary
Maintain intra-aortic balloon pumps	N	X	Glossary
Provide routine care for patient with urinary catheter	S	C	46

Provide routine care for patient with ostomy drainage system	A	S	46
Provide routine care for patient with non-catheter urinary drainage system	A	A	46
Monitor chest tubes	X	X	Glossary
Conduct needle thoracostomy	X	S	25, Glossary
Conduct oral and nasal gastric tube insertion	X	S	41, 42, 46
Conduct urinary catheterization	X	A	46, Glossary

General Competency 5.6 Provide basic care for soft tissue injuries

Treat soft tissue injuries	P	P	19, 20
Treat burn	S	S	21, 42, 43
Treat eye injury	S	S	23
Treat penetration wound	S	S	18 20 25 42
Treat local cold injury	S	S	36

General Competency 5.7 Immobilize actual and suspected fractures

Immobilize suspected fractures involving appendicular skeleton	S	S	17, 22, 42, 43
Immobilize suspected fractures involving axial skeleton	P	P	17, 22, 24, 42

General Competency 5.8 Administer medications

Recognize principles of pharmacology as applied to the medications listed in Appendix 5 of the profiles	A	A	14, 22, 23, 27a, 24, 28, 30, 31, 41, 42, Drug cards
Follow safe process for responsible medication administration	S	P	14, 15
Administer medication via subcutaneous route	S	C	14, 15
Administer medication via intramuscular route	S	C	14, 15
Administer medication via intravenous route	X	P	14, 15, 42
Administer medication via intraosseous route	X	S	14, 15, 42
Administer medication via endotracheal route	X	S	14, 15
Administer medication via sublingual route	S	C	14, 15
Administer medication via topical route	X	S	14, 15
Administer medication via oral route	S	C	14, 15
Administer medication via rectal route	X	A	14, 15
Administer medication via inhalation	S	C	14, 15

AREA 6 INTEGRATION

Specific Competency	PCP	ACP	Reference Chapter(s)

General Competency 6.1 Utilize differential diagnosis skills, decision-making skills, and psychomotor skills in providing care to patients

Provide care to patient experiencing illness or injury primarily involving cardiovascular system	P	P	17, 18, 25, 42, 43
Provide care to patient experiencing illness or injury primarily involving neurological system	P	P	17, 18, 19, 29, 42, 43
Provide care to patient experiencing illness or injury primarily involving respiratory system	P	P	17, 18, 20, 21, 25, 27, 27a, 42, 43, 46
Provide care to patient experiencing illness or injury primarily involving genitourinary/reproductive systems	S	S	33, 39, 43
Provide care to patient experiencing illness or injury primarily involving gastrointestinal system	P	P	7, 18, 20, 26, 32, 42, 43
Provide care to patient experiencing illness or injury primarily involving integumentary system	P	P	17, 18, 20, 42, 43
Provide care to patient experiencing illness or injury primarily involving musculoskeletal system	P	P	17, 18, 20, 22, 24, 42, 43
Provide care to patient experiencing illness or injury primarily	S	S	31, 42

involving immune system

Specific Competency	PCP	ACP	Reference Chapter(s)
Provide care to patient experiencing illness or injury primarily involving endocrine system	S	S	30, 40, 42, 43
Provide care to patient experiencing illness or injury primarily involving the eyes, ears, nose, or throat	S	S	18, 19, 20, 42
Provide care to patient experiencing illness or injury due to poisoning or overdose	S	P	34, 42, 43
Provide care to patient experiencing non-urgent medical problem	P	P	11, 46
Provide care to patient experiencing terminal illness	S	S	29, 45, 46
Provide care to patient experiencing illness or injury due to extremes of temperature or adverse environments	S	S	36, 41, 43
Provide care to patient based on understanding of common physiological, anatomical, incident- and patient-specific field trauma criteria that determine appropriate decisions for triage, transport, and destination	P	P	7, 16
Provide care for patient experiencing psychiatric crisis	S	P	43, 38
Provide care for patient in labour	S	C	40

General Competency 6.2 Provide care to meet the needs of unique patient groups

Specific Competency	PCP	ACP	Reference Chapter(s)
Provide care for neonatal patient	S	C	40, 41
Provide care for pediatric patient	C	C	6, 23, 26, 27a, 42, 44
Provide care for geriatric patient	C	C	38, 44
Provide care for physically-challenged patient	S	S	42, 45
Provide care for mentally-challenged patient	S	S	45

General Competency 6.3 Conduct ongoing assessments and provide care

Specific Competency	PCP	ACP	Reference Chapter(s)
Conduct ongoing assessments based on patient presentation and interpret findings	P	P	11, 7, 10
Re-direct priorities based on assessment findings	P	P	7, 10, 11

AREA 7 TRANSPORTATION

Specific Competency	PCP	ACP	Reference Chapter(s)

General Competency 7.1 Prepare ambulance for service

Specific Competency	PCP	ACP	Reference Chapter(s)
Conduct vehicle maintenance and safety check	P	P	3
Recognize conditions requiring removal of vehicle from service	A	A	3
Utilize all vehicle equipment and vehicle devices within ambulance	S	S	3

General Competency 7.2 Drive ambulance or similar type vehicle

Specific Competency	PCP	ACP	Reference Chapter(s)
Utilize defensive driving techniques	A	A	1, 3
Utilize safe emergency driving techniques	A	A	1, 3
Drive in a manner that ensures patient comfort and a safe environment for all passengers	A	A	1, 3

General Competency 7.3 Transfer patient to air ambulance

Specific Competency	PCP	ACP	Reference Chapter(s)
Create safe landing zone for rotary-wing aircraft	A	A	3
Safely approach stationary rotary-wing aircraft	A	A	3
Safely approach stationary fixed-wing aircraft	A	A	3

General Competency 7.4 Transport patient in air ambulance

Specific Competency	PCP	ACP	Reference Chapter(s)
Prepare patient for air medical transport	A	A	3
Recognize the stressors of flight on patient, crew, and equipment, and the implications for patient care	A	A	3, 16

Glossary

ABCs airway, breathing, and circulation.

aberrant conduction conduction of the electrical impulse through the heart's conductive system in an abnormal fashion.

abortion termination of pregnancy before the 20th week of gestation. The term "abortion" refers to both miscarriage and induced abortion. Commonly, "abortion" is used for elective termination of pregnancy and "miscarriage" for the loss of a fetus by natural means. A miscarriage is sometimes called a "spontaneous abortion."

abrasion scraping or abrading away of the superficial layers of the skin; an open soft-tissue injury.

abruptio placentae a condition in which the placenta separates from the uterine wall.

absence seizure type of generalized seizure with sudden onset, characterized by a brief loss of awareness and rapid recovery.

absolute refractory period the period of the cardiac cycle when stimulation will not produce any depolarization whatever.

acceleration the rate at which speed or velocity increases.

acclimatization the reversible changes in body structure and function by which the body becomes adjusted to a change in environment.

acid a substance that liberates hydrogen ions (H+) when in solution.

acquired immunity immunity that develops over time and results from exposure to an antigen.

acrocyanosis cyanosis of the extremities.

activated charcoal a powder, usually premixed with water, that will adsorb (bind) some poisons and help prevent them from being absorbed by the body.

active immunity acquired immunity that occurs following exposure to an antigen and results in the production of antibodies specific for the antigen.

acute arterial occlusion the sudden occlusion of arterial blood flow.

acute gastroenteritis sudden onset of inflammation of the stomach and intestines.

acute pulmonary embolism blockage that occurs when a blood clot or other particle lodges in a pulmonary artery.

acute renal failure (ARF) the sudden onset of severely decreased urine production.

acute respiratory distress syndrome (ARDS) respiratory insufficiency marked by progressive hypoxemia, due to severe inflammatory damage and fluid accumulation in the alveoli of the lungs.

acute retinal artery occlusion a nontraumatic occlusion of the retinal artery resulting in a sudden, painless loss of vision in one eye.

acute tubular necrosis a particular syndrome characterized by the sudden death of renal tubular cells.

addiction compulsive and overwhelming dependence on a drug; an addiction may be physiological, psychological, or both.

Addison's disease endocrine disorder characterized by adrenocortical insufficiency. Symptoms may include weakness, fatigue, weight loss, and hyperpigmentation of skin and mucous membranes.

Addisonian crisis form of shock associated with adrenocortical insufficiency and characterized by profound hypotension and electrolyte imbalances.

adhesion union of normally separate tissue surfaces by a fibrous band of new tissue.

adult respiratory distress syndrome (ARDS) respiratory insufficiency marked by progressive hypoxemia, due to severe inflammatory damage and fluid accumulation in the alveoli of the lungs.

affect visible indicators of mood.

afterbirth the placenta and accompanying membranes that are expelled from the uterus after the birth of a child.

ageism discrimination against aged or elderly people.

aggregate to cluster or come together.

airborne transmitted through the air by droplets or particles.

alkali a substance that liberates hydroxyl ions (OH⁻) when in solution; a strong base.

allergen a substance capable of inducing allergy of specific hypersensitivity. Allergens may be protein or nonprotein, although most are protein.

allergic reaction an exaggerated response by the immune system to a foreign substance.

allergy a hypersensitive state acquired through exposure to a particular allergen.

alpha radiation low level form of nuclear radiation; a weak source of energy that is stopped by clothing or the first layers of skin.

Alzheimer's disease a degenerative brain disorder; the most common cause of dementia in the elderly.

amniotic fluid clear, watery fluid that surrounds and protects the developing fetus.

amniotic sac the membranes that surround and protect the developing fetus throughout the period of intrauterine development.

ampere basic unit for measuring the strength of an electric current.

amputation severance, removal, or detachment, either partial or complete, of a body part.

amyotrophic lateral sclerosis (ALS) progressive degeneration of specific nerve cells that control voluntary movement characterized by weakness, loss of motor control, difficulty speaking, and cramping. Also called *Lou Gehrig's disease*.

anabolism the constructive or "building up" phase of metabolism.

anaerobic able to live without oxygen.

anaphylaxis a life-threatening allergic reaction; also called *anaphylactic shock*; an unusual or exaggerated allergic reaction to a foreign protein or other substance. Anaphylaxis means the opposite of "phylaxis," or protection.

anemia a reduction in the hemoglobin content in the blood to a point below that required to meet the oxygen requirements of the body.

aneurysm a weakening or ballooning in the wall of a blood vessel.

anger hostility or rage to compensate for an underlying feeling of anxiety.

angina pectoris chest pain that results when the blood supply's oxygen demands exceed the heart's.

angioneurotic edema marked edema of the skin that usually involves the head, neck, face, and upper airway; a common manifestation of severe allergic reactions and anaphylaxis.

anorexia nervosa psychological disorder characterized by voluntary refusal to eat.

anoxia the absence or near-absence of oxygen.

anoxic hypoxemia an oxygen deficiency due to disordered pulmonary mechanisms of oxygenation.

antepartum before the onset of labor.

anterior cord syndrome condition that is caused by bony fragments or pressure compressing the arteries of the anterior spinal cord and resulting in loss of motor function and sensation to pain, light touch, and temperature below the injury site.

anterograde amnesia inability to remember events that occurred after the trauma that caused the condition.

antibiotic-resistant infection an infection by an organism that has become resistant to common forms of antibiotics.

antibody principal agent of a chemical attack of an invading substance.

antidote a substance that will neutralize a specific toxin or counteract its effect on the body.

antigen any substance that is capable, under appropriate conditions, of inducing a specific immune response;

protein on the surface of a donor's red blood cells that the patient's body recognizes as "not self."

anuria no elimination of urine.

anxiety disorder condition characterized by dominating apprehension and fear.

anxiety state of uneasiness, discomfort, apprehension, and restlessness.

aortic dissection a degeneration of the wall of the aorta.

APGAR score a numerical system of rating the condition of a newborn. It evaluates the newborn's heart rate, respiratory rate, muscle tone, reflex irritability, and colour.

aphasia absence or impairment of the ability to communicate through speaking, writing, or signing as a result of brain dysfunction; occurs when the individual suffers brain damage due to stroke or head injury.

apnea absence of breathing.

apneustic respiration breathing characterized by a prolonged inspiration unrelieved by expiration attempts, seen in patients with damage to the upper part of the pons.

appendicitis inflammation of the vermiform appendix at the juncture of the large and small intestines.

arrhythmia the absence of cardiac electrical activity; often used interchangeably with dysrhythmia.

arterial gas embolism (AGE) an air bubble, or air embolism, that enters the circulatory system from a damaged lung.

arterial line monitoring placement of a catheter, usually into the radial artery. Used to obtain frequent arterial blood samples and to monitor arterial pressures.

arteriosclerosis a thickening, loss of elasticity, and hardening of the walls of the arteries from calcium deposits.

arthritis inflammation of a joint.

artifact deflection on the ECG produced by factors other than the heart's electrical activity.

asphyxia a decrease in the amount of oxygen and an increase in the amount of carbon dioxide as a result of some interference with respiration.

asthma a condition marked by recurrent attacks of dyspnea with wheezing due to spasmodic constriction of the bronchi, often as a response to allergens or mucous plugs in the arterial walls.

ataxic respiration poor respirations due to CNS damage, causing ineffective thoracic muscular coordination.

atherosclerosis a progressive, degenerative disease of the medium-sized and large arteries.

attention deficit disorder impulsiveness and short or poor attention span that is inappropriate for the child's age. May also include hyperactive behaviour. Features may be present as early as 4–7 years of age but do not usually impair academic or social functioning until middle school.

augmented leads another term for unipolar leads, reflecting the fact that the ground lead is disconnected, which increases the amplitude of deflection on the ECG tracing.

autistic disorder developmental disorder in which language develops abnormally or not at all, and the child may display ritualistic, compulsive behaviour.

autoimmune disorders disorders in which the body's immune system attacks normal body tissues, resulting in destruction of some types of body tissues, abnormal organ growth, or altered organ function.

autonomic dysfunction an abnormality of the involuntary aspect of the nervous system.

autonomic hyperreflexia syndrome condition associated with the body's adjustment to the effects of neurogenic shock; presentations include sudden hypertension, bradycardia, pounding headache, blurred vision, and sweating and flushing of the skin above the point of injury.

autonomic neuropathy condition that damages the autonomic nervous system, which usually senses changes in core temperature and controls vasodilation and perspiration to dissipate heat.

avulsion forceful tearing away or separation of body tissue; an avulsion may be partial or complete.

axial loading application of the forces of trauma along the axis of the spine; this often results in compression fractures of the spine.

bacteria microscopic, single-celled organisms that range in length from 1 to 20 micrometres.

bacterial tracheitis bacterial infection of the airway, subglottic region; in children, most likely to appear after episodes of croup.

bactericidal capable of killing bacteria.

bacteriostatic capable of inhibiting bacterial growth or reproduction.

bag-valve mask ventilation device consisting of a self-inflating bag with two one-way valves and a transparent plastic face mask.

ballistics the study of projectile motion and its interactions with the gun, the air, and the object it contacts.

baroreceptor sensory nerve ending, found in the walls of the atria of the heart, vena cava, aortic arch, and carotid sinus, that is stimulated by changes in pressure.

barotrauma injury caused by pressure within an enclosed space; when occuring during a diving descent is commonly called *the squeeze.*

basal metabolic rate (BMR) rate at which the body consumes energy just to maintain stability; the basic metabolic rate (measured by the rate of oxygen consumption) of an awake, relaxed person 12 to 14 hours after eating and at a comfortable temperature.

basophil type of white blood cell that participates in allergic responses.

behaviour a person's observable conduct and activity.

behavioural emergency situation in which a patient's behaviour becomes so unusual that it alarms the patient or another person and requires intervention.

Bell's palsy one-sided facial paralysis with an unknown cause characterized by the inability to close the eye, pain, tearing of the eyes, drooling, hypersensitivity to sound, and impairment of taste.

bend fractures fractures characterized by angulation and deformity in the bone without an obvious break.

benign prostatic hypertrophy a noncancerous enlargement of the prostate associated with aging.

bereavement death of a loved one.

beta radiation medium-strength radiation that is stopped with light clothing or the uppermost layers of skin.

bilateral periorbital ecchymosis black-and-blue discoloration of the area surrounding the eyes. It is usually associated with basilar skull fracture. (Also called raccoon eyes.)

biological/organic related to disease processes or structural changes.

BiPAP bilevel positive airway pressure.

bipolar disorder condition characterized by one or more manic episodes, with or without periods of depression.

bipolar leads electrocardiogram leads applied to the arms and legs that contain two electrodes of opposite (positive and negative) polarity; leads I, II, and III.

birth injury avoidable and unavoidable mechanical and anoxic trauma incurred by the newborn during labor and delivery.

blast wind the air movement caused as the heated and pressurized products of an explosion move outward.

blepharospasm twitching of the eyelids.

bloodborne transmitted by contact with blood or body fluids.

blunt trauma injury caused by the collision of an object with the body in which the object does not enter the body.

body surface area (BSA) amount of a patient's body affected by a burn.

bowel obstruction blockage of the hollow space within the intestines.

bradycardia a slow heart rate; a heart rate of fewer than 60 beats per minute.

bradypnea slow respiration.

brain abscess a collection of pus localized in an area of the brain.

brain ischemia injury to brain tissues caused by an inadequate supply of oxygen and nutrients.

bronchiectasis chronic dilation of a bronchus or bronchi, with a secondary infection typically involving the lower portion of the lung.

bronchiolitis viral infection of the medium-sized airways, occurring most frequently during the first year of life.

Brown-Séquard's syndrome condition caused by partial cutting of one side of the spinal cord resulting in sensory and motor loss to that side of the body.

Brudzinkis's sign physical exam finding in which flexion of the neck causes flexion of the hips and knees.

bruit sound of turbulent blood flow around a partial obstruction; usually associated with atherosclerotic disease.

buckle fractures fractures characterized by a raised or bulging projection at the fracture site.

bulimia nervosa recurrent episodes of binge eating.

bundle branch block a kind of interventricular heart block in which conduction through either the right or left bundle branches is blocked or delayed.

bundle of Kent an accessory AV conduction pathway that is thought to be responsible for the ECG findings of pre-excitation syndrome.

bursitis acute or chronic inflammation of the small synovial sacs.

calibre the diameter of a bullet expressed in hundredths of an inch (.22 calibre = 0.22 inches); the inside diameter of the barrel of a handgun, shotgun, or rifle.

callus thickened area that forms at the site of a fracture as part of the repair process.

cancer a group of cells (usually derived from a single cell) that have lost their normal control mechanisms and thus have unregulated growth. Cancerous (malignant) cells can develop from any tissue within any organ. As cancerous cells grow and multiply, they form a mass of cancerous tissue—called a tumour—that invades and destroys normal adjacent tissues. The term "tumour" refers to an abnormal growth or mass; tumours can be cancerous or noncancerous. Cancerous cells from the primary (initial) site can spread (metastasize)

capnography the measurement of exhaled carbon dioxide concentrations.

cardiac arrest the absence of ventricular contraction.

cardiac tamponade accumulation of excess fluid inside the pericardium.

cardiogenic shock the inability of the heart to pump enough blood to perfuse all parts of the body, resulting in inadequate tissue perfusion.

cardiovascular disease (CVD) disease affecting the heart, peripheral blood vessels, or both.

catabolism the destructive or "breaking down" phase of metabolism.

cataracts medical condition in which the lens of the eye loses its clearness.

catatonia condition characterized by immobility and stupor, often a sign of schizophrenia.

catecholamine a hormone, such as epinephrine or norepinephrine, that strongly affects the nervous and cardiovascular systems, metabolic rate, temperature, and smooth muscle.

cavitation the outward motion of tissue due to a projectile's passage, resulting in a temporary cavity and vacuum.

cellular immunity immunity resulting from a direct attack of a foreign substance by specialized cells of the immune system.

cellulitis inflammation of cellular or connective tissue.

central cord syndrome condition usually related to hyperflexion of the cervical spine that results in motor weakness, usually in the upper extremities, and possible bladder dysfunction.

central IV line intravenous line placed into the superior vena cava for the administration of long-term fluid therapy.

central neurogenic hyperventilation hyperventilation caused by a lesion in the central nervous system, often characterized by rapid, deep, noisy respirations.

central pain syndrome condition resulting from damage or injury to the brain, brainstem, or spinal cord characterized by intense, steady pain described as burning, aching, tingling, or a "pins and needles" sensation.

central venous pressure monitoring placement of a catheter into the superior vena cava. Central venous pressure reflects the pressure in the right atrium when filled.

cerumen earwax.

chain of evidence legally retaining items of evidence and accounting for their whereabouts at all times to prevent loss or tampering.

chancroid highly contagious sexually transmitted ulcer.

chemotactic factors chemicals released by white blood cells that attract more white blood cells to an area of inflammation.

chest tube tube placed through chest wall to allow drainage of air or fluid from the pleural space. Used in managing pneumothorax, hemothorax, or pleural effusion.

Cheyne-Stokes respiration a breathing pattern characterized by a period of apnea lasting 10-60 seconds, followed by gradually increasing depth and frequency of respirations; respiratory pattern of alternating periods of apnea and tachypnea.

child abuse physical or emotional violence or neglect toward a person from infancy to eighteen years of age.

chlamydia group of intracellular parasites that cause sexually transmitted diseases.

choanal atresia congenital closure of the passage between the nose and pharynx by a bony or membranous structure.

chronic gastroenteritis non-acute inflammation of the gastric mucosa.

chronic obstructive pulmonary disease (COPD) a disease characterized by a decreased ability of the lungs to perform the function of ventilation.

chronic renal failure permanently inadequate renal function due to nephron loss.

cirrhosis degenerative disease of the liver.

claudication severe pain in the calf muscle due to inadequate blood supply. It typically occurs with exertion and subsides with rest.

cleft lip congenital vertical fissure in the upper lip.

cleft palate congenital fissure in the roof of the mouth, forming a passageway between oral and nasal cavities.

clonic phase phase of a seizure characterized by alternating contraction and relaxation of muscles.

closed fracture a broken bone in which the bone ends or the forces that caused it do not penetrate the skin.

clotting the body's three-step response to stop the loss of blood.

coagulation necrosis the process in which an acid, while destroying tissue, forms an insoluble layer that limits further damage.

coagulation third step in the clotting process, which involves the formation of a protein called fibrin that forms a network around a wound to stop bleeding, ward off infection, and lay a foundation for healing and repair of the wound.

colicky abdominal pain acute pain associated with cramping or spasms in the abdominal organs.

collagen tough, strong protein that comprises most of the body's connective tissue.

colostomy a surgical diversion of the large intestine through an opening in the skin where the fecal matter is collected in a pouch; may be temporary or permanent.

coma a state of unconsciousness from which the patient cannot be aroused.

comminuted fracture fracture in which a bone is broken into several pieces.

communicable period time when a host can transmit an infectious agent to someone else.

communicable capable of being transmitted to another host.

community-acquired infection an infection occurring in a nonhospitalized patient who is not undergoing regular medical procedures, including the use of instruments such as catheters.

co-morbidity associated disease process.

compartment syndrome muscle ischemia that is caused by rising pressures within an anatomic fascial space.

compensated shock hemodynamic insult to the body in which the body responds effectively. Signs and symptoms are limited, and the human system functions normally.

compensatory pause the pause following an ectopic beat where the SA node is unaffected and the cadence of the heart is uninterrupted.

complex partial seizure type of partial seizure usually originating in the temporal lobe characterized by an aura and focal findings such as alterations in mental status or mood.

compliance the stiffness or flexibility of the lung tissue.

concussion a transient period of unconsciousness. In most cases, the unconsciousness will be followed by a complete return of function.

conduction moving electrons, ions, heat, or sound waves through a conductor or conducting medium.

conductive deafness deafness caused when there is a blocking of the transmission of the sound waves through the external ear canal to the middle or inner ear.

confusion state of being unclear or unable to make a decision easily.

congenital present at birth.

congestive heart failure (CHF) condition in which the heart's reduced stroke volume causes an overload of fluid in the body's other tissues.

contamination presence of an agent only on the surface of the host without penetrating it.

contrecoup injury occurring on the opposite side; an injury to the brain opposite the site of impact.

contusion closed wound in which the skin is unbroken, although damage has occurred to the tissue immediately beneath.

convection transfer of heat via currents in liquids or gases.

cor pulmonale hypertrophy of the right ventricle resulting from disorders of the lung; congestive heart failure secondary to pulmonary hypertension.

core temperature the body temperature of the deep tissues, which usually does not vary more than a degree or so from its normal 37°C.

coup injury an injury to the brain occurring on the same side as the site of impact.

coupling interval distance between the preceding beat and a premature ventricular contraction (PVC).

CPAP continuous positive airway pressure.

cramping muscle pain resulting from overactivity, lack of oxygen, and accumulation of waste products.

crepitus crunching sounds of unlubricated parts in joints rubbing against each other; crackling sounds.

cricothyrostomy the introduction of a needle or other tube into the cricothyroid membrane, usually to provide an emergency airway.

cricothyrotomy a surgical incision into the cricothyroid membrane, usually to provide an emergency airway.

Crohn's disease idiopathic inflammatory bowel disorder associated with the small intestine.

croup viral illness characterized by inspiratory and expiratory stridor and a seal-bark-like cough.

crowning the bulging of the fetal head past the opening of the vagina during a contraction. Crowning is an indication of impending delivery.

crumple zone the region of a vehicle designed to absorb the energy of impact.

crush injury mechanism of injury in which tissue is locally compressed by high-pressure forces.

crush syndrome systemic disorder of severe metabolic disturbances resulting from the crush of a limb or other body part.

Cullen's sign ecchymosis over the umbilicus.

current the rate of flow of an electric charge.

Cushing's reflex response due to cerebral ischemia that causes an increase in systemic blood pressure, which maintains cerebral perfusion during increased ICP; a collective change in vital signs (increased blood pressure and temperature and decreased pulse and respirations) associated with increasing intracranial pressure.

Cushing's syndrome pathological condition resulting from excess adrenocortical hormones. Symptoms may include changed body habitus, hypertension, vulnerability to infection.

cyanosis bluish discoloration of the skin due to significantly reduced hemoglobin in the blood. The condition is directly related to poor ventilation.

cystic medial necrosis a death or degeneration of a part of the wall of an artery.

cystitis an infection and inflammation of the urinary bladder.

cytochrome oxidase enzyme complex, found in cellular mitochondria, that enables oxygen to create the adenosine triphosphate (ATP) required for all muscle energy.

deafness the inability to hear.

deceleration the rate at which speed or velocity decreases.

decerebrate posture sustained contraction of extensor muscles of the extremities resulting from a lesion in the brainstem. The patient presents with stiff and extended extremities and retracted head.

decompensated shock continuing hemodynamic insult to the body in which the compensatory mechanisms break down. The signs and symptoms become very pronounced, and the patient moves rapidly toward death.

decompression illness development of nitrogen bubbles within the tissues due to a rapid reduction of air pressure when a diver returns to the surface; also called "the bends."

decontaminate to destroy or remove pathogens.

decontamination the process of minimizing toxicity by reducing the amount of toxin absorbed into the body.

decorticate posture characteristic posture associated with a lesion at or above the upper brainstem. The patient presents with the arms flexed, fists clenched, and legs extended.

deep frostbite freezing involving epidermal and subcutaneous tissues resulting in a white appearance, hard (frozen) feeling on palpation, and loss of sensation.

deep venous thrombosis a blood clot in a vein.

defamation an intentional false communication that injures another person's reputation or good name.

defibrillation the process of passing an electrical current through a fibrillating heart to depolarize a critical mass of myocardial cells. This allows them to depolarize uniformly, resulting in an organized rhythm.

degenerative neurological disorders a collection of diseases that selectively affect one or more functional systems of the central nervous system.

degloving injury avulsion in which the mechanism of injury tears the skin off the underlying muscle, tissue, blood vessels, and bone.

delayed hypersensitivity reaction a hypersensitivity reaction that takes place after the elapse of some time following reexposure to an antigen. Delayed hypersensitivity reactions are usually less severe than immediate reactions.

DeLee suction trap a suction device that contains a suction trap connected to a suction catheter. The negative pressure that powers it can come either from the mouth of the operator or, preferably, from an external vacuum source.

delirium tremens (DTs) disorder found in habitual and excessive users of alcoholic beverages after cessation of drinking for 48–72 hours. Patients experience visual, tactile, and auditory disturbances. Death may result in severe cases.

delirium condition characterized by relatively rapid onset of widespread disorganized thought.

delusions fixed, false beliefs not widely held within the individual's cultural or religious group.

demand valve device a ventilation device that is manually operated by a push button or lever.

dementia condition involving gradual development of memory impairment and cognitive disturbance.

demylenation destruction or removal of the myelin sheath of nerve tissue; found in Guillain–Barré syndrome.

denature alter the usual substance of something.

dental abscess a collection of pus, usually from an infection, that spreads from a tooth to the tissues surrounding the tooth.

depersonalization feeling detached from yourself.

depression profound sadness or feeling of melancholy.

diabetes mellitus disorder of inadequate insulin activity, due either to inadequate production of insulin or to decreased responsiveness of body cells to insulin.

diabetic ketoacidosis complication of Type I diabetes due to decreased insulin intake. Marked by high blood glucose, metabolic acidosis, and, in advanced stages, coma. Ketoacidosis is often called diabetic coma.

diabetic retinopathy slow loss of vision as a result of damage done by diabetes.

dialysate the solution used in dialysis that is hypo-osmolar to many of the wastes and key electrolytes in blood.

dialysis a procedure that replaces some lost kidney functions.

diaphoresis sweatiness.

diaphragmatic hernia protrusion of abdominal contents into the thoracic cavity through an opening in the diaphragm.

diffuse axonal injury (DAI) type of brain injury characterized by shearing, stretching, or tearing of nerve fibres with subsequent axonal damage.

diffusion the movement of molecules through a membrane from an area of greater concentration to an area of lesser concentration.

diplopia double vision.

direct pressure method of hemorrhage control that relies on the application of pressure to the actual site of the bleeding.

disease period the duration from the onset of signs and symptoms of disease until the resolution of symptoms or death.

disinfection destroying certain forms of microorganisms, but not all.

dislocation complete displacement of a bone end from its position in a joint capsule.

dissecting aortic aneurysm aneurysm caused when blood gets between and separates the layers of the arterial wall.

disseminated intravascular coagulation (DIC) a disorder of coagulation caused by systemic activation of the coagulation cascade.

dissociative disorder condition in which the individual avoids stress by separating from his core personality.

distributive shock marked decrease in peripheral vascular resistance with resultant hypotension; examples include septic shock, neurogenic shock, and anaphylactic shock.

diuresis formation and passage of a dilute urine, decreasing blood volume.

diverticula small outpouchings in the mucosal lining of the intestinal tract.

diverticulitis inflammation of diverticula.

diverticulosis presence of diverticula, with or without associated bleeding.

domestic elder abuse physical or emotional violence or neglect when an elder is being cared for in a home-based setting.

down time duration from the beginning of the cardiac arrest until effective CPR is established.

drag the forces acting on a projectile in motion to slow its progress.

drowning asphyxiation resulting from submersion in liquid with death occurring within 24 hours of submersion.

drug overdose poisoning from a pharmacological substance in excess of that usually prescribed or that the body can tolerate.

ductus arteriosus channel between the main pulmonary artery and the aorta of the fetus.

dysmenorrhea painful menstruation.

dyspareunia painful sexual intercourse.

dysphagia inability to swallow or difficulty swallowing.

dysphoria an exaggerated feeling of depression or unrest, characterized by a mood of general dissatisfaction, restlessness, discomfort, and unhappiness.

dyspnea laboured or difficult breathing.

dysrhythmia any deviation from the normal electrical rhythm of the heart.

dystonias a group of disorders characterized by muscle contractions that cause twisting and repetitive movements, abnormal postures, or freezing in the middle of an action.

dysuria painful urination often associated with cystitis.

ecchymosis blue-black discoloration of the skin due to leakage of blood into the tissues.

ectopic beat cardiac depolarization resulting from depolarization of ectopic focus.

ectopic focus nonpacemaker heart cell that automatically depolarizes; *pl.* ectopic foci.

ectopic pregnancy the implantation of a developing fetus outside of the uterus, often in fallopian tubes.

effacement the thinning and shortening of the cervix during labour.

Einthoven's triangle the triangle around the heart formed by the bipolar leads.

elderly a person age 65 or older.

electrical alternans alternating amplitude of the P, QRS, and T waves on the ECG rhythm strip as the heart swings in a pendulum-like fashion within the pericardial sac during tamponade.

electrocardiogram (ECG) the graphic recording of the heart's electrical activity. It may be displayed either on paper or on an oscilloscope.

emboli undissolved solid, liquid, or gaseous matter in the bloodstream that may cause blockage of blood vessels.

emergent phase first stage of the burn process that is characterized by a catecholamine release and pain-mediated reaction.

emesis vomitus.

encephalitis acute infection of the brain, usually caused by a virus.

endocarditis inflammation of the endocardium (lining of the heart) and heart valves.

endocrine gland gland that secretes chemical substances directly into the blood; also called a *ductless gland*.

endometriosis condition in which endometrial tissue grows outside of the uterus.

endometritis infection of the endometrium.

endometrium the inner layer of the uterine wall where the fertilized egg implants.

endotoxin toxic products released when bacteria die and decompose.

end-stage renal failure an extreme failure of kidney function due to nephron loss.

energy the capacity to do work in the strict physical sense.

enterotoxin an exotoxin that produces gastrointestinal symptoms and diseases such as food poisoning.

enucleation removal of the eyeball after trauma or illness.

environmental emergency a medical condition caused or exacerbated by the weather, terrain, atmospheric pressure, or other local factors.

epidural hematoma accumulation of blood between the dura mater and the cranium.

epiglottitis infection and inflammation of the epiglottis.

epiphyseal fracture disruption in the epiphyseal plate of a child's bone.

epistaxis bleeding from the nose resulting from injury, disease, or environmental factors; a nosebleed.

epithelialization early stage of wound healing in which epithelial cells migrate over the surface of the wound.

erythema general reddening of the skin due to dilation of the superficial capillaries.

eschar hard, leathery product of a deep full thickness burn; it consists of dead and denatured skin.

Esophageal Tracheal CombiTube dual-lumen airway with a ventilation port for each lumen.

esophageal varicies (*singular* **varix**) enlarged and tortuous esophageal veins.

estimated date of confinement (EDC) the approximate day the infant will be born. This date is usually set at 40 weeks after the date of the mother's last menstrual period (LMP).

ETT endotracheal tube.

evaporation change from liquid to a gaseous state.

evisceration a protrusion of organs from a wound.

exertional metabolic rate rate at which the body consumes energy during activity. It is faster than the basic metabolic rate.

exocrine gland gland that secretes chemical substances to nearby tissues through a duct; also called a *ducted gland*.

exocrine disorder involving external secretions.

exotoxin a soluble poisonous substance secreted during growth of a bacterium.

exsanguination the draining of blood to the point at which life cannot be sustained.

extrauterine outside the uterus.

extravascular space the volume contained by all the cells (intracellular space) and the spaces between the cells (interstitial space).

extubation removing a tube from a body opening.

factitious disorder condition in which the patient feigns illness in order to assume the sick role.

fascia a fibrous membrane that covers, supports, and separates muscles and may also unite the skin with underlying tissue.

fasciculations involuntary contractions or twitchings of muscle fibres.

fatigue fracture break in a bone associated with prolonged or repeated stress.

fatigue condition in which a muscle's ability to respond to stimulation is lost or reduced through overactivity.

fear feeling of alarm and discontentment in the expectation of danger.

febrile seizures seizures that occur as a result of a sudden increase in temperature; occur most commonly between ages six months and six years.

fecal-oral route transmission of organisms picked up from the gastrointestinal tract (e.g., feces) into the mouth.

fibrin protein fibres that trap red blood cells as part of the clotting process.

fibroblasts specialized cells that form collagen.

fibrosis the formation of fiber-like connective tissue, also called scar tissue in an organ.

flail chest defect in the chest wall that allows for free movement of a segment; one or more ribs fractured in two or more places, creating an unattached rib segment. Breathing will cause paradoxical chest wall motion.

flat affect appearance of being disinterested, often lacking facial expression.

flechettes arrow-shaped projectiles found in some military ordnance.

fluid shift phase stage of the burn process in which there is a massive shift of fluid from the intravascular to the extravascular space.

food poisoning nonspecific term often applied to gastroenteritis that occurs suddenly and that is caused by the ingestion of food containing preformed toxins.

foreign body airway obstruction (FBAO) blockage or obstruction of the airway by an object that impairs respiration; in the case of pediatric patients, tongues, abundant secretions, and deciduous (baby) teeth are most likely to block airways.

French unit of measurement approximately equal to one-third of a millimetre.

frostbite environmentally induced freezing of body tissues causing destruction of cells.

fugue state condition in which an amnesiac patient physically flees.

full thickness burn burn that damages all layers of the skin; characterized by areas that are white and dry; also called third-degree burn.

functional impairment decreased ability to meet daily needs on an independent basis.

fungus plant-like microorganism.

gamma radiation powerful electromagnetic radiation emitted by radioactive substances with powerful penetrating properties; it is stronger than alpha and beta radiation.

gangrene death of tissue or bone, usually from an insufficient blood supply; deep space infection usually caused by the anaerobic bacterium *Clostridium perfringens*.

gastric lavage removing an ingested poison by repeatedly filling and emptying the stomach with water or saline via a gastric tube; also known as "pumping the stomach."

gastroenteritis generalized disorder involving nausea, vomiting, gastrointestinal cramping or discomfort, and diarrhea. *See also* acute gastroenteritis.

generalized seizures seizures that begin as an electrical discharge in a small area of the brain but spread to involve the entire cerebral cortex, causing widespread malfunction.

genitourinary system the male organ system that includes reproductive and urinary structures.

geriatric abuse a syndrome in which an elderly person is physically or psychologically injured by another person.

geriatrics the study and treatment of diseases of the aged.

gerontology scientific study of the effects of aging and of age-related diseases on humans.

Glasgow Coma Scale scoring system for monitoring the neurological status of patients with head injuries.

glaucoma medical condition where the pressure within the eye increases; group of eye diseases that results in increased intraocular pressure on the optic nerve; if left untreated, can lead to blindness.

global aphasia a combination of motor and sensory aphasia.

glomerulonephritis a form of nephritis, or inflammation of the kidneys; primarily involves the glomeruli, one of the capillary networks that are part of the renal corpuscles in the nephrons.

glottic function opening and closing of the glottic space.

glucose intolerance the body cells' inability to take up glucose from the bloodstream.

glycosuria glucose in urine, which occurs when blood glucose levels exceed the kidney's ability to reabsorb glucose.

Golden Hour the 60-minute period after a severe injury; it is the maximum acceptable time between the injury and initiation of surgery for the seriously injured trauma patient.

gonorrhea sexually transmitted disease caused by a gram-negative bacterium.

gout inflammation of joints and connective tissue due to buildup of uric acid crystals.

Gram stain method of differentiating types of bacteria according to their reaction to a chemical stain process.

granulocytes white blood cells charged with the primary purpose of neutralizing foreign bacteria.

Graves' disease endocrine disorder characterized by excess thyroid hormones resulting in body changes associated with increased metabolism; primary cause of *thyrotoxicosis*.

Gray a unit of absorbed radiation dose equal to 100 rads.

greenstick fracture partial fracture of a child's bone.

Grey-Turner's sign ecchymosis in the flank.

growth plate the area just below the head of a long bone in which growth in bone length occurs; the epiphyseal plate.

guarding protective tensing of the abdominal muscles by a patient suffering abdominal pain; may be a voluntary or involuntary response.

Guillain–Barré syndrome acute viral infection that triggers the production of autoantibodies, which damage the myelin sheath covering the peripheral nerves; causes rapid, progressive loss of motor function, ranging from muscle weakness to full-body paralysis.

gynecology the branch of medicine that deals with the health maintenance and the diseases of women, primarily of the reproductive organs.

hairline fracture small crack in a bone that does not disrupt its total structure.

half-life time required for half of the nuclei of a radioactive substance to lose activity by undergoing radioactive decay. In biology and pharmacology, the time required by the body to metabolize and inactivate half the amount of a substance taken in.

hallucinations sensory perceptions with no basis in reality.

hantavirus family of viruses that are carried by the deer mouse and transmitted by ticks and other arthropods.

heart failure clinical syndrome in which the heart's mechanical performance is compromised so that cardiac output cannot meet the body's needs.

heat cramps acute painful spasms of the voluntary muscles following strenuous activity in a hot environment without adequate fluid or salt intake.

heat exhaustion a mild heat illness; an acute reaction to heat exposure.

heat illness increased core body temperature due to inadequate thermolysis.

heatstroke acute, dangerous reaction to heat exposure, characterized by a body temperature usually above 40.6°C and central nervous system disturbances. The body usually ceases to perspire.

hematemesis vomiting blood.

hematochezia passage of stools containing red blood.

hematoma collection of blood beneath the skin or trapped within a body compartment.

hematomegaly enlarged liver.

hematuria blood in the urine.

hemodialysis a dialysis procedure relying on vascular access to the blood and on an artificial membrane.

hemoglobin the transport protein that carries oxygen in the blood.

hemophilia a blood disorder in which one of the proteins necessary for blood clotting is missing or defective.

hemopneumothorax condition where air and blood are in the pleural space.

hemoptysis expectoration of blood from the respiratory tract.

hemorrhoid small mass of swollen veins in the anus or rectum.

hemostasis the body's natural ability to stop bleeding, the ability to clot blood.

hemothorax blood within the pleural space.

hepatitis inflammation of the liver characterized by diffuse or patchy tissue necrosis.

hernia protrusion of an organ through its protective sheath.

herniation protrusion or projection of an organ or part of an organ through the wall of the cavity that normally contains it.

herpes simplex virus organism that causes infections characterized by fluid-filled vesicles, usually in the oral cavity or on the genitals.

herpes zoster an acute eruption caused by a reactivation of latent varicella virus (chicken pox) in the dorsal root ganglia; also known as shingles.

hiatal hernia protrusion of the stomach upward into the mediastinal cavity through the esophageal hiatus of the diaphragm.

high-pressure regulators are used to transfer oxygen at high pressures from tank to tank.

histamine a product of mast cells and basophils that causes vasodilation, capillary permeability, bronchoconstriction, and constriction of the gut.

homeostasis the natural tendency of the body to maintain a steady and normal internal environment.

hookworm parasite that attaches to the host's intestinal lining.

hormone chemical substance released by a gland that controls or affects processes in other glands or body systems.

hospice program of palliative care and support services that addresses the physical, social, economic, and spiritual needs of terminally ill patients and their families.

human immunodeficiency virus (HIV) organism responsible for acquired immune deficiency syndrome (AIDS).

humoral immunity immunity resulting from attack of an invading substance by antibodies.

hydrostatic pressure the pressure of liquids in equilibrium; the pressure exerted by or within liquids.

Hymenoptera any of an order of highly specialized insects such as bees and wasps.

hyperbaric oxygen chamber recompression chamber used to treat patients suffering from barotrauma.

hyperbilirubinemia an excessive amount of bilirubin—the orange-coloured pigment associated with bile—in the blood. In newborns, the condition appears as jaundice. Precipitating factors include maternal Rh or ABO incompatibility, neonatal septicemia, anoxia, hypoglycemia, and congenital liver or gastrointestinal defects.

hyperglycemia excessive blood glucose.

hyperglycemic hyperosmolar nonketotic (HHNK) coma complication of Type II diabetes due to inadequate insulin activity. Marked by high blood glucose, marked dehydration, and decreased mental function. Often mistaken for ketoacidosis.

hypermetabolic phase stage of the burn process in which there is increased body metabolism in an attempt by the body to heal the burn.

hypersensitivity an unexpected and exaggerated reaction to a particular antigen. It is used synonymously with the term *allergy*.

hypertensive emergency an acute elevation of blood pressure that requires the blood pressure to be lowered within one hour; characterized by end-organ changes such as hypertensive encephalopathy, renal failure, or blindness.

hypertensive encephalopathy a cerebral disorder of hypertension indicated by severe headache, nausea, vomiting, and altered mental status. Neurological symptoms may include blindness, muscle twitches, inability to speak, weakness, and paralysis.

hyperthermia unusually high core body temperature.

hyperthyroidism excessive secretion of thyroid hormones resulting in an increased metabolic rate.

hypertrophy an increase in the size or bulk of an organ.

hyphema blood in the anterior chamber of the eye, in front of the iris.

hypochondriasis an abnormal concern with one's health, with the false belief of suffering from some disease, despite medical assurances to the contrary; commonly known as hypochondria.

hypoglycemia deficiency of blood glucose. Sometimes called *insulin shock*. Hypoglycemia is a medical emergency.

hypoglycemic seizure seizure that occurs when brain cells aren't functioning normally due to low blood glucose.

hypothalamus portion of the diencephalon producing neurosecretions important in the control of certain metabolic activities, including regulation of body temperature.

hypothermia state of low body temperature, particularly low core body temperature.

hypothyroidism inadequate secretion of thyroid hormones resulting in a decreased metabolic rate.

hypovolemic shock decreased amount of intravascular fluid in the body; often due to trauma that causes blood loss into a body cavity or frank external hemorrhage; in children, can be the result of vomiting and diarrhea.

hypoxia state in which insufficient oxygen is available to meet the oxygen requirements of the cells.

immediate hypersensitivity reaction a hypersensitivity reaction that occurs swiftly following reexposure to an antigen. Immediate hypersensitivity reactions are usually more severe than delayed reactions. The swiftest and most severe of such reactions is anaphylaxis.

immune response complex cascade of events within the body that works toward the destruction or inactivation of pathogens, abnormal cells, or foreign molecules.

immune senescence diminished vigour of the immune response to the challenge and rechallenge by pathogens.

immune system the body system responsible for combating infection.

immunoglobulins (Igs) alternative term for antibody.

impacted fracture break in a bone in which the bone is compressed on itself.

impaled object foreign body embedded in a wound.

impetigo infection of the skin caused by staphylococci or streptococci.

impulse control disorder condition characterized by the patient's failure to control recurrent impulses.

incendiary an agent that combusts easily or creates combustion.

incision very smooth or surgical laceration, frequently caused by a knife, scalpel, razor blade, or piece of glass.

incontinence inability to retain urine or feces because of loss of sphincter control or cerebral or spinal lesions.

incubation period the time between a host's exposure to an infectious agent and the appearance of the first symptoms.

index case the individual who first introduced an infectious agent to a population.

index of suspicion the anticipation of injury to a body region, organ, or structure based on analysis of the mechanism of injury.

induced active immunity immunity achieved through vaccination given to generate an immune response that results in the development of antibodies specific for the injected antigen; also called *artificially acquired immunity*.

inertia tendency of an object to remain at rest or remain in motion unless acted upon by an external force.

infarction area of dead tissue caused by lack of blood.

infection presence of an agent within the host, without necessarily causing disease.

infestation presence of parasites that do not break the host's skin.

inflammation complex process of local cellular and biochemical changes as a consequence of injury or infection; an early stage of healing.

influenza disease caused by a group of viruses.

inhalation entry of a substance into the body through the respiratory tract.

injection entry of a substance into the body through a break in the skin.

institutional elder abuse physical or emotional violence or neglect when an elder is being cared for by a person paid to provide care.

insufflate to blow into.

integumentary system skin, consisting of the epidermis, dermis, and subcutaneous layers.

intermittent mandatory ventilation (IMV) respirator setting where a patient-triggered breath does not result in assistance by the machine.

interpolated beat a premature ventricular contraction (PVC) that falls between two sinus beats without effectively interrupting this rhythm.

interstitial nephritis an inflammation within the tissue surrounding the nephrons.

intra-aortic balloon pump an inflatable balloon inserted into the aortic arch. It is used in patients with unstable angina or pump failure; inflation of the balloon reduces cardiac work by decreasing afterload and also increases coronary blood flow.

intracerebral hemorrhage bleeding directly into the tissue of the brain.

intractable resistant to cure, relief, or control.

intrapartum occurring during childbirth.

intrarenal abscess a pocket of infection within kidney tissue.

intravascular space the volume contained by all the arteries, veins, capillaries, and other components of the circulatory system.

intussusception condition that occurs when part of an intestine slips into the part just distal to itself.

ionization the process of changing a substance into separate charged particles (ions).

ionizing radiation electromagnetic radiation (e.g., x-ray) or particulate radiation (e.g., alpha particles, beta particles, and neutrons) that, by direct or secondary processes, ionizes materials that absorb the radiation. Ionizing radiation can penetrate the cells of living organisms, depositing an electrical charge within them. When sufficiently intense, this form of energy kills cells.

irreversible shock final stage of shock in which organs and cells are so damaged that recovery is impossible.

ischemia a blockage in the delivery of oxygenated blood to the cells.

isolette also known as an *incubator*; a clear plastic enclosed bassinet used to keep prematurely born infants warm. The temperature of an isolette can be adjusted regardless of the room temperature. Some isolettes also provide humidity control.

isosthenuria the inability to concentrate or dilute urine relative to the osmolarity of blood.

J wave ECG deflection found at the junction of the QRS complex and the ST segment. It is associated with hypothermia and seen at core temperatures below 32°C, most commonly in leads II and V_6; also called an *Osborn wave*.

Jackson's theory of thermal wounds explanation of the physical effects of thermal burns.

Joule's law principle identifying that the rate of heat production is directly proportional to the resistance of the circuit and the square of the current.

keloid a formation resulting from overproduction of scar tissue.

Kernig's sign inability to fully extend the knees with hips flexed.

ketone bodies compounds produced during the catabolism of fatty acids, including acetoacetic acid, β-hydroxybutyric acid, and acetone.

ketosis the presence of significant quantities of ketone bodies in the blood.

kidney transplantation implantation of a kidney into a person without functioning kidneys.

kinetic energy the energy an object has while it is in motion. It is related to the object's mass and velocity.

kinetics the branch of physics that deals with motion, taking into consideration mass and force.

Korsakoff's psychosis psychosis characterized by disorientation, muttering delirium, insomnia, delusions, and hallucinations. Symptoms include painful extremities, bilateral wrist drop (rarely), bilateral foot drop (frequently), and pain on pressure over the long nerves.

Kussmaul's respiration rapid, deep respirations caused by severe metabolic and CNS problems.

kyphosis exaggeration of the normal posterior curvature of the spine.

labour the time and processes that occur during childbirth; the physiologic and mechanical process in which the baby, placenta, and amniotic sac are expelled through the birth canal.

labrynthitis inner ear infection that causes vertigo, nausea, and an unsteady gait.

laceration an open wound, normally a tear with jagged borders.

lactic acid compound produced from pyruvic acid during anerobic glycolysis.

laryngoscope instrument for lifting the tongue and epiglottis in order to see the vocal cords.

latent period time when a host cannot transmit an infectious agent to someone else.

Le Fort criteria classification system for fractures involving the maxilla.

leukemia a cancer of the hematopoietic cells.

leukocytosis too many white blood cells.

leukopenia too few white blood cells.

lice parasitic infestation of the skin of the scalp, trunk, or pubic area.

ligament of Treitz ligament that supports the duodenojejunal junction.

liquefaction necrosis the process in which an alkali dissolves and liquefies tissue.

lower gastrointestinal bleeding bleeding in the gastrointestinal tract distal to the ligament of Treitz.

lumen opening, or space, within a needle, artery, vein, or other hollow vessel.

Lyme disease recurrent inflammatory disorder caused by a tick-borne spirochete.

lymphangitis inflammation of the lymph channels, usually as a result of a distal infection.

lymphoma a cancer of the lymphatic system.

maceration process of softening a solid by soaking in a liquid.

macrophage immune system cell that has the ability to recognize and ingest foreign antibodies.

Magill forceps scissor-style clamps with circular tips.

malaria infection caused by parasite *Plasmodium*, carried by mosquitoes. Also spread through blood-to-blood contact, such as in blood transfusion or sharing needles. Symptoms include fever, chills, anemia, and enlarged spleen.

Mallory-Weiss tear esophageal laceration, usually secondary to vomiting.

mammalian diving reflex a complex cardiovascular reflex, resulting from submersion of the face and nose in water, that constricts blood flow everywhere except to the brain.

manic characterized by excessive excitement or activity (mania).

Marfan's syndrome hereditary condition of connective tissue, bones, muscles, ligaments, and skeletal structures characterized by irregular and unsteady gait, tall lean body type with long extremities, flat feet, stooped shoulders. The aorta is usually dilated and may become weakened enough to allow an aneurysm to develop.

mask a device for protecting the face.

mass a measure of the matter that an object contains; the property of a physical body that gives the body inertia.

mast cell specialized cell of the immune system that contains chemicals that assist in the immune response.

McBurney's point common site of pain from appendicitis, four to five centimetres above the anterior iliac crest in a direct line with the umbilicus.

measles highly contagious, acute viral disease characterized by a reddish rash that appears on the fourth or fifth day of illness.

mechanism of injury the processes and forces that cause trauma.

meconium dark green material found in the intestine of the full-term newborn. It can be expelled from the intestine into the amniotic fluid during periods of fetal distress.

melena dark, tar-like feces due to gastrointestinal bleeding.

Meniere's disease a disease of the inner ear characterized by vertigo, nerve deafness, and a roar or buzzing in the ear.

meningitis inflammation of the meninges, usually caused by an infection.

meningomyelocele hernia of the spinal cord and membranes through a defect in the spinal column.

menorrhagia excessive menstrual flow.

mental status examination (MSE) a structured exam designed to quickly evaluate a patient's level of mental functioning.

mental status the state of the patient's cerebral functioning.

mesenteric infarct death of tissue in the peritoneal fold (mesentery) that encircles the small intestine; a life-threatening condition.

metabolism the total changes that take place in an organism during physiological processes; the sum of cellular processes that produce the energy and molecules needed for growth and repair.

microangiopathy a disease affecting the smallest blood vessels.

miscarriage commonly used term to describe a pregnancy that ends before 20 weeks gestation; may also be called spontaneous abortion.

mononucleosis acute disease caused by the Epstein-Barr virus.

mood disorder pervasive and sustained emotion that colours a person's perception of the world.

motion the process of changing place; movement.

motor aphasia occurs when the patient cannot speak but can understand what is said.

mucoviscidosis cystic fibrosis of the pancreas resulting in abnormally viscous mucoid secretion from the pancreas.

multiple myeloma a cancerous disorder of plasma cells.

multiple personality disorder manifestation of two or more complete systems of personality.

multiple sclerosis disease that involves inflammation of certain nerve cells followed by demyelination, or the destruction of the myelin sheath, which is the fatty insulation surrounding nerve fibres.

mumps acute viral disease characterized by painful enlargement of the salivary glands.

Murphy's sign pain caused when an inflamed gallbladder is palpated by pressing under the right costal margin.

muscular dystrophy a group of genetic diseases characterized by progressive muscle weakness and degeneration of the skeletal or voluntary muscle fibres.

mylasthania gravis disease characterized by episodic muscle weakness triggered by an autoimmune attack of the acetylcholine receptors.

myocardial infarction (MI) death and subsequent necrosis of the heart muscle caused by inadequate blood supply; also *acute myocardial infarction (AMI)*.

myocarditis inflammation of the myocardium (muscle of the heart).

myoclonus temporary, involuntary twitching or spasm of a muscle or group of muscles.

myxedema coma life-threatening condition associated with advanced myxedema, with profound hypothermia, bradycardia, and electrolyte imbalance.

myxedema condition that reflects long-term exposure to inadequate levels of thyroid hormones with resultant changes in body structure and function.

nasal cannula catheter placed at the nares.

nasal flaring excessive widening of the nares with respiration.

nasogastric tube/orogastric tube a tube that runs through the nose or mouth and esophagus into the stomach; used for administering liquid nutrients or medications or for removing air or liquids from the stomach.

nasopharyngeal airway uncuffed tube that follows the natural curvature of the nasopharynx, passing through the nose and extending from the nostril to the posterior pharynx.

nasotracheal route through the nose and into the trachea.

natural immunity genetically predetermined immunity that is present at birth; also called *innate immunity*.

naturally acquired immunity immunity that begins to develop after birth and is continually enhanced by exposure to new pathogens and antigens throughout life.

near-drowning an incident of potentially fatal submersion in liquid that did not result in death or in which death occurred more than 24 hours after submersion.

necrosis tissue death, usually from ischemia.

necrotizing fasciitis severe form of bacterial skin infection reaching deep to the fascia of the muscles. Blood flow to the affected tissues is blocked, leading to death of the surrounding tissues. Skin over the affected area is initially pale but becomes red, warm, and swollen. Blisters may form, filled with watery, brownish fluid. As toxins build, the patient may become feverish, ill, and tachycardic, with a decreased level of consciousness. The death rate from necrotizing fasciitis is about 30 percent.

needle cricothyrostomy surgical airway technique that inserts a 14-gauge needle into the trachea at the cricothyroid membrane.

needle thoracostomy creation of a hole in the chest wall using a needle, usually to obtain samples or drain fluid from the pleural space.

negative feedback homeostatic mechanism in which a change in a variable ultimately inhibits the process that led to the shift.

neonatal abstinence syndrome (NAS) a generalized disorder presenting a clinical picture of CNS hyperirritability, gastrointestinal dysfunction, respiratory distress, and vague autonomic symptoms. It may be due to intrauterine exposure to heroin, methadone, or other less potent opiates. Nonopiate central nervous system depressants may also cause NAS.

neonate newborn infant; an infant from the time of birth to one month of age.

neoplasm literally meaning "new form"; a new or abnormal formation; a tumour.

neovascularization new growth of capillaries in response to healing.

nephrology the medical specialty dealing with the kidneys.

nephron the functional units of the kidneys.

neutron radiation powerful radiation with penetrating properties between that of beta and gamma radiation.

neutropenia a reduction in the number of neutrophils.

neutropenic a condition that results from an abnormally low neutrophyl count in the blood (less than $2000/mm^3$).

nitrogen narcosis a state of stupor that develops during deep dives due to nitrogen's effect on cerebral function; also called "raptures of the deep."

nocturia excessive urination during the night.

noncardiogenic shock types of shock that result from causes other than inadequate cardiac output.

noncompensatory pause pause following an ectopic beat when the SA node is depolarized and the underlying cadence of the heart is interrupted.

normal flora organisms that live inside our bodies without ordinarily causing disease.

normal sinus rhythm the normal heart rhythm.

nosocomial infection an infection acquired in a medical setting.

obligate intracellular parasite organism that can grow and reproduce only within a host cell.

oblique fracture break in a bone running across it at an angle other than 90 degrees.

oblique having a slanted position or direction.

obstetrics the branch of medicine that deals with the care of women throughout pregnancy.

ohm basic unit for measuring the strength of electrical resistance.

Ohm's law the physical law identifying that the current in an electrical circuit is directly proportional to the voltage and inversely proportional to the resistance.

oliguria decreased urine elimination to 400–500 ml or less per day.

omphalocele congenital hernia of the umbilicus.

open cricothyrotomy surgical airway technique that places an endotracheal or tracheostomy tube directly into the trachea through a surgical incision at the cricothyroid membrane.

open fracture a broken bone in which the bone ends or the forces that caused it penetrate the surrounding skin.

opportunistic pathogen ordinarily nonharmful bacterium that causes disease only under unusual circumstances.

ordnance military weapons and munitions.

organophosphates phosphorus-containing organic pesticides.

oropharyngeal airway semicircular device that follows the palate's curvature.

orthopnea difficulty in breathing while lying supine.

orthostatic hypotension a decrease in blood pressure that occurs when a person moves from a supine to a sitting or upright position.

osmotic diuresis greatly increased urination and dehydration that results when high levels of glucose cannot be reabsorbed into the blood from the kidney tubules and the osmotic pressure of the glucose in the tubules also prevents water reabsorption.

osteoarthritis inflammation of a joint resulting from wearing down of the articular cartilage; a degenerative joint disease, characterized by a loss of articular cartilage and hypertrophy of bone.

osteomyelitis an infection of the bone or bone marrow usually caused through infected blood, direct infection, or infection of surrounding tissues. Sources of infection may include surgery, trauma, kidney dialysis, and intravenous drug use. Often occurs in long bones of children and vertebrae of adults. Symptoms include increasing continuous pain and tenderness in the bone, muscle spasm, and generalized fever. The area around the infection may be red and swollen and have pain with movement.

osteoporosis weakening of bone tissue due to loss of essential minerals, especially calcium.

otitis media middle ear infection.

overdrive respiration positive pressure ventilation supplied to a breathing patient.

overpressure a rapid increase and then decrease in atmospheric pressure created by an explosion.

ovulation the release of an egg from the ovary.

oxidizer an agent that enhances combustion of a fuel.

pallor paleness.

pancolitis ulcerative colitis spread throughout the entire colon.

panic attack extreme period of anxiety resulting in great emotional distress.

paradoxical breathing assymetrical chest wall movement that lessens respiratory efficiency.

parasite organism that lives in or on another organism.

Parkinson's disease chronic and progressive motor system disorder characterized by tremor, rigidity, bradykinesia, and postural instability.

paroxysmal nocturnal dyspnea (PND) short attacks of dypsnea that occur at night and interrupt sleep.

partial seizures seizures that remain confined to a limited portion of the brain, causing localized malfunction. Partial seizures may spread and become generalized.

partial thickness burn burn in which the epidermis is burned through and the dermis is damaged; characterized by redness and blistering; also called a second-degree burn.

partner abuse physical or emotional violence from a man or woman toward a domestic partner.

passive immunity acquired immunity that results from administration of antibodies either from the mother to the infant across the placental barrier (natural passive immunity) or through vaccination (induced passive immunity).

pathogen disease-producing agent or invading substance.

PEEP positive end expiratory pressure.

pelvic inflammatory disease (PID) an acute infection of the reproductive organs that can be caused by a bacteria, virus, or fungus.

penetrating trauma injury caused by an object breaking the skin and entering the body.

peptic ulcer erosion caused by gastric acid.

perfusion the circulation of blood through the capillaries.

pericardial tamponade filling of the pericardial sac with fluid, which in turn limits the filling and function of the heart.

pericarditis inflammation of the pericardium (outer covering of the heart). May be linked to cancer, injury, or heart attack.

perinephric abscess a pocket of infection in the layer of fat surrounding the kidney.

peripheral arterial atherosclerotic disease a progressive degenerative disease of the medium-sized and large arteries.

peripheral neuropathy any malfunction or damage of the peripheral nerves. Results may include muscle weakness, loss of sensation, impaired reflexes, and internal organ malfunctions.

peritoneal dialysis a dialysis procedure relying on the peritoneal membrane as the semipermeable membrane.

peritonitis inflammation of the peritoneum caused by chemical or bacterial irritation.

peritonsillar abscess a collection of pus in the tonsils and surrounding tissues.

persistent fetal circulation condition in which blood continues to bypass the fetal respiratory system, resulting in ongoing hypoxia.

personality disorder condition that results in persistently maladaptive behaviour.

pertussis disease characterized by severe, violent coughing.

phagocytosis process in which a cell surrounds and absorbs a bacterium or other particle.

pharyngitis infection of the pharynx and tonsils.

pharyngo-tracheal lumen airway (PtL) a two-tube airway system.

phobia excessive fear that interferes with functioning.

phototherapy exposure to sunlight or artificial light for therapeutic purposes. In newborns, light is used to treat hyperbilirubinemia or jaundice.

Pierre Robin syndrome unusually small jaw, combined with a cleft palate, downward displacement of the tongue, and an absent gag reflex.

pill-rolling motion an involuntary tremor, usually in one hand or sometimes in both, in which fingers move as if they were rolling a pin back and forth.

pinworm parasite that is 3–10 mm long and lives in the distal colon.

placenta the organ that serves as a lifeline for the developing fetus. The placenta is attached to the wall of the uterus and the umbilical cord.

platelet phase second step in the clotting process in which platelets adhere to blood vessel walls and to each other.

pleuritic sharp or tearing, as a description of pain.

pneumatic antishock garment (PASG) garment designed to produce uniform pressure on the lower extremities and abdomen; used with shock and hemorrhage patients in some EMS systems.

pneumomediastinum the presence of air in the mediastinum.

pneumonia acute infection of the lung, including alveolar spaces and interstitial tissue.

pneumothorax a collection of air in the pleural space between the chest wall and lungs, causing a loss of the negative pressure that binds the lung to the chest wall. In an *open pneumothorax*, air enters the pleural space through an injury to the chest wall. In a *closed pneumothorax*, air enters the pleural space through an opening in the pleura that covers the lung. A *tension pneumothorax* develops when air in the pleural space cannot escape, causing a buildup of pressure and collapse of the lung.

poliomyelitis (polio) infectious, inflammatory viral disease of the central nervous system that sometimes results in permanent paralysis.

polycythemia an excess of red blood cells. In a newborn, the condition may reflect hypovolemia or prolonged intrauterine hypoxia.

polymorphonuclear cells *see* granulocytes.

polypharmacy multiple drug therapy in which there is a concurrent use of a number of drugs.

portal pertaining to the flow of blood into the liver.

positive end expiratory pressure (PEEP) a method of holding the alveoli open by increasing expiratory pressure. Some bag-valve units used in EMS have PEEP attachments. Also, EMS personnel sometimes transport patients who are on ventilators with PEEP attachments.

postpartum depression the "let down" feeling experienced during the period following birth occurring in 70–80 percent of mothers.

postrenal acute renal failure acute renal failure due to obstruction distal to the kidney.

posttraumatic stress syndrome reaction to an extreme stressor.

posture position, attitude, or bearing of the body.

PPD purified protein derivative, the substance used in a test for tuberculosis.

precordial leads electrocardiogram leads applied to the chest in a pattern that permits a view of the horizontal plane of the heart; leads V1, V2, V3, V4, V5, and V6.

precordium area of the chest wall overlying the heart.

prerenal acute renal failure acute renal failure due to decreased blood perfusion of kidneys.

presbycusis progressive hearing loss that occurs with aging.

pressure ulcer ischemic damage and subsequent necrosis affecting the skin, subcutaneous tissue, and often the muscle; result of intense pressure over a short time or low pressure over a long time; also known as pressure sore or bedsore.

pressure wave area of overpressure that radiates outward from an explosion.

preventive strategy a management plan to minimize further damage to vital tissues.

primary response initial, generalized response to an antigen.

Prinzmetal's angina variant of angina pectoris caused by vasospasm of the coronary arteries; not blockage per se. Also called *vasopastic angina* or *atypical angina.*

prions particles of protein folded in such a way that protease enzymes cannot act upon them.

proctitis ulcerative colitis limited to the rectum.

profile the size and shape of a projectile as it contacts a target; it is the energy exchange surface of the contact.

prognosis the anticipated outcome of a disease or injury.

prolonged QT interval QT interval greater than .44 seconds.

prostatitis infection and inflammation of the prostate gland.

protozoan single-celled parasitic organism with flexible membranes and the ability to move.

pruritus itching; often occurs as a symptom of some systemic change or illness.

psychogenic amnesia failure to recall, as opposed to inability to recall.

psychosis extreme response to stress characterized by impaired ability to deal with reality.

psychosocial related to a patient's personality style, dynamics of unresolved conflict, or crisis management methods.

puerperium the time period surrounding delivery.

pulmonary embolism blood clot in one of the pulmonary arteries.

pulmonary overpressure expansion of air held in the lungs during ascent. If not exhaled, the expanded air may cause injury to the lungs and surrounding structures.

pulse oximetry a measurement of hemoglobin oxygen saturation in the peripheral tissues.

pulse pressure difference between the systolic and diastolic blood pressures.

pulsus paradoxus drop of greater than 10 mmHg in the systolic blood pressure during the inspiratory phase of respiration that occurs in patients with pericardial tamponade.

puncture specific soft-tissue injury involving a deep, narrow wound to the skin and underlying organs that carries an increased danger of infection.

pyelonephritis an infection and inflammation of the kidney.

pyrexia fever, or above-normal body temperature.

pyrogen any substance causing a fever, such as viruses and bacteria or substances produced within the body in response to infection or inflammation.

QT interval period from the beginning of the QRS to the end of the T wave.

rabies viral disorder that affects the nervous system.

rad basic unit of absorbed radiation dose.

radiation transfer of energy through space or matter.

rape usually defined as penile penetration of the genitalia or rectum (however slight) without the consent of the victim.

rapid sequence intubation giving medications to sedate (induce) and temporarily paralyze a patient and then performing orotracheal intubation.

rebound tenderness pain on release of the examiner's hands, allowing the abdominal wall to return to its normal position; associated with peritoneal irritation.

recompression resubmission of a person to a greater pressure so that gradual decompression can be achieved; often used in the treatment of diving emergencies.

reduced nephron mass the decrease in number of functional nephrons that causes chronic renal failure.

reduced renal mass the decrease in kidney size associated with chronic renal failure.

referred pain pain that originates in a region other than where it is felt.

refractory period the period of time when myocardial cells have not yet completely repolarized and cannot be stimulated again.

relative refractory period the period of the cardiac cycle when a sufficiently strong stimulus may produce depolarization.

remodelling stage in the wound healing process in which collagen is broken down and relaid in an orderly fashion.

renal acute renal failure ARF due to pathology within kidney tissue itself.

renal calculi kidney stones.

renal dialysis artificial replacement of some critical kidney functions.

renal pertaining to the kidneys.

reservoir any living creature or environment (water, soil, etc.) that can harbour an infectious agent.

resiliency the connective strength and elasticity of an object or fabric.

resistance (1) a host's ability to fight off infection. (2) property of a conductor that opposes the passage of an electric current.

resolution phase final stage of the burn process in which scar tissue is laid down and the healing process is completed.

respiration the exchange of gases between a living organism and its environment.

respirator an apparatus worn that cleanses or qualifies the air.

respiratory syncytial virus (RSV) common cause of pneumonia and bronchiolitis in children.

restraint asphyxia death from positioning that prevents sufficient intake of oxygen.

resuscitation provision of efforts to return a spontaneous pulse and breathing.

retinal detachment condition that may be of traumatic origin and present with patient complaint of a dark curtain obstructing a portion of the field of view.

retinopathy any disorder of the retina.

retroauricular ecchymosis black-and-blue discoloration over the mastoid process (just behind the ear) that is characteristic of a basilar skull fracture. (Also called Battle's sign.)

retrograde amnesia inability to remember events that occurred before the trauma that caused the condition.

retropharyngeal abscess a collection of pus in the pharyngeal walls caused by suppuration of inflamed retropharyngeal lymph nodes. Most common in children.

return of spontaneous circulation resuscitation results in the patient's having a spontaneous pulse.

rhabdomyolysis acute disease that involves the destruction of skeletal muscle.

rheumatoid arthritis chronic disease that causes deterioration of peripheral joint connective tissue.

rhythm strip electrocardiogram printout.

rouleaux group of red blood cells that are stuck together.

rubella (German measles) systemic viral disease characterized by a fine pink rash that appears on the face, trunk, and extremities and fades quickly.

rule of nines method of estimating amount of body surface area burned by a division of the body into regions, each of which represents approximately 9 percent of total BSA (plus 1 percent for the genital region).

rule of palms method of estimating amount of body surface area burned that sizes the area burned in comparison to the patient's palmar surface.

scabies skin disease caused by mite infestation and characterized by intense itching.

schizophrenia common disorder involving significant change in behavior often including hallucinations, delusions, and depression.

scuba acronym for *self-contained underwater breathing apparatus*. Portable apparatus that contains compressed air, which allows the diver to breathe underwater.

secondary response response by the immune system that takes place if the body is exposed to the same antigen again; in secondary response, antibodies specific for the offending antigen are released.

seizure a temporary alteration in behaviour due to the massive electrical discharge of one or more groups of neurons in the brain. Seizures can be clinically classified as generalized or partial.

Sengstaken-Blakemore tube three-lumen tube used in treating esophageal bleeding.

senile dementia general term used to describe an abnormal decline in mental functioning seen in the elderly; also called "organic brain syndrome" or "multi-infarct dementia."

sensitization initial exposure of a person to an antigen that results in an immune response.

sensorineural deafness deafness caused by the inability of nerve impulses to reach the auditory centre of the brain because of nerve damage either to the inner ear or to the brain.

sensorium sensory apparatus of the body as a whole; also that portion of the brain that functions as a centre of sensations.

sensory aphasia occurs when the patient cannot understand the spoken word.

seroconversion creation of antibodies after exposure to a disease.

serous fluid a cellular component of blood, similar to plasma.

sexual assault unwanted oral, genital, rectal, or manual sexual contact.

sexually transmitted disease (STD) illness most commonly transmitted through sexual contact.

shunt surgical connection that runs from the brain to the abdomen for the purpose of draining excess CNS fluid and preventing increased intracranial pressure.

Shy-Drager syndrome chronic orthostatic hypotension caused by a primary autonomic nervous system deficiency.

sick sinus syndrome a group of disorders characterized by dysfunction of the sinoatrial node in the heart.

sickle cell anemia an inherited disorder of red blood cell production so named because the red blood cells become sickle-shaped when oxygen levels are low.

silent myocardial infarction a myocardial infarction that occurs without exhibiting obvious signs and symptoms.

simple partial seizure type of partial seizure that involves local motor, sensory, or autonomic dysfunction of one area of the body. There is no loss of consciousness.

sinusitis inflammation of the paranasal sinuses. Most common causes include allergy, dental infection, and upper respiratory infection, such as a common cold.

slow-reacting substance of anaphylaxis (SRS-A) substance released from basophils and mast cells that causes spasm of the bronchiole smooth muscle, resulting in an asthma-like attack and occasionally asphyxia.

sociocultural related to the patient's actions and interactions within society.

somatic pain sharp, localized pain that originates in walls of the body such as skeletal muscles.

somatoform disorder condition characterized by physical symptoms that have no apparent physiological cause and are attributable to psychological factors.

spasm intermittent or continuous contraction of a muscle.

spina bifida (SB) a neural defect that results from the failure of one or more of the fetal vertebrae to close properly during the first month of pregnancy.

spiral fracture a curving break in a bone as may be caused by rotational forces.

spondylosis a degeneration of the vertebral body.

spontaneous pneumothorax a pneumothorax (collection of air in the pleural space) that occurs spontaneously, in the absence of blunt or penetrating trauma.

sprain tearing of a joint capsule's connective tissues.

status epilepticus series of two or more generalized motor seizures without any intervening periods of consciousness.

stenosis narrowing or constriction.

sterilization destroying all microorganisms.

Stokes-Adams syndrome a series of symptoms resulting from heart block, most commonly syncope. The symptoms result from decreased blood flow to the brain caused by the sudden decrease in cardiac output.

stoma opening in the anterior neck that connects the trachea with ambient air; a permanent surgical opening in the neck through which the patient breathes.

strain injury resulting from overstretching of muscle fibres.

stroke injury or death of brain tissue resulting from interruption of cerebral blood flow and oxygenation; caused by either ischemic or hemorrhagic lesions to a portion of the brain, resulting in damage or destruction of brain tissue. Commonly also called a cerebrovascular accident or "brain attack."

stylet plastic-covered metal wire used to bend the endotracheal tube into a J or hockey-stick shape.

subarachnoid hemorrhage bleeding that occurs between the arachoid and dura mater of the brain.

subcutaneous emphysema presence of air in the subcutaneous tissue.

subdural hematoma collection of blood directly beneath the dura mater.

subendocardial infarction myocardial infarction that affects only the deeper levels of the myocardium; also called non-Q-wave infarction because it typically does not result in a significant Q wave in the affected lead.

subglottic referring to the lower airway.

subluxation partial displacement of a bone end from its position in a joint capsule.

substance abuse use of a pharmacological substance for purposes other than medically defined reasons.

suction to remove with a vacuum-type device.

sudden death death within one hour after the onset of symptoms.

sudden infant death syndrome (SIDS) illness of unknown etiology that occurs during the first year of life, with the peak at ages 2–4 months.

superficial burn a burn that involves only the epidermis; characterized by reddening of the skin; also called a first-degree burn.

superficial frostbite freezing involving only epidermal tissues resulting in redness followed by blanching and diminished sensation; also called *frostnip*.

supraglottic referring to the upper airway.

surface absorption entry of a substance into the body directly through the skin or mucous membrane.

surfactant a compound secreted by cells in the lungs that regulates the surface tension of the fluid that lines the alveoli, important in keeping the alveoli open for gas exchange.

survival when a patient is resuscitated and survives to be discharged from the hospital.

synchronized cardioversion the passage of an electric current through the heart during a specific part of the cardiac cycle to terminate certain kinds of dysrhythmias.

syncope transient loss of consciousness due to inadequate flow of blood to the brain with rapid recovery of consciousness on becoming supine; fainting.

syphilis bloodborne sexually transmitted disease caused by the spirochete *Treponema pallidum.*

tachycardia rapid heart rate; a heart rate of more than 100 beats per minute.

tachypnea rapid respiration.

tactile fremitus vibratory tremours felt through the chest by palpation.

tendinitis inflammation of a tendon and/or its protective sheath.

tension lines natural patterns in the surface of the skin revealing tensions within.

tension pneumothorax buildup of air under pressure within the thorax. The resulting compression of the lung severely reduces the effectiveness of respirations.

tetanus acute bacterial infection of the central nervous system.

therapeutic index the maximum tolerated dose divided by the minimum curative close of a drug; the range between curative and toxic dosages; also called *therapeutic window.*

therapy regulators are used for delivering oxygen to patients.

thermal gradient the difference in temperature between the environment and the body.

thermogenesis the production of heat, especially within the body.

thermoregulation the maintenance or regulation of a particular temperature of the body.

thrombocytopenia an abnormal decrease in the number of platelets.

thrombocytosis an abnormal increase in the number of platelets.

thyrotoxic crisis toxic condition characterized by hyperthermia, tachycardia, nervous symptoms, and rapid metabolism; also known as *thyroid storm.*

thyrotoxicosis condition that reflects prolonged exposure to excess thyroid hormones with resultant changes in body structure and function.

tidal volume average volume of gas inhaled or exhaled in

tilt test drop in the systolic blood pressure of 20 mmHg or an increase in the pulse rate of 20 beats per minute when a patient is moved from a supine to a sitting position; a finding suggestive of a relative hypovolemia.

tinnitus subjective ringing or tingling sound in the ear.

tocolysis the process of stopping labour.

tolerance the need to progressively increase the dose of a drug to reproduce the effect originally achieved by smaller doses.

tonic phase phase of a seizure characterized by tension or contraction of muscles.

tonic-clonic seizure type of generalized seizure characterized by rapid loss of consciousness and motor coordination, muscle spasms, and jerking motions.

tonsillitis an infection of the tonsils and their surrounding tissues, characterized by pain on swallowing. Patient may complain of feeling unwell, fever, redness and swelling of the uvula and soft palate, and swelling above the tonsil. Spasm of muscles of chewing may lead to trismus.

total down time duration from the beginning of the arrest until the patient's delivery to the emergency department.

tourniquet a constrictor used on an extremity to apply circumferential pressure on all arteries to control bleeding.

toxicology study of the detection, chemistry, pharmacological actions, and antidotes of toxic substances.

toxic shock syndrome a syndrome of symptoms caused by toxins produced by staphylococcal or streptococcal bacteria. Symptoms include high fever, severe headache, vomiting, diarrhea, confusion, and skin rash (erythroderma). May progress to severe hypotension and shock. Most cases of toxic shock syndrome are associated with menstruating women who use high-absorbency tampons. Less common causes include postpartum or postoperative infections.

toxidrome a toxic syndrome; a group of typical signs and symptoms consistently associated with exposure to a particular type of toxin.

toxin any chemical (drug, poison, or other) that causes adverse effects on an organism that is exposed to it; any poisonous chemical secreted by bacteria or released following destruction of the bacteria.

tracheal deviation any position of the trachea other than midline.

tracheal tugging retraction of the tissues of the neck due to airway obstruction or dyspnea.

tracheobronchial tree the structures of the trachea and the bronchi.

tracheostomy a surgical incision that a surgeon makes from the anterior neck into the trachea held open by a metal or plastic tube.

trajectory the path a projectile follows.

transection a cutting across a long axis; a cross-sectional cut.

transient ischemic attack (TIA) temporary interruption of blood supply to the brain; often seen as a precursor to a stroke.

transmural infarction myocardial infarction that affects the full thickness of the myocardium and almost always results in a pathological Q wave in the affected leads.

transvenous pacing insertion of a wire through the jugular vein to the right ventricle. The wire is connected to an external pacemaker. Transvenous pacing is indicated for patients who require ongoing pacing, or in those high-risk patients requiring pacing.

transverse fracture a break that runs across a bone perpendicular to the bone's orientation.

trauma centre medical facility that has the capability of caring for acutely injured patients; trauma centres must meet strict criteria to use this designation.

trauma registry a data retrieval system for trauma patient information, used to evaluate and improve the trauma system.

trauma triage criteria guidelines to aid prehospital personnel in determining which trauma patients require urgent transportation to a trauma centre.

trauma a physical injury or wound caused by external force or violence.

trichinosis disease resulting from an infestation of *Trichinella spriralis*.

trichomoniasis sexually transmitted disease caused by the protozoan *Trichomonas vaginalis*.

trismus difficulty opening the mouth or jaw. Causes include arthritis, tonsillitis, and tetanus.

tumour (vascular) a mass or abnormal growth of cells. A tumour may be cancerous or noncancerous. In a cancerous tumour, the cells lose their normal control mechanisms and grow in an unregulated manner, invading and destroying the tissues and organs around the tumour.

turgor ability of the skin to return to normal appearance after being subjected to pressure.

two-pillow orthopnea the number of pillows—in this case, two—needed to ease the difficulty of breathing while lying down; a significant factor in assessing the level of respiratory distress.

umbilical cord structure containing two arteries and one vein that connects the placenta and the fetus.

unipolar leads electrocardiogram leads applied to the arms and legs, consisting of one polarized (positive) electrode and a nonpolarized reference point that is created by the ECG machine combining two additional electrodes; also called augmented leads; leads aVR, aVL, and aVF.

upper airway obstruction an interference with air movement through the upper airway.

upper gastrointestinal bleeding bleeding within the gastrointestinal tract proximal to the ligament of Treitz.

urea waste derived from ammonia produced through protein metabolism.

uremia the syndrome of signs and symptoms associated with chronic renal failure.

urethritis an infection and inflammation of the urethra.

urinary catheterization generally indicated to collect uncontaminated urine samples, monitor urinary output, and manage acute urinary retention and in chronically bedridden patients. Equipment required to insert a urinary catheter includes a catheter tray, appropriately sized Foley catheter, drainage bag, and topical anaesthetic.

urinary stasis a condition in which the bladder empties incompletely during urination.

urinary system the group of organs that produces urine, maintaining fluid and electrolyte balance for the body.

urinary tract infection (UTI) an infection, usually bacterial, at any site in the urinary tract.

urine the fluid made by the kidney and eliminated from the body.

urology the surgical specialty dealing with the urinary/genitourinary system.

urosepsis septicemia originating from the urinary tract.

urostomy surgical diversion of the urinary tract to a stoma, or hole, in the abdominal wall.

urticaria the raised areas, or weals, that occur on the skin, associated with vasodilation due to histamine release; commonly called "hives."

vagal response stimulation of the vagus nerve causing a parasympathetic response.

valsalva maneuvre forced exhalation against a closed glottis, such as with coughing. This maneuvre stimulates the parasympathetic nervous system via the vagus nerve, which in turn slows the heart rate.

varicella viral disease characterized by a rash of fluid-filled vesicles that rupture, forming small ulcers that eventually scab; commonly called *chicken pox.*

varicose veins dilated superficial veins, usually in the lower extremity.

varicosities *see* **varicose veins.**

vascular phase first step in the clotting process in which smooth blood vessel muscle contracts, reducing the vessel lumen and the flow of blood through it.

vasculitis inflammation of blood vessels.

velocity the rate of motion in a particular direction in relation to time.

ventilation the mechanical process of moving air in and out of the lungs.

venturi mask high-flow face mask that uses a venturi system to deliver relatively precise oxygen concentrations.

vertigo the sensation of faintness or dizziness; may cause a loss of balance.

virulence an organism's strength or ability to infect or overcome the body's defences.

virus disease-causing organism that can be seen only with an electron microscope.

visceral pain dull, poorly localized pain that originates in the walls of hollow organs.

voltage the difference of electric potential between two points with different concentrations of electrons.

volvulus twisting of the intestine on itself.

von Willebrand's disease condition in which the vWF component of factor VIII is deficient.

washout release of accumulated lactic acid, carbon dioxide (carbonic acid), potassium, and rouleaux into the venous circulation.

Wernicke's syndrome condition characterized by loss of memory and disorientation, associated with chronic alcohol intake and a diet deficient in thiamine.

whole bowel irrigation administration of polyethylene glycol continuously at 1–2 L/hr through a nasogastric tube until the effluent is clear or objects are recovered.

window phase time between exposure to a disease and seroconversion.

withdrawal referring to alcohol or drug withdrawal in which the patient's body reacts severely when deprived of the abused substance.

yaw swing or wobble around the axis of a projectile's travel.

Zollinger-Ellison syndrome condition that causes the stomach to secrete excessive amounts of hydrochloric acid and pepsin.

zone of coagulation area in a burn nearest the heat source that suffers the most damage and is characterized by clotted blood and thrombosed blood vessels.

zone of hyperemia area peripheral to a burn that is characterized by increased blood flow.

zone of stasis area in a burn surrounding the zone of coagulation and that is characterized by decreased blood flow.

Index

ABCs, 372–373, 618, 665, 1019
abdominal aortic aneurysm, 560, 561f
abdominal pain
    E. coli O157:H7, 820
    gastrointestinal emergencies. *See* gastrointestinal (GI) emergencies
    gynecological emergencies, 858, 861–863
    hematopoietic emergencies, 731
    miscarriage, 863
    pregnancy complications, 879
    urological emergencies. *See* urological emergencies
abdominal trauma
    abdominal wall injury, 312–313
    abnormal pulsation, 322
    assessment, 318–324
    blast injuries, 39–40, 312
    blunt injuries, 311–312, 319
    bowel injury, 315
    child abuse, 1083
    children, 318
    described, 310
    evisceration, 313
    guarding, 316
    gunshot wounds, 320
    hidden hemorrhage, signs of, 324
    high-velocity weapons, 320
    hollow organ injuries, 313
    hypoperfusion, 320
    impaled objects, 325
    index of suspicion, 319
    management of, 324–326
    mechanism of injury, 310–312
    mesentery, 315
    ongoing assessment, 324
    pathophysiology, 310–318
    pediatric trauma, 1010
    pelvic injury, 316
    penetrating injuries, 57, 311, 313, 319–320, 322–323, 325
    peritoneum injury, 315–316
    peritonitis, 315–316
    positioning of patient, 324–325
    pregnant women, 316–318, 323–324, 326
    prevention, 310
    primary assessment, 321
    rapid trauma assessment, 321–324
    relative mortality and morbidity, 310
    scene assessment, 318–321
    shotgun, 311
    soft-tissue injury management, 132
    solid organ injuries, 314–315
    thoracic injury, and co-morbidity, 277
    vascular structures, 315
abdominal wall injury, 312–313
aberrant conduction, 507
abnormal breath sounds, 343–344
abnormal delivery presentations
    breech presentation, 896–897, 897f, 898f
    limb presentation, 897–898
    occiput posterior position, 898
    other abnormal presentations, 898–899
    prolapsed cord, 897, 899f, 900f
abnormal scar formation, 108–109
abortion, 880
abortion (A), 859
abrasions, 97, 97f
abruptio placentae, 318, 318f, 323, 882–883, 882f
abscess, 107
absence seizure, 591
absent cardiac rhythm, 992–994
absolute refractory period, 462
absorbent dressings, 112
abuse
    bruises, colouring and age of, 1082t
    burns, 150–151
    child abuse, 150–151, 1005, 1012–1016
    crime of, 1086
    domestic elder abuse, 1078, 1079
    elder abuse, 150–151, 1069–1070, 1078–1079, 1080f
    emotional abuse, 1083–1084
    institutional elder abuse, 1078
    mandatory reporting, 1015, 1070, 1084, 1087
    men, abuse by women, 1075
    partner abuse, 1075–1078
    pregnancy complications, and physical abuse, 878
    sexual abuse, 1013
    statistics, 1075
abusers' characteristics
    child abuse, 1080–1081
    elder abusers, 1079, 1080f
    partner abuse, 1077
acalculus cholecystitis, 653
accelerated idioventricular rhythm, 496
accelerated junctional rhythm, 492–493, 492f
acceleration, 15
accessory organ diseases
    appendicitis, 652–653
    cholecystitis, 653–654
    hepatitis, 655–656
    pancreatitis, 654–655
acclimatization, 748
ace bandages, 113
acetaminophen, 753
acetaminophen overdose, 702
acetazolamide, 773
acetylcholinesterase inhibition, 692t
acid stimulators, 644
acids, 696–697
acinar tissue destruction, 654
acini, 654
acquired immune deficiency syndrome (AIDS), 798
acquired immunity, 625
acrocyanosis, 895, 933
action potential, 451
activated charcoal, 686, 703
active immunity, 625
active labour, 877
active rewarming, 757
activity limitations, 515
acute appendicitis, 652
acute arterial occlusion, 561, 563
acute bacteria prostatitis, 677
acute coronary syndrome, 544f
acute cystitis, 677
acute gastroenteritis, 642–643
acute hemodynamic compromise, 727
acute hemorrhage, 72
acute interventions. *See* home care patients
acute lymphocytic leukemia, 736
acute mountain sickness (AMS), 773–774
acute myeologenous leukemia, 736
acute pancreatitis, 654
acute pulmonary embolism, 561
acute renal failure (ARF)
    anuria, 665
    assessment, 667–668
    causes, 666t
    defined, 665
    focused secondary assessment, 668
    glomerular injury, 667
    interstitial nephritis, 667
    management, 669
    microangiopathy, 667
    mortality, 665
    oliguria, 665
    pathophysiology, 666–667
    postrenal ARF, 667
    prerenal ARF, 666
    prevention strategies, 669
    renal ARF, 667
    tubular cell death, 667
acute retinal artery occlusion, 222–223
acute tubular necrosis, 667
acyclovir, 811, 817
addiction, 715
Addisonian crisis, 620
Addison's disease, 619, 620
adenosine (Adenocard), 479, 494
adherent dressings, 112
adhesions, 650, 651f
adhesive bandages, 113
adolescents, 944–945
adrenal gland disorders
    Addison's disease, 619, 620
    adrenal insufficiency, 620
    Cushing's syndrome, 619–620
    hyperadrenalism, 619–620
adrenal insufficiency, 620
adult-onset diabetes, 611–612
adult respiratory distress syndrome (ARDS)
    assessment, 350–351
    defined, 349
    geriatric trauma, 1068

management, 351
mortality, 350
near-drowning, 764
pathophysiology, 350
PEEP ventilator option, 1127
positive end expiratory pressure (PEEP), 351
pulse oximetry, 351
and SARS, 808
symptoms, 350
ventilation, 440
Advair®, 341
advanced airway management
described, 387
endotracheal intubation. *See* endotracheal intubation
Esophageal Tracheal CombiTube (ETC), 417–419, 417f, 418f
field extubation, 416–417
foreign body removal under direct laryngoscopy, 422, 423f
laryngeal mask airway, 419–420, 420f
nasotracheal intubation, 414–417, 415f
orotracheal intubation, 396–414
pharyngo-tracheal lumen airway (PtL), 420–422, 421f
surgical airways, 422–430
advanced care paramedic (ACP) competencies
assessment and diagnostics, 1143–1144
communication, 1142–1143
health and safety, 1143
integration, 1146–1147
professional responsibilities, 1141–1142
therapeutics, 1145–1146
transportation, 1147
advanced directives, 558–559
advanced life support (ALS), 521, 964–970, 1108, 1138–1140
Advanced Pediatric Life Support (APLS), 939
adventitious sounds, 519
AEIOU-TIPS, 582–583
aerosol inhalation, 690
affect, 837
afterbirth, 869
afterload, 450
ageism, 1024
aggregate, 66
aggressive fluid therapy, 68
aging. *See* geriatric patients
agnosia, 841
agonal respirations, 375
air embolism, 767, 770
air hunger, 86
air medical transport, and Golden Hour, 8
air pressure, effects of, 764–765
air splint, 186–187, 193, 194
airbags, 19–20, 1004f
airborne route, 788
airway
asphyxia, 296, 340
assessment, 339–340
bacterial tracheitis, 982–983
edema, 335
evaluation, 226
pediatric assessment, 951
thermal burn, 144–146
trauma, 224
airway adjuncts, pediatric care, 961–963

airway management
see also ventilation
advanced airway management, 387
anaphylaxis, 629
central nervous system injuries, 574
children. *See* pediatric airway management
conscious adult, 348–349
endotracheal intubation. *See* endotracheal intubation
Esophageal Tracheal CombiTube (ETC), 417–419, 417f, 418f
field extubation, 416–417
foreign body removal under direct laryngoscopy, 422, 423f
gastric decompression, 434
head, facial, and neck injury management, 232–234
head-tilt/chin-lift manoeuvre, 373, 380–382, 952
home care patients, 1108
jaw-thrust manoeuvre, 373, 382, 952, 1006f
laryngeal mask airway, 419–420, 420f
lower-airway distress, 983–986
lower-airway foreign-body obstruction, 986
manual airway manoeuvres, 380–383
mechanical airways, basic, 383–386
nasopharyngeal airways, 233–234, 384–385, 385f
nasotracheal intubation, 414–417, 415f
newborns, 912
oropharyngeal airway, 233–234, 385–386, 387f
orotracheal intubation, 396–414
oxygenation, 435–436
patient positioning, 233
pediatric care. *See* pediatric airway management
pediatric trauma, 1006
pharyngo-tracheal lumen airway (PtL), 420–422, 421f
Sellick's manoeuvre, 234, 235, 382–383, 383f, 408
shock, 89
stoma sites, patients with, 431–432
suctioning, 233, 432–433
surgical airways, 422–430
unconscious adult, 348–349
upper airway obstruction, 348–349, 370, 979–980
visualized endotracheal intubation, 131
airway obstruction
aspiration, 372
assessment, 348
complete obstruction, 370
conscious adult, 348–349
foreign bodies, 371
laryngeal spasm and edema, 371
management, 348–349
partial obstruction, 370
relaxed tongue, 348
signs of impending, 146
tongue, 371
trauma, 371
unconscious adult, 348–349
upper airway obstruction, 348–349, 370

alcohol, 335, 642, 644, 654, 716, 717t
alcohol abuse
chronic alcoholism, 583–584, 721f
consequences of chronic alcohol ingestion, 720–722
delirium tremens (DTs), 721
dry mouth syndrome, 719
general alcoholic profile, 720
geriatric patients, 1065–1066
"green tongue syndrome," 720
incidence of, 719
management, 722
physiological effects, 719
rum fits, 721
seizures, 721
withdrawal symptoms, 720–721
alcohol coma, 200
alcohol dependence syndrome, 719
alcohol-induced cellular dehydration, 719
alcohol-related accidents, 29
alcoholism. *See* alcohol abuse
alkalinization, 716
alkalis, 696–697
all-terrain vehicles (ATVs), 34
allergen, 626
allergic reaction
allergen, 626
anaphylaxis. *See* anaphylaxis
angioneurotic edema, 627
assessment, 631
body systems affected by, 624
common allergens, 626
described, 623
histamine, 627
and immune system, 624–626
management, 631–632
medications, 629–631, 632
pathophysiology, 624–627
pediatric emergencies, 990
process, 627
psychological support, 631
severe. *See* anaphylaxis
signs and symptoms, 631t
skin, 628
urticaria, 628, 628f
allergies
defined, 626
delayed hypersensitivity reaction, 626
hypersensitivity, 626
immediate hypersensitivity reactions, 626
to medications, 341, 515
sensitization, 626
alpha particles, 775
alpha radiation, 141
altered mental status, 582–584, 1109–1110
Alzheimer's disease, 599, 1052, 1053
Amanita mushrooms, 706, 706f
amantadine, 814
American College of Surgeons, 4
American Heart Association, 556, 759
American Psychiatric Association (APA), 840
American Sign Language (ASL), 1092
aminophylline, 631
amiodarone (Cordarone), 500
amnesia, 217
amniotic fluid, 870, 879
amniotic sac, 870

ampere, 138
amphetamines, 716, 718*t*
ampulla of Vater, 654
amputations, 101, 101*f*, 125–126, 126*f*
amyotrophic lateral sclerosis (ALS), 295, 335, 601
anabolism, 609
anaerobic metabolites, 69
analgesics, 200, 679, 1008, 1064
anaphylactic shock, 990
anaphylaxis
    agents causing, 624*t*
    airway, protection of, 629
    angioneurotic edema, 627, 628
    antihistamines, 630
    assessment, 628–629
    beta agonists, 630
    bronchospasm, 630
    circulatory shock, 627
    corticosteroids, 630
    described, 623
    epinephrine, 630
    fatal reactions, 626–627
    histamine, 627, 629
    and injection, 627
    insect stings, 626–627
    laryngeal edema, 628, 630
    management of, 629–631
    medications, 629–631
    monitoring devices, 629
    oxygen administration, 630
    parenteral penicillin injections, 626–627
    pathophysiology, 627
    psychological support, 631
    risk of, 623
    signs and symptoms, 631*t*
    skin, 628
    slow-reacting substance of anaphylaxis (SRS-A), 627
    urticaria, 628, 628*f*
    vasopressors, 630
    vital signs, 629
anemia, 72, 337, 670, 733–735
aneurysm, 293, 560–561, 586, 1048
anger, 843
angina pectoris
    angina, 537, 733
    defined, 537
    described, 537
    ECG tracing, 538
    field assessment, 538–539
    geriatric patients, 1046
    management, 539
    Prinzmetal's angina, 537
    S-T segment depression, 539
    stable angina, 537
    unstable angina, 537
angioedema, 627
angioneurotic edema, 627, 628
angiotensin-converting enzyme (ACE) inhibitors, 1063
angiotensin II capillary microcirculation, 84
anguished facial expression, 515
angular impact, 31
angulated knee dislocations, 196*f*
animal bites, 684, 821–823
ankle bandage, 123*f*, 125
ankle dislocations, 196–197

ankle injuries, 196–197
anorexia nervosa, 847, 1030
anoxic hypoxemia, 1037
antepartum, 875
antepartum factors, 908
anterior cord syndrome, 254
anterior descending artery, 448
anterior fascicles, 451
anterior hip dislocations, 191–192, 195
anterior knee dislocations, 195
anterograde amnesia, 217
anti-inflammatory agents, 1064
antibiotics, 106, 341, 861–862
antibodies, 624, 790
anticholinergic agents, 243, 692*t*, 752
anticoagulant therapy, 1130–1131
anticoagulants, 107, 482
anticonvulsant medications, 593
antidepressants, 698–699, 700–701, 1064
antidiuretic hormone (ADH), 888
antidotes, 687–688, 687*t*
antidysrhythmic drugs, 500, 526*t*
antiemetics, 821
antigen, 624, 725, 790
antihistamines, 630
antihypertensives, 1063
antiparkinsonion agents, 1064
antipsychotics, 748, 856, 1064
antipyretics, 753
antiseizure medications, 1064
antivenin, 709, 710, 713
ants. *See* fire ants (*Formicoidea*)
anuria, 665
anxiety, 514, 842
anxiety disorders
    described, 842
    panic attack, 842–843
    phobias, 843
    posttraumatic stress syndrome, 843
aorta, 294, 448
aortic aneurysm, 293, 306
aortic dissection, 1048
aortic rupture, 293–294, 294*f*
aortic valve, 448
APGAR scoring, 895, 896*t*, 911–912, 919
aphasia, 841, 1093–1094
apnea, 336, 593, 909, 928
apnea monitors, 1017
apneustic respiration, 336, 576
appendicitis, 635, 636, 652–653, 879
appendix, 652
apraxia, 841
ARDS. *See* adult respiratory distress syndrome (ARDS)
arm bone fractures, 194
arrhythmia, 465
    see also dysrhythmias
arrows, 51
arsenic, 703
arterial blood pressure, 670
arterial gas embolism (AGE), 767, 770
arterial hemorrhage, 66, 68, 79–80
arteries, 315, 448
arteriosclerosis, 560
arteriovenous malformations, 586
arthritis, 177, 1099
articulation disorders, 1094
artifacts, 452

artificial airways, 1124–1126
artificial monitors, home, 1018
artificial pacemaker rhythm, 505–506, 506*f*
artificially acquired immunity, 625
aseptic meningitis, 817
Asherman chest seal, 132
asphyxia, 296, 340
aspiration, 349, 372, 689
aspirin, 68, 350, 642, 644, 701
assault rifle, 51
assessment
    abdominal trauma, 318–324
    abortion, 880
    abruptio placentae, 883
    acute renal failure (ARF), 667–668
    adult respiratory distress syndrome (ARDS), 350–351
    Addison's disease (adrenal insufficiency), 620
    allergic reaction, 631
    altered mental status, 583
    anaphylaxis, 628–629
    angina pectoris, 538–539
    asthma, 356–357, 984
    AVPU method, 573
    back pain, 604
    bacterial tracheitis, 982
    behavioural emergencies, 836–840
    birth injuries, 935–936
    blast injuries, 37–39
    brochiolitis, 985
    carbon monoxide inhalation, 364
    cardiac arrest, 555
    cardiac tamponade, 549
    cardiogenic shock, 552–553
    cardiovascular emergencies, 511–520
    central nervous system dysfunction, 368
    chemical burns, 161–164
    child abuse, 1015
    chronic bronchitis, 355
    chronic renal failure (CRF), 670–672
    chronic respiratory disorders, 1128–1129
    croup, 980
    Cushing's syndrome, 620
    degenerative neurological disorders, 601
    diabetic ketoacidosis, 614
    diving emergencies, 767
    ectopic pregnancy, 881
    electrical burns, 160–161
    emotional status, 573–574
    emphysema, 352–353
    epiglottitis, 981
    extremities, 180–182
    facial injuries, 225–232
    foreign body aspiration, 983
    fractures, 177–183
    gastrointestinal (GI) emergencies, 636–638
    geriatric patients, 1030–1034
    geriatric trauma, 1069–1070
    gestational diabetes, 886–887
    Graves' disease, 616
    head injuries, 225–232
    headache, 595–596
    heart failure, 547–548
    hematopoietic emergencies, 727–732
    hemorrhage, 74–79
    home care patients, 1114–1118

hyperadrenal crisis, 620
hyperglycemia, 1000
hyperglycemic hyperosmolar nonketotic (HHNK) coma, 615
hypertensive disorders of pregnancy, 884–885
hypertensive emergencies, 551
hyperventilation syndrome, 368
hypoglycemia (insulin shock), 615–616, 998–999
hypothyroidism, 618–619
infectious diseases, 795–797
ingested toxins, 688–689
inhaled toxins, 690
joint injuries, 177–183
lower-airway foreign-body obstruction, 986
lung cancer, 362
meningitis, 997
mental status, 573
muscular injury, 177–183
musculoskeletal trauma, 177–183
myocardial infarction (MI), 541–542
myxedema, 618–619
neck injuries, 225–232
neglected child, 1015
neonatal resuscitation, 918–919
neoplasms, 597–598
nerve dysfunction, 369
neurological emergencies, 572–581
neurovascular function, 185
newborns, 911–912
obstetric patient, 875–878
pediatric anatomy and physiology, 945–949
pediatric hyperglycemia, 1000
pediatric hypoglycemia, 998–999
pediatric patients, 950–959
pediatric poisoning, 1001
pediatric seizures, 996
peripheral vascular emergencies, 562–563
placenta previa, 882
pneumonia, 360–361, 807, 985
poisoning, 1001
pregnant patients, 323–324
preterm labour, 888
pulmonary embolism, 365
radiation burns, 164–165
renal calculi (kidney stones), 676
respiratory muscle dysfunction, 369
respiratory problems, 372–380
respiratory system, 338–347
seizures, 591–592, 996
sexual assault victims, 864–865
shock, 86–89
soft-tissue trauma, 113–118
special-needs children and infants, 1019–1020
spinal cord dysfunction, 369
spinal injury, 256–261
spontaneous abortion, 880
spontaneous pneumothorax, 366
stroke, 587–588
sudden infant death syndrome (SIDS), 1012
suicidal patients, 849
supine-hypotensive syndrome, 885, 886f

surface-absorbed toxins, 691
syncope, 594
thermal burns, 151–156
thoracic trauma, 296–302
thyrotoxic crisis (thyroid storm), 617
toxic inhalation, 363
upper airway obstruction, 348
upper respiratory infection (URI), 359
urinary tract infection (UTI), 678
urological emergencies, 661–664
"weak and dizzy," 596
assessment competencies, 1143–1144
assessment techniques
    inquiry, 117
    inspection, 117–118
    palpation, 118
    soft-tissue trauma, 117–118
asthma
    assessment, 356–357, 984
    children, 351, 358
    defined, 983
    focused history and secondary assessment, 357
    home care patients, 1120–1121
    incidence, 356
    management, 358, 984
    medications, 356
    mortality rate, 356
    pathophysiology, 356, 983–984
    patient history of, 341
    peak expiratory flow rate (PEFR), 357
    pediatric respiratory emergencies, 983–984
    presenting signs, 356
    second phase reaction, 356
    special cases, 358
    status asthmaticus, 358, 984
    triggers, 356, 984
    vital signs, 357
asystole, 503, 503f, 504f, 542, 993–994
ataxia, 1101
ataxic respirations, 336, 576
atelectasis, 287, 762
atherosclerosis, 559–560, 828, 1048
atherosclerotic heart disease (ASHD), 493, 539
athetosis, 1101
athletes. See sports injuries
atracurium (Tracrium), 408
atria, 448
atria, dysrhythmias originating in. See dysrhythmias
atrial depolarization, 456
atrial fibrillation, 481–482, 481f, 585
atrial flutter, 479–481, 480f
atrial syncytium, 450
atrioventricular (AV) bundle, 450
atrioventricular (AV) junction
    accelerated junctional rhythm, 492–493, 492f
    AV blocks, 483–489
    AV node, organization of, 483f
    dysrhythmias sustained or originating in, 489–495
    junctional escape complexes and rhythms, 491–492, 491f
    paroxysmal junctional tachycardia (PJT), 493–495, 494f

premature junctional contractions (PJCs), 489–490, 490f
atrioventricular (AV) sequential pacemakers, 505
atrioventricular blocks (AV blocks)
    classification, 484
    complete block, 487–489, 488f
    described, 483–484
    dysrhythmias, 483–489
    first-degree AV block, 484, 485f
    third-degree AV block, 487–489, 488f
    type I second-degree AV block, 484–485, 486f
    type II second-degree AV block, 486–487, 487f
atropine, 274, 408, 503
atropine sulphate, 556
Atrovent®, 341
attackers' characteristics, 54
atypical angina, 537
augmented leads, 453
aura, 590
auscultation
    cardiovascular emergencies, 518–519
    respiratory problems, 375–377
    respiratory status, 343
auto impacts. See vehicular collisions
auto rollover, 26–27
automatic transport ventilator, 440–441
automaticity of cardiac cells, 451
automobile collisions. See vehicular collisions
automobile restraints, 19–21, 27
autonomic dysfunction, 1049
autonomic hyperreflexia syndrome, 255
autonomic nervous system, 571
autonomic nervous system disorders, 572
autonomic neuropathy, 748
AV blocks. See atrioventricular blocks (AV blocks)
AV junction. See atrioventricular (AV) junction
AV sequential pacemakers, 505
AVPU method, 573, 729
avulsions, 100–101, 100f, 209, 244
axial loading, 24, 251
axial stress, 251–252
axonal disruptions, 213
azithromycin, 500, 828
azole antifungal agents, 500
aztemizole, 500

B cells, 624
Babinski's sign, 260, 260f
back pain
    assessment, 604
    causes of, 603–604
    cysts and tumours, 604
    disc injury, 603
    low back pain, 602–603
    management, 605
    other medical causes, 604
    vertebral injury, 603
bacteria, 784–785, 784f
bacterial gastrointestinal infections, 820
bacterial peritonitis, 315–316
bacterial pneumonia, 360
bacterial spores, 794
bacterial tracheitis, 982–983
bactericidal antibiotics, 785

bacteriostatic antibiotics, 785
bag of waters, 870
bag-valve mask, 438–439, 438f, 921
bag-valve-mask ventilation (BVM
    ventilation), 373, 373f, 382, 394, 439, 920
ballistics
    cavitation, 46
    defined, 46
    drag, 46
    expansion, 48
    fragmentation, 48
    profile, 47
    secondary impacts, 48–49
    shape of bullet, 49
    stability, 47
    trajectory, 46
bandaging
    ace bandages, 113
    adhesive bandages, 113
    anatomical considerations, 122–125
    ankle, 123f, 125
    complications, 125
    cravats, 113
    ears, 123f, 124
    elastic bandages, 113
    elbow, 124
    facial wounds, 123–124
    finger injuries, 124–125
    foot, 123f, 125
    gauze bandages, 113
    groin, 124
    hemorrhage control, 119f, 120–121
    hip, 124
    immobilization, 122
    improvised restraints, 854
    knee, 124
    neck wounds, 124
    objectives of, 118–122
    scalp, 122–123, 123f
    self-adherent roller bandages, 113
    shoulder, 123f, 124
    sterility, 121–122
    triangular bandages, 113
    trunk wounds, 124
    types of, 112
barbiturates, 335, 716, 717t
bark scorpion, 709
barotrauma
    arterial gas embolism (AGE), 770
    decompression illness, 767–769, 768f
    defined, 424
    described, 766
    hyperbaric oxygen chamber, 768
    and needle cricothyrostomy, 424
    nitrogen narcosis, 770–771
    pneumomediastinum, 770
    pulmonary overpressure accidents, 769
    recompression, 768
barrel chest, 353
basal metabolic rate (BMR), 747
basic life support manoeuvres, pediatric, 960t
basilar skull fracture, 210, 221, 222f
basophils, 627
bat rabies, 822
battered patients. See abuse; partner abuse
beclomethasone, 341
Beclovent®, 341
bed sores, 1057, 1058, 1111f

bee stings, 623, 707
behaviour, 834
behavioural change, 515
behavioural emergencies
    see also psychiatric disorders
    assessment, 836–840
    continuum of patient responses, 852f
    defined, 834
    emotional response, 837
    focused history and secondary
        assessment, 837–839
    geriatric patients, 1066–1068
    management, 851–853
    medical care, 852
    mental status examination (MSE), 839
    primary assessment, 837
    psychiatric medications, 839–840
    psychological care, 852–853
    scene assessment, 836–837
    transport considerations, 853–854
    violent patients and restraint, 853–856
belladonna alkaloids, 692t
Bell's palsy, 600
Benadryl, 630
bend fractures, 1010
"the bends," 766
benign prostatic hypertrophy, 660
benign tumours, 597
benzocaine, 243
benzodiazepines, 335, 716, 718t
bereavement, 844
Bernoulli effect, 806
beta-adrenergic blockers, 616, 617
beta agonists, 630
beta-blockers, 480, 482, 716, 748, 1063
beta particles, 776
beta radiation, 142
bigeminy, 497
bilateral periorbital ecchymosis, 210, 210f
bilirubin, 729–730
biological, 835
Biot's respirations, 336, 375
BiPAP (bilevel positive airway pressure),
    1120, 1128
bipolar disorder, 701, 845
bipolar frame device, 187, 188f, 192
bipolar leads, 453, 453t
birds, deaths of, 809
birth injuries, 935–936
black clap, 825
black widow spider bites, 709, 710f
blast injuries
    abdominal injuries, 39–40, 312
    assessment, 37–39
    blast debris, 36
    blast wind, 36
    burns, 37, 40
    causes of, 34
    confined space explosions, 36–37
    disaster triage, 38
    ears, 40
    emergency care, 39–40
    explosion, 35
    flechettes, 36
    incendiary, 37
    magnitude of, 34
    ordnance, 36
    overpressure, 35–36

    oxidizer mixes, 34
    penetrating wounds, 40
    personnel displacement, 36
    phases, 37
    pressure wave, 35–36
    primary blast injuries, 37
    projectiles, 36
    pulmonary injuries, 38, 39
    secondary blast injuries, 37
    structural collapses, 37
    tertiary blast injuries, 37
    thoracic trauma, 278
    underwater detonation, 35
blast wind, 36
blastocyst, 869
bleeding. See hemorrhage
bleeding gums, 731
blepharospasm, 163
blind orotracheal intubation, 402f
blindness, 1031
blocked pancreatic duct, 645
blood
    anemia, 72
    clotting, 66–68
    fluid resuscitation, 89
    hematoma, 71, 97
    transfusion, 83
blood clotting disorders
    thrombocytopenia, 738
    thrombocytosis, 737–738
blood-doping, 772
blood glucometer, 581
blood glucose, regulation of, 610–611
blood glucose test, 999
blood pressure
    arterial blood pressure, 670
    diastolic pressure, 1048
    maintenance, 238–239
    orthostatic hypotension, 78
    pediatric assessment, 957–958
    pulsus paradoxus, 293
    systolic pressure, 1048
    tilt test, 78
blood products, 725–726
blood transfusion, 725–726, 726t
blood transfusion reactions, 726–727
    see also hematopoietic emergencies
blood typing, 725–726
blood vessel trauma, 223–224
bloodborne diseases, 788
blowout fractures, 220
blue bloaters, 355
blunt mediastinal injury, 300
blunt trauma
    abdominal injury, 311–312, 319
    automobile collisions, 16–30
    blast injuries, 34–40
    crush injuries, 43
    defined, 3
    described, 13, 15, 16f
    effects of, 15
    facial injuries, 206–207
    falls, 40–42
    head injuries, 206–207
    heart, effect on, 15
    kinetics of, 13–15
    liver, effect on, 15
    motorcycle collisions, 30–32

neck injuries, 206–207
pedestrian accidents, 32
pediatric trauma, 1009
pregnant women, 315, 318
recreational vehicle accidents, 33–34
sports injuries, 42–43
thoracic injury, 277, 278–279, 299–300
body armour, 48–49
body cavity injuries, 29
body dysmorphic disorder, 846
body lice, 829–830
body substance isolation (BSI) precautions, 75–76, 225, 392, 727–728, 822
body surface area (BSA), 147–148, 157, 948
body temperatures, comparative, 745
bone
    see also fractures
    callus, 176
    osteoporosis, 175
    pediatric considerations, 174–175
    penetrating trauma, 56
    reduction, 190
bone repair cycle, 176
bony fish poisoning, 705
Bordetella pertussis, 816
Borrelia burgdorferi, 824
botulism, 705, 820
bovine spongiform encephalitis (BSE), 786
bowel infarction, 650
bowel injury, 315
bowel obstruction, 650–651, 650f, 1056–1057
Boyle's law, 764
bradycardia, 464, 469, 929, 993f
bradydysrhythmias, 992
bradykinesia, 600
bradypnea, 345
brain abscess, 598
brain attack. *See* stroke
brain injury
    anterograde amnesia, 217
    brainstem pressure, 217
    cerebral contusion, 212
    Cheyne-Stokes respirations, 217
    concussion, 214
    contrecoup injuries, 212, 212f
    coup injuries, 211–212, 212f
    Cushing's reflex, 217
    defined, 211
    diffuse axonal injury (DAI), 214
    diffuse injuries, 213–214
    direct injury, 211–214
    epidural hematoma, 212–213, 213f
    focal injuries, 212–213
    hypotension, 215
    hypoxia, 215
    indirect injury, 214–216
    intracerebral hemorrhage, 213
    intracranial hemorrhage, 212–213
    intracranial perfusion, 214–215
    intracranial pressure, 217f
    moderate diffuse axonal injury, 214
    pathway of deterioration, 216f
    pediatric trauma, 1008
    pressure and structural displacement, 215–216
    retrograde amnesia, 217
    severe diffuse axonal injury, 214

signs and symptoms, 216–218
    subdural hematoma, 213, 213f
brain ischemia, 1050
brainstem pressure, 217
branding, 150
Braxton-Hicks contractions, 887
breathing
    see also respiration
    abnormal breath sounds, 343–344
    adventitious sounds, 519
    assessment of, 340, 518–519
    dyspnea, 39, 285, 340
    management, 89, 237–238
    normal breathing sounds, 343
    orthopnea, 340
    paradoxical breathing, 373
    paroxysmal nocturnal dyspnea, 340
    pediatric assessment, 951–954
    sounds, 376
breech presentation, 896–897, 897f, 898f, 935
brochiolitis, 985
bronchial asthma, 331
bronchitis, 1119–1120
bronchopulmonary dysplasia (BPD), 1121–1122
bronchospasm, 351, 440, 630
Broselow Tape, 439
Broviac catheters, 1130
brown recluse spider bite, 708–709, 709f
Brown-Séquard's syndrome, 254
Brudzinski's sign, 812
bruises, colouring and age of, 1082t
bruit, 477, 577
buckle fractures, 1010
bulimia nervosa, 847
bullet entry wounds, 59
bullets. *See* ballistics; penetrating trauma
bull's eye rash, 824
bundle branch block, 507
bundle of His, 451
bundle of Kent, 510
burn surface area (BSA), 1010
burns
    airway edema, 335
    assessment of chemical burns, 161–164
    assessment of electrical burns, 160–161
    assessment of radiation injury, 164–165
    assessment of thermal burns, 151–156
    blast injuries, 37, 40
    body surface area (BSA), 147–148
    burn surface area (BSA), 1010
    car seat burns, 1081
    caustic substances, 696
    characteristics of various depths of burns, 155t
    chemical burns, 140–141, 141f, 161–164, 163f
    child abuse, 1014f, 1082
    depth of, 146–147, 146f, 153–154
    described, 136
    dressings, 157
    duration of exposure, 137
    electrical burns, 138–140, 139f, 140f, 160–161
    emergent phase, 137
    eschar, 149, 149f, 154–155
    first-degree burn, 146

fluid accumulation in lungs, 349
fluid administration, 158
fluid resuscitation, 158–159
fluid shift phase, 138
focused history and secondary assessment, 153–156
full thickness burns, 147
geriatric trauma, 1072–1073
hydrofluoric (HF) acid, 697–698
hypermetabolic phase, 138
hypothermia, 148–149
hypovolemia, 149, 158
incendiary, 37
infection, 149, 156, 158
inhalation injury, 144–146, 159
injuries that benefit from burn centre care, 156
intravenous routes, establishing, 158
Jackson's theory of thermal wounds, 137
lightning strikes, 160
local burns, 156–157
management of thermal burns, 156–159
minor burns, 156–157
moderate burns, 157–159
ongoing assessment, 156, 166
organ failure, 150
pain of, 158
partial thickness burn, 147
pathophysiology, 136–151
pediatric trauma, 1005, 1010–1011
physical abuse, 150–151, 1014f
primary assessment, 152–153
radiation injury, 141–144, 142f, 164–165
rapid trauma assessment, 153–156
resolution phase, 138
rule of nines, 147, 148f, 153, 1010–1011, 1011f
rule of palms, 148, 148f, 1011
scene assessment, 151–152
second-degree burn, 147
severe burns, 157–159
severity, 155t
special factors affecting treatment and transport, 150
sunburn, 147
superficial burn, 146
systemic complications, 148–151
thermal burns, 136–138, 151–156
third-degree burns, 147
types of, 136–146
zone of coagulation, 137
zone of hyperemia, 137
zone of stasis, 137
zones of injury, 138f
bursitis, 177

C-grip, 439
café coronary, 348, 371
calcium channel blockers, 888–889
calcium fluoride, 697
calcium stones, 675–676
callus, 176
calories, 747
Campylobacter, 820
Campylobacter jejuni, 643, 819
Canadian Institute for Health Information (CIHIs), 248

Canadian Public Health Laboratory Network, 783
cancer, 1099–1100
cancer, lung. *See* lung cancer
cancer of the larynx, 1094
Candida, 678
Candida albicans, 784
capillaries, 448
capillary hemorrhage, 66
capillary microcirculation, 84
capillary refill, 957
capillary washout, 84
capnography, 346, 379–380
capnometry, 346–347, 347
caput succedaneum, 935
car seat burns, 1081
car-*versus*-pedestrian injuries. *See* pedestrian accidents
carbamazepine, 600
carbon dioxide, 332, 334, 346
carbon monoxide (CO) poisoning, 695
carbon monoxide inhalation, 363–364, 364
carbon monoxide poisoning, 6, 144
cardiac arrest, 350, 555–559
cardiac conductive system, 451, 452f
cardiac contusion, 291
cardiac cycle, 450
cardiac decompensation, 1109
cardiac depolarization, 450–451
cardiac dysrhythmias. *See* dysrhythmias
cardiac enzymes, 545
cardiac medication overdose, 696
cardiac output, 450
cardiac physiology, 450
cardiac syncope, 1049
cardiac tamponade, 549–550
cardinal positions of gaze, 575–576
cardiogenic pulmonary edema, 349, 440
cardiogenic shock, 552–553, 554f, 988, 990–994
cardiology
    arrhythmia, 465
    cardiac conductive system, 451, 452f
    cardiac depolarization, 450–451
    cardiac physiology, 450
    cardiovascular anatomy, 448, 449f
    dysrhythmias. *See* dysrhythmias
    electrocardiographic monitoring, 452–465
    electrophysiology, 450–452
    normal sinus rhythm, 465
cardiomyopathy, 991
cardiopulmonary arrest, 955
cardiopulmonary bypass, 350
cardiopulmonary resuscitation (CPR)
    asystole, pediatric, 993–994
    cardiac arrest, 555, 556
    hemorrhage, 79
    impaled objects, removal of, 127
cardiovascular anatomy, 448, 449f
cardiovascular diseases (CVD)
    defined, 447
    incidence of, 447
    mortality rate, 447
    public education, 447–448
    risk factors, 447
cardiovascular emergencies
    acute arterial occlusion, 561, 563

acute pulmonary embolism, 561
advanced life support, 521
aneurysm, 560–561, 1048
angina pectoris, 537–539, 1046
aortic dissection, 1048
assessment. *See* cardiovascular emergency assessment
atherosclerosis, 559–560
basic life support, 521
cardiac arrest, 555–559
cardiac tamponade, 549–550
cardiogenic shock, 552–553, 554f
carotid sinus massage, 536
deep venous thrombosis, 562
defibrillation, 527–528, 529f, 530f
defibrillator pads, 524
dysrhythmias. *See* dysrhythmias
ECG monitoring in the field, 521–525, 522f, 523f
geriatric disorders, 1045–1049
geriatric trauma, 1070
heart failure, 545–549, 1046–1047
home care patients, 1131–1132
hypertensive emergencies, 550–552, 1048–1049
myocardial infarction, 539–545, 1046
noncritical peripheral vascular conditions, 562
peripheral arterial atherosclerotic disease, 562
peripheral vascular emergencies, 559–564
pharmacological interventions, 525, 526t
post-cardiac-arrest management, 556
precordial thump, 525, 525f
prehospital 12-lead ECG monitoring, 564–567, 565f, 566f
resuscitation, 555
return of spontaneous circulation (ROSC), 555
support and communication, 536
survival, 555
synchronized cardioversion, 531, 532f
syncope, 1049
transcutaneous cardiac pacing (TCP), 533, 534f, 535f
vagal manoeuvres, 525
varicose veins, 562
vasculitis, 562
walking and, 1037
withholding resuscitation, 558–559
cardiovascular emergency assessment
    allergies, 515
    auscultation, 518–519
    breath sounds, 518–519
    carotid artery bruit, 519
    chest pain, 512, 513
    common symptoms, 512–515
    coughing, 514
    described, 511–512
    dyspnea, 513–514
    epigastrium, 518, 520
    focused history, 512–517
    heart sounds, 519
    inspection, 517–518
    last oral intake, 516
    medications, and respiratory status, 341
    medications, history of, 515–516

OPQRST questions, 513
other related signs and symptoms, 514–515
palpation, 520
past medical history, 516
peripheral edema, 518
preceding events, 517
presacral edema, 518
primary assessment, 512
pulse rate, 520
scene assessment, 512
secondary assessment, 517–520
skin, changes in, 518
subtle signs of cardiac disease, 518
thorax, 517–518, 520
tracheal position, 517
cardiovascular injuries
    aortic aneurysm, 293
    aortic rupture, 293–294, 294f
    cardiac contusion, 291
    myocardial aneurysm, 293
    myocardial contusion, 290–291, 291f
    myocardial rupture, 293
    other vascular injuries, 294
    pericardial tamponade, 291–293, 292f
    traumatic aneurysm, 293–294
    traumatic rupture, 293–294, 294f
cardiovascular status, 576–577
cardiovascular syphilis, 826
cardiovascular system
    geriatric patients, 1037–1038
    pediatric care, 948–949
    and pregnancy changes, 871–872
carotid artery bruit, 519
carotid artery massage, 477
carotid sinus massage, 536
carpal tunnel syndrome, 572
carpopedal spasm, 344, 367
catabolism, 609
cataracts, 1031, 1032f
catarrhal phase of pertussis, 816
catatonia, 841
catatonic schizophrenia, 842
catecholamine, 73
cations, 697
caustic ingestion, 642
caustic substances, 696–697
cavitation, 46, 53
ceftriaxone, 812
cellular asphyxiant, 694
cellular hypoxia, 83
cellular immunity, 624, 626
cellular ischemia, 83
cellular respiration, 334
cellulitis, 1110
Centers for Disease Control, 799, 800, 808, 813, 822
central cord syndrome, 254
central cyanosis, 921
central IV line, 1018
central nervous system disorders, 570–571
    see also neurological emergencies
central nervous system dysfunction, 368–369
central neurogenic hyperventilation, 336, 375
central pain syndrome, 600
Centre for Emergency Preparedness and Response (CEPR), 783

Centre for Infectious Disease Prevention and Control (CIDPC), 783
Centre for Surveillance Coordination (CSC), 783
cephalopelvic disproportion, 900, 935
cerebral contusion, 212
cerebral homeostasis, 571
cerebral hypoxia, 764. *See* hypoxia
cerebral palsy, 1100–1101
cerebral thrombus, 585
cerebrospinal fluid (CSF), 210
cerebrovascular disease, 1050–1051
cerumen, 1090
cervical collar, 226, 257
cervical collar application, 264
cervical immobilization device (CID), 272
cervical spine immobilization, 975
cervical spine trauma, 224
cesarean section, 890
chain of evidence, 1087
challenged patients
    arthritis, 1099
    cancer, 1099–1100
    cerebral palsy, 1100–1101
    chronic-care patients, 1098–1104
    colostomy, 1096
    cystic fibrosis, 1101–1102
    developmental disabilities, 1096–1098
    Down syndrome, 1097–1098
    emotional impairments, 1096
    fetal alcohol spectrum disorder (FASD), 1098
    hearing impairments, 1090–1092
    mental challenges, 1096
    multiple sclerosis (MS), 1102
    muscular dystrophy (MD), 1102
    myasthenia gravis, 1104
    neutropenic, 1100
    obesity, 1094–1095
    paralysis, 1096
    pathological challenges, 1098–1104
    physical disabilities, 1089–1096
    poliomyelitis (polio), 1102–1103
    postpolio syndrome, 1103
    previous head injuries, 1103
    speech impairments, 1093–1094
    spina bifida (SB), 1103–1104
    visual impairments, 1092–1093
chancroid, 828
chemical burns, 140–141, 141f, 161–164, 163f
chemical peritonitis, 316
chemical restraint, 856
chemotactic factors, 104
chest, pediatric, 947–948
chest compressions, newborns, 922, 923f
chest injuries. *See* chest wall injuries; thoracic trauma
chest pain, 512, 513, 541, 663
chest wall injuries
    blunt injury, 300
    contusion, 281
    described, 280–281
    flail chest, 283–284, 284f, 303, 335
    hypoventilation, 281
    rib fractures, 281–282, 302–303
    sternal fracture and dislocations, 282–283, 303

ventilation disruption, 335
chest wounds
    care of, 62
    heart injuries, assessment of, 62
Cheyne-Stokes respirations, 217, 335–336, 375, 576
chickenpox, 810–811, 1081
child abuse
    abdominal injuries, 1083
    abused children, characteristics of, 1081
    abusers, characteristics of, 1080–1081
    alerting factors, 1013
    assessment, 1015
    bruises, colouring and age of, 1082t
    burns, 150–151, 1014f, 1082
    common conditions mistaken for abuse, 1081
    death in infants, 1013
    defined, 1079
    documentation, 1084
    effects of, 1015f
    emotional abuse, 1083–1084
    forms of, 1080f
    fractures, 1082
    head injuries, 1082
    identification of abused child, 1081–1084
    index of suspicion, 1015
    management, 1015–1016
    mandatory reporting, 1015, 1084, 1087
    marks of, 1014f
    neglect. *See* neglect
    perpetrators of, 1013
    physical abuse, 1005
    resources, 1016
    scalds, 1082
    secondary assessment, 1082–1083
    sexual abuse, 1013, 1085
    shaken baby syndrome, 1082–1083
    types of abuse, 1013
child growth and development
    adolescents, 944–945
    infants, 942–943
    neonates, 942
    newborns, 942
    preschoolers, 943–944
    school-aged children, 944
    toddlers, 943
child safety seats, 21
childbirth. *See* puerperium
children. *See* pediatric care
chlamydia, 827–828, 861
Chlamydia, 678
Chlamydia pneumoniae, 828
Chlamydia trachomatis, 827–828, 861
chlamydial infections, 825
chloracetophenon, 162
chlorpromazine, 856
choanal atresia, 911
cholecystitis, 653–654
cholinergic, 692t
Christmas disease, 738
chronic alcoholism, 583–584
chronic bronchitis
    airway, establishment of, 355
    assessment, 355
    blue bloaters, 355
    described, 354, 354f

    incidence, 351
    management, 355
    pathophysiology, 355
chronic-care patients. *See* home care patients
chronic cholecystitis, 653
chronic gastroenteritis, 643–644
chronic hemorrhage, 72
chronic hypertension, 884
chronic hypertension superimposed with preeclampsia, 884
chronic lymphocytic leukemia, 736
chronic myelogenous leukemia, 736, 738
chronic obstructive pulmonary disease (COPD)
    asthma. *See* asthma
    bronchitis, 1119–1120
    chronic bronchitis, 354–355
    clubbing of fingers, 344
    cor pulmonale, 546
    defined, 331
    described, 1043
    emphysema, 1119–1120. *See* emphysema
    geriatric patients, 1043–1044
    home respiratory support, 1119–1121
    oxygenation, 435
    primary hypertension, 546
    statistics, 351
    upper respiratory infection (URI), 360
chronic renal failure (CRF)
    abdominal assessment, 672
    assessment, 670–672
    causes of, 669t
    described, 669
    disruption of renal functions, 670
    end-stage renal failure, 669
    hemodialysis, 673–674, 673f
    immediate management, 672
    interstitial nephritis, 669
    isosthenuria, 670
    long-term management, 673–674
    management, 672–674
    microangiopathy, 669
    neuromuscular abnormalities, 672
    pathophysiology, 669–670
    peritoneal dialysis, 674, 674f
    prevention strategies, 672
    reduced nephron mass, 670
    reduced renal mass, 670
    renal dialysis, 673
    tubular cell death, 669
    uremia, 670–671, 671t
    uremic frost, 671
chronic respiratory disorders
    artificial airways, 1124–1126
    assessment considerations, 1128–1129
    asthma, 1120–1121
    BiPAP (bilevel positive airway pressure), 1120, 1128
    bronchitis, 1119–1120
    bronchopulmonary dysplasia (BPD), 1121–1122
    chronic obstructive pulmonary disease (COPD), 1119–1121
    congestive heart failure (CHF), 1121
    CPAP (continuous positive airway pressure), 1120, 1128
    cystic fibrosis, 1121
    emphysema, 1119–1120

Guillain-Barré syndrome, 1122
home oxygen therapy, 1123–1124
lung transplantation, awaiting, 1123
management considerations, 1129
muscular dystrophy (MD), 1122
myasthenia gravis, 1122–1123
negative-pressure ventilators, 1127
neuromuscular degenerative diseases,
    1122–1123
PEEP (positive end-expiratory pressure),
    1120, 1127–1128
poliomyelitis (polio), 1122
positive-pressure ventilators, 1127
sleep apnea, 1123
tracheostomy, 1124–1126
ventilators, 1126–1129
chrontotropy, 450
ciguatera (bony fish) poisoning, 705
ciprofloxacin, 812
circulation
    head, facial, and neck injury
        management, 238–239
    pediatric assessment, 954–955
    pediatric emergencies, 970–974
    peripheral circulation, 954
    peripheral circulation, alterations in,
        1109
circumflex artery, 448
cirrhosis, 641–642
clarithramycin, 500
classic heatstroke, 751
clavicular fractures, 193
clean accident, 777
cleft lip, 911
cleft palate, 911
clonic phase, 590
closed fracture, 173, 173f
closed wounds
    see also soft-tissue trauma
    compartment syndrome, 108
    contusions, 96, 97f
    crush injuries, 97, 97f
    epidemiology, 95
    hematoma, 97
    types of, 95, 96–97
Clostridium botulinum, 705, 789, 820, 821
Clostridium tetani, 107, 823
clothesline impact, 207
Clotridium perfringens, 107
clots, 585
clotting, 66–68, 103, 107–108
Cluster A personality disorders, 848
Cluster B personality disorders, 848
Cluster C personality disorders, 848
cluster headaches, 595
CNS disease, 826
co-morbidity, 277
coagulation, 66
coagulation necrosis, 140
cocaine, 716, 717t
cognitive deficits, 841
cognitive disorders
    delirium, 840–841, 1052, 1052t
    dementia, 841, 1052, 1052t, 1053
colchicine, 106
cold disorders
    deep frostbite, 760

frostbite, 759–761, 760f
hypothermia, 753–759
pathophysiology, 744–747
superficial frostbite, 760
cold diuresis, 757
colicky abdominal pain, 647
collagen, 105
Colles' fracture, 194, 198
collisions. See vehicular collisions
colon lesions, 646
colonic diverticula, 649
colostomy, 1096, 1133–1134, 1136f
coma, 570
combative patients, 274
Combivent®, 341
comfort care, 1138–1140
comminuted fracture, 174, 174f, 209
common cold influenza, 814
communicable, 789
communicable disease. See infectious disease
communicable period, 790
communication, 536, 940–942
communication challenges, 1028, 1028t,
    1031–1033
communication competencies, 1142–1143
community-acquired infections, 678
comorbidity, 1026
compact ventilator, 440–441
comparative body temperatures, 745
compartment syndrome
    closed wounds, 108
    crush injuries, 170
    early indicators, 181
    fractures, 170
    muscular injury, 170
    musculoskeletal trauma, 181
    open wounds, 108
    soft-tissue injury management, 130–131
    soft-tissue trauma, 108
compensated hypothermia, 754
compensated shock, 84–85, 85f, 987
compensatory pause, 489
complete block, 487–489, 488f
complex partial seizures, 591
compliance, 377, 1026–1027
compression of spinal cord, 253
concussion, 214
concussion of spinal cord, 253
conduction, 744
conduction disorders
    preexcitation syndromes, 509–510
    ventricular conduction disturbances,
        507–509
    Wolff-Parkinson-White syndrome,
        509–510
conductive deafness, 1090
conductivity of cardiac cells, 451
condyloma acuminatum, 827
confidentiality, 795
confined space explosions, 36–37
confusion, 837, 841, 1025, 1033
congenital aneurysms, 560
congenital anomalies, 910–911
congenital heart disease, 990, 991
congestive heart failure (CHF), 541,
    546–547, 547, 1121
connective tissue, 55, 190, 199
consciousness, 570

consent, 853
conservation of energy, 14, 46
consolidation, 807
contaminated food, 704–705
contamination, 789
continence, 1028–1029
contraception, 859
contractility of cardiac cells, 451
contrecoup injuries, 212, 212f
contusion
    cardiac contusion, 291
    cerebral contusion, 212
    chest wall, 281
    closed wounds, 96, 97f
    muscular injury, 170
    myocardial contusion, 290–291, 291f,
        306
    pulmonary contusion, 289–290
    soft-tissue trauma, 96, 97f
    of spinal cord, 253
convalescent phase of pertussis, 816
convection, 744, 912
conversion disorder, 846
copperheads, 711
cor pulmonale, 352, 546, 1121
coral snake bites, 711, 713–714
core body temperatures (CBT), 746, 747
core temperature, 745
coronary arteries, 448
coronary artery bypass graft (CABG), 545
coronary artery lesions, 545
coronary circulation, 449f
corticosteroids, 630, 817, 888, 1064
cortisone, 106
cottonmouths, 711
coughing, 374, 514
coughing up blood, 340
Council of Chief Medical Officers of Health,
    783
countercurrent heat exchange, 747
coup injuries, 211–212, 212f
coupling interval, 497
CPAP (continuous positive airway pressure),
    1120, 1128
crabs, 829–830
crackles, 343, 376
cramping, 170–171
cranial injury, 209–211, 209f
cranial nerves status, 579
cravats, 113, 188, 854
creatine phosphokinase (CK), 545
crepitus, 282, 342
Creutzfeldt-Jakob disease, 786
cricoid cartilage, 382
cricothyrostomy, 62
cricothyrotomy, 62, 236–237
Crohn's disease, 648
cromolyn sodium, 631
Crotalidae, 711
Crotalus viridis, 711
Crotalus viridis oreganos, 711
Crotus virdidis virdis, 711
croup, 818, 980, 980f
crow die-offs, 809
crowing sounds, 146
crowning, 878
crumple zones, 24, 24f
crush injuries, 97f

associated injuries, 110
blunt trauma, 43
closed soft-tissue wounds, 97
compartment syndrome, 170
defined, 97
described, 109–110
hemorrhage, 82, 110
and normal bleeding control measures, 120
soft-tissue injury management, 128–130
and soft-tissue trauma, 109–110
thoracic trauma, 278
crush syndrome, 97, 110, 128–130
Cryptosporidium parvum, 643, 819
Cullen's sign, 638
culturally diverse patients, 1104–1105
current, 138
Cushing's reflex, 217, 580
Cushing's syndrome, 619–620
cyanide poisoning, 159, 694
cyanosis, 339, 930–931, 954
cyclopeptide mushrooms, 706
Cyclospora cayetansis, 819
Cyclosporidium cayetenis, 643, 644
cystic fibrosis, 1101–1102, 1121
cystic medical necrosis, 560–561
cystine stones, 676
cystitis, 677, 862
cysts, 604, 862
cytomegalovirus (CMV), 1092

Dalton's Law, 765, 771
data, and trauma registry, 10
date rape drug, 716
deafness, 1031, 1090
    see also hearing impairments
death
    regulations pertaining to, 559
    stages of, 1140
deceleration, 15, 40, 278, 289
decerebrate posturing, 578, 578f
decision to transport, 9–10
decompensated shock, 85–86, 987–988
decompression illness, 766, 767–769, 768f
decontaminate, 794
decontamination, 686–687, 794
decorticate posturing, 578, 578f
decubitus ulcers, 1058
deep frostbite, 760
deep suctioning, 916
deep venous thrombosis, 562
deer, 824
deer mouse, 818–819
defibrillation, 527–528, 529f, 530f
defibrillator, 527
defibrillator pads, 524
degenerative conditions, 176–177
degenerative joint disease, 177
degenerative neurological disorders
    Alzheimer's disease, 599
    amyotrophic lateral sclerosis (ALS), 601
    anxiety, 602
    assessment, 601
    Bell's palsy, 600
    central pain syndrome, 600
    communication, 602
    defined, 598
    dystonias, 599

management, 602
mobility, 602
multiple sclerosis (MS), 599
muscular dystrophy (MD), 599
myoclonus, 601
Parkinson's disease, 599–600
poliomyelitis (polio), 601
respiratory compromise, 602
spina bifida (SB), 601
types of, 599–601
degloving injury, 100–101, 101f
degranulation, 627
dehydration, 752, 797, 998t
deja vu, 591
delayed healing, 108
delayed hypersensitivity reaction, 626
DeLee suction trap, 912
delirium, 840–841, 1052, 1052t
delirium tremens (DTs), 721
delivery. *See* puerperium
delivery complications
    breech presentation, 896–897, 897f, 898f
    cephalopelvic disproportion, 900
    limb presentation, 897–898
    maternal complications, 901–903
    meconium staining, 901
    multiple births, 899–900
    occiput posterior position, 898
    other abnormal presentations, 898–899
    precipitous delivery, 900–901
    prolapsed cord, 897, 899f, 900f
    shoulder dystocia, 901
delta hepatitis, 803
delta wave, 510, 510f
delusions, 841
demand pacemaker, 505
dementia, 841, 1052, 1052t, 1053
demographics, 1023–1025
demylenation, 1122
denature, 137
dental injury, 220
dependence, 715, 846
depersonalization, 847
depolarized, 450
depression, 843–844, 1067
detailed secondary assessment
    facial injuries, 232
    head injuries, 232
    musculoskeletal trauma, 182
    neck injuries, 232
    shock, 88
    soft-tissue trauma, 117
developmental disabilities
    accommodations for, 1097
    causes of, 1096–1097
    described, 1096
    Down syndrome, 1097–1098
    fetal alcohol spectrum disorder (FASD), 1098
dexamethasone, 616, 630
dextrose, 243, 615, 931
diabetes mellitus
    blood glucose, regulation of, 610–611
    described, 608
    diabetic emergencies, 612t, 613t
    diabetic retinopathy, 1092
    geriatric patients, 1038, 1054–1055

gestational diabetes, 876, 886–887
glucose metabolism, 609–610, 609t
glycosuria, 611
hyperglycemia, 610, 611
incidence of, 608–609
influenza vaccination, 814
osmotic diuresis, 611
Type I diabetes mellitus, 611
Type II diabetes mellitus, 611–612
diabetic coma. *See* diabetic ketoacidosis
diabetic emergencies
    diabetic ketoacidosis (diabetic coma), 610, 612–614, 1000
    diagnostic signs by system, 613t
    hyperglycemia, 1000, 1000t
    hyperglycemic hyperosmolar nonketotic (HHNK) coma, 612, 614–615
    hypoglycemia (insulin shock), 615–616, 998–999
    pediatric emergencies, 998
    types of, described, 612t
diabetic ketoacidosis (diabetic coma)
    assessment, 614
    defined, 612
    ketosis, 610
    Kussmaul's respirations, 613
    management, 614
    pathophysiology, 613
    pediatric emergencies, 1000
    signs and symptoms, 613–614
diabetic retinopathy, 1092
diabetogenic effect of pregnancy, 886
Diagnostic and Statistical Manual of Mental Disorders, Fourth Edition *(DSM-IV)*, 840
diagnostic testing
    capnography, 379–380
    capnometry, 346–347
    end-tidal CO_2 detector, 347f, 379, 379f
    esophageal detector device, 380, 381f
    peak expiratory flow rate (PEFR), 346, 346f, 380
    pulse oximetry, 345, 345f, 377–379, 378f
    respiratory status, 345–347
diagnostics competencies, 1143–1144
dialysate, 673
dialysis, 659, 673–674
dialysis shunts, 1130
diaphoresis, 339, 514
diaphragm
    tears, 313
    traumatic rupture or perforation of, 295, 335
    ventilation disruption, 335
diaphragmatic hernia, 910, 928–929, 929f
diarrhea
    food poisoning, 820–821
    gastroenteritis, 820
    gastrointestinal emergencies, 637, 662
        see also gastrointestinal (GI) emergencies
    neonatal emergencies, 934–935
    pediatric emergencies, 998
    urological emergencies. *See* urological emergencies
diastole, 450
diastolic pressure, 1048
diazepam (Valium®), 200, 235, 241–242, 716, 843, 996

diet-induced thermogenesis, 744
diffuse axonal injury (DAI), 214
diffuse injuries, 213–214
diffusion, 332, 337
digital intubation, 234–235, 258, 402–404, 403f, 404f
digitalis, 553, 1064
digoxin, 480, 482, 553
dilation stage, 889–890
diltiazem (Cardizem), 480, 482
dino-flagellate-contaminated shellfish, 705
diphenhydramine, 630
diphenhydramine hydrochloride, 707
diphtheria-pertussis-tetanus (DTP) vaccine, 816
diplopia, 220
direct injury (brain), 211–214
direct injury (projectile), 52–53
direct pressure, 68, 79–80, 120, 131
directed intubation, 235
dirty accident, 778
disaster triage, in blast injuries, 38
disc injury, 603
disease period, 790
disinfection, 794
dislocations
    angulated knee dislocations, 196f
    ankle dislocations, 196–197
    anterior hip dislocations, 191–192, 195
    defined, 172
    facial injuries, 219–221
    knee dislocation, 172f
    knee dislocation reduction, 196f
    mandibular dislocation, 219
    patellar dislocations, 195
    posterior hip dislocation, 195
    posterior knee dislocations, 196
    reduction, 190
    sternal dislocations, 282–283
    sternoclavicular dislocation, 303
dislodged teeth, 246
disopyramide, 500
disorganized schizophrenia, 842
disorganized speech, 841
disruption, 295–296, 306
dissecting abdominal aortic artery, 635–636
dissecting aortic aneurysms, 560–561
disseminated intravascular coagulation (DIC), 727, 739
dissociative disorders, 847
distal neurovascular function, 198
distention, 635
distraction, 251–252
distressed newborns. See neonatal distress
distributive shock, 989–990
district trauma centre (DTC), 5
disturbance in executive functioning, 841
diuresis, 611, 716
diuretics, 240, 748, 1063
Divers Alert Network (DAN), 771
diverticula, 649
diverticulitis, 649
diverticulosis, 646, 649
diving emergencies
    air embolism, 767
    air pressure, effects of, 764–765
    arterial gas embolism (AGE), 767, 770
    ascent, injuries during, 766–767

assessment, 767
    barotrauma, 766, 767–771
    "the bends," 766
    the bottom, injuries on, 766
    Boyle's law, 764
    classification of diving injuries, 766–767
    Dalton's Law, 765
    decompression illness, 766, 767–769, 768f
    descent, injuries during, 766
    diving injury immobilization, 272–273
    Henry's Law, 765
    nitrogen narcosis, 766, 770–771
    pathophysiology, 765
    pneumomediastinum, 767, 770
    pneumothorax, 767
    pressure disorders, 766, 767–771
    pulmonary overpressure, 766–767
    pulmonary overpressure accidents, 769
    "the squeeze," 766
    surface injuries, 766
dizziness, 1051
dizzy, 596–597
do not resuscitate (DNR) order, 1108, 1118
dobutamine (Dobutrex), 548, 553, 556, 975
documentation of sexual assault, 866
domestic elder abuse, 1078, 1079
dopamine (Intropin®), 273, 548, 553, 556, 630, 925t, 975
down-and-under pathway, 22
Down syndrome, 1097–1098
down time, 555
doxycycline, 828
drag, 46
dressings
    see also bandaging
    absorbent/nonabsorbent dressings, 112
    adherent/nonadherent dressings, 112
    burns, 157
    hemorrhage control, 119f, 120–121
    objectives of, 118–122
    occlusive/nonocclusive dressings, 111f, 112, 132
    size of, 125
    sterile/nonsterile dressings, 111–112, 111f
    sterility, 121–122
    types of, 112
    wet/dry dressings, 112–113
dromotrophy, 450
drowning
    defined, 761
    dry, 761–762
    fresh-water, 762
    incidence, 761
    pathophysiology, 761–763, 762f
    pediatric trauma, 1004–1005
    saltwater, 762–763
    survival, factors affecting, 763
    wet, 761–762
drug abuse, 1065
    see also substance abuse
drug overdose. See overdose
drug resistance, 804
drugs. See medications; pharmacological interventions
drugs of abuse
    commonly abused drugs, 716, 717–718t

sexual purposes, drugs used for, 716
dry dressings, 112–113
dry drowning, 761–762
dry lime, 162, 163f
dual-chambered pacemakers, 505
Duchenne, 599
ductus arteriosus, 874, 909
ductus venosus, 874
duodenal ulcers, 644, 645
$D_{50}W$, 716
dysarthria, 1094
dysmenorrhea, 858
dyspareunia, 858, 863
dysphagia, 1026
dysphoria, 1067
dyspnea, 39, 285, 340, 374, 513–514, 1042f
dysrhythmias
    absent cardiac rhythm, 992–994
    accelerated idioventricular rhythm, 496
    accelerated junctional rhythm, 492–493, 492f
    artificial pacemaker rhythm, 505–506, 506f
    asystole, 503, 503f, 504f, 542, 993–994
    atrial fibrillation, 481–482, 481f
    atrial flutter, 479–481, 480f
    atrioventricular blocks, 483–489
    bradycardia, 469, 993f
    bradydysrhythmias, 992
    causes of, 465
    classification, 466
    complete block, 487–489, 488f
    defined, 465
    ECG changes due to electrolyte abnormalities and hypothermia, 510
    ectopic beat, 466
    ectopic foci, 466
    enhanced automaticity, 466
    first-degree AV block, 484, 485f
    geriatric patients, 1047–1048
    in healthy heart, 465
    heart failure and, 545
    importance of, 483
    junctional escape complexes and rhythms, 491–492, 491f
    mechanism of impulse formation, 465–466
    multifocal atrial tachycardia (MAT), 474–475, 474f
    myocardial contusion and, 291
    and myocardial infarction (MI), 540, 542
    originating in atria, 472–482
    originating in SA node, 466–472
    originating in ventricles, 495–507
    originating within AV junction (AV blocks), 483–489
    paroxysmal junctional tachycardia (PJT), 493–495, 494f
    paroxysmal supraventricular tachycardia (PSVT), 476–479, 477f
    pediatric shock, 991–994
    preexcitation syndromes, 509–510
    premature atrial contractions (PACs), 475, 476f
    premature junctional contractions (PJCs), 489–490, 490f
    premature ventricular contractions (PVC), 497–499, 498f

pulseless electrical activity (PEA), 507, 508f, 994
pulseless ventricular tachycardia (VF/VT), 994
reentry, 466
resulting from conduction disorders, 507–510
sinus arrest, 471–472, 472f
sinus bradycardia, 467–468, 467f, 469f
sinus dysrhythmia, 470, 471f
sinus tachycardia, 468, 470f
supraventricular tachycardia, 992
sustained or originating in AV junction, 489–495
tachycardia, 478f
tachydysrhythmias, 991
third-degree AV block, 487–489, 488f
torsade de pointes, 500–501, 501f
type I second-degree AV block, 484–485, 486f
type II second-degree AV block, 486–487, 487f
ventricular conduction disturbances, 507–509
ventricular escape complexes and rhythms, 295–296
ventricular fibrillation, 501–502, 502f, 994
ventricular tachycardia (VT), 499–501, 500f
ventricular tachycardia (VT) with a pulse, 992
wandering atrial pacemaker, 473–474, 473f
Wolff-Parkinson-White syndrome, 509–510, 510f
dystonias, 599
dysuria, 862

ears
bandaging, 123f, 124
blast injuries, 40
hearing impairments. See hearing impairments
injuries, 221
pinnal injury, 244–245
earwax, 1090
eating disorders, 847
ecchymosis, 96, 640
ecchymosis in the flank, 638
ECG graph paper, 455–456, 456f
ECG leads, 453
eclampsia, 883–884, 885
Ecstasy, 716
ectopic beat, 466
ectopic foci, 466
ectopic pregnancy, 863, 880–881
edema
airway edema, 335
angioedema, 627
angioneurotic edema, 627
cardiogenic pulmonary edema, 349, 440
control, and soft-tissue injury management, 122
extremities, 514
of feet, and acute renal failure (ARF), 669f

high-altitude cerebral edema (HACE), 774–775
high-altitude pulmonary edema (HAPE), 774
laryngeal edema, 371, 628, 630
noncardiogenic pulmonary adult/edema respiratory distress syndrome, 349–351
peripheral edema, 518
presacral edema, 514, 518
pulmonary edema, 546, 547, 548, 554f
sacral edema, 514
effacement, 887, 889
egophony, 361
Einthoven's triangle, 453, 454, 454f
ejection, 24, 27, 31
ejection fraction, 450
Elapidae, 711
elastic bandages, 113
elbow
bandaging, 124
injuries, 198
elder abuse, 150–151, 1069–1070, 1078–1079, 1080f
the elderly
see also geriatric emergencies; geriatric patients
ageism, 1024
defined, 1023
demographics, 1023–1025
epidemiology, 1023–1025
geriatrics, 1024
gerontology, 1024
old-old, 1026
population characteristics, 1023–1024
prevention, 1025, 1025t
self-help, 1025
societal issues, 1024
women, 1024
electrical alternans, 293
electrical burns, 138–140, 139f, 140f, 160–161
electrical mechanical dissociation, 507
electrical therapy
atrial fibrillation, 482
atrial flutter, 480
paroxysmal junctional tachycardia (PJT), 494
paroxysmal supraventricular tachycardia (PSVT), 479
pediatric emergencies, 974
electrocardiogram (ECG)
absolute refractory period, 462
amplitude of deflection, 455
analyzing rate, 464
analyzing rhythm, 464
artifacts, 452
atrial contraction, 458f
atrial depolarization, 456
atrial excitation, 459f
augmented leads, 453
bipolar leads, 453, 453t
bradycardia, 464
chest electrodes, 524
defibrillator pads, 524
defined, 452
ECG graph paper, 455–456, 456f
ECG lead groupings, 463t

ECG leads, 453
ECG rhythm, changes to, 576–577
Einthoven's triangle, 453, 454, 454f
electrical events of the heart, relationship to, 456–463, 457f
electrical excitation of ventricles, 460f
electrocardiogram (ECG), 452–456
field monitoring of, 521–525, 522f, 523f
heart rate calculatory rulers, 464
hyperkalemia, signs of, 668f
impulse delay at AV junction, 460f
impulse initiation in SA node, 458f
isoelectric line, 452
Lead II, 454
lead systems and heart surfaces, 463
modified chest lead 1 (MCL$_1$), 454
negative impulses, 452
normal interval durations, 461
P-R interval (PRI), 460f, 461, 465
P wave, 456, 458f, 459f, 464–465
pediatric assessment, 958–959
poor signals, 524
poor tracings, 524
positive impulses, 452
precordial leads, 453
prehospital 12-lead ECG monitoring, 564–567, 565f, 566f
prolonged QT interval, 461
Q wave, 456
QRS complex, 456, 460f, 465
QRS interval, 461
QT interval, 461
R-R interval, 464
R wave, 456
refractory period, 462, 462f
relative refractory period, 462
rhythm strips, interpretation of, 452, 463–465
routine ECG monitoring, 454–455
S-T segment, 461, 462
S wave, 456
six-second method, 464
T wave, 456, 461f
tachycardia, 464
time intervals, 461
triplicate method, 464
U wave, 456
unipolar leads, 453
ventricular depolarization, 456, 461
ventricular repolarization, 456, 461f
electrocardiographic monitoring. See electrocardiogram (ECG)
electrocution, 252
electrolyte abnormalities, 510, 997
electrolyte administration, 90
electrolyte balances, 450
electrons, 775
electrophysiology
cardiac conductive system, 451, 452f
cardiac depolarization, 450–451
described, 450
elimination problems, 1029, 1029t
emboli, 39, 350, 1137
embolic strokes, 585
embolus, 585
embryonic stage, 872
emergent phase, 137

emesis, 1115
emotional abuse, 1083–1084
emotional impairments, 1096
emotional response, 837
emotional status, assessment of, 573–574
emotional support, 244
emphysema
    acute respiratory infections, 352
    airway, establishment of, 355
    assessment, 352–353
    barrel chest, 353
    cardiac dysrhythmias, 352
    cigarette smoking and, 352
    home care patients, 1119–1120
    management, 353
    pathophysiology, 352
    pink puffers, 353
    secondary assessment, 353
    typical patient appearance, 354f
empyema, 335
EMS system, and injury prevention, 10
encephalitic phase of rabies, 822
encephalomyelitis, 822
end-organ perfusion, 954
end-stage renal failure, 659, 669
end-tidal CO$_2$ detector, 347f, 379, 379f, 392, 581
endobronchial intubation, 395
endocardium, 448
endocrine glands, 607–608, 608t
endocrine system, 607, 1038–1039
endocrinological emergencies
    Addison's disease, 619, 620
    adrenal gland disorders, 619–620
    adrenal insufficiency, 620
    Cushing's syndrome, 619–620
    diabetes mellitus, 608–612, 1054–1055
    diabetic emergencies, 612t, 613t
    diabetic ketoacidosis (diabetic coma), 610, 612–614
    geriatric disorders, 1054–1055
    Graves' disease, 616
    hyperadrenalism, 619–620
    hyperglycemic hyperosmolar nonketotic (HHNK) coma, 612, 614–615
    hypoglycemia, 615–616
    hypothyroidism, 616, 618–619
    Marfan's syndrome, 1039
    myxedema, 616, 618–619
    myxedema coma, 618
    pancreas, disorders of, 608–616
    pediatric emergencies, 998–1001
    thyroid gland disorders, 616–619, 1055
    thyrotoxic crisis, 617
endometriosis, 862–863
endometritis, 862
endotoxins, 785
endotracheal intubation
    additional airways, 392
    advantages of, 393
    blind orotracheal intubation, 402f
    complications of, 393–395
    confirmation of tube placement, 236
    described, 388
    digital intubation, 234–235, 402–404, 403f, 404f
    directed intubation, 235
    disadvantages of, 393

end-tidal CO$_2$ detector, 392
endobronchial intubation, 395
endotracheal tubes (ETT), 389–391, 390f, 391f, 394, 399–400
epiglottitis, presence of, 393
equipment, 388–392
equipment malfunctions, 393
esophageal intubation, 394
Esophageal-Tracheal CombiTubes (ETC), 965
hypoxia, 394
illustration of, 397f
with in-line stabilization, 406f
indications, 392–393
infant/child endotracheal tubes, 966t
laryngoscope, 388–389, 388f, 389f, 390f, 394
lighted stylet, 400f
lubricants, 392
Magill forceps, 392, 392f
nasotracheal intubation, 235
neonatal resuscitation, 920f
neuromuscular blockers, 408
orotracheal intubation, 234, 396–414
paralytic agents, 407
pediatric intubation, 410–414, 411t, 413f, 965–969, 968f
protective equipment, 392
rapid sequence intubation (RSI), 235–236, 405–410
retrograde intubation, 410
Sellick's manoeuvre, 234, 235, 382–383
soft-tissue lacerations, 393–394
stylet, 391, 391f, 400f
suction unit, 392
syringe, 391, 391f
teeth breakage, 393–394
tension pneumothorax, 395
transillumination intubation, 400–402, 401f
trauma patient intubation, 405
tube-holding devices, 391–392
verification of proper ETT placement, 399–400
endotracheal tubes (ETT), 389–391, 390f, 391f, 394, 399–400
energy, 14
Engerix B, 802
enhanced automaticity, 466
entero-hepatic circulation, 703
Enterobacter, 643
Enterobacter aerogenes, 819
Enterobacteriaceae, 783
enterotoxins, 705
enteroviruses, 811
entrance wounds, 58–59
enucleation, 1092
environment, 836
environmental emergencies
    cold disorders, 753–760
    defined, 743
    diving emergencies, 764–771
    drowning, 761–764
    and environmental factors, 743
    fever (pyrexia), 752–753
    frostbite, 759–761, 760f
    geriatric emergencies, 1061–1062
    heat disorders, 747–753

    heat exhaustion, 749–750
    heat illness, 747
    heat (muscle) cramps, 749
    heatstroke, 750–752, 1061
    high-altitude illness, 771–775
    homeostasis, 743–744
    hyperthermia, 747–749, 1061, 1062
    hypothermia, 753–759, 1061–1062
    near-drowning, 761–764
    nuclear radiation, 775–778
    pathophysiology, 744–747
    thermal gradient, 744
environmental factors, 743
epidural hematoma, 212–213, 213f
epiglottitis, 335, 393, 817–818, 980–982, 980f
epilepsy, 590. *See* seizures
epinephrine, 351–352, 503, 507, 556, 630, 925t, 975, 984
epiphyseal fracture, 175, 202
epistaxis, 71, 221, 1048
epithelialization, 104
Epstein-Barr virus (EBV), 817
equipment malfunction (home care), 1111–1112
erythema, 96
erythema migrans, 824
Erythroblastosis fetalis, 726
erythromycin (PCE), 500, 828
eschar, 149, 149f, 154–155, 696
Escherichia coli, 643, 705, 819, 821
Escherichia coli O157:H7, 820
esophageal detector device, 380, 381f
esophageal intubation, 394
esophageal rupture, traumatic, 295
Esophageal Tracheal CombiTube (ETC), 417–419, 417f, 418f, 965
esophageal varices, 72, 641–642, 641f
estimated date of confinement (EDC), 872
ethylene glycol, 719
evaporation, 745
evisceration, 313
excessive rotation, 251
excitability of cardiac cells, 451
exclusion criteria for termination of resuscitation, 558
executive functioning, disturbance in, 841
exertional heatstroke, 751
exertional metabolic rate, 747
exit wounds, 59
exocrine disorder, 1121
exocrine glands, 607
exotoxins, 705, 785
expansion (bullets), 48
expiration, 332
explosions, 34, 35
    see also blast injuries
expulsion stage, 890
exsanguination, 15
external cardiac pacing, 533, 534f, 535f
external hemorrhage, 68–69
extraocular movement, 575–576
extrapyramidal, 693t
extrauterine life, 909
extravascular space, 138
extremes of motion, 249–251
extremities
    acrocyanosis, 933

assessment, 180–182
distal extremity, evaluation of, 181
edema, 514
fractures. *See* fractures
pediatric care, 948
pediatric trauma, 1010
penetrating trauma, 56–57
peripheral cyanosis, 344
physical examination of, 344
potential upper extremity injury, 181
six Ps, 180
extubation, 371
eyes
acute retinal artery occlusion, 222–223
assessment, 575–576
blepharospasm, 163
cardinal positions of gaze, 575–576
chemical burns and, 163
diplopia, 220
and expanding cranial lesion, 218
head injury, 218–219
hyphema, 222
injuries, 222–223
injury management, 245–246, 245f
retinal detachment, 223
subconjunctival hemorrhage, 222
visual impairments. *See* visual impairments

face, assessment of, 575
facial injuries
airway evaluation, 226
assessment, 225–232
blowout fractures, 220
blunt injury, 206–207
breathing, monitoring, 226–227
circulation, evaluation of, 227
dental injury, 220
detailed secondary assessment, 232
dislocations, 219–221
ear injuries, 221
eye injuries, 222–223
focused history and secondary assessment, 231
fractures, 219–221
Glasgow Coma Scale (GCS), 230–231, 230t
Le Fort criteria, 219–220, 220f
management. *See* head, facial, and neck injury management
mandible fractures, 219
mandibular dislocation, 219
maxillary fractures, 219–220
mechanisms of injury, 206–207
nasal injury, 221
ongoing assessment, 232
orbital fractures, 220
pathophysiology, 219–223
penetrating trauma, 207
primary assessment, 225–227
rapid trauma assessment, 227–231
respiration and, 219
scene assessment, 225
soft-tissue injuries, 219
suicide attempts, 220–221
vital signs, monitoring of, 231
zygomatic fractures, 220

facial wounds
bandaging, 123–124
care of, 61–62
cricothyrostomy, 62
cricothyrotomy, 62
soft-tissue injury management, 131, 131f
factitious disorders, 846–847
falls
blunt trauma, 40–42
common fractures, 41
evaluation of, 42
geriatric patients, 42, 1027–1028, 1071–1072
pediatric trauma, 1003, 1003f
false labour, 887
fascia, 71
fasciculations, 241
fatal familial insomnia, 786
fatigue, 514
fatigue fracture, 174, 174f
fatigue (muscle), 170
fear, 837
febrile nonhemolytic reaction, 727
febrile seizures, 996
fecal-oral transmission, 643–644, 788, 803, 819, 820
femur fractures, 191–192
fentanyl analgesia, 157
fentanyl (Sublimaze®), 201, 242–243
fetal alcohol spectrum disorder (FASD), 1098
fetal circulation, 873–874, 874f
fetal development, 872–873, 873f
fetal heart tones (FHTs), 872
fetal stage, 872
fever (pyrexia), 752–753, 932
fibrin, 66
fibrin formation cascade, 108
fibroblasts, 105
fibula fractures, 192–193
field assessment. *See* assessment
field delivery, 891–894
field extubation, 416–417
field intubation, 153
fingers
bandaging, 124–125
clubbing, 344, 344f, 353
fractures, 198–199
fire, 151
see also burns
fire ants *(Formicoidea)*, 627, 707
firearms. *See* weapons
first-degree AV block, 484, 485f
first-degree burn, 146
fish, toxins in, 705
fixed-rate pacemakers, 505
flail chest, 283–284, 284f, 303, 335, 373
flashover danger, 151
flat affect, 841
flechettes, 36
Flovent®, 341
flu, 813–814
fluency disorders, 1094
fluid administration, 689–690, 1007
fluid resuscitation, 89–90, 158–159, 239, 614, 617, 620, 821
fluid shift phase, 138
fluid therapy, 973
flumazenil, 716

flunitrazepam, 716
fluticasone, 341
flutter valve, 304f
focal clonic seizures, 932
focal injuries, 212–213
focused history and secondary assessment
asthma, 357
behavioural emergencies, 837–839
cardiovascular emergencies, 512–517
facial injuries, 231
head injuries, 231
hematopoietic emergencies, 728–732
hemorrhage, 77–79
home care patients, 1116–1118
musculoskeletal trauma, 179–182
neck injuries, 231
neurological emergencies, 574–581
pediatric assessment, 956–959
respiratory problems, 373–380
respiratory status, 340–347
shock, 87–89
soft-tissue trauma, 115–117
thermal burns, 153–156
focused trauma assessment
hemorrhage, 78
soft-tissue trauma, 116–117
folk medicine, 1104
follicle stimulating hormone (FSH), 868
food, contaminated, 704–705
food poisoning, 704–705, 820–821
foodborne illnesses, 788
foot bandage, 123f, 125
foot injuries, 197
foramen ovale, 874
force, 15, 40
foreign bodies, 371
foreign body airway obstruction (FBAO), 960, 964–965
foreign body aspiration, 335, 983
foreign body removal under direct laryngoscopy, 422, 423f
formable splints, 186, 194f
fracture care
see also fractures
arm bone fractures, 194
clavicular fractures, 193
Colles' fracture, 194
femur fractures, 191–192
fibula fractures, 192–193
fingers, 198–199
generally, 191–195
humerus fractures, 193–194
leg bone fractures, 192–193
long spine board, 192
pelvic fracture, 191
pelvic ring fractures, 191
proximal fractures, 191
radius fractures, 194
silver fork deformity, 194
tibia fractures, 192–193
ulna fractures, 194
wrist fractures, 198
fractures
see also fracture care
assessment, 177–183
basilar skull fracture, 210, 221, 222f
bend fractures, 1010
blowout fractures, 220

bone repair cycle, 176
buckle fractures, 1010
callus, 176
causes of, 172
child abuse, 1082
closed fracture, 173, 173*f*
Colles' fracture, 198
comminuted fracture, 174, 174*f*
compartment syndrome, 170
described, 172–173
epiphyseal fracture, 175, 202
facial injuries, 219–221
falls, 41
fatigue fracture, 174, 174*f*
fracture care, 189
geriatric considerations, 175, 1072
greenstick fracture, 175, 202, 1010
hairline fracture, 173
hypovolemia, 179
impacted fracture, 173, 174*f*
Le Fort criteria, 219–220, 220*f*
long bone fracture, 176
mandible, 219
maxillary fractures, 219–220
oblique fracture, 174, 174*f*
open fracture, 173, 173*f*
orbital fractures, 220
pathological fractures, 175, 740
pediatric considerations, 174–175
pelvic fracture, 179, 316
rib fractures, 281–282, 302–303
shaft fractures, 176
silver fork deformity, 198
skull fractures, 209–211, 209*f*
spiral fracture, 174, 174*f*
and stability, 176
sternal fractures, 282–283
subcapital femoral neck fracture, 1072*f*
transverse fracture, 174, 174*f*
types of, 173, 174*f*
zygomatic fractures, 220
fragmentation (bullets), 48
Frank-Starling reflex, 255
French, 384
fresh-water drowning, 762
frontal impact, 278*f*
axial loading, 24
crumple zones, 24, 24*f*
down-and-under pathway, 22
ejection, 24
motorcycles, 31
"paper bag" syndrome, 22, 23*f*
up-and-over pathway, 22–24, 23*f*
frostbite, 759–761, 760*f*
frostnip, 760
fugue state, 847
full thickness burns, 147
fulminant meningitis, 997
functional impairment, 1025
fundal height, 877
fungal pneumonia, 360
fungi, 786–787
furosemide (Lasix®), 240, 548, 553, 726–727

Galerina mushrooms, 706, 706*f*
gallbladder, 313, 654
see also abdominal trauma
gallstones, 653, 879

gambling, pathological, 849
gamma radiation, 143
gamma rays, 776
gangrene, 107, 1109
gas exchange processes, 331–334
gas gangrene, 823
gastric decompression, 434
gastric feeding tubes, 1018–1019
gastric lavage, 686
gastric ulcers, 644, 645
gastritis, 639, 642
gastroenteritis, 642, 819–820, 997
gastrointestinal bacteria, 372
gastrointestinal bleeding, 72
gastrointestinal (GI) emergencies
    accessory organ diseases, 652–656
    acute gastroenteritis, 642–643
    appendicitis, 652–653
    assessment, 636–638
    bowel obstruction, 650–651, 650*f*,
        1056–1057
    cholecystitis, 653–654
    chronic gastroenteritis, 643–644
    Crohn's disease, 648
    Cullen's sign, 638
    distention, 635
    diverticulitis, 649
    esophageal varices, 641–642, 641*f*
    fluid loss, signs of, 638
    geriatric emergencies, 1055–1057
    GI bleeding, 1056
    Grey-Turner's sign, 638
    hemorrhoids, 649–650
    hepatitis, 655–656
    history, 636–638
    home care patients, 1110, 1132–1135
    inflammation, 635
    intravenous therapy, 638
    ischemia, 635
    lower gastrointestinal bleeding, 646–647
    lower gastrointestinal diseases, 646–652
    lower GI bleed, 1056
    melena, 1056
    mesenteric infarct, 1057
    OPQRST-ASPN history, 636–637
    pain, 635
    palpation of abdomen, 638
    pancreatitis, 654–655
    past medical history, 637–638
    pathophysiology, 635–636
    pediatric emergencies, 997–998
    peptic ulcers, 644–646, 645*f*
    primary assessment, 636
    referred pain, 635–636, 637
    SAMPLE history, 636, 637
    scene assessment, 636
    secondary assessment, 638
    somatic pain, 635
    statistics, 634
    treatment (general), 638–639
    ulcerative colitis, 647–648
    upper gastrointestinal bleeding, 639–641
    upper gastrointestinal disease, 639–646
    upper GI bleed, 1056
    visceral pain, 635
gastrointestinal system
    food poisoning, 820–821
    gastroenteritis, 819–820

geriatric patients, 1039
    and histamine, 629
    infections, 819–821
    pregnancy, changes during, 872
gastrointestinal tract devices, 1133–1135
gastrostomy tubes, 1018–1019
gauze bandages, 113
Geiger counter, 776
generalized antibodies, 625
generalized seizures, 590–591
genital herpes, 827
genital warts, 827
genitourinary system, 659, 1041, 1132–1135
geriatric abuse, 1069–1070
    see also elder abuse
geriatric emergencies
    see also geriatric trauma
    alcohol abuse, 1065–1066
    Alzheimer's disease, 1052, 1053
    analgesic toxicity, 1064
    aneurysm, 1048
    angina pectoris, 1046
    angiotensin-converting enzyme (ACE)
        inhibitor toxicity, 1063
    anti-inflammatory agent toxicity, 1064
    antidepressant toxicity, 1064
    antihypertensive toxicity, 1063
    antiparkinsonion agents, toxicity of,
        1064
    antipsychotic toxicity, 1064
    antiseizure medication toxicity, 1064
    aortic dissection, 1048
    atherosclerosis, 1048
    behavioural disorders, 1066–1068
    beta-blocker toxicity, 1063
    bowel obstruction, 1056–1057
    cardiovascular disorders, 1045–1049
    cerebrovascular disease, 1050–1051
    chronic obstructive pulmonary disease,
        1043–1044
    corticosteroid toxicity, 1064
    delirium, 1052, 1052*t*
    dementia, 1052, 1052*t*, 1053
    depression, 1067
    diabetes mellitus, 1054–1055
    digitalis toxicity, 1064
    diuretic toxicity, 1063
    dizziness, 1051
    drug abuse, 1065
    dysphoria, 1067
    dysrhythmias, 1047–1048
    endocrine disorders, 1054–1055
    environmental emergencies, 1061–1062
    falls, 42
    fractures, 175
    gastrointestinal disorders, 1055–1057
    GI hemorrhage, 1056
    Glasgow Coma Scale (GCS), 1050–1051
    glomerulonephritis, 1060
    heart failure, 1046–1047
    heatstroke, 1062
    hemorrhage, 74
    hepatomegaly, 1047
    herpes zoster, 1057
    hypertension, 1048–1049
    hyperthermia, 1061, 1062
    hypochondriasis, 1067
    hypothermia, 1061–1062

lidocaine toxicity, 1063
lower GI bleed, 1056
lung cancer, 1045
mesenteric infarct, 1057
metabolic disorders, 1054–1055
musculoskeletal disorders, 1058–1060
neurological disorders, 1049–1054
neurological emergencies, assessment
    of, 581
nocturia, 1047
osteoarthritis, 1058, 1059
osteoporosis, 1058, 1059–1060
Parkinson's disease, 1053–1054
pneumonia, 1042–1043
polypharmacy, and side effects, 1063
pressure ulcers, 1057, 1058
pruritus, 1057
psychological disorders, 1066–1068
pulmonary disorders, 1042–1045
pulmonary edema, 1045
pulmonary embolism, 1044–1045
renal disorders, 1060
respiratory disorders, 1042–1045
secondary depression, 1066
seizures, 1051
silent myocardial infarction, 1046
skin disorders, 1057–1058
stroke, 1050–1051
substance abuse, 1064–1066
suicide, 1067–1068
syncope, 1049
thyroid disorders, 1055
toxicological emergencies, 1062–1064
two pillow orthopnea, 1047
upper GI bleed, 1056
urinary disorders, 1060–1061
urinary tract infection (UTI),
    1060–1061
vertigo, 1051
geriatric patients
    see also the elderly
    altered mental status, 1033
    anorexia nervosa, 1030
    anoxic hypoxemia, 1037
    assessment considerations, 1030–1034
    blindness, 1031
    cardiovascular system, 1037–1038
    cataracts, 1031, 1032f
    common age-related systemic changes,
        1036t
    communication difficulties, 1028,
        1028t, 1031–1033
    comorbidity, 1026
    compliance, 1026–1027
    concluding the history, 1033–1034
    confusion, 1025, 1033
    diabetes mellitus, 1038
    diminished liver function, 1039
    domestic elder abuse, 1078, 1079
    dysphagia, 1026
    elder abuse, 150–151, 1069–1070,
        1078–1079, 1080f
    elimination problems, 1029, 1029t
    endocrine system, 1038–1039
    falls, 1027–1028
    functional impairment, 1025
    gastroenteritis, 819
    gastrointestinal system, 1039

general health assessment, 1030
genitourinary system, 1041
glaucoma, 1031
head injuries, risk of, 206
hearing, 1031
hematological system, 1041
hiatal hernias, 1039
history, 1031–1034
hypertrophy, 1037
immune system, 1041
incontinence, 1028–1029
institutional elder abuse, 1078
integumentary system, 1040
kyphosis, 1036
lidocaine, and toxicity, 1039
malnutrition, by-products of, 1030
management considerations,
    1034–1035
Marfan's syndrome, 1039
medical history, 1027
Meniere's disease, 1031
mobility problems, 1027–1028
multiple-system failure, 1026
musculoskeletal system, 1040
nervous system, 1038
osteoporosis, 175
pathophysiology, 1026–1029,
    1030–1031
pharmacology, 1026–1027
physical abuse, and burns, 150–151
pneumonia, risk of, 807
polypharmacy, 1026, 1063
psychiatric disorders, 850–851
renal system, 1040–1041
respiratory distress, 1037
respiratory system, 1035–1037
rib fractures, 282
secondary assessment, 1034
stroke, 1038
system pathophysiology, 1035–1041
tenting skill, assessment of, 1040
thermal burns, 155
thermoregulatory system, 1039–1040
thyroid gland disorders, 139
tinnitus, 1031
and tuberculosis (TB), 805
vaccination, 1041
vaccination against pneumonia, 808
vision, 1031
geriatric trauma
    adult respiratory distress syndrome
        (ARDS), 1068
    assessment, 1069–1070
    burns, 1072–1073
    cardiovascular considerations, 1070
    common fractures, 1072
    contributing factors, 1068
    geriatric abuse, 1069–1070
    head injuries, 1073
    management, 1070–1071
    neglect, 1069–1070
    othorpedic injuries, 1071–1072
    renal considerations, 1070
    respiratory conditions, 1070
    spinal injury, 1073
    subcapital femoral neck fracture, 1072f
    transport considerations, 1071
geriatrics, 1024

German measles, 815, 1100
gerontology, 1024
gestation, 875
gestational diabetes, 876, 886–887
Giardia lamblia, 643, 819
gingivitis, 731
Glasgow Coma Scale (GCS), 218, 230–231,
    230t, 579–580, 579f, 957, 958t,
    1050–1051
glaucoma, 1031, 1092
global aphasia, 1094
glomerular injury, 667
glomerulonephritis, 1060
glottic function, 922
Glucagon, 999
glucocorticoid therapy, 616, 617
glucose intolerance, 670
glucose loss in urine, 611
glucose metabolism, 609–610, 609t
glycosuria, 611, 668
Golden Hour, 8
gonorrhea, 825, 861
goose bumps, 753
gout, 177
gradual ascent, 772
Gram stain, 784
grand mal seizure, 590
grand multiparity, 875
granules, 627
granulocytes, 104, 627
graph paper, ECG, 455–456, 456f
Graves' disease, 616
gravida (G), 858–859
gravidity, 875
Gray (gy), 143–144
greenstick fracture, 175, 202, 1010
Grey-Turner's sign, 638
grief, 1140
groin, bandaging, 124
Groshong catheter, 1100, 1130
Group A Streptococcus, 359
growth plate, 948
grunting, 375
guarding, 316
Guillain-Barré syndrome, 572, 1109, 1122
gummas, 826
gunshot wounds, 207, 316, 320
gurgling, 376
gynecological emergencies
    abdominal pain, 858
    abortion (A), 859
    assessment, 858–860
    contraception, 859
    cystitis, 862
    dysmenorrhea, 858
    dyspareunia, 858
    ectopic pregnancy, 863
    endometriosis, 862–863
    endometritis, 862
    gravida (G), 858–859
    gynecological history, 859
    history, 858–859
    internal vaginal exam, 860
    last menstrual period (LMP), 859
    last normal menstrual period (LNMP),
        859
    living (L), 859
    management, 860–861

medical gynecological emergencies, 861–863
mittelschmerz, 862
most common emergency complaints, 858
nontraumatic vaginal bleeding, 863
obstetric history, 858–859
para/parity (P), 859
pelvic inflammatory disease (PID), 861–862
professional demeanour, 859
psychological support, 861
ruptured ovarian cyst, 862
secondary assessment, 859–860
sexual assault injuries, 864–866
term (T), 859
traumatic gynecological emergencies, 863–866
vaginal bleeding, 858, 860
vaginal discharge, 860
gynecological history, 859
gynecology, 858

habituation, 715
Haemophilus ducreyi, 828
Haemophilus influenzae, 807, 811, 818
hairline fracture, 173
hairy cell leukemia, 736
half-life, 775
hallucinations, 841
hallucinogens, 716, 718*t*
halo sign, 210
halo test, 211*f*
haloperidol, 716, 856
handgun, 49–50
hands
    amputation, 126*f*
    bandaging of, 123*f*, 124–125
    fractures, 198
    injuries, 198
handwashing, 793, 813, 829, 831
hanging, 251–252
hantavirus, 818–819
hantavirus pulmonary syndrome (HPS), 819
hard measles, 814
hard/rigid catheters, 432, 432*t*
Hare traction splint, 187
hazardous material, 782
head, facial, and neck injury management
    airway, 232–234
    atropine, 243
    avulsions, 244
    blood pressure maintenance, 238–239
    breathing, 237–238
    circulation, 238–239
    cricothyrotomy, 236–237
    dextrose, 243
    diazepam (Valium®), 241–242
    digital intubation, 234–235
    directed intubation, 235
    dislodged teeth, 246
    diuretics, 240
    emotional support, 244
    endotracheal intubation, 234–236
    eye injuries, 245–246, 245*f*
    fentanyl (Sublimaze®), 242–243
    fluid resuscitation, 239
    furosemide (Lasix®), 240

hemorrhage control, 238
hypotension, 239
hypovolemia, 239
hypoxia, 239
impaled objects, 246
mannitol, 240
medications, 239–244
midazolam (Versed®), 242
morphine sulphate, 242
naloxone hydrochloride (Narcan®), 242
nasopharyngeal airways, 233–234
nasotracheal intubation, 235
needle cricothyrostomy, 236–237
oropharyngeal airway, 233–234
orotracheal intubation, 234
oxygen administration, 237, 239–240
pancuronium (Pavulon®), 241
paralytic agents, 240–241
patient positioning, 233
pediatric trauma, 1009
pinnal injury, 244–245
rapid sequence intubation, 235–236
sedatives, 241–243
special injury care, 244–246
succinylcholine (Anectine®), 241
suctioning, 233
surgical cricothyrotomy, 236–237
thiamine, 243
topical anesthetic spray, 243–244
transport considerations, 244
vecuronium (Norcuron®), 241
ventilations, 238
vitamin B_1, 243
head injuries
    airway evaluation, 226
    assessment, 225–232
    at-risk population, 206
    avulsions, 209
    bandaging, 122–123, 123*f*
    basilar skull fracture, 210, 221, 222*f*
    bilateral periorbital ecchymosis, 210, 210*f*
    blunt injury, 206–207
    brain injury. *See* brain injury
    breathing, monitoring, 226–227
    bullet impacts, 210–211
    child abuse, 1082
    circulation, evaluation of, 227
    cranial injury, 209–211, 209*f*
    detailed secondary assessment, 232
    eye signs, 218–219
    fluid accumulation in lungs, 350
    focused history and secondary assessment, 231
    geriatric trauma, 1073
    Glasgow Coma Scale (GCS), 218, 230–231, 230*t*
    hemorrhage, 80–81
    hypoxia, 239
    impaled objects, 211
    index of suspicion, 7–8
    management. *See* head, facial, and neck injury management
    mechanisms of injury, 206–207
    ongoing assessment, 232
    pathophysiology, 208–219
    pediatric head trauma, 218
    pediatric patients, 946–947

penetrating trauma, 58, 207
previous head injuries, 1103
primary assessment, 225–227
rapid trauma assessment, 227–231
retroauricular ecchymosis, 210, 210*f*
scalp injuries, 208–209, 208*f*
scene assessment, 225
skull fractures, 209–211, 209*f*
and trauma death, 206
vehicular collisions, 29
vital signs, monitoring of, 231
head lice, 829–830
head-on impact, 31
head-protection airbags, 20
head-tilt/chin-lift manoeuvre, 373, 380–382, 952
headache, 514–515, 595–596
health and safety competencies, 1143
Health Canada, 783, 800, 809, 813
hearing impairments
    accommodations for deaf patients, 1091–1092
    children and infants, 1090–1091
    conductive deafness, 1090
    deafness, 1090
    labrynthitis, 1091
    presbycusis, 1091
    recognition of deafness, 1091
    sensorineural deafness, 1090–1091
    sign language, 1092
    types of, 1090–1091
heart
    see also cardiology; cardiovascular injuries
    autonomic control of, 450
    electrical events of, and electrocardiogram (ECG), 456–463, 457*f*
    exsanguination, 15
    penetrating trauma, 301
    pericardial tamponade, 55
    regulation of function, 450
    sounds, 519
    tachycardia, 340
heart disease, and pregnancy, 876
heart failure
    congestive heart failure (CHF), 546–547, 547
    cor pulmonale, 546
    current medications, 547
    defined, 545
    described, 541
    and dysrhythmias, 545
    field assessment, 547–548
    geriatric patients, 1046–1047
    laboured breathing, 547
    left ventricular failure, 546
    management, 548–549
    OPQRST questions, 547
    pharmacological interventions, 548
    pulmonary edema, 547, 548
    pulmonary embolism, 546
    pulmonary hypertension, 546
    right ventricular failure, 546
    skin colour, 547
    Starling's law of the heart, 546
    transport considerations, 548–549
heart rate, 576

heart rate calculatory rulers, 464
heat conservation mechanisms, 753
heat disorders
    dehydration, role of, 752
    fever (pyrexia), 752–753
    heat exhaustion, 749–750
    heat illness, 747
    heat (muscle) cramps, 749
    heatstroke, 750–752
    hyperthermia, 747–749
    pathophysiology, 744–747
heat exhaustion, 749–750
heat generation, 744
heat illness, 747
heat loss, 744–745, 745f, 753, 912–914, 949
heat (muscle) cramps, 749
heatstroke, 750–752, 1061, 1062
heavy metals, 703
Helicobacter pylori bacillus, 643, 644, 645
helmet removal, 266–267
helmets, 31–32, 42–43, 226
hematemesis, 313, 640, 642
hematochezia, 78, 313, 643
hematocrit, 668
hematological crises, 735
hematology
    blood products, 725–726
    blood transfusion, 725–726
    blood typing, 725–726
    defined, 724
hematoma, 71, 97, 1090
hematopoietic disorders
    anemia, 733–735
    disseminated intravascular coagulation (DIC), 739
    easy bruising, and mistaken child abuse, 1081–1082
    hemophilia, 738–739
    leukocytosis, 736
    leukopenia, 735–736
    lymphomas, 737
    multiple myeloma, 739–740
    neutropenia, 735–736
    platelet/blood clotting disorders, 737–739
    polycythemia, 735
    red blood cell diseases, 733–735
    sickle cell anemia, 734–735
    thrombocytopenia, 738
    thrombocytosis, 737–738
    von Willebrand's disease, 739
    white blood cell disorders, 735–737
hematopoietic emergencies
    see also hematopoietic disorders
    abdominal pain, 731
    acute hemodynamic compromise, 727
    assessment, 727–732
    AVPU method, 729
    bleeding gums, 731
    cardiorespiratory system, assessment of, 732
    febrile nonhemolytic reaction, 727
    focused history and secondary assessment, 728–732
    gastrointestinal system, assessment of, 730–731
    genitourinary effects, 732
    geriatric patients, 1041

lymphatic system, assessment of, 730
    management, 732
    musculoskeletal system, assessment of, 731–732
    nervous system, evaluation of, 729
    primary assessment, 728
    SAMPLE history, 728–729
    scene assessment, 727–728
    secondary assessment, 729–732
    skin, observation of, 729–730
    transfusion reactions, 726–727
hematuria, 313
hemodialysis, 350, 673–674, 673f
hemodilution, 762
hemoglobin, 333
hemoglobinopathies, 693t
hemolytic disease of the newborn, 726
hemolytic reaction, 727
hemolytic uremic syndrome, 820
hemophilia, 738–739
hemopneumothorax, 288
hemoptysis, 39, 340, 1121
hemorrhage
    abdominal injuries, 324
    acute hemorrhage, 72
    aggressive fluid therapy, 68
    arterial hemorrhage, 66, 68, 79–80
    assessment, 74–79
    body substance isolation (BSI) precautions, 75–76
    body's response to blood loss, 83–84
    capillary hemorrhage, 66
    chronic hemorrhage, 72
    control, 68–72, 69f, 89, 119f, 120–121, 238
    crush injuries, 82, 110
    defined, 65
    direct pressure, 68, 79–80
    dissecting abdominal aortic artery, 635–636
    effects of, 72
    epistaxis, 71
    external hemorrhage, 68–69
    focused history, 77–79
    focused secondary assessment, 78
    gaping wounds, 82
    gastric hemorrhage, 72
    head injuries, 80–81
    hemothorax, 288–289, 289f
    hyphema, 222
    injuries causing significant blood loss, 77
    internal hemorrhage, 66, 69–72, 76, 78
    intracranial hemorrhage, 212–213, 584–588
    lungs, 72
    management of hemorrhage, 79–82
    mechanism of injury evaluation, 76
    microhemorrhage, 290
    neck wounds, 81
    ongoing assessment, 79
    pediatric care, 949
    postpartum hemorrhage, 902
    primary assessment, 76–77
    pulmonary hemorrhage, 1121
    rapid trauma assessment, 77–78
    rebleeding, 108
    respiratory system, 72

scene assessment, 75–76
secondary assessment, 77–79
shock. *See* shock
soft-tissue trauma, 102, 102f
specific wound considerations, 80–82
spinal cord, 254
stages of hemorrhage, 72–74, 73t
subarachnoid hemorrhages, 586f
subconjunctival hemorrhage, 222
tourniquet, use of, 69, 70f, 121
transport considerations, 82
types of, 66
upper gastrointestinal bleeding, 639–641
vaginal hemorrhage, 72
venous hemorrhage, 66
hemorrhagic pneumonitis, 762
hemorrhagic strokes, 585–586
hemorrhoids, 649–650
hemostasis, 102–104
hemostasis, impaired, 107–108
hemothorax, 288–289, 289f, 305, 335
Henry's Law, 765
HEPA filtration, 806
HEPA respirators, 806f
heparin, 68, 107, 482
hepatitis, 655–656, 801–804
hepatitis A (HAV), 655, 801–802
hepatitis B (HBV), 655, 789, 802–803
hepatitis C (HCV), 655, 803
hepatitis D (HDV), 655, 803
hepatitis E (HEV), 656, 803–804
hepatomegaly, 1047
herd immunity, 811
hernias, 650, 651f, 1039
herniation, 585, 928
herpes simplex Type 1, 817
herpes simplex Type 2, 827
herpes simplex virus, 817
herpes zoster, 1057
hiatal hernias, 1039
hiccoughing, 374–375
Hickman catheter, 1100, 1130
high-altitude cerebral edema (HACE), 774–775
high-altitude illness
    acetazolamide, 773
    acute mountain sickness (AMS), 773–774
    blood changes, 772
    cardiovascular changes, 772
    described, 771–772
    extreme altitude, 772
    and fluid accumulation in lungs, 350
    gradual ascent, 772
    high altitude, 772
    high-altitude cerebral edema (HACE), 774–775
    high-altitude pulmonary edema (HAPE), 774
    high-carbohydrate diet and, 773
    limited exertion, 773
    medications for prevention, 773
    nifedipine, 773
    prevention, 772–773
    sleeping altitude, 773
    types of, 773–775
    ventilatory changes, 772
    very high altitude, 772

high-altitude pulmonary edema (HAPE), 774
high-level disinfection, 794
high-pressure regulators, 435
high-velocity weapons, 320
hip
    bandaging, 124
    dislocation, 195
histamine, 104, 627, 629
histamine poisoning, 705
histamine receptors, 627
history
    gastrointestinal (GI) emergencies,
      636–638
    geriatric patients, 1031–1034
    gynecological emergencies, 858–859
    ingested toxins, 688
    medication use, 341
    neurological emergencies, 574–575
    obstetric patient, 875–877
    pediatric assessment, 956
    pneumonia, 807
    respiratory problems, 373–374
    respiratory status, 340–341
    SAMPLE history. See SAMPLE history
    toxicological emergencies, 685–686
    urological emergencies, 661–663
HIV. See human immunodeficiency virus
    (HIV)
hives, 628, 628f
hobble restraint, 855
Hodgkin's lymphoma, 737
hog-tie restraint, 855
hold-up position, 260
hollow organs, 55, 313, 635
home artificial ventilators, 1018
home care patients
    acute infections, 1135–1136
    airway complications, 1108
    ALS intervention, 1138–1140
    ALS response to, 1108
    altered mental status, 1109–1110
    anticoagulant therapy, 1130–1131
    arthritis, 1099
    artificial airways, 1124–1126
    assessment, 1114–1118
    asthma, 1120–1121
    BiPAP (bilevel positive airway pressure),
      1120, 1128
    bronchitis, 1119–1120
    bronchopulmonary dysplasia (BPD),
      1121–1122
    cancer, 1099–1100
    cardiac conditions, 1131–1132
    cardiac decompensation, 1109
    cerebral palsy, 1100–1101
    chronic obstructive pulmonary disease
      (COPD), 1119–1121
    colostomy, 1136f
    comfort care, 1138–1140
    congestive heart failure (CHF), 1121
    CPAP (continuous positive airway
      pressure), 1120, 1128
    cystic fibrosis, 1101–1102, 1121
    do not resuscitate (DNR) order, 1108,
      1118
    emphysema, 1119–1120
    environment, evaluation of, 1115–1116
    epidemiology, 1107–1113

equipment malfunction, 1111–1112
focused history, 1116–1118
gastrointestinal tract devices,
    1133–1135
GI/GU crises, 1110, 1132–1135
Guillain-Barré syndrome, 1122
home health-care practitioners,
    intervention by, 1112–1113
home oxygen therapy, 1123–1124
hospice, 1113, 1138–1140
indwelling devices, 1110
infections, 1110–1111
injury control and prevention, 1113
lung transplantation, awaiting, 1123
management treatment plan, 1118
maternal care, 1136–1138
medical devices, commonly found, 1112
mental status, 1116–1117
multiple sclerosis (MS), 1102
muscular dystrophy (MD), 1102, 1122
myasthenia gravis, 1104, 1122–1123
nasogastric intubation, 1134f
negative-pressure ventilators, 1127
neuromuscular degenerative diseases,
    1122–1123
neutropenic, 1100
newborns, 1136–1138
open wounds, 1135–1136
other medical disorders, 1112
PEEP (positive end-expiratory pressure),
    1120, 1127–1128
peripheral circulation, alterations in,
    1109
physicians, intervention by, 1112–1113
poliomyelitis (polio), 1102–1103, 1122
positive-pressure ventilators, 1127
postpolio syndrome, 1103
pressure disorders, 1111f
previous head injuries, 1103
primary assessment, 1116–1118
respiratory disorders, 1119–1129
respiratory failure, 1109
scene assessment, 1114–1116
scene safety, 1114–1115
secondary assessment, 1116–1118
septic complications, 1110–1111
sleep apnea, 1123
spina bifida (SB), 1103–1104
tracheostomy, 1124–1126
transport considerations, 1118
typical responses, 1108–1112
urinary tract devices, 1132, 1132f,
    1133f
vascular access devices (VADs),
    1129–1131
ventilators, 1126–1129
homeostasis, 65, 82, 249, 608, 610, 743–744
honey bees (Apoidea), 627
hookworms, 787
hormones, 607–608
hornets (Vespidae), 627, 707
hospice, 1113, 1138–1140
hospital acquired diseases, 830–831
host defences, 783
household plants, poisonous, 705–706
huffers, 690
human immunodeficiency virus (HIV)
    clinical presentation, 799

described, 798
general public, risk to, 799
health-care workers, risk to, 799
pathogenesis, 798
postexposure prophylaxis, 800
summary of, 800
universal (standard) precautions,
    800–801
vector transmission, 799
human papillomavirus (HPV), 827
humerus fractures, 193–194
humoral immunity, 624
hydration, 957
hydrocarbons, 690, 698
hydrochloric acid, 644
hydrocortisone, 630
hydrofluoric (HF) acid, 697–698
hydrophobia, 822
hydrostatic pressure, 84
hydroxyzine, 630
Hymenoptera, 623, 627, 684, 707, 708
hyperadrenalism, 619–620
hyperbaric chamber, 695f, 769f
hyperbaric oxygen chamber, 768
hyperbaric oxygenation, 6, 159
hyperbilirubinemia, 914
hypercapnia, 771
hyperextension, 249–251
hyperflexion, 249–251
hyperglycemia, 610, 611, 1000, 1000t
hyperglycemic hyperosmolar nonketotic
    (HHNK) coma, 612, 614–615
hyperkalemia, 510, 666, 668f, 672, 751
hypermetabolic phase, 138
hypersensitivity
    see also allergies
    delayed hypersensitivity reaction, 626
    immediate hypersensitivity reactions,
      626
hypertension, 550, 876, 885
hypertensive disorders of pregnancy, 883–885
hypertensive emergencies, 550–552,
    1048–1049
hypertensive encephalopathy, 550
hyperthermia, 747–749, 1061, 1062
hyperthyroidism, 616
hypertonic phase, 590
hypertrophic scar formation, 109
hypertrophy, 1037, 1109
hyperventilation syndrome, 367–368, 367t,
    771
hyphema, 222
hypocalcemia, 670
hypochondriasis, 846, 1067
hypoglycemia (insulin shock), 610, 615–616,
    620, 933–934, 998–999
hypoglycemic seizure, 615
hypokalemia, 931
hypoperfusion, 320, 666, 879
    see also shock (hypoperfusion)
hypotension
    brain injury, 215
    fluid accumulation in lungs, 350
    following verapamil administration, 494
    head, facial, and neck injury
      management, 239
    infectious disease and, 797
    management, 554f

orthostatic hypotension, 78, 640
pediatric emergencies, 958
hypothalamus
  cold diuresis, 757
  defined, 746
  resuscitation, 759
  thermoregulation, 746, 746f
hypothermia
  active rewarming, 757
  acute exposure, 754
  adult respiratory distress syndrome
    (ARDS), 350
  advanced care paramedics, 759
  burns, 148–149
  causes of, 755
  chronic exposure, 754
  clinical findings at different degrees, 756t
  compensated hypothermia, 754
  critical care paramedics, 759
  defined, 753
  degrees of, 754–755
  ECG changes due to, 510
  geriatric emergencies, 1061–1062
  J waves, 755, 757f
  management, 755–757, 758f
  mechanisms of heat conservation and
    loss, 753
  mild hypothermia, 754
  neonatal emergencies, 932–933
  predisposing factors, 754
  preventive measures, 754
  primary care paramedic, 759
  rewarming shock, 757
  severe hypothermia, 754
  signs and symptoms, 755, 756t
  subacute exposure, 754
  transport, 759
hypothyroidism, 616, 618–619, 844
hypoventilation, 281, 282
hypovolemia, 149, 158, 179, 224, 239, 317,
  408, 931
hypovolemic shock, 989
hypoxemia, 762
hypoxia
  in adult respiratory distress syndrome
    (ARDS), 351
  anemia and, 733
  arterial interruption and, 224
  bradycardia in newborn, 929
  cerebral hypoxia, 764
  defined, 337
  disruption in diffusion and, 337
  dyspnea, 344
  and endotracheal intubation, 394
  fetal hypoxic incident, 901
  fluid accumulation in lungs, 350
  frequent monitoring, 239
  head injury, effect on, 215
  inhaled toxins, 690
  neonatal cardiac arrest, 936
  neonatal distress, 923, 927
  ongoing assessment for, 232
  persistent fetal circulation, 909
  in restrained patients, 855
  rib fracture and, 282
  sleep, and high altitude, 773
  status epilepticus, 593
  suctioning, complications of, 433

hypoxic injury, 109
hypoxic ventilatory response (HVR), 772
hysterical seizures, 591

ibuprofen, 702, 753
idiopathic epilepsy, 589
idiopathic thrombocytopenia purpura (ITP),
  738
idioventricular rhythm, 495
immediate hypersensitivity reactions, 626
immobilization
  see also specific injuries
  bandaging, 122
  cervical immobilization device (CID),
    272
  diving injury immobilization, 272–273
  manual cervical immobilization,
    263–264
  manual immobilization, 257, 259f
  muscular and connective tissue injuries,
    190
  musculoskeletal injury management,
    185
  pediatric trauma, 1006–1007, 1007f
  soft-tissue injury management, 122
  wound immobilization. See splinting
immune response, 624
immune senescence, 1041
immune system, 624–626, 1041
immunity
  acquired immunity, 625
  active immunity, 625
  artificially acquired immunity, 625
  cellular immunity, 624, 626
  chickenpox, 810–811
  humoral immunity, 624
  induced active immunity, 625
  induced passive immunity, 625
  innate immunity, 625
  natural immunity, 625
  natural passive immunity, 625
  naturally acquired immunity, 625
  passive immunity, 625
immunization
  see also vaccination
  influenza, 813–814
  keeping immunizations current, 831
  measles, 814
  meningitis, 812
  pneumonia, 808
immunoglobulins (Igs), 624
immunosuppressant medications, 106
impacted fracture, 173, 174f
impacts, auto. See vehicular collisions
impaired hemostasis, 107–108
impaired mentation, 672
impaled objects
  abdominal injuries, 325
  cardiopulmonary resuscitation (CPR),
    and removal of, 127
  described, 62–63
  head, facial, and neck injury
    management, 246
  head injuries, 211
  open wounds, 100, 100f
  soft-tissue injury management, 126–127,
    127f
impending doom, 514

impetigo, 829
impulse control disorders, 849
IN SAD CAGES, 844
inadequate tissue perfusion, 541
inadequate ventilation, 372
incendiary, 37
incidential anticholinergics, 692t
incisions, 98
inclusion criteria for termination of
  resuscitation, 558
incomplete bundle branch block, 509
incontinence, 1028–1029
incubation period, 790
index case, 782
index of suspicion, 7–8, 25, 831, 1015
indirect injury (brain), 214–216
indomethacin, 702, 888
induced active immunity, 625
induced passive immunity, 625
induced vomiting, 686, 690
induction agents, 409t
inertia, 13–14
infants
  see also pediatric care
  anatomy, 945–949
  bronchopulmonary dysplasia (BPD),
    1121–1122
  child abuse. See child abuse
  of diabetic mothers, 876
  Glasgow Coma Scale (GCS), 958t
  growth and development, 942–943
  head injuries, risk of, 206
  hemolytic disease of the newborn, 726
  hemorrhage, 74
  herpes simplex virus Type 2, 827
  herpes simplex virus Type I, 817
  meningococcemia, 812
  neonatal care. See neonatal care
  neonates. See neonates
  newborn. See newborns
  peripheral oxygen saturation, 377
  physiology, 945–949
  premature infants, 1090–1091
  rule of nines, 147
  shaken baby syndrome, 1082–1083
  with special needs, 1016–1020
  sudden infant death syndrome (SIDS),
    943, 1011–1012
  thoracic trauma, 279
infarct, 224
infarction, 584–585, 650
infection control
  decontaminate, 794
  decontamination methods and
    procedures, 794
  hand washing, 793
  high-level disinfection, 794
  intermediate-level disinfection, 794
  low-level disinfection, 794
  patient contact, 792
  phases of, 790
  preparation for response, 791–792
  recovery, 793–794
  response, 792
  sterilization, 794
infections
  see also infectious disease
  abscess, 107

airway edema, 335
and antibiotics, 106
bacterial tracheitis, 982–983
brochiolitis, 985
burns, 149, 156, 158
cellulitis, 1110
common skin and soft-tissue infections, 105
community-acquired urinary tract infection (UTI), 678
cystitis, 677
cytomegalovirus (CMV), 1092
defined, 789
drugs, effect of, 106
encephalitis, 821
epiglottitis, 980–982
food poisoning, 820–821
gangrene, 107
gastroenteritis, 819–820
gastrointestinal bacteria, 372
gastrointestinal system infections, 819–821
Guillain-Barré syndrome, 1109
home care patients, 1110–1111, 1135–1136
interstitial tissue, 667
Lyme disease, 824–825
lymphangitis, 105
management of, 107
nervous system infections, 821–825
nosocomial urinary tract infection (UTI), 678
pediatric emergencies, 976–977
pharyngitis, 818
prostatitis, 677
rabies, 821–823
risk factors, 106
as serious complication, 105
soft-tissue trauma, 105–107
tetanus, 107, 823–824
treatment and, 106
upper airway structures, 335
upper respiratory infection (URI), 358–360
and wound location, 106
infectious acute gastroenteritis, 642
infectious agents, 782
infectious crises, 735
infectious disease
    airborne route, 788
    assessment, 795–797
    bacteria, 784–785, 784f
    bloodborne diseases, 788
    challenging situation, 1105
    chancroid, 828
    chickenpox, 810–811
    chlamydia, 827–828
    common cold influenza, 814
    communicable, 789
    communicable period, 790
    confidentiality, 795
    contamination, 789
    contraction, 787–790
    correct mode of entry, 789
    croup, 818
    decontamination methods and procedures, 794
    defined, 782

dehydration, 797
disease period, 790
diseases of immediate concern to EMS providers, 797
dose, 789
encephalitis, 821
epiglottitis, 817–818
factors affecting transmission, 789–790
fecal-oral transmission, 788
food poisoning, 820–821
gastroenteritis, 819–820
gastrointestinal system infections, 819–821
genital warts, 827
gonorrhea, 825
handwashing, 813
hantavirus, 818–819
hepatitis, 801–804
herd immunity, 811
herpes simplex Type 2, 827
herpes simplex virus, 817
human immunodeficiency virus (HIV), 798–801
impetigo, 829
incubation period, 790
index case, 782
infection control, 790–795
infectious respiratory conditions, 817–819
influenza, 813–814
latent period, 790
lice, 829–830
Lyme disease, 824–825
measles, 814
measurable transmission, 788
meningitis, 811–812
microorganisms, 783–787
mononucleosis, 817
mumps, 814–815
nervous system infections, 821–825
Norwegian scabies, 830
nosocomial infections, 830–831
past medical history, 796
patient contact, 792
pediatric emergencies, 976–977
penetration of host, 789
pertussis, 816
pharyngitis, 818
phases of infectious process, 790
pneumonia, 807–808
poliomyelitis (polio), 601, 1102–1103
postexposure, 795
preparation for response, 791–792
prevention of disease transmission, 831–832
public health agencies, 783
public health principles, 782–783
rabies, 821–823
recovery, 793–794
reporting exposures, 795
reservoir, 788
resistance, 789–790
respiratory syncytial virus (RSV), 815–816
response, 792
rubella (German measles), 815
SARS (severe acute respiratory syndrome), 808–809

scabies, 830
secondary assessment, 796–797
seroconversion, 790
sexually transmitted diseases, 825–828
sinusitis, 818
skin diseases, 828–830
stages of disease, 787–790
syphilis, 826–827
tetanus, 823–824
theoretical transmission, 788
transmission, 787–790, 789t
transmission routes, 813
trichomoniasis, 828
tuberculosis, 804–807
viral diseases transmitted by contact, 816–817
virulence, 789
viruses, 785–786, 786f
West Nile virus, 809–810
window phase, 790
infectious respiratory conditions
    croup, 818
    epiglottitis, 817–818
    hantavirus, 818–819
    pharyngitis, 818
    sinusitis, 818
inferior venae cavae, 448
infestation, 829
inflammation
    arthritis, 177
    Bell's palsy, 600
    bursitis, 177
    chemotactic factors, 104
    cystitis, 677
    defined, 104
    epiglottitis, 817–818, 980–982
    gastrointestinal (GI) emergencies, 635
    gout, 177
    granulocytes, 104
    interstitial tissue, 667
    lymphangitis, 105
    osteoarthritis, 177
    peritonitis, 315–316
    prostatitis, 677
    rheumatoid arthritis, 177
    sinusitis, 818
    tendinitis, 177
    urethritis, 677
    vasculitis, 562
    wound healing, 104
inflammatory bowel disorders, 646, 647–648
inflammatory conditions, 176–177
influenza, 813–814
infranodal, 486
ingested toxins
    aspiration, prevention of, 689
    assessment, 688–689
    fluid administration, 689–690
    history, 688
    intravenous therapy, 689–690
    management, 689–690
    patient features, 689
    secondary assessment, 688–689
ingestion, 683–684
inhalation injury
    airway thermal burn, 144–146
    carbon monoxide poisoning, 144
    fluid accumulation in lungs, 349

intubation, 159
toxic inhalation, 144
inhalation (poison), 684
inhaled toxins, 690–691
injected toxins
black widow spider bites, 709, 710f
brown recluse spider bite, 708–709, 709f
coral snake bites, 711, 713–714
general management principles, 707
insect bites and stings, 707–710
marine animal injection, 714–715
pit viper bites, 711–713
scorpion stings, 709–710, 710f
snakebites, 711–714, 711f
injection injury, 110–111, 111f
injection (toxic agent), 684
injury prevention, 10
innate immunity, 625
inotropy, 450
inquiry, 117
insect bites and stings, 626–627, 684, 707–710
inspection
cardiovascular emergencies, 517–518
respiratory problems, 374–375
respiratory system, 342
soft-tissue trauma, 117–118
inspiration process, 219, 332
institutional elder abuse, 1078
insulin, 611, 612, 614
insulin-dependent diabetes mellitus (IDDM), 611
insulin shock, 615–616
integration competencies, 1146–1147
integumentary system, 95, 1040
intercalated discs, 450
intermediate-level disinfection, 794
intermittent explosive disorder, 849
Intermittent Mandatory Ventilation (IMV), 1121
internal hemorrhage, 66, 69–72, 76, 78
internodal atrial pathways, 451
interpolated beat, 497
interstitial nephritis, 667, 669
intoxication suspicions, 29
intracerebral hemorrhage, 213, 586f, 1050
intracranial hemorrhage, 212–213, 584–588
intracranial perfusion, 214–215
intracranial pressure, 210, 217f, 227, 584
intractable vertigo, 1051
intraosseous (IO) infusion, 972–973, 973f
intrapartum factors, 908
intrarenal abscesses, 678
intrathoracic injuries, 131
intrauterine devices (IUDs), 859
intrauterine pregnancy, 860
intravascular space, 138
intravenous therapy
anaphylaxis, 629
burns, 158
central IV line, 1018
chronic bronchitis, 355
dopamine (Intropin®), 273
fluid administration, 689–690, 1007
fluid therapy, 973
gastrointestinal (GI) emergencies, 638
heatstroke, 751

infusions, preparation of (pediatric), 975t
ingested toxins, 689–690
insulin, 614
intraosseous (IO) infusion, 972–973, 973f
leukemia, 737
pediatric emergencies, 970–974
renal calculi (kidney stones), 676
spinal injury management, 273
thoracic trauma management, 302, 304–305
transfusion reactions, 726–727
upper gastrointestinal bleeding, 641
intubation
see also airway management
advanced care paramedics, 387
blind orotracheal intubation, 402f
critical care paramedics, 387
digital intubation, 234–235, 258, 402–404, 403f, 404f
directed intubation, 235
endobronchial intubation, 395
endotracheal intubation, 234–236
see also endotracheal intubation
esophageal intubation, 394
field extubation, 416–417
field intubation, 153
inhalation injury, 159
meconium, removal of, 913f
myxedema coma, 618
nasogastric intubation, 969–970, 971f, 1134f
nasotracheal intubation, 235, 414–417, 415f
neonatal emergencies, 927, 927f
neonatal resuscitation, 922
orotracheal intubation, 234, 258, 396–414
pediatric intubation, 410–414, 411t, 413f, 965–970, 968f
rapid sequence intubation (RSI), 235–236, 405–410, 970
retrograde intubation, 410
Sellick's manoeuvre, 234, 235
transillumination intubation, 400–402, 401f
trauma patient intubation, 405
visualized endotracheal intubation, 131
intussusception, 650, 651f
ionization effects, 143, 165f
ionizing radiation, 775
ipratropium, 341
ipratropium bromide, 341
iron, 704
irreversible shock, 86, 988
ischemia, 83, 462, 584–585, 635
ischemic brain injury, 931
isoelectric line, 452
isoproterenol, 556
isosthenuria, 670
isotopes, 775

J waves, 755, 757f
Jackson's theory of thermal wounds, 137
jaw-thrust manoeuvre, 373, 382, 952, 1006f
jet skis, 33–34
jet ventilation, 426f

joint care
see also fractures
ankle injuries, 196–197
anterior hip dislocations, 195
elbow injuries, 198
fingers, 198–199
foot injuries, 197
generally, 189–190
hand injuries, 198
hip dislocation, 195
knee injuries, 195–196
posterior hip dislocation, 195
posterior knee dislocations, 196
shoulder injuries, 197–198
sprains, 196–197
wrist injuries, 198
joint injuries
see also joint care
anterior hip dislocations, 191–192
areas around the joints, 176
assessment, 177–183
dislocation, 172, 190
knee dislocation, 172f
sprains, 171
subluxation, 171–172
types of, 171
joint reduction, 190
Joule's law, 139
jugular vein distention, 287
jugular venous distention (JVD), 577
junctional escape complexes and rhythms, 491–492, 491f
juvenile-onset diabetes, 611

Kaposi's sarcomi, 799
keloid, 108
Kendrick extrication device (KED), 226
Kernig's sign, 812
ketone bodies, 610
see also diabetic ketoacidosis
ketorolac, 702
ketosis, 610
Kevlar™ fabric, 48–49
kidney stones, 659–660, 675–676
kidney transplantation, 659
kidneys
see also nephrology; renal disorders; renal emergencies
dialysis, 659, 673–674
injury to, 314
kidney disease, 659
renal function, 668
kinetic energy, 14–15
kinetics of trauma
acceleration, 15
blunt trauma, 13–15
conservation of energy, 14
deceleration, 15
defined, 13
described, 13
force, 15
inertia, 13–14
kinetic energy, 14–15
mass, 14
penetrating trauma, 45–46
velocity, 14
King Snake, 711
Kisselbach's plexus, 221

Klebsiella pneumoniae, 643, 678, 807, 819
kleptomania, 849
knee
    bandaging, 124
    dislocation, 172f
    dislocation reduction, 196f
    injuries, 195–196
knives, 51, 207
Korsakoff's psychosis, 584
Kuru, 786
Kussmaul's respirations, 336, 375, 576, 613
kyphosis, 1036
kyphotic deformity, 1054

labour
    defined, 889
    described, 889
    dilation stage, 889–890
    expulsion stage, 890
    management of patient in labour,
      890–891
    maternal complications, 901–903
    placental stage, 890
    prolonged labour, 935
    rupture of the membranes (ROM), 889
    stage one, 889–890
    stage three, 890
    stage two, 890
    vertex position, 890
labrynthitis, 1091
laceration of spinal cord, 254
lacerations, 98, 98f
lactate dehydrogenase (LDH), 545
lactic acid, 69
ladder splint, 186
language disorders, 1093–1094
lap belts, 19
laparoscopic surgery, 653
large bowel, 313
    see also abdominal trauma
laryngeal edema, 371, 628, 630
laryngeal mask airway, 419–420, 420f, 965
laryngeal spasm, 371
laryngectomy, 431
laryngoscope, 388–389, 388f, 389f, 390f,
    394, 967f
laryngoscopy, 422
laryngospasm, 416, 822
laryngotracheobronchitis, 818
last menstrual period (LMP), 859
last normal menstrual period (LNMP), 859
last oral intake, 516
latent period, 790
latent syphilis (third stage), 826
lateral bending, 251
lateral impact
    crumple zones, 24, 24f
    described, 25, 25f
    index of suspicion, 25
lateral-impact airbags, 20
Lawrence Berkeley National Laboratory,
    821
"laying the bike down," 31
Le Fort criteria, 219–220, 220f
lead, 703, 704
Lead II, 454
left atrium, 448
left bundle branch, 451

left coronary artery, 448
left ventricular failure, 546
leg bone fractures, 192–193
Legionella, 807
lesions, 826–827, 829
leukemia, 736–737
leukocytosis, 735, 736
leukopenia, 735–736
level of consciousness, 663, 860, 951
lice, 829–830
lidocaine, 408, 499, 556, 975, 1063
life-threatening problems, 3–4
ligament of Treitz, 639
light sensitivity, 229
lightning strikes, 160
limb alignment, 184
limb positioning, 184, 185f
limbs. *See* extremities
lindane, 830
linear skull fractures, 209
lip lesions, 817
liquefaction necrosis, 141
liquid oxygen, 1124
lithium, 701
liver
    blood clotting and, 731
    and blunt trauma, 15
    cirrhosis, 641–642
    hepatitis, 655–656
    hepatomegaly, 1047
    injury to, 314–315
living (L), 859
Lloyd's sign, 678
local burns, 156–157
log roll, 267–268, 268f
long bone fracture, 176
long padded board splints, 193f, 194
long spine board, 189, 192, 271–272, 272f
lorazepam, 843
Lou Gehrig's disease, 295, 335, 601
low back pain, 602–603
low-level disinfection, 794
low-velocity wounds, 54
lower airway distress, 983–986
lower-airway foreign-body obstruction, 986
lower airway obstruction, 335
lower gastrointestinal bleeding, 646–647,
    1056
lower gastrointestinal diseases
    bowel obstruction, 650–651, 650f
    Crohn's disease, 648
    diverticulitis, 649
    diverticulosis, 646
    hemorrhoids, 649–650
    lower gastrointestinal bleeding, 646–647
    pancolitis, 647
    proctitis, 647
    ulcerative colitis, 647–648
lower GI bleed, 646–647, 1056
lower GI tract, 646
lower respiratory tract, 335
lumen, 417
lung cancer
    assessment, 362
    cigarette smoking, 361
    described, 361
    geriatric patients, 1045
    management, 362

    pathophysiology, 362
    types of, 361
lung transplantation, awaiting, 1123
lungs
    see also pulmonary injuries; respiratory
      system
    blast injuries, 39
    compliance, 377
    cor pulmonale, 352
    diffusion, 332
    dyspnea, 39
    emboli, 39
    hemoptysis, 39
    hemorrhage in, 72
    pediatric care, 947–948
    penetrating trauma, 56
    perfusion, 333–334
    pneumothorax, 39
    pressure shock wave, 53
    ventilation, 332
luteinizing hormone (LH), 868
Lyme disease, 824–825
lymphangitis, 105
lymphomas, 737

mace, 162
maceration, 1058
machine pistols, 50
macrolide antibiotics, 500
macrophage, 104
mad cow disease, 786
Magill forceps, 388, 392, 392f
magnets, 506
major depression, 844
malignant lymphomas, 737
malignant tumours, 597
malleable splint, 186, 194f
Mallory-Weiss tear, 639, 640
malnutrition, 1030
mammalian diving reflex, 763
management
    see also specific conditions and injuries
    abdominal trauma, 324–326
    abnormal delivery presentations,
      898–899
    abortion, 880
    abruptio placentae, 883
    acetaminophen overdose, 702
    acute coronary syndrome, 544f
    acute mountain sickness (AMS), 774
    acute renal failure (ARF), 669
    adult respiratory distress syndrome
      (ARDS), 351
    Addison's disease (adrenal insufficiency),
      620
    airway management. *See* airway
      management
    airway obstruction, 348–349
    alcohol abuse, 722
    allergic reactions, 631–632
    altered mental status, 583–584
    anaphylaxis, 629–631
    angina pectoris, 539
    antidepressant overdose, 699, 700–701
    anxiety disorders, 843
    arterial gas embolism (AGE), 770
    asthma, 358, 984
    back pain, 605

bacterial tracheitis, 982–983
behavioural emergencies, 851–853
bipolar disorder, 845
birth injuries, 936
black widow spider bites, 709
breathing, 89, 237–238
breech presentation, 897
brochiolitis, 985
brown recluse spider bite, 708–709, 709f
carbon monoxide (CO) poisoning, 695
carbon monoxide inhalation, 364
cardiac arrest, 555–556
cardiac medication overdose, 696
cardiac tamponade, 550
cardiogenic shock, 553, 554f
cardiovascular emergencies. *See* cardiovascular emergency management
caustic substances, 697
central nervous system dysfunction, 368–369
cephalopelvic disproportion, 900
child abuse, 1015–1016
chronic bronchitis, 355
chronic renal failure (CRF), 672–674
chronic respiratory disorders, 1129
compartment syndrome, 130–131
coral snake bites, 714
croup, 980
crush injuries, 128–130
Cushing's syndrome, 620
cyanide poisoning, 694
decompression illness, 768–769
degenerative neurological disorders, 602
diabetic ketoacidosis, 614
ectopic pregnancy, 881
edema control, 122
emphysema, 353
epiglottitis, 982
eye injury, 245–246, 245f
facial wounds, 131, 131f
foreign body aspiration, 983
gastrointestinal (GI) emergencies, 638–639
geriatric patients, 1034–1035
geriatric trauma, 1070–1071
gestational diabetes, 887
Graves' disease, 616
gynecological abdominal pain, 863
gynecological emergencies, 860–861
head, facial, and neck injury management. *See* head, facial, and neck injury management
headache, 596
heart failure, 548–549
heat exhaustion, 750
heat (muscle) cramps, 749
heatstroke, 751–752
hematopoietic emergencies, 732
hemorrhage, 79–82
high-altitude cerebral edema (HACE), 774–775
high-altitude pulmonary edema (HAPE), 774
home care patients, 1118
hydrocarbons, 698
hydrofluoric (HF) acid, 697–698

Hymenoptera stings, 708
hyperadrenal crisis, 620
hyperglycemia, 1000
hyperglycemic hyperosmolar nonketotic (HHNK) coma, 615
hypertensive disorders of pregnancy, 884–885
hypertensive emergencies, 551–552
hyperventilation syndrome, 368
hypoglycemia (insulin shock), 615–616, 999
hypotension, 554f
hypothermia, 755–757, 758f, 933
hypothyroidism, 618–619
infection, 107
influenza, 813
ingested toxins, 689–690
inhaled toxins, 691
injected toxins, 707
iron overdose, 704
labour, patient in, 890–891
lead overdose, 704
limb presentation during delivery, 897–898
lithium overdose, 701
lower-airway foreign-body obstruction, 986
lung cancer, 362
marine animal injection, 715
meconium staining, 901
meningitis, 997
mercury, 704
musculoskeletal injury management in children, 202
myocardial infarction (MI), 543–545
myxedema, 618–619
near-drowning, 763–764
neglected child, 1015–1016
neonatal hypothermia, 933
neonatal vomiting, 934
neoplasms, 598
nerve dysfunction, 369
neurological emergencies. *See* neurological emergencies
newborns, 912–914
nitrogen narcosis, 771
nontraumatic vaginal bleeding, 863
NSAIDs overdose, 703
obstetric patient, 878
pediatric burns, 1011
pediatric emergencies, generally, 959–976
pediatric hyperglycemia, 1000
pediatric hypoglycemia, 999
pediatric poisonings, 1002–1003
pediatric seizures, 996–997
peripheral vascular emergencies, 563–564
phobias, 843
pit viper bites, 712–713
placenta previa, 882
pneumomediastinum, 770
pneumonia, 361, 808, 986
poisonings, 1002–1003
poisonous plants and mushrooms, 706
post-cardiac-arrest management, 556
postpartum hemorrhage, 902
posttraumatic stress syndrome, 843

precipitous delivery, 900–901
pregnant women, 326
preterm labour, 888–889
prolapsed cord, 897
pulmonary edema, 554f
pulmonary embolism, 366, 903
pulseless ventricular tachycardia (VF/VT), 557f
radioactive emergencies, 778
renal calculi (kidney stones), 676
respiratory compromise (pediatric), 979
respiratory disorders, management principles, 347–348
respiratory muscle dysfunction, 369
resuscitation, 555
return of spontaneous circulation (ROSC), 555
salicylate overdose, 702
scorpion stings, 710
seizures, 592–593, 996–997
sexual assault injuries, 865–866
shock, 89–92
shoulder dystocia, 901
soft-tissue injury, 132
soft-tissue injury management. *See* soft-tissue injury management
special-needs children and infants, 1019–1020
spinal cord dysfunction, 369
spinal injury management. *See* spinal injury management
spontaneous abortion, 880
spontaneous pneumothorax, 368
stroke, 588, 589f
sudden infant death syndrome (SIDS), 1012
supine-hypotensive syndrome, 885, 886f
surface-absorbed toxins, 691
survival, 555
syncope, 594–595
theophylline overdose, 703
thermal burns, 156–159
thoracic trauma management. *See* thoracic trauma management
thyrotoxic crisis (thyroid storm), 617
toxic inhalation, 363
toxicological emergencies, 686–688
tracheostomy patient, 1126
traumatic gynecological emergencies, 864
tricyclic antidepressants, 699
tuberculosis (TB), 806–807
upper respiratory infection (URI), 359–360
urinary tract infection (UTI), 678–679
urological emergencies, 664–665
uterine inversion, 903
uterine rupture, 902
ventricular fibrillation, 557f
"weak and dizzy," 596–597
mandatory reporting, 1015
mandible fractures, 219
mandibular dislocation, 219
manic-depressive, 701, 845
mannitol, 240
manual airway manoeuvres
head-tilt/chin-lift manoeuvre, 373, 380–382, 952

jaw-thrust manoeuvre, 373, 382, 952, 1006f
    Sellick's manoeuvre, 234, 235, 382–383, 383f, 408
manual cervical immobilization, 263–264
manual immobilization, 257, 259f
manual stabilization, 257
MAO inhibitors, 699–700
Marfan's syndrome, 560, 1039
marginal artery, 448
marijuana, 718t
marine animal injection, 684, 714–715
masks, 806, 822
mass, 14
Massassauga, 711
MAST, 91–92
mast cells, 627
mastoid bandaging, 124
maternal care, 1136–1138
maternal complications of labour and delivery
    postpartum hemorrhage, 902
    pulmonary embolism, 903
    uterine inversion, 902–903
    uterine rupture, 902
maternal-fetal circulation, 873–874, 874f
maternal mortality, 316
maternal narcotic use, 924–926
maxillary fractures, 219–220
McBurney's point, 652
MDMA, 716
measles, 814
mechanisms of injury
    abdominal trauma, 310–312
    analysis, 7
    blunt injury, 206–207
    defined, 7
    facial injuries, 206–207
    head injuries, 206–207
    hemorrhage, 76
    internal hemorrhage, significant, 71
    neck injuries, 206–207
    pediatric emergencies, 950
    pediatric trauma, 1003–1005
    soft-tissue trauma, 115–116
    spinal injury, 249–252, 250f
meconium, 912, 915
meconium-stained amniotic fluid, 926–927
meconium staining, 901
Medi-Port, 1130
mediastinal displacement, 295, 300
mediastinum, 448
medical antishock trouser (MAST), 91–92
medical emergencies
    allergic reactions. See allergic reaction; anaphylaxis
    cardiovascular emergencies. See cardiovascular emergencies
    endocrinological emergencies. See endocrinological emergencies
    gastrointestinal (GI) emergencies. See gastrointestinal (GI) emergencies
    gynecological emergencies. See gynecological emergencies
    hematopoietic emergencies. See hematopoietic emergencies
    neurological emergencies. See neurological emergencies

pulmonary emergencies. See respiratory disorders
renal emergencies. See renal emergencies
respiration. See respiratory disorders
toxicological emergencies. See toxicological emergencies
urological emergencies. See urological emergencies
medical gynecological emergencies
    cystitis, 862
    ectopic pregnancy, 863
    endometriosis, 862–863
    endometritis, 862
    gynecological abdominal pain, 861–863
    mittelschmerz, 862
    nontraumatic vaginal bleeding, 863
    pelvic inflammatory disease (PID), 861–862
    ruptured ovarian cyst, 862
medication allergies, 341
medications
    infection, effect on, 106
    as interventions. See pharmacological interventions
    toxicity of. See toxicological emergencies
melena, 72, 78, 1056
men, abuse by women, 1075
Meniere's disease, 1031
meningitis, 595, 811–812, 826, 932, 997
meningocele, 601
meningococcal meningitis, 811–812
meningoencephalitis, 815, 817
meningomyelocele, 911
menopause, 1039
menorrhagia, 863
mental challenges, 1096
mental status
    altered mental status, 582–584, 1109–1110
    and AVPU method, 573
    defined, 837
    determination of, 837
    geriatric patients, 1033
    home care patients, 1116–1117
mental status examination (MSE), 839
meperidine hydrochloride (Demerol®), 201–202
mercury, 703, 704
mesenteric infarct, 1056, 1057
mesentery, 315
metabolic acidosis, 666, 672
metabolic disorders. See endocrinological emergencies
metabolic rate, 747
metabolism, 82, 608, 609
metal fume fever, 693t
metal sheet splint, 186
metastasize, 597
methamphetamines, 716
methanol, 719
methemoglobin, 694
methicillin-resistant Staphylococcus aureus (MRSA), 830
methylprednisolone, 630
microangiopathy, 667, 669
microhemorrhage, 290

microorganisms
    bacteria, 784–785, 784f
    fungi, 786–787
    hookworms, 787
    normal flora, 783
    opportunistic pathogens, 784
    parasites, 787
    pathogens, 783
    pinworms, 787
    prions, 786
    protozoa, 787
    trichinosis, 787
    viruses, 785–786, 786f
midazolam (Versed®), 200, 235, 242
migraines, 595
mild hypothermia, 754
minor burns, 156–157
miscarriage, 862, 863, 880
mites, 830
mitral valve, 448
mittelschmerz, 862
MMR vaccination, 815
Mobitz I, 484–485, 486f
Mobitz II, 486
moderate burns, 157–159
moderate diffuse axonal injury, 214
modified chest lead 1 (MCL$_1$), 454
monomorphic VT, 499
mononeuropathy, 571–572
mononucleosis, 817
mood disorders
    bipolar disorder, 845
    defined, 843
    depression, 843–844
    major depression, 844
    IN SAD CAGES, 844
Moraxella catarrhalis, 807
Morbilli, 814
morphine sulphate, 157, 201, 235, 242, 548, 553
mosquito bites, 809–810
motor aphasia, 1093
motor system status, 578–579
motor-vehicle collisions (MVCs). See vehicular collisions
motorcycle collisions, 30–32, 266–267
motorcycle helmets, 31–32
mouth, assessment of, 576
mouth-to-mask ventilation, 437–438
mouth-to-mouth ventilation, 437
mouth-to-nose ventilation, 437
movement of spinal injury patient
    cervical immobilization device (CID), 272
    diving injury immobilization, 272–273
    final patient positioning, 271
    log roll, 267–268, 268f
    long spine board, 271–272, 272f
    orthopedic stretcher, 269
    rapid extrication, 270–271, 271f
    short spine board, 269–270
    straddle slide, 268–269
    vest-type immobilization device, 269–270, 269f
Mucomyst, 702
mucoviscidosis, 1101
multifocal atrial tachycardia (MAT), 474–475, 474f

multifocal seizures, 932
multigravidas, 875, 898
multipara, 875
multiple births, 899–900
multiple myeloma, 739–740
multiple personality disorder, 847
multiple sclerosis (MS), 335, 599, 876, 1102
multiple-system failure, 1026
mumps, 814–815
Munchausen syndrome, 847
mural emboli, 561
Murphy's sign, 654
muscle cramps, 749
muscular dystrophy (MD), 335, 599, 1102, 1122
muscular injury
    assessment, 177–183
    compartment syndrome, 170
    contusion, 170
    cramping, 170–171
    damaged tendons, 170
    described, 169
    fatigue (muscle), 170
    hypovolemia, 179
    muscular and connective tissue care, 190, 199
    penetrating injury, 170
    spasm, 171, 176, 282
    strain, 171
    types of, 169
musculoskeletal compartments, 109f
musculoskeletal disorders
    geriatric patients, 1058–1060
    osteoarthritis, 1058, 1059
    osteoporosis, 1058, 1059–1060
musculoskeletal injury management
    see also fractures
    analgesics, 200
    ankle injuries, 196–197
    arm bone fractures, 194
    clavicular fractures, 193
    diazepam (Valium®), 200
    elbow injuries, 198
    femur fractures, 191–192
    fentanyl (Sublimaze®), 201
    fibula fractures, 192–193
    foot injuries, 197
    fracture care, 189, 191–195
    general principles, 183–185
    hip dislocation, 195
    humerus fractures, 193–194
    immobilization, 185
    joint care, 189–190, 195–199
    knee injuries, 195–196
    leg bone fractures, 192–193
    limb positioning, 184, 185f
    medications, 199–202
    meperidine hydrochloride (Demerol®), 201–202
    midazolam (Versed®), 200
    morphine sulphate, 201
    muscular and connective tissue care, 190
    muscular and connective tissue injuries, 199
    naloxone hydrochloride (Narcan®), 201
    neurovascular function, evaluation of, 185
    nitrous oxide (Nitronox®), 200

open wounds, protection of, 184
patient refusals, 203
pediatric considerations, 202
pelvic fractures, 191
proximal fractures, 191
psychological support, 203
radius fractures, 194
sedatives, 200
shoulder injuries, 197–198
splinting devices, 186–189
sports injuries, 202
sprains, 196–197
tibia fractures, 192–193
ulna fractures, 194
musculoskeletal system, and pregnancy, 872
musculoskeletal trauma
    see also fractures
    assessment, 177–183
    bone injuries, 172–175
    classification, 178
    compartment syndrome, 181
    degenerative conditions, 176–177
    described, 168–169
    detailed secondary assessment, 182
    focused history and secondary assessment, 179–182
    general considerations, 175–176
    inflammatory conditions, 176–177
    joint injury, 171–172
    management of musculoskeletal injury. See musculoskeletal injury management
    muscular injury, 169–171
    ongoing assessment, 182
    pathophysiology, 169–177
    prevention strategies, 169
    primary assessment, 178–179
    rapid trauma assessment, 179
    scene assessment, 178
    secondary assessment, 182
    six Ps, 180
    sports injury considerations, 183
mushrooms, poisonous, 705–706
MVCs. See vehicular collisions
myalgia, 705
myasthenia gravis, 1104, 1109, 1122–1123
Mycobacterium, 785, 804
Mycobacterium tuberculosis, 794, 799, 804
    see also tuberculosis (TB)
Mycoplasma pneumoniae, 807
myelin, 599
myelomeningocele, 601
myocardial aneurysm, 293
myocardial contusion, 290–291, 291f, 306
myocardial infarction (MI)
    and angina pectoris, 537
    asystole, 542
    chest pain, 541
    congestive heart failure, 546
    and congestive heart failure (CHF), 541
    defined, 539
    dysrhythmias and, 540, 542
    field assessment, 541–542
    geriatric patients, 1046
    heart failure, 541
    in-hospital management, 544–545
    inadequate tissue perfusion, 541
    management, 543–545

non-Q-wave infarction, 540
OPQRST questions, 541
pathological Q wave, 542
pump failure, 541
reperfusion, 537
silent myocardial infarction, 1046
subendocardial infarction, 540
thrombus, 540
transmural infarction, 540
transport considerations, 543
ventricular aneurysm, 541
myocardial ischemia, 526t
myocardial rupture, 293
myocardium, 448
myoclonic seizures, 932
myoclonus, 601
myotomes, evaluation of, 260
myxedema, 616, 618–619
myxedema coma, 618

N. gonorrhoeae, 678
N-acetylcysteine, 702
N95 respirators, 806, 806f
NAC, 702
naloxone, 716, 924–925
naloxone hydrochloride (Narcan®), 201, 242
naproxen sodium, 702
narcan neonatal, 925t
narcotic, 693t
narcotics, 716, 717t
nasal cannula, 436
nasal flaring, 339
nasal injury, 221
nasogastric intubation, 969–970, 971f, 1134f
nasogastric tube, 922
nasogastric tube placement, 434
nasopharyngeal airways, 233–234, 384–385, 385f, 963
nasotracheal intubation, 235, 414–417, 415f
nasotracheal route, 414
natal, 875
National Advisory Committee on Immunization, 822
National Head Injury Foundation, 211
National Institute for Occupational Safety and Health (NIOSH), 806
natural immunity, 625
natural passive immunity, 625
naturally acquired immunity, 625
nature of the illness (NOI), 950
nausea, 514, 637, 662, 997–998
    see also gastrointestinal (GI) emergencies; urological emergencies
near-drowning
    adult respiratory distress syndrome (ARDS), 350, 764
    defined, 761
    incidence, 761
    mammalian diving reflex, 763
    management, 763–764
    pathophysiology, 761–763
    pediatric trauma, 1004–1005
    sequelae, 764
    survival, factors affecting, 763
neck, and soft-tissue infections, 335
neck injuries
    airway evaluation, 226
    airway trauma, 224

assessment, 225–232

blood vessel trauma, 223–224

blunt injury, 206–207

breathing, monitoring, 226–227

cervical spine trauma, 224

circulation, evaluation of, 227

deep penetrating trauma, 224

detailed secondary assessment, 232

focused history and secondary assessment, 231

Glasgow Coma Scale (GCS), 230–231, 230t

laceration, 224f

management. *See* head, facial, and neck injury management

mechanisms of injury, 206–207

ongoing assessment, 232

pathophysiology, 223–224

penetrating trauma, 207

primary assessment, 225–227

rapid trauma assessment, 227–231

scene assessment, 225

subcutaneous emphysema, 224

vital signs, monitoring of, 231

neck wounds

bandaging, 124

hemorrhage, 81

penetrating trauma, 58

soft-tissue injury management, 131

necrosis, 110, 462

needle cricothyrostomy, 131, 236–237, 422, 423–427, 425f, 426f, 965

negative feedback, 746

negative impulses, 452

negative-pressure ventilators, 1127

negative symptoms, 841

neglect

alerting factors, 1013

assessment, 1015

effects of, 1015f

geriatric patients, 1069–1070

index of suspicion, 1015

management of neglected child, 1015–1016

perpetrators of, 1013

resources, 1016

signs of, 1083

Neisseria gonorrhoeae, 825, 861

Neisseria meningitidis, 785, 811

neonatal abstinence syndrome (NAS), 935

neonatal care

see also newborns

APGAR scoring, 895, 896t, 911–912

resuscitation, 896

routine care, 894–895

stimulation of infant, 895f

neonatal distress

see also neonatal emergencies

aspiration of meconium, 915

central cyanosis, 921

fetal heart rate, 915

maternal narcotic use, 924–926

naloxone, 924–925

particulate meconium, 915

resuscitation, 915–924

transport considerations, 926

vagal response, 916

vital signs, 915

neonatal emergencies

see also neonatal distress

acrocyanosis, 933

apnea, 928

aspiration of meconium, 927

birth injuries, 935–936

bradycardia, 929

caput succedaneum, 935

cardiac resuscitation. *See* neonatal resuscitation

cranial injuries, 935

cyanosis, 930–931

diaphragmatic hernia, 928–929, 929f

diarrhea, 934–935

fever, 932

focal clonic seizures, 932

hypoglycemia, 933–934

hypothermia, 932–933

hypovolemia, 931

intubation, 927, 927f

meconium-stained amniotic fluid, 926–927

meningitis, 932

multifocal seizures, 932

myoclonic seizures, 932

neonatal abstinence syndrome (NAS), 935

phototherapy, 935

pneumothorax, 927

post resuscitation, 936

premature infants, 929–930, 930f, 933

respiratory distress, 930–931

seizures, 931–932

small-for-gestational-age (SGA) newborns, 933

stabilization, 936

subtle seizures, 931

thyrotoxicosis, 935

tonic seizures, 931–932

vomiting, 934

neonatal intensive care unit (NICU), 926

neonatal resuscitation

APGAR score, 919

assessment parameters, 918–919

chest compressions, 922, 923f

colour, 919

depth of insertion, 919t

drying, 916–920

endotracheal intubation, 920f

equipment, 916–917

face masks, 921

heart rate, 918

intubation, 922

inverted pyramid for, 916–924, 916f

medications, 923–924, 925t

nasogastric tube, 922

neonatal cardiac arrest, incidence of, 936

opening the airway, 919f

orogastric tube, 922

oxygen concentration, guidelines for estimating, 921f

positioning, 916–920

potential interventions, 918f

procedure, illustrated, 917f

respiratory effort, 918

suctioning, 916–920

supplemental oxygen, 921

tactile stimulation, 916–920

tracheal suctioning, 920f

tracheal tube sizes, 919t

vascular access for fluid and drug administration, 923–924, 924f

ventilation, 921–922

warming, 916–920

neonates

acrocyanosis, 895

defined, 894, 907

growth and development, 942

newborn, 907

see also newborns

resuscitation. *See* neonatal resuscitation

neoplasms, 597–598

neoplastic agents, 106

neovascularization, 104–105

nephrology, 659

see also renal disorders

nerve dysfunction, 369

nerve root injury, 260

nervous system

central nervous system disorders, 570–571

see also neurological emergencies

central nervous system dysfunction, 368–369

disorders. *See* neurological emergencies

emergencies. *See* neurological emergencies

geriatric patients, 1038

overview, 570f

pediatric care, 949

status, 577–579

nervous system infections

encephalitis, 821

Lyme disease, 824–825

rabies, 821–823

tetanus, 823–824

neurogenic shock, 224, 255, 273–274, 990

neurological emergencies

AEIOU-TIPS, 582–583

airway and breathing, 582

alteration in cognitive systems, 570

altered mental status, 582–584

Alzheimer's disease, 1053

autonomic nervous system disorders, 572

back pain, 602–605

brain abscess, 598

central nervous system disorders, 570–571

cerebral homeostasis, 571

cerebrovascular disease, 1050–1051

chronic alcoholism, 583–584

circulatory support, 582

degenerative neurological disorders, 598–602

delirium, 1052, 1052t

dementia, 1052, 1052t, 1053

described, 569

dizziness, 1051

epilepsy, 589–594

geriatric disorders, 1049–1054

headache, 595–596

intracranial hemorrhage, 584–588

intracranial pressure, 584

Korsakoff's psychosis, 584

neoplasms, 597–598
nontraumatic spinal disorders, 602–605
Parkinson's disease, 1053–1054
pathophysiology, 570–572
pediatric emergencies, 994–997
peripheral nervous system disorders, 571–572
peripheral neuropathy, 571–572
pharmacological interventions, 582
psychological support, 582
seizures, 589–594, 1051
stroke, 584–588, 1050–1051
supportive treatment, 581–582
symptoms, reduction of, 582
syncope, 594–595
transport considerations, 582
vertigo, 1051
"weak and dizzy," 596–597
Wernicke's syndrome, 583
neurological emergency assessment
additional assessment tools, 580–581
airway, monitoring, 574
AVPU method, 573
blood glucometer, 581
cardiovascular status, 576–577
cranial nerves status, 579
Cushing's reflex, 580
decerebrate posturing, 578, 578f
decorticate posturing, 578, 578f
difficulty of, 572
emotional status, assessment of, 573–574
end-tidal CO_2 detector, 581
eyes, 575–576
face, 575
focused history and secondary assessment, 574–581
geriatric considerations, 581
Glasgow Coma Scale (GCS), 579–580, 579f
history, 574–575
mental status assessment, 573, 579
motor system status, 578–579
nervous system status, 577–578
nose/mouth, 576
ongoing assessment, 581
primary assessment, 572–574
pulse oximeter, 581
respiratory status, 576, 577f
scene assessment, 572–574
secondary assessment, 575–580
sensorimotor evaluation, 577–578
vital signs, 580, 580f
neurological neoplasms, 597
neuromuscular blockers, 241, 408
neuromuscular degenerative diseases, 1122–1123
neuromuscular disorders, 876
neurosyphilis, 826
neurovascular function, 185, 198
neutral, in-line positioning, 257, 262–263
neutron radiation, 143
neutrons, 775, 776
neutropenia, 735–736
neutropenic, 1100
newborns
airway management, 912
antepartum factors, 908
APGAR scale, 911–912
assessment, 911–912
bronchopulmonary dysplasia (BPD), 1121–1122
choanal atresia, 911
cleft lip, 911
cleft palate, 911
common complications, 1137–1138
congenital anomalies, 910–911
defined, 907
DeLee suction trap, 912
diaphragmatic hernia, 910
distressed newborns. See neonatal distress
drying, 912, 914f
epidemiology, 908–909
first breaths, 909
growth and development, 942
heat loss, prevention of, 912–914
hemodynamic changes at birth, 910
home care, 1136–1138
hyperbilirubinemia, 914
intrapartum factors, 908
intubation, 913f
meconium, 912
meningomyelocele, 911
normal vital signs, 919
omphalocele, 911
pathophysiology, 909–911
persistent fetal circulation, 909
Pierre Robin syndrome, 911
polycythemia, 914
postterm, 926
premature infants, 929–930, 930f, 933
primary apnea, 909
risk factors for complications, 908t
secondary apnea, 909
small-for-gestational-age (SGA) newborns, 926, 933
spinal cord defects, 911
suctioning, 912, 913f
syndromes, 910
treatment, 912–914
umbilical cord, cutting, 914
umbilicus area defects, 911
newly born infant, 907
see also neonates
Newton's first law, 13–14
Newton's second law, 15, 40
nicotine, 642, 644
nifedipine, 773, 888–889
nitrogen narcosis, 766, 770–771
nitroglycerine, 539, 548, 553
nitrous oxide (Nitronox®), 200, 563
nocturia, 1047
non-Hodgkin's lymphoma, 737
non-insulin-dependent diabetes mellitus (NIDDM), 611–612
non-Q-wave infarction, 540
nonabsorbent dressings, 112
nonadherent dressings, 112
noncardiogenic pulmonary adult/edema respiratory distress syndrome, 349–351
noncardiogenic shock, 988–989
noncompensatory pause, 475, 489
nongonococcal urethritis (NGU), 827
nonocclusive dressings, 112
nonprescription medications, 515–516
nonrebreather mask, 436
nonsterile dressings, 111–112
nonsteroidal anti-inflammatory drugs. See NSAIDs (nonsteroidal anti-inflammatory drugs)
nontraumatic vaginal bleeding, 863
norepinephrine (Levophed), 553, 556, 630
normal breathing sounds, 343
normal delivery, 892f, 893f
normal flora, 783
normal sinus rhythm, 465
northern Pacific rattlesnake, 711
Norwalk virus, 643, 819
Norwegian scabies, 830
nose, assessment of, 576
nosebleed, 71, 221
nosocomial infections, 678, 830–831
NSAIDs (nonsteroidal anti-inflammatory drugs), 68, 106, 642, 644, 702–703, 817, 1099
nuclear radiation, 141–144, 142f, 775–778
nulligravida, 875
nullipara, 875

obese patients
accommodations, 1095
children, 1094–1095
diabetes, 611
etiologies, 1095
and hemorrhage, 74
statistics, 1094–1095
obligate intracellular parasites, 785
oblique angle, 26
oblique fracture, 174, 174f
obstetric history, 858–859
obstetric patients
see also pregnancy; pregnancy complications
active labour, 877
afterbirth, 869
aggravated medical conditions, 876
amniotic fluid, 870, 879
amniotic sac, 870
anatomy of, 868–870
assessment, 875–878
childbirth. See puerperium
delivery. See puerperium
general information from, 875
gestational diabetes, 876
heart disease, 876
history, 875–877
hypertension, 876
management, 878
neuromuscular disorders, 876
pain, 876–877
physiology, 868–870
placenta, 869, 870f
preexisting medical conditions, 876
primary assessment, 875
rupture of the membranes (ROM), 870
secondary assessment, 877–878
seizure disorders, 876
shock, 879
umbilical cord, 869–870, 894f, 897, 899f, 900f
vaginal bleeding, 877
vital signs, 877
obstetric terminology, 874–875

obstetrics, 858
obstructive lung disease
    abnormal ventilation, 351–352
    air trapping distal to the obstruction, 352
    asthma, 356–358
    chronic bronchitis, 354–355
    chronic obstructive pulmonary disease (COPD), 331, 341, 344, 351, 352–355
    emphysema, 352–353
    types of, 351
occiput posterior position, 898
occlusive dressings, 111f, 112, 132
occlusive strokes, 584–585
occulta, 601
Occupational Safety and Health Administration (OSHA) standards, 806
ohm, 138
Ohm's law, 139
old-old, 1026
oleoresin capsicum, 162
oliguria, 665
omphalocele, 911
ongoing assessment
    abdominal trauma, 324
    burns, 166
    cardiovascular emergencies, 511
    facial injuries, 232
    head injuries, 232
    hemorrhage, 79
    musculoskeletal trauma, 182
    neck injuries, 232
    neurological emergencies, 581
    pediatric assessment, 959
    shock, 89
    soft-tissue trauma, 118
    spinal injury, 261
    thermal burns, 156
    thoracic trauma, 301–302
    toxicological emergencies, 685–686
open cricothyrotomy, 422, 427, 428f–430f
open-ended questions, 837–838
open fracture, 173, 173f
open pneumothorax, 286–287, 286f, 303, 335
open wounds
    see also soft-tissue trauma
    abrasions, 97, 97f
    amputations, 101, 101f
    avulsions, 100–101, 100f
    compartment syndrome, 108
    degloving injury, 100–101, 101f
    epidemiology, 95
    home care patients, 1135–1136
    impaled objects, 100, 100f
    incisions, 98
    lacerations, 98, 98f
    protection of, 184
    punctures, 98–99, 99f
    ring injury, 101, 101f
    types of, 96f
opiates, 350, 716
opportunistic pathogens, 784
OPQRST questions, 340, 513, 541, 547, 636–637, 661–663
oral contraceptives, 859
oral fluid therapy, 751

orbital fractures, 220
ordnance, 36
organ failure, and burns, 150
organic, 835
organic brain syndrome, 1053
organic headaches, 595
organophsophates, 692t
organs
    abdominal injuries, 313, 314–315
    accessory organ diseases. See accessory organ diseases
    end-organ perfusion, 954
    hematemesis, 313
    hematochezia, 313
    hematuria, 313
    hollow organs, 55, 313, 635
    internal hemorrhage, 71
    penetrating trauma, 55
    solid organs, 55, 314–315
orogastric tube, 434, 922
oropharyngeal airway, 233–234, 385–386, 387f, 962, 962f
orotracheal intubation, 234, 258, 396–414
orthopedic injuries, 1071–1072
orthopedic stretcher, 269
orthopnea, 340
orthostatic hypotension, 78, 640
orthostatic syncope, 1049
Osborn waves, 510f, 755
oseltamivir, 814
osmosis, 611
osmotic diuresis, 611
osteoarthritis, 177, 1058, 1059
osteoporosis, 175, 1058, 1059–1060, 1071–1072
otitis media, 811
ovarian cysts, 862
overdose
    see also substance abuse; toxicological emergencies
    acetaminophen, 702
    antidepressants, 698, 700–701
    cardiac medications, 696
    defined, 681, 715
    iron, 704
    lead, 704
    lithium, 701
    MAO inhibitors, 699–700
    metals, 703–704
    salicylates, 701–702
    theophylline, 703
overdrive respiration, 89
overpressure, 35–36
ovulation, 868
oxidizer mixes, 34
oxygen administration, 237, 239–240, 331, 630, 632, 751, 820–821
    see also oxygenation
oxygen concentrators, 1124
oxygen cylinders, 1124
oxygen delivery devices, 435–436
oxygen dissociation curve, 333, 333f
oxygen humidifier, 436
oxygen saturation percentage, 378
oxygen supply and regulators, 435
oxygen toxicity, 350, 771
oxygenation
    see also oxygen administration

chronic obstructive pulmonary disease (COPD), 435
    described, 435
    heart failure, 548
    high-pressure regulators, 435
    home oxygen therapy, 1123–1124
    nasal cannula, 436
    neonatal resuscitation, 921
    nonrebreather mask, 436
    oxygen delivery devices, 435–436
    oxygen humidifier, 436
    oxygen supply and regulators, 435
    partial rebreather mask, 436
    pediatric airway management, 961
    simple face mask, 436
    small-volume nebulizer, 436
    therapy regulators, 435
    thyrotoxic crisis (thyroid storm), 617
    venturi mask, 436
oxytocin, 888

P-Q interval (PQI), 461
P-R interval (PRI), 460f, 461, 465
P wave, 456, 458f, 459f, 464–465
pacemaker
    artificial pacemaker rhythm, 505–506, 506f
    AV sequential pacemakers, 505
    battery failure, 505
    demand pacemaker, 505
    dual-chambered pacemakers, 505
    fixed-rate pacemakers, 505
    insertion, 487, 488–489
    magnets, 506
    problems with, 505–506
    runaway pacemaker, 505
    wandering atrial pacemaker, 473–474, 473f
padded board splint, 199f
pain
    abdominal pain. See abdominal pain
    central pain syndrome, 600
    chest pain, 512, 513, 541, 663
    control, and soft-tissue injury management, 122
    gastrointestinal (GI) emergencies, 635
    headache, 595–596
    Murphy's sign, 654
    musculoskeletal trauma, 180
    obstetric patients, 876–877
    pathophysiological basis of pain, 660–661
    pleuritic, 360
    referred pain, 635–636, 637, 661
    somatic pain, 635
    tic douloureux, 600
    trigeminal neuralgia, 600
    urological disorders, 660–661
    visceral pain, 635, 661
pain disorder, 846
paint sniffing, 690
pallor, 180, 339
palpation
    abdomen, 638
    cardiovascular emergencies, 520
    respiratory problems, 377
    respiratory system, 342–343
    soft-tissue trauma, 118

palpitations, 514
pancolitis, 647
pancreas
    injury to, 314
    mucoviscidosis, 1101
pancreas disorders
    diabetes mellitus, 608–612
    diabetic emergencies, 612t, 613t
    diabetic ketoacidosis (diabetic coma),
        610, 612–614
    hyperglycemic hyperosmolar nonketotic
        (HHNK) coma, 612, 614–615
    hypoglycemia (insulin shock), 615–616
pancreatic duct, blocked, 645
pancreatitis, 350, 654–655
pancuronium (Pavulon®), 235, 241, 408
panic attack, 842–843
"paper bag" syndrome, 22, 23f
para/parity (P), 859
paracetamol, 702
paradoxical breathing, 373
paralysis, 180, 1096
paralytic agents, 235, 240–241, 407
paralytic shellfish poisoning, 705
paramedics
    competencies. See advanced care
        paramedic (ACP) competencies;
        primary care paramedic (PCP)
        competencies
    Golden Hour, 8
    index of suspicion, 7–8
    injury prevention, support of, 10
    mechanism of injury analysis, 7
    seat belt use, 19
    transport decision, 9–10
    trauma system, role in, 6–11
    trauma triage criteria, 6
Paramyxovirus, 814
paranoid schizophrenia, 842
paraplegia, 248, 1096
parasites, 787, 819
parenteral penicillin injections, 626–627
paresthesia, 180, 260, 705
parity, 875
Parkinson's disease, 599–600, 1053–1054
paroxysmal junctional tachycardia (PJT),
    493–495, 494f
paroxysmal nocturnal dyspnea (PND), 340,
    547
paroxysmal phase of pertusis, 816
paroxysmal supraventricular tachycardia
    (PSVT), 476–479, 477f, 493
paroxysms, 493
partial ejection, 27
partial rebreather mask, 436
partial seizures, 591
partial thickness burn, 147
particulate meconium, 915
partner abuse
    abused partners, characteristics of, 1077
    abusers, characteristics of, 1077
    assessment of battered patient,
        1077–1078
    defined, 1075
    generic risk factors, 1076–1077
    identification of, 1076–1077
    potential for, 1075
    reasons for not reporting, 1076

same-sex couples, 1076
    sexual abuse, 1076
    verbal abuse, 1076
    victim characteristics, 1084–1085
PASG, 91–92
passenger airbags, 20
passive immunity, 625
past medical history, 516
Pasteurella multocida, 105
patellar dislocations, 195
pathogens, 624, 783
pathological fractures, 175, 740
pathological gambling, 849
pathological Q wave, 542
pathophysiology
    abdominal trauma, 310–318
    acute renal failure (ARF), 666–667
    adult respiratory distress syndrome
        (ARDS), 350
    adrenal insufficiency (Addison's disease),
        620
    allergic reaction, 624–627
    anaphylaxis, 627
    asthma, 356, 983–984
    burns, 136–151
    carbon monoxide inhalation, 364
    cardiovascular emergencies, specific. See
        cardiovascular emergency
        management
    central nervous system dysfunction, 368
    chronic bronchitis, 355
    chronic renal failure (CRF), 669–670
    cold disorders, 744–747
    diabetic ketoacidosis, 613
    diving emergencies, 765
    drowning, 761–763, 762f
    emphysema, 352
    environmental emergencies, 744–747
    facial injuries, 219–223
    gastrointestinal (GI) emergencies,
        635–636
    geriatric patients, 1026–1029,
        1030–1031, 1035–1041
    Graves' disease, 616
    head injuries, 208–219
    heat disorders, 744–747
    hyperadrenalism (Cushing's syndrome),
        619
    hyperglycemic hyperosmolar nonketotic
        (HHNK) coma, 614
    hyperventilation syndrome, 367
    hypoglycemia (insulin shock), 615
    hypothyroidism, 618
    kidney stones, 675–676
    lung cancer, 362
    musculoskeletal trauma, 169–177
    near-drowning, 761–763
    neck injuries, 223–224
    nerve dysfunction, 369
    neurological emergencies, 570–572
    newborns, 909–911
    pain, 660–661
    pneumonia, 360
    psychiatric disorders, 835–836
    pulmonary embolism, 365
    renal calculi, 675–676
    respiratory disorders, 334–337
    respiratory muscle dysfunction, 369

soft-tissue trauma, 95–96
    spinal cord dysfunction, 369
    spinal injury, 249–255
    spontaneous pneumothorax, 366
    thoracic trauma, 278–296
    thyrotoxic crisis (thyroid storm), 617
    toxic inhalation, 363
    Type I diabetes mellitus, 611
    upper respiratory infection (URI),
        358–359
    urinary tract infection (UTI), 677–678
    urological disorders, 660–661
patient positioning, 233
patient refusals, 203
peak expiratory flow rate (PEFR), 346, 346f,
    357, 380
pedestrian accidents, 32, 32f, 33f, 1004
Pediatric Advanced Life Support (PALS), 939
pediatric airway management
    advanced, 964–970
    airway adjuncts, 961–963
    basic, 959–964, 960t
    endotracheal intubation, 965–969, 968f
    equipment guidelines, 963t
    foreign body airway obstruction
        (FBAO), 960, 964–965
    general, 947, 952f
    infant/child endotracheal tubes, 966t
    laryngeal mask airway, 965
    laryngoscope placement, 967f
    manual positioning, 959
    nasogastric intubation, 969–970, 971f
    nasopharyngeal airways, 963
    needle cricothyrostomy, 965
    newborns, 912
    oropharyngeal airways, 962, 962f
    oxygenation, 961
    rapid sequence intubation (RSI), 970
    suction catheter sizes, 961f, 961t
    suctioning, 960–961
    ventilation, 964
pediatric assessment
    airway, 951
    basic considerations, 950
    breathing, 951–954
    capillary refill, 957
    cardiopulmonary arrest, anticipation
        of, 955
    circulation, 954–955
    colour, 954
    cyanosis, 954
    electrocardiogram (ECG), 958–959
    end-organ perfusion, 954
    focused assessment, 956–957
    focused history and secondary
        assessment, 956–959
    general impression, 951
    Glasgow Coma Scale (GCS), 957, 958t
    head-tilt/chin-lift manoeuvre, 952
    heart rate, 954
    history, 956
    hydration, 957
    jaw-thrust manoeuvre, 952
    level of consciousness, 951
    noninvasive monitoring, 958–959
    ongoing assessment, 959
    opening the airway, 952f
    pediatric assessment triangle, 951

peripheral circulation, 954
primary assessment, 951–956
pulse oximetry, 957
pupils, 957
respiratory effort, 954, 954t
respiratory rate, 952
scene assessment, 950
secondary assessment, 956–959
transitional phase, 955–956
transport priority, 955
triangle, 951
vital functions, 951–955, 953t
vital signs, 957–958
Pediatric Basic Trauma Life Support (PBTLS), 939
pediatric care
abdomen, assessment of, 948
abdominal injuries, 318
acute appendicitis, 652
airway management, 947
anatomy of infants and children, 945–949
asthma, 351, 358
bag-valve-mask ventilation (BVM ventilation), 439
bag-valve masks, 439
bend fractures, 1010
body surface area (BSA), 948
Brudzinski's sign, 812
buckle fractures, 1010
cardiovascular system, 948–949
chancroid lesions, 828
chest, evaluation of, 947–948
chickenpox vaccine, 810
continuing education and training, 939–940
croup, 818
elbow injuries, 198
endotracheal intubation, 410–414, 411t, 413f
epiglottitis, 359
epiphyseal fracture, 175, 202
extremities, assessment of, 948
febrile seizures, 589, 753
fetal alcohol spectrum disorder (FASD), 1098
fever, 753
fever, tachypnea and retraction triad, 807
fractures, 174–175
gastroenteritis, 819
greenstick fracture, 175, 202, 1010
growth and development, 942–945
growth plate, 948
head, 946–947
head injuries, risk of, 206
head lice, 829
head trauma, 218
heat loss, prevention of, 949
hemorrhage, 74, 949
hepatitis A (HAV), 801
Kernig's sign, 812
leukemia, 736
lungs, evaluation of, 947–948
measles, 814
meningococcemia, 812
metabolic differences, 949
musculoskeletal injury management, 202

nervous system, 949
obesity, 1094–1095
paramedics, role of, 939–940
pedestrian accidents, 32, 33f
pertussis, 814
physical abuse, and burns, 150–151
physiology of infants and children, 945–949, 945t
poisoning, 682
psychiatric disorders, 851
respiratory syncytial virus (RSV), 815–816
respiratory system, 948
rib fractures, 281–282
rule of nines, 147
self-study, 940
sensorineural deafness, 1090–1091
sickle cell anemia, 731
skin, 948
thermal burns, 155
thoracic trauma, 279
tracheal shift, 287
vaccination against pneumonia, 808
ventilation, 439–440
pediatric emergencies
ABCs, 1019
adolescents, 944–945
airway management. See pediatric airway management
allergic reaction, 990
apnea monitors, 1017
assessment. See pediatric assessment
cannula problems, 1125
caregivers, responding to, 941–942
central IV line, 1018
cervical spine immobilization, 975
child abuse, 1012–1016
circulation, 970–974
communication, 940–942
dehydration, 997, 998t
diabetes mellitus, 998
diabetic ketoacidosis (diabetic coma), 1000
diarrhea, 998
electrical therapy, 974
electrolyte abnormalities, 997
febrile seizures, 996
fluid therapy, 973
fulminant meningitis, 997
gastric feeding tubes, 1018–1019
gastroenteritis, 997
gastrointestinal emergencies, 997–998
gastrostomy tubes, 1018–1019
general approach, 940–949
home artificial ventilators, 1018
hyperglycemia, 1000, 1000t
hypoglycemia, 998–999
hypotension, 958
infants, 942–943
infections, 976–977
infusions, preparation of, 975t
ingested poisoning, indications of, 1002f
intraosseous (IO) infusion, 972–973, 973f
management, generally, 959–976
medications, 973–974, 974t
meningitis, 997
metabolic emergencies, 998–1001

nausea, 997–998
neglect, 1012–1016
neonates, 942
neurological emergencies, 994–997
newborns, 942
parents, responding to, 941–942
patient needs, responding to, 940–941
poisonings, 1001–1003, 1002f
preschoolers, 943–944
psychological support, 940–942, 976
rapid cardiopulmonary collapse, 997
respiratory emergencies. See pediatric respiratory emergencies
school-aged children, 944
seizures, 994–997
sepsis, 989–990
shock (hypoperfusion), 986–994
    see also pediatric shock
shunts, 1019
special-needs children and infants, 1016–1020
status epilepticus, 996
stoma, 1017
sudden infant death syndrome (SIDS), 1011–1012
toddlers, 943
toxic exposure, 1001–1003, 1002f
tracheostomy tubes, 1016–1017, 1017t
transport guidelines, 975–976
trauma emergencies. See pediatric trauma
vascular access, 970–974
vomiting, 997–998
warming techniques, emphasis on, 949
pediatric intubation, 410–414, 411t, 413f
pediatric patients. See pediatric care
pediatric pulseless arrest treatment algorithm, 995f
pediatric respiratory emergencies
asthma, 983–984
bacterial tracheitis, 982–983
brochiolitis, 985
croup, 980, 980f
epiglottitis, 980–982, 980f
foreign body aspiration, 983
lower-airway distress, 983–986
lower-airway foreign-body obstruction, 986
management of respiratory compromise, 979
pneumonia, 985–986
respiratory arrest, 978
respiratory distress, 977–978
respiratory failure, 978
severity of respiratory compromise, 977
upper-airway obstruction, 979–980
pediatric shock
absent cardiac rhythm, 992–994
anaphylactic shock, 990
asystole, 993–994
bradycardia, 993f
bradydysrhythmias, 992
cardiogenic shock, 988, 990–994
cardiomyopathy, 991
categories of shock, 988–990
compensated shock, 987
congenital heart disease, 990, 991
decompensated shock, 987–988

distributive shock, 989–990
dysrhythmias, 991–994
hypovolemic shock, 989
irreversible shock, 988
life-threatening nature of, 986–987
neurogenic shock, 990
noncardiogenic shock, 988–989
pulseless electrical activity (PEA), 994
pulseless ventricular tachycardia
(VF/VT), 994
septic shock, 989–990
severity of shock, 987–988
signs and symptoms, 988f
supraventricular tachycardia, 992
tachydysrhythmias, 991
ventricular fibrillation, 994
ventricular tachycardia (VT) with a
pulse, 992
pediatric trauma
abdominal injuries, 1010
airbags, 1004f
airway management, 1006
analgesia, 1008
brain injury, 1008
burn surface area (BSA), 1010
burns, 1005, 1010–1011
chest injuries, 1009–1010
drowning, 1004–1005
extremities, 1010
falls, 1003, 1003f
fluid management, 1007
head, face, and neck injuries, 1009
immobilization, 1006–1007, 1007f
jaw-thrust/spine stabilization
manoeuvre, 1006f
mechanisms of injury, 1003–1005
near-drowning, 1004–1005
pedestrian accidents, 1004
penetrating trauma, 1005
physical abuse, 1005
pulmonary contusion, 1009
rule of nines, 1010–1011, 1011f
rule of palms, 1011
sedation, 1008
special considerations, 1006–1008
tension pneumothorax, 1010
vehicular collisions, 1004
Pediculus humanus var. capitis, 829
PEEP (positive end-expiratory pressure), 922,
1120, 1127–1128
pelvic fracture, 179, 191, 316
pelvic inflammatory disease (PID), 825,
861–862, 881
pelvic injury, 316
pelvic ring fractures, 191
penetrating trauma
see also penetrating wounds, specific
abdominal injury, 311, 313, 319–320,
322–323, 325
arrows, 51
assault rifle, 51
attackers' characteristics, 54
ballistics, 46–49
blast injuries, 40
bullet entry wounds, 59
cranial fracture, and bullet impacts,
210–211
damage pathway, 52–54

defined, 3
described, 16, 16f, 45
direct injury, 52–53
energy exchange between projectile and
body tissue, 46–49
exit wounds, 59
facial injuries, 207
fluid administration and, 90–91
handgun, 49–50
head injuries, 58, 207
heart, 301
kinetics of, 45–46
knives, 51
low-velocity wounds, 54
mortality, 57
muscular injury, 170
neck injuries, 207
organ injuries, specific, 55–59
pediatric trauma, 1005
permanent cavity, 54
pregnant women, mortality of, 316
pressure shock wave, 53
projectile injury process, 52
rifles, 50
safety issues, 59–61
scene assessment, 59–61
shotgun, 51
simple pneumothorax, 300
special emergency concerns, 59–63
specific wounds. *See* penetrating
wounds, specific
spinal injury, 252
temporary cavity, 53
thoracic injury, 277, 279–280, 280t,
300–301
tissue injuries, specific, 55–59
vascular injuries, 315
victims' characteristics, 54
weapon characteristics, 49–51
wound assessment, 61
wound care, 61–63
zone of injury, 54
penetrating wounds, specific
abdomen, 57
assessment, 61
bone, 56
chest wounds, 62
connective tissue, 55
entrance wounds, 58–59
exit wounds, 59
extremities, 56–57
facial wounds, 61–62
general body regions, 56–59
head, 58
hollow organs, 55
impaled objects, 62–63
lungs, 56
neck, 58
organs, 55
solid organs, 55
thorax, 58
wound care, 61–63
penicillinase-producing *N. gonorrhoeae*
(PPNG), 825
penicillins, 107, 623, 626–627
pepper spray, 162
peptic ulcer disease, 639, 640
peptic ulcers, 644–646, 645f

percussion, 343
percutaneous transluminal coronary
angioplasty (PTCA), 545
perfusion
defined, 333
disruption in, 337
process of, 333–334
pulmonary embolism, 334
pericardial tamponade, 55, 291–293, 292f,
306
pericardium, 448
perinephric abscesses, 678
perineum tears, 894
peripheral access device, 1100
peripheral arterial atherosclerotic disease,
562
peripheral circulation, 954
peripheral cyanosis, 344
peripheral edema, 518
peripheral nervous system disorders, 571–572
peripheral neuropathy, 571–572
peripheral oxygen saturation, 377
peripheral vascular emergencies
acute arterial occlusion, 561, 563
acute pulmonary embolism, 561
aneurysm, 560–561
assessment, 562–563
atherosclerosis, 559–560
deep venous thrombosis, 562
management, 563–564
noncritical conditions, 562
peripheral arterial atherosclerotic
disease, 562
transport considerations, 563–564
varicose veins, 562
vasculitis, 562
peripheral vasoconstriction, 753
peripherally inserted central catheters (PICC
lines), 1130
peritoneal dialysis, 674, 674f
peritoneum injury, 315–316
peritonitis, 315–316, 635, 650, 652
peritonsillar abscess, 335
periumbilical ecchymosis, 638
permanent cavity, 54
permethrin agents, 829
pernicious anemia, 729
persistent fetal circulation, 909
personality disorders, 847–848
perspiration, 514
pertussis, 816
petechia, 932
petit mal seizure, 591
phagocytosis, 104
pharmacological interventions
see also medications
allergic reactions, 629–631, 632
amyotrophic lateral sclerosis (ALS), 601
analgesics, 200, 679, 1008
anaphylaxis, 629–631
anticholinergic agents, 243, 752
antidysrhythmic drugs, 500, 526t
asystole, 503
atrial fibrillation, 482
atrial flutter, 480–481
bactericidal antibiotics, 785
bacteriostatic antibiotics, 785
Bell's palsy, 600

cardiac arrest, 556
cardiogenic shock, 553
cardiovascular emergencies, 525, 526t
central pain syndrome, 600
combative patients, 274
dextrose, 243
diuretics, 240
geriatric patients, 1026–1027, 1062–1064
head, facial, and neck injury management, 239–244
heart failure, 548
induction agents, 409t
medication allergies, 341
mononucleosis, 817
musculoskeletal injury management, 199–202
myocardial ischemia, 526t
myoclonus, 601
neonatal resuscitation, 925t
neurological emergencies, 582
neuromuscular blockers, 241, 408
paralytic agents, 235, 240–241, 407
paroxysmal junctional tachycardia (PJT), 494
paroxysmal supraventricular tachycardia (PSVT), 479
pediatric emergencies, 973–974, 974t, 1008
pelvic inflammatory disease (PID), 861–862
peptic ulcers, 645, 646
polypharmacy, 1026
preterm labour, 888
psychiatric medications, 839–840
rapid sequence intubation, 235
renal calculi (kidney stones), 676
for restraint, 856
sedatives, 200, 241–243, 409t, 1008
shock, 92
spinal injury management, 273–274
sympathomimetic agents, 526t
thrombolytic agents, 526t, 584
topical anesthetic spray, 243–244
trigeminal neuralgia, 600
urinary tract infection (UTI), 679
urological emergencies, 665
vascular emergencies, 563
pharyngitis, 818
pharyngo-tracheal lumen airway (PtL), 420–422, 421f
pharynx, and abscess formation, 335
phenol, 162
phenothiazines, 748
phobias, 843
photophobia, 229
phototherapy, 935
phrenic nerve, 337
physical abuse. See abuse
physical dependence, 846
physical disabilities
    effect of, 1089–1090
    hearing impairments, 1090–1092
    obesity, 1094–1095
    paralysis, 1096
    speech impairments, 1093–1094
    visual impairments, 1092–1093
physical evidence, preservation of, 865–866

physics. See kinetics of trauma
physiological dependence, 715
pica, 733
Pierre Robin syndrome, 911
"the pill," 859
pill rolling, 600
pill-rolling motion, 1054
pillow splint, 187
piloerection, 753
pink puffers, 353
pinnal injury, 244–245
pinworms, 787
pipe bombs, 36
pit viper bites, 711–713
placenta, 869, 870f
placenta previa, 881–882
placental stage, 890
plants, poisonous, 705–706
platelet/blood clotting disorders
    thrombocytopenia, 738
    thrombocytosis, 737–738
platelet phase, 66
pleural friction rub, 343
pleuritic, 360
pneumatic antishock garment (PASG), 91–92
Pneumocystis carinii, 784, 798, 799, 807
pneumomediastinum, 767, 770
pneumonia
    vs. acute pulmonary edema, 807
    adult respiratory distress syndrome (ARDS), 349
    assessment, 360–361, 807, 985
    bacterial, 360
    vs. congestive heart failure, 807
    consolidation, 807
    described, 360, 807
    egophony, 361
    fungal, 360
    geriatric emergencies, 1042–1043
    highest risk of, 807
    history, 807
    immunization, 808
    management, 361, 808, 986
    pathophysiology, 360
    pediatric respiratory emergencies, 985–986
    primary atypical pneumonia, 807
    risk factors, 360
    SARS (severe acute respiratory syndrome), 808–809
    secondary assessment, 361
    signs and symptoms, 807, 1043
    systemic symptoms, 361
    viral, 360
pneumothorax
    defined, 39, 285, 335, 767
    diving emergencies, 767
    hemopneumothorax, 288
    neonatal emergency, 927
    open pneumothorax, 286–287, 286f, 303, 335
    simple pneumothorax, 285–286, 285f, 300
    spontaneous pneumothorax, 366–367
    tension pneumothorax, 287–288, 288f, 304–305, 304f, 335, 343, 367, 395, 1010

ventilations and, 39
pocket mask, 437
Poison Control Centres, 682, 685, 705
poisonings
    see also toxicological emergencies
    accidental, 682
    animal bites, 684
    carbon monoxide (CO) poisoning, 695
    children, 682
    ciguatera (bony fish) poisoning, 705
    cyanide poisoning, 159
    defined, 681
    food poisoning, 704–705, 820–821
    hydrocarbons, 698
    insect stings, 684
    intentional, 682
    paralytic shellfish poisoning, 705
    pediatric emergencies, 1001–1003
    Poison Control Centres, 682
    rapid sequence intubation (RSI), 689
    scombroid (histamine) poisoning, 705
    ten most common poisons, 683t
poisonous plants and mushrooms, 705–706
poliomyelitis (polio), 601, 1102–1103, 1122
polycythemia, 352, 733, 735, 914, 1051
polymerase chain reaction (PCR) test, 807
polymorphic VT, 499
polyneuropathy, 571, 572
polypharmacy, 1026, 1063
Population and Public Health Branch (PPHB), 783
Port-A-Cath, 1130
portal hypertension, 641
portal pressure, 641
positive end expiratory pressure (PEEP), 351, 352
positive impulses, 452
positive pressure ventilation, 284
positive-pressure ventilators, 1127
post-cardiac-arrest management, 556
posterior descending artery, 448
posterior fascicles, 451
posterior hip dislocation, 195
posterior knee dislocations, 196
postexposure, 795
postexposure prophylaxis, 800
postictal state, 590
postnasal drip, 818
postpartum, 875
postpartum depression, 1137
postpartum hemorrhage, 902
postpolio syndrome, 1103
postrenal ARF, 667
postterm newborns, 926
posttraumatic stress syndrome, 843
postural instability, 600
posture, 837
PPD, 792
Prairie rattlesnake, 711
pre-formed splint, 186
precipitous delivery, 900–901
precordial leads, 453
precordial thump, 525, 525f
precordium, 291
prednisone, 106
preeclampsia, 550, 883–884, 885
preembryonic stage, 872
preexcitation syndromes, 509–510

pregnancy
  see also obstetric patient
  abruptio placentae, 318, 318*f*, 323
  abuse during, 1077
  active labour, 877
  assessment considerations, 323–324
  asymmetrical uterus, 324
  blunt trauma, 318
  cardiovascular system, changes in, 871–872
  childbirth. *See* puerperium
  complications. *See* pregnancy complications
  crowning, 878
  delivery. *See* puerperium
  diabetogenic effect of pregnancy, 886
  due date, 872
  ectopic pregnancy, 863, 880–881
  estimated date of confinement (EDC), 872
  fetal circulation, 873–874, 874*f*
  fetal development, 872–873, 873*f*
  fundal height, 877
  gastrointestinal system, changes in, 872
  hemorrhage, reaction to, 74
  hypovolemia, 317
  injury during, 316–318
  intrauterine pregnancy, 860
  late-term, 317, 323
  management of, 326
  miscarriage, 862, 863
  musculoskeletal system, changes in, 872
  normal duration of, 872
  obstetric terminology, 874–875
  open wound to uterus, 318
  physiological changes, 870–872
  preeclampsia, 550
  prolapsed cord, 877–878
  reproductive system, changes in, 870–871
  respiratory system, changes in, 871
  rubella, impact of, 815
  trauma as number one killer, 316
  trimesters, 872
  urinary system, changes in, 872
  uterine changes, 871*f*
  uterus, 317, 317*f*
pregnancy complications
  abdominal pain, 879
  abortion, 880
  abruptio placentae, 882–883, 882*f*
  appendicitis, 879
  bleeding, 879–883
  Braxton-Hicks contractions, 887
  chronic hypertension, 884
  chronic hypertension superimposed with preeclampsia, 884
  eclampsia, 883–884, 885
  ectopic pregnancy, 880–881
  gallstones, 879
  gestational diabetes, 886–887
  hypertensive disorders, 883–885
  maternal shock, 879
  medical complications, 883–887
  medical conditions, 879
  miscarriage, 880
  painless bleeding, 882
  physical abuse, 878

placenta previa, 881–882
preeclampsia, 883–884, 885
preterm labour, 887–889
supine-hypotensive syndrome, 885
transient hypertension, 884
trauma, 878–879
vaginal bleeding, 879–883
pregnant patient. *See* obstetric patient; pregnancy
prehospital 12-lead ECG monitoring, 564–567
prehospital infection control. *See* infection control
preload, 450
premature atrial contractions (PACs), 475, 476*f*
premature infants, 929–930, 930*f*, 933, 1090–1091
premature junctional contractions (PJCs), 489–490, 490*f*
premature ventricular contractions (PVC), 497–499, 498*f*
premethrin cream, 830
prenatal, 875
prenatal period, 868
  see also obstetric patient
prerenal ARF, 666, 666*t*
presacral edema, 514, 518
presbycusis, 1091
preservation of physical evidence, 865–866
pressure, 180
pressure disorders. *See* barotrauma
pressure injuries, 109
pressure shock wave, 53
pressure sores, 1111*f*
pressure ulcers, 1057, 1058
pressure wave, 35–36, 289
preterm labour, 887–889
prevention
  abdominal trauma, 310
  acute renal failure (ARF), 669
  chronic renal failure (CRF), 672
  disease transmission, 831–832
  the elderly, 1025, 1025*t*
  firearms, and thoracic injury, 277
  foodborne illness, 821
  high-altitude illness, 772–773
  hyperthermia, 748–749, 1062
  hypothermia, 754, 1062
  injury, and home care patients, 1113
  injury prevention programs and developments, 10
  musculoskeletal trauma, 169
  osteoarthritis, 1059
  preventable injuries, 3
  strokes, 1051
  suicide, among elderly, 1068
preventive strategies, 660
priapism, 260
primary apnea, 909
primary assessment
  ABCs, 372–373
  abdominal trauma, 321
  behavioural emergencies, 837
  cardiovascular emergencies, 512
  facial injuries, 225–227
  gastrointestinal (GI) emergencies, 636
  head injuries, 225–227

hematopoietic emergencies, 728
hemorrhage, 76–77
home care patients, 1116–1118
musculoskeletal trauma, 178–179
neck injuries, 225–227
neurological emergencies, 572–574
obstetric patient, 875
pediatric emergencies, 951–956
respiratory problems, 372–373
respiratory system, 338–340
shock, 86–87
soft-tissue trauma, 115
spinal injury, 257–258
thermal burns, 152–153
thoracic trauma, 297
toxicological emergencies, 685
urological emergencies, 661
primary blast injuries, 37
primary care paramedic (PCP) competencies
  assessment and diagnostics, 1143–1144
  communication, 1142–1143
  health and safety, 1143
  integration, 1146–1147
  professional responsibilities, 1141–1142
  therapeutics, 1145–1146
  transportation, 1147
primary response, 624
primary syphilis (first stage), 826
primary trauma centre (PTC), 5
primigravida, 875, 898
primipara, 875
Prinzmetal's angina, 537
prions, 786
procainamide, 480, 482, 500, 556
proctitis, 647
prodrome phase of rabies, 822
professional responsibilities, 1141–1142
profile (bullet), 47
prognosis, 62
projectile injury process, 52
projectile wounds. *See* penetrating trauma
projectiles, 36
prolapsed cord, 877–878, 897, 899*f*, 900*f*
prolonged QT interval, 461
promethazine, 630
propellants, sniffing of, 690
propranolol, 616
prostaglandin inhibitors, 888
prostate gland, and benign prostatic hypertrophy, 660
prostatitis, 677
protective respirator, 805–806
proteinuria, 668
Proteus, 678
protons, 775
protozoa, 787
proximal fractures, 191
pruritus, 1057
pryogens, 752
Pseudomonas aeruginosa, 105, 678
pseudoseizures, 591
psychiatric disorders
  see also behavioural emergencies
  age-related conditions, 850–851
  anorexia nervosa, 847
  anxiety disorders, 842–843
  biological, 835
  bipolar disorder, 845

body dysmorphic disorder, 846
bulimia nervosa, 847
catatonic schizophrenia, 842
cognitive disorders, 840–841
conversion disorder, 846
delirium, 840–841
dementia, 841
depersonalization, 847
depression, 843–844, 1067
disorganized schizophrenia, 842
dissociative disorders, 847
dysphoria, 1067
eating disorders, 847
factitious disorders, 846–847
fugue state, 847
geriatric emergencies, 1066–1068
geriatric patients, 850–851
hypochondriasis, 846, 1067
impulse control disorders, 849
intermittent explosive disorder, 849
kleptomania, 849
major depression, 844
mood disorders, 843–845
multiple personality disorder, 847
organic, 835
pain disorder, 846
panic attack, 842–843
paranoid schizophrenia, 842
and partner abuse, 1077
pathological gambling, 849
pathophysiology, 835–836
pediatric patients, 851
personality disorders, 847–848
phobias, 843
posttraumatic stress syndrome, 843
psychogenic amnesia, 847
psychosocial, 836
pyromania, 849
IN SAD CAGES, 844
schizophrenia, 841–842
sociocultural, 836
somatization disorder, 846
somatoform disorders, 846
substance-related disorders, 845–846
suicide, 849–850, 1067–1068
trichotillomania, 849
undifferentiated schizophrenia, 842
psychiatric medications, 839–840
psychogenic amnesia, 847
psychological dependence, 715
psychological support, 203, 582, 631, 861, 940–942, 976
psychosocial, 836
psychotropics, 748
pubic live, 829–830
public health agencies, 783
public health principles, 782–783
puerperium
abnormal delivery situations, 896–898
breech presentation, 896–897, 897f, 898f
cephalopelvic disproportion, 900
cesarean section, 890
clamp and cut cord, 894f
defined, 889
field delivery, 891–894
labour, 889–891
limb presentation, 897–898

maternal blood loss, usual, 894
maternal complications of labour and delivery, 901–903
meconium staining, 901
multiple births, 899–900
neonatal care, 894–896
normal delivery, 892f, 893f
occiput posterior position, 898
perineum tears, inspection for, 894
postpartum hemorrhage, 902
precipitous delivery, 900–901
prolapsed cord, 897, 899f, 900f
pulmonary embolism, 903
shoulder dystocia, 901
uterine inversion, 902–903
uterine rupture, 902
vaginal birth after cesarean (VBAC), 890
pulmonary artery, 448
pulmonary contusion, 440, 1009
pulmonary disorders. See respiratory disorders
pulmonary edema, 546, 547, 548, 554f, 1045
pulmonary embolism, 334, 364–366, 546, 903, 1044–1045
pulmonary hemorrhage, 1121
pulmonary hypertension, 546
pulmonary injuries
see also lungs
blast injuries, 38, 39
contusion, 289–290
fluid accumulation in lungs, 349
hemopneumothorax, 288
hemothorax, 288–289, 289f
magnitude of, 290
microhemorrhage, 290
open pneumothorax, 286–287, 286f
simple pneumothorax, 285–286, 285f
sucking chest wound, 286–287, 286f
tension pneumothorax, 287–288, 288f
pulmonary overpressure, 766–767
pulmonary overpressure accidents, 769
pulmonary respiration, 334
pulmonary shunting, 337
pulmonary valve, 448
pulmonary veins, 448
pulse oximeter, 581
pulse oximetry, 345, 345f, 351, 377–379, 378f, 957
pulse pressure, 73
pulse rate, 76, 520
pulseless electrical activity (PEA), 507, 508f, 994
pulseless ventricular tachycardia (VF/VT), 557f, 994
pulses, 180
pulsus alternans, 548
pulsus paradoxus, 293, 344, 375, 548
pump failure, 541
pumping the stomach, 686
punctures, 98–99, 99f
purified protein derivative (PPD) skin test, 804–805
Purkinje system, 451
pyelonephritis, 661, 678
pyrethrin agents, 829
pyrexia, 752–753
pyromania, 849

Q wave, 456
QRS complex, 456, 460f, 465, 755
QRS interval, 461
QT interval, 461
quadrigemini, 497
quadriplegia, 248, 1096
quality factor (QF), 776
quality improvement (QI), 10–11
quality management (QM), 10
quiet breathing sounds, 376
quinidine, 480, 482, 500

R-R interval, 464
R wave, 456
rabies, 821–823
rad, 143
radiation, 744–745
radiation absorbed dose (RAD), 776
radiation injury, 141–144, 142f, 164–165
radioactive emergencies
basic nuclear physics, 775–776
beta particles, 776
biological effects, 776
clean accident, 777
dirty accident, 778
distance, 777
dose-effect relationships to ionizing radiation, 777t
gamma rays, 776
half-life, 775
ionizing radiation, 775
management, 778
neutrons, 776
radiation effects on the body, 776
radioactive substances, 775–776
safety principles, 777–778
shielding, 777
time, 777
radioactive warning labels, 164f, 778f
radioisotope, 775
radionuclide, 775
radius fractures, 194
rales, 343, 376
rape, 1084
see also sexual assault
rapid cardiopulmonary collapse, 997
rapid sequence intubation (RSI), 235–236, 405–410, 689, 970
rapid trauma assessment
abdominal trauma, 321–324
face, 228–229
facial injuries, 227–231
Glasgow Coma Scale (GCS), 230–231, 230t
head, 227–228
head injuries, 227–231
hemorrhage, 77–78
musculoskeletal trauma, 179
neck, 229–230
neck injuries, 227–231
shock, 87–88
soft-tissue trauma, 115–116
spinal injury, 258–261
thermal burns, 153–156
thoracic trauma, 297–301
transport decision, 231
vital signs, monitoring of, 231
rattlesnakes, 711

reactive airway disease. *See* asthma
rear-end impact
　　crumple zones, 24, 24*f*
　　described, 26
　　effects, 27*f*
rebleeding, 108
rebound tenderness, 316
Recombivax HB, 802
recompression, 768
recovery, 793–794
recreational vehicle accidents, 33–34
rectal lesions, 646
rectum, 313
　　see also abdominal trauma
recurrent HSV labialis, 817
red blood cell diseases
　　anemias, 733–734, 734*t*
　　polycythemia, 735
　　sickle cell disease, 734–735
reduced nephron mass, 670
reduced renal mass, 670
reduction, 190, 196*f*
reentry, 466
referral/release incidents, 132–133, 203
referred pain, 635–636, 637, 661
refractory period, 462, 462*f*
relative refractory period, 462
relaxed tongue, 348
remodelling, 105
renal, 659
renal ARF, 666*t*, 667
renal calculi, 659–660, 675–676
renal dialysis, 673–674
renal disorders
　　end-stage renal failure, 659
　　geriatric disorders, 1060
　　incidence of, 659
　　kidney disease, 659
　　renal calculi, 659–660
　　risk factors, 665
renal emergencies
　　acute renal failure (ARF), 665–669
　　chronic renal failure (CRF), 669–674
　　common renal emergencies, 665
　　geriatric patients, 1040–1041
　　geriatric trauma, 1070
　　glomerulonephritis, 1060
　　renal calculi, 675–676
renal function, 668
reperfusion, 539
repetitive PVCs, 497
repolarization, 451
reporting exposures, 795
reproductive system changes, in obstetric
　　patient, 870–871
rescuer safety. *See* safety issues
reservoir, 788
resiliency, 55
resistance, 138, 789–790
resolution phase, 138
Respi-Gam, 816
respiration, 806*f*
　　see also breathing
　　abnormal respiratory patterns, 375
　　agonal respirations, 375
　　apnea, 336
　　apneustic respiration, 336, 576
　　ataxic respirations, 336, 576

Biot's respirations, 336, 375
bradypnea, 345
central neurogenic hyperventilation,
　　336, 375
Cheyne-Stokes respirations, 217,
　　335–336, 375, 576
coughing, 374
defined, 334, 745
grunting, 375
hiccoughing, 374–375
Kussmaul's respirations, 336, 375, 576,
　　613
modified forms of, 374–375
sighing, 375
sneezing, 374
tachypnea, 86, 345
respirators, 806
respiratory disorders
　　adult respiratory distress syndrome
　　　　(ARDS), 349–351
　　asthma, 356–358
　　carbon monoxide inhalation, 363–364
　　central nervous system dysfunction,
　　　　368–369
　　chest wall, 335
　　chronic bronchitis, 354–355
　　chronic obstructive pulmonary disease
　　　　(COPD), 331, 1043–1044
　　described, 331
　　diffusion, disruption in, 337
　　emphysema, 352–353
　　genetic influences, 331
　　geriatric emergencies, 1042–1045
　　home care patients, 1119–1129
　　hyperventilation syndrome, 367–368,
　　　　367*t*
　　lower respiratory tract, 335
　　lung cancer, 361–362
　　management principles, 347–348
　　nerve dysfunction, 369
　　nervous system, and ventilation
　　　　disruption, 335–337
　　obstructive lung disease, 351–358
　　OPQRST questions, 340
　　pathophysiology, 334–337
　　perfusion, disruption in, 337
　　pneumonia, 360–361, 1042–1043
　　pulmonary edema, 1045
　　pulmonary embolism, 364–366,
　　　　1044–1045
　　respiratory muscle dysfunction, 369
　　risk factors, 331
　　spinal cord dysfunction, 369
　　spontaneous pneumothorax, 366–367
　　toxic inhalation, 363
　　upper airway obstruction, 348–349
　　upper respiratory infection (URI),
　　　　358–360
　　upper respiratory tract, 335
　　ventilation, disruption in, 335–337
respiratory distress
　　anoxic hypoxemia, 1037
　　fever, tachypnea and retraction triad in
　　　　children, 807
　　geriatric patients, 1037
　　home care patients, 1109
　　neonatal emergencies, 930–931
　　pediatric, 977–978

signs of, 339
two pillow orthopnea, 1047
respiratory emergencies
　　ABCs, 372–373
　　airway management. *See* airway
　　　　management
　　airway obstruction, 370–372
　　assessment of respiratory system,
　　　　372–380
　　auscultation, 375–377
　　capnography, 379–380
　　esophageal detector device, 380, 381*f*
　　focused history and secondary
　　　　assessment, 373–380
　　geriatric trauma, 1070
　　inadequate ventilation, 372
　　inspection, 374–375
　　noninvasive respiratory monitoring,
　　　　377–380
　　palpation, 377
　　peak expiratory flow rate (PEFR), 380
　　pediatric emergencies. *See* pediatric
　　　　respiratory emergencies
　　primary assessment, 372–373
　　pulse oximetry, 377–379, 378*f*
　　secondary assessment, 374–377
respiratory involvement
　　Cheyne-Stokes respirations, 217
　　facial injuries, 219
　　field intubation, 153
　　spinal injury, 258
　　thermal burns, 153
respiratory membrane, 332
respiratory muscle dysfunction, 369
respiratory status
　　ability to speak, 339
　　abnormal breath sounds, 343–344
　　airway, 339–340
　　assessment, 338–347
　　breathing, 340
　　capnometry, 346–347
　　colour, 339
　　diagnostic testing, 345–347
　　focused history and secondary
　　　　assessment, 340–347
　　general impression of respiratory status,
　　　　338–339
　　history, 340–341
　　medication allergies, 341
　　medication use, 341
　　mental status, 339
　　nasal flaring, 339
　　neurological emergencies, 576, 577*f*
　　normal breathing sounds, 343
　　OPQRST questions, 340
　　peak expiratory flow rate (PEFR), 346,
　　　　346*f*
　　position of patient, 338–339
　　primary assessment, 338–340
　　pulse oximetry, 345, 345*f*
　　reassessment, 344
　　respiratory effort, 339
　　SAMPLE history, 340
　　scene assessment, 338
　　signs of respiratory distress, 339
　　tracheal tugging, 339
　　tripod position, 339, 339*f*
　　vital signs, 344–345

respiratory syncytial virus (RSV), 815–816
respiratory system
    and anaphylactic reaction, 628
    assessment. *See* respiratory status
    diffusion, 332
    gas exchange processes, 331–334
    geriatric patients, 1035–1037
    hemorrhage, 72
    kyphosis, 1036
    in obstetric patient, 871
    pediatric care, 948
    perfusion, 333–334
    physical examination of, 342–343
    physiological processes, 331–334
    ventilation, 332
resting potential, 451
restless legs syndrome, 672
restlessness, 514
restraint asphyxia, 855
restraints (automobile), 19–21, 27
restraints (patient)
    chemical restraint, 856
    hobble, 855
    hog-tie, 855
    improvised, 854
    methods, 854–855
    positioning for transport, 855
    steps, 854–855
resuscitation, 555, 558–559, 759, 896,
    915–924
reticular activating system (RAS), 570
retinal detachment, 223
retroauricular ecchymosis, 210, 210f
retrograde amnesia, 217
retrograde intubation, 410
retropharyngeal abscess, 335
return of spontaneous circulation (ROSC),
    555
reverse transcriptase, 798
rewarming shock, 757
rhabdomyolysis, 110
rheumatic heart disease, 493
rheumatoid arthritis, 177
rhonchi, 343, 376
rhythm strips, 452, 463–465
rib fractures, 281–282, 302–303
ribavirin, 816
RICE acronym, 202
rifampin, 812
rifles, 50
right bundle branch, 451
right coronary artery, 448
right ventricular failure, 546
right ventricular hypertrophy, 1121
rigid splints, 186, 193
rigidity, 600
riluzole, 601
rimantadine, 814
ring injury, 101, 101f
Ringer's Lactate, 89–90, 164, 273, 689, 726,
    737, 989
riot control agents, 162
risus sardonicus, 823
rodents, and hantavirus, 818–819
roentgen equivalent in man (REM), 776
rohypnol, 716
roller bandages, 113, 854
rollover, 26–27, 28

rotational impact, 26
rotavirus, 643, 819
rouleaux, 84
roundworms, 787
RSV immune globulin, 816
rubella (German measles), 815, 1100
rubeola, 814
Rubivirus, 815
rule of nines, 147, 148f, 153, 1010–1011,
    1011f
rule of palms, 148, 148f, 1011
rum fits, 721
runaway pacemaker, 505
rupture of the membranes (ROM), 870, 889
ruptured ovarian cyst, 862

S-T segment, 461, 462
S wave, 456
SA node
    cessation of activity, 472
    dysrhythmias originating in. *See*
        dysrhythmias
sacral edema, 514
safety issues
    burn scenes, 152
    disease transmission, prevention of,
        831–832
    HBV transmission, prevention of, 793
    HIV transmission, prevention of, 793
    home care patients, 1114–1115
    ionizing radiation, 777–778
    penetrating trauma scene assessment,
        59–61
    radiation hazards, 164
    radioactive emergencies, 777–778
    sexually transmitted diseases (STDs),
        825
    toxicological emergencies, 685
    tuberculosis (TB), 805–806
Sager traction splint, 187
salbutamol, 341, 351–352, 356, 630
salicylates, 701–702
salmeterol, 341
Salmonella, 643, 705, 819, 820
salmonellosis, 642
saltwater drowning, 762–763
same-sex couples, abuse and, 1076
SAMPLE history
    gastrointestinal (GI) emergencies, 636,
        637
    hematopoietic emergencies, 728–729
    respiratory status, 340
Sarcoptes scabiei, 830
SARS (severe acute respiratory syndrome),
    808–809
scabies, 830
scalds, 1082
scalp avulsions. *See* avulsions
scalp bandaging, 122–123, 123f
scalp hematoma, 935
scalp injuries, 208–209, 208f
scene assessment
    abdominal trauma, 318–321
    behavioural emergencies, 836–837
    cardiovascular emergencies, 512
    facial injuries, 225
    gastrointestinal (GI) emergencies, 636
    head injuries, 225

    hematopoietic emergencies, 727–728
    hemorrhage, 75–76
    home care patients, 1114–1116
    musculoskeletal trauma, 178
    neck injuries, 225
    neurological emergencies, 572–574
    pediatric emergencies, 950
    penetrating trauma, 59–61
    respiratory system, 338
    shock, 86
    soft-tissue trauma, 114
    spinal injury, 256–257
    thermal burns, 151–152
    thoracic trauma, 297
    toxicological emergencies, 685
    urological emergencies, 661
    vehicular collisions, 27–30
scene safety. *See* safety issues
schizophrenia, 841–842
school-aged children, 944
sciatica, 603
scombroid (histamine) poisoning, 705
scorpion stings, 709–710, 710f
SCUBA (self-contained underwater breathing
    apparatus) diving, 6, 764
    see also diving emergencies
seat belts, 19
second-degree burn, 147
secondary apnea, 909
secondary assessment
    acute renal failure (ARF), 668
    cardiovascular emergencies, 517–520
    child abuse, 1082–1083
    emphysema, 353
    gastrointestinal (GI) emergencies, 638
    geriatric patients, 1034
    gynecological emergencies, 859–860
    hematopoietic emergencies, 729–732
    hemorrhage, 77–79
    home care patients, 1116–1118
    infectious diseases, 796–797
    ingested toxins, 688–689
    musculoskeletal trauma, 182
    neurological emergencies, 575–580
    obstetric patient, 877–878
    pediatric assessment, 956–959
    pneumonia, 361
    renal calculi (kidney stones), 676
    respiratory problems, 374–377
    respiratory status, 342–344
    seizures, 592
    shock, 87–89
    spinal injury, 260
    spontaneous pneumothorax, 366
    toxicological emergencies, 685–686
    urinary tract infection (UTI), 678
    urological emergencies, 663–664
secondary blast injuries, 37
secondary depression, 1066
secondary impacts, 48–49
secondary response, 625
secondary syphilis (second stage), 826
sedatives, 200, 241–243, 409t, 718t, 1008
seizures
    absence seizure, 591
    alcohol, withdrawal from, 721
    assessment, 591–592
    complex partial seizures, 591

defined, 589
eclampsia, 883, 885
febrile seizures, 589, 996
focal clonic seizures, 932
generalized seizures, 590–591
geriatric patients, 1051
grand mal seizure, 590
hypoglycemic seizure, 615
hysterical seizures, 591
idiopathic epilepsy, 589
management, 592–593
multifocal seizures, 932
myoclonic seizures, 932
neonatal emergencies, 931–932
obstetric patients, 876
partial seizures, 591
pediatric emergencies, 994–997
petit mal seizure, 591
pseudoseizures, 591
secondary assessment, 592
simple partial seizures, 591
status epilepticus, 593–594, 996
subtle seizures, 931
vs. syncope, 592, 592*t*
syncopes, 1049
tonic-clonic seizure, 590
tonic seizures, 931–932
types of, 590–591
self-adherent roller bandages, 113
Sellick's manoeuvre, 234, 235, 382–383,
    383*f*, 408
Sengstaken-Blakemore tube, 641, 642
senile dementia, 1053
sensitization, 626
sensorimotor evaluation, 577–578
sensorineural deafness, 1090–1091
sensorium, 1110
sensory aphasia, 1093
sepsis, 349, 731, 989–990
septic arthritis, 825
septic complications, 1110–1111
septic shock, 989–990
sequelae, 764
seroconversion, 790
serous fluid, 108
seven-year itch, 830
severe allergic reaction. *See* anaphylaxis
severe burns, 157–159
severe diffuse axonal injury, 214
severe hypothermia, 754
sexual abuse
    child sexual abuse, 1013, 1085
    partner abuse, 1076
sexual assault
    assessment of victims, 864–865
    chain of evidence, 1087
    children and, 1085
    crime of, 1084, 1086
    defined, 1084
    documentation, 866, 1087
    emotional support, 1086
    EMS responsibilities, 1086
    injuries, 316, 864–866
    legal considerations, 1086–1087
    rape, 1084
    sexual assailants, characteristics of,
        1085–1086
sexual purposes, drugs used for, 716

sexually transmitted diseases (STDs)
    chancroid, 828
    chlamydia, 827–828
    described, 825
    genital warts, 827
    gonorrhea, 825
    herpes simplex Type 2, 827
    syphilis, 826–827
    trichomoniasis, 828
shaft fractures, 176
shaken baby syndrome, 1082–1083
shaking palsy, 599
shear forces, 311–312
shellfish poisoning, paralytic, 705
shielding, 143
Shigella, 643, 705, 819, 820
shigellosis, 820
shivering, 746, 753
shock (hypoperfusion)
    air hunger, 86
    airway management, 89
    anaphylactic shock, 990
    anaphylaxis and circulatory shock, 627
    anemia and, 733
    assessment, 86–89
    blood loss, body's response to, 83–84
    blood vessel trauma, 224
    breathing management, 89
    cardiogenic shock, 552–553, 554*f*, 988,
        990–994
    categories of shock, 988–990
    compensated shock, 84–85, 85*f*, 987
    decompensated shock, 85–86, 987–988
    defined, 65, 82
    detailed secondary assessment, 88
    distributive shock, 989–990
    electrolyte administration, 90
    fight or flight response, 92
    fluid resuscitation, 89–90
    focused history and secondary
        assessment, 87–89
    hemorrhage control, 89
    hypoglycemia (insulin shock), 610,
        615–616, 620, 933–934
    hypovolemic shock, 989
    index of suspicion, 7–8
    irreversible shock, 86, 988
    management of shock, 89–92
    midazolam (Versed®), 200
    neurogenic shock, 224, 255, 990
    noncardiogenic shock, 988–989
    obstetric patients, 879
    ongoing assessment, 89
    overdrive respiration, 89
    pediatric emergencies, 986–994
        see also pediatric shock
    pharmacological interventions, 92
    pneumatic antishock garment (PASG),
        91–92
    primary assessment, 86–87
    process, 83–84
    pulse rate and, 76
    rapid trauma assessment, 87–88
    rewarming shock, 757
    scene assessment, 86
    septic shock, 989–990
    severity of shock, 987–988
    signs of, 76

spinal shock, 254
stages of shock, 84–86, 85*t*
tachypnea, 86
temperature control, 91
volemic patients, 92
shootings. *See* penetrating trauma
short spine board, 269–270
shotgun, 51, 280, 311
shoulder bandage, 123*f*, 124
shoulder dystocia, 901
shoulder injuries, 197–198
shoulder straps, 19
shunt failure, 1019
shunts, 1019, 1130
Shy-Drager syndrome, 1054
sick sinus syndrome, 1049
sickle cell anemia, 729, 731, 734–735
sickle cell trait, 734–735
sighing, 375
sign language, 1092
silent myocardial infarction, 1046
silver fork deformity, 194, 198
simple face mask, 436
simple partial seizures, 591
simple pneumothorax, 285–286, 285*f*, 300
sinus arrest, 471–472, 472*f*
sinus bradycardia, 467–468, 467*f*, 469*f*
sinus dysrhythmia, 470, 471*f*
sinus tachycardia, 468, 470*f*
sinusitis, 818
Sistrurus catenus, 711
situational causes, 836
six Ps in limb injury evaluation, 180
six-second method, 464
skin
    see also soft-tissue trauma
    and allergic reactions, 628
    and anaphylaxis, 628
    described, 95
    ecchymosis, 96
    erythema, 96
    eschar, 149, 149*f*, 154–155
    geriatric patients, 1040
    lesions, 826–827, 829
    pediatric care, 948
    purified protein derivative (PPD) skin
        test, 804–805
    tension lines, 98, 99*f*
    uremic frost, 671
    urticaria, 628, 628*f*
skin diseases
    genetic patients, 1057–1058
    impetigo, 829
    lice, 829–830
    Norwegian scabies, 830
    pruritus, 1057
    scabies, 830
skull fractures, 209–211, 209*f*
sleep, and high altitude, 773
sleep apnea, 1123
sliding impact, 31
sling and swathe, 193
slow-reacting substance of anaphylaxis (SRS-
    A), 627
small bowel, 313
    see also abdominal trauma
small-for-gestational-age (SGA) newborns,
    926, 933

small-volume nebulizer, 436
snakebites, 711–714, 711*f*
sneezing, 374
snoring, 343, 376
snowmobile collisions, 33
societal issues, and the elderly, 1024
sociocultural, 836
sodium, 162
sodium bicarbonate, 503, 553, 556, 925*t*
soft catheters, 432, 432*t*
soft splints, 186–187
soft-tissue injury management
    abdominal injuries, 132
    amputations, 125–126, 126*f*
    anatomical considerations of bandaging, 122–125
    compartment syndrome, 130–131
    complications of bandaging, 125
    crush syndrome, 128–130
    direct pressure, 120
    edema control, 122
    facial wounds, 131, 131*f*
    hemorrhage control, 119*f*, 120–121
    immobilization, 122
    impaled objects, 126–127, 127*f*
    neck wounds, 131
    objectives of wound dressing and bandaging, 118–122
    pain control, 122
    referral/release, 132–133
    sterility, 121–122
    thorax, 131–132
    treatment, 132–133
    wounds requiring transport, 132
soft-tissue trauma
    abnormal scar formation, 108–109
    abrasions, 97, 97*f*
    amputations, 101, 101*f*
    assessment, 113–118
    assessment techniques, 117–118
    avulsions, 100–101, 100*f*
    bandage materials, 113
    burns. *See* burns
    closed wounds, 95, 96–97
    common nature of, 95
    compartment syndrome, 108
    complications, 107–109
    contusions, 96, 97*f*
    crush injuries, 97, 97*f*, 109–110
    crush syndrome, 110
    degloving injury, 100–101, 101*f*
    delayed healing, 108
    described, 95
    detailed secondary assessment, 117
    dressings, 111–113
    from endotracheal intubation, 393–394
    epidemiology, 95
    facial injuries, 219
    focused history and secondary assessment, 115–117
    focused trauma assessment, 116–117
    hematoma, 97
    hemorrhage, 102, 102*f*
    hypertrophic scar formation, 109
    impaired hemostasis, 107–108
    impaled objects, 100, 100*f*
    incisions, 98
    infection, 105–107

injection injury, 110–111
inquiry, 117
inspection, 117–118
keloid, 108
lacerations, 98, 98*f*
management of. *See* soft-tissue injury management
mechanism of injury, 115–116
necrosis, 110
ongoing assessment, 118
open wounds, 95, 96*f*
palpation, 118
pathophysiology, 95–96
pressure injuries, 109
primary assessment, 115
punctures, 98–99, 99*f*
rapid trauma assessment, 115–116
rebleeding, 108
ring injury, 101, 101*f*
scene assessment, 114
and serious internal injury, 115*f*
serous fluid, 108
skin. *See* skin
wound healing, 102–105
solid organs, 55, 314–315
somatic pain, 635
somatization disorder, 846
somatoform disorders, 846
sotolol, 500
spasm (muscle), 171, 176, 282
spastic paralysis, 1101
special-needs children and infants
    apnea monitors, 1017
    assessment, 1019–1020
    central IV line, 1018
    "disability," avoiding use of term, 1019
    gastric feeding tubes, 1018–1019
    gastrostomy tubes, 1018–1019
    home artificial ventilators, 1018
    management, 1019–1020
    shunts, 1019
    stoma, 1017
    tracheostomy tubes, 1016–1017, 1017*t*
specialty centres, 5–6
speech impairments
    accommodations for, 1094
    aphasia, 1093–1094
    articulation disorders, 1094
    dysarthria, 1094
    fluency disorders, 1094
    global aphasia, 1094
    language disorders, 1093–1094
    motor aphasia, 1093
    sensory aphasia, 1093
    types of, 1093–1094
    voice production disorders, 1094
speed splints, 193
sphincter of Oddi, 653
sphygmomanometer, 121
spina bifida cystica, 1103
spina bifida occulta, 1103
spina bifida (SB), 601, 1103–1104
spinal alignment, 262–263
spinal column injury, 253
spinal cord dysfunction, 369
spinal cord injury
    anterior cord syndrome, 254
    Brown-Séquard's syndrome, 254

central cord syndrome, 254
compression, 253
concussion of the cord, 253
contusion, 253
devastation of, 248–249
hemorrhage, 254
laceration, 254
transection, 254
types of, 253–254
spinal injury
    see also spinal injury management
    assessment, 256–261
    autonomic hyperreflexia syndrome, 255
    axial stress, 251–252
    Babinski's sign, 260, 260*f*
    cervical collar, 257
    cervical spine immobilization (pediatric), 975
    coccygeal region, 252
    column injury, 253
    cord injury. *See* spinal cord injury
    described, 248–249
    digital intubation, 258
    direct injury, 252
    electrocution, 252
    excessive rotation, 251
    extension injury, 249–251
    extremes of motion, 249–251
    geriatric trauma, 1073
    hanging, 251–252
    hold-up position, 260
    hyperextension, 249–251
    hyperflexion, 249–251
    incidence of, 248
    lateral bending, 251
    limb sensation, 259–260
    manual immobilization, 257, 259*f*
    mechanism of injury, 249–252, 250*f*
    motorcycle helmets and, 32
    movement of patient. *See* movement of spinal injury patient
    nerve root injury, 260
    neurogenic shock, 255
    neurological dysfunction, 255
    neutral, in-line positioning, 257
    ongoing assessment, 261
    orotracheal intubation, 258
    pediatric emergencies, 975
    penetrating trauma, 252
    priapism, 260
    primary assessment, 257–258
    rapid trauma assessment, 258–261
    respiratory involvement, 258
    results of trauma on spinal column, 252–255
    scene assessment, 256–257
    secondary assessment, 260
    signs and symptoms, 253
    spinal shock, 254
    spondylosis, 1073
    vital signs, 261
spinal injury management
    atropine, 274
    cervical collar application, 264
    cervical immobilization device (CID), 272
    combative patients, 274
    contraindications in movement, 263

diving injury immobilization, 272–273
dopamine (Intropin®), 273
final patient positioning, 271
helmet removal, 266–267
log roll, 267–268, 268f
long spine board, 271–272, 272f
manual cervical immobilization,
 263–264
medications, 273–274
movement of spinal injury patient,
 267–273
neurogenic shock, 273–274
neutral, in-line positioning, 262–263
orthopedic stretcher, 269
precautions, 261–262
rapid extrication, 270–271, 271f
short spine board, 269–270
spinal alignment, 262–263
standing takedown, 265–266
straddle slide, 268–269
vest-type immobilization device,
 269–270, 269f
spinal shock, 254
spine stabilization manoeuvre, 1006f
spinothalamic tract, 260
spiral fracture, 174, 174f
spleen injury, 314
splenomegaly, 817
splinting
 air splint, 186–187, 193, 194
 bipolar frame device, 187, 188f, 192
 clotting and, 68
 cravats, 188
 devices, 186–189
 formable splints, 186, 194f
 fracture care, 189
 Hare traction splint, 187
 internal hemorrhage, 71
 joint care, 189
 ladder splint, 186
 long padded board splints, 193f, 194
 malleable splint, 186, 194f
 metal sheet splint, 186
 pillow splint, 187
 pre-formed splint, 186
 rigid splints, 186, 193
 Sager traction splint, 187
 sling and swathe, 193
 soft splints, 186–187
 speed splints, 193
 Thomas traction splint, 187
 traction splint, 187, 192f
 traction splinting, 191
 unipolar traction device, 187, 188f, 192
 vacuum splints, 187, 188f
 Velcro® straps, 188
spondylosis, 1073
spontaneous abortion, 880
spontaneous pneumothorax, 366–367
sports injuries
 blunt trauma, 42–43
 causes, 42
 helmet removal, 266–267
 hemorrhage, 74
 musculoskeletal injury management,
  202
 musculoskeletal trauma, 183
 protective gear, 42–43

RICE acronym, 202
 trainers, knowing, 202
sprains, 171, 196–197
"the squeeze," 766
stabbings. See penetrating trauma
stability (bullets), 47
stable angina, 537
stages of hemorrhage, 72–74, 73t
stages of shock, 84–86, 85t
standing takedown, 265–266
staphylococcal scalded skin syndrome, 1081
Staphylococcus, 105, 642, 783
Staphylococcus aureus, 785, 807, 818
Starling's law of the heart, 450, 546
status asthmaticus, 358, 984
status epilepticus, 593–594, 996
STDs. See sexually transmitted diseases (STDs)
steady-state metabolism, 746
steering wheel impact, 22
stenosis, 423, 431
stent, 545
sterile dressings, 111–112, 111f
sterilization, 794
sternal fracture and dislocations, 282–283
sternoclavicular dislocation, 303
Stokes-Adams' syndrome, 1049
stoma, 431, 1017
stoma sites, patients with, 431–432
stomach, 313
 see also abdominal trauma
straddle injury, 864
straddle slide, 268–269
strain, 171
strep throat, 359
Streptococcus, 105, 783, 818
Streptococcus pneumoniae, 807, 811, 818
streptokinase, 107
stridor, 153, 343, 376
stroke
 assessment, 587–588
 atrial fibrillation, 482
 brain hemorrhage, 1050
 brain ischemia, 1050
 categories of, 584–585
 cerebral thrombus, 585
 defined, 584
 embolic strokes, 585
 geriatric patients, 1038, 1050–1051
 Glasgow Coma Scale (GCS),
  1050–1051
 hemorrhagic strokes, 585–586
 intracerebral hemorrhage, 1050
 management, 588, 589f
 mortality rates, 584
 occlusive strokes, 584–585
 prevention, 1051
 signs and symptoms, 587
 subarachnoid hemorrhages, 1050
 thrombotic strokes, 585
 tissue plasminogen activator (tPA), 584
 vs. transient ischemic attack (TIA), 587
stroke volume, 450
structural collapses, 37
structural lesions, 570
struvite stones, 676
stuttering, 1094
stylet, 391, 391f, 400f
subarachnoid hemorrhages, 586, 586f, 1050

subcapital femoral neck fracture, 1072f
subconjunctival hemorrhage, 222
subcutaneous emphysema, 224, 342
subdural hematomas, 213, 213f, 1083
subendocardial infarction, 540
subglottic structures, 145
subluxation, 171–172
substance abuse
 see also overdose
 addiction, 715
 alcohol abuse, 719–722, 1065–1066
 defined, 715, 1064
 dependence, 715
 drug abuse, 1065
 geriatric patients, 1064–1066
 habituation, 715
 and partner abuse, 1077
 physiological dependence, 715
 as psychiatric disorders, 845–846
 psychological dependence, 715
 tolerance, 715
 withdrawal, 715
subtle seizures, 931
succinylcholine (Anectine®), 235, 241, 407
sucking chest wound, 286–287, 286f
suction, 432
suction catheters, 432, 432t
suction unit, 392
suctioning
 catheters, types of, 432, 432t
 complications, 433
 deep suctioning, 916
 equipment, 432–433
 head, facial, and neck injury
  management, 233
 limiting attempts, 433
 newborns, 912, 913f
 pediatric airway management, 960–961
 preparation, 432
 techniques, 433
 tracheal suctioning, 920f
 tracheobronchial suctioning, 433
sudden death, 555
sudden infant death syndrome (SIDS), 943,
 1011–1012
suicide
 assessment of potentially suicidal
  patients, 849
 common methods of, 849
 cyanide salt, 694
 described, 849
 facial damage, 58, 220–221
 geriatric patients, 1067–1068
 poisonings, 682
 rates, 849
 risk factors, 850
 transport considerations, 853–854
sunburn, 147
superficial burn, 146
superficial frostbite, 760
superheated steam, 145
superior vena cava syndrome, 362
superior venae cavae, 448
supine-hypotensive syndrome, 885, 886f
supplemental restraint systems (SRS), 19–20
support, 536
supraglottic structures, 145
supraventricular tachycardia, 992

surface-absorbed toxins, 691
surface absorption, 684
surfactant, 762
surgical cricothyrotomy
    complications, 424, 427
    indications, 423
    jet ventilation, 426f
    as life-saving measure, 131
    needle cricothyrostomy, 131, 236–237,
        422, 423–427, 425f, 426f
    open cricothyrotomy, 422, 427,
        428f–430f
    procedure, 236–237
surgically implanted medication delivery
    systems, 1130
survival, 555
sweating, 746
swimmer's ear, 1090
sylvatic rabies, 822
sympathomimetic agents, 526t, 693t
synchronized cardioversion, 531, 532f
syncope, 515, 592, 592t, 594–595, 1049
syncytium, 450
synthetic anticholinergics, 692t
syphilis, 826–827
syphilitic meningitis, 826
syringe, 391, 391f
syrup of ipecac, 686
systole, 450
systolic pressure, 1048

T wave, 456, 461f
tachycardia, 340, 464, 478f
tachydysrhythmias, 466, 991
tachypnea, 86, 345, 952
tactile fremitus, 343
tear gas, 162
teeth, dislodged, 246
teeth breakage, and endotracheal intubation,
    393–394
temperature control, and shock, 91
temporary cavity, 53
tendinitis, 177
tension headaches, 595
tension lines, 98, 99f
tension pneumothorax, 287–288, 288f,
    304–305, 304f, 335, 343, 367, 395, 1010
terbutaline, 984
terfenadine, 500
term, 872
term (T), 859
terminally ill patients, 1105, 1138–1140
termination of resuscitation, 558–559
tertiary blast injuries, 37
tertiary syphilis (fourth stage), 826
tertiary trauma centre (TTC), 5
tetanus, 107, 823–824
tetanus vaccination, 625–626
tetracycline, 828
Tetralogy of Fallot, 991
theophylline, 703
therapeutic index, 698
therapeutics competencies, 1145–1146
therapy regulators, 435
thermal burns
    see also burns
    assessment, 151–156
    described, 136–138

focused history and secondary
    assessment, 153–156
    local burns, 156–157
    management of, 156–159
    minor burns, 156–157
    moderate burns, 157–159
    ongoing assessment, 156
    primary assessment, 152–153
    rapid trauma assessment, 153–156
    scene assessment, 151–152
    severe burns, 157–159
thermal gradient, 744
thermogenesis, 744
thermolysis, 744–745, 745f
thermoreceptors, 747
thermoregulation, 745–746, 1039–1040
thermoregulatory thermogenesis, 744
thiamine, 243, 716
thiosulphate, 694
third-degree AV block, 487–489, 488f
third-degree burns, 147
Thomas traction splint, 187
thoracic trauma
        see also thoracic trauma management
        abdominal injuries, and co-morbidity,
        277
        assessment, 296–302
        ausculation, 299
        blast injuries, 278
        blunt thoracic trauma, 277, 278–279
        blunt trauma assessment, 299–300
        cardiovascular injuries, 290–294
        chest wall injuries, 280–284
        children, 279
        crush injuries, 278
        deceleration, 278
        described, 277
        diaphragm, traumatic rupture or
            perforation of, 295
        esophageal rupture, traumatic, 295
        frontal impact, 278f
        high-energy wounds, 279–280
        infants, 279
        low-energy wounds, 279
        observation, 297–298
        ongoing assessment, 301–302
        palpation, 298–299
        pathophysiology, 278–296
        pediatric trauma, 1009–1010
        penetrating trauma, 58, 277, 279–280,
            280t
        penetrating trauma assessment, 300–301
        primary assessment, 297
        pulmonary injuries, 284–294
        questions, 298
        rapid trauma assessment, 297–301
        scene assessment, 297
        shotgun, 280
        simple pneumothorax, 300
        soft-tissue injury management, 131–132
        stab wound to chest, 279f
        tracheobronchial injury (disruption),
            295–296
        tracheobronchial tree, 277
        traumatic asphyxia, 296
thoracic trauma management
        aortic aneurysm, 306
        flail chest, 303

hemothorax, 305
intravenous fluid infusion, 302,
    304–305
myocardial contusion, 306
open pneumothorax, 303
oxygenation, 302
pericardial tamponade, 306
respiratory volume and rate, 302
rib fractures, 302–303
sternoclavicular dislocation, 303
tension pneumothorax, 304–305, 304f
tracheobronchial injury (disruption),
    306
traumatic asphyxia, 306–307
thrombocytopenia, 737, 738
thrombocytosis, 737–738
thromboemboli, 585
thrombolitics, 107
thrombolytic agents, 526t, 584
thrombophlebitis, 561
thrombotic strokes, 585
thrombus, 540
thyroid gland disorders
    geriatric disorders, 1055
    geriatric patients, 139
    Graves' disease, 616
    hyperthyroidism, 616
    hypothyroidism, 616, 618–619
    myxedema, 616, 618–619
    myxedema coma, 618
    thyrotoxic crisis, 617
    thyrotoxicosis, 616
thyroid storm, 617
thyrotoxic crisis, 617
thyrotoxicosis, 616, 935
TIAs (transient ischemic attack), 587
tibia fractures, 192–193
tic douloureux, 600
ticks, 824
tilt test, 78, 640
tinnitus, 1031
tissue injuries
    connective tissue, 55
    resiliency, 55
tocolysis, 888–889
toddlers, 943
tolerance, 715
tongue, 371
tonic-clonic seizure, 590
tonic phase, 590
tonic seizures, 931–932
tonsil tip catheters, 432
tonsillitis, 335
topical anesthetic spray, 243–244
torsade de pointes, 499, 500–501, 501f
total down time, 555
tourniquet, 69, 70f, 121
toxic gas build-up, 151–152
toxic inhalation, 144, 363
toxic-metabolic states, 571
toxic syndromes, 692–693t
toxicological emergencies
    acetaminophen, 702
    activated charcoal, 686, 703
    aerosol inhalation, 690
    analgesic toxicity, 1064
    angiotensin-converting enzyme (ACE)
        inhibitor toxicity, 1063

anti-inflammatory agent toxicity, 1064
antidepressant toxicity, 1064
antidepressants, 700–701
antidotes, 687–688, 687t
antihypertensive toxicity, 1063
antiparkinsonion agents, toxicity of, 1064
antipsychotic toxicity, 1064
antiseizure medication toxicity, 1064
assessment, 685–686
beta-blocker toxicity, 1063
carbon monoxide (CO), 695
cardiac medications, 696
caustic substances, 696–697
corticosteroid toxicity, 1064
cyanide, 694
decontamination, 686–687
described, 681
digitalis toxicity, 1064
diuretic toxicity, 1063
entero-hepatic circulation, 703
epidemiology, 681–682
food poisoning, 704–705
gastric lavage, 686
geriatric emergencies, 1062–1064
history, 685–686
hydrocarbons, 698
hydrofluoric (HF) acid, 697–698
and induced vomiting, 686, 690
ingested toxins, 688–690
ingestion, 683–684
inhalation, 684
inhaled toxins, 690–691
injected toxins, 707–715
injection, 684
insect bites and stings, 707–710
lidocaine toxicity, 1063
lithium, 701
management, 686–688
MAO inhibitors, 699–700
marine animal injection, 714–715
metals, 703–704
NSAIDs (nonsteroidal anti-inflammatory drugs), 702–703
ongoing assessment, 685–686
overdose. See overdose
pediatric emergencies, 1001–1003
poisonings. See poisonings
poisonous plants and mushrooms, 705–706
primary assessment, 685
pumping the stomach, 686
rapid sequence intubation (RSI), 689
rescuer safety, 685
routes of toxic exposure, 682–684
salicylates, 701–702
scene assessment, 685
secondary assessment, 685–686
snakebites, 711–714, 711f
specific toxins, 691–706
standard toxicological emergency procedures, 685
substance abuse. See substance abuse
surface-absorbed toxins, 691
surface absorption, 684
syrup of ipecac, non-acceptability of, 686
ten most common poisons, 683t

theophylline, 703
toxic syndromes, 692–693t
tricyclic antidepressants, 698–699
whole bowel irrigation, 687
toxicology, 681
toxins
acetaminophen, 702
antidepressants, 700–701
carbon monoxide (CO), 695
cardiac medications, 696
caustic substances, 696–697
cyanide, 694
defined, 681
in fish, 705
food poisoning, 704–705
hydrocarbons, 698
hydrofluoric (HF) acid, 697–698
ingested toxins, 688–690
inhaled toxins, 690–691
injected toxins, 707–715
insect bites and stings, 707–710
lithium, 701
MAO inhibitors, 699–700
marine animal injection, 714–715
metals, 703–704
NSAIDs (nonsteroidal anti-inflammatory drugs), 702–703
poisonous plants and mushrooms, 705–706
salicylates, 701–702
snakebites, 711–714, 711f
surface-absorbed toxins, 691
theophylline, 703
tricyclic antidepressants, 698–699
TPA (tissue plasminogen activator), 107
trachea, 224
tracheal deviation, 343
tracheal shift, 287
tracheal suctioning, 920f
tracheal tugging, 339
tracheobronchial injury (disruption), 295–296, 306
tracheobronchial suctioning, 433
tracheobronchial tree, 277
tracheostomy, 1016–1017, 1017t, 1124–1126
tracheostomy cannulae, 431f
traction splint, 187, 192f
traction splinting, 191
trajectory, 46
transcient ischemic attack (TIA), 1029
transcutaneous cardiac pacing (TCP), 533, 534f, 535f
transection, 254
transfusion, 83, 725–726, 726t
transfusion reactions, 726–727
see also hematopoietic emergencies
transient hypertension, 884
transient ischemic attack (TIA), 587, 1049
transillumination intubation, 400–402, 401f
transitional phase, pediatric care, 955–956
translaryngeal cannula. See needle cricothyrostomy
transmural infarction, 540
transport considerations
behavioural emergencies, 853–854
field labour, 891
geriatric trauma, 1071

head, facial, and neck injury management, 244
heart failure, 548–549
hemorrhage, 82
home care patients, 1118
hypothermia, 759
labour, 890–891
movement of spinal injury patient. See movement of spinal injury patient
myocardial infarction (MI), 543
neonatal distress, 926
neurological emergencies, 582
newborns, 909
pediatric assessment, 955
pediatric emergencies, 975–976
peripheral vascular emergencies, 563–564
rapid trauma assessment, end of, 231
restraint, 855
spinal injury patients. See movement of spinal injury patient
suicidal elderly patients, 1068
transport decision, 9–10
urological emergencies, 665
wounds requiring transport, 132
transport decision, 9–10
transportation competencies, 1147
transverse fracture, 174
trauma
abdominal. See abdominal trauma
airway obstruction, 371
blunt trauma, 3
see also blunt trauma
and cardiovascular emergencies, 515
categories of, 3
defined, 3, 15
geriatric emergencies. See geriatric trauma
Golden Hour, 8
gynecological emergencies. See traumatic gynecological emergencies
kinetics. See kinetics of trauma
as leading killer, 3
and life-threatening conditions, 3–4
musculoskeletal trauma. See musculoskeletal trauma
pediatric emergencies. See pediatric trauma
penetrating trauma, 3
see also penetrating trauma
pregnancy complications, 878–879
soft-tissue trauma. See soft-tissue trauma
spinal trauma. See spinal injury
surgical disease, serious trauma as, 4
thoracic trauma. See thoracic trauma
types of, 15–16
Trauma Care Systems Planning and Development Act of 1990, 4
trauma centre
defined, 5
designation, 5–6
district trauma centre (DTC), 5
levels of, 5
primary trauma centre (PTC), 5
specialty centres, 5–6
tertiary trauma centre (TTC), 5
trauma patient intubation, 405

trauma registry, 10
trauma system
    described, 4
    paramedics, role of, 6–11
    quality improvement (QI), 10–11
trauma triage criteria
    application of, 10
    defined, 6
    described, 4
    immediate transport needs, 9t
    "over-triage" of trauma patients, 10
traumatic aneurysm, 293–294
traumatic asphyxia, 296, 306–307
traumatic diaphragmatic rupture, 295
traumatic esophageal rupture, 295
traumatic gynecological emergencies
    blunt trauma, 864
    causes of gynecological trauma, 864
    management, 864
    sexual assault injuries, 864–866
    straddle injury, 864
traumatic rhabdomyolysis, 110
traumatic rupture, 293–294, 294f
treatment. See management
tremor, 600
Treponema pallidum, 826
triangular bandages, 113, 854
trichinosis, 787
Trichomonas vaginalis, 828
trichomoniasis, 828
trichotillomania, 849
tricuspid valve, 448
tricyclic antidepressants, 698–699
trigeminal neuralgia, 600
trigeminy, 497
trimesters, 872
triplicate method, 464
tripod position, 339, 339f, 374
trunk wounds, bandaging, 124
tube-holding devices, 391–392
tuberculosis (TB)
    described, 804
    EMS response, 805–806
    and geriatric patients, 805
    incubation period, 805
    management, 806–807
    multdrug-resistant tuberculosis (MDR-TB), 804
    pathogenesis, 805
    personal safety, 805–806
    polymerase chain reaction (PCR) test, 807
    postexposure identification, 806–807
    respiration, 806f
    respirators, 806
    signs and symptoms, 805
    skin testing, 804–805
    transmission of, 804
tubular cell death, 667, 669
tumour destruction, 350
tumours, 604
two pillow orthopnea, 1047
Tylenol, 702
tympanic injuries, 221
Type I diabetes mellitus, 611
type I second-degree AV block, 484–485, 486f
Type II diabetes mellitus, 611–612

type II second-degree AV block, 486–487, 487f
tyramine, 699

U wave, 456
ulcerative colitis, 647–648
ulna fractures, 194
umbilical cord, 869–870, 894f, 897, 899f, 900f, 914, 923–924, 924f
uncuffed endotracheal tube, 922
underwater detonation, 35
undifferentiated schizophrenia, 842
unipolar leads, 453
unipolar traction device, 187, 188f, 192
universal donors, 725
universal recipient, 725
unstable angina, 537
up-and-over pathway, 22–24, 23f
upper airway obstruction, 348–349, 370, 979–980
upper airway trauma, 335
upper gastrointestinal bleeding, 639–641, 1056
upper gastrointestinal diseases
    acute gastroenteritis, 642–643
    chronic gastroenteritis, 643–644
    esophageal varices, 641–642, 641f
    gastritis, 639, 642
    gastroenteritis, 642
    hematemesis, 640
    Mallory-Weiss tear, 639, 640
    peptic ulcer disease, 639, 640
    peptic ulcers, 644–646, 645f
    tilt test, 640
    upper gastrointestinal bleeding, 639–641
    Zollinger-Ellison syndrome, 645
upper GI bleed, 639–641, 1056
upper GI tract, 639
upper respiratory infection (URI)
    assessment, 359
    described, 358
    locations, symptoms and signs, 359t
    management, 359–360
    pathophysiology, 358–359
    patients with asthma or COPD, 360
    viruses, 359
upper respiratory tract, 335
urban rabies, 821–822
urea, 659
uremia, 670–671, 671t
uremic frost, 671
uremic syndrome, 671t
urethritis, 677
uric acid stones, 676
urinary bladder, 313
    see also abdominal trauma
urinary stasis, 677
urinary system, 659, 872
urinary tract devices, 1132, 1132f, 1133f
urinary tract infection (UTI)
    assessment, 678
    community-acquired infections, 678
    cystitis, 677
    described, 677
    geriatric patients, 1060–1061
    intrarenal abscesses, 678
    lower UTIs, 678

    management, 678–679
    morbidities, 677
    nosocomial infections, 678
    pathophysiology, 677–678
    perinephric abscesses, 678
    prostatitis, 677
    pyelonephritis, 661, 678
    secondary assessment, 678
    upper UTIs, 678
    urinary stasis, 677
urinary tract obstruction, 667
urine
    alkalinization, 716
    defined, 659
    dysuria, 862
    glucose loss in, 611
    nocturia, 1047
urological disorders
    geriatric disorders, 1060–1061
    incidence of, 659
    nontraumatic tissue problems, general mechanisms of, 660
    pathophysiological basis of pain, 660–661
urological emergencies
    ABCs, 665
    abdominal assessment, 664
    apparent state of health, 663–664
    appearance, 663
    assessment, 661–664
    focused history, 661–663
    level of consciousness, 663
    management, 664–665
    nonpharmacological interventions, 665
    OPQRST questions, 661–663
    pain, types of, 661
    pharmacological interventions, 665
    posture, 663
    preventive strategies, 660
    primary assessment, 661
    referred pain, 661
    renal emergencies. See renal emergencies
    scene assessment, 661
    secondary assessment, 663–664
    skin colour, 664
    urinary tract infection (UTI), 677–679
    visceral pain, 661
    vital signs, 664
urology, 659
urostomies, 1132
urticaria, 628, 628f
uterine atony, 902
uterine bleeding, abnormal, 863
uterine inversion, 902–903
uterine rupture, 902

vaccination
    see also immunization
    diphtheria-pertussis-tetanus (DTP) vaccine, 816
    geriatric patients, 1041
    Lyme disease, 825
    MMR vaccination, 815
    mumps, 815
    poliomyelitis (polio), 1103
    rubella, 815
vacuum splints, 187, 188f

vagal manoeuvres
    cardiovascular emergencies, 525
    paroxysmal junctional tachycardia
        (PJT), 494
    paroxysmal supraventricular
        tachycardia (PSVT), 477
vagal response, 916
vaginal birth after cesarean (VBAC), 890
vaginal bleeding, 858, 860, 863, 877,
    879–883
vaginal hemorrhage, 72
vagotomy, 645
valsalva manoeuvre
    cardiovascular emergencies, 525
    defined, 1049
    paroxysmal junctional tachycardia
        (PJT), 494
    paroxysmal supraventricular
        tachycardia (PSVT), 477
vancomycin-resistant enterococcus (VRE),
    830
varicella, 810
varicella-zoster immune globulin (VZIG), 811
varicose veins, 562
varicosities, 1049
Varivax, 810, 811
vascular access devices (VADs)
    anticoagulant therapy, 1130–1131
    Broviac catheters, 1130
    complications, 1131
    described, 1129
    dialysis shunts, 1130
    Groshong catheter, 1130
    Hickman catheter, 1130
    peripherally inserted central catheters
        (PICC lines), 1130
    surgically implanted medication delivery
        systems, 1130
    types of, 1130
vascular emergencies. See peripheral vascular
    emergencies
vascular headaches, 595
vascular phase, 66
vascular structures, 315
vasculitis, 562
vaso-occlusive crises, 735
vasoconstriction, 746
vasodepressor syncope, 1049
vasodilation, 746
vasopressin, 556, 719
vasopressors, 553, 630, 752
vasospastic angina, 537
vasovagal syncope, 1049
vecuronium (Norcuron®), 235, 241, 407–408
vehicular collisions
    additional impacts, 19
    airbags, 19–20
    alcohol and, 719
    analysis, 27–30
    angular impact, 31
    axial loading, 24
    blunt thoracic trauma, 277
    blunt trauma, 16
    body cavity injuries, 29
    body collision, 17–18, 17f
    child safety seats, 21
    collision evaluation, 30
    crumple zones, 24, 24f

down-and-under pathway, 22
ejection, 24, 27, 31
events of impact, 16–19
extension injury, 249–251
frontal impact, 22–24, 31, 278f
head injuries, 29
incidence of impacts, 21, 21f
injuries, incidence by body area, 30
intoxication, 29
lateral impact, 25–26
myocardial aneurysm or rupture, 293
oblique angle, 26
organ collision, 18, 18f
"paper bag" syndrome, 22, 23f
partial ejection, 27
pediatric trauma, 1004
rear-end impact, 26
restraints, 19–21
rollover, 26–27
rotational impact, 26
scene assessment, 27–30
seat belts, 19
secondary collisions, 18–19, 18f
signs of impacts, 28
sliding impact, 31
types of impact, 21–27
up-and-over pathway, 22–24, 23f
vehicle collision, 17, 17f
vehicular trauma, 29–30
veins, 315, 448
Velcro® straps, and splints, 188
velocity, 14
venomous stings, 684
venous hemorrhage, 66
venous thromboembolism, 903
ventilation
    see also airway management
    artificial monitors, home, 1018
    automatic transport ventilator, 440–441
    bag-valve devices, 438–439, 438f
    bag-valve mask, 921
    bag-valve-mask ventilation (BVM
        ventilation), 373, 373f, 382, 394,
        439, 920
    chest wall, 335
    compact ventilator, 440–441
    defined, 332
    described, 437
    diaphragm, 335
    disruption in, 335–337
    gastric decompression, 434
    head, facial, and neck injury
        management, 238
    home ventilation, 1126–1129
    inadequate, 372
    jet ventilation, 426f
    lower respiratory tract, 335
    mouth-to-mask ventilation, 437–438
    mouth-to-mouth ventilation, 437
    mouth-to-nose ventilation, 437
    myxedema coma, 618
    neonatal resuscitation, 921–922
    nervous system and, 335–337
    pediatric airway management, 964
        see also pediatric airway management
    pediatric ventilation, 439–440
    phrenic nerve, 337
    pop-off valve, 440

positive pressure ventilation, 284
positive-pressure ventilators, 1127
requirements, 437
stages of, 332
thyrotoxic crisis (thyroid storm), 617
upper respiratory tract, 335
ventilation systems, 806
ventricles, 448
ventricles, dysrhythmias originating in
    accelerated idioventricular rhythm, 496
    artificial pacemaker rhythm, 505–506,
        506f
    asystole, 503, 503f, 504f
    premature ventricular contractions
        (PVC), 497–499, 498f
    ventricular escape complexes and
        rhythms, 295–296
    ventricular fibrillation, 501–502, 502f
    ventricular tachycardia (VT), 499–501,
        500f
ventricular aneurysm, 541
ventricular conduction disturbances, 507–509
ventricular depolarization, 456, 461
ventricular ectopic, 497–499
ventricular escape beat, 495
ventricular escape rhythm, 495
ventricular fibrillation, 501–502, 502f, 557f,
    755, 974, 992, 994
ventricular repolarization, 456, 461f
ventricular synctium, 450
ventricular tachycardia (VT), 499–501, 500f
ventricular tachycardia (VT) with a pulse,
    992
venturi mask, 436
verapamil, 479, 480, 482, 494
vertebral injury, 603
vertigo, 1051
vest-type immobilization device, 269–270,
    269f
Vibrio cholerae, 643, 819, 820
victims' characteristics, 54
violent crime, 277
violent patients, 853–856
viral (aseptic) meningitis, 811
viral diseases transmitted by contact,
    816–817
viral gastrointestinal infections, 820
viral pneumonia, 360
viral rhinitis, 814
virulence, 789
visceral pain, 635, 661
visual impairments
    accommodation of, 1093
    causes of, 1092
    congenital disorders, 1092
    degenerative disorders, 1092
    diabetic retinopathy, 1092
    enucleation, 1092
    etiologies, 1092
    glaucoma, 1092
    previous injury, 1092
    recognition of, 1093
visualized endotracheal intubation, 131
vital signs
    anaphylaxis, 629
    asthma, 357
    facial injuries, 231
    head injuries, 231

monitoring of, 200–201
neck injuries, 231
neonatal distress, 915
neurological emergencies, 580, 580*f*
newborns, 919
obstetric patient, 877
pediatric assessment, 951–955, 953*t*,
957–958
pulse oximetry, 378
rapid trauma assessment, 231
respiratory status, 344–345
spinal injury, 261
urological emergencies, 664
vitamin B₁, 243
voice production disorders, 1094
voltage, 138
volume expanders, 925*t*
volvulus, 650, 651*f*
vomiting
abdominal pain, 662
bulimia nervosa, 847
cardiovascular events and, 514
food poisoning, 820–821
gastroenteritis, 819–820
gastrointestinal emergencies, 637
see also gastrointestinal (GI)
emergencies
induced, 686, 690
neonatal emergencies, 934
pediatric emergencies, 997–998
urological emergencies. *See* urological
emergencies
vomitus, 372
von Willebrand's disease, 739

wandering atrial pacemaker, 473–474, 473*f*
warfarin (Coumadin), 68, 107, 482
washing hands. *See* handwashing
washout, 84
wasp stings, 623, 627, 707

water, contaminated, 643–644
water moccasins, 711
watercraft accidents, 33–34
"weak and dizzy," 596–597
weapons
arrows, 51
assault rifle, 51
the elderly and suicide, 1068
handgun, 49–50
high-velocity weapons, 320
knives, 51
rifles, 50
shotgun, 51
and thoracic injury, 277
Wenckebach, 484–485, 486*f*
Wernicke's syndrome, 583
West Nile virus, 809–810
Western rattlesnake, 711
wet dressings, 112–113
wet drowning, 761–762
wheezing, 343, 376
whistle tip catheters, 432
white blood cell disorders
hemophilia, 738–739
leukemia, 736–737
leukocytosis, 735
leukopenia, 735–736
lymphomas, 737
neutropenia, 735–736
von Willebrand's disease, 739
whole bowel irrigation, 687
whooping cough, 816
wild animals, and rabies, 822
window phase, 790
withdrawal, 693*t*, 715, 720–721, 846
Wolff-Parkinson-White syndrome, 482, 493,
509–510, 510*f*
women. *See* gynecological emergencies;
partner abuse; pregnancy
work-induced thermogenesis, 744

World Health Organization (WHO), 813,
820
wound assessment, 113
see also penetrating trauma; soft-tissue
trauma
wound dressing and bandaging. *See*
bandaging; dressings
wound healing
abnormal scar formation, 108–109
collagen synthesis, 105
epithelialization, 104
hemostasis, 102–104
hypertrophic scar formation, 109
inflammation, 104
keloid, 108
neovascularization, 104–105
process, 103*f*
remodelling, 105
wound immobilization. *See* splinting
wound infections. *See* infection
Wright Spirometer, 346, 346*f*
wrist injuries, 198

xylocaine, 243

Yankauer catheters, 432
yellow jackets, 627

zanamavir, 814
Zollinger-Ellison syndrome, 645
zone of coagulation, 137
zone of hyperemia, 137
zone of injury, 54
zone of stasis, 137
zygomatic fractures, 220